Beauty Therapy

THE FOUNDATIONS

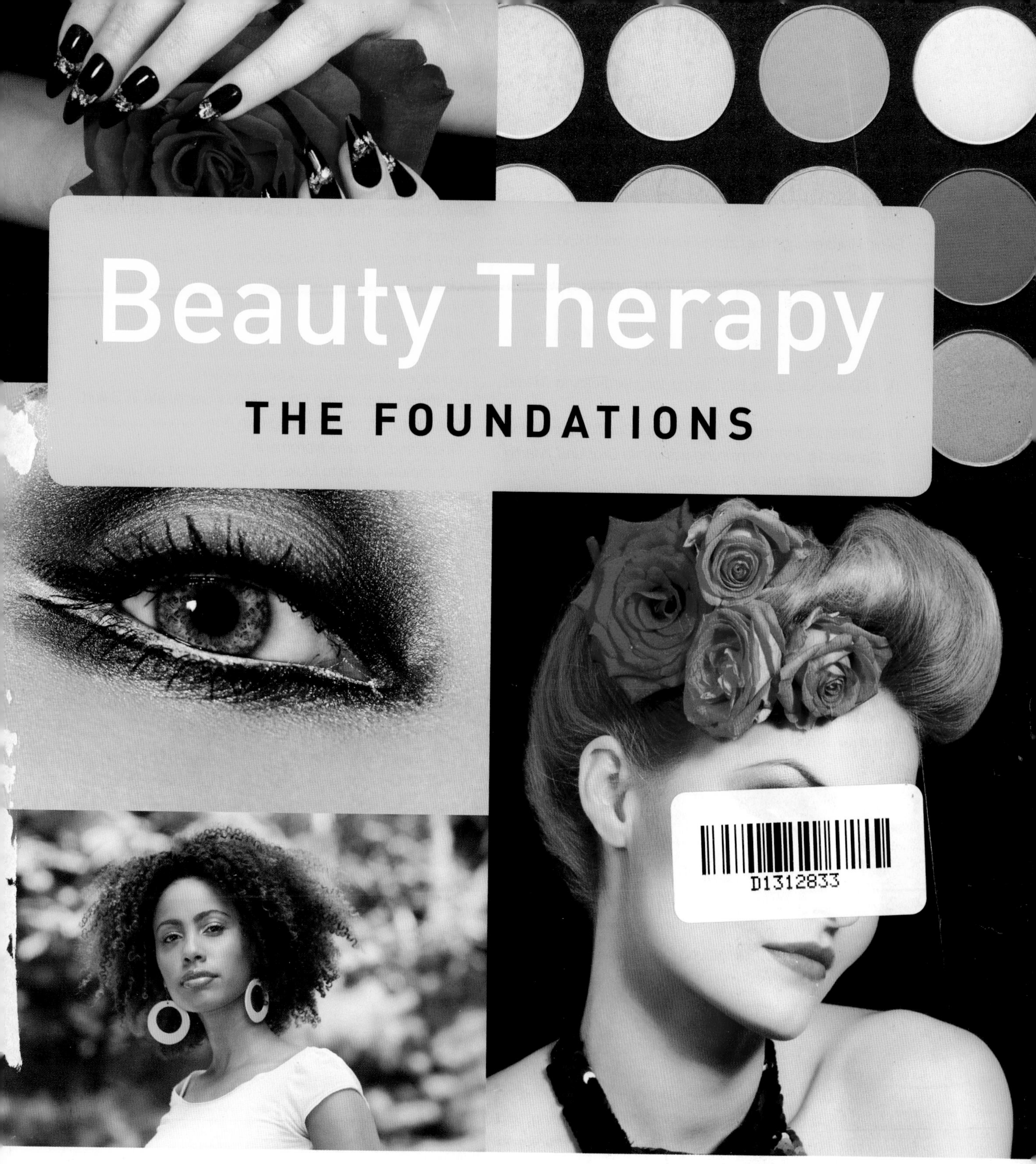

HABIA SERIES LIST

Hairdressing

Student textbooks

Begin Hairdressing: The Official Guide to Level 1 REVISED 2e *Martin Green*

Hairdressing – The Foundations: The Official Guide to Level 2 REVISED 6e *Leo Palladino and Martin Green*

Professional Hairdressing: The Official Guide to Level 3 REVISED 6e *Martin Green and Leo Palladino*

The Pocket Guide to Key Terms for Hairdressing *Martin Green*

The Official Guide to the City & Guilds Certificate in Salon Service 1e *John Armstrong with Anita Crosland, Martin Green and Lorraine Nordmann*

The Colour Book: The Official Guide to Colour for NVQ Levels 2 & 3 1e *Tracey Lloyd with Christine McMillan-Bodell*

eXtensions: The Official Guide to Hair Extensions 1e *Theresa Bullock*

Salon Management *Martin Green*

Men's Hairdressing: Traditional and Modern Barbering 2e *Maurice Lister*

African-Caribbean Hairdressing 2e *Sandra Gittens*

The World of Hair Colour 1e *John Gray*

The Cutting Book: The Official Guide to Cutting at S/NVQ Levels 2 and 3 *Jane Goldsbro and Elaine White*

Professional Hairdressing titles

Trevor Sorbie: The Bridal Hair Book 1e *Trevor Sorbie and Jacki Wadeson*

The Art of Dressing Long Hair 1e *Guy Kremer and Jacki Wadeson*

Patrick Cameron: Dressing Long Hair 1e *Patrick Cameron and Jacki Wadeson*

Patrick Cameron: Dressing Long Hair 2 1e *Patrick Cameron and Jacki Wadeson*

Bridal Hair 1e *Pat Dixon and Jacki Wadeson*

Professional Men's Hairdressing: The Art of Cutting and Styling 1e *Guy Kremer and Jacki Wadeson*

Essensuals, the Next Generation Toni and Guy: Step by Step 1e *Sacha Mascolo, Christian Mascolo and Stuart Wesson*

Mahogany Hairdressing: Step to Cutting, Colouring and Finishing Hair 1e *Martin Gannon and Richard Thompson*

Mahogany Hairdressing: Advanced Looks 1e *Martin Gannon and Richard Thompson*

The Total Look: The Style Guide for Hair and Make-up Professional 1e *Ian Mistlin*

Trevor Sorbie: Visions in Hair 1e *Trevor Sorbie, Kris Sorbie and Jacki Wadeson*

The Art of Hair Colouring 1e *David Adams and Jacki Wadeson*

Beauty therapy

Beauty Basics: The Official Guide to Level 1 3e *Lorraine Nordmann*

Beauty Therapy – The Foundations: The Official Guide to Level 2 5e *Lorraine Nordmann*

Professional Beauty Therapy – The Official Guide to Level 3 4e *Lorraine Nordmann*

The Pocket Guide to Key Terms for Beauty Therapy *Lorraine Nordmann and Marian Newman*

The Official Guide to the City & Guilds Certificate in Salon Services 1e *John Armstrong with Anita Crosland, Martin Green and Lorraine Nordmann*

The Complete Guide to Make-Up 1e *Suzanne Le Quesne*

The Encyclopedia of Nails 1e *Jacqui Jefford and Anne Swain*

The Art of Nails: A Comprehensive Style Guide to Nail Treatments and Nail Art 1e *Jacqui Jefford*

Nail Artistry 1e *Jacqui Jefford*

The Complete Nail Technician 3e *Marian Newman*

Manicure, Pedicure and Advanced Nail Techniques 1e *Elaine Almond*

The Official Guide to Body Massage 2e *Adele O'Keefe*

An Holistic Guide to Massage 1e *Tina Parsons*

Indian Head Massage 2e *Muriel Burnham-Airey and Adele O'Keefe*

Aromatherapy for the Beauty Therapist 1e *Valerie Worwood*

An Holistic Guide to Reflexology 1e *Tina Parsons*

An Holistic Guide to Anatomy and Physiology 1e *Tina Parsons*

The Essential Guide to Holistic and Complementary Therapy 1e *Helen Beckmann and Suzanne Le Quesne*

The Spa Book 1e *Jane Crebbin-Bailey, Dr John Harcup, and John Harrington*

SPA: The Official Guide to Spa Therapy at Levels 2 and 3, *Joan Scott and Andrea Harrison*

Nutrition: A Practical Approach 1e *Suzanne Le Quesne*

Hands on Sports Therapty 1e *Keith Ward*

Encyclopedia of Hair Removal: A Complete Reference to Methods, Techniques and Career Opportunities, *Gill Morris and Janice Brown*

The Anatomy and Physiology Workbook: For Beauty and Holistic Therapies Levels 1–3. *Tina Parsons*

The Anatomy and Physiology CD-Rom

Beautiful Selling: The Complete Guide to Sales Success in the Salon *Rath Langley*

The Official Guide to the Diploma in Hair and Beauty Studies at Foundation Level 1e *Jane Goldsbro and Elaine White*

The Official Guide to the Diploma in Hair and Beauty Studies at Higher Level 1e *Jane Goldsbro and Elaine White*

The Official Guide to Foundation Learning in Hair and Beauty 1e *Jane Goldsbro and Elaine White*

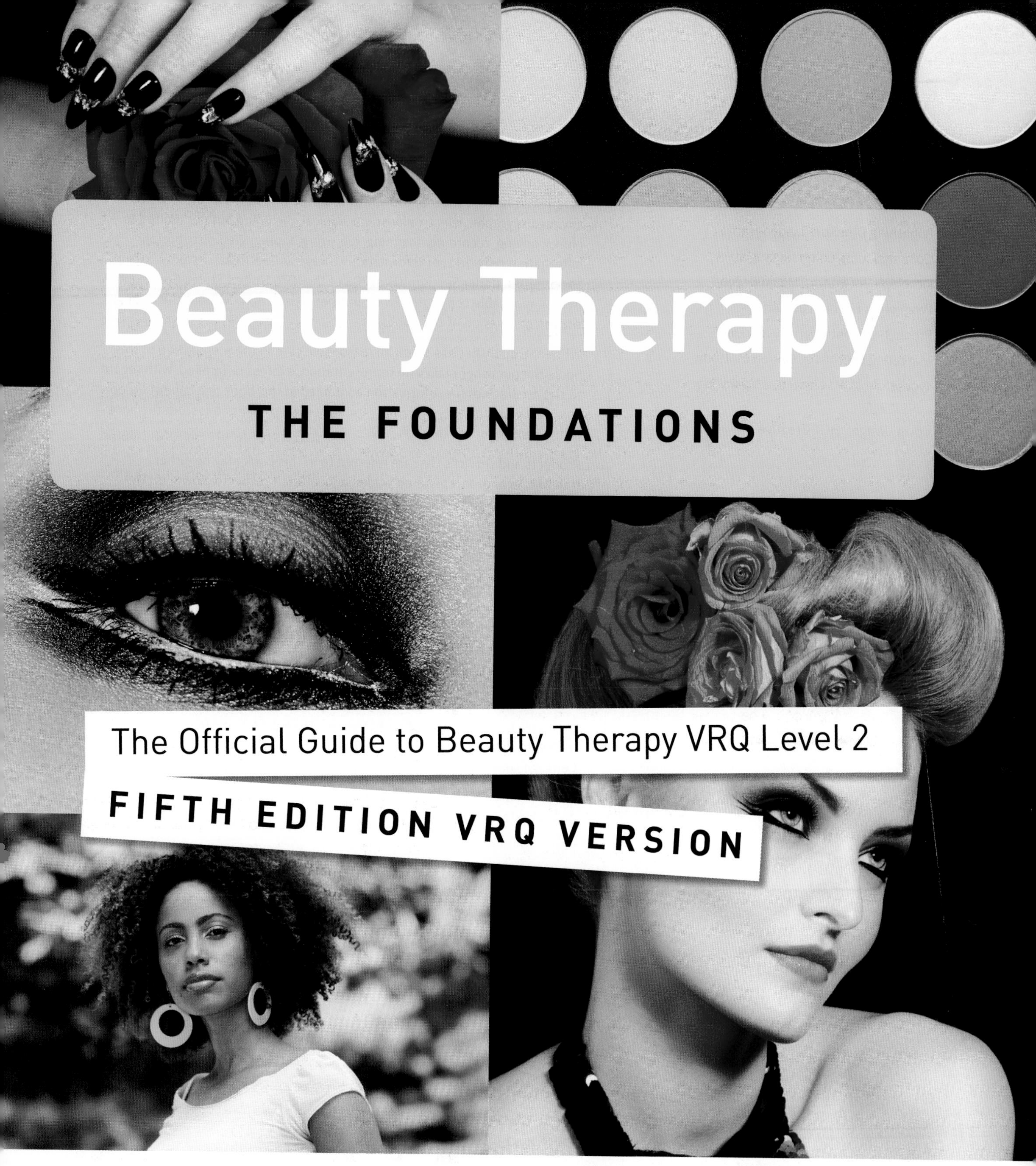

Beauty Therapy

THE FOUNDATIONS

The Official Guide to Beauty Therapy VRQ Level 2

FIFTH EDITION VRQ VERSION

LORRAINE NORDMANN AND MARIAN NEWMAN

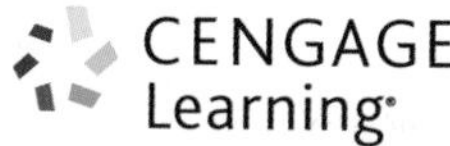

Australia • Brazil • Japan • Korea • Mexico • Singapore • Spain • United Kingdom • United States

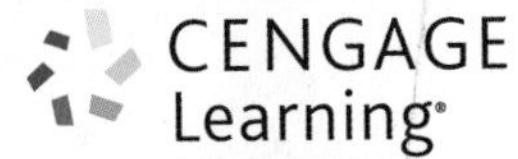

Beauty Therapy The Foundations: The Official Guide to VRQ Level 2
Lorraine Nordmann and Marian Newman

Publishing Director: Linden Harris
Commissioning Editor: Lucy Mills
Development Editor: Helen Green
Production Editor: Lucy Arthy
Production Controller: Eyvett Davis
Marketing Executive: Lauren Mottram
Typesetter: MPS Limited, a Macmillan Company
Cover design: HCT Creative

For product information and technology assistance, contact **emea.info@cengage.com**.

For permission to use material from this text or product, and for permission queries, email **emea.permissions@cengage.com.**

This work is adapted from *Beauty Therapy: The Foundations: The Official Guide to Beauty Therapy at Level 2, fifth edition* by Lorraine Nordmann published by Cengage Learning, Inc. © 2010.

British Library Cataloguing-in-Publication Data
A catalogue record for this book is available from the British Library.

ISBN: 978-1-4080-5496-3

Cengage Learning EMEA
Cheriton House, North Way, Andover, Hampshire, SP10 5BE
United Kingdom

Cengage Learning products are represented in Canada by Nelson Education Ltd.

For your lifelong learning solutions, visit **www.cengage.co.uk**

Purchase your next print book, e-book or e-chapter at **www.cengagebrain.com**

Printed in China by RR Donnelley
1 2 3 4 5 6 7 8 9 10 – 14 13 12

Contents

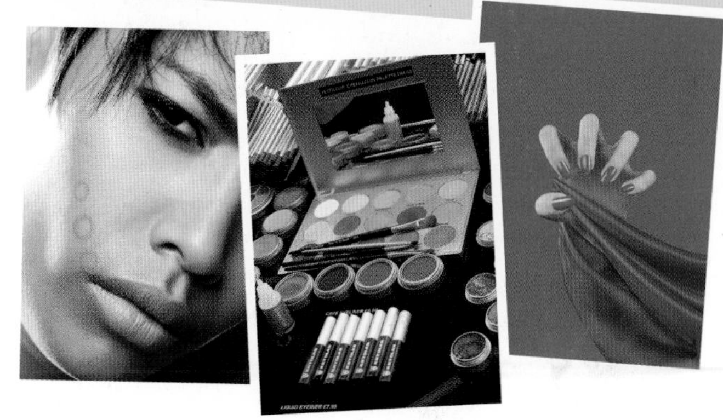

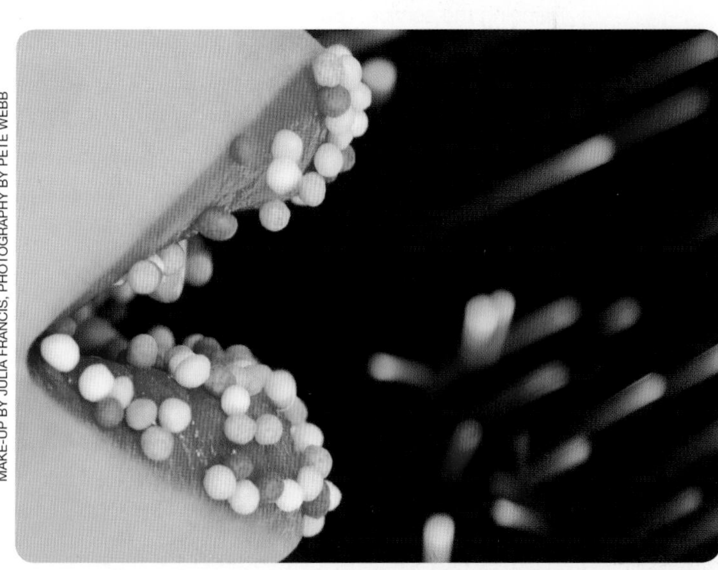

MAKE-UP BY JULIA FRANCIS, PHOTOGRAPHY BY PETE WEBB

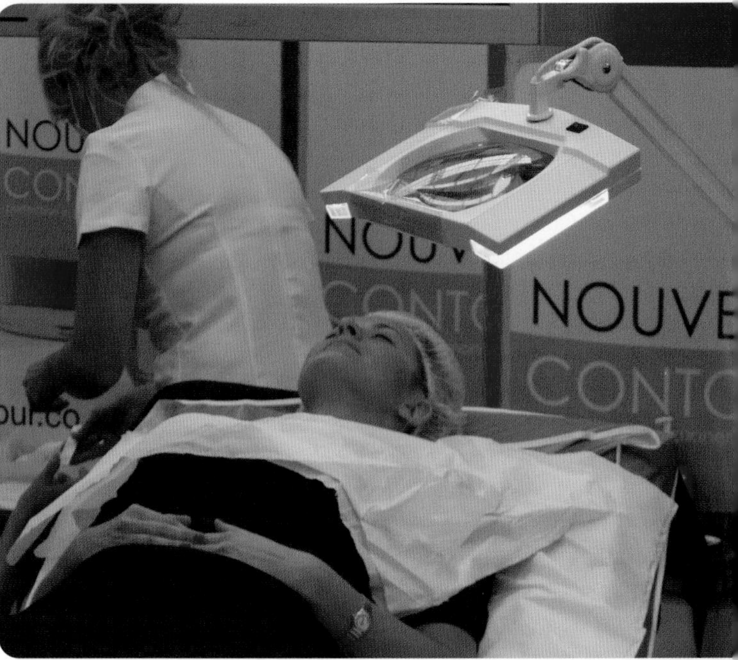

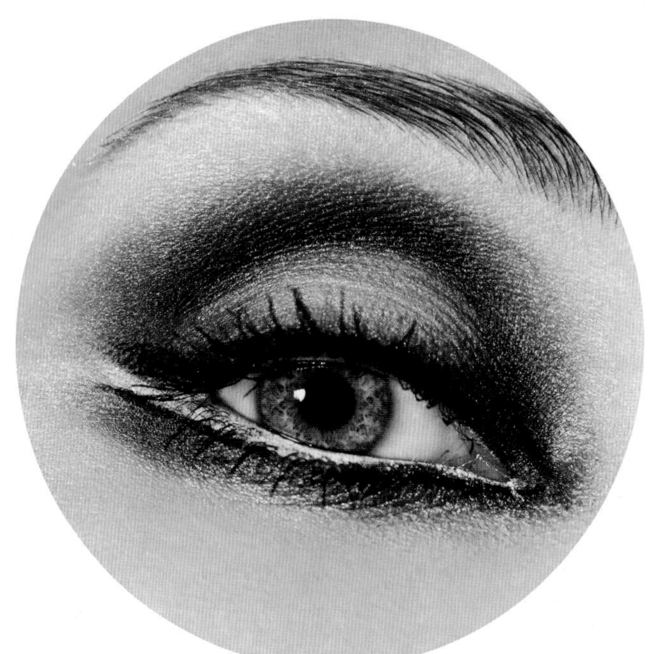

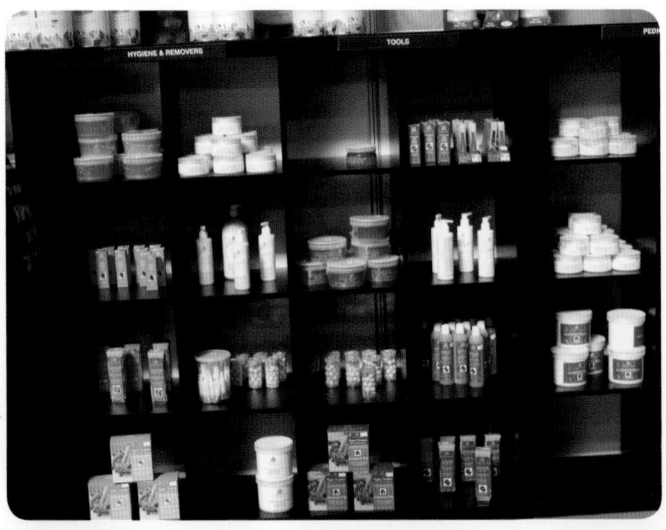
HYGIENE & REMOVERS
TOOLS

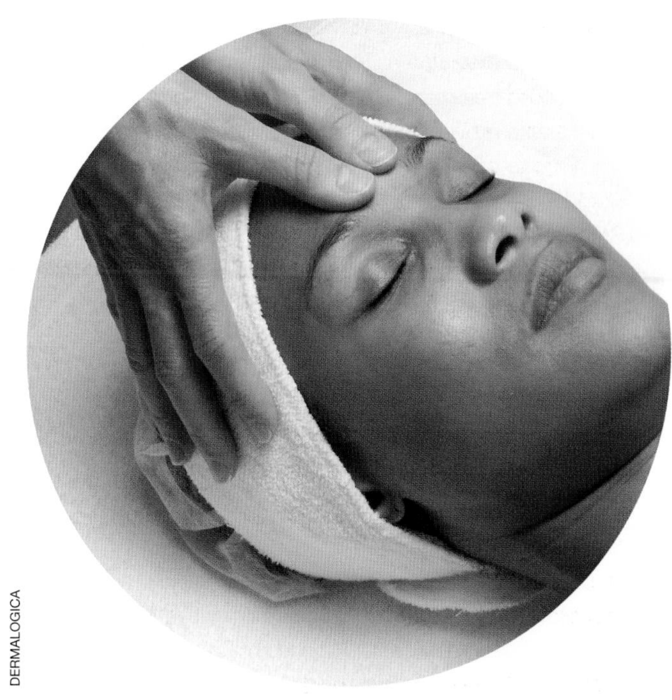
DERMALOGICA

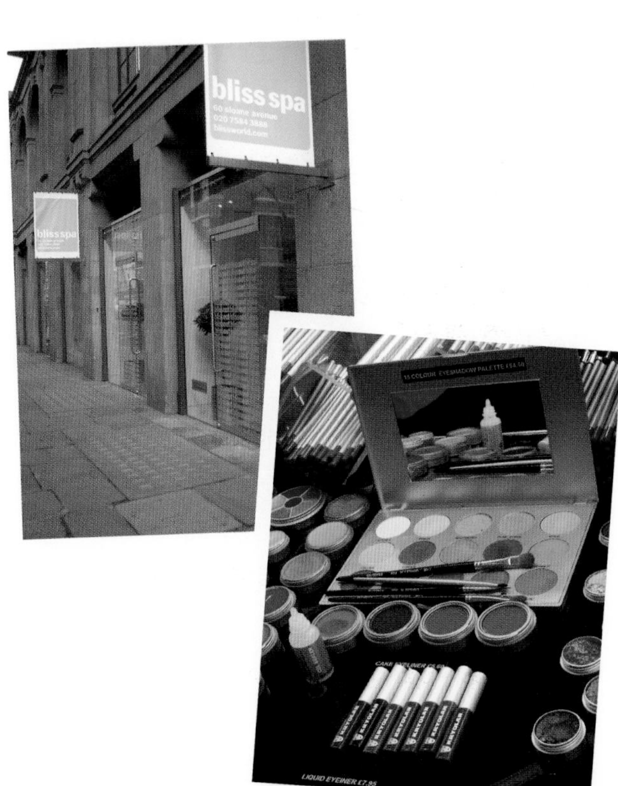

Foreword

I can scarcely believe that it has been 16 years since I wrote the foreword for the second edition of Lorraine Nordmann's excellent book *Beauty Therapy – The Foundations*.

Since then, the beauty industry has gone from strength to strength, advancing in professionalism, technology and capability. The new national occupational standards incorporate all that has been achieved in the industry since the millennium and there have been many exciting changes over this time. I have also seen a real shift in the way that consumers of both genders invest in their appearance and well-being.

UK standards are widely considered the best in the world and I am certain that Lorraine has played a huge role in pushing the development of beauty therapy to the quality we now see. With her dedication, expertise and passion, she has helped to make the industry the success it is today.

If you've never had the opportunity of meeting Lorraine, her passion for the industry and keeping her skills up to date is overwhelming. She is also a good straight talker and knows exactly what is needed from a trainer, college or salon perspective.

The fact that this VRQ edition has now been published is testament to the popularity of her books and the depth and knowledge that they provide to year after year of students. Her commitment to the development and introduction of innovative learning support and guidance is clearly reflected in her work.

Without doubt, *Beauty Therapy – The Foundations, Fifth Edition VRQ Version,* is the must-have book to cover the Level 2 Beauty Therapy Standards as laid down by Habia.

Alan Goldsbro
Chief Executive Officer, Habia

About this book

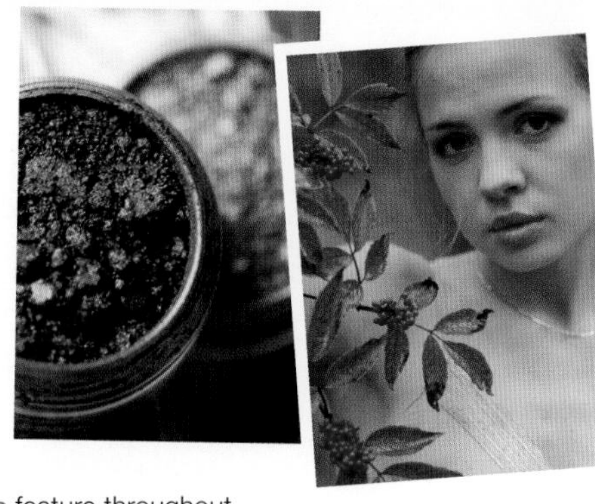

Industry role models feature throughout the book and are your insight into the exciting beauty industry. Their profile is included at the start of the chapter and they provide subject specific tips that are both practical and inspiring.

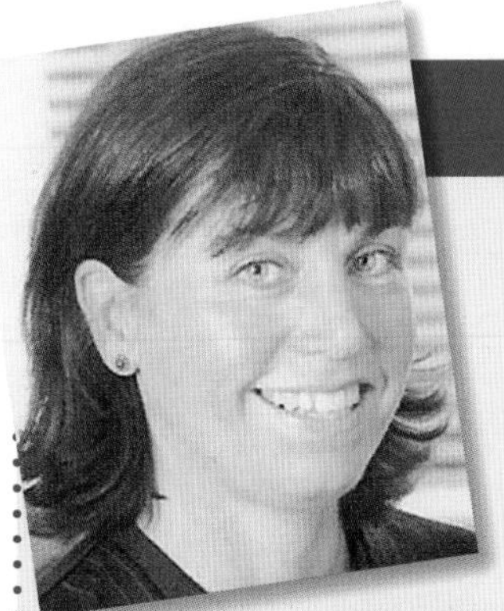

ROLE MODEL

Janice Brown

Director of HOF Beauty (House of Famuir Ltd)

My career journey has taken me from working in and later managing a group of salons, through sales, teaching, training, research and development and I am currently director of HOF Beauty Ltd. Along the way I have specialized in electrolysis and hair removal. I am the co-author of *Practical Electrolysis: The Official Guide to Electro-epilation* along with Gill Morris. I am proud to say that I have been able to make a real difference to people's lives by helping to correct skin, body and hair growth issues. I hope I have also been able to inspire and encourage fellow beauty therapists through the training I have provided. In the course of my career I have been fortunate enough to travel the world and work with wonderful people. Beauty therapy for me is not only a career but is a true passion.

ACTIVITY

Reception role play

With colleagues, act out the following situations, which may occur when working as a receptionist. You may wish to video the role plays for review and discussion later.

1. A client arrives very late for an appointment but insists that she be treated.
2. A client questions the bill.
3. A client comes in to complain about a service given previously (choose a particular service).

Alternatively you may choose to do this as a written activity with a discussion of your answers.

Activity boxes feature within all chapters and provide additional tasks for you to further your understanding.

Selling is a vital part of the role of a therapist. It is important that the client gets the right treatment and products in order to get the results they are after. Clients do not buy our treatments or products, they buy the benefits and results. It is your job to help them imagine how using the products and treatments will make them look and feel. Remember that we all hate to be sold to but love to buy; so practise and perfect your selling skills.

Janice Brown

Role model quotes are included throughout a number of core chapters. Each quote provides valuable insight into the world of work, providing helpful and practical advice about working in such a varied and innovative industry.

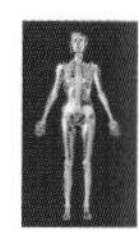

A&P icons highlight essential anatomy and physiology knowledge needed for the unit

Anatomy and physiology essential knowledge for unit	
Provide facial skincare	Chapter 7
Provide eyelash and brow treatments	Chapter 8
Provide eyelash perming	Chapter 8
Provide threading services for hair removal	Chapter 9
Apply make-up	Chapter 10
Provide manicure treatments	Chapter 11

BEST PRACTICE

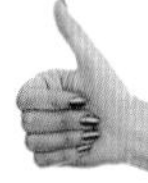

Promotion

All staff should be aware of any promotions that their business is offering so that they can build on a client's initial interest in a product or service and turn it into a sale. Always know about your products and services.

Best practice boxes suggest good working practice and help you develop your skills and awareness during your training.

ALWAYS REMEMBER

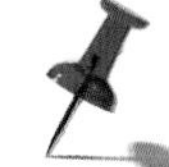

Emotional effect

Because clients relax with head massage they may then wish to talk about their problems.

If this happens, *listen* – but unless qualified you should not *counsel*.

Always remember boxes draw your attention to key information or helpful hints that will help you prepare for assessment.

TOP TIP

Foot spa

Foot spas help to relax the feet by a combination of massage provided by an integral vibration feature, aeration of the water, creating a bubbling effect, and heating of the water.

Top tips share the author's experience and provide positive suggestions to improve knowledge and skills for each unit.

PRODUCTS, TOOLS AND EQUIPMENT

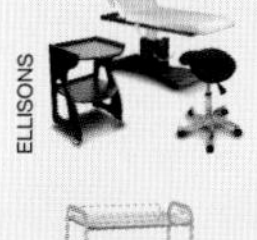

Couch or chair
With sit-up and lie-down positions and an easy-to-clean surface

Trolley
On which to place everything

Eye make-up remover (non-oily)
To cleanse the eye area before treatment application

YOU WILL ALSO NEED:

Disposable tissue roll Such as bedroll

Towels (2) Freshly laundered for each client

Flat mask brushes (3) Disinfected

Trolley To display all facial treatment products to be used in the facial service

Client's record card To record all the details relevant to the client's service

Facial toning lotions (a selection) To suit various types of skin

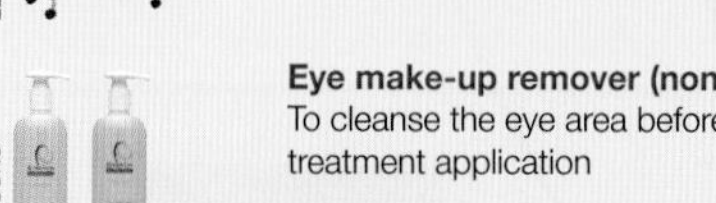

Products, tool and equipment lists help you prepare for each practical treatment and show you the tools, materials and products required.

HEALTH & SAFETY

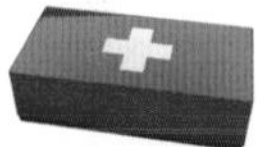

Follow manufacturers' instructions

Always read the manufacturer's instructions carefully and follow them exactly. For tools, it is usual that a fresh disinfectant solution must be made every day. When dealing with any disinfectant solution you should wear protective equipment as they are always irritants.

Health & Safety boxes draw your attention to related health and safety information essential for each technical skill.

Sample client record card

<table>
<tr><td>Date</td><td colspan="2">Beauty therapist</td></tr>
<tr><td colspan="2">Client name</td><td>Date of birth (identifying client age group)</td></tr>
<tr><td colspan="2">Home address</td><td>Postcode</td></tr>
<tr><td>Email address</td><td>Landline</td><td>Mobile phone number</td></tr>
<tr><td>Name of doctor</td><td colspan="2">Doctor's address and phone number</td></tr>
<tr><td colspan="3">Related medical history (conditions that may restrict or prohibit treatment application)</td></tr>
<tr><td colspan="3">Are you taking any medication? (this may affect the appearance of the skin or skin sensitivity)</td></tr>
</table>

Client record cards illustrate what you need to assess and gain from the client at consultation and also provide guidance on information following a treatment.

Step-by-step: Deep cleansing

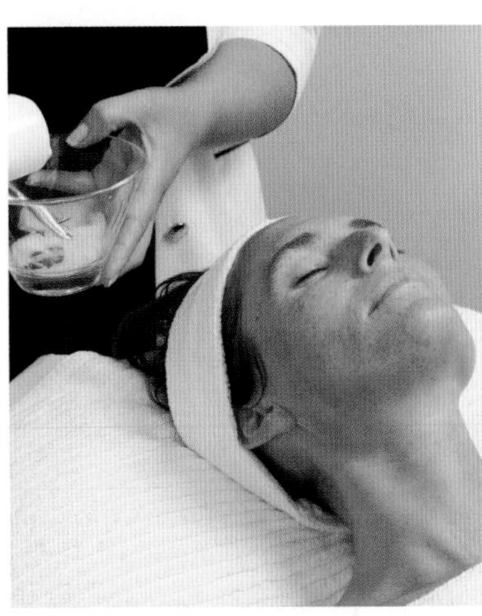

1 Select a cleansing medium to suit your client's skin type. The procedure for application is the same as that for the superficial cleanse.

Step-by-step sequences demonstrate the featured practical skills using colour photographs to enhance your understanding.

ASSESSMENT OF KNOWLEDGE AND UNDERSTANDING

You have now learnt about health and safety in the beauty therapy workplace. To test your level of knowledge, answer the following short questions. These will prepare you for your summative (final) assessment.

1. Cleaning agents that are formulated for use on skin are:
   a. disinfectants
   b. antiseptics
   c. sterilizers
   d. sanitizers
2. The hygiene control method of sterilization:
   a. is the destruction of most living organisms
   b. is the cleaning method using a disinfectant cleaning agent
   c. is the total destruction of all living micro-organisms
   d. uses ultra-violet light (UVL) to minimize harmful micro-organisms
3. What is a disinfectant?
   a. a chemical solution that destroys most micro-organisms
   b. a solution that prevent the multiplication of micro-organisms
   c. a type of distilled water to avoid damaging the autoclave
   d. a physical agent that destroys most micro-organisms

Assessment of knowledge and understanding questions are provided at the end of all core chapters. You can use the questions to prepare for oral and written assessments and help test your own knowledge throughout. Seek guidance from your supervisor/ assessor if there are areas you are unsure of.

Beauty Therapy
E-Teaching Website

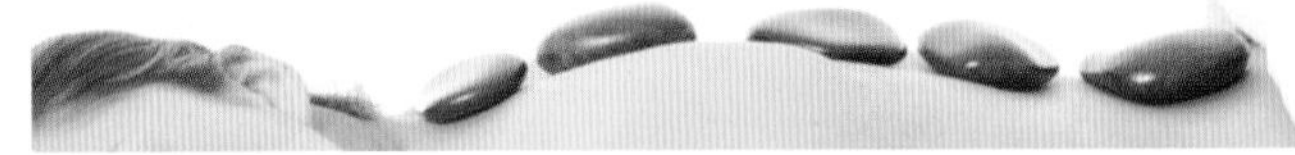

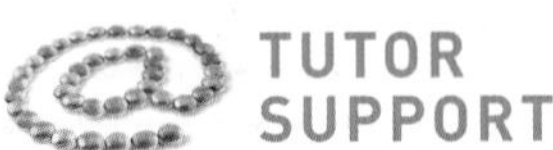

TUTOR SUPPORT

Links to the E-Teach resources are flagged throughout the text. If your trainer subscribes to one E-Teaching website, they will be able to download these and use them in class.

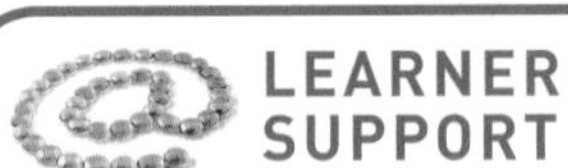

LEARNER SUPPORT

Free online Student Resources are available wherever you see this red symbol.

E-Teaching website

A **new E-Teaching website for trainers** accompanies this textbook. This resource includes **handouts, PowerPoint™ slides, interactive assessments, an image bank and videoclips** – all carefully designed to help trainers make classroom delivery more interactive and to provide extra materials for lesson planning.

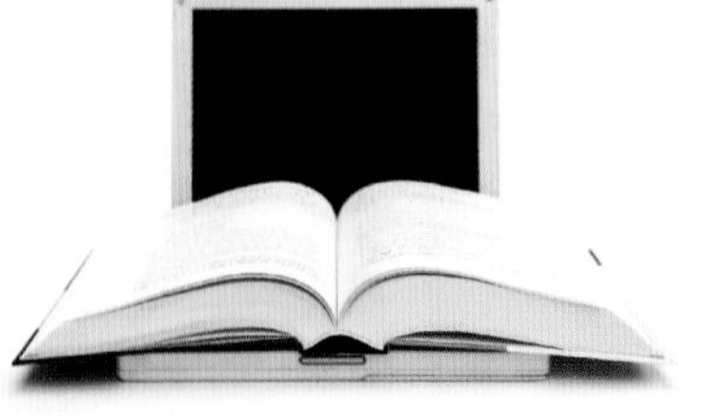

Please visit **www.eteachbeautytherapy.co.uk** for more information or contact your Cengage Learning sales representative at emea.fesales@cengage.com.

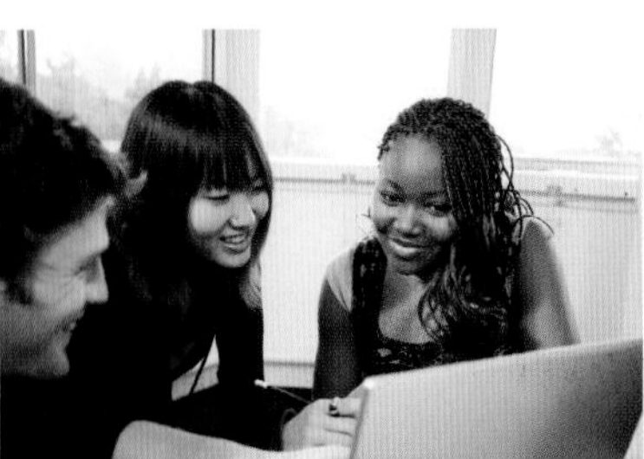

Students! Access your FREE online resources by following the Level 2 student links on **www.eteachbeautytherapy.co.uk** and entering your password 'bronzing'.

From the authors

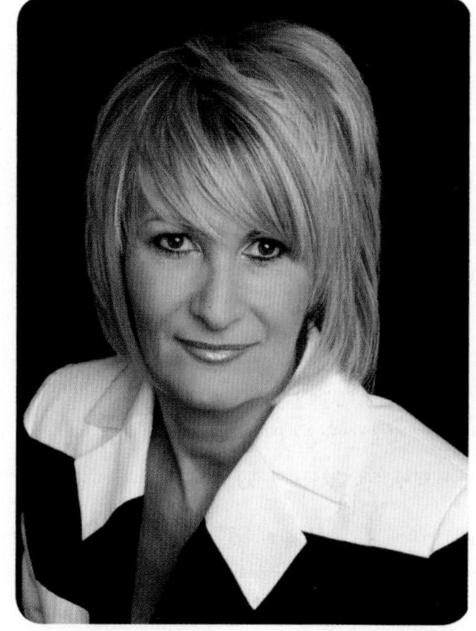

I am proud to have worked in beauty therapy for the past 30 years and am amazed at the technological advances that have been made. The beauty therapy industry is never boring, offers immense job satisfaction, clear progression opportunities and is increasingly diverse allowing you to specialize in what has effectively become micro-industries within what was traditionally termed beauty therapy, i.e. nails, make-up, massage and spa. This allows you to excel in the area of the industry that you feel passionate about, which ultimately raises the profile of our industry. Industry role models feature in each chapter to share their experiences offering practical advice throughout.

This VRQ Level 2 book aims to support you as you develop the capability and knowledge required when preparing to gain employment and work in the beauty therapy industry.

Enjoy your training and I wish you great success in the industry.

Lorraine Nordmann

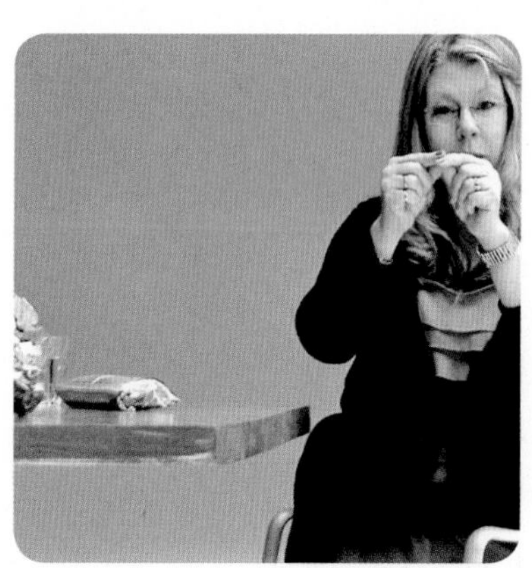

I was delighted to be invited to contribute to the VRQ edition of Lorraine's book, *Beauty Therapy – The Foundations*. I feel very strongly about the standards of education and skills of nail technicians working in the professional industry.

Hopefully these nail chapters provide many answers but also encourage further research. For those interested in a career as a nail technician I recommend the third edition of my book *The Complete Nail Technician* as the next step.

Marian Newman

About the contributor

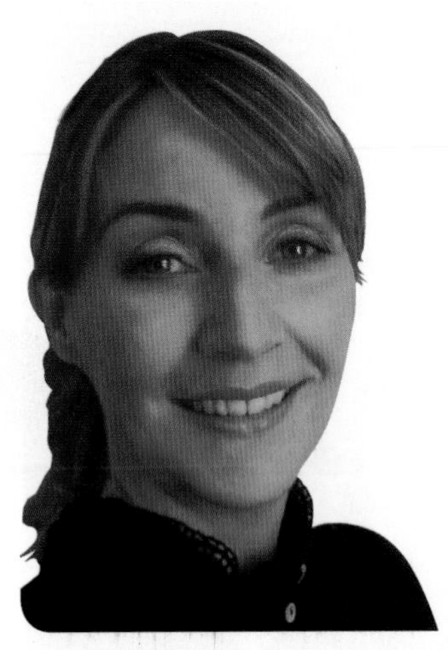

Following a career in nursing, I entered the beauty industry in 1995. After many years as a therapist and salon owner I decided to follow my passion for education and began to lecture at a Further Education college in Surrey.

In the following six years I gained further professional skills and qualifications including writing examination questions for CIBTAC (Confederation of International Beauty Therapy and Cosmetology), achieving the Cert.Ed. teaching qualification and embarking on training to become a beauty therapy examiner.

I set up my first training company, The National School of Threading, in 2006 in response to a growing demand for experienced threading teachers and have since performed many demonstrations and exhibitions in London and participated in the World Skills Championships.

As the leading expert and role model in this field, I have been privileged to work alongside some high profile businesses to provide both training and consultative work including NAILS INC – trade testing, training and launching their 'Get Lashed' brand, GMTTEC Training Education Consultancy and more recently, Boots UK, where I was commissioned as a consultant to assist in the development of a new brand concept.

Since 2007, I have been working closely with the ASA (Asian Style Awards) to assist the regulation of South Asian treatments and training, in particular threading, with a view to raising standards and protect other businesses and our consumers. I was selected to judge at their 2008 awards ceremony in London and will be writing a feature in their trade journal.

In 2009–10 I worked with Habia – the government recognized body that sets the National Occupational Standards for hair and beauty – to develop threading standards for a new industry qualification in threading, which was introduced in September 2010.

My plan for the future is to offer a wide range of short courses with my new training company – The Surrey School of Beauty & Complementary Health – to provide training for both new and practising therapists across many therapies, and to expand my threading expertise into Europe where the skill is still relatively unknown.

Lorraine Onorato

Acknowledgements

The author and publishers would like to thank the following:

For providing the cover image:

Photograph courtesy of Claire Harrison, www.claireharrisonphotography.com

For providing pictures for the book:

Absolute Aesthetics, www.absoluteaesthetics.co.uk
Alamy
Aquadome Ireland, www.aquadome.ie
Aqua Sana, Centre Parcs, www.aquasana.co.uk
Australian Bodycare
Babor
Beauty Express Ltd
Bliss Spa, www.blisslondon.co.uk
Caflon Ltd, www.caflon.com
Caress, www.caressmanufacturing.co.uk
Corbis
Covermark, Farmeco, www.farmeco.com
Daylight Company Ltd
Dermalogica, The International Dermal Institute, www.dermalinstitute.co.uk
Dorling Kindersley Ltd
Dr A L Wright
Dr John Gray, *The World of Skincare*
Dr M H Beck
Ellisons
Everlash
Gloss Communications
Gorgeous PR
Guinot
Habia
Health and Safety Executive
Helinova Ltd
House of Famuir, www.hofbeauty.co.uk
Intercontinental Hotel Group, Holiday Inn Hotel, Newton-le-Willows, Spirit Health Club, http://www.spirit-fit.com/clubs/haydock
Istock photo
Jane Iredale, www.janeiredaleuk.eu
Jessica Cosmetics, www.jessicacosmetics.co.uk
Korres Natural Products, www.korres.com
Mavala
Mediscan
Moom waxing, www.moom-uk.com
Wellcome Photo Library
Naissance, www.enaissance.co.uk
National Cancer Institute
NHF inspire, photography by Simon Powell
Salon Iris, www.saloniris.co.uk
Simon Jersey Ltd, www.simonjersey.com
Sister PR
Studex UK Ltd, www.studex.com
The Colour Wheel Company, www.colourwheelco.com
Thalgo UK Ltd, www.thalgo.com
The Beauty Lounge
The Sanctuary at Covent Garden Ltd, www.thesanctuary.co.uk
Unilever
www.shavata.co.uk
World of Beauty by Katy, Park Road, London

For their help with the photoshoot:

Mike Turner, www.miketurner-photography.co.uk

For their contribution as industry role models:

Jacqui Jefford
Jade Rogers
Janice Brown
Julia Francis
Lorraine Onorato
Pamela Linforth
Ruth Langley
Sally Biles
Sally Penford
Sally-Anne Braithwaite
Shavata Singh
Vicky Kennedy
Wendy Turner

For their help with the review process:

Debbie Le Grave, Newham College London
Joanne Mackinnon, London College of Beauty Therapy
Anita Crosland, Product Manager for Beauty, Nails Services, Spa and Complementary Therapies, City & Guilds

The author would personally like to thank:

Elizabeth and Norman Whiteside
Kathryn Leach
Shane Noden – personal trainer, The Personal Training People, Kenyons Lane South, Haydock, St Helens, Merseyside
Clare Kirkman
Christine Berry
Mike Turner – Photographer
Helen Eastwood
Chloe Eastwood
Gemma Hanlon
Vicky Kennedy – salon owner and beauty therapist, New Woman, New Man and Evolve, Westhoughton
Jacqueline Davi

1 Introduction

This book covers the essential practical skills and underpinning knowledge required to become a beauty therapist qualified at Diploma Level 2, VRQ (Vocationally Related Qualification), a *preparation for work qualification*.

What is a Beauty Therapy VRQ?

The VRQ is a nationally recognized Vocationally Related Qualification with its content based on the Beauty Therapy National Occupational Standards (NOS). It assesses the skills and abilities required for the beauty therapy workplace, in particular the knowledge and understanding requirements, preparing you for your career in the beauty therapy sector. VRQs are known as 'preparation for work qualifications' and may take place in a simulated, although realistic, beauty therapy learning environment abiding by all relevant health and safety legislation. This may include schools, colleges, training providers, the workplace and through distance learning. Practical assessment is not always performed on a client and can include colleagues, friends and family and even yourself!

Each awarding organization is required to cover the same standards in the design of their qualification. The National Occupational Standards are provided by the government-approved standards-setting body for hairdressing, beauty therapy, nails and spa therapy, **Habia** (Hairdressing and Beauty Therapy Industry Authority). This ensures that a future employer or training provider can be confident of the skills you will have acquired in accordance with the VRQ level you have achieved, whichever awarding body has accredited it. When you have successfully qualified, your diploma will bear the logo of the awarding body you registered and qualified with, as well as the Habia logo to show that Habia approves the qualification.

The Habia website provides a list of the qualifications that can be studied. See www.habia.org.

A list of approved training centres can also be found on the Habia website.

The aim of the VRQ is to develop the skills and knowledge required when preparing to gain employment and work in the beauty therapy industry. Another beauty therapy vocational qualification available is the NVQ (National Vocational Qualification). The main difference between a VRQ and an NVQ is that an NVQ is a 'job ready qualification', meaning that an NVQ assessment identifies your competence and capability and readiness for work. If competent, you are said to be ready to perform your skill, meeting both the industry's, and the clients' commercial expectations. A VRQ does not assess competence', but capability and knowledge. With further experience you will become 'job ready'.

Judgment is made upon your level of practical skills and underpinning knowledge. Commercial competence requirements are less important as it is recognized that these will be achieved with experience.

Units and learning outcomes

Your qualification is made up of a number of **units.** Each unit describes a specific activity or skill.

Each unit is divided into **learning outcomes,** which list the practical skills and underpinning knowledge requirements to carry out the activity or skill.

Each awarding organization will specify a structure (rules of combination) for their own Level 2 Beauty Therapy VRQ Diploma(s). There will be mandatory units which must be studied and achieved and there may be further optional units to select from. Refer to your qualification handbook for details on which units are mandatory and which are optional for your particular qualification.

This book covers the following list of units which includes all the mandatory units across all the awarding organizations and the most popular optional units. Anatomy and physiology underpinning knowledge is required for all treatment units and is covered in Chapter 2.

Unit	Chapter
Working in beauty related industries	Chapter 1
Follow health and safety practice in the salon	Chapter 3
Promote products and services to clients in the salon	Chapter 4
Client care and communication in beauty related industries	Chapter 5
Salon reception duties	Chapter 6
Provide facial skincare	Chapter 7
Provide eyelash and brow treatments	Chapter 8
Shaping and colouring eyebrows	Chapter 8
Provide eyelash perming	Chapter 8
Provide threading services for hair removal	Chapter 9
Apply make-up	Chapter 10
Create an image based on a theme	Chapter 10
Provide manicure treatments	Chapter 11
Provide pedicure treatments	Chapter 12
Provide and maintain nail enhancements	Chapter 13
Provide nail art	Chapter 14
Remove hair using waxing techniques	Chapter 15
Provide ear piercing	Chapter 16
Head massage	Chapter 17
Apply skin tanning techniques	Chapter 18

ALWAYS REMEMBER

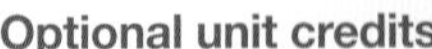

Optional unit credits

Units carry a credit weighting and the optional units you can select from must achieve the required total credit figure for the qualification.

Practical skills – what you can do

The practical skills are a list of practical activities to be carried out or tasks to demonstrate your practical skills and capabilities to the assessor.

Range – what you must cover

Range statements are identified for each outcome. The range relates to what you must cover and the different conditions under which a skill or knowledge of the unit must be demonstrated.

Where evidence has been achieved, this is cross-referenced (directed) in the portfolio (a place where you store your evidence) to where the evidence can be found.

To achieve each unit, all practical skills and underpinning knowledge requirements must have been met and evidence presented as necessary. Evidence is provided by completion of practical and written tasks or knowledge tests which may often be completed electronically with an on-line test. Evidence is usually provided in your assessment book and portfolio and may be paper-based or electronic.

This edition of *Beauty Therapy – The Foundations* follows the Beauty Therapy VRQ Beauty Therapy Level 2 Diploma practical skills and underpinning knowledge requirements for both the mandatory and optional units.

When you qualify and receive your VRQ Level 2 Diploma you may gain employment in the beauty therapy workplace and study towards an NVQ, although this is not an essential requirement.

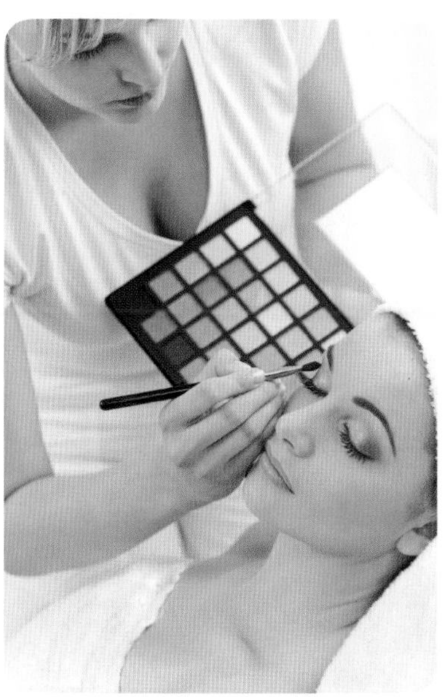

Professional beauty therapist/make-up artist

Working in beauty related industries

Learning Objectives

This chapter covers the **VRQ Unit Working in beauty related industries.**

This unit informs you about the requirements for working in the beauty related industries, helping you to learn about key features and working practices required.

There are **two** learning outcomes for this unit which you much achieve:

1. Know the key characteristics of the beauty related industries
2. Know the working practices associated in the beauty related industries

From the range statement, you must show that you can:

- **source information** to learn more about employment, education and training opportunities
- describe the different **organizations** and their functions
- describe the **main services** available in the beauty industry
- describe the different industry **occupational roles** and the opportunities to transfer to other sectors and industries
- describe the **employment characteristics** working in beauty related industries
- describe the **legislation** affecting the beauty related industries
- describe the **principles of finance and selling**
- describe the **forms of marketing and publicity** used in beauty related industries
- describe **good working practices**
- describe industry **personal presentation** requirements
- describe industry **employment rights and employer responsibilities**

Outcome 1: Know the key characteristics of the beauty related industries

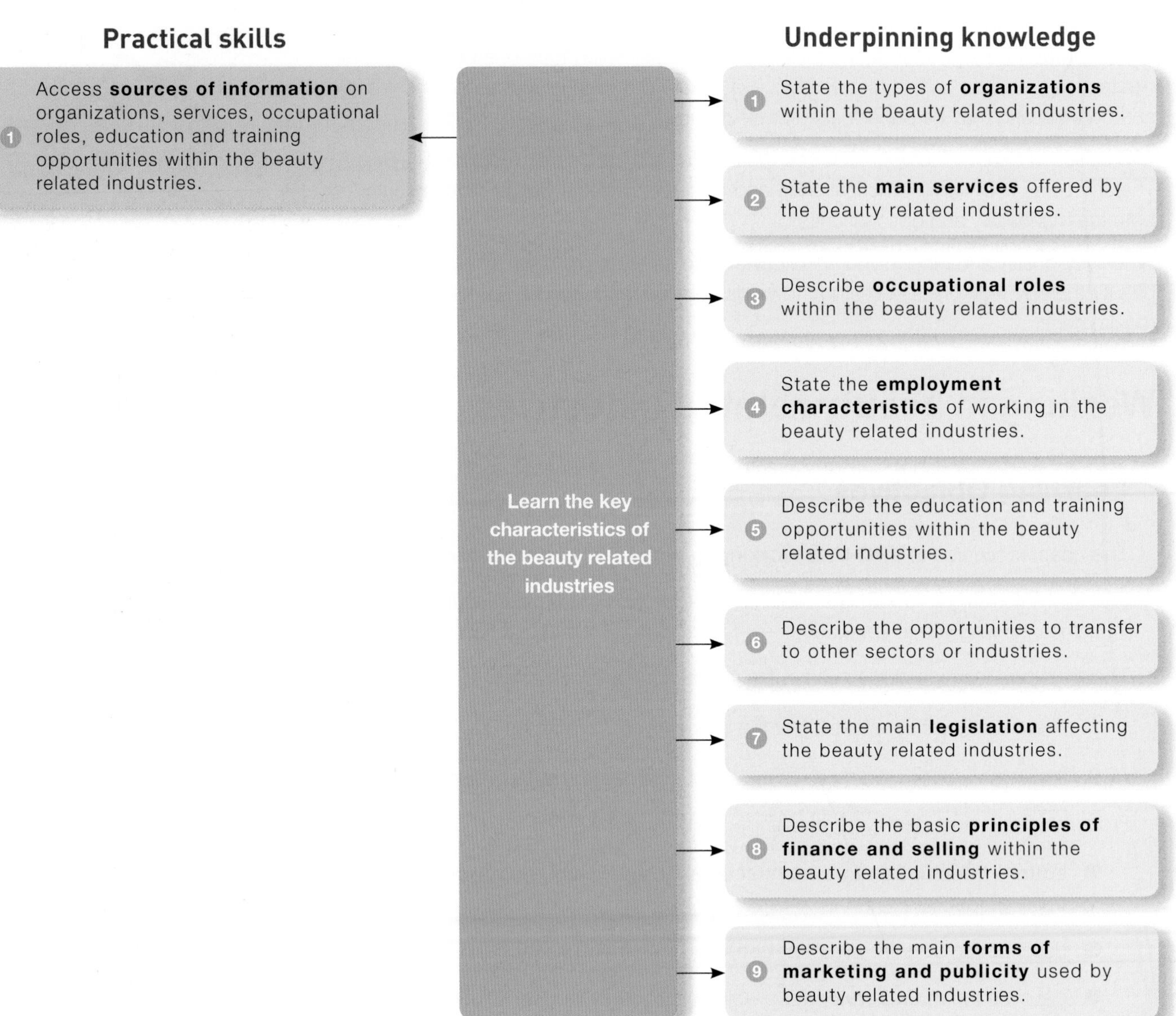
Practical skills
Underpinning knowledge
1 Access **sources of information** on organizations, services, occupational roles, education and training opportunities within the beauty related industries.
Learn the key characteristics of the beauty related industries
1 State the types of **organizations** within the beauty related industries.
2 State the **main services** offered by the beauty related industries.
3 Describe **occupational roles** within the beauty related industries.
4 State the **employment characteristics** of working in the beauty related industries.
5 Describe the education and training opportunities within the beauty related industries.
6 Describe the opportunities to transfer to other sectors or industries.
7 State the main **legislation** affecting the beauty related industries.
8 Describe the basic **principles of finance and selling** within the beauty related industries.
9 Describe the main **forms of marketing and publicity** used by beauty related industries.

Sources of information

You can access the following to supply you with the information about working in the beauty related industries through:

- the internet
- professional beauty therapy journals
- Habia: www.habia.org.uk
- training providers
- further education colleges
- awarding bodies
- career guidance providers, e.g. Connexions.

The beauty industry

Different types of organisations within the beauty related industries are listed below.

Beauty organization	Description
Manufacturer	These are different companies who make or supply the different tools, products and equipment that you work with. 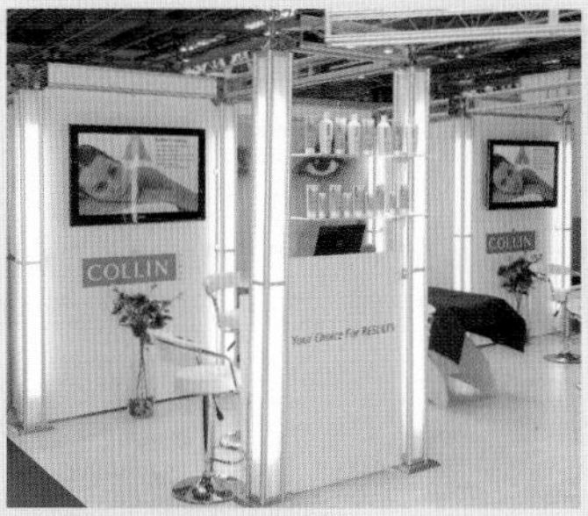
Salon	Salons employ staff to deliver beauty therapy services to meet the needs of their clients. Some salons choose to specialize in particular areas of beauty therapy, for example hair removal services. It is popular for hairdressing salons to offer a variety of beauty therapy services too. 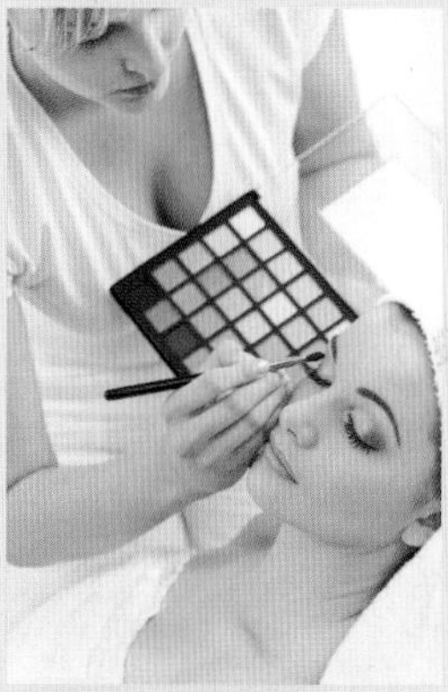
Health spa	Health spas provide health and well-being services in a relaxing environment. Specialist products and services achieve different therapeutic effects. 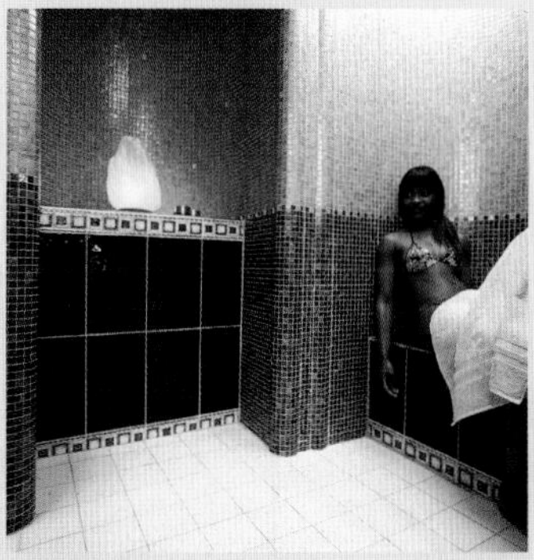
Hotel	Some hotels offer onsite a range of beauty services, which often include spa. 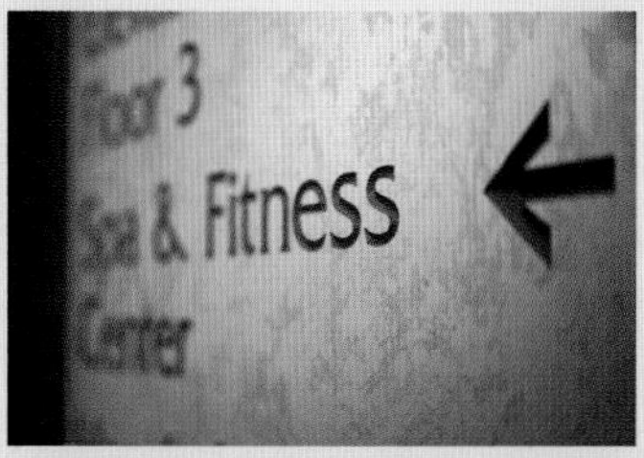
Cruise liners	Cruise liners employ beauty therapists to provide services and promotional activities to cruise liner passengers whilst on their holiday vacation. Retail of both products and services is a key work target, so good selling skills are essential. 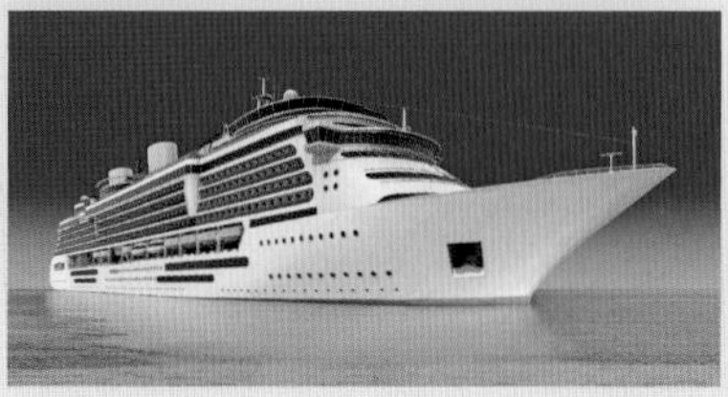

Collin UK

istock/© Lauri Wiberg

Dale Sauna Ltd, www.dalessauna.co.uk

Beauty organization	Description	
Fitness and leisure providers	Some fitness and leisure centres offer onsite a range of beauty services to support the total achievement of health and well-being.	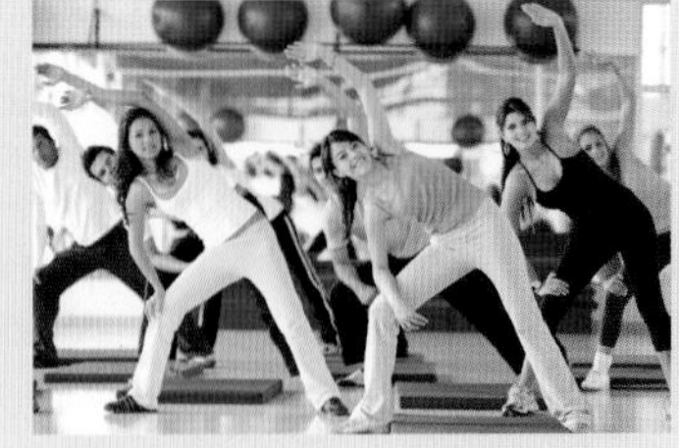
Professional membership organizations	As a professional beauty therapist, it is important that you adhere to a code of ethical practice and keep current in your skills and knowledge. You may wish to become a member of professional organization or body, which will issue you with a copy of its agreed standards and provide industry updates. Some membership organizations offer insurance benefits also.	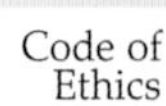 Code of Ethics 1. Towards BABTAC a) By not bringing the profession as a whole into disrepute b) By protecting collective morality. Members should not professionally associate themselves with any person or premises which may be deemed to be unprofessional or disreputable, as such an Association which may put the good name of the therapist and of BABTAC at risk. 2. Towards clients (concerned with the individual therapist/client relationship) a) Appointments must be kept. If unforeseen circumstances arise every effort must be made to make the client aware of the treatment cancellation. b) Client confidentiality - personal information should be kept private and only used for the specific purpose for which it is given, namely, to enable the therapist to carry out a safe and effective treatment. c) Information concerning the client and views formed must be kept confidential. The member should make every effort to ensure that this same level of confidence is upheld by receptionists and assistants where applicable. d) Client treatment details should remain confidential. Possible exceptions are the following: i) The client's knowledge and written consent are obtained. ii) There is a necessity for the information to be given for example if the client is being referred on to another professional. The exceptions are: iii) If the therapist is required by law to disclose the information. iv) If the therapist considers it their duty for the protection of the public. If a therapist has information of a criminal nature the member is advised to take legal advice. BABTAC, The British Association of Beauty Therapy and Cosmetology
Suppliers	Suppliers provide you with all the resources you need to carry out your services. These range from general consumables, such as cottonwool etc., to specialist suppliers or products, tools and equipment.	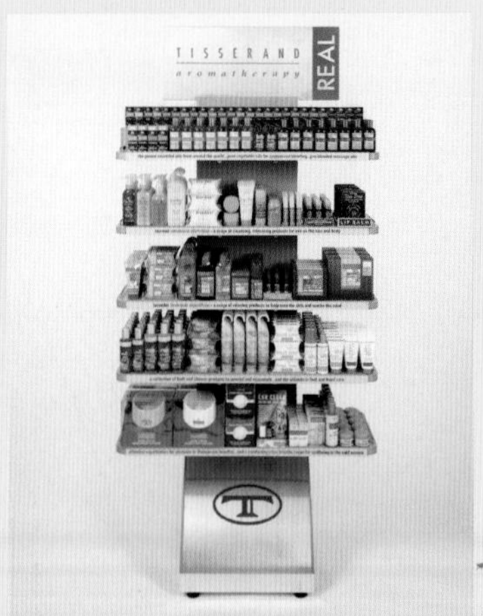 Tisserand
Industry leading bodies	Habia is the government-appointed standards-setting body for hair, beauty, nails, spa therapy, barbering and African type hair, and creates the standards that form the basis of all qualifications including NVQs, SVQs, apprenticeships, diplomas and foundation degrees, as well as industry codes of practice. Habia provides guidance on careers, business development, legislation, salon safety and equal opportunities, and is responsible to government on industry issues such as education and skills. Habia raises the profile of its industries through the press and media, and is the first port of call for news organizations and broadcasters on news items and background information. www.habia.org	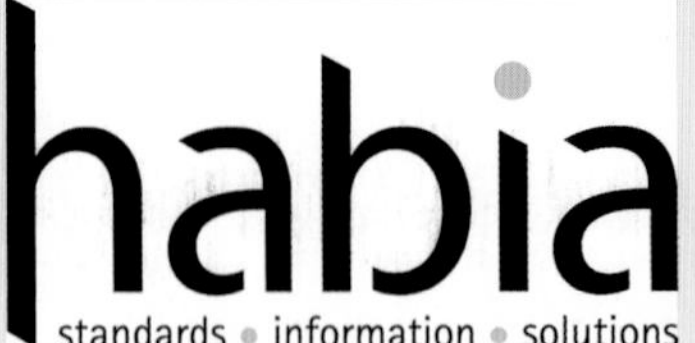

Beauty services

Some of the **main services** offered by the beauty related industries are listed below.

Beauty service	Description
Manicures	A treatment to care for and improve the condition and appearance of the hands and nails. 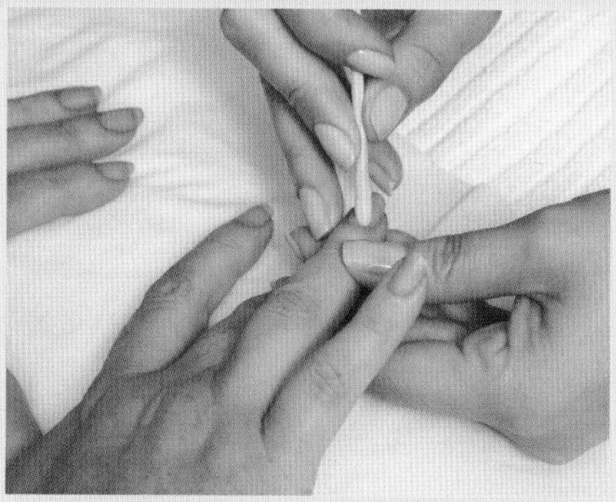
Pedicure	A treatment to care for and improve the condition and appearance of the skin and nails of the feet. 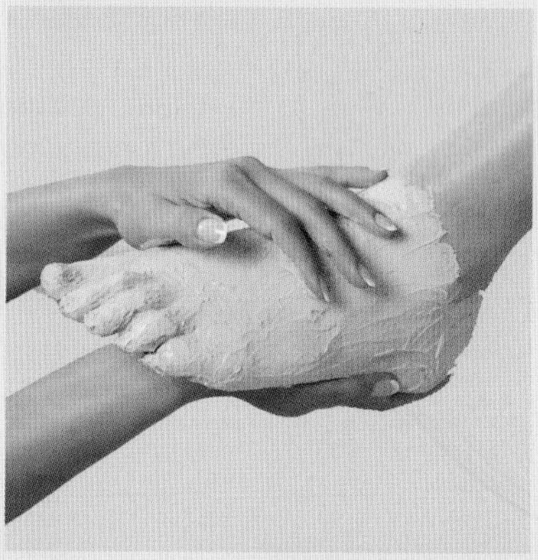
Waxing	The temporary removal of excess or unwanted hair from a body part using wax. 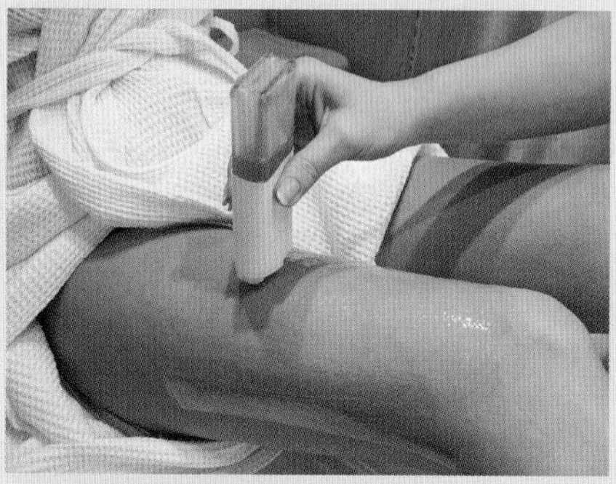
Nail enhancement	Artificial nail structures are applied to enhance the natural nail by: increasing its length; improving overall appearance and to strengthen and repair. 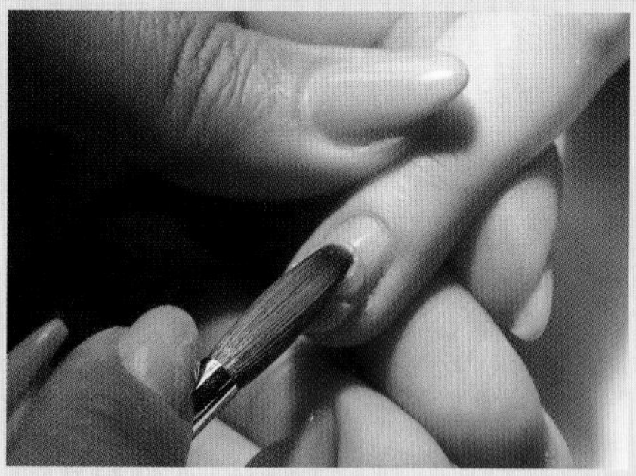

Australian Bodycare

Beauty service	Description
Make-up	Cosmetics applied to the skin of the face to enhance and accentuate, or to minimize facial features. Make-up products create balance in the face. 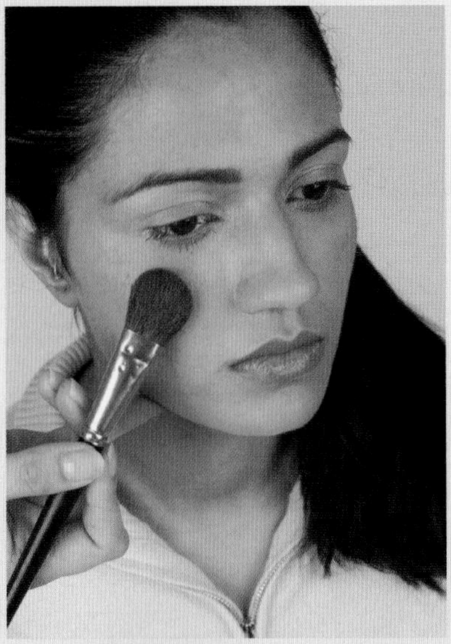
Basic facial	A treatment used to improve the appearance, condition and functioning of the skin and underlying structures. 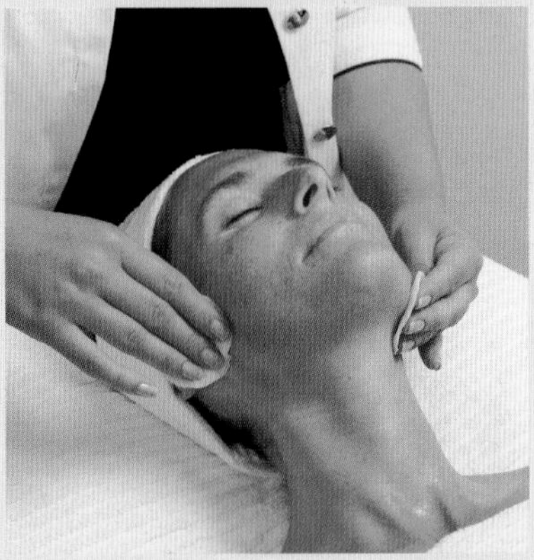
Electrical facial	Also referred to as **electrotherapy**. Mechanical or electrical equipment Is used to improve the condition and appearance of the face and neck area. Each piece of equipment creates specific effects. 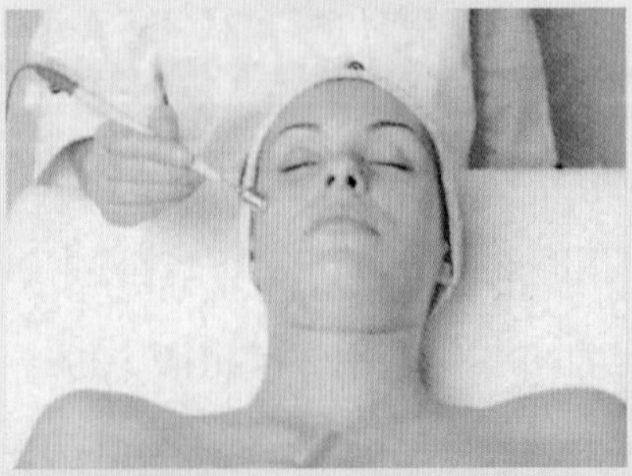
Electrolysis	Total destruction of the hair follicle using an electric current to permanently stop hair growth. 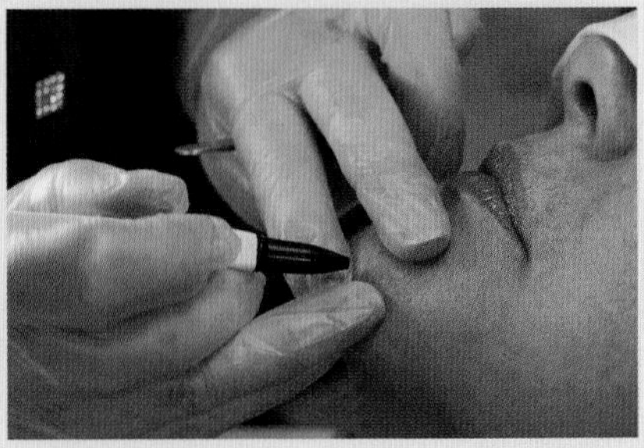

Smart Buy

Beauty service	Description
Eyelash and eyebrow treatments	Treatments applied to enhance the eye area including eyebrow shaping; permanent eyelash and eyebrow services and artificial eyelash application. 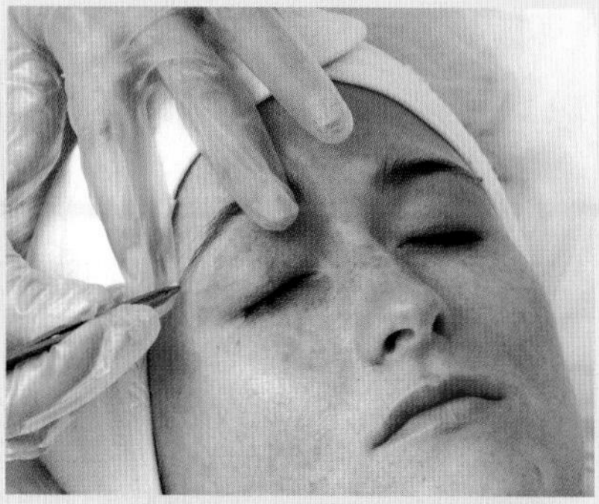
Body massage	Manipulation of the soft tissues of the body, producing heat in the area of application stimulating the bodies muscular, circulatory and nervous systems. 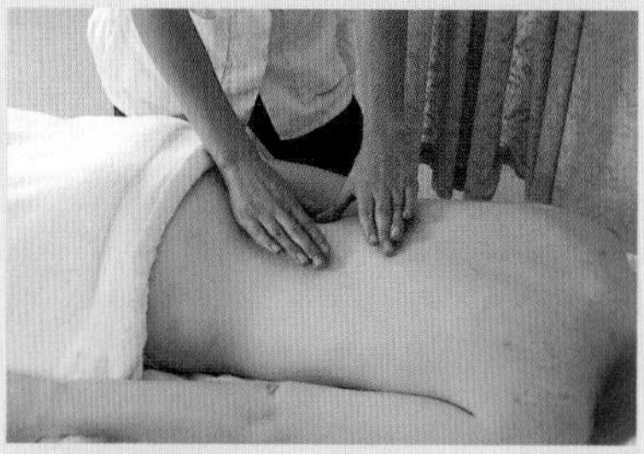
Aromatherapy	The use of essential oils – aromatic substances that have a vast range of aromas extracted from flowers, seeds, roots, fruits and bark. Usually combined with massage to influence the client's mood and create a feeling of well-being. 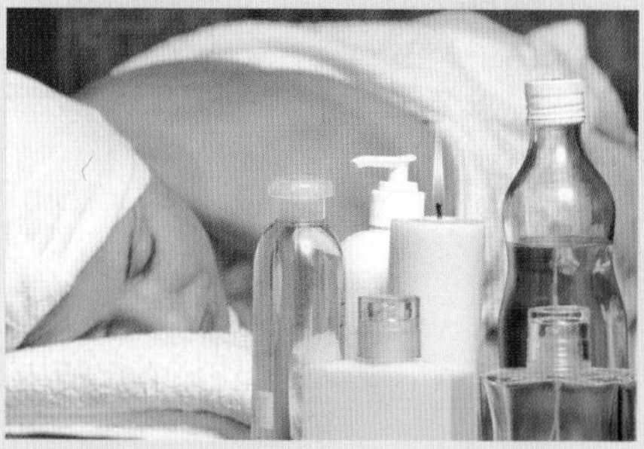
Reflexology	A treatment using finger point pressure applied to the zones of the feet and hands to enhance energy flow through the body. Derived from Ancient Chinese, Egyptian and Indian techniques. 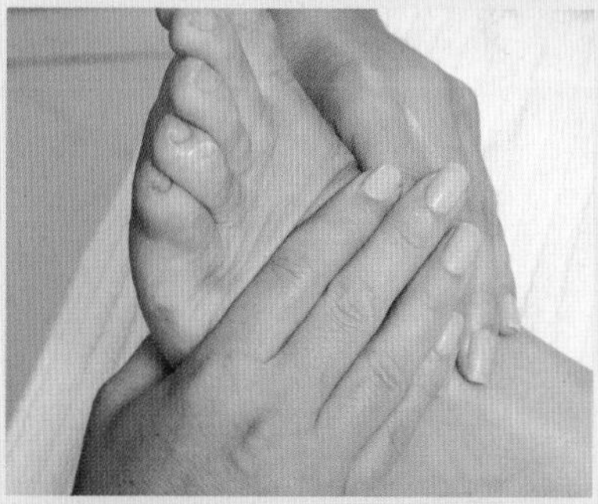
Heat and water therapy	Heat therapy – skin warming treatments including the use of moist and dry heat. Treatments include sauna, and steam treatments. Water therapy – also known as hydrotherapy (derived from the Greek *hydor* 'water' and *therapia* 'therapy' meaning 'the theraputic use of water'). Treatments include: hydrotherapy baths; water jet tunnel and wet flotation treatments; spa pools; pools and showers.

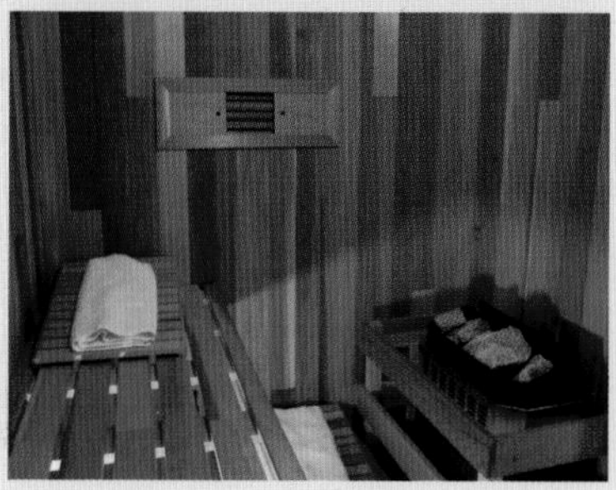

© Leah-Anne Thompson/Shutterstock

Dale Sauna Ltd, www.dalessauna.co.uk

Beauty service	Description
Hot stone therapy	Massage usually using a variety of volcanic stones, which may be cold or heated to stimulate or relax; used in conjunction with massage they help to restore the flow of energy in the body by using a variety of application techniques.
Indian head massage	A massage treatment traditionally practised in India. It is applied to the upper body using the hands. The massage helps to relieve stress and tension, creating a feeling of well-being. Oils may be applied to the scalp and hair to improve their condition.
Electrical body treatments	Also referred to as **electrotherapy**. Mechanical or electrical equipment Is used to improve the condition and appearance of the limbs and trunk areas or overall appearance of the body. Each piece of equipment creates specific effects.
Body wrapping	A body treatment where the body is wrapped in bandages, plastic sheets or thermal blankets to achieve different therapeutic effects.
Tanning	Also known as **UV tanning** or **self tanning**. In UV tanning the skin is exposed to artificially produced UV and the skin darkens creating a tan. Self tanning uses cosmetic products containing an ingredient which gives a healthy, tanned appearance to the skin. Different methods can be used to apply self-tan products including automated spray, manual and airbrush application.

Depilex

Spa Find www.spafindskincare.com

Beauty related work roles

There are a wide range of different job opportunities available in the beauty related industries. A brief explanation of the various occupational beauty related work roles are described below.

Occupational work role	Description of activities
Beauty therapist	Beauty therapists provide beauty treatments and services which, if qualified to Level 3 (VRQ or NVQ), may include those listed in the chart on pages 7–11. They also give advice to clients and promote retail beauty products to support the services they offer. Beauty therapists may work in a salon, in their own home or travel to clients' homes. 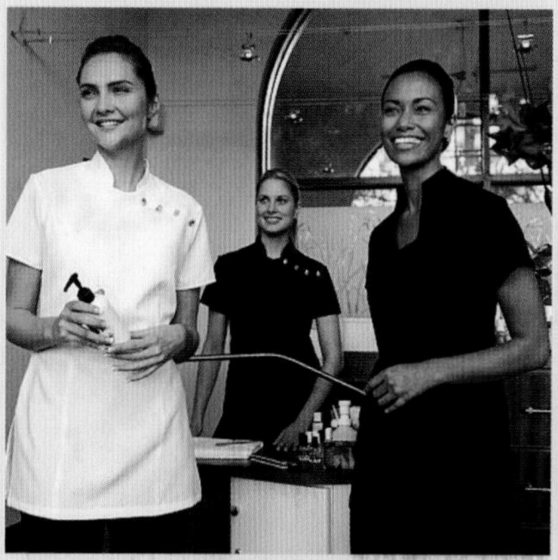
Make-up artist	Make-up artists apply make-up and often also style the hair of performers and presenters for TV, film, theatre, fashion shows, live performances and photo shoots. 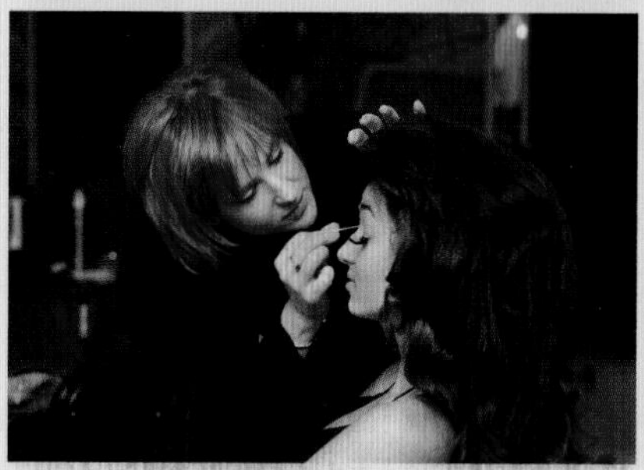
Electrologist	A specialist in hair removal who uses electrolysis to permanently destroy the hair follicle to stop hair growth. A sterile needle is used to apply an electric current with galvanic or short wave diathermy electrical equipment. 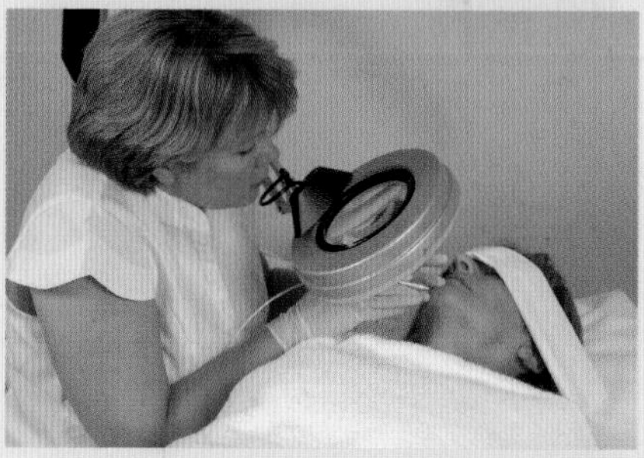
Nail technician	A specialist in nail treatments including care of the natural nail with manicures and pedicures, nail art application and artificial nail enhancement techniques. 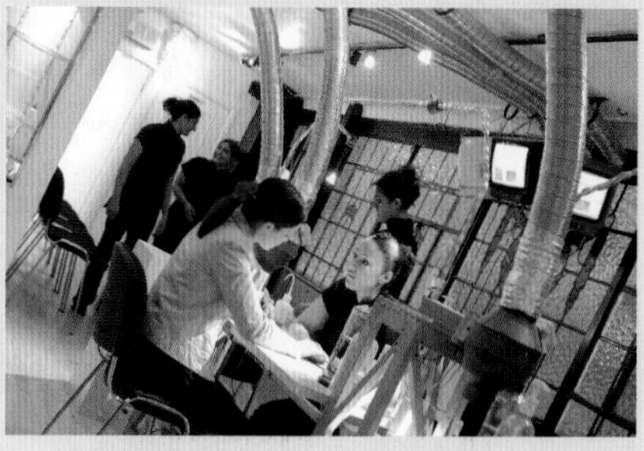

www.simonjersey.com

ISTOCK/ © LISE GAGNE

Marco Benito

Occupational work role	Description of activities	
Manicurist/pedicurist	A specialist manicurist/pedicurist specializes treatments for the hands (manicure) and feet in (pedicure) with the aim to improve or maintain their health and appearance through the provision of specialized tretaments.	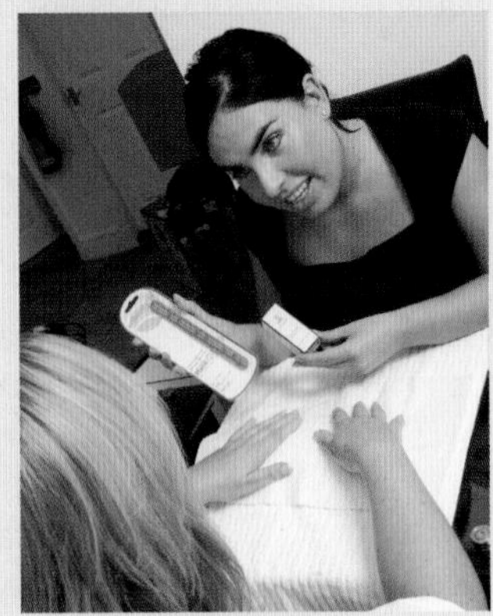
Massage therapist	The massage therapist provides massage treatments to the face, head and body. This may be performed *manually*, where the beauty therapist's hands manipulate the client's skin, tissue and underlying muscles, or *mechanically* using a machine. Massage techniques can achieve a relaxing or stimulating effect and create a feeling of well-being.	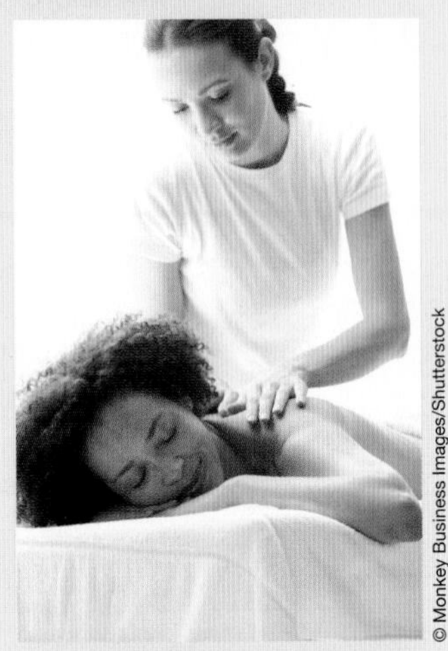 © Monkey Business Images/Shutterstock
Aromatherapist	Aromatherapists treat a variety of physical conditions and psychological disorders using essential aromatic oils that are extracted from flowers, trees, fruit and herbs, selected for their therapeutic properties.	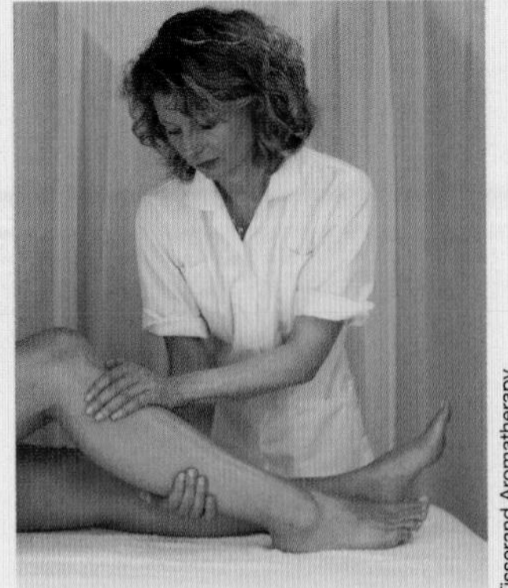 Tisserand Aromatherapy
Reflexologist	In reflexology every part of the body is reflected in a precise area, or reflex point, on the feet and hands. The reflexologist works on the foot or the hand as appropriate, using a precise technique based upon the application of finger point pressure on the reflex zones of the feet and hands to restore the flow of energy through the body.	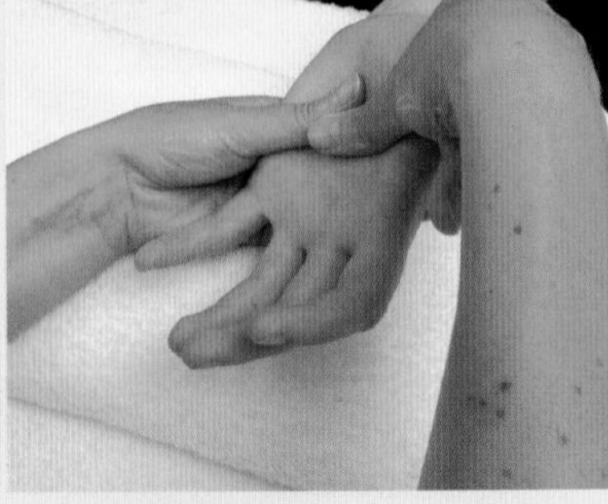

Occupational work role	Description of activities
Complementary therapist	A practitioner providing treatment alongside or in addition to conventional medicine. This is referred to as 'complementary medicine' as the two practices *complement* each other. The practitioner treats the client's body and mind as a whole and this is often referred to as an 'holistic approach'. 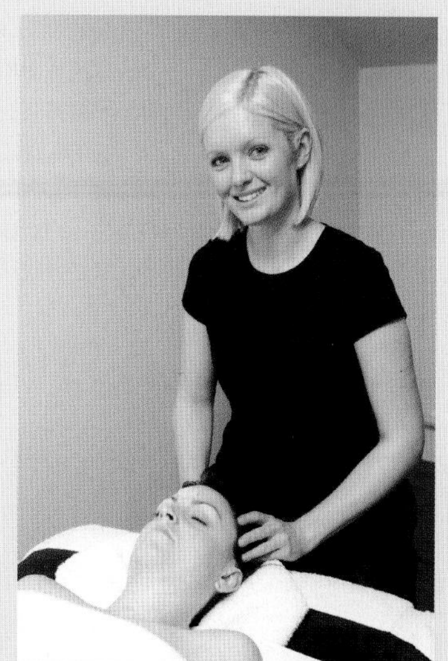
Cosmetic consultant	Usually employed by a cosmetic company in a retail environment or freelanc, cosmetic consultants sell cosmetics and advise customers on the right products to meet their requirements. 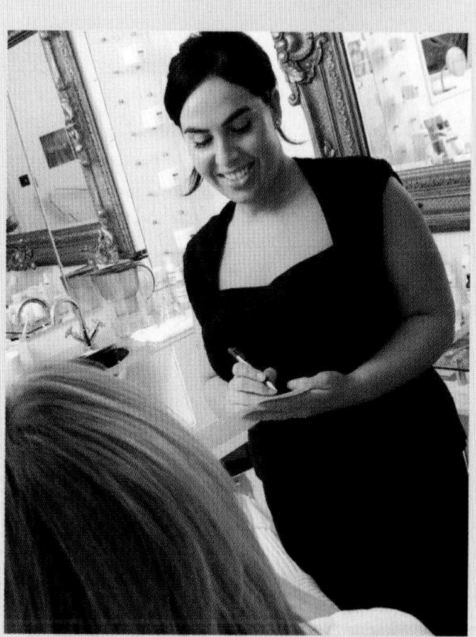
Sales representative	Promotes a particular product, service or company "brand". They are often experts in their field and can offer technical support and training within the beauty related industries through continuing professional development (CPD). 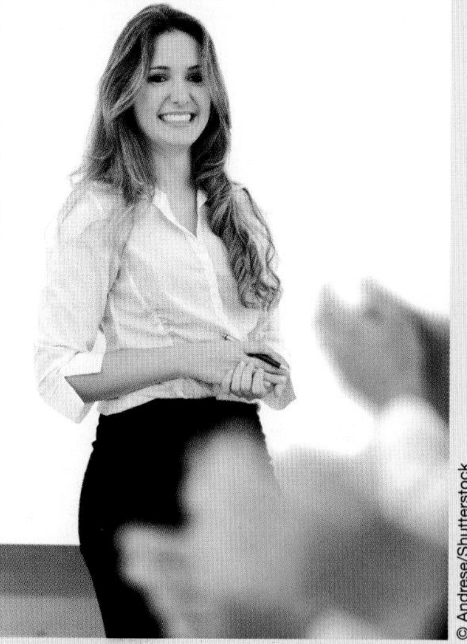

Occupational work role	Description of activities	
Receptionist	The receptionist and receives people entering the beauty work area, handles enquiries, makes appointments, deals with client payments and maintains the appearance of the reception area. The receptionist should always deal with people in a polite, efficient manner particularly while questioning them to find out what they require.	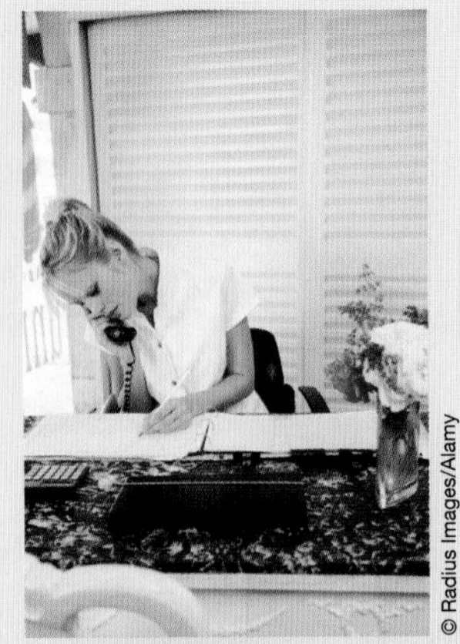 © Radius Images/Alamy
Salon manager	The salon manager and supports other colleagues with additional responsibilities for the day to day running of the business, complying with all workplace legislation and monitoring performance and attainment towards any specific targets.	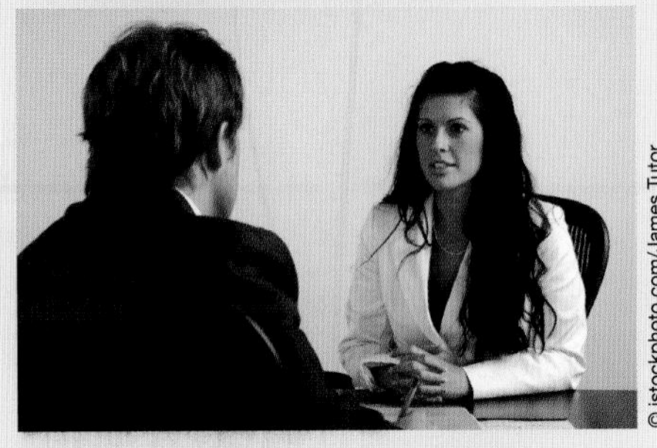 © istockphoto.com/James Tutor
Teacher	Teachers are qualified and trained to teach their occupational skills and assess their learners' competence or capability across a variety of courses and levels.	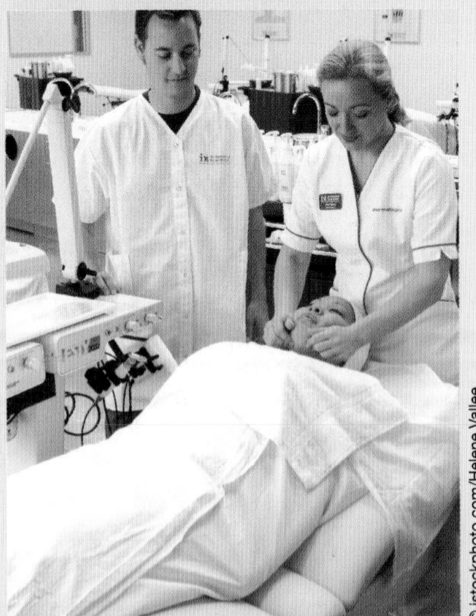 © istockphoto.com/Helene Vallee
Trainer	Trainers are qualified to train learners in a variety of courses, often in specific, continuing professional development (CPD) courses.	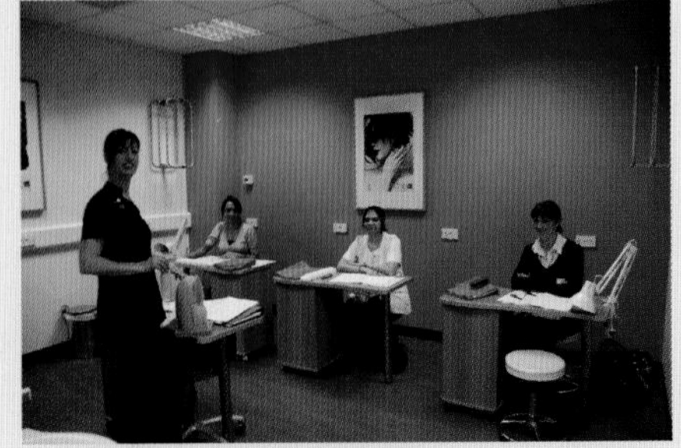 Ellisons

Legislation

There is a great deal of legislation affecting the beauty related industries.

To find out more about the following legislation, refer to Chapter 3 Health and Safety and Chapter 4 Selling Skills

- Equal Opportunity and Discrimination Acts
- Working Time Regulations
- National Minimum Wage
- Employment Rights Act
- Employment Act
- Health and Safety at Work Act
- Performing Rights Regulations
- Data Protection Act
- Trade Description Act
- Consumer Protection Act

ALWAYS REMEMBER

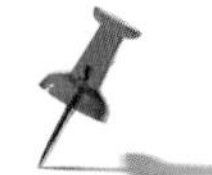

Continuing professional development (CPD)
This is a term used to refer to knowledge and technical development, after qualifying, to ensure the most up-to-date knowledge.

You are required to be able to describe the basic principles of finance and selling. This includes knowing how to inform clients about products and services and the importance of good product knowledge; knowing when and how to promote a product using effective communication skills; following through the stages of the selling process identifying the need for the product; the most appropriate product to meet the need and demonstrating the product's features and benefits, overcoming any obstacles presented by the client and finally closing the sale.

To help your research on techniques selling refer to Chapter 4 Selling Skills. When you have achieved a sale, you need to know how to handle the different types of payments. Find out more about this in Chapter 6 Salon Reception. The pricing of products and services are covered by different legislation that you need to comply with. Find out more about consumer protection legislation in Chapter 4 Selling Skills. Finally, for a business to be successful it is essential that clients are aware of your business and what services and products you provide.

Business marketing and publicity

Marketing and publicity is essential to raise client awareness of product or services and create or maintain interest. These activities let existing and potential clients know what you have to offer. A budget is allocated for marketing and the choice of advertising will depend upon how much money is available to spend and which is most cost-effective. Marketing activities such as promotional activities can occur internally at the business premises or off site at an external venue. Promotions are essential to the success of the business. An annual business plan should identify what promotions are intended to be implemented – an event list. This will be based upon a promotion strategy (which will involve all staff) to reach target markets in order to achieve a specific objective(s).

There may be a contribution from sponsors, such as skincare companies, who will play a part in supporting the success of a promotional event or sponsor advertising. Ideas from staff are important and appraisals provide a good opportunity for you to offer ideas such as how a new client target group can be reached or how the profile of the services that are on offer can be raised.

Methods of marketing and publicity include using signage in the business, fliers, direct mailings, email, text phone messaging, website advertisement and media such as advertisements in papers, commercial journals, radio and television. The advertising campaign needs a specific goal. This could be a short-term goal, e.g., the launch of a new product, discounted services, etc. or a long-term goal such as establishing the business name and familiarity with its product and services, "the brand". This would be achieved through repeat advertising. The best advert is your clients who if happy advertise through positive word-of-mouth.

Where possible, videos and photographic images of marketing activities may be shown on the business website or as an information medium in the reception area to maintain interest and awareness.

Never miss any marketing opportunities for the business when holding a promotion. Te local press can be informed, if invited advice them of the best time to be there and who to contact.

ALWAYS REMEMBER

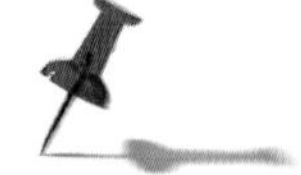

Only ever work within your job role in any activity.

The *trade press* can also be used who will feature new developmental areas within the sector and commentary on items such as charity-based events. If there is something new and innovative this could be reviewed by the *consumer press* who will then put it into the public domain, so the potential to raise the business profile from this opportunity is much higher.

Outcome 2: Know the working practices associated with the beauty related industries

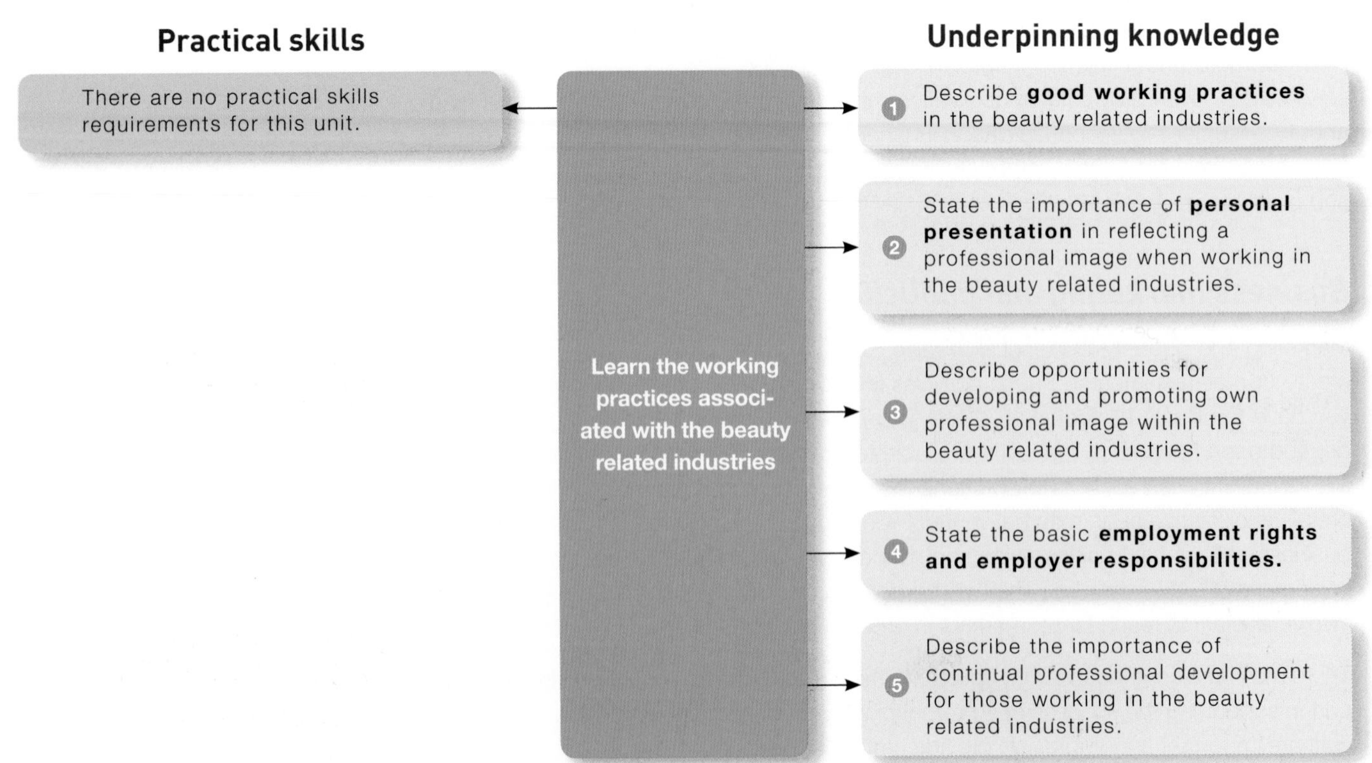

Practical skills
There are no practical skills requirements for this unit.
Learn the working practices associated with the beauty related industries
Underpinning knowledge
1 Describe good working practices in the beauty related industries.
2 State the importance of personal presentation in reflecting a professional image when working in the beauty related industries.
3 Describe opportunities for developing and promoting own professional image within the beauty related industries.
4 State the basic employment rights and employer responsibilities.
5 Describe the importance of continual professional development for those working in the beauty related industries.

A successful career in beauty therapy

To gain employment within the beauty related industries, as well as having received the necessary training and qualifications you must also have good employability skills. An employer regards these as being just as important as your qualification.

An employer would expect you to adopt good working practices at all times:

Professional – presenting a consistent, positive image of yourself and the workplace.

Courteous – clients should be treated with respect in all communication and contact, both verbal and non-verbal and during each stage of service delivery.

Discreet – you must be careful and tactful in how you communicate and express yourself at all times in the working environment. Certain conversation topics may not be suitable and cause embarrassment. Always 'think before you speak'. Avoid passing on personal opinions which may cause offence. In compliance with the legislation of the Data Protection Act (1998), never pass on client or staff information unless agreement has been given.

Personable – a successful business requires employees who are personable or pleasant and have people skills. These would mean having a positive attitude, being able to work well, co-operate and communicate with others – a team player.

Enthusiastic – employers want employees to have high aspirations and be willing to work hard to achieve them.

Responsible – your employer will expect you to think carefully when performing any tasks to avoid unnecessary error. Self-discipline is a good attribute to ensure all tasks are completed competently and meet the required deadline.

When you have successfully completed your VRQ in Beauty Therapy at Level 2 you can gain employment or progress your training, gaining a further technical awards or certificates or higher qualification.

ACTIVITY

List some examples of what being courteous means to you, when dealing with a client. Consider the scenarios below and state how you would deal with each in a courteous manner:

- A client arriving at reception when you are already busy with another client
- A client arriving late for a service
- A client receiving a service for the first time

BEST PRACTICE

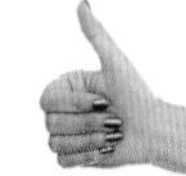

Good working practices
These include completing services to the best of your ability and following all relevant legislation, codes of practice and work-related policies and procedures.

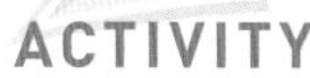

ACTIVITY

Write a list of the personal strengths you feel you have that would make you successful as a beauty therapist.

Write a list of any weaknesses you have e.g. poor punctuality, which need improvement to improve your personal employability skills?

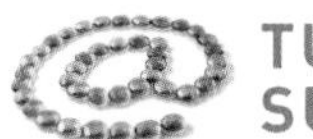

TUTOR SUPPORT

Activity 1: Professional appearance poster

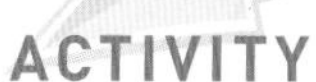

ACTIVITY

If a client could not receive a service because she had a skin disorder that could not be treated, how would you deal with this discreetly?

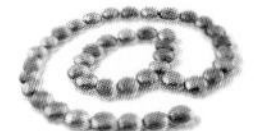

TUTOR SUPPORT

Activity 2: Professional approach report

KNOWLEDGE CHECK

What do you understand by the requirements of the legislation and codes of practice listed below and how do you comply with them in your everyday work?

Personal Protective Equipment(PPE) (2002)
Control of Substances Hazardous to Health (COSHH) (2002)
Manual Handling Operations Regulations (1992)
Electricity at Work Regulations (1989)
Habia Code of Practice for Waxing

Need more help? Refer to Chapter 3 Health and Safety, to find out more about the legislation and how it applies to you.

ACTIVITY

List further employability skills you think are important and explain why.

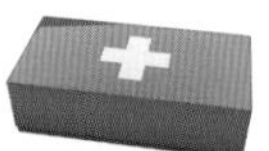

HEALTH & SAFETY

Aprons and the Personal Protective Equipment (PPE) at Work Regulations (1992)
For certain services, such as waxing services, it is necessary to wear a protective apron over the overall to protect the overall and keep it clean.

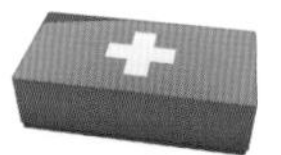

HEALTH & SAFETY

Control of substances hazardous to health (COSHH) (2002)

Essential information for beauty therapists is available on the HSE website in a section called COSHH and your industry. You will be able to find out more about how COSHH affects you? See www.hse.gov.uk.

Personal health, hygiene and presentation

Your appearance enables the client to make their first judgment about both you and the workplace, so make sure that you create the correct impression! Employees in the work-place should always reflect the most desirable image of the profession that they work in. The following general rules apply:

Due to the nature of many of the services offered, the beauty therapist must wear protective, hygienic work wear. A cotton overall is ideal; air can circulate, allowing perspiration to evaporate and discouraging unpleasant stale body smells referred to as body odour. The wearing of a colour such as white immediately shows the client that you are clean. An overall might comprise a dress, in a length suited to a work role, a jumpsuit or a tunic top, with coordinating trousers. Overalls should be laundered regularly and a fresh, clean overall worn each day. Flesh coloured tights may be worn to protect the leg area if exposed.

Make-up If worn, wear attractive make-up, and use the correct skincare cosmetics to suit your skin type. A healthy complexion will be a positive advertisement for your work.

Jewellery Keep jewellery to a minimum, such as a wedding ring, a fob watch and small stud earrings. This prevents scratching the client accidentally during the service and for reasons of hygiene.

Nails Nails, both natural and artificial if worn, should be short, neatly manicured and free of nail polish unless the employee's main duties involve nail services or reception duties. Nail polish contains ingredients which can cause an allergic response in some people.

Shoes Wear flat, well-fitting, comfortable shoes that enclose the feet fully. This will provide protection if you accidentally drop anything on your feet, e.g. hot paraffin wax. Remember that you will be on your feet for most of the day: they need to support your feet properly!

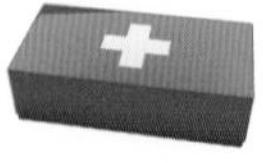

HEALTH & SAFETY

Workplace policy
Employers will advise you on personal presentation requirements in relation to facial piercings, nail length and if nail polish may be worn.

Employment opportunities

Employment opportunities in beauty therapy include:

- Business owner
- Freelance working for yourself
- Junior therapist in a salon
- Retail in cosmetics and skincare, referred to as a make-up consultant
- Specializing in a particular area of beauty therapy such as skincare or waxing hair removal
- Employment in a spa or leisure centre providing beauty therapy services.

TOP TIP

Visiting trade shows and subscribing to professional trade magazines provide an excellent opportunity to keep up to date with new products, equipment and services. The internet also allows you to follow current and future trends.

TOP TIP

While training for your VRQ, completing work placements, voluntary or paid, is vital to improve your confidence and help you gain a greater understanding of the requirements for working in the beauty related industries 'on the job'. This will increase your CV, helping you to build an impressive work experience related portfolio.

Employment rights and responsibilities

It is important to have a basic understanding of employment law that protects you and which employers must abide by. These laws and regulations are designed to ensure that you are not exploited or treated unfairly.

ACTIVITY

Why is employee image important to a business?

Give examples of professional best practice in your work role as a beauty therapist.

Contract of employment

Because there are so many ways that a person may be employed each person should have a contract of employment which states the 'terms and conditions' of their employment. This is regulated by the Employment Rights Act (1996). It may be referred to in the case of a dispute as evidence of an employee's 'terms and conditions'.

A contract of employment should be issued by the employer to the employee within eight weeks of start of work. It will include important information such as the date your employment began; your hours of work; when and how you will be paid and your hours of work including your holiday entitlement. Also, it will include your job title and job description; your place of work; whether it is a permanent or fix termed post (also known as contractual) and details of sickness and pension entitlements. The disciplinary and grievance procedures should always be included in your contract of employment. Finally, it must include the address of the place of work as you need to be informed if you are working in more than one place.

National Minimum Wage Act (1998)

Since 1998 it has been illegal to pay less than the national minimum hourly rate of pay. Every year the government amends the national minimum hourly rate to allow for inflation and average increases in wages.

TOP TIP

To find out more about aspects of employment law visit www.direct.gov.uk/en/Employment/index.htm.

Working safely

There is a good deal of legislation relating to health and safety in the workplace. It is there to provide safe working environment for all. You will need to know the laws relating to beauty therapy – your responsibilities and your rights. If you cause harm to your client or put them at risk you will be liable for prosecution. The same applies to an employer who does not provide a safe working environment for their employees.

The Health and Safety at Work Act (1974) (HASAWA) states the minimum standards of health, safety and welfare required in each area of the workplace. Refer to Chapter 3 Health and Safety, to find out more about health, safety and welfare in the workplace.

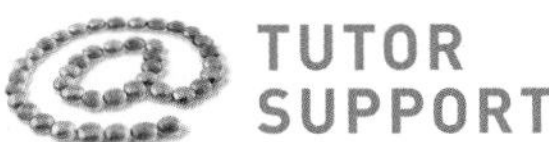

TUTOR SUPPORT

Activity 3: Employability skills and recruitment

Progression opportunities

When qualified at VRQ Level 2 you can continue to develop your skills and knowledge as follows:

- VRQ or NVQ Level 3 Beauty Therapy or Make-up
- Other associated industry qualifications in hairdressing, nails, massage or spa
- Further training to gain advanced practical techniques to maintain continuous professional development (CPD). CPD is important to keep yourself up to date and meet the emerging trends of the industry. This may include further VRQ awards or certificates.
- On achievement of Level 3 qualifications you may find employment dependent upon your training route as a:
    - business owner
    - college lecturer and assessor
    - salon trainer and assessor
    - technician for a manufacturer providing training on products, equipment and services
    - salon manager
    - senior therapist or make-up artist
    - sales and marketing manager
    - cruise ship or airline beauty therapist
- Other routes include:
    - working in the media – magazines, advertisements and television
    - specializing in a particular area such as electrolysis or photographic make-up
    - working as a make-up artist working on film sets, in television studio, theatre, music videos and fashion providing fashion runway make-up

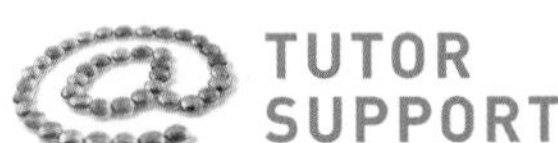

TUTOR SUPPORT

Activity 4: Personal development plan

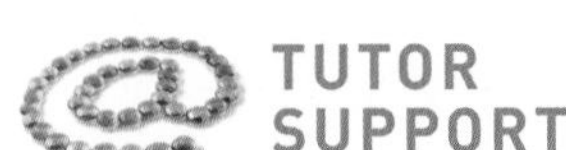

TUTOR SUPPORT

Activity 5: Beauty sector roles research

Again when you achieve your Level 3 qualification in beauty therapy or make-up you can continue to update and advance your skills as relevant to your career path/goals.

STUDENT CASE STUDY

Name: Verity Eden

Title of Qualification:
VRQ Level 2 Beauty Therapy (nearly completed VRQ Level 3 Beauty Therapy)

What did you enjoy most about studying, and what did you find most challenging?

I have really enjoyed carrying out treatments in the college salon as this has enabled me to perfect my practical skills without the pressure of a real work environment. The anatomy and physiology knowledge is definitely the most challenging part of the course but I know how important it is so I don't mind studying hard to get it right.

What are your next steps in your career development, and where would you like to see yourself in the future?

I am due to finish my VRQ Level 3 Beauty Therapy Diploma in a couple of months. Once this has been completed, I look forward to working in a salon and building up my skills further. In the future I would like have my own salon, specializing in dermatology and facial treatments.

What inspires and motivates you?

My college tutors are inspirational; they have such a passion for the subjects they teach, you can't help but feel passionate too. I am also inspired by some of the leading professionals in the beauty therapy world such as the role models in this book.

I feel motivated when I receive good feedback from a client, whether it's a family member, friend or someone who has come into the college salon. It is a really nice feeling when a client tells you that you have made them feel better and that they will come back to see you again.

What is the most important thing you have learnt from your beauty therapy qualifications?

The consultation process is the most important part of any treatment so one of most important things I have learnt is how to communicate effectively and professionally with clients. If you can get the consultation right, the treatment should be successful, so good communication skills are the key.

What would you say to a new student starting their Level 2 qualification?

Go for it! The theory side of the course, especially the anatomy and physiology, is a lot harder than Level 1 but it all seems worth it when you're practising your treatments and getting it right. If you have any choices, make sure you choose your optional units carefully and don't just do what your friends are doing.

What do you think makes a good beauty therapist?

I think to be good beauty therapist you need to be polite and professional with your clients, and also be able to show empathy where necessary. The hygiene and appearance of the therapist is also extremely important.

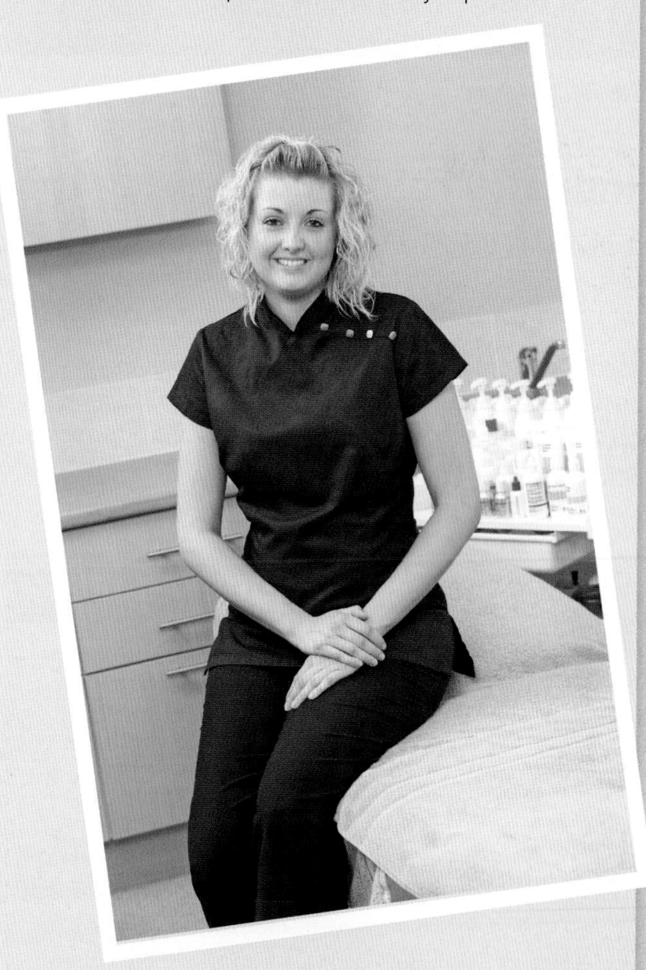

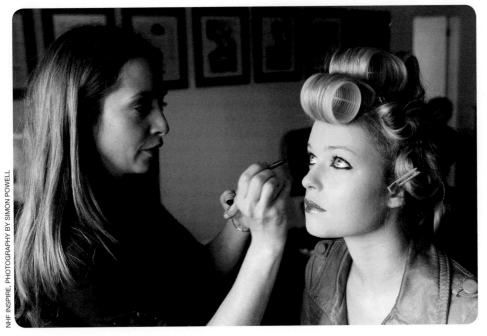

NHF INSPIRE, PHOTOGRAPHY BY SIMON POWELL

Fashion photo shoot

ACTIVITY

What would you consider your 'dream job'. Using professional journals/magazines or online job advertisements search for a vacancy and obtain a job description so you can see the qualifications, experience and personal attributes that you will need to have. You can then draw up a plan of what you will need to achieve when and how to gain the necessary evidence and experience. This is your career path, the journey required to achieve your career goal.

Industry role models

In the beauty therapy and make-up industry there are many role models who have extensive experience which has helped raise the industry profile, and a passion for their work which is inspirational to our beauty therapists and make-up artists of the future.

Industry role models have contributed 'tips of the trade' in this book sharing their expertise and valued knowledge. On successful completion of your Level 2 qualification you will be able to work in a rewarding job full of variety with career possibilities that are endless!

TOP TIP

Beauty therapy is one of the UK's 20 happiest sectors to work in, according to City & Guilds, scoring 8 out of 10.

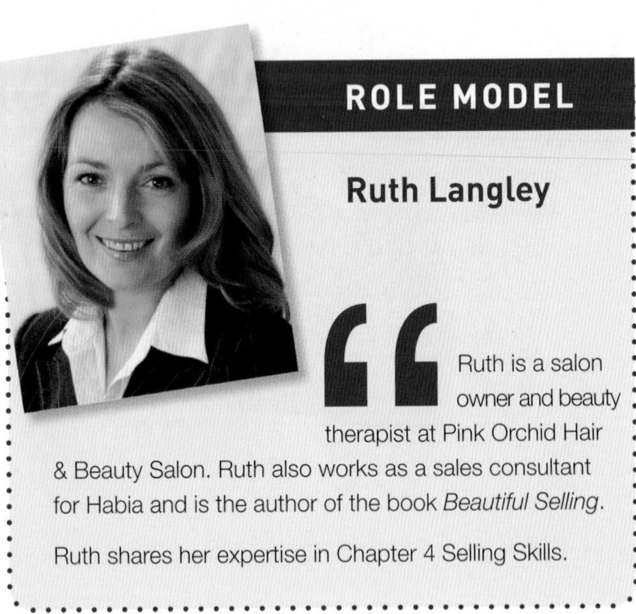

ROLE MODEL

Ruth Langley

Ruth is a salon owner and beauty therapist at Pink Orchid Hair & Beauty Salon. Ruth also works as a sales consultant for Habia and is the author of the book *Beautiful Selling*.

Ruth shares her expertise in Chapter 4 Selling Skills.

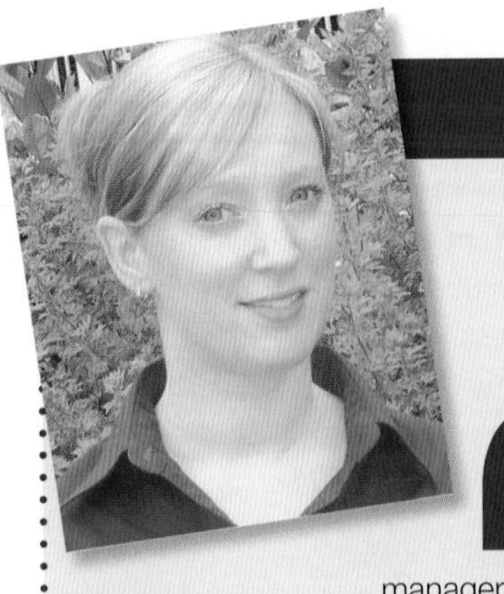

ROLE MODEL

Sally-Anne Braithwaite

Sally-Anne is front of house manager at Oxley's at Ambleside – Blue Fish Spa. Sally-Anne's responsibilities include running reception, meeting and greeting customers, product sales and helping with marketing and accounts.

Sally-Anne shares her expertise in Chapter 6 Salon Reception.

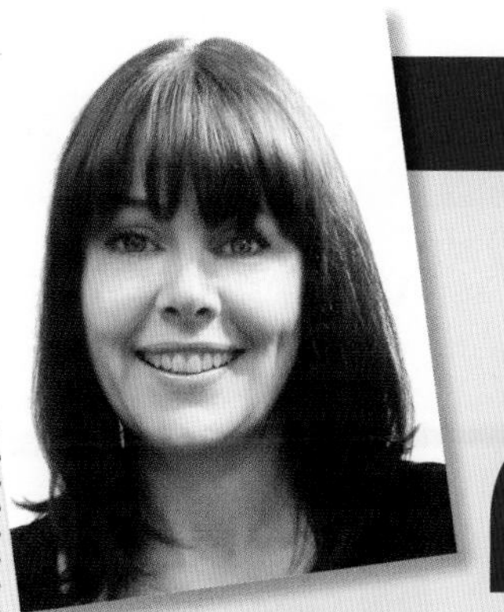

ROLE MODEL

Sally Penford

“ As Education Manager for the International Dermal Institute in the UK, Sally Penford is responsible for training and development of a highly specialized team of lecturers, along with overall operations for the education division in training centres located across the country.

Sally shares her expertise in Chapter 7 Facial Skincare.

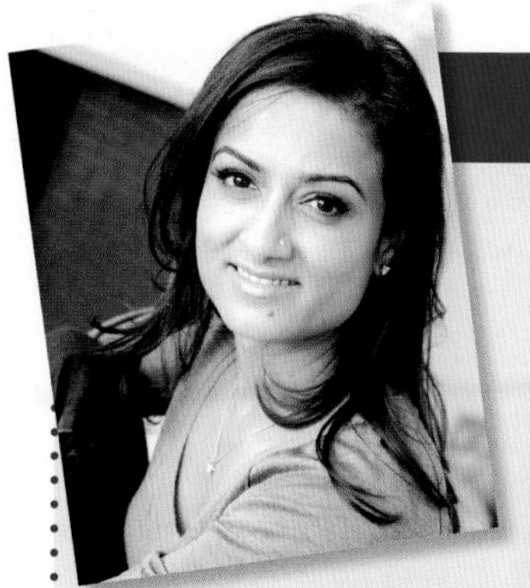

ROLE MODEL

Shavata Singh

“ Shavata Singh is Brand Director of Shavata UK (encompassing Shavata Brow Studio and LASH LOUNGE by Shavata).

Shavata shares her expertise in Chapter 8 Eyelash and Brow Treatments.

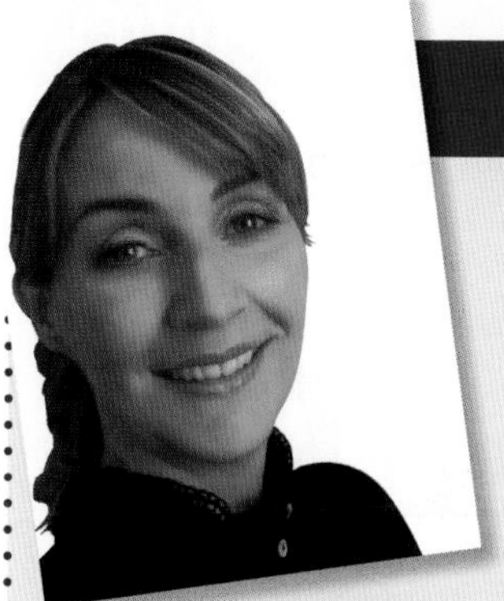

ROLE MODEL

Lorraine Onorato

“ Lorraine is an industry authority on threading and travels the world giving demonstrations and lectures. As Principal of The Surrey School of Beauty & Complementary Health, Lorraine is working with Habia to develop threading standards for a new industry qualification in threading which will be introduced in September 2010.

Lorraine shares her expertise in Chapter 9 Threading.

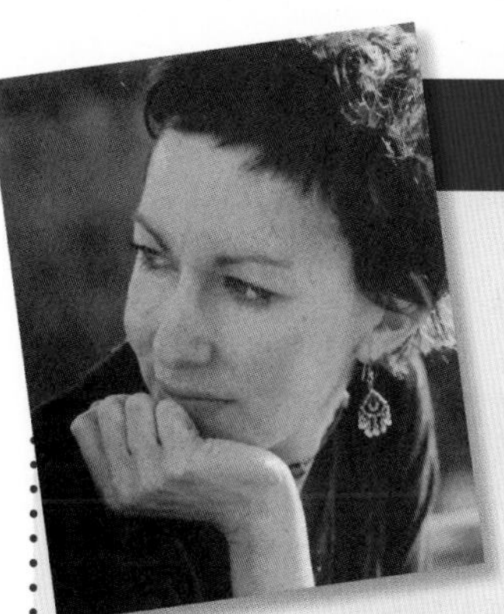

ROLE MODEL

Julia Francis

“ Julia is a professional make-up artist and body painter. Julia is also an experienced teacher and make-up consultant and has been conducting workshops for many years.

Julia shares her expertise in Chapter 10 Make-up Treatments.

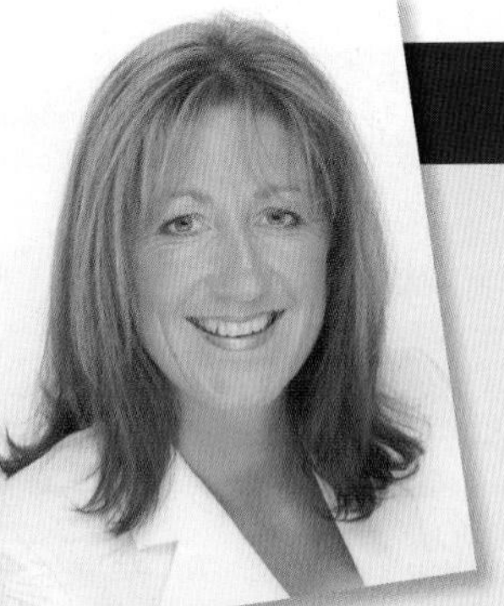

ROLE MODEL

Jacqui Jefford

"Jacqui has been in the nail and beauty industry for over 25 years, and is one of the leading figures in the industry in the UK and internationally. Her work has taken her to many countries as a consultant in education, competitions (winning, designing and judging them), taking educational seminars and working in PR, TV and with the consumer press. Jacqui has previously run her own salon, school and distribution company, and continues to work with many FE colleges as a tutor, assessor and internal verifier. Jacqui has also worked at London and Paris Fashion Weeks as well as decorating the covers of top magazines such as Vogue. Her passion has always been good education and she has worked alongside Habia on many projects over the years. Jacqui is author of four successful books and five DVDs.

Jacqui shares her expertise in Chapter 11 Manicure Treatments.

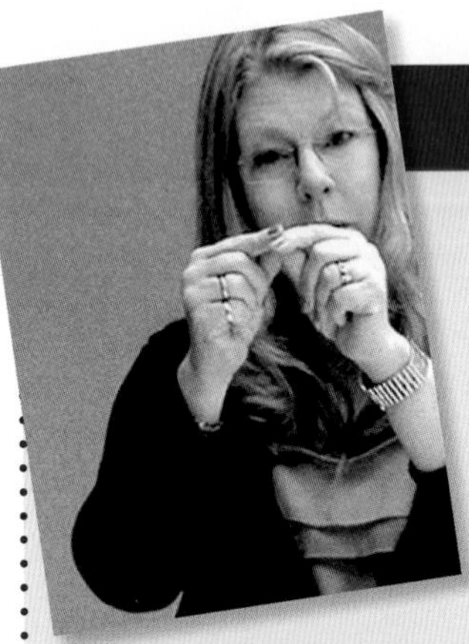

ROLE MODEL

Marian Newman

"Contributing author to this book, Marian is one of the leading professionals in the beauty therapy industry. Marian has worked in the professional nail industry since 1986 and comes from a scientific background. After working with several product companies, she now works independently within the media and fashion sector. Marian has a close association with Habia in the development of educational standards and skills and is the Chairperson of the Nail Services Forum.

Marian shares her expertise in Chapter 13 Nail Enhancement and Chapter 14 Nail Art.

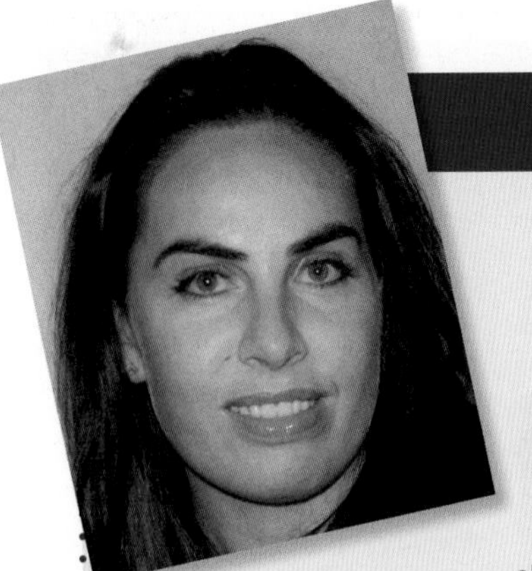

ROLE MODEL

Vicky Kennedy

"Vicky is a paramedical skin practitioner and beauty therapist and has been the principle owner of a very successful beauty therapy salon since 1991.

Vicky shares her expertise in Chapter 12 Pedicure Treatments.

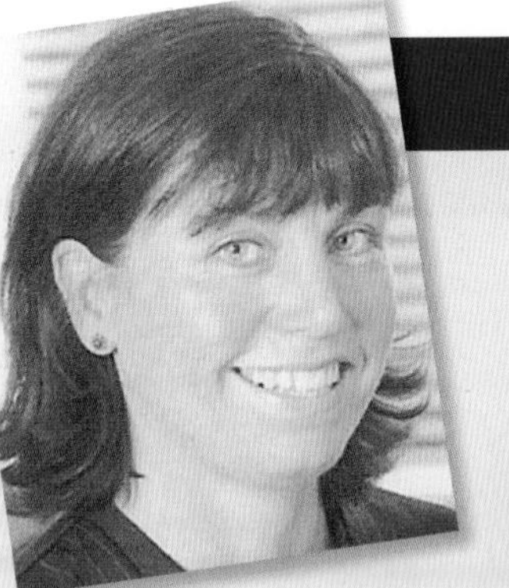

ROLE MODEL

Janice Brown

"Janice is Director of Beauty (House of Famuir Ltd). Her career journey has taken her from working in and later managing a group of salons, through sales, teaching, training, research and development. Janice is co-author of the two books – *The Encyclopaedia of Hair Removal* and *Practical Electrolysis: The Official Guide to Electro-epilation* – with Gill Morris.

Janice shares her expertise in Chapter 15 Waxing Treatments.

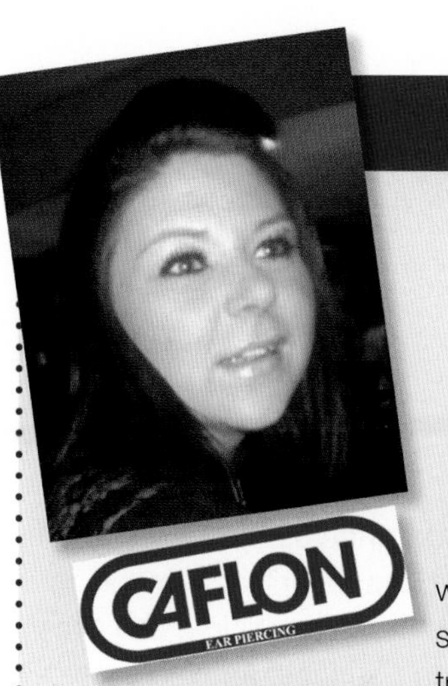

ROLE MODEL

Jade Rogers

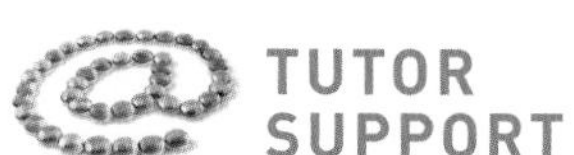

Jade is a Sales Technician with Caflon Ltd in the UK. Jade spends 70 per cent of her time training people in how to pierce ears and the remainder of the time she visits Caflon customers throughout the UK. Jade's customers come from the world of hair and beauty, others from the medical field and a core of clients from the jewellery industry.

Jade shares her expertise in Chapter 16 Ear Piercing.

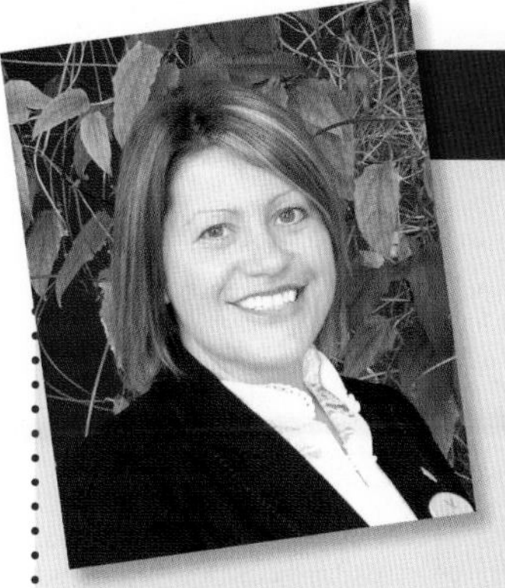

ROLE MODEL

Zoe Crowley

Zoe is Manager of the Aqua Sana spa at Elveden Forest Center Parcs resort. After qualifying as a beauty therapist in 1996, Zoe worked on cruise ships working her way up from beauty therapist to Spa Director before returning to dry land to work for Molton Brown and then relocating to work for Center Parcs.

Zoe shares her expertise in Chapter 17 Head Massage.

TUTOR SUPPORT

Activity 6: Develop a professional CV

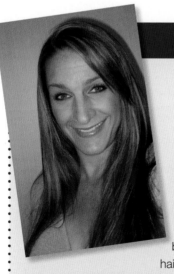

ROLE MODEL

Tammy Baker

Tammy is Education and Events Manager for St Tropez. Tammy has been working in the beauty, hair and wellness industry for over 17 years with involvement in the television industry and working as a personal trainer for clients including Robbie Williams. As Education and Events Manager, Tammy is responsible for the continuous improvement of teaching material, techniques and training of the education team.

Tammy shares her expertise in Chapter 18 Skin Tanning.

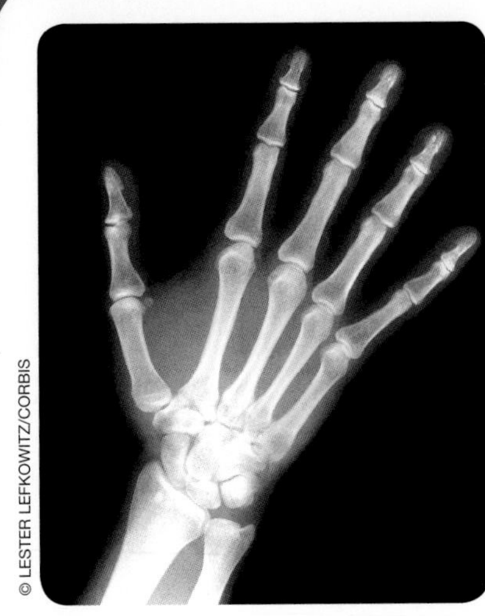

© LESTER LEFKOWITZ/CORBIS

2 Anatomy and Physiology

As a beauty therapist it is important that you have a good understanding of anatomy and physiology, as many of your services aim to improve the particular functioning of the different systems of the body. For example, a facial massage will improve **blood** and **lymph** circulation in the area as you massage the skin's surface, and increase cellular renewal as you improve nutrition to the living cells, while removing dead skin cells. The result is healthier looking skin.

Knowledge and understanding requirements

It is necessary for you to have knowledge and understanding of the anatomy and physiology relevant to and required for each unit you are studying as part of your VRQ qualification. You may be assessed through written questions or assignments. To guide you in your study and revision the anatomy and physiology you need to know and understand for each unit has been identified with an A&P symbol in each chapter. As you study each unit, look for the A&P symbol to remind you to check back here for your essential anatomy and physiology knowledge!

Anatomy and physiology underpinning knowledge	
The beauty therapy units with anatomy and physiology knowledge requirements are:	
Provide facial skincare	Chapter 7
Provide eyelash and brow treatments	Chapter 8
Provide eyelash perming	Chapter 8
Provide threading services for hair removal	Chapter 9
Apply make-up	Chapter 10
Provide manicure treatments	Chapter 11
Provide pedicure treatments	Chapter 12
Provide and maintain nail enhancements	Chapter 13
Provide nail art	Chapter 14
Remove hair using waxing techniques	Chapter 15
Provide ear piercing	Chapter 16
Head massage	Chapter 17
Apply skin tanning techniques	Chapter 18

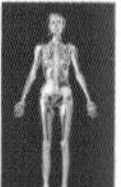

Anatomy and physiology knowledge requirements for each for VRQ unit

	Provide facial skincare	*Remove hair using waxing techniques*	*Provide manicure treatment*	*Provide pedicure treatment*	*Provide eyelash and eyebrow treatments*	*Apply make-up*	*Provide and maintain nail enhancement*	*Provide nail art*	*Provide ear piercing*	*Eyelash perming*	*Provide threading services for hair removal*	*Head massage*	*Apply skin tanning techniques*	*Facial care for men*
Skin structure and function	✓	✓	✓	✓	✓	✓	✓	✓	✓	✓	✓	✓	✓	✓
Structure of hair and types of hair growth		✓			✓					✓	✓	✓		
Hair growth cycle		✓			✓					✓	✓	✓		
Nail structure and function			✓	✓			✓	✓						
Nail growth			✓	✓			✓	✓						
Muscle groups in the treatment area of the body, position and action	✓		✓	✓		✓			✓			✓		✓
Bones in the treatment area of the body, position, structure and function	✓		✓	✓		✓			✓			✓		✓
Composition and function of blood and lymph	✓	✓	✓	✓		✓	✓		✓			✓		✓
Blood and lymphatic system circulation	✓	✓	✓	✓		✓	✓		✓			✓		✓
External ear structure									✓					

Anatomical terminology

Anatomical terminology is used to describe the location, function and description of a body part. It is useful to know these terms, as it will assist your anatomy understanding. As you read through this chapter you will notice those terms.

Activity 1: Anatomical terms handout

Anterior	Front (usually refers to front of the body)	**Superficial**	Near the surface
Posterior	Back (usually refers to the back of the body)	**Superior**	Above
Proximal	Nearest to	**Inferior**	Below
Medial	Middle	**Plantar**	Front surface
Distal	Furthest away	**Dorsal**	Back surface
Lateral	Side		

The skin

The skin varies in appearance according to our race, gender and age. It also alters from season to season and from year to year, and reflects our general health, lifestyle and diet.

The outer layer of the epidermis, the **stratum corneum** is up to 20 per cent thicker in men than women. Male skin also contains more collagen, a skin protein providing strength. Collagen production in females slows at the menopause which can result in sudden skin ageing. As such, skin ageing appears faster in females than males. Males produce more of the skin's natural oil sebum making their skin appear oilier, and they have fewer **sweat glands**.

More information on how race, gender and age affects skin's appearance can be found in Chapter 7 Facial Skincare.

At puberty the chemical substances (**hormones**) that control many of our bodies' activities become very active. Among other effects, this activity causes the skin to become more oily, and often blemishes appear on the skin's surface. Seven out of ten teenagers find that their skin becomes blemished with blackheads (**comedones**), inflamed angry spots (**pustules** and **papules**) and even scars at this time: a skin disorder called **acne vulgaris.**

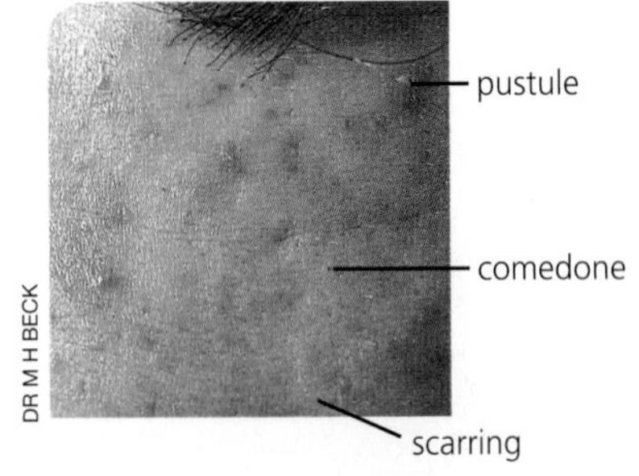

The skin disorder acne vulgaris

During our twenties our skin should look its best; any hormonal imbalance that occurred at puberty should by now have stabilized. As we grow older, the skin ages too. In our late twenties and early thirties we will see fine lines appearing on the skin's surface, especially around the eyes where the skin is thinner and gradually becomes drier as the production of the skin's natural oil, sebum, slows.

At around the age of 40, hormone activity in the body becomes slower and the skin begins to lose its strength and elasticity. The skin becomes increasingly drier, and lines and wrinkles appear on the surface. In our late fifties brown patches of discoloured skin (**lentigines**) may appear: these are commonly seen at the temple region of the face and on the backs of the hands and are caused by ultra-violet light damage.

Fortunately, help is at hand to care for the skin: there is an ever-increasing number of skin-care products from a vast and highly profitable cosmetics industry, and there are the skill and expertise of the qualified beauty therapist.

If it is your intention to become a qualified beauty professional, you need to learn about **skin types** and construction, its function, and how and why skin is changed by both internal and external influences.

Types of tissue and general functions

Name of tissue	Examples	General functions
Epithelial 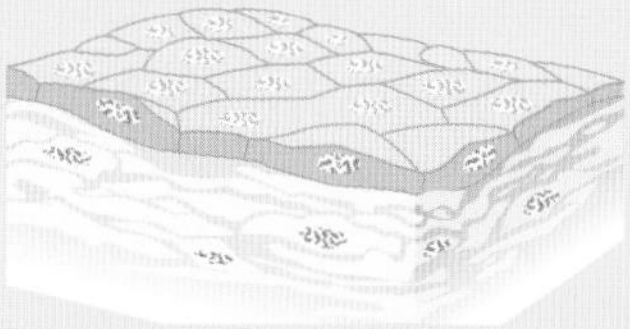	Epidermis outer layer of skin	Forms surface and linings for protection.
Connective 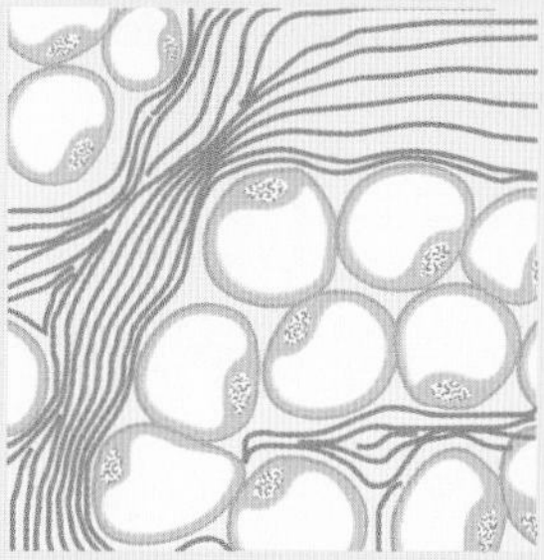	Dermis layer of skin Collagen fibres Bone Ligaments Tendons	A structural tissue that supports, surrounds and connects different parts of the body.
Muscular 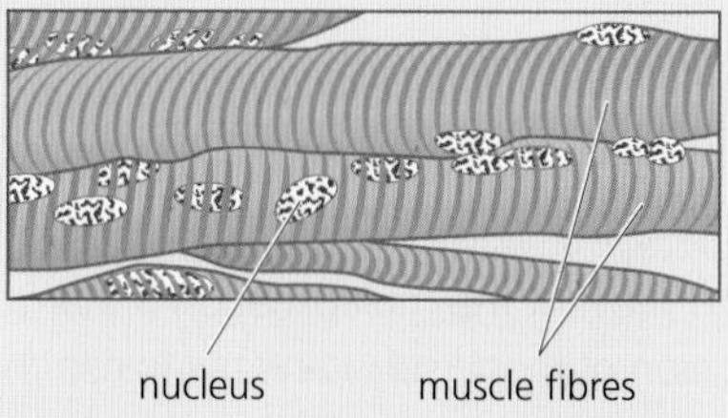 nucleus muscle fibres	Voluntary or skeletal, muscle tissue Involuntary or smooth muscle tissue	Contracts and shortens producing movement. Skeletal muscle tissue moves the body and maintains posture. Smooth muscle tissue moves substances through the body.
Nervous 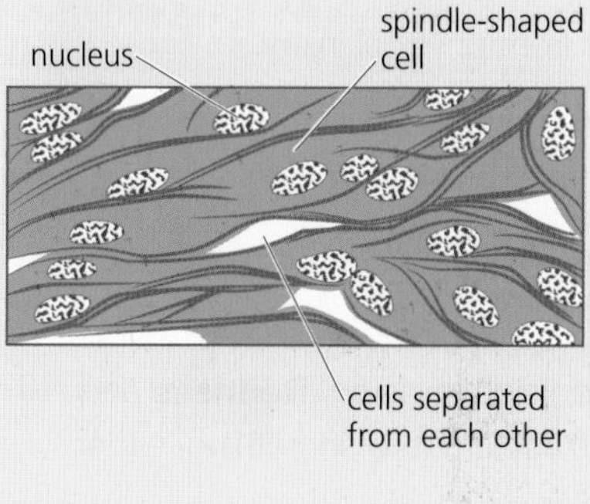 nucleus spindle-shaped cell cells separated from each other	**Neurones** (nerve cells)	Forms a communication system between different parts of the body, controlling and co-ordinating most body processes.

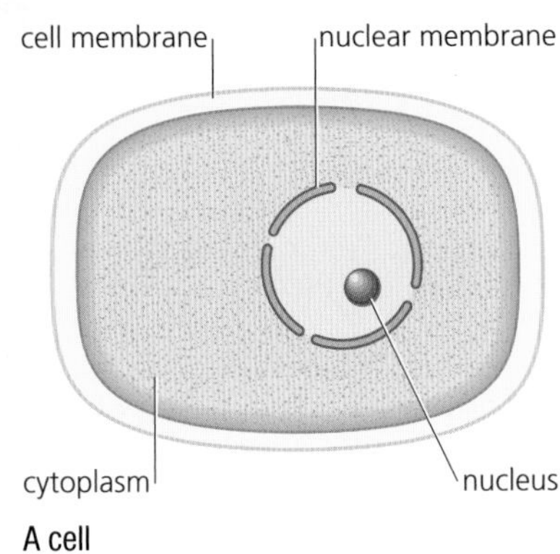

A cell

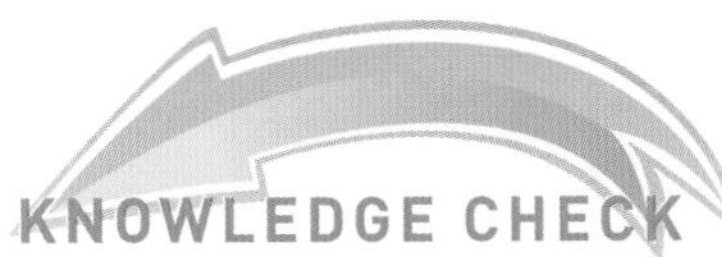

What are the effects of ageing on the skin?

Need more time... refer to page 28 to help you.

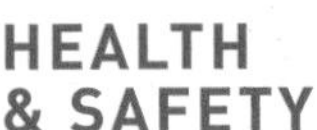

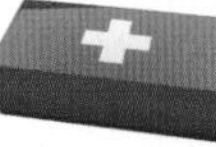

Skin protection
Although the skin is structured to avoid penetration of harmful substances by absorption, certain chemicals can be absorbed through the skin. Always protect the skin when using potentially harmful substances, and wear gloves when using harsh chemical cleaning agents.

TOP TIP

Did you know?
Although the skin has a waterproof property it allows approximately 500ml of water to be lost from the tissues through evaporation every day.

Cells

The human body consists of many trillions of microscopic **cells**. Each cell contains a chemical substance called **protoplasm**, which contains various specialized structures whose activities are essential to our health. If cells are unable to function properly, a disorder results.

Surrounding the cell is the **cell membrane**. This forms a boundary between the cell contents and their environment. The membrane has a porous surface that permits food to enter and waste materials to leave.

In the centre of the cell is the **nucleus**, which contains the **chromosomes**. On these are the genes we have inherited from our parents. The **genes** are ultimately responsible for cell reproduction and cell functioning.

The liquid within the cell membrane and surrounding the nucleus is called **cytoplasm**. Scattered throughout this are other small bodies, the **organelles** or 'little organs'; each has a specific function within the cell.

Cells in the body tend to specialize in carrying out particular functions. Groups of cells which share function, shape, size or structure are called **tissues**.

Tissues

If the tissues are damaged, for example if the skin is accidentally broken, the tissue cells divide to repair the damage – called **regeneration**. The body is composed of four basic tissues. These are described in the table on the previous page.

Tissues may be grouped to form the larger functional and structural units we know as **organs**, such as the heart.

Functions of the skin

The human skin is an organ – the largest of the body. It provides a tough, flexible covering, with many different important functions. The main functions are listed below.

Protection

The skin protects the body from potentially harmful substances and conditions.

- The outer surface is **bactericidal**, helping to prevent the multiplication of harmful microorganisms. It also prevents the absorption of many substances (unless the surface is broken), because of the construction of the cells on its outer surface, which form a chemical and physical barrier.
- The skin cushions the underlying structures from physical injury.
- The skin provides a **waterproof coating**. Its natural oil, **sebum**, prevents the skin from losing vital water, and thus prevents skin dehydration.
- The skin contains a pigment called **melanin**. This absorbs harmful rays of ultra-violet light.
- The skin affords a warning system against outside invasion. **Redness** and **irritation** of the skin indicate that the skin is intolerant to something, either external or internal.

Heat regulation

Humans maintain a normal body **temperature** of 36.8–37°C. Body temperature is controlled in part by heat loss through the skin and by sweating. If the temperature of the body is increased by 0.25–0.5°C, the sweat glands secrete sweat on to the skin's surface. The body is cooled by the loss of heat used to evaporate the sweat from the skin's surface. If the body becomes too warm there is an increase in blood flow into the blood capillaries in the skin. The blood capillaries widen (dilate) and heat is lost from the skin. Hair limits heat loss from the scalp.

Secretion

The skin secretes its natural oil, **sebum**, which is a mixture of fats and waxes and covers the skin's entire surface except the palms and the soles and helps to protect the skin.

Excretion

Small amounts of certain **waste products**, such as urea, water and salt, are removed from the body in sweat by excretion from sweat glands through the surface of the skin from the skin's pores.

Sensation

The skin is a sensory organ and the sensations of **touch, pressure, pain, heat** and **cold** are identified by sensory nerves and receptors in the skin. It also allows us to recognize objects by their feel and shape.

TOP TIP

Did you know?

The skin accounts for one-eighth of the body's total weight. It measures approximately 1.5m² in total, depending on body size. It is thinnest on the eye lids (0.05mm), and thickest on the soles of the feet (approximately 5mm).

Nutrition

The skin provides storage for fat, which provides an energy reserve. It is also responsible for producing a significant proportion of our vitamin D, which is created by a chemical reaction when sunlight is in contact with the skin.

Moisture control

The skin controls the movement of moisture from within the deeper layers of the skin.

The structure of the skin

If we looked within the skin using a microscope, we would be able to see two distinct layers: the epidermis and the dermis. Between these layers is a specialized membrane which acts like a 'glue', sticking the two layers together: this is the **basement membrane**. If the epidermis and dermis become separated, body fluids fill the space, creating a **blister**.

Situated below the epidermis and dermis is a further layer, the subcutaneous layer or fat layer. The fat layer consists of cells containing fatty deposits, called adipose cells. The thickness of the subcutaneous layer varies according to the body area, and is, for example, very thin around the eyes.

TOP TIP

Functions of the skin

By remembering the word *SHAPES* this will help you remember the functions of the skin:

Sensation
Heat regulation
Absorption
Protection
Excretion
Secretion

HEALTH & SAFETY

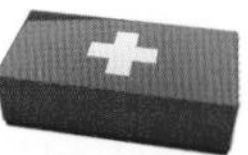

If the external temperature becomes low, blood flow nearer the skin's surface is decreased and the blood capillaries narrow (constrict), preventing heat loss and conserving heat.

ALWAYS REMEMBER

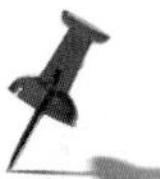

The skin's correct functioning is essential to life. It becomes darker to protect against excessive UV exposure but can also produce vitamin D. A fatty substance in the skin is converted to vitamin D with UV light from the sun. This circulates in the blood and with the mineral salts calcium and phosphorus helps the formation and maintenance of the health of the body's bones. Lack of vitamin D can lead to bone softening disease.

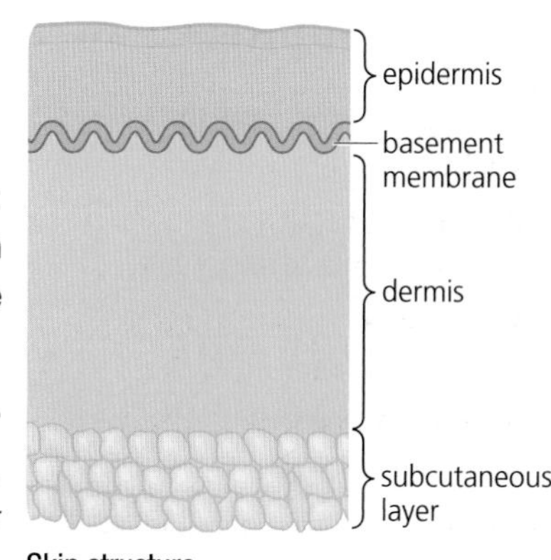

Skin structure

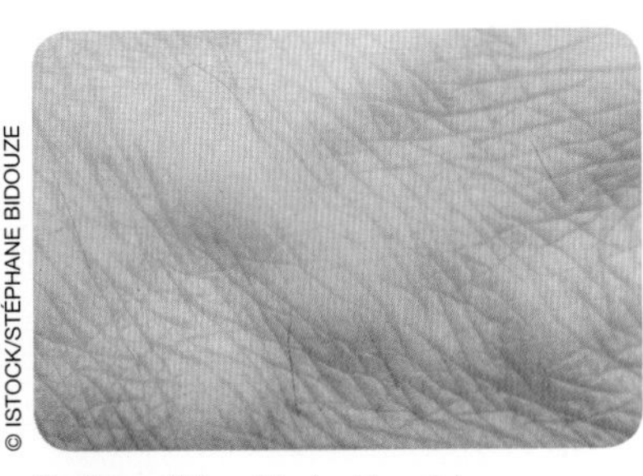

Surface of the skin (epidermis)

TOP TIP

The epidermis
The epidermis is the most significant layer of the skin with regard to the external application of skincare cosmetics and make-up due to the effect on its appearance.

TOP TIP

Did you know?
Every five days we shed a complete surface layer of skin cells. About 80 per cent of household dust is composed of dead skin cells.

ALWAYS REMEMBER

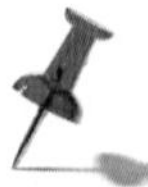

Psoriasis
In the skin disorder psoriasis, cell division occurs much more quickly, resulting in clusters of dead skin cells appearing on the skin's surface.

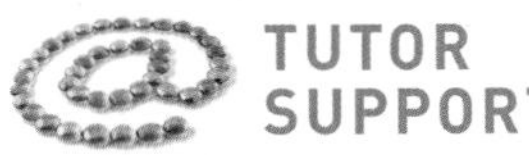

TUTOR SUPPORT

Activity 2: Epidermis label the diagram

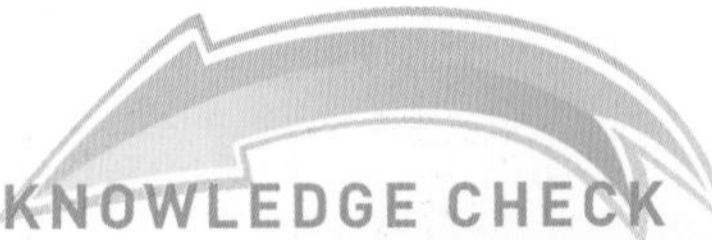

KNOWLEDGE CHECK

Name seven functions of the skin.

Need more time... refer to pages 30–31 to help you.

The epidermis

The epidermis is located directly above the dermis. It is composed of five layers, with the surface layer forming the outer skin – what we can see and touch. The main function of the epidermis is to protect the deeper living structures from invasion and harm from the external environment.

There is no blood supply in the epidermis. Nourishment of the epidermis, essential for growth is received from a liquid called the **interstitial fluid** formed from blood plasma. This acts as a link between the blood and cells.

Each layer of the epidermis can be recognized by its shape and by the function of its cells. The main type of cell found in the epidermis is the **keratinocyte**, which produces the protein **keratin**. It is keratin that makes the skin tough and that reduces the passage of substances into or out of the body.

Over a period of about four weeks, cells move from the bottom layer of the epidermis to the top layer, the skin's surface, changing in shape and structure as they progress. The process of cellular change takes place in stages:

- *The cell is formed* – by division of an earlier cell. This type of cell division is called mitosis.
- *The cell matures* – it changes structure and moves upwards and outwards.
- *The cell dies* – it moves upwards and becomes an empty shell, which is eventually shed.

The layers of the epidermis There are five layers or **strata** that makeup the epidermis. The thickness of these layers varies over the body's surface. Each layer is found either in the germinative zone or keratinization zone. This is illustrated and described below:

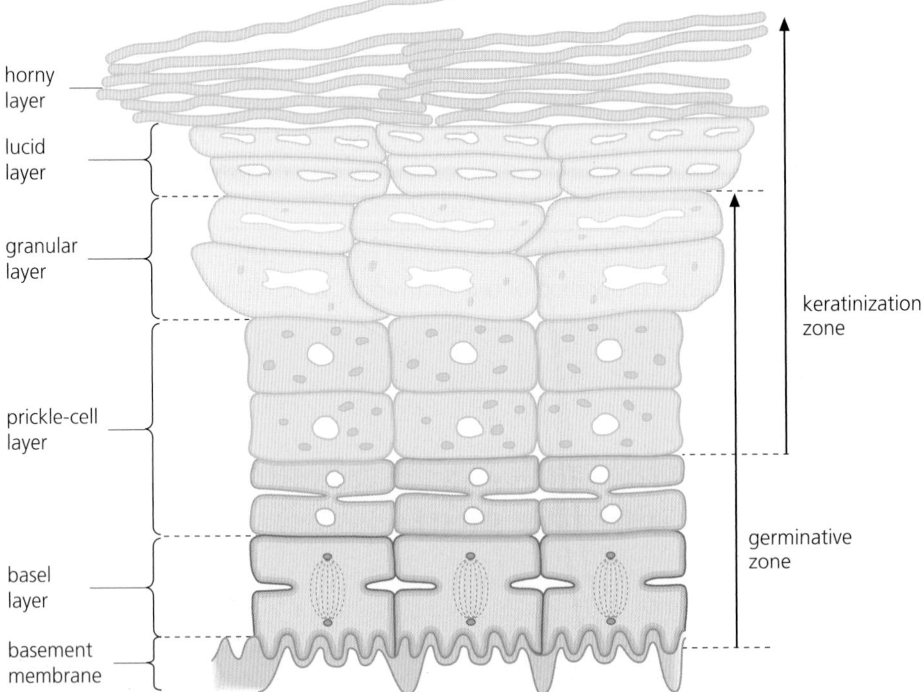

The layers of the epidermis

The germinative zone In the **germinative zone** the cells of the epidermis layers are living cells. The germinative zone layers of the epidermis are the **stratum germinativum, stratum spinosum** and **stratum granulosum**.

Stratum germinativum The **stratum germinativum**, or **basal layer**, is the lowermost layer of the epidermis. It is formed from a single layer of column-shaped cells joined to the basement membrane. These cells divide continuously and produce new epidermal cells (keratinocytes), a process known as mitosis.

Stratum spinosum The **stratum spinosum**, or **prickle-cell layer**, is formed from two to six rows of elongated cells; these have a surface of spiky spines which connect to surrounding cells. Each cell has a large nucleus and is filled with fluid.

Two other important cells are found in the germinative zone of the epidermis: langerhan cells and melanocyte cells.

ALWAYS REMEMBER

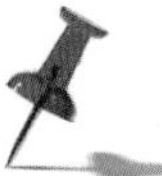

When the epidermis cell dies and is eventually shed from the skin's surface this is termed desquamation.

ALWAYS REMEMBER

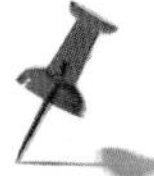

Stratum is the Latin word for layer.

Langerhan cells

Special defence cells absorb and remove foreign bodies that enter the skin. They then move from the epidermis to the dermis below, and finally enter the lymph system (the body's waste-transport system) where the foreign bodies are made safe by neutralizing them.

Melanocyte cells

Produce the skin pigment **melanin**, which contributes to our skin colour. About one in every ten germinative cells is a melanocyte. Melanocytes are stimulated to produce melanin by ultra-violet rays, and their main function is to protect the other epidermal cells in this way from the harmful effects of ultra-violet.

The quantity and distribution of melanocytes differs according to race. In a white Caucasian person the melanin tends to be destroyed when it reaches the granular layer. With stimulation from artificial or natural ultra-violet light, however, melanin will also be present in the upper epidermis.

TOP TIP

Every time the stratum corneum cells are removed through desquamation, the basal cell makes new cells to replace those removed. The dermis also makes more collagen and elastin. This is good news for your client!

TOP TIP

Artificial skin tanning

Self-tanning products contain an ingredient called dihydroxyacetone (DHA). This provides an artificial tanned appearance to the skin. DHA reacts with the skin's amino acids, chemical protein chains in the stratum corneum. Through desquamation the colour is lost as the skin's surface cells are removed.

ALWAYS REMEMBER

Allergic reactions

Most people will be unaware that a foreign body has invaded the skin. Sometimes, however, the skin's surface intolerance to a substance is apparent. It shows as an allergic reaction, in which the skin becomes red, itchy and swollen.

In contrast a black skin has melanin present in larger quantities throughout *all* the epidermal layers, a level of protection that has evolved to deal with bright ultra-violet light. This increased protection allows less ultra-violet to penetrate the dermis below, reducing the possibility of premature ageing from exposure to ultra-violet light. The more even quality and distribution of melanin also means that people with dark skins are less at risk of developing skin cancer.

Another pigment, **carotene**, which is yellowish, also occurs in epidermal cells. Its contribution to skin colour lessens in importance as the amount of melanin in the skin increases.

Skin colour also increases when the skin becomes warm. This is because the **blood capillaries** at the surface dilate, bringing blood nearer to the surface so that heat can be lost – this is called vasodilation. If the temperature is cold the blood capillaries become

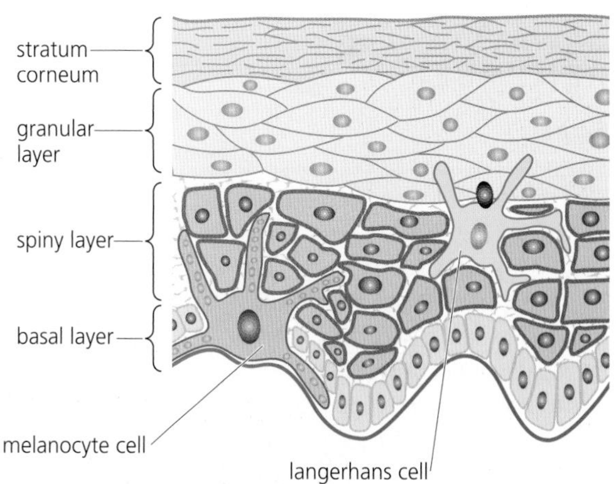

Melanocyte and langerhan cells in the skin

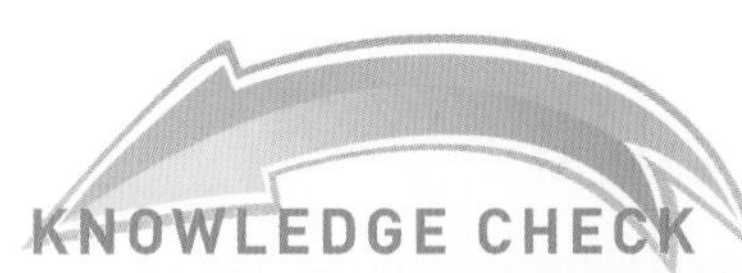

KNOWLEDGE CHECK

What are the three main layers of the skin?

Need more time... refer to page 31 to help you.

HEALTH & SAFETY

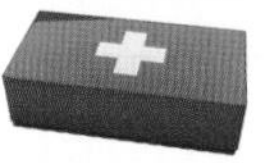

Vitiligo

Lack of skin pigment is called *vitiligo* or *leucoderma*. It can occur with any skin colour, but is more obvious on dark skin. Avoid exposing such skin to ultra-violet light as it does not have melanin protection.

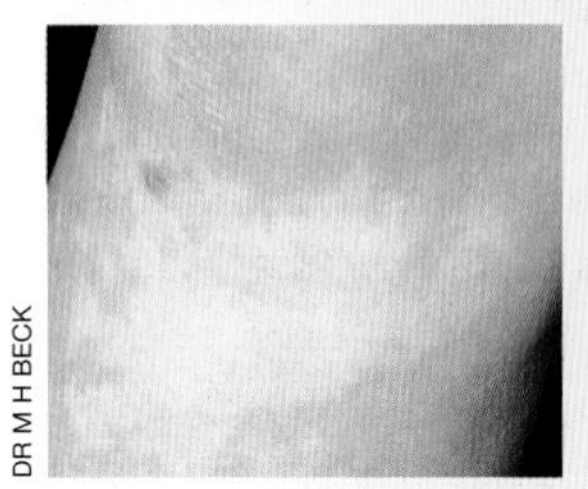

DR M H BECK

HEALTH & SAFETY

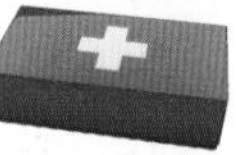

Sunburn

If the skin becomes red on exposure to sunlight, this indicates that the skin has been over-exposed to ultra-violet. It will often blister and shed itself.

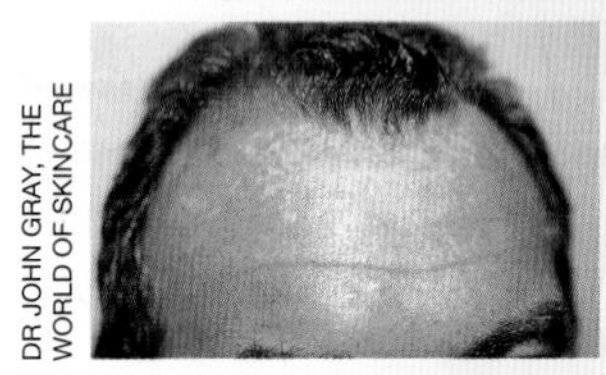

DR JOHN GRAY, THE WORLD OF SKINCARE

ALWAYS REMEMBER

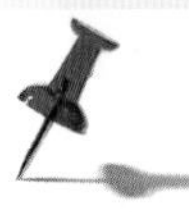

Scars

When the surface has been broken, the skin at the site of the injury is replaced but may leave a scar. This initially appears red, due to the increased blood supply to the area, required while the skin heals. When healed, the redness will fade. If the skin's healing process continues for longer than necessary, too much scar tissue will be formed, resulting in a raised scar called a 'keloid' scar.

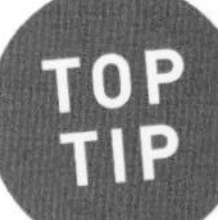

TOP TIP

Cosmetic sunscreens

Many hair and skincare products and cosmetics, including lipsticks and mascaras, now contain sunscreens. This is because research has shown that ultra-violet exposure is the principal cause of skin ageing and can also cause the hair to become dry.

narrower so less blood is brought to the skin's surface to conserve heat – this is called vaso-constriction and the skin will lose colour.

Stratum granulosum

The **stratum granulosum**, or **granular layer**, is composed of one, two or three layers of cells that have become much flatter. The nucleus of the cell has begun to break up, creating what appear to be granules within the cell cytoplasm. These are known as **keratohyaline granules** and later form keratin. At this stage the cells form a new, combined layer.

The keratinization zone The **keratinization zone**, or **cornified zone**, is where the cells begin to die and where finally they will be shed from the skin. The cells at this stage become progressively flatter, and the cell cytoplasm is replaced with the hard protein keratin.

Stratum lucidum

The **stratum lucidum**, **clear layer** or **lucid layer**, is only seen in non-hairy areas of the skin such as the palms of the hands and the soles of the feet. The cells here lack a nucleus and are filled with a clear substance called eledin produced at a further stage of keratinization.

Stratum corneum

The **stratum corneum**, **cornified** or **horny layer**, is formed from several layers of flattened, scale-like overlapping cells, composed mainly of keratin. These help to reflect ultra-violet light from the skin's surface; black skin, which evolved to withstand strong ultra-violet, has a thicker stratum corneum than does Caucasian skin.

It takes about three weeks for the epidermal cells to reach the stratum corneum from the stratum germinativum. The cells are then shed, a process called **desquamation.**

The dermis

The dermis is the inner portion of the skin, situated underneath the epidermis and composed of dense **connective tissue** containing other structures such as the lymphatic system, **blood vessels** and nerves. It is much thicker than the epidermis.

The papillary layer Near the surface of the dermis are tiny projections called **papillae**; these contain both **nerve** endings and blood capillaries. This part of the dermis is known as the **papillary layer**, and it also supplies the upper epidermis with its nutrition.

The reticular layer The dermis contains a dense network of protein fibres called the reticular layer. These fibres allow the skin to expand, to contract, and to perform intricate, supple movements. The reticular layer contains sweat glands, blood vessels, hair follicles, lymph vessels, the arrector pili muscles and sebaceous glands.

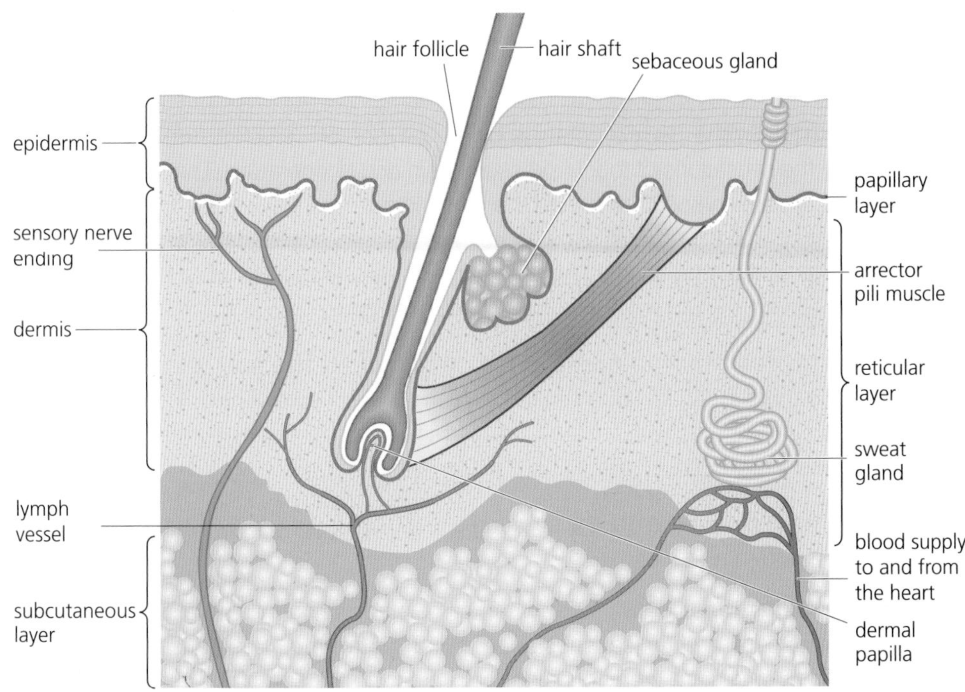

The skin

This network is composed of two sorts of protein fibre: yellow **elastin** fibres and white **collagen** fibres. Elastin fibres give the skin its elasticity, and collagen fibres give it its strength. The fibres are produced by specialized cells called **fibroblasts**, and are held in a gel called the **ground substance**.

While this network is strong, the skin will appear youthful and firm. As the fibres harden and fragment, however, the network begins to collapse, losing its elasticity. The skin then begins to show visible signs of ageing.

A major cause of damage to this network is unprotected exposure of the skin to ultraviolet light and to weather. Sometimes, too, the skin loses its elasticity because of a sudden increase in body weight, for example at puberty or pregnancy. This results in the appearance of **stretch marks**, streaks of thin skin are a different colour from the

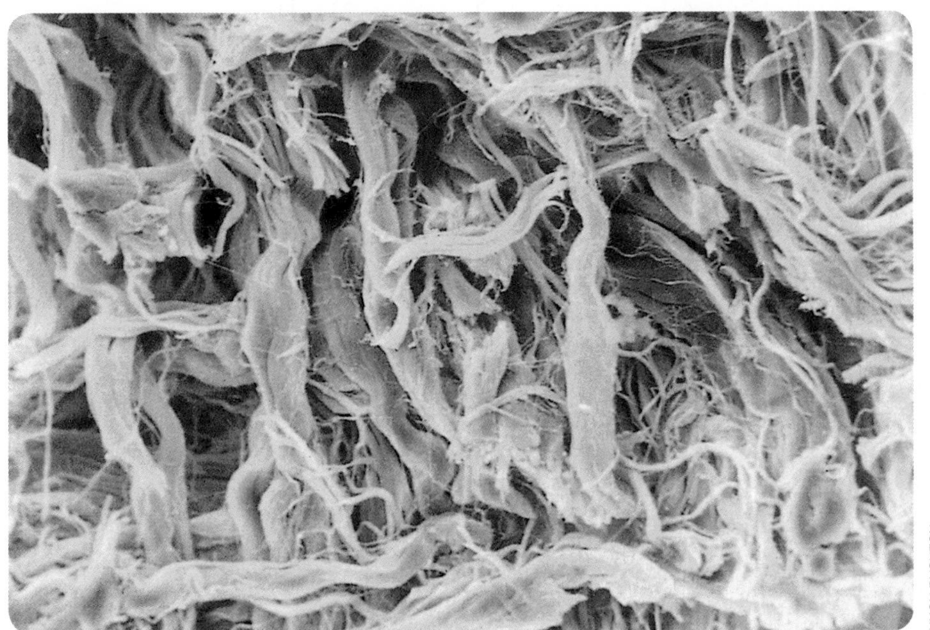

Collagen and elastin fibres in the dermis

KNOWLEDGE CHECK

What is the main function of the following cells found in the germinative zone of the epidermis?

- langerhan cells
- melanocyte cells

Need more time... refer to page 33 to help you.

TOP TIP

Calluses

The skin will become much thicker in response to friction. A client with a manual occupation may therefore develop hard skin (calluses) on their hands. The skin condition can be treated with an emollient preparation, which will moisturise and soften the dry skin.

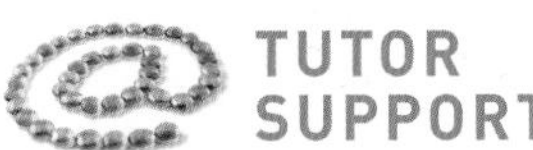

TUTOR SUPPORT

Activity 3: Label cross section of the skin

TOP TIP

The formation of the papillae ridges in the dermis are unique to each individual, and this provides our fingerprint.

TOP TIP

Massage

Appropriate external massage movements can be used to increase the blood supply within the dermis, bringing extra nutrients and oxygen to the skin and to the underlying muscle. At the same time, the lymphatic circulation is increased, improving the removal of waste products that may have accumulated.

HEALTH & SAFETY

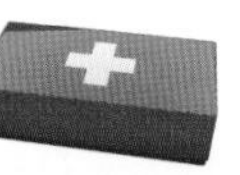

Sunbathing

When sunbathing, always protect the skin with an appropriate protective sunscreen product, and always use an emollient aftersun preparation to minimize the cumulative effects of premature ageing, by rehydrating and soothing the skin.

KNOWLEDGE CHECK

How many layers form the epidermis of the skin?

Names these layers in order. starting with the outermost layer.

Need more time... refer to pages 32–33 to help you.

ALWAYS REMEMBER

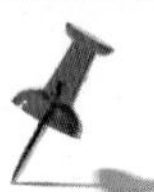

Sensory nerve endings

Sensory nerve endings are most numerous in sensitive parts of the skin, such as the finger tips and the lips.

KNOWLEDGE CHECK

What is the function of fibroblast cells?

Name two protein fibres found in the skin.

What does each protein provide the skin with?

In the dermis, what is this dense network of protein fibres called?

Need more time... refer to page 35 to help you.

TOP TIP

Moisturisers

Cosmetic moisturisers mimic sebum in providing an oily covering for the skin's surface to reduce moisture loss.

surrounding skin: on white skin they appear as thin reddish streaks; on black skin they appear slightly lighter than the surrounding skin. The lost elasticity cannot be restored. Cosmetic treatments can be applied to improve their appearance.

Nerve endings The dermis contains different types of **sensory nerve endings**, which register the sensations of touch, pressure, pain and temperature. These send messages to the central nervous system and the brain, informing us about the outside world and what is happening on the skin's surface. The appearance of each of these nerve endings is quite varied. The sensory nerve endings in the skin cause us to have a reflex action to unpleasant stimuli protecting the skin from injury.

Growth and repair The body's blood system of arteries and veins continually brings blood to the capillary networks in the skin and takes it away again. The blood carries the nutrients and oxygen essential for the skin's health, maintenance and growth, and takes away waste products.

Defence Within the dermis are the structures responsible for protecting the skin from harmful foreign bodies and irritants.

One set of cells, the **mast cells**, burst when stimulated during inflammation or allergic reactions, and release a chemical substance called **histamine**. This causes the blood vessels nearby to enlarge, thereby bringing more blood to the site of the irritation to limit skin damage and begin repair.

In the blood, and also in the lymph and the connective tissue, are another group of cells: the **macrophages** or 'big eaters'. These destroy microorganisms and engulf dead cells and other unwanted particles. When necessary, they travel to an area where they are needed, for example, the site of an infection. They form a role in the immune system that protects the body from disease-causing microorganisms.

Collecting waste Lymph vessels in the skin carry a fluid called **lymph**, a straw-coloured fluid similar in composition to blood plasma. Plasma is the liquid part of the blood that disperses from the blood capillaries into the tissue spaces. Lymph is composed of water, lymphocytes (a type of white blood cell that plays a key role in the immune system), oxygen, nutrients, hormones, salts and waste products. The waste products are eliminated and usable protein is recycled for further use by the body. It acts as a link between the blood and the cells.

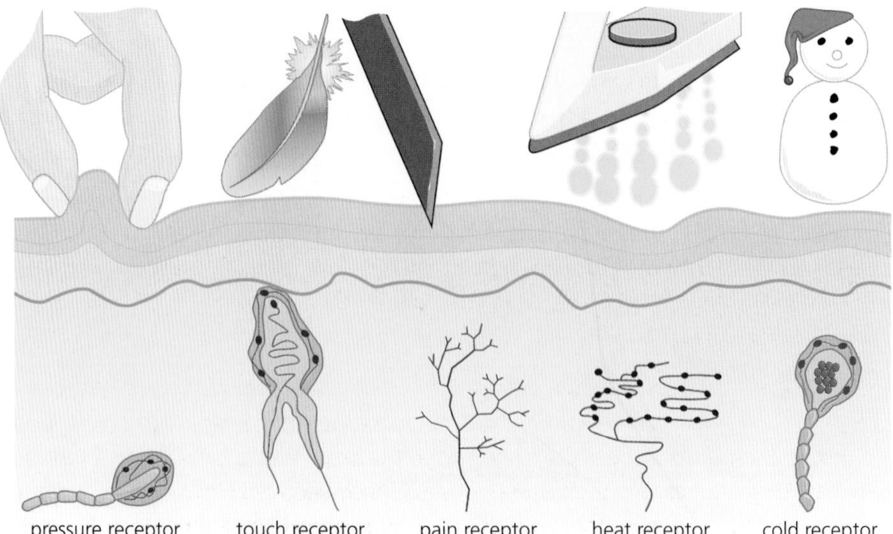

Sensory nerves

Control of skin functioning **Hormones** are chemical messengers transported in the blood. They control the activity of many organs in the body, including the cells and glands in the skin. These include **melanosomes**, which produce skin pigment, and the **sweat glands** and **sebaceous glands**.

Hormone imbalance at different times of our life may disturb the normal functioning of these cells and structures, causing various **skin disorders**.

Skin appendages Within the dermis are structures called **skin appendages**. These include:

- sweat glands
- sebaceous glands
- hair follicles, which produce **hair**
- nails

Sweat glands **Sweat glands** or **sudoriferous glands** are composed of **epithelial tissue**, a specialized lining tissue which extends from the epidermis into the dermis. These glands are found all over the body, but are particularly abundant on the palms of the hands and the soles of the feet. Their function is to regulate body temperature through the evaporation of sweat from the surface of the skin. Fluid loss and control of body temperature are important to prevent the body overheating, especially in hot, humid climates. For this reason, perhaps, sweat glands are larger and more abundant in black skins than white skins.

There are two types of sweat glands: *eccrine glands* and *apocrine glands*. **Eccrine glands** are simple sweat-producing glands, found over most of the body, appearing as tiny tubes (**ducts**). The eccrine glands are responsive to heat. They are straight in the epidermis, and coiled in the dermis. The duct opens directly onto the surface of the skin through an opening called a **pore**.

Eccrine glands continuously secrete small amounts of sweat, even when we appear not to be perspiring. In this way they maintain the body temperature at a constant 36.8–37°C.

TOP TIP

Pores

Pores allow the absorption of some facial cosmetics into the skin. Many facial treatments are therefore aimed at cleansing the pores, some with a particularly deep cleansing action, as with *cosmetic cleansers* and *facial masks*.

The pores may become enlarged due to congestion caused by dirt, dead skin cells, cosmetics and ageing. The application of an *exfoliating* and *astringent* skincare preparation creates deep cleansing and a tightening effect upon the skin's surface, slightly reducing the size of the pores.

Apocrine glands are found in the underarm, the nipples and the groin area. This kind of gland is larger than the eccrine gland, and is attached to a hair follicle. Apocrine glands are controlled by hormones, becoming active at puberty. They also increase in activity when we are excited, nervous or stressed. The fluid they secrete is thicker than that from the eccrine glands, and may contain urea, fats, sugars and small amounts of protein. Also present are traces of aromatic molecules called **pheromones**, which are thought to cause sexual attraction between individuals.

ALWAYS REMEMBER

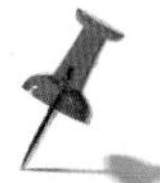

If the skin is damaged, it repairs itself. Blood transports repair cells to the site of the injury. These blood cells then form a clot, which dries and prevents infection from germs entering the skin. Collagen fibres are secreted by fibroblast cells in the dermis, which bind the surface of the wound together. Epithelial cells of the dermis cover the wound underneath the clot. The clot or scab is lost. The cells of the dermis grow upwards until the skin's thickness is restored.

KNOWLEDGE CHECK

What happens at the keratinization zone of the epidermis?

Which three layers of the skin make-up this zone?

Need more time... refer to page 34 to help you.

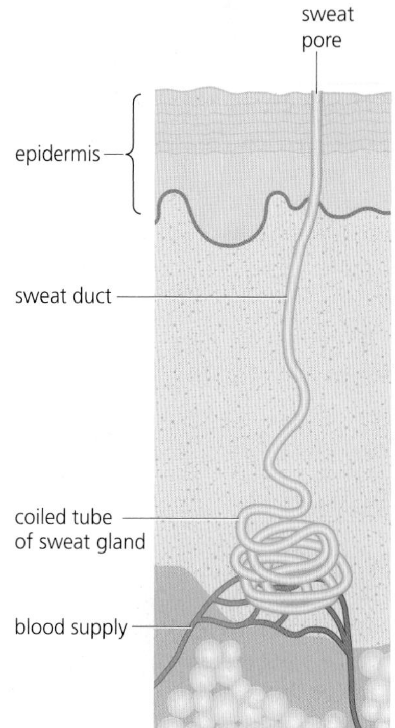

An eccrine sweat gland

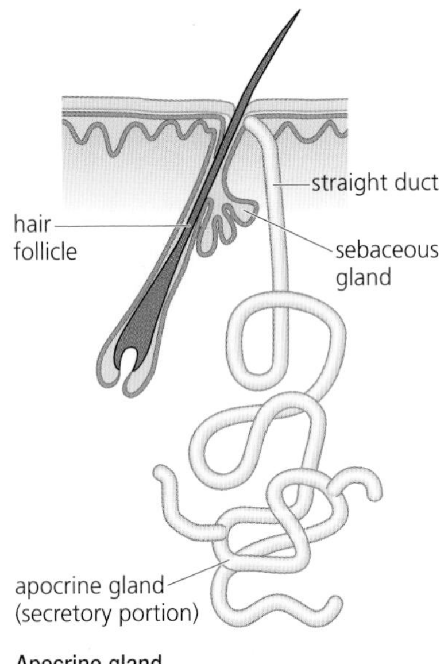

Apocrine gland

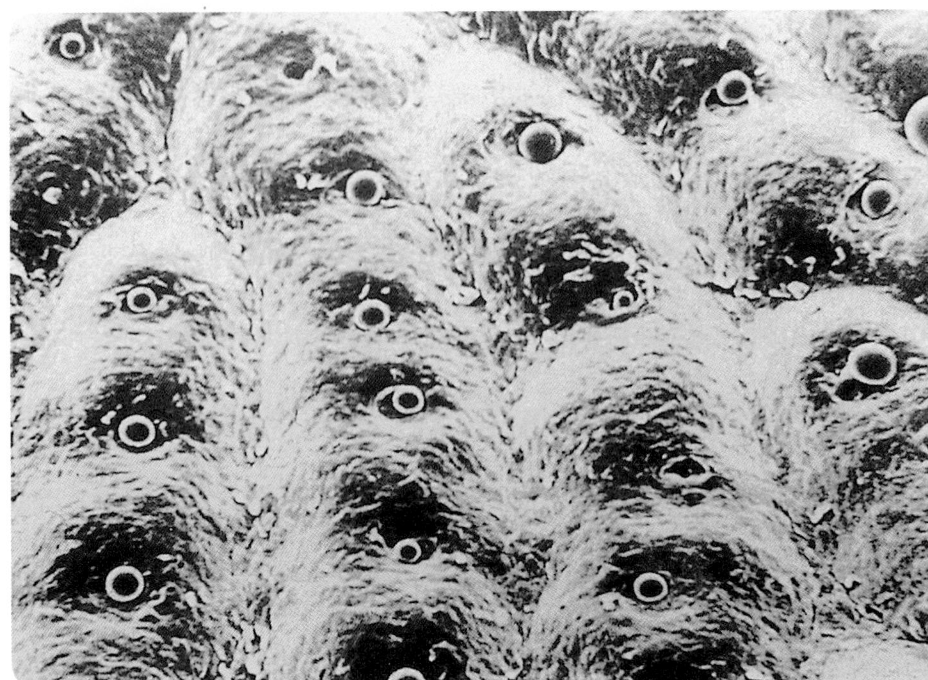

Sweat pores on the skin's surface

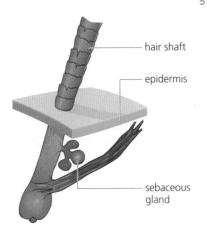

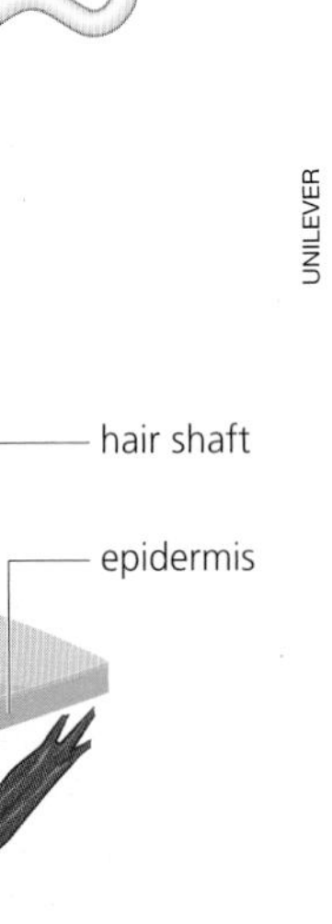

Sebaceous gland

An unpleasant smell – **body odour** – develops when apocrine sweat is broken down by skin bacteria. Good habits of personal hygiene will prevent this.

Cosmetic perspiration control To extend hygiene protection during the day, apply either a deodorant or an antiperspirant. **Antiperspirants** reduce the amount of sweat that reaches the skin's surface: they have an astringent action which closes the pores. **Deodorants** contain an active antiseptic ingredient which reduces the skin's bacterial activity, thereby reducing the risk of odour from stale sweat.

Sebaceous glands The **sebaceous gland** appears as a minute sac-like organ. Usually it is associated with the hair follicle with which it forms the **pilosebaceous unit,** but the two can appear independently.

HEALTH & SAFETY

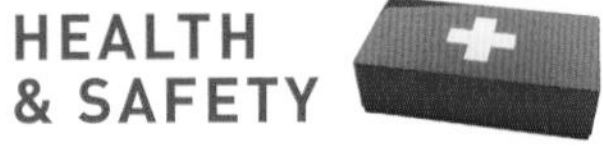

Antiperspirants

The active ingredient in most antiperspirant products is aluminium chlorohydrate. This is known to cause contact dermatitis in some people, especially if the skin has been damaged by recent removal of unwanted hair. Bear this in mind if you are performing an under arm depilatory wax service. (See the aftercare instructions, pages 509–510.)

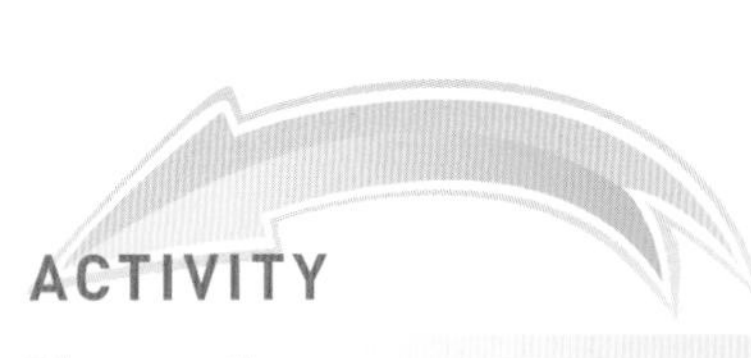

ACTIVITY

The emotions

Emotions can affect blood supply to the skin: blood vessels in the dermis may enlarge or constrict. Think of different emotions, and how these might affect the appearance of the skin.

Sebaceous glands are found all over the body, except on the palms of the hands and the soles of the feet. They are particularly numerous on the scalp, the forehead, and in the back and chest region. The cells of the glands decompose, producing the skin's natural oil, **sebum**. This empties directly into the hair follicle.

The activity of the sebaceous gland increases at puberty, when stimulated by the male hormone **androgen**. In adults, activity of the sebaceous gland gradually decreases again. Men secrete slightly more sebum than women; and on black skin the sebaceous glands are larger and more numerous than on white skin.

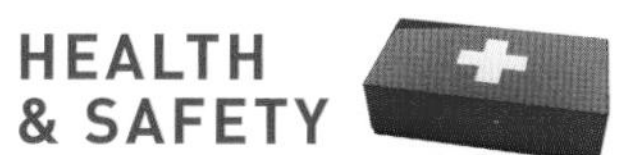

HEALTH & SAFETY

Skin problems are common at puberty when changes in hormone levels cause sebaceous glands to produce excess sebum and the skin's surface becomes oily. Growth of skin bacteria can increase in the sebum causing inflammation of the surrounding tissues. This can lead to the skin disorder acne vulgaris see page 28. The skin should always be kept clean and handled with clean hands.

Sebum is composed of fatty acids and waxes. These have **bactericidal** and **fungicidal** properties, and so discourage the multiplication of microorganisms on the surface of the skin. Sebum also reduces the evaporation of moisture from the skin, and so prevents the skin from drying out.

Acid mantle Sweat and sebum combine on the skin's surface, creating an acid film. This is known as the **acid mantle** and discourages the growth of bacteria and fungi.

Acidity and alkalinity are measured by a number called the pH. An *acidic solution* has a pH of 0–6.9; a *neutral solution* has a pH of 7; and an *alkaline solution* has a pH of 7.1–14. The acid mantle of the skin has a pH of 5.5–5.6.

Subcutaneous layer Beneath the dermis lies the subcutaneous layer made up of adipose (fat) tissue. It is supplied with a network of arteries that run parallel to the skin's surface. Fat cells are called adipocytes and contain droplets of fat.

The fatty layer has a protective function and:

- acts as an insulator to conserve body heat, keeping you warm
- cushions muscles and bones below from injury
- acts as an energy source, as excess fat is stored in this layer.

KNOWLEDGE CHECK

Name each part of the skin's structure numbered below.

Need more time... refer to page 32 to help you.

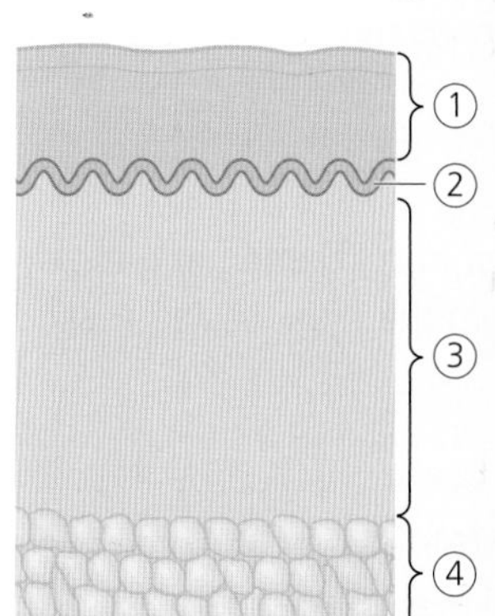

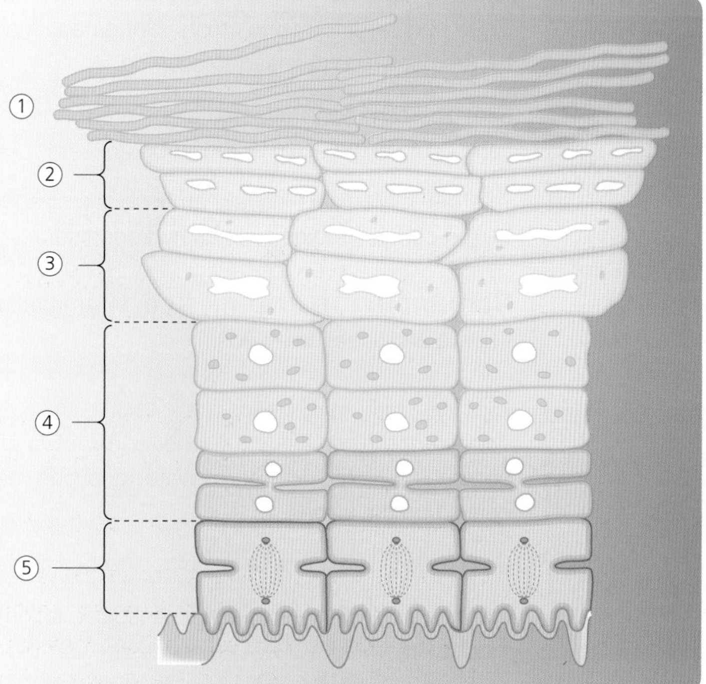

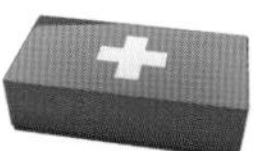

HEALTH & SAFETY

Moisture balance

Excessive sweating, which can occur through exposure to high temperatures or during illness, can lead to *skin dehydration* – insufficient water content. Fluid intake must be increased to rebalance the body fluids.

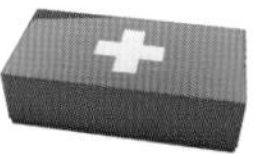

HEALTH & SAFETY

The lips

Sebaceous glands are not present on the surface of the lips. For this reason the lips should be protected with a lip emollient preparation to prevent them from becoming dry and chapped.

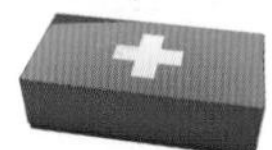

HEALTH & SAFETY

Using alkaline products

Because the skin has an acid pH, if alkaline products are used on it the acid mantle will be disturbed. It will take several hours for this protective film to be restored; during this time, the skin will be irritated and sensitive.

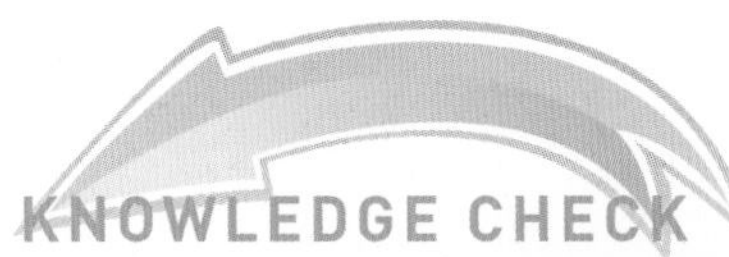

KNOWLEDGE CHECK

How do the following structures help to defend the skin from harm?

- mast cells
- macrophages

Need more time... refer to page 36 to help you.

Skin diseases and disorders

Having learnt about the skin the beauty therapist must be able to distinguish a healthy skin from one suffering from a skin disease or disorder. Certain skin disorders and diseases prevent treatment: proceeding would expose the beauty therapist and other clients to the risk of cross-infection through contact. It is therefore vital that you are familiar with the skin diseases and disorders with which you might come into contact in the workplace, those that are a risk and those that are not, and the correct action to take. Relevant skin diseases and disorders are also discussed in each treatment chapter.

HEALTH & SAFETY

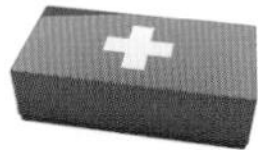

Skin problems
If you are unable to identify a skin condition with confidence, so that you are uncertain whether or not you should treat the client, don't! Tactfully refer them to their GP before proceeding with the planned treatment.

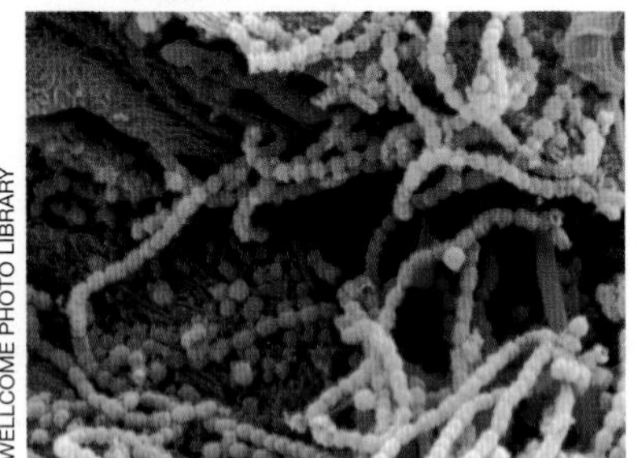

WELLCOME PHOTO LIBRARY

Example of a microscopic bacteria – streptococcus bacteria on the tongue

Bacterial infections

Bacteria are minute single-celled organisms of varied shapes. Large numbers of bacteria inhabit the surface of the skin and are harmless (**non-pathogenic**); indeed some play an important positive role in the health of the skin. Others, however, are harmful (**pathogenic**) and can cause skin diseases.

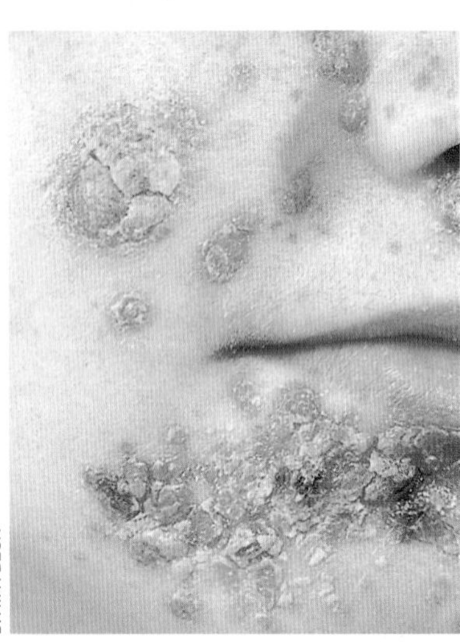

DR M H BECK

Impetigo

Impetigo An inflammatory disease of the surface of the skin, usually appearing on exposed areas.

Infectious? Yes.

Appearance: Initially the skin appears red and is itchy. Small thin-walled blisters appear; these burst and form into crusts. Untreated small pus-filled ulcers can occur with a dark, thick crust which can lead to scarring.

Site: The commonly affected areas are the nose, the mouth and the ears, but impetigo can occur on the scalp or the limbs.

Treatment: Medical – usually an antibiotic or an antibacterial ointment is prescribed containing corticosteroids such as hydrocortisone.

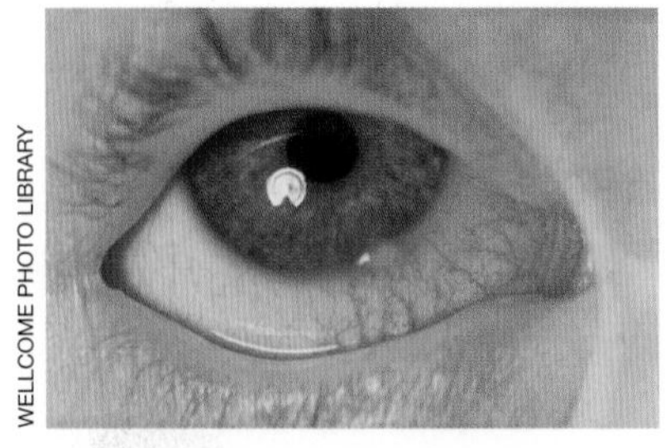

WELLCOME PHOTO LIBRARY

Conjunctivitis or pink eye

Conjunctivitis or pink eye Inflammation of the mucous membrane that covers the eye and lines the eyelids.

Infectious? Yes.

Appearance: The skin of the inner conjunctiva of the eye becomes inflamed and the eye becomes very red and sore. Water and pus may exude from the area leaving a sticky coating on the lashes.

Site: The eyes, either one or both, may be infected.

Treatment: Medical – usually an antibiotic lotion is prescribed. However, in some cases medical treatment will not be necessary and the infection will heal independently.

Hordeola or styes Infection of the sebaceous glands of eyelash hair follicles. It can be an effect of blepharitis (inflammation of the eyelids).

Infectious? Yes.

Appearance: Small red, inflamed lumps containing pus, a sign of infection.

Site: The inner rim of the eyelid.

Treatment: Medical – usually an antibiotic is prescribed.

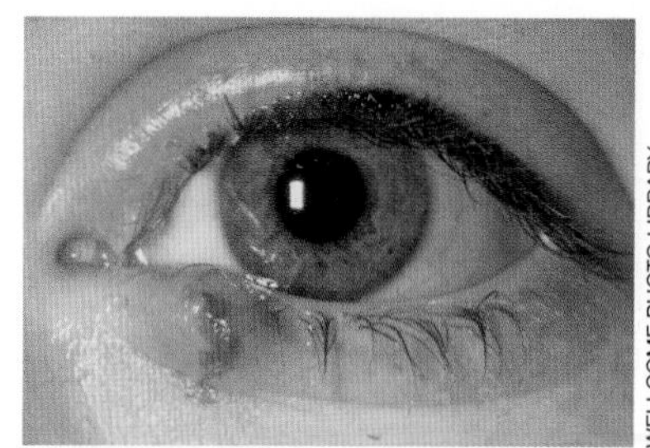
WELLCOME PHOTO LIBRARY

Hordeola or styes

Furuncles or boils Red, painful lumps, extending deeply into the skin.

Infectious? Yes.

Appearance: A localized red lump occurs around a hair follicle; it then develops a core or pus. Scarring of the skin often remains after the boil has healed.

Site: The back of the neck, the armpits and buttocks and thighs are common areas, but furuncles can occur anywhere.

Treatment: Medical – Antibiotics may help to control infection.

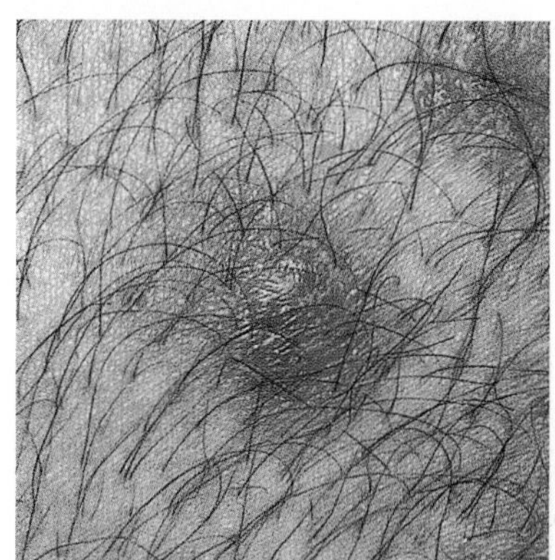
DR A L WRIGHT

Furuncle or boil

Carbuncles Infection of numerous hair follicles.

Infectious? Yes.

Appearance: A hard, round abscess, larger than a boil, which oozes pus from several points upon its surface. Scarring often occurs after the carbuncle has healed.

Site: In particular where there is friction, such as the back of the neck, or on the thighs. However, they can occur anywhere.

Treatment: Medical – usually involving incision, drainage of the pus, and a course of antibiotics.

HEALTH & SAFETY

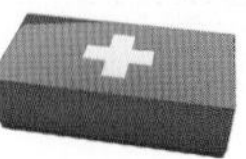

Boils

Boils occurring on the upper lip or in the nose should be referred immediately to a GP. Boils can be dangerous when near to the eyes or brain.

Paronychia Infection of the skin tissue surrounding the nail (the nail fold). If left untreated, the nail bed may become infected.

Infectious? Yes.

Appearance: Swelling, redness and pus in the nail fold and the area of the nail wall.

Site: The skin surrounding the nail plate.

Treatment: Medical – usually a course of antibiotics, incision and drainage of pus is necessary if it collects next to the nail.

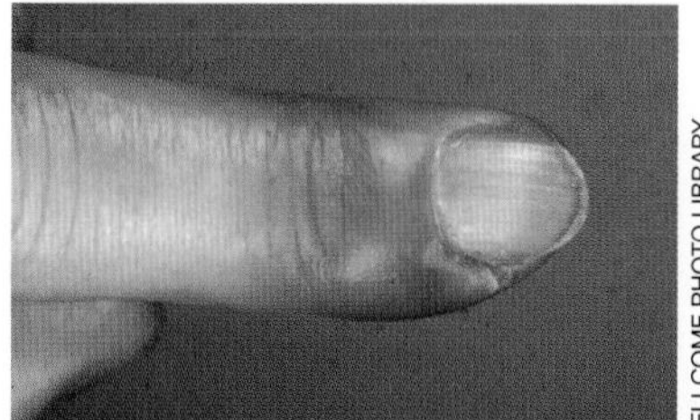
WELLCOME PHOTO LIBRARY

Paronychia

Viral infections

Viruses are minute entities, too small to see even under an ordinary microscope. They are considered to be **parasites**, as they require living tissue in order to survive. Viruses invade healthy body cells and multiply within the cell: in due course the cell walls break down, liberating new viral particles to attack further cells, and thus the infection spreads.

Herpes simplex This is commonly referred to as a cold sore and a recurring skin condition, appearing at times when the skin's resistance is lowered through ill health or stress. It may also be caused by exposure of the skin to extremes of temperature or to ultra-violet light.

Infectious? Yes.

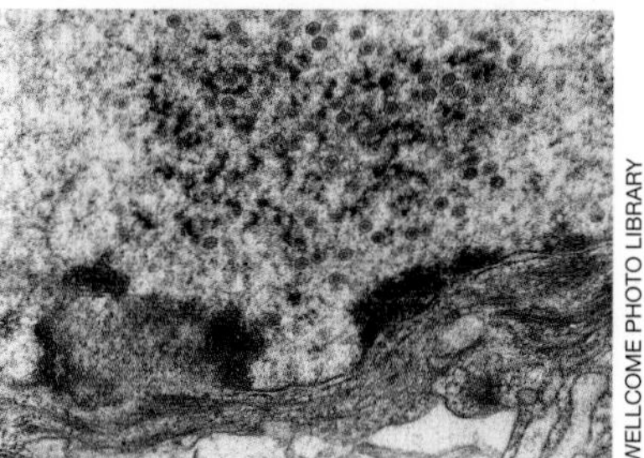
WELLCOME PHOTO LIBRARY

Example of a microscopic virus – herpes simplex virus particles (orange) in the nucleus of an epithelial cell

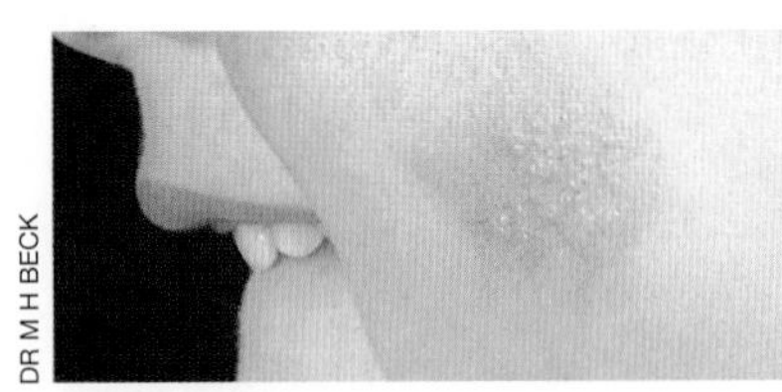

Herpes simplex

Appearance: Inflammation of the skin occurs in localized areas. As well as being red, the skin becomes itchy and small vesicles appear. These are followed by a crust, which may crack and weep tissue fluid.

Site: The mucous membranes of the nose or lips; herpes can also occur on the skin generally.

Treatment: There is no specific treatment, they usually clear in 7–10 days. A proprietary brand of anti-inflammatory antiseptic drying cream is usually prescribed, which must be applied in the early stages of the condition when a tingling, itching sensation is experienced.

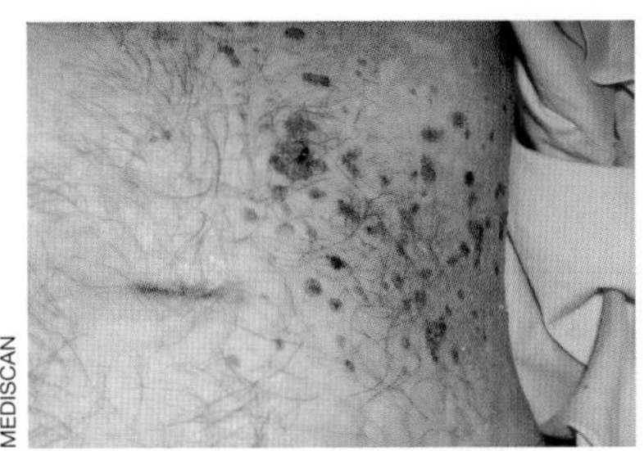

Shingles

Herpes zoster or shingles In this painful disease from the virus that causes chicken pox, the virus attacks the sensory nerve endings and is thought to lie dormant in the body and be triggered when the body's defences are at a low ebb.

Infectious? Yes.

Appearance: Redness of the skin occurs along a line of the affected nerves. Blisters develop and form crusts, leaving purplish-pink pigmentation.

Site: Commonly the chest and the abdomen.

Treatment: Medical – usually including anti-viral medicines. Calamine lotion can soothe the irritation. If there are complications with bacterial infection, antibiotics will be prescribed.

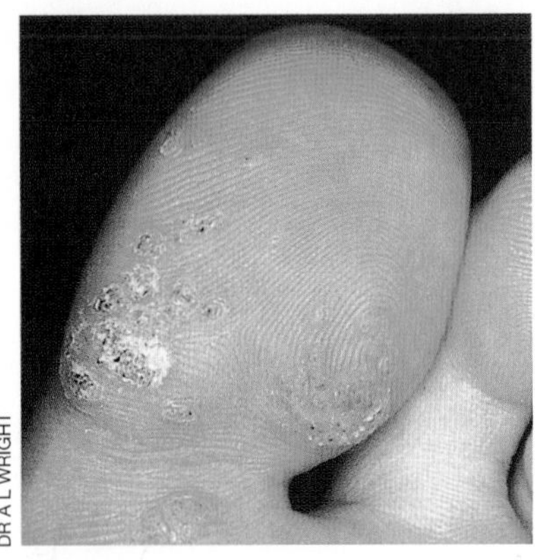

Verruca

Verrucae or warts Small epidermal skin growths. Warts can be raised or flat, depending upon their position. There are several types of wart: plane, common, plantar and mosaic.

Infectious? Yes.

Appearance: Warts vary in size, shape, texture and colour. Usually they have a rough surface and are raised. If a wart occurs on the sole of the foot it grows inwards, due to the pressure of body weight.

Site:

- plane wart (flat wart): the fingers, either surface of the hand, face and legs
- common wart (verruca vulgaris): the hands, elbows and knees
- plantar wart (verrucae): the sole of the foot and toes
- mosaic (palmar warts): hands and feet

Treatment: Medical – using acids, i.e. salicylic acid, solid carbon dioxide (cryotherapy) or electrocautery.

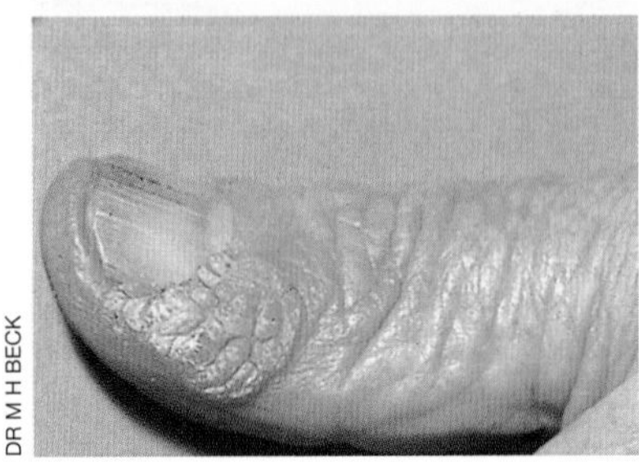

A wart

Infestations

Scabies or itch mites (sarcoptes scabiei) A condition in which an **infestation** of a tiny mite parasite burrows beneath the skin and invades the hair follicles. The mite feeds on tissue and fluid as it burrows into the skin.

Infectious? Yes.

Appearance: At the onset, minute papules and wavy greyish lines appear, where dirt has entered the burrows. Secondary bacterial infection may occur as a result of scratching.

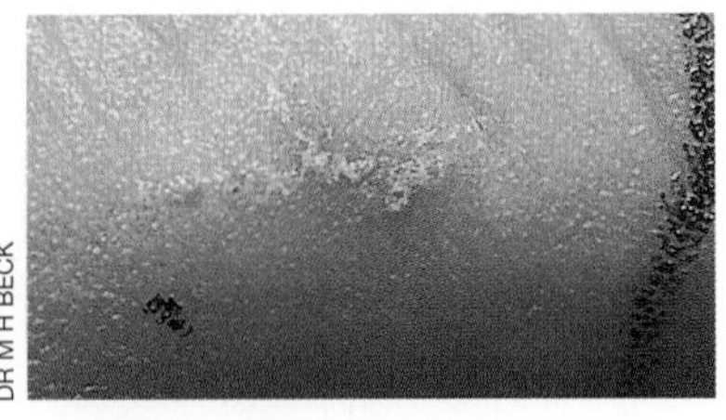

A scabies burrow

Site: Usually seen in warm areas of loose skin, such as the webs of the fingers, under the fingernails and the creases of the elbows.

Treatment: Medical – an anti-scabetic lotion containing an insecticide.

Pediculosis capitis or head lice A condition in which small lice parasites infest scalp hair.

Infectious? Yes.

Appearance: The lice cling to the hair of the scalp. Eggs are laid, attached to the hair close to the skin. The lice bite the skin to draw nourishment from the blood; this creates irritation and itching of the skin, which may lead to secondary bacterial infection.

Site: The hair of the scalp.

Treatment: Medical – an appropriate medicated insecticide lotion or rinse.

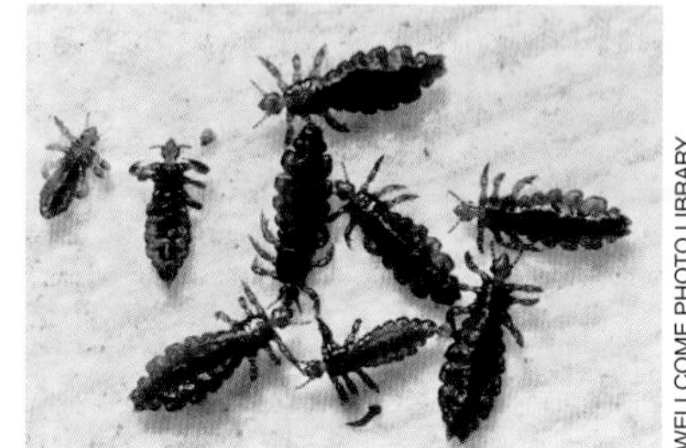

WELLCOME PHOTO LIBRARY

Head lice

Pediculosis pubis or pubic lice A condition in which small lice parasites infest body hair.

Infectious? Yes.

Appearance: The lice cling to the hair of the body. Eggs are laid, attached to the hair close to the skin. The lice bite the skin to draw nourishment from the blood; this creates irritation and itching of the skin, which may lead to secondary bacterial infection.

Site: Pubic hair, eyebrows and eyelashes.

Treatment: Medical – an appropriate insecticidal lotion.

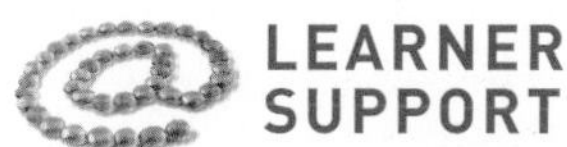

Health multiple choice quiz

Pediculosis corporis or body lice A condition in which small parasites live and feed on body skin.

Infectious? Yes.

Appearance: The lice cling to the hair of the body. Eggs are laid, attached to the hair close to the skin. The lice bite the skin to draw nourishment from the blood; this creates irritation and itching of the skin, which may lead to secondary bacterial infection. Where body lice bite the skin, small red marks can be seen.

Site: Body hair.

Treatment: Medical – an appropriate insecticidal lotion.

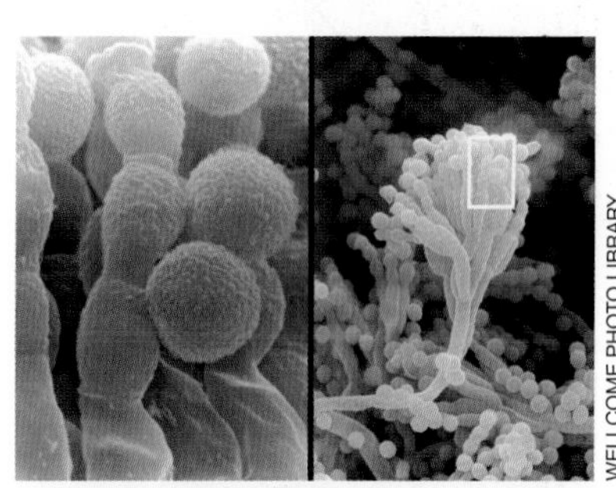

WELLCOME PHOTO LIBRARY

Example of a microscopic fungi – penicillium mould producing spores, plus very close up view of spore formulation

Fungal diseases

Fungi are microscopic plants. They are parasites, dependent upon a host for their existence. Fungal diseases of the skin feed off the waste products of the skin. Some fungi are found on the skin's surface; others attack the deeper tissues. Reproduction of fungi is by means of simple cell division or by the production of spores.

Tinea pedis or athlete's foot A common fungal foot infection.

Infectious? Yes.

Appearance: Small blisters form, which later burst. The skin in the area can then become dry, giving a scaly appearance.

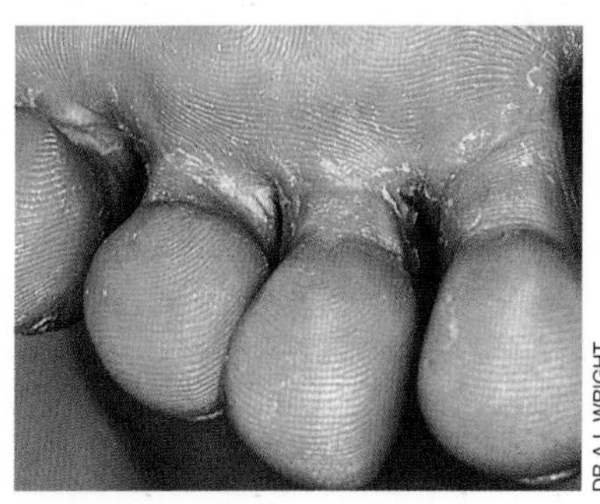

DR A L WRIGHT

Tinea pedis or athlete's foot

Site: Commonly affects the webs of skin between the toes.

Treatment: Thorough cleansing of the area. Medical application of fungicides. Untreated, infections such as bacterial infections may occur. It can also lead to infection of the toe and fingernails.

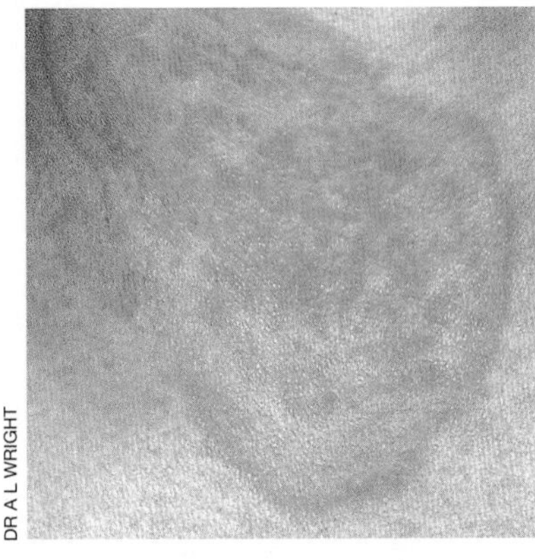
DR A L WRIGHT

Tinea corporis or body ringworm

Tinea corporis or body ringworm A fungal infection of the skin.

Infectious? Yes.

Appearance: Small scaly red patches, which spread outwards and then heal from the centre, leaving a ring.

Site: The trunk of the body, the limbs and the face.

Treatment: Medical – using a fungicidal cream. Oral anti-fungal medication is necessary if there are several infection sites.

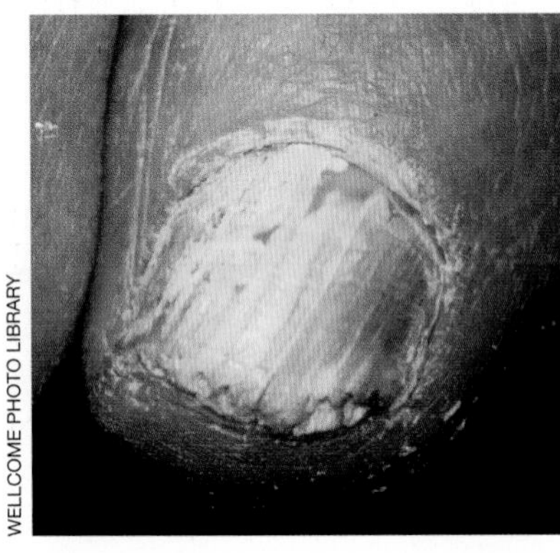
WELLCOME PHOTO LIBRARY

Tinea unguium

Tinea unguium or onychomycosis Ringworm infection of the fingernails.

Infectious? Yes.

Appearance: The nail plate is white and opaque. Eventually the nail plate becomes brittle and separates from the nail bed.

Site: The nail plate.

Treatment: Medical application of fungicides.

HEALTH & SAFETY

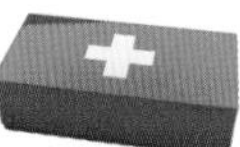

Artificial nails

Artificial nails increase the risk of developing infection due to the natural nail plate being roughened and if not maintained correctly moisture can collect between the artificial nail and the natural nail plate which provides ideal growth for fungi.

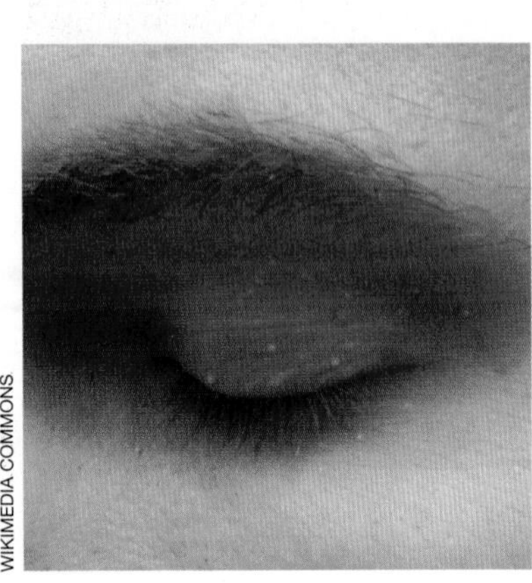
WIKIMEDIA COMMONS

Milia on the eyelid

Sebaceous gland disorders

Milia Keratinization of the skin over the hair follicle occurs, causing sebum to accumulate in the hair follicle. This condition usually accompanies dry skin.

Infectious? No.

Appearance: Small, hard, pearly white cysts.

Site: The upper face or close to the eyes.

Treatment: The milium may be removed by a beauty therapist (if qualified to do so) or by a GP, depending on the location. A sterile lancet is used to pierce the skin of the overlying cuticle and thereby free the milium. Micro-dermabrasion may be used to avoid their development. Also retinoid creams may be applied which remove the outer epidermal layers.

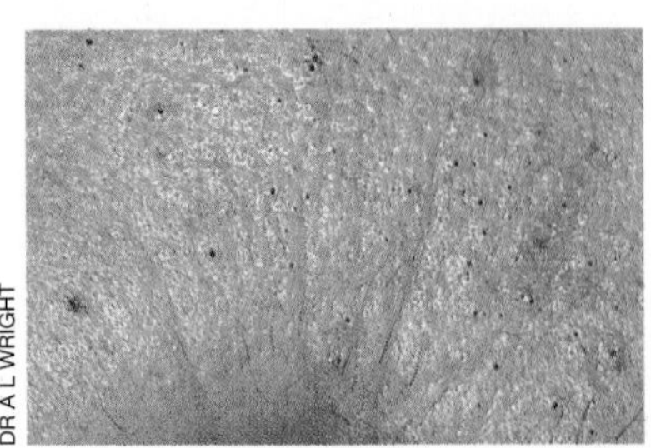
DR A L WRIGHT

Comedones or blackheads

Comedones or blackheads Excess sebum and keratinized cells block the mouth of the hair follicle.

Infectious? No.

Site: The face (the chin, nose and forehead), the upper back and chest.

Treatment: The area should be cleansed and an electrical vapour treatment or other pre-heating treatment should be given to relax the mouth of the hair follicle; a sterile comedo extractor should then be used to remove the blockage. A regular cleansing treatment should be recommended by the beauty therapist to limit the production of comedones.

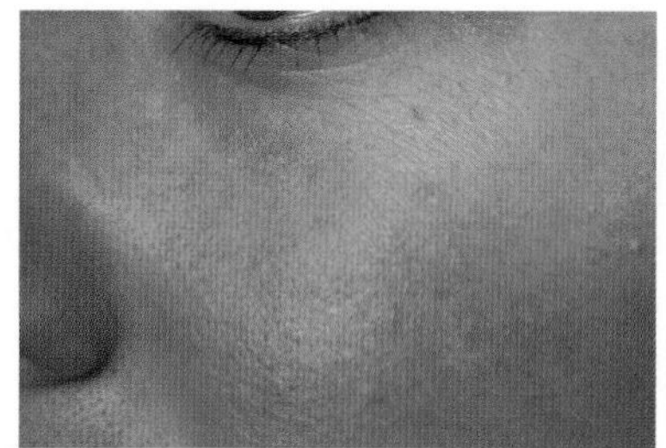

MEDISCAN

Seborrhoeic skin

Seborrhoea Excessive secretion of sebum from the sebaceous gland. This usually occurs during puberty, as a result of hormonal changes in the body.

Infectious? No.

Appearance: The follicle openings enlarge and excessive sebum is secreted. The skin appears coarse and oily; comedones, pustules and papules are present.

Site: The face and scalp. Seborrhoea may also affect the back and the chest.

Treatment: The area should be cleansed to remove excess oil. Medical treatment may be required – this would use locally applied steroid creams.

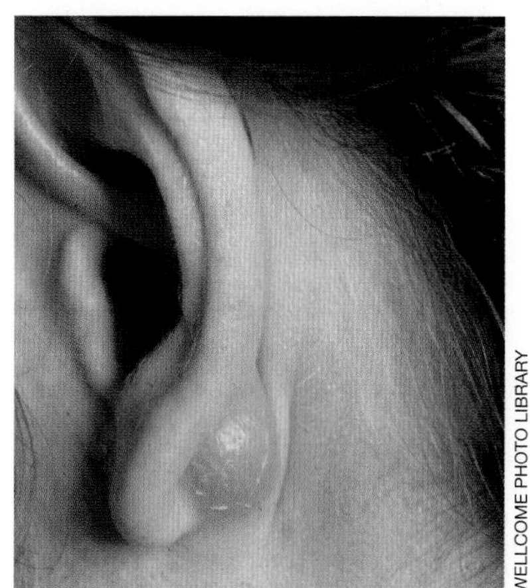

WELLCOME PHOTO LIBRARY

Sebaceous cyst

Steatomas, sebaceous cysts or wens Localized pockets or sacs of sebum, which form in hair follicles or under the sebaceous glands in the skin. The sebum becomes blocked, the sebaceous gland becomes distended and a lump forms.

Infectious? No.

Appearance: Semi-globular in shape, either raised or flat and hard or soft. The cysts are the same colour as the skin, or red if secondary bacterial infection occurs. A comedo can often be seen at the original mouth of the hair follicle.

Site: If the cyst appears on the upper eyelid, it is known as a **chalazion** or **meibomian cyst**.

Treatment: Medical – often a GP will remove the cyst under local anaesthetic. Small inflamed cysts can be medically treated with steroid medications or antibiotics.

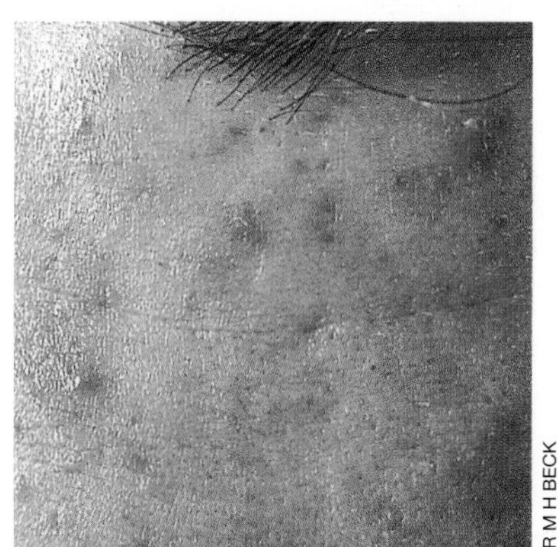

DR M H BECK

Acne vulgaris

Acne vulgaris Hormone imbalance in the body at puberty influences the activity of the sebaceous gland, causing an increased production of sebum. The sebum may be retained within the sebaceous ducts, causing congestion and bacterial infection of the surrounding tissues.

Infectious? No.

Appearance: Inflammation of the skin, accompanied by comedones, pustules and papules.

Site: Commonly on the face, the nose, the chin and the forehead. Acne may also occur on the chest and back.

Treatment: Medical – oral antibiotics may be prescribed, as well as medicated creams. With medical approval, regular salon treatments may be given to cleanse the skin deeply and also to stimulate the blood circulation.

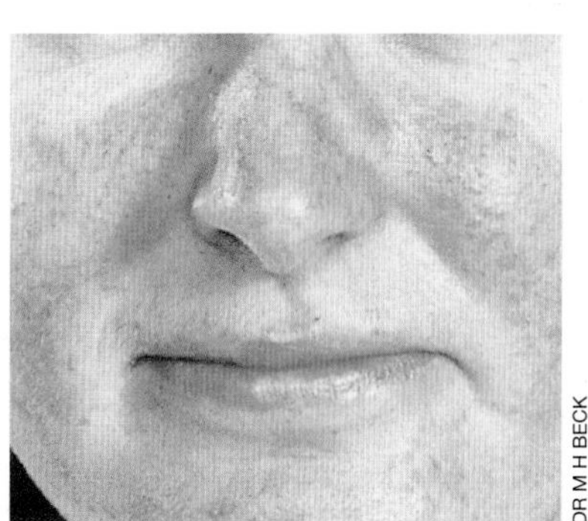

DR M H BECK

Rosacea

Rosacea Excessive sebum secretion combined with a chronic inflammatory condition, caused by dilation of the blood capillaries.

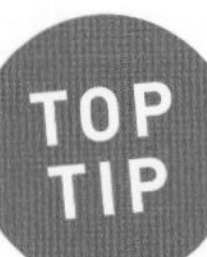

TOP TIP

Hypopigmentation

Hypopigmentation may result from certain skin injuries, disorders or diseases.

Infectious? No.

Appearance: The skin becomes coarse, the pores enlarge and the cheek and nose area become inflamed, sometimes swelling and producing a butterfly pattern. Blood circulation slows in the dilated capillaries, creating a purplish appearance.

Treatment: Medical – usually including antibiotics.

Pigmentation disorders

Pigmentation of the skin varies, according to the person's genetic characteristics. In general, the darker the skin, the more pigment is present, but some abnormal changes in skin pigmentation can occur.

- **Hyperpigmentation** – increased pigment production
- **Hypopigmentation** – loss of pigmentation in the skin

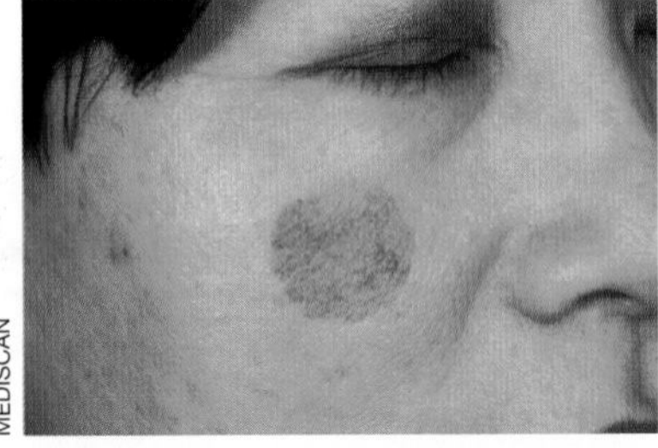

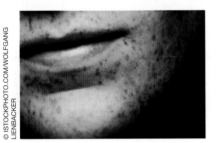

Ephelides or freckles

Ephelides or freckles Multiple, small hyperpigmented areas of the skin. Exposure to ultra-violet light (as in sunlight) stimulates the production of melanin, intensifying their appearance.

Infectious? No.

Appearance: Small, flat, pigmented areas, darker that the surrounding skin.

Site: Commonly the nose and cheeks of fair-skinned people. Freckles may also occur on the shoulders, arms, hands and back.

Treatment: Freckles may be concealed with cosmetics if required. A sun block should be recommended, to prevent them intensifying in colour.

Lentigo

Lentigo (plural, lentigines) Hyperpigmented areas of skin, slightly larger than freckles. Lentigo simplex occur in childhood. Actinic (solar) lentigines occur in middle age as a result of sun exposure.

Infectious? No.

Appearance: Brown, slightly raised, pigmented patches of skin, of variable size.

Site: The face, hands and shoulders.

Treatment: Application of cosmetic concealing products.

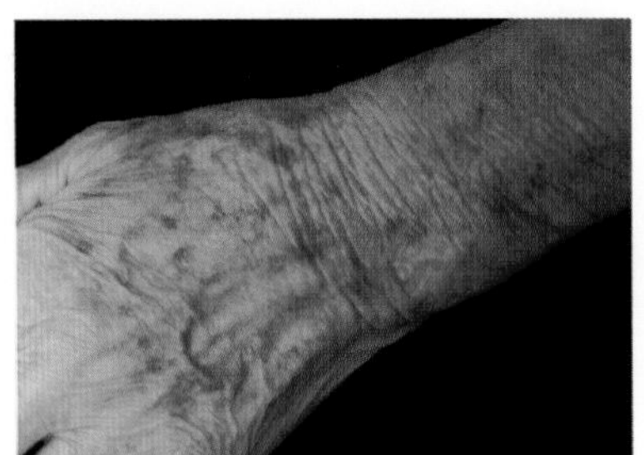

Chloasmata or liver spots

Chloasmata or liver spots Hyperpigmentation in specific areas, stimulated by a skin irritant such as ultra-violet light, usually affecting women and darkly pigmented skins. The condition often occurs during pregnancy and usually disappears soon after the birth of the baby. It may also occur as a result of taking the oral contraceptive pill. The female hormone oestrogen is thought to stimulate melanin production.

Infectious? No.

Appearance: Flat, smooth, irregularly shaped, pigmented areas of skin, varying in colour from light tan to dark brown. Chloasmata are larger than ephelides, and of variable size.

Site: The back of the hands, the forearms, the upper part of the chest, the temples and the forehead.

Treatment: A barrier cream or a total sun-block will reduce the risk of the chloasmata increasing in size or number and thereby becoming more apparent.

Dermatosis papulosa nigra Often called flesh moles, these are characterized by multiple benign, small brown to black hyperpigmented papules, common among dark-skinned people.

Infectious? No.

Appearance: Raised pigmented markings resembling moles.

Site: Usually seen on the cheeks and forehead, although they may appear on the neck, upper chest and back.

Treatment: Medical by medication or surgery.

Vitiligo or leucoderma Patches of completely white skin which have lost their pigment, or which were never pigmented.

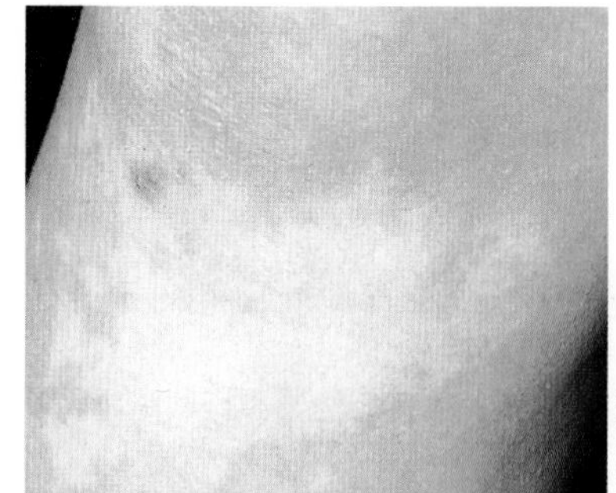

DR M H BECK

Vitiligo or leucoderma

Infectious? No.

Appearance: Well-defined patches of white skin, lacking pigment.

Site: The face, the neck, the hands, the lower abdomen and the thighs. If vitiligo occurs over the eyebrows, the hairs in the area will also lose their pigment.

Treatment: Camouflage cosmetic concealer can be applied to give even skin colour; or skin-staining preparations can be used in the de-pigmented areas. Care must be taken when the skin is exposed to ultra-violet light, as the skin will not have the same protection in the areas lacking pigment.

Albinism The skin is unable to produce the melanin pigment and the skin, hair and eyes lack colour.

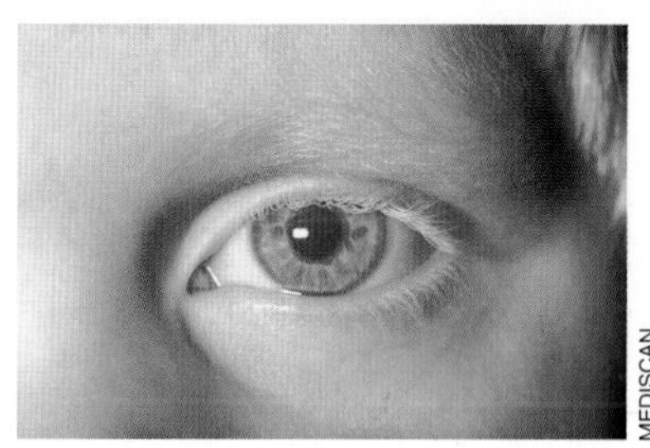

MEDISCAN

Albinism

Infectious? No.

Appearance: The skin is usually very pale pink and the hair is white. The eyes also are pink and extremely sensitive to light.

Site: The entire skin.

Treatment: There is no effective treatment. Maximum skin protection is necessary when the client is exposed to ultra-violet light and sunglasses should be worn to protect the eyes.

Vascular naevi There are two types of naevus of concern to beauty therapists: vascular and cellular. **Vascular naevi** are skin conditions in which small or large areas of skin pigmentation are caused by the permanent dilation of blood capillaries.

> **TOP TIP**
>
> **Vascular disorders**
>
> **If there is a vascular skin disorder, avoid over stimulating the skin or the problem will become more noticeable and the treatment may even cause further damage.**

Erythema An area of skin in which blood capillaries have dilated, due either to injury or inflammation.

Infectious? No.

Appearance: The skin appears red.

Site: Erythema may affect one area (locally) or all of the skin (generally).

Treatment: The cause of the inflammation should be identified. In the case of a **skin allergy**, the client must not be brought into contact with the irritant again. If the cause is unknown, refer the client to their GP.

Dilated capillaries Capillaries near the surface of the skin that are permanently dilated.

Infectious? No.

Appearance: Small red visible blood capillaries.

Site: Areas where the skin is neglected, dry or fine, such as the cheek area.

Treatment: Dilated capillaries can be concealed using a green corrective camouflage cosmetic, or removed by qualified electrologist using diathermy.

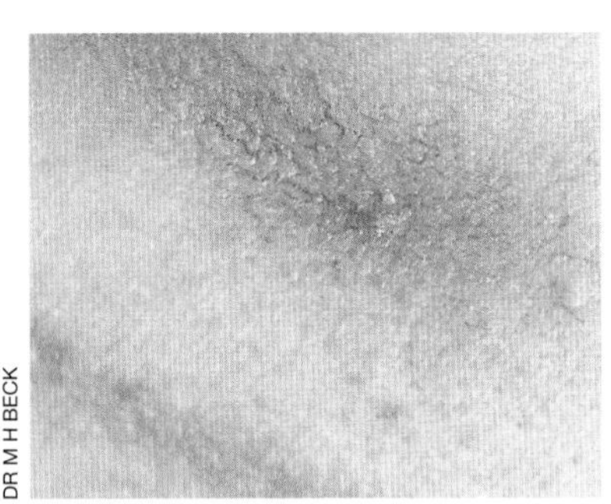

DR M H BECK

Spider naevus or stellate haemangiomas

Spider naevi or stellate haemangiomas Dilated blood vessels, with smaller dilated capillaries radiating from them.

Infectious? No.

Appearance: Small red capillaries, radiating like a spider's legs from a central point.

Site: Commonly the cheek area, but may occur on the upper body, the arms and the neck. Spider naevi are usually caused by an injury to the skin.

Treatment: Spider naevi can be concealed using a camouflage cosmetic, or treated by a qualified electrologist with diathermy.

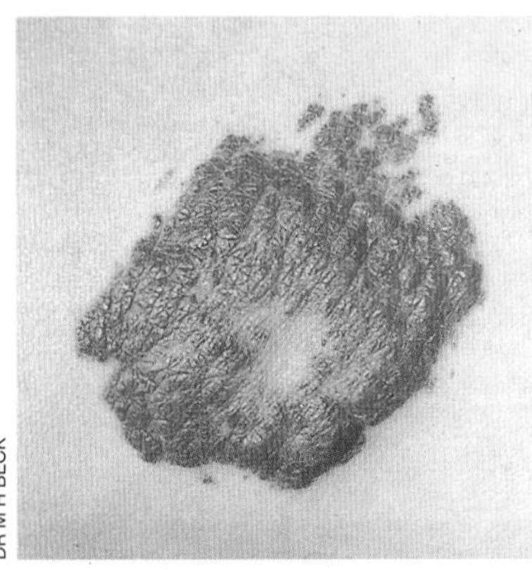

DR M H BECK

Naevi vasculosis or strawberry marks

Naevi vasculosis or strawberry marks Red or purplish raised marks which appear on the skin at birth.

Infectious? No.

Appearance: Red or purplish lobed mark, of any size.

Site: Any area of the skin.

Treatment: About 60 per cent disappear by the age of six years. Treatment is not usually necessary; concealing cosmetics can be applied if desired.

Capillary naevi or port-wine stains Large areas of dilated capillaries that contrast noticeably with the surrounding areas.

Infectious? No.

Appearance: The naevus has a smooth flat surface.

Site: Some 75 per cent occur on the head; they are probably formed at the foetal stage. Naevi may also be found on the neck and face.

Treatment: Camouflage cosmetic creams can be applied to disguise the area.

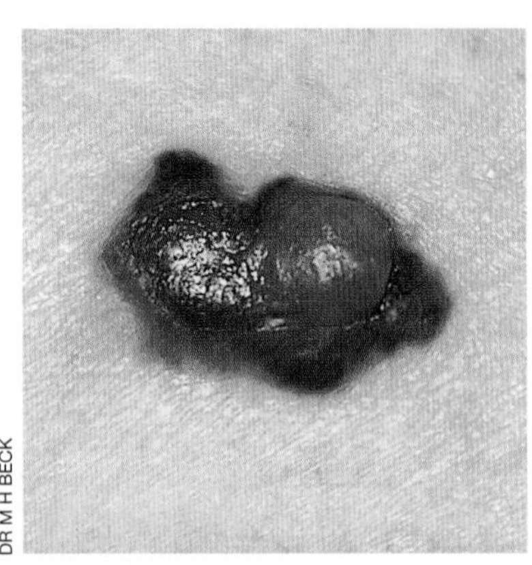

DR M H BECK

Malignant melanoma

Cellular naevi or moles **Cellular naevi** are skin conditions in which changes in the cells of the skin result in skin malformations.

Malignant melanomas or malignant moles Rapidly-growing skin cancers, usually occurring in adults.

Infectious? No.

Appearance: Each melanoma commences as a bluish-black mole, which enlarges rapidly, darkening in colour and developing a halo of pigmentation around it. It later becomes raised, bleeds and ulcerates. Secondary growths will develop in internal organs if the melanoma is not treated.

Normal Mole	Melanoma	Sign	Characteristic
		Asymmetry	When half of the mole does not match the other half.
		Border	When the border (edges) of the mole are ragged or irregular.
		Colour	When the colour of the mole varies throughout.
		Diameter	If the mole's diameter is larger than a pencil's eraser.

PERMISSION OF THE NATIONAL CANCER INSTITUTE

Guidance images for moles

HEALTH & SAFETY

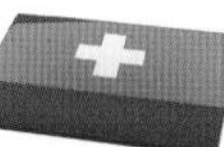

Moles

If moles change in shape or size, if they bleed or form crusts, seek medical attention.

HEALTH & SAFETY

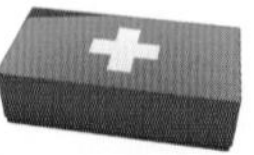

Malignant melanoma risk

The risk of melanoma increases as the number of naevi increases. Therefore clients with lots of naevi or moles are at highest risk.

Site: Usually the lower abdomen, legs or feet.

Treatment: Medical – always recommend that a client has a mole checked if it is changing in size, structure or colour, or if it becomes itchy or bleeds.

Junction naevi Localized collections of naevoid cells that arise from the mass production locally of pigment-forming cells (melanocytes).

Infectious? No.

Appearance: In childhood junction naevi appear as smooth or slightly raised pigmented marks. They vary in colour from brown to black.

Site: Any area.

Treatment: None.

Dermal naevi Localized collections of naevoid cells.

Infectious? No.

Appearance: About 1cm wide, dermal naevi appear smooth and dome-shaped. Their colour ranges from skin tone to dark brown. Frequently one or more hairs may grow from the naevus.

Site: Usually the face.

Treatment: None.

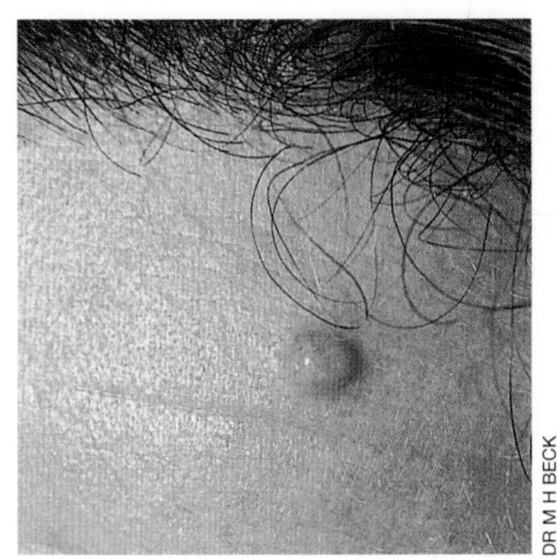

DR M H BECK

Benign naevus

TOP TIP

Naevi numbers and skin colour

Caucasian skin normally has up to four times as many naevi than black skin.

HEALTH & SAFETY

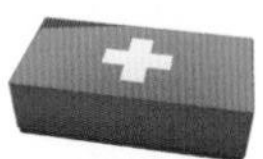

Skin tags

Skin tags often occur under the arms. In case they are present, take care when carrying out a wax depilation service in this area: do not apply wax over tags.

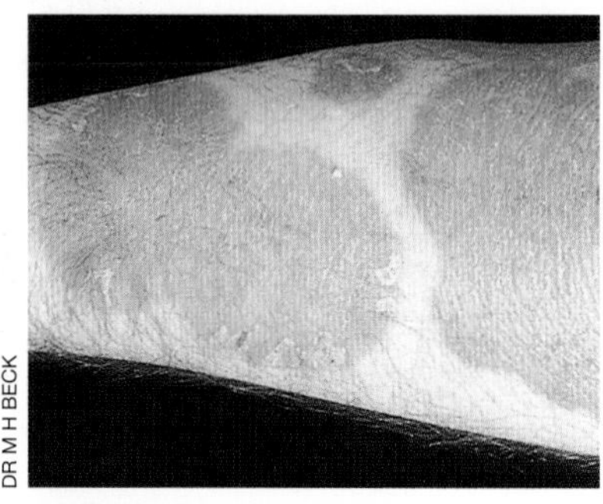

DR M H BECK

Psoriasis

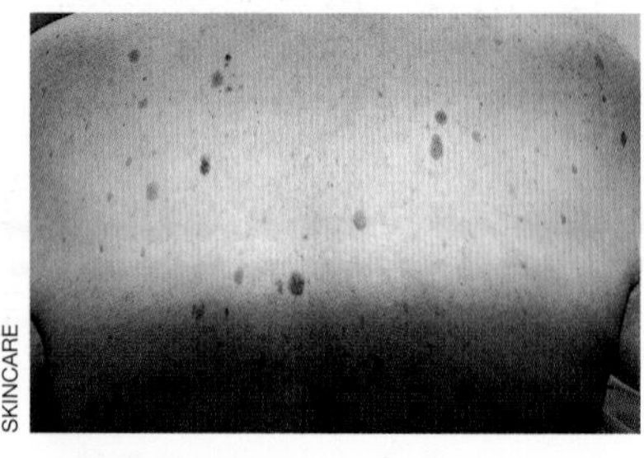

DR JOHN GRAY, THE WORLD OF SKINCARE

Seborrhoeic or senile warts

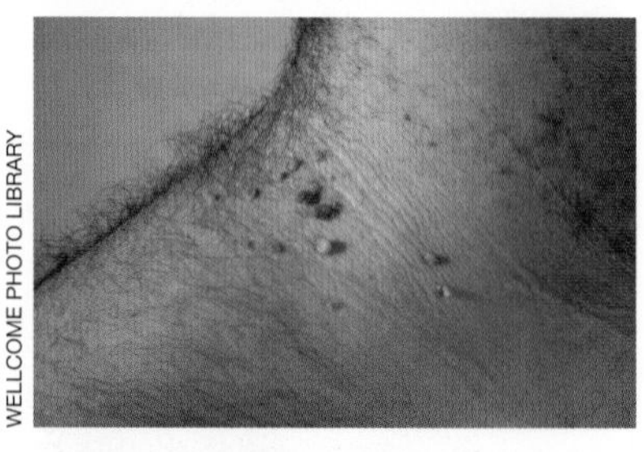

WELLCOME PHOTO LIBRARY

Verrucae filliformis or skin tags

Hairy naevi Moles exhibiting coarse hairs from their surface.

Infectious? No.

Appearance: Slightly raised moles, varying in size from 3cm to much larger. Colour ranges from fawn to dark brown.

Site: Anywhere on the skin.

Treatment: Hairy naevi may be surgically removed where possible and this is often done for cosmetic reasons. Hair growing from a mole should be cut, not plucked: if plucked, the hair will become coarser and the growth of further hairs may be stimulated.

Skin disorders involving abnormal growth

Psoriasis Patches of itchy, red, flaky skin, the cause of which is unknown.

Infectious? No. Secondary infection with bacteria can occur if the skin becomes broken and dirt enters the skin.

Appearance: Red patches of skin appear, covered in waxy, silvery scales. Bleeding will occur if the area is scratched and scales are removed.

Site: The elbows, the knees, the lower back and the scalp.

Treatment: There is no known treatment. Medication including steroid creams can bring relief to the symptoms.

Seborrhoeic or senile warts: Raised, pigmented, benign tumours occurring in middle age.

Infectious? No.

Appearance: Slightly raised, brown or black, rough patches of skin. Such warts can be confused with pigmented moles.

Site: The trunk, the scalp and the temples.

Treatment: Medical – the warts can be cauterized by a GP.

Verrucae filliformis or skin tags These verrucae appear as threads projecting from the skin.

Infectious? No.

Appearance: Skin-coloured threads of skin 3–6mm long.

Site: Mainly seen on the neck and the eyelids, but may occur in other areas such as under the arms.

Treatment: Medical – cauterization with diathermy, either by a GP or by a qualified electrologist.

Xanthomas Small yellow growths appearing upon the surface of the skin made up of cholesterol deposits.

Infectious? No.

Appearance: A yellow flat or raised area of skin with distinct edges.

Site: Common on the eyelids, but can appear anywhere on the body.

Treatment: Medical – the growth is thought to be connected with certain medical diseases, such as diabetes or high or low blood pressure. Sometimes a low-fat diet can correct the condition.

Keloids Keloids occur following skin injury and are overgrown abnormal scar tissue which spreads, characterized by excess deposits of collagen. To avoid skin discoloration the keloid must be protected from UV exposure.

Infectious? No.

Appearance: The skin tends to be red, raised, shiny and ridged.

Site: Located over the site of a wound or other lesion.

Treatment: Medical by drug therapy, such as cortisone injection, or surgery.

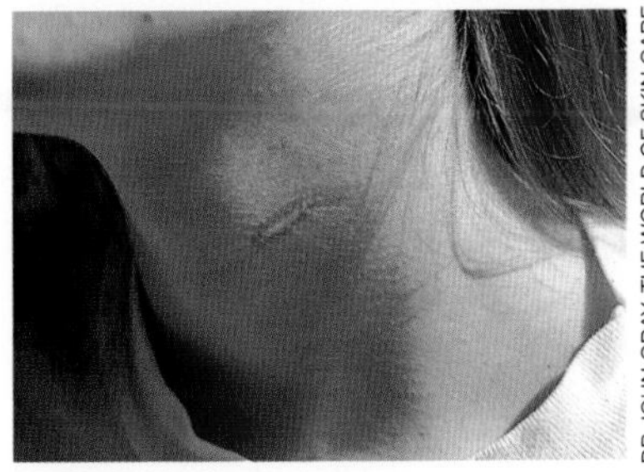
DR JOHN GRAY, THE WORLD OF SKIN CARE

Keloid

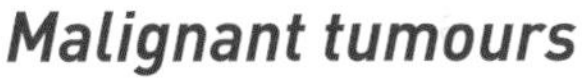

Malignant tumours

Squamous cell carcinomas or prickle-cell cancers Malignant growths originating in the epidermis.

Infectious? No.

Appearance: When fully formed, the carcinoma appears as a raised area of skin.

Site: Anywhere on the skin.

Treatment: Includes surgical removal also radiotherapy (treatment with x-ray) or treatment with drugs as necessary.

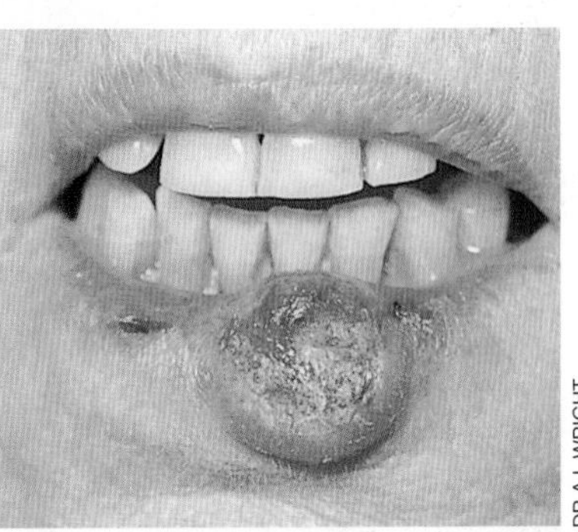
DR A L WRIGHT

Squamous cell carcinoma

Basal cell carcinomas or rodent ulcers Slow-growing malignant tumours, occurring in middle age.

Infectious? No.

Appearance: A small, shiny, waxy nodule with a depressed centre. The disease extends, with more nodules appearing on the border of the original ulcer.

Site: Usually on the face.

Treatment: Includes surgical removal also radiotherapy (treatment with x-ray) or treatment with drugs as necessary.

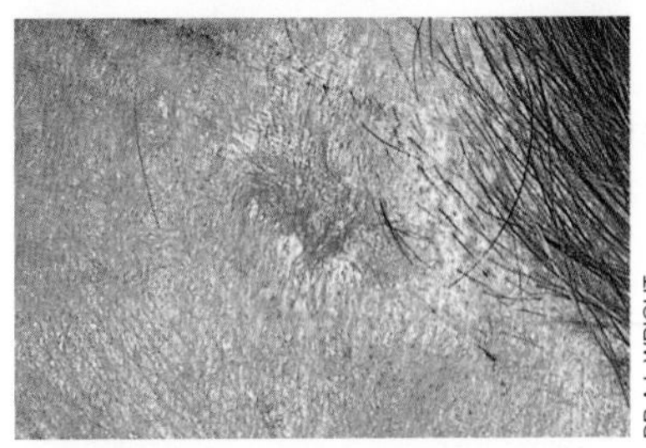
DR A L WRIGHT

Basal cell carcinomas

Skin allergies

The skin can protect itself to some degree from damage or invasion. **Mast cells** detect damage to the skin; if damage occurs, the mast cells burst, releasing the chemical **histamine** into the tissues. Histamine causes the blood capillaries to dilate, giving the reddening we call 'erythema'. The increased blood flow transports materials in blood which tend to limit the damage and begin repair.

If the skin is sensitive to and becomes inflamed on contact with a particular substance, this substance is called an **allergen**. Allergens may be animal, chemical or vegetable substances, and they can be inhaled, eaten or absorbed following contact with the skin. An **allergic skin reaction** appears as irritation, itching and discomfort, with reddening and swelling (as with nettle rash). If the allergen is removed, the allergic reaction subsides.

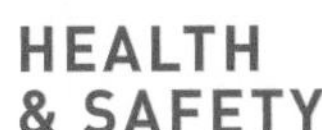

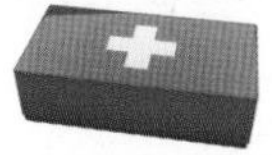

Record any known allergies
When completing the client record card, always ask whether your client has any known allergies.

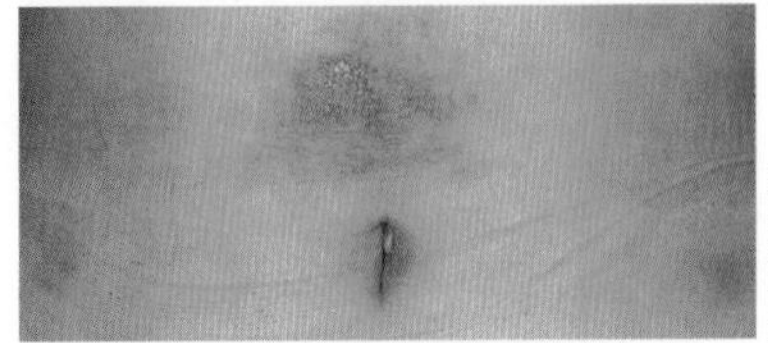
DR M H BECK

Allergic reaction to a nickel button

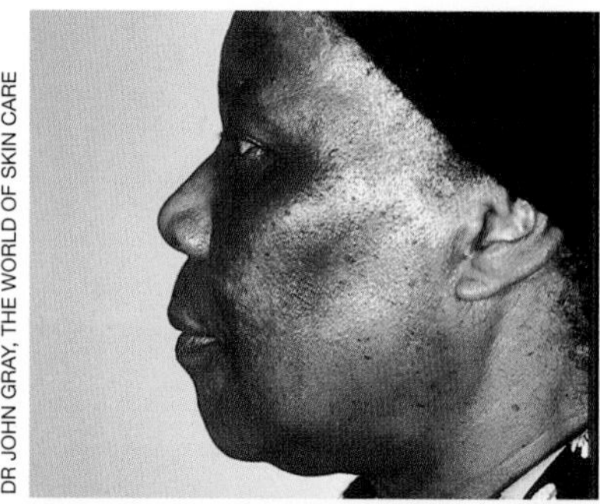
DR JOHN GRAY, THE WORLD OF SKIN CARE

Allergic reaction to an ingredient in hair dye

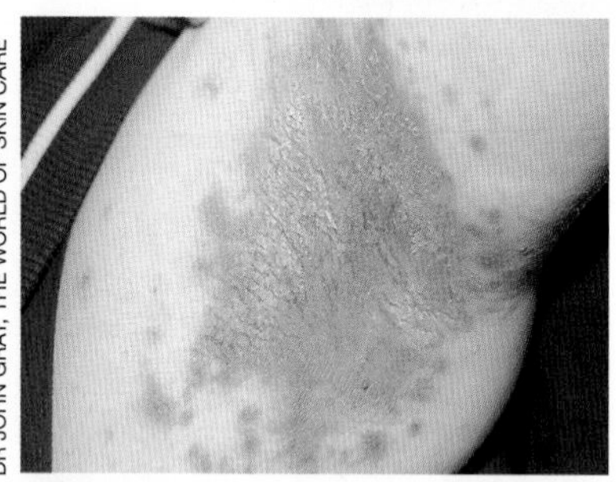
DR JOHN GRAY, THE WORLD OF SKIN CARE

Allergic reaction to an antiperspirant

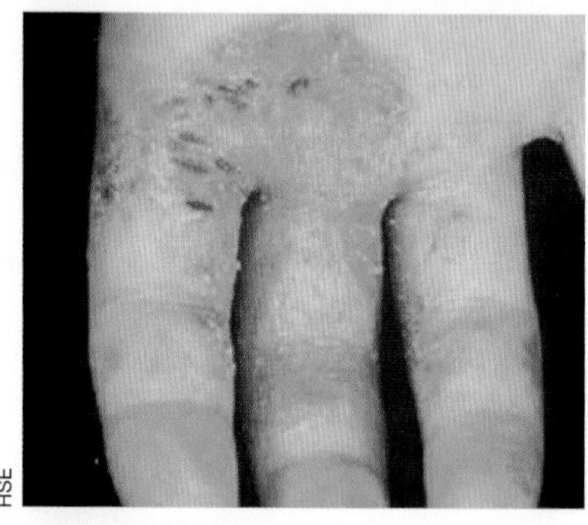
HSE

Contact dermatitis

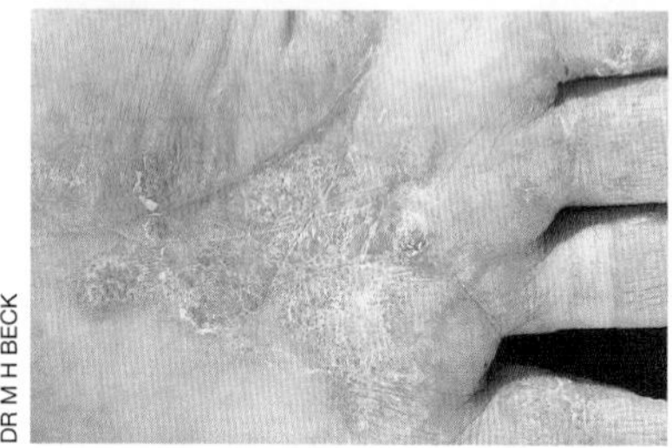
DR M H BECK

Dermatitis

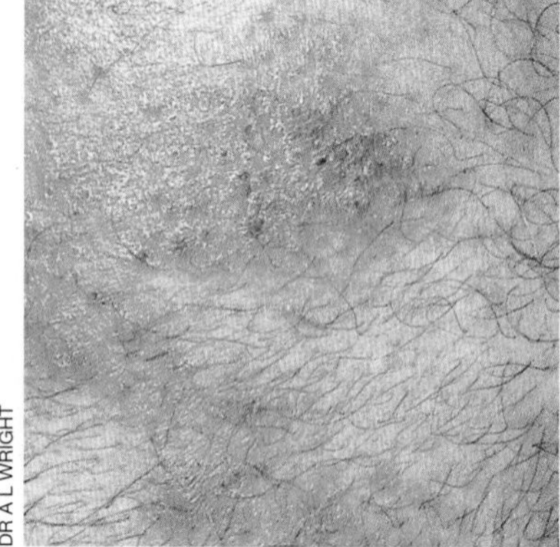
DR A L WRIGHT

Eczema

Each individual has different tolerances to the various substances we encounter in daily life. What causes an allergic reaction in one individual may be perfectly harmless to another.

Here are just a few examples of allergens known to cause allergic skin reactions in some people:

- metal objects containing nickel
- sticking plaster
- rubber
- lipstick containing eosin dye
- nail polish containing formaldehyde resin
- hair and eyelash dyes
- lanolin, the skin moisturizing agent
- detergents that dry the skin
- foods – well-known examples are peanuts, cow's milk, lobster, shellfish and strawberries
- plants such as tulips and chrysanthemums

Dermatitis An inflammatory skin disorder in which the skin become red, itchy and swollen. There are two types of dermatitis. In *primary dermatitis* the skin is irritated by the action of a substance on the skin, and this leads to skin inflammation. In *allergic contact dermatitis*, the problem is caused by intolerance of the skin to a particular substance or groups of substances. On exposure to the substance the skin quickly becomes irritated and an allergic reaction occurs.

Infectious? No.

Appearance: Reddening and swelling of the skin, with the possible appearance of blisters.

Site: If the skin reacts to a skin irritant outside the body, the reaction is localized. Repeated contact with the allergen will lead to a general hypersensitivity. If the irritant gains entry to the body it will be transported in the bloodstream and may cause a general allergic skin reaction.

Treatment: Moisturizing cream can be used to help prevent drying of the skin. Personal protective equipment should be worn in the case of occupational hazards, i.e. gloves should be worn by a hairdresser to avoid developing contact dermatitis due to the hazards in the nature of the work, like contact with water for long periods. When an allergic dermatitis reaction occurs, the only 'cure' is the absolute avoidance of the substance. Steroid creams such as hydrocortisone are usually prescribed, to soothe the damaged skin and reduce the irritation.

Eczema Inflammation of the skin caused by contact, internally or externally, with an irritant.

Infectious? No.

Appearance: Reddening of the skin, with swelling and blisters. The blisters leak tissue fluid which later hardens, forming scabs.

Site: The face, the neck and the skin, particularly at the inner creases of the elbows and behind the knees.

Treatment: Refer the client to their GP. Eczema may disappear if the source of irritation is identified and removed. Steroid cream may be prescribed by the GP and special diets may help.

Urticaria (nettle rash) or hives A minor skin disorder caused by contact with an allergen, either internally (food or drugs) or externally (insect bites).

Infectious? No.

Appearance: Erythema with raised round whitish skin wheals. In some cases the lesions can cause intense burning or itching, a condition known as pruritis. Pruritis is a symptom of a disease (such as diabetes), not a disease itself.

Site: At the point of contact.

Treatment: Antihistamines may be prescribed to reduce the itching. The visible skin reaction usually disappears quickly leaving no trace. Complete avoidance of the allergen 'cures' the problem.

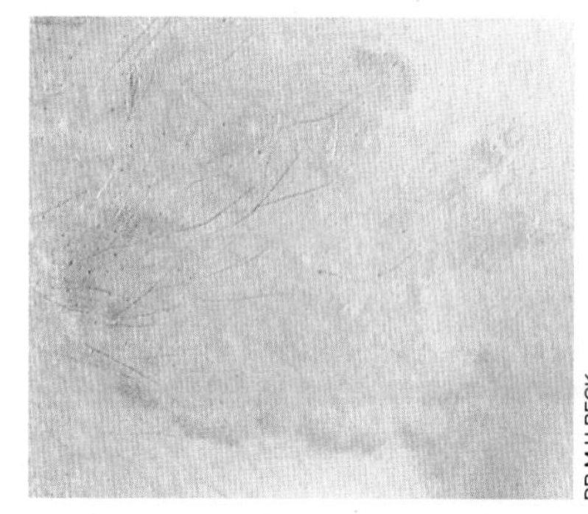

DR M H BECK

Urticaria (nettle rash) or hives

HEALTH & SAFETY

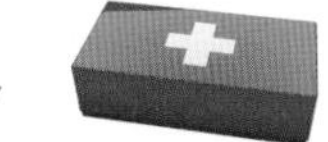

Hypoallergenic products
The use of hypoallergenic products minimizes the risk of skin contact with likely irritants.

Allergies
You may suddenly become allergic to a substance that has previously been perfectly harmless. Equally, you may over time cease to be allergic to something.

Infection following allergy
Following an allergic skin reaction in which the skin's surface has become itchy and broken, scratching may cause the skin to become infected with bacteria.

ALWAYS REMEMBER

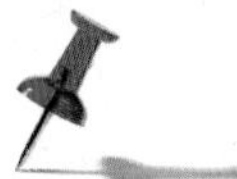

Cosmetic piercing
Skin piercing of the earlobe and cosmetic body piercing are classified in the single term cosmetic piercing.

The ears

The structure and function of the earlobe

The external ear collects sound waves and directs these to the inner ear. The part of the ear that is commonly seen pierced is called the **pinna**, which comprises the **helix** and **lobule**. The helix is composed of cartilage, which does not heal quickly, can be painful and can form lumpy scar tissue; it is therefore considered unsuitable for piercing. The lobule, in contrast, consists of fibrous and fatty tissue with no cartilage, and is therefore suitable for piercing.

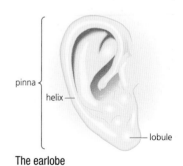

The earlobe

The hair

The structure and function of hair and the surrounding tissues

A hair is a long, slender structure which grows out of, and is part of, the skin. Each hair is made up of dead skin cells, which contain the protein called keratin. Hairs cover the whole body, except for the palms of the hands, the soles of the feet, the lips, and parts of the sex organs.

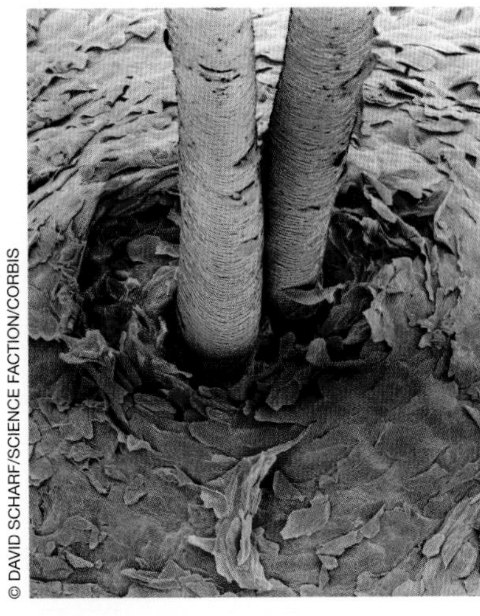

Hair extending from the scalp

Hair has many functions:

- *scalp hair* insulates the head against cold, protects it from the sun, and cushions it against bumps
- *eyebrows* cushion the brow bone from bumps, and prevent sweat from running into the eyes
- *eyelashes* help to prevent foreign particles entering the eyes
- *nostril hair* traps dust particles inhaled with the air
- *ear hair* helps to protect the ear canal. Hair cells in the inner ear send signals to the brain when the head moves, this information is used to help the body maintain balance.
- *body hair* helps to provide an insulating cover (though this function is almost obsolete in humans), has a valuable sensory function, and is linked with the secretion of sebum onto the surface of the skin.

Hair also plays a role in social communication.

TOP TIP

Did you know?
There are approximately 100,000 hairs on the scalp.

TOP TIP

Did you know?
A strand of hair is stronger than an equivalent strand of nylon or copper.

The structure of hair Most **hairs** are made up of three layers of different types of epithelial cells: the *medulla*, the *cortex* and the *cuticle*.

The **medulla** is the central core of the hair. The cells of the medulla contain soft keratin, and sometimes some pigment granules. The medulla only exists in medium to coarser hair – there is usually no medulla in thinner hair.

The **cortex** is the thickest layer of the hair, and is made up of several layers of closely packed, elongated cells. These contain pigment granules and hard keratin.

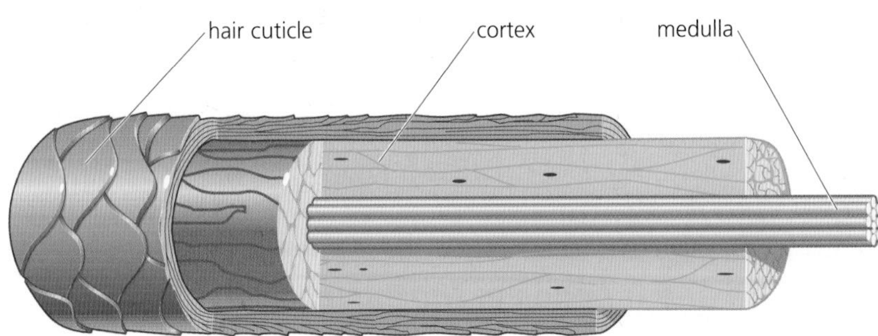

Cross-section of the hair

It is the **pigment** in the cortex that gives hair its colour. When this pigment is no longer made, the hair appears white. As the proportion of white hairs rises, the hair seems to go 'grey'; in fact, however, each individual hair is either coloured as before, or white.

The **cuticle** is the protective outer layer of the hair, and is composed of a layer of thin, unpigmented, flat, scale-like cells. These contain hard keratin, and overlap each other from the base to the tip of the hair.

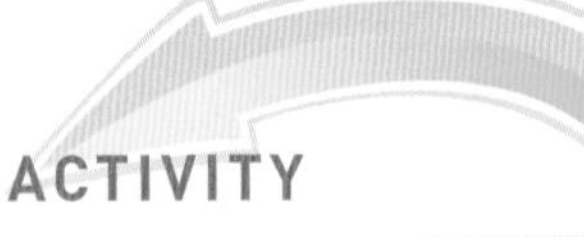

ACTIVITY

The function of hair
Humans are not very hairy but their hairs sometimes stand on end! How does the appearance of skin change? What is the purpose of hair standing on end?

The parts of the hair and related skin Each **hair** is recognized by three parts: the **root**, the **bulb** and the **shaft**:

- the **root** is the part of the hair that is in the follicle
- the **bulb** is the enlarged base of the root
- the **shaft** is the part of the hair that can be seen above the skin's surface

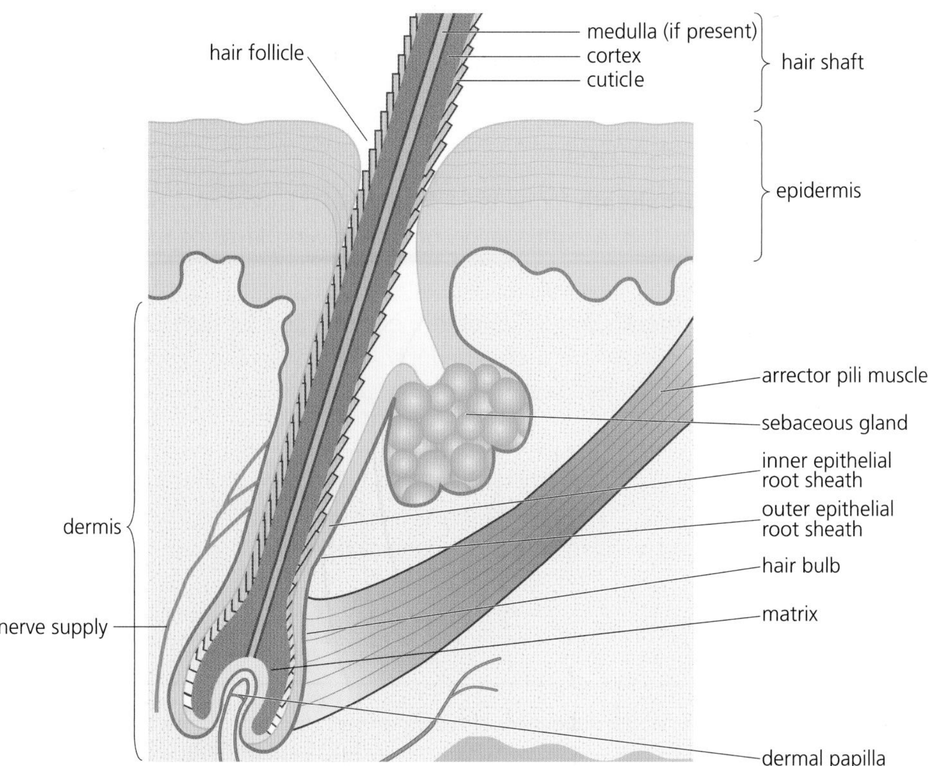

Cross-section of the skin and hair follicle

TOP TIP

Eyelash perm lotion and the eyelash/eyebrow tint mixed with hydrogen peroxide swell and penetrate the cuticle so that the products can enter the cortex. The coarser the hair the more resistant it is! Eyelash and eyebrow tints and perming make the permanent chemical changes to the hair's natural appearance in the cortex.

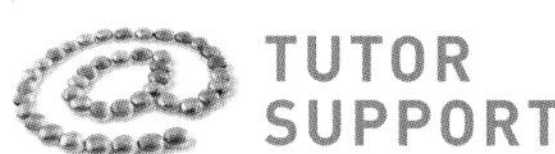

Activity 4: Label the hair follicle

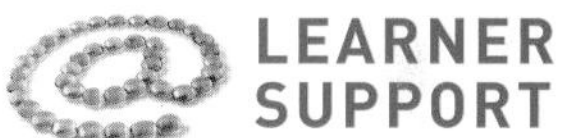

Label the hair follicle

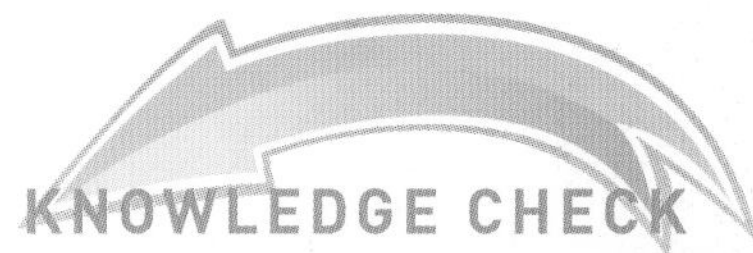

Name the three layers that make up the hair shaft structure.

Need more time... refer to page 54 to help you.

Each hair grows out of a tube-like indentation in the epidermis, the **hair follicle**. The walls of the follicle are a continuation of the epidermal layer of the skin.

The **arrector pili muscle** is attached at an angle to the base of the follicle. Cold, aggression or fright stimulates this muscle to contract, pulling the follicle and the hair upright.

The **sebaceous gland** is attached to the upper part of the follicle; from it, a duct enters directly into the hair follicle. The gland produces an oily substance, **sebum**, which is secreted into the follicle. Sebum waterproofs, lubricates and softens the hair and the surface of the skin; it also protects the skin against bacterial and fungal infections. The contraction of the arrector pili muscle aids the secretion of sebum.

The **dermal papilla**, a connective tissue sheath, is surrounded by the hair bulb. It provides an excellent blood supply, necessary for the growth of the hair. It is not itself part of the follicle, but a separate tiny organ which transports blood to the follicle.

The **bulb** is the expanded base of the hair root. A gap at the base leads to a cavity inside, which houses the papilla. The bulb contains in its lower part the dividing cells that create the hair. The hair continues to develop as it passes through the regions of the upper bulb and the root.

The **matrix** is the name given to the lower part of the bulb, which comprises actively dividing cells from which the hair is formed.

The hair follicle The **hair follicle** extends into the dermis, and is made up of three sheaths: the *inner epithelial root sheath*, the *outer epithelial root sheath* and the surrounding *connective-tissue sheath.*

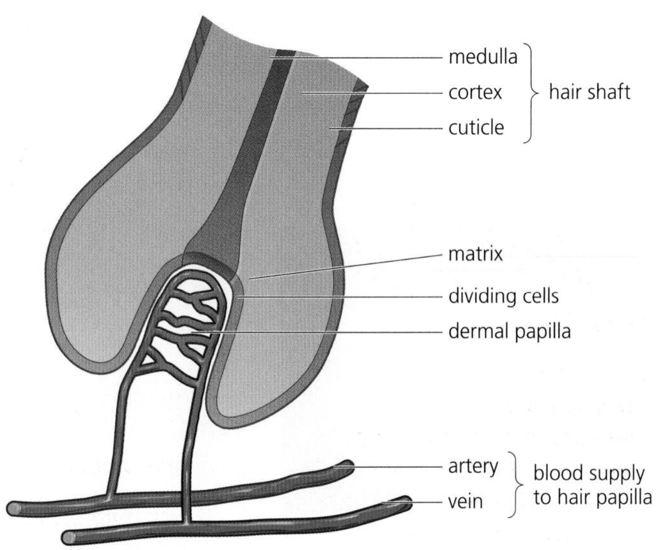

The hair bulb

TOP TIP

Broken hairs

When hairs break off due to incorrect waxing technique, they will break at the level at which they are locked into the follicle by the cells of the inner root sheath.

The **inner epithelial root sheath** grows from the bottom of the follicle at the papilla; both the hair and the inner root sheath grow upwards together. The inner surface of this sheath is covered with cuticle cells, in the same way as the outer surface of the hair: these cells lock together, anchoring the hair firmly in place. The inner root sheath ceases to grow when level with the sebaceous gland.

The **outer epithelial root sheath** forms the follicle wall. This does not grow up with the hair, but is stationary. It is a continuation of the growing layer of the epidermis of the skin.

The **connective-tissue sheath** surrounds both the follicle and the sebaceous gland, providing both a sensory supply and a blood supply. The connective-tissue sheath includes, and is a continuation of, the papilla.

The *shape* of the hairs is determined by the shape of the hair follicle – an angled or bent follicle will produce an oval or flat hair, whereas a straight follicle will produce a round hair. Flat hairs are curly, oval hairs are wavy, and round hairs are straight. As a general rule, during waxing curly hairs break off more easily than straight hairs.

TOP TIP

An angled follicle may cause the hair to be broken off at the angle during waxing, instead of being completely pulled out with its root. If this happens, broken hairs will appear at the skin's surface within a few days.

By causing damage to the follicle and changing its shape, waxing can cause the regrowth of hairs to be frizzy or curled where previously the hairs have been straight.

Curly	Wavy	Straight
Flat ribbon-like	Oval	Round

Hair shapes

The nerve supply The number, size and type of nerve endings associated with hair follicles is related to the size and type of follicle. The follicles of vellus hairs (see page 57) have the fewest nerve endings; those of terminal hairs have the most.

The nerve endings surrounding hair follicles respond mainly to rapid movements when the hair is moved. Nerve endings that respond to touch can also be found around the surface openings of some hair follicles, as well as just below the epidermis.

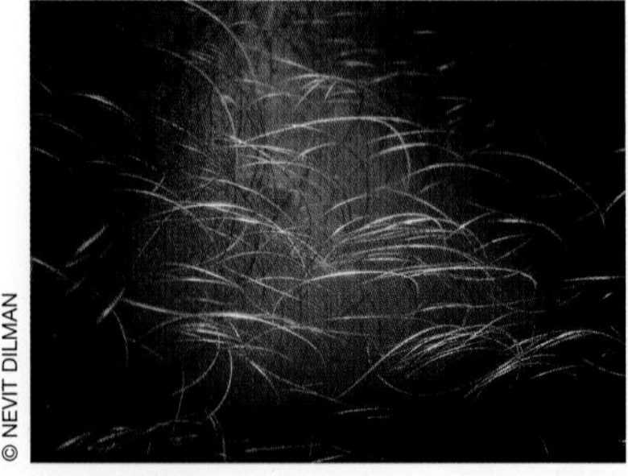

lanugo hairs

The three types of hair

There are three main types of hair: *lanugo*, *vellus* and *terminal*.

Lanugo hairs are found on the body prior to birth. They are fine and soft, do not have a medulla, and are often unpigmented. They grow from around the third to the fifth month of pregnancy, and are shed to be replaced by the secondary vellus hairs around the seventh to the eighth month of pregnancy. Lanugo hairs on the scalp, eyebrows and eyelashes are replaced by terminal hairs.

Vellus hairs are fine, downy and soft, and are found on the face and body. They are often unpigmented, rarely longer than 20mm, and do not have a medulla or a well-formed bulb. The base of these hairs is very close to the skin's surface. If stimulated, the shallow follicle of a vellus hair can grow downwards and become a follicle that produces terminal hairs.

Terminal hairs are longer and coarser than vellus hairs, and most are pigmented. They vary greatly in shape, in diameter and length, and in colour and texture. The follicles from which they grow are set deeply in the dermis and have well-defined bulbs. Terminal hair is the coarse hair of the scalp, eyebrows, eyelashes, pubic and underarm regions. It is also present on the face, chest and sometimes the back of males.

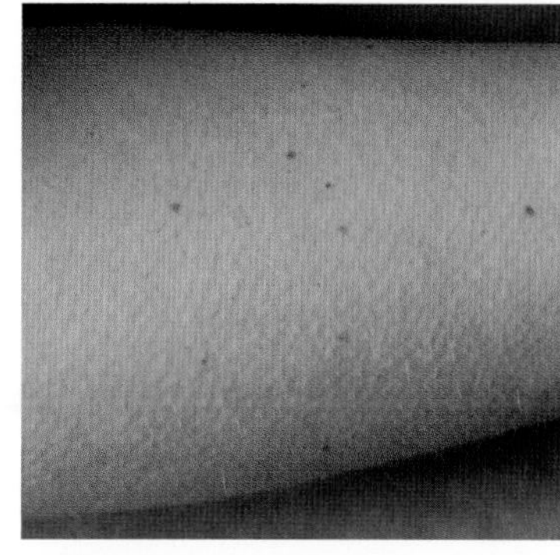

Vellus hairs

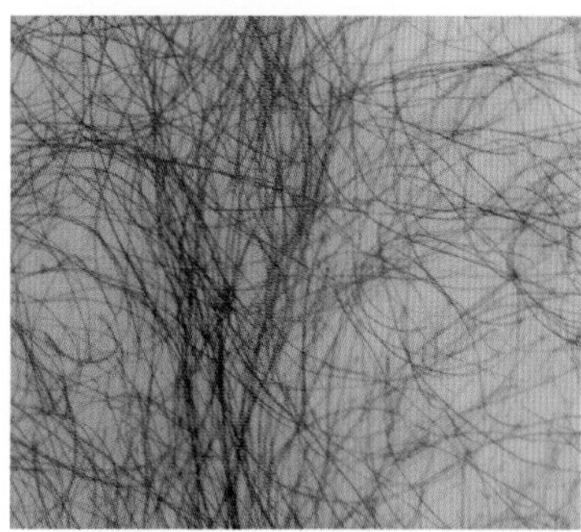

Terminal hairs

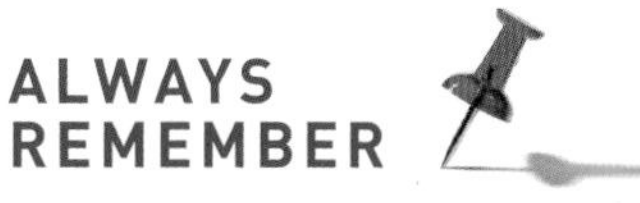

Waxing terminal hair

Some areas of the body – for example, the bikini line and underarm areas – often have terminal hairs with very deep follicles. When these hairs are removed, the resulting tissue damage may cause minor bleeding from the entrance of the follicle. Removal of these deep-seated hairs is obviously more uncomfortable than the removal of shallower, finer hairs.

Hair growth

All hair has a **cyclical pattern of growth**, which can be divided into three phases: *anagen, catagen and telogen.*

Anagen is the actively growing stage of the hair – the follicle has re-formed; the hair bulb is developing, surrounding the life-giving dermal papilla; and a new hair forms, growing from the matrix in the bulb.

Catagen is the changing stage when the hair separates from the papilla. Over a few days it is carried by the movement of the inner root sheath, up the follicle to the base of the sebaceous gland. Here it stays until it either falls out or is pushed out by a new hair growing up behind it.

This stage can be very rapid, with a new hair growing straight away; or slower, with the papilla and the follicle below the sebaceous gland degenerating and entering a resting stage, telogen.

Telogen is a resting stage. Many hair follicles do not undergo this stage, but start to produce a new hair immediately. During resting phases, hairs may still be loosely inserted in the shallow follicles.

TOP TIP

Vellus hairs

Vellus hairs grow slowly and take two to three months to return after waxing. They can remain dormant in the follicle for six to eight months before shedding.

TOP TIP

A hair pulled out at the anagen stage will be surrounded by the inner root sheath and have a properly formed bulb.

TOP TIP

Because of the cyclical nature of hair growth, the follicles are always at different stages of their growth cycle. When the hair is removed, therefore, the hair will not all grow back at the same time. For this reason, waxing or threading can appear to reduce the quantity of hair growth. This is not so; given time, all the hair will regrow. Waxing and threading are classed as a temporary means of hair removal.

TOP TIP

A hair pulled out at the catagen or telogen stage can be recognized by the brush-like appearance of the root.

Name the basic hair types and say where they can be found.

Need more time... refer to pages 56–57 to help you.

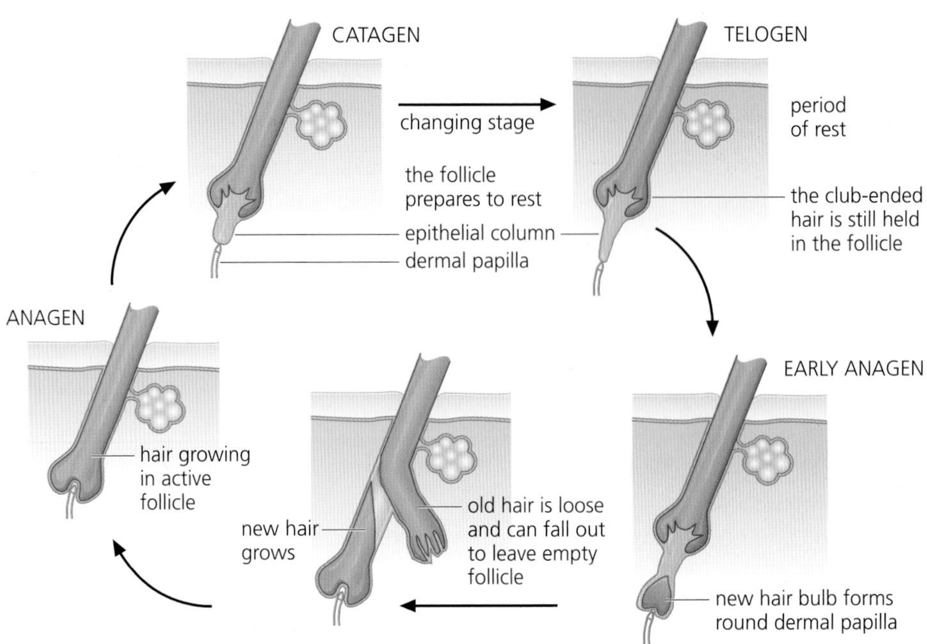

The hair growth cycle

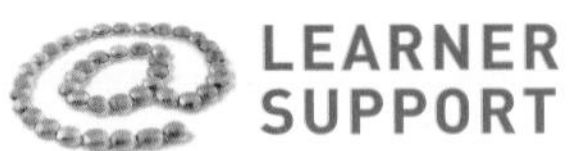

Skin and hair true or false

TOP TIP

Male facial hair grows at a rate of approximately 10mm a month.

Speed of growth The anagen, catagen and telogen stages last for different lengths of time in different hair types and in different parts of the body:

- *scalp hair* grows for two to seven years, and has a resting stage of three to four months
- *eyebrow hair* grows for one to two months, and has a resting stage of three to four months
- *eyelashes* grow for three to six weeks, and have a resting stage of three to four months.

After a waxing service, body hair will take approximately six to eight weeks to return.

Because hair growth cycles are not all in synchronization, we always have hair present at any given time. On the scalp, at any one time for example, 85 per cent of hairs may be in the anagen phase. This is why hair growth after waxing starts within a few days: what is seen is the appearance of hairs that were already developing in the follicle at the time of waxing.

Types of hair growth **Hirsutism** is a term used to describe a pattern of hair growth that is abnormal for that person's sex, such as when a woman's hair growth follows a man's hair-growth pattern. The hair growth is usually terminal when it should be of a vellus type.

Hypertrichosis is an abnormal growth of excess hair for a person's sex, age and race. It is usually due to abnormal conditions brought about by disease or injury.

Superfluous hair (excess hair) is perfectly normal at certain periods in a woman's life, such as during puberty or pregnancy. Terminal hairs formed at these times usually disappear once the normal hormonal balance has returned. Those newly formed during the menopause are often permanent unless treated with a permanent method of hair removal, such as electrical epilation or laser treatment.

ALWAYS REMEMBER

Alopecia
This is often caused by a nervous disorder and is where there are round patches of smooth scalp as the hair follicles are not producing new hairs.

Factors affecting the growth rate and quantity of hair Hair does not always grow uniformly:

- *Time of day* – Hair grows faster at night than during the day.
- *Weather* – Hairs grow faster in warm weather than in cold.
- *Pregnancy* – In women, hairs grow faster and during mid-pregnancy.
- *Age* – Hairs grow faster between the ages of 16 and 24. The rate of hair growth slows down with age. In women, however, facial hair growth continues to increase in old age, while trunk and limb hair increases into middle age and then decreases.
- *Colour* – Hairs of different colour grow at different speeds – for example, coarse black hair grows more quickly than fine blonde hair.
- *Part of the body* – Hair in different areas of the body grows at different rates, as do different types and thicknesses of hair. The weekly growth rate varies from approximately 1.5mm (fine hair) to 2.8mm (coarse hair), when actively growing.
- *Heredity* – Members of a family may have inherited growth patterns, such as excess hair that starts to grow at puberty and increases until the age of 20–25.
- *Health and diet* – Health and a varied, balanced diet are crucial in the rate of hair growth and appearance.
- *Stress* – Emotional stress can cause a temporary hormonal imbalance within the body, which may lead to a temporary growth of excess hair.
- *Medical conditions* – A sudden unexplained increase of body hair growth may indicate a more serious medical problem, such as malfunction of the ovaries, or result from the taking of certain drugs, such as corticosteroids and certain birth control and high blood pressure medications.

The quantity as well as the type of hair present may vary with race:

- *People of Latin extraction* tend to possess heavier body, facial and scalp hair, which is relatively coarse and straight.
- *People of East Asian extraction* tend to possess very little or no body and facial hair growth, and usually their scalp hair growth is relatively coarse and straight. This gives the appearance of greater hair density by they actually have a lower hair density than Caucasian and Latin African-Caribbean people.
- *People of Northern European and Caucasian extraction* tend to have light to medium body and facial hair growth, with their scalp hair growth being wavy, loosely curled or straight.
- *People of African-Caribbean extraction* tend to have little body and facial hair growth, but usually their scalp hair growth is relatively coarse and tightly curled.

HEALTH & SAFETY 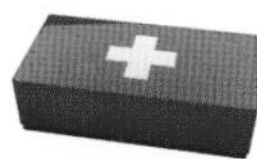

African-Caribbean clients
The body hair of African-Caribbean clients is prone to breaking during waxing, and to ingrowing after waxing. Skin damage can result in the loss of pigmentation (hypopigmentation).

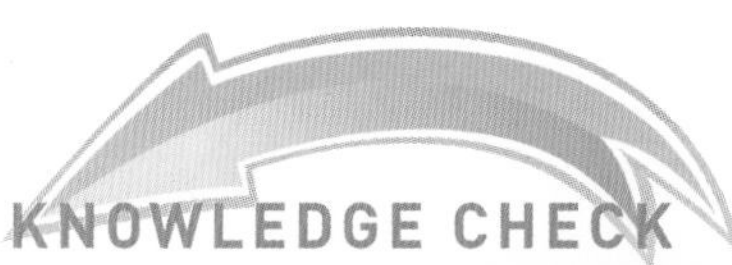

KNOWLEDGE CHECK

What are the different stages of the hair growth cycle called? What happens to the hair at each stage?

Need more time... refer to pages 57–58 to help you.

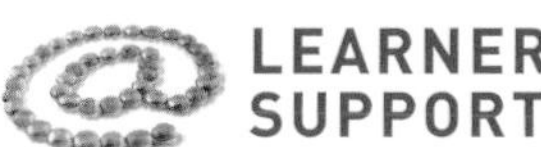

LEARNER SUPPORT

Nails true or false

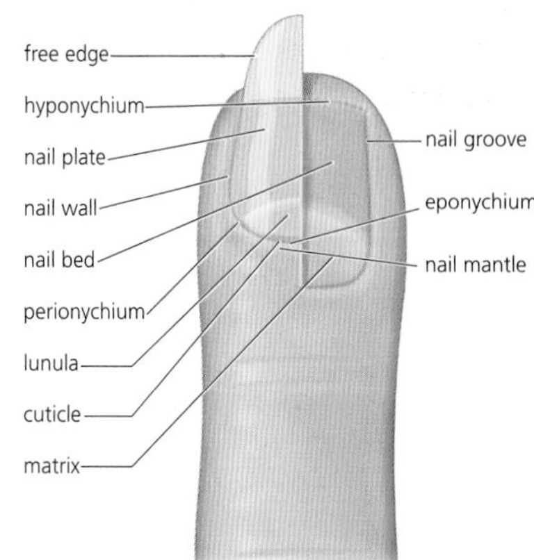

The structure of the nail

The nails

The structure and function of the nail

Nails grow from the ends of the fingers and toes and serve as a form of protection. They also help when picking up small objects. The different components of the nails and surrounding tissues are discussed below.

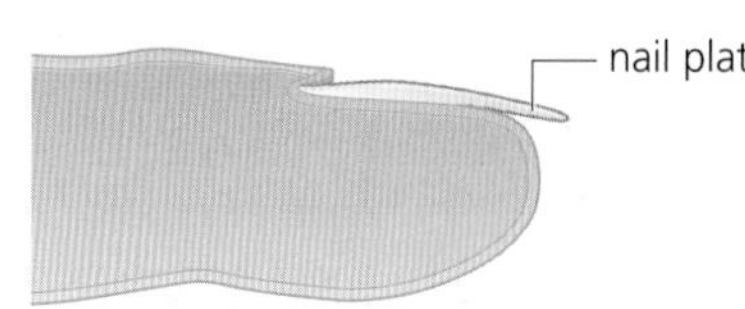

The nail plate

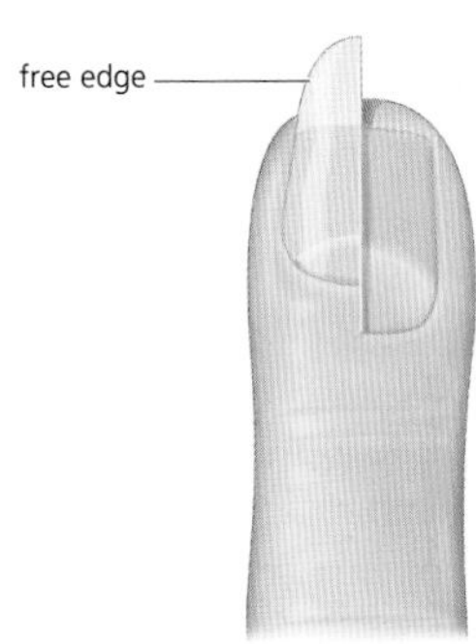

The free edge

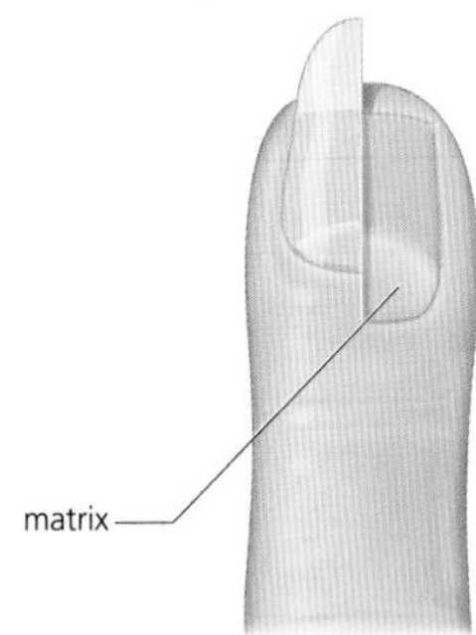

The matrix

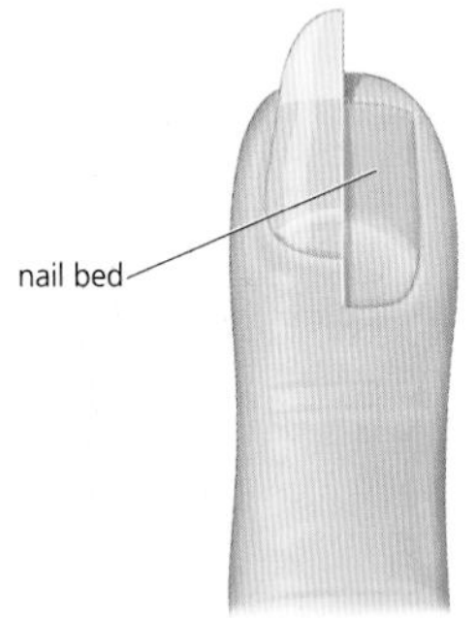

The nail bed

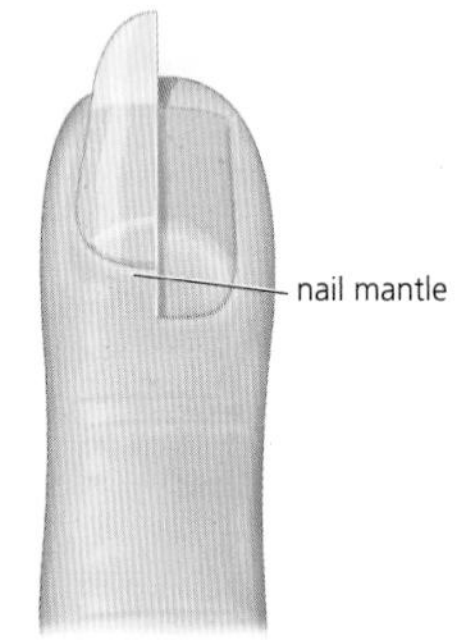

The nail mantle

The nail plate The **nail plate** is composed of compact translucent layers of keratinized epidermal cells: it is this that makes up the main body of the nail. The layers of cells are packed very closely together, with fat but very little moisture.

The nail gradually grows forward over the nail bed, until finally it becomes the free edge. The underside of the nail plate is grooved by longitudinal ridges and furrows, which help to keep it in place.

In normal health the plate curves in two directions:

- **transversely** – from side to side across the nail
- **longitudinally** – from the base of the nail to the free edge

There are no blood vessels or nerves in the nail plate: this is why the nails, like hair, can be cut without pain or bleeding. The pink colour of the nail plate derives from the blood vessels that pass beneath it – the nail bed.

Function: To protect the living nail bed of the fingers and toes.

The free edge The **free edge** is the part of the nail that extends beyond the fingertip; this is the part that is filed. It appears white as there is no nail bed underneath.

Function: To protect the tip of the fingers and toes and the hyponychium (see page 61). The free edge when filed can be shaped into a variety of shapes; find out what these are by turning to page 377.

The matrix The **matrix**, sometimes called the nail root, is the growing area of the nail. It is formed by the division of cells in this area, called mitosis, and is part of the stratum germinativum layer of the epidermis. It lies under the eponychium (see page 61), at the base of the nail. The process of keratinization takes place in the epidermal cells of the matrix, forming the hardened tissue of the nail plate.

Function: To produce new nail cells.

The nail bed The **nail bed** is the portion of skin upon which the nail plate rests. It has a pattern of grooves and furrows corresponding to those found on the underside of the nail plate; these interlock, keeping the nail in place, but separate at the end of the nail to form the free edge. The nail bed is liberally supplied with blood vessels, which provide the nourishment necessary for continued growth; and sensory nerves, for protection.

Function: To supply nourishment and protection.

The nail mantle The **nail mantle** is the layer of epidermis at the base of the nail above the matrix, before the cuticle. It appears as a deep fold of skin.

Function: To protect the matrix from physical damage.

The lunula The crescent-shaped **lunula** is located at the base of the nail. These cells gradually harden through keratinization. It is white, relative to the rest of the nail, and there are two theories to account for this:

- newly formed nail plates may be more opaque than mature nail plates
- the lunula may indicate the extent of the underlying matrix – the matrix is thicker than the epidermis of the nail bed, and the capillaries beneath it would not show through as well.

Function: None.

ALWAYS REMEMBER

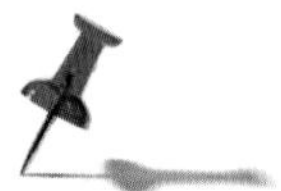

If the nail bed is pink this means the blood circulation to the nail bed is good. Poor health disorders such as respiratory illness and anaemia can affect the appearance of the nail colour called 'blue nail'.

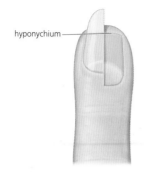

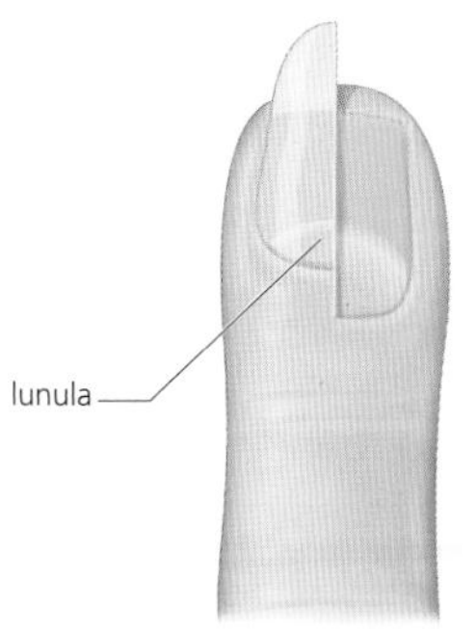

Lunula

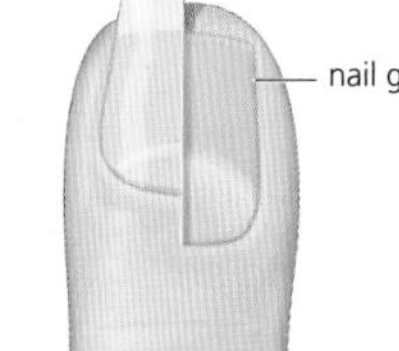

Hyponychium

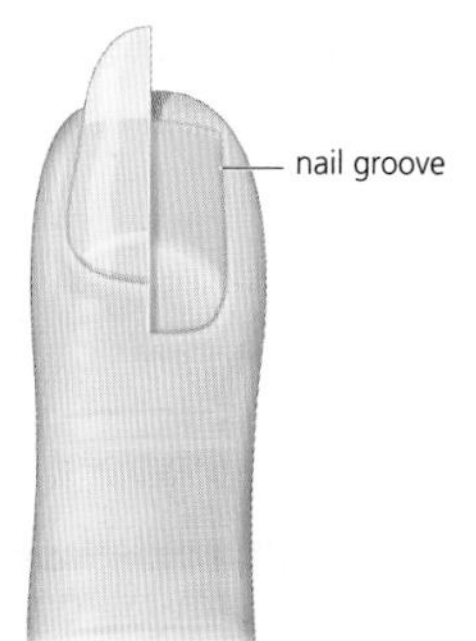

Nail grooves

TOP TIP

Did you know?
Fingernails grow more quickly than toenails. Fingernails grow about 0.1mm each day, 3–4mm per month (4cm per year), and grow faster in summer than in winter.

The hyponychium The **hyponychium** is part of the epidermis under the free edge of the nail.

Function: To protect the nail bed from infection by preventing dirt and bacteria gathering underneath the nail plate by forming a waterproof barrier.

The nail grooves The **nail grooves** run alongside the edge of the nail plate.

Function: To guide the body of the nail plate as it grows forward over the nail bed.

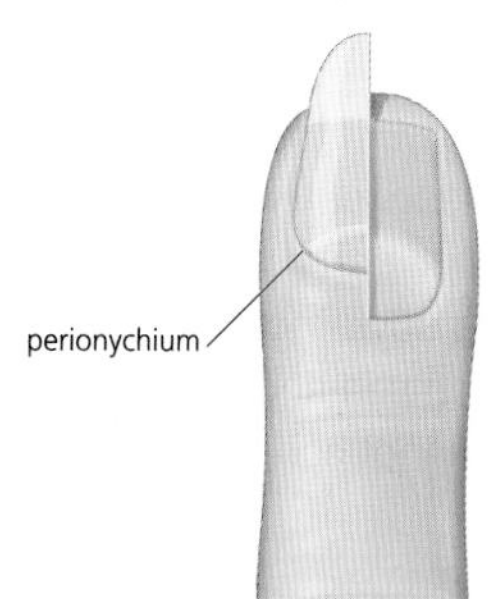

Perionychium

The perionychium The **perionychium** is the collective name given to the cuticle at the sides of the nail.

Function: To protect the nail bed from infection by preventing dirt and bacteria getting underneath the nail plate by forming a waterproof barrier.

The nail walls The **nail walls** are the folds of skin overlapping the sides of the nails.

Function: To cushion and protect the nail plate and grooves from damage.

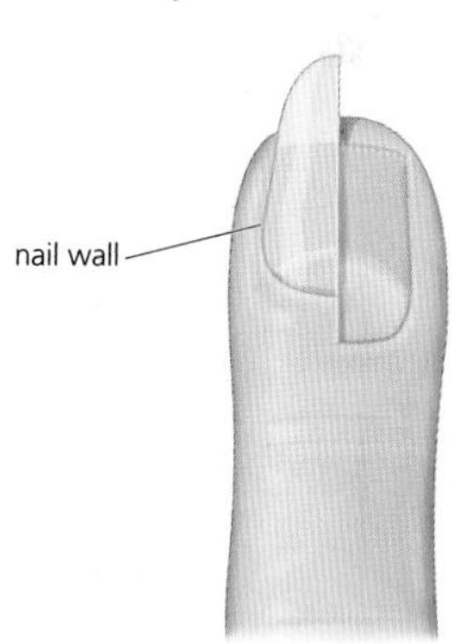

Nail wall

The eponychium The **eponychium** is the extension of the cuticle at the base of the nail plate, under which the nail plate emerges from the matrix.

Function: To protect the matrix from infection by preventing dirt and bacteria getting underneath the nail plate by forming a waterproof barrier.

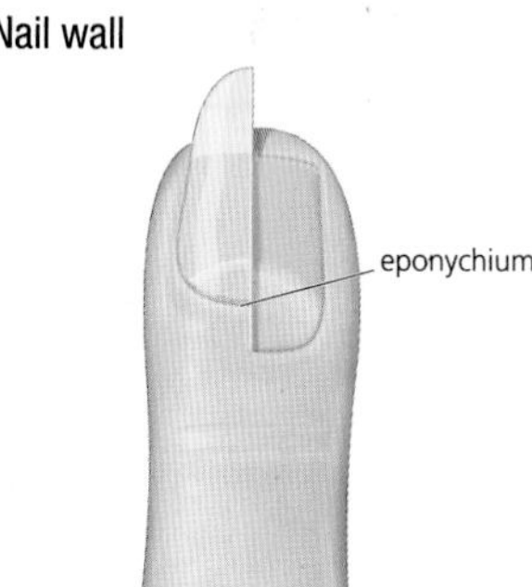

Eponychium

The cuticle The **cuticle** is the overlapping epidermis around and extending onto the base of the nail, developing from the stratum corneum. When in good condition, it is soft and loose.

Function: To protect the matrix and nail bed from infection by preventing dirt and bacteria getting underneath the nail plate by forming a waterproof barrier.

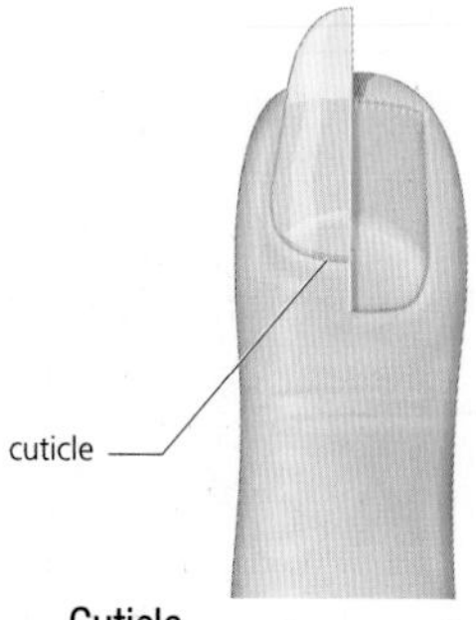

Cuticle

Nail growth

When **nail growth** occurs the cells divide in the matrix and the nail grows forward over the nail bed, guided by the nail grooves, until it reaches the end of the finger or toe, where it becomes the free edge. As they first emerge from the matrix the translucent cells are plump and soft, but they get harder and flatter as they move toward the free edge. The top two layers of the epidermis form the nail plate; the remaining three form the nail bed.

The nails' cells die in a process called keratinization where the cells become filled with a protein called keratin.

KNOWLEDGE CHECK

What are the functions of the nails?

Need more time... refer to pages 59–61 to help you.

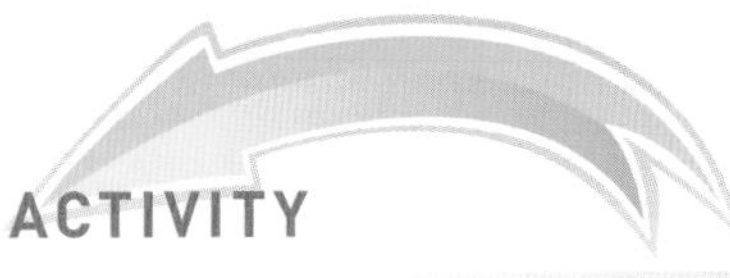

ACTIVITY

Recognizing nail structure
With a colleague, try to identify the structural parts of each other's nails. Write down both the parts that you can see and the parts that you cannot see.

The nail bed has a pattern of grooves and furrows corresponding to those found on the underside of the nail plate: the two surfaces interlock, holding the nail in place.

Fingernails grow at approximately twice the speed of toenails. It takes about six months for a fingernail to grow from cuticle to free edge, but about 12 months for a toenail to do so.

The beauty therapist must be able to distinguish a healthy nail and surrounding skin from one suffering from a nail/skin disease or disorder. Certain nail/skin diseases and disorders prevent treatment: proceeding would expose the beauty therapist and other clients to the risk of cross-infection through contact. It is therefore vital that you are familiar with the nail/skin diseases and disorders with which you might come into contact in the workplace and those that are a risk and those that are not and the correct action to take. Related nail/skin diseases and disorders are discussed in each treatment Chapter 11 Manicure Treatments and Chapter 12 Pedicure Treatments.

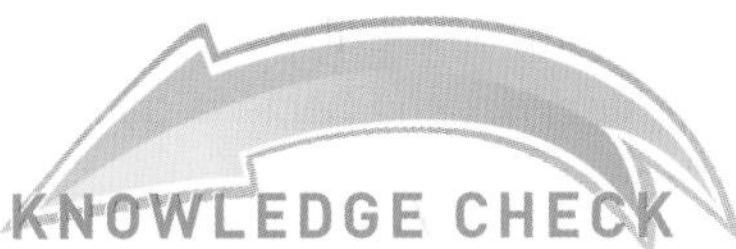

KNOWLEDGE CHECK

In what part of the nail structure do the cells divide to form the nail?

As they nail cells grow forward they harden; what is this process called?

How long does it take the finger nails and toe nails to grow from cuticle to free edge?

Need more time... refer to page 61 to help you.

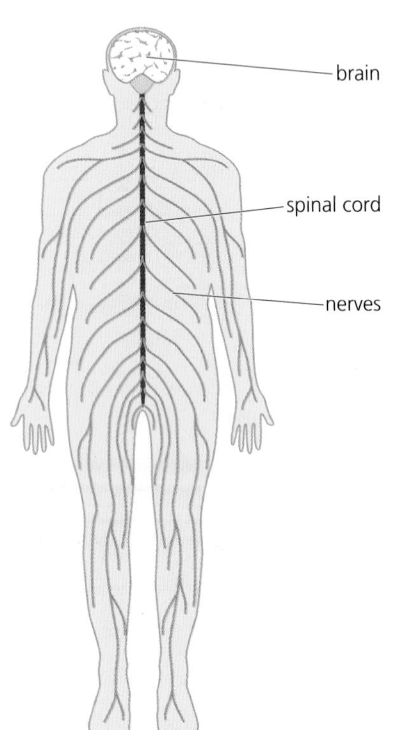

Central nervous system

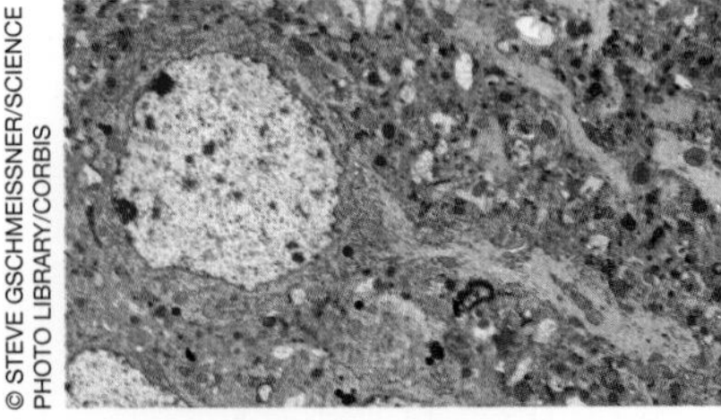

A nerve cell

The nervous system

The **nervous system** transmits messages between the brain and other parts of the body and is vast and complex. It controls everything that the body does with another body system, the endocrine system. The nervous system is made up of a network of nerve cells, called neurones. They transmit messages to and from the central nervous system (CNS) in the form of impulses. The nervous system of the body has two main divisions:

1. The central nervous system.
2. The autonomic nervous system.

The central nervous system

The central nervous system (CNS) is composed of the brain and spinal cord. The CNS co-ordinates the activities of the entire body.

The brain transmits impulses to all parts of the body in order to stimulate other organs to act and is protected by the bones of the cranium. The spinal cord runs along inside the vertebral column and is protected by the bones (vertebrae) of the spinal column. The brain is composed of several parts, each of which performs special functions.

Nerves

A nerve is a whitish bundle of fibres made up of neurones (nerve cells) that transmits impulses of sensations between the brain or spinal cord and other parts of the body. Nerve cells are long, narrow and delicate. They are made up of a cell body containing a large central nucleus and nerve fibres that transmit messages to other neurones.

Kinds of nerves There are two types of nerve: *sensory nerves* and *motor nerves*. Both are composed of white fibres enclosed in a sheath.

- **Sensory or afferent nerves** These receive information from receptors in the sense organs and relay it to the brain and spinal cord. They are found near to the skin's surface and respond to touch, pressure, temperature and pain.
- **Motor or efferent nerves** These are situated in muscle tissue and act on information received from the brain or spinal cord to a muscle or gland, causing a particular response, typically muscle movement.

All nerves emerge from the CNS. Sensory (receptor) nerves are linked to sensory receptors, while motor (effector) nerves end in a muscle or gland. Twelve pairs of cranial nerves emerge from the brain; 31 pairs of spinal nerves emerge from between the vertebrae of the spinal column.

HEALTH & SAFETY

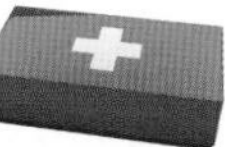

Nerve damage
Nerve cells do not reproduce; when damaged, only a limited repair occurs.

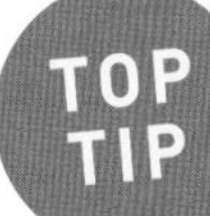

TOP TIP

Massage
Appropriate massage manipulations, when applied to the skin, produce a stimulating or relaxing effect on nerves.

Nerves of the face and neck These nerves link the brain with the muscles of the head, face and neck.

Cranial nerves control muscles in the head and neck region, or carry nerve impulses from sense organs to the brain. Those of concern to the beauty therapist when performing a facial treatment are as follows:

- the 5th cranial nerve, or **trigeminal** controls the muscles involved in mastication (chewing) and passes on sensory information from the face such as the eyes
- the 7th cranial nerve, or **facial** controls the muscles involved in facial expression
- the 11th cranial nerve, or **accessory** controls muscles involved in moving the head, the sternocleidomastoid and trapezius muscle.

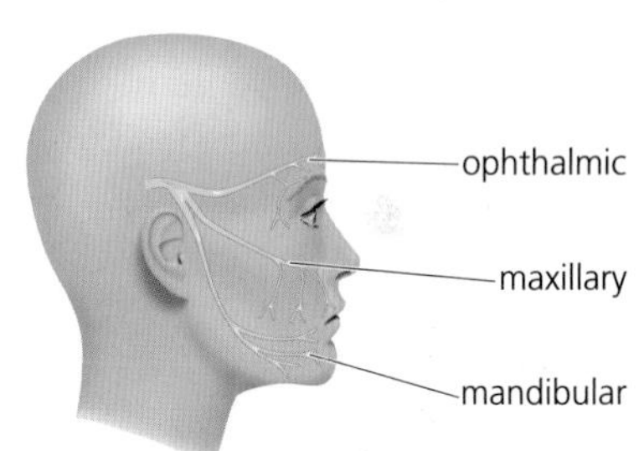

5th cranial nerve

5th cranial nerve This nerve carries messages to the brain from the sensory nerves of the skin, the teeth, the nose and the mouth. It also stimulates the motor nerve to create the chewing action when eating. The 5th cranial nerve has three branches:

- the **ophthalmic nerve** serves the tear glands of the eye, the skin of the forehead, and the upper cheeks
- the **maxillary nerve** serves the upper jaw and the mouth
- the **mandibular nerve** serves the lower jaw muscle, the teeth and the muscle involved with chewing.

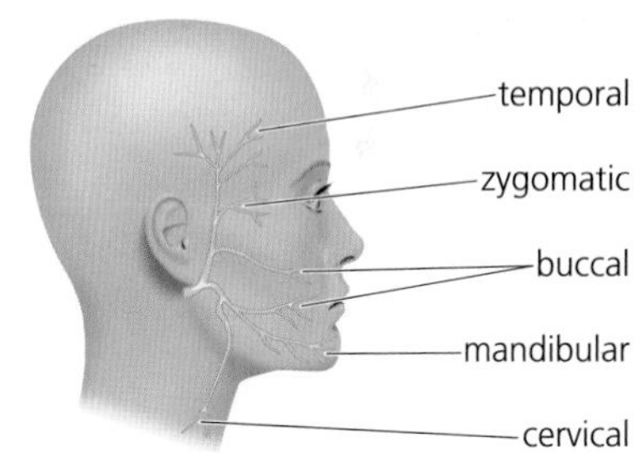

7th cranial nerve

7th cranial nerve This nerve passes through the temporal bone and behind the ear, and then divides. It serves the ear muscle and the **muscles of facial expression**, the tongue and the palate.

The 7th cranial nerve has five branches:

- the **temporal nerve** serves the orbicularis oculi and the frontalis muscles
- the **zygomatic nerve** serves the eye muscles
- the **buccal nerve** serves the upper lip and the sides of the nose
- the **mandibular nerve** serves the lower lip and the mentalis muscle of the chin
- the **cervical nerve** serves the platysma muscle of the neck

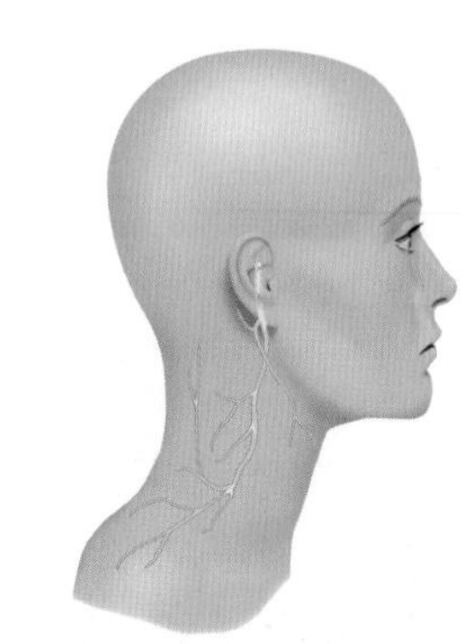

11th cranial nerve

TOP TIP

Botox® botulinum toxin A

Botox® has been developed as a cosmetic treatment from its previous use medically to treat eye spasms and disorders of the central nervous system. A purified protein called botulinum toxin A is injected into the face, where it binds to the nerve endings, which prevent the release of the neuro-transmitter substance that stimulates the muscle fibres to contract. The result is a paralysis of the muscle preventing expressions that may lead to visible expression lines on the face, such as frown lines.

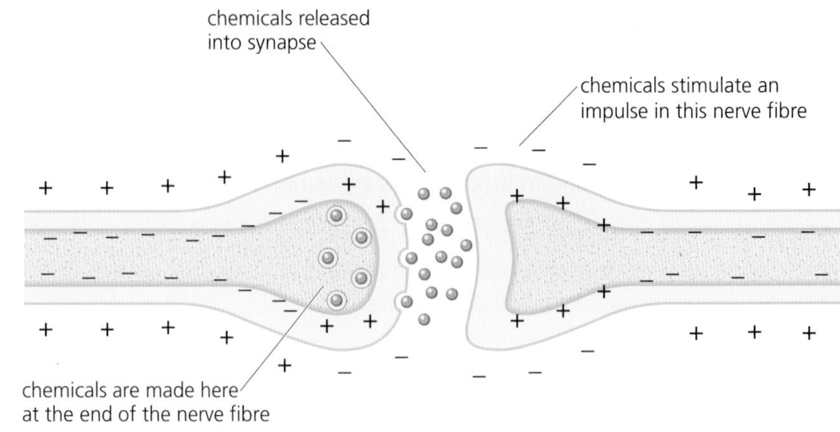

Passage of an impulse across a synapse

11th cranial nerve This nerve serves the sternomastoid and trapezius muscles of the neck, which move the head and shoulders.

Nerve impulses The CNS transmits instructions to organs through nerve impulses – tiny electrical signals – that pass along a neurone. Each nerve consists of a nerve cell and its parts, axons and dendrites. Axons carry nerve impulses away from the cell; dendrites carry impulses towards the cell.

When an impulse reaches the end of a nerve fibre, a chemical called a *neurotransmitter substance* is released. This chemical passes across a tiny gap called a *synapse* and is taken up by an adjacent neurone, generating an electrical impulse in the neurone.

When neuro-transmitters land at their receptor sites they can stimulate or inhibit the receiving cell. Both responses are important to relay the correct message through the nervous system.

Neurones can stimulate muscle fibres to contract. The *motor point* is where a motor nerve enters a muscle. When stimulated by a motor nerve, muscle contraction occurs.

TOP TIP

Lifestyle factors affect the nervous system

Caffeine is a stimulant and will increase the release of the neurotransmitter chemical across the synapse between adjacent neurones.

Alcohol is a sedative and will slow the release of the neurotransmitter chemical across the synapse between adjacent neurones.

Can you think of other substances that affect the nervous system?

The autonomic nervous system

The other nervous system division is the autonomic nervous system. The main function being to maintain constant conditions within the body called *homeostasis*.

The autonomic nervous system controls those body structures over which there is no conscious control – the involuntary activities. It regulates the functioning of organs such as the heart, the stomach, the lungs and the secretion of most glands. There are two divisions of the autonomic nervous system – the *sympathetic* and *parasympathetic nervous systems*.

TOP TIP

Memory aid

The sympathetic division is associated with stress. The parasympathetic system is associated with peace.

sympathetic = stress
parasympathetic = peace

Many organs receive a supply from each division. Fibres from one division stimulate the organ while fibres from the other division inhibit it, thus ensuring balance in the body.

The sympathetic nervous system is stimulated in periods of stress or danger and prepares the body for physical activity. Fibres of the sympathetic division increase blood flow by causing the heart to beat faster and the blood vessels in the muscles to widen. Activities that are not essential in this stressful situation are inhibited.

The parasympathetic nervous system is associated with resting and causes the blood flow to slow by causing the heart to beat slower and the blood vessels in the muscles to contract (go smaller). Fibres of this division stimulate digestion and absorption of food.

The nervous system therefore co-ordinates the activities of the body by responding to stimuli received by sense organs, including the nose, tongue, eyes, ears and skin.

The muscular system

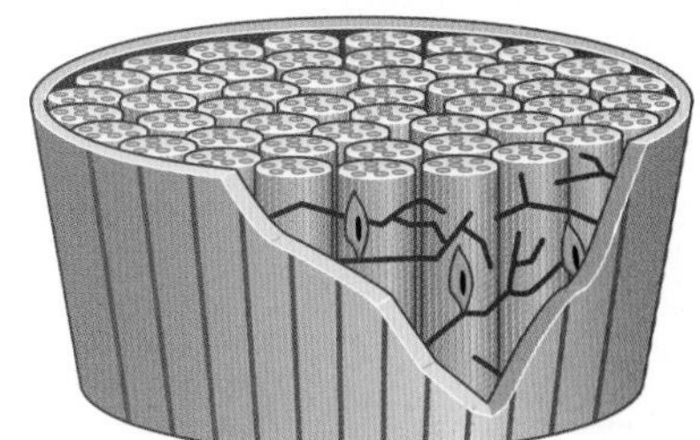
Muscle tissue

Muscles are responsible for the movement of body parts. Each is made up of a bundle of elastic fibres bound together in a sheath, the **fascia**. Muscular tissue contracts (shortens) and produces movement. Muscles never completely relax – there are always a few contracted fibres in every muscle. These make the muscles slightly tense and this tension is called **muscle tone**.

Muscle tissue has the following properties:

- it has the ability to contract
- it is extensible (when the extensor muscle in a joint contracts the corresponding flexor muscle will be stretched or lengthened)
- it is elastic – following contraction or extension it returns to its original length
- it is responsive – it contracts in response to nerve stimulation

A muscle is usually anchored by a strong tendon to one bone: the point of attachment is known as the muscle's **origin**. The muscle is likewise joined to a second bone: the attachment in this case is called the muscle's **insertion.** It is this second bone that is moved: the muscle contracts, pulling the two bones towards each other. (A different muscle, on the other side of the bone, has the contrary effect.) Not all muscles attach to bones, however: some insert into an adjacent muscle, or into the skin itself. The muscles with which we are concerned here are those of the face, the neck and the shoulders.

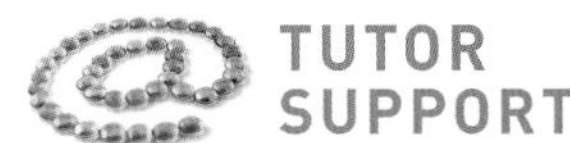

Activity 10: Label the muscles that move the head

Facial muscles

Many of the muscles located in the face are very small and are attached to (insert into) another small muscle or the facial skin. When the muscles contract, they pull the facial skin in a particular way; this creates facial expressions.

With age, the facial expressions that we make every day produce lines on the skin – frown lines. The amount of tension, or **tone**, also decreases with age. When performing facial massage, the aim is to improve the general tone of the facial muscles.

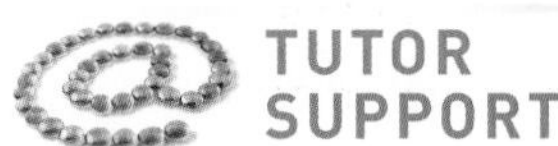

Activity 11: Label the muscles of the face and neck

To balance and move the head and facial features the muscles of the head, face and neck work together.

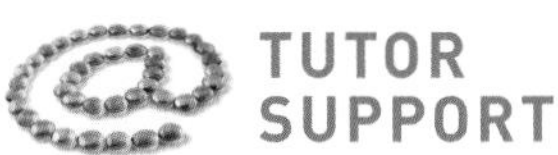

TUTOR SUPPORT

Activity 12: Facial muscles handout

ALWAYS REMEMBER

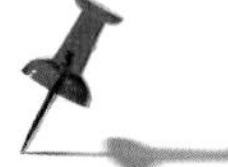

Nerves of the face
Almost all facial muscles are controlled by the 7th cranial or facial nerve.

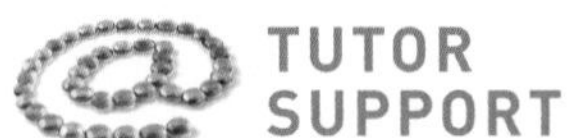

TUTOR SUPPORT

Activity 18: Label the 5th and 7th cranial nerves

TOP TIP

Terminology for action

Flexor **– bends a joint** ***Extensor*** **– straightens a joint**

If a muscle has 'flexor' or 'extensor' in front of the muscle name you will know what the action of the muscle is!

Abduction **– 'move away'** ***Adduction*** **– 'move towards'**

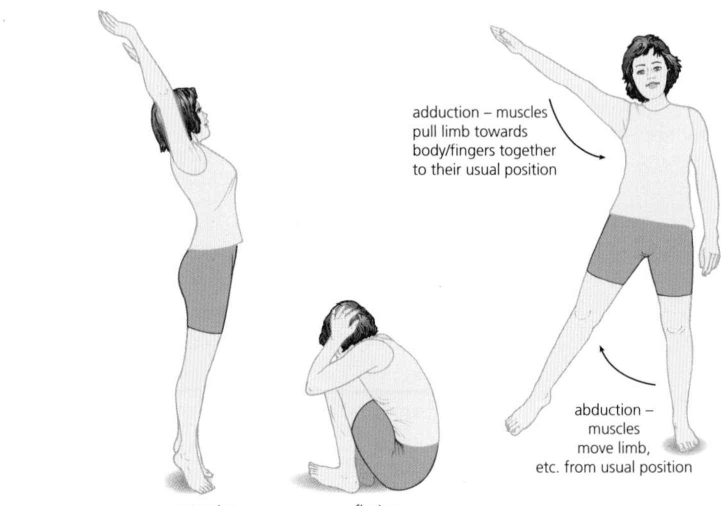
adduction – muscles pull limb towards body/fingers together to their usual position
abduction – muscles move limb, etc. from usual position
extension
flexion

Muscles of facial expression

Muscle	Expression	Location	Action
Frontalis	Surprise	The forehead.	Raises the eyebrows, causes wrinkling across forehead.
Corrugator corrugator	Frowning	Between the eyebrows.	Draws the eyebrows down and together.
Orbicularis oculi orbicularis oculi	Winking	Surrounds the eyes.	Closes the eyelid.

Muscle	Expression	Location	Action
Risorius 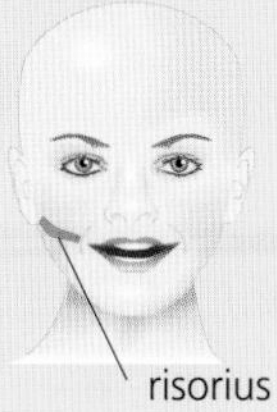	Smiling, grinning 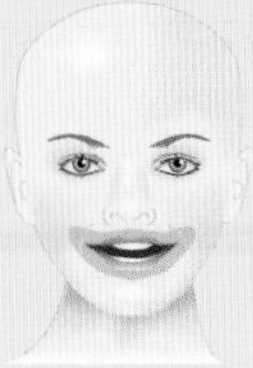	Extends diagonally from the masseter muscle to the corners of the mouth.	Draws mouth corners outwards and backwards in a grinning action.
Buccinator 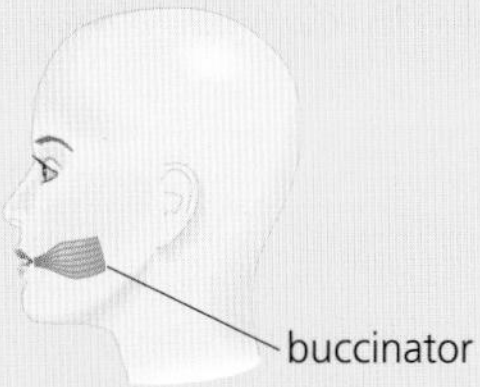	Blowing 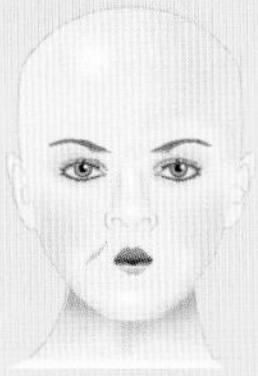	Inside the cheeks, between upper jaw and lower jaw.	Compresses the cheeks.
Zygomaticus (made up of major and minor muscles) 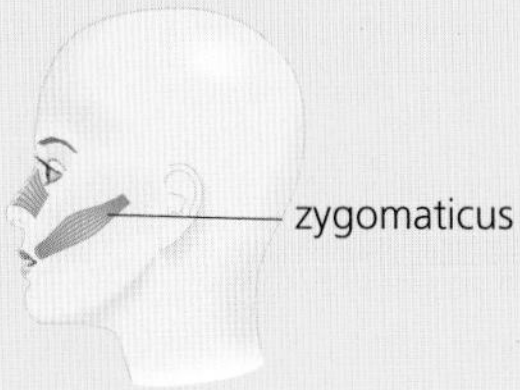	Smiling, laughing 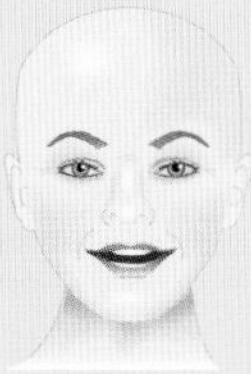	Extend diagonally from the zygomatic (cheekbone) to the corners of the mouth.	Lifts the corners of the mouth backwards and upwards.
Procerus 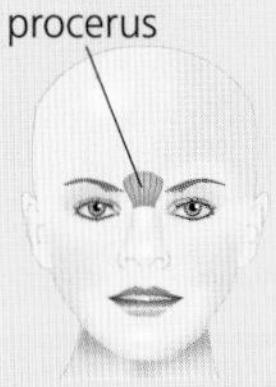	Distaste 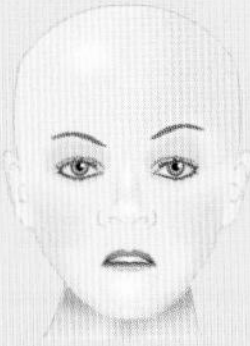	Covers the bridge of the nose.	Draws down eyebrows and wrinkles the skin over the bridge of the nose.
Nasalis (made up of several small muscles) 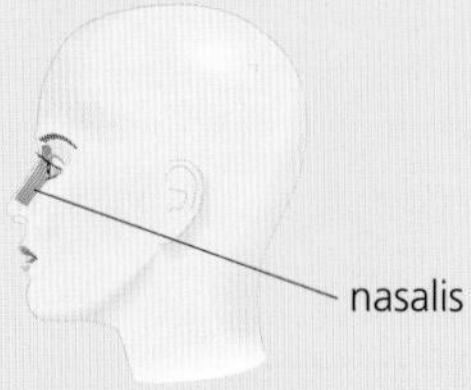	Anger 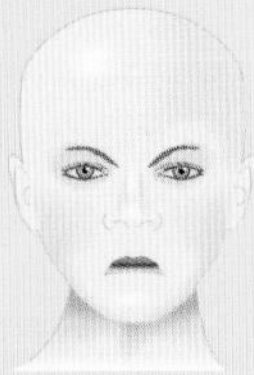	Covers the front of the nose and surrounds nostrils.	Opens and closes the nasal openings.
Levator labii 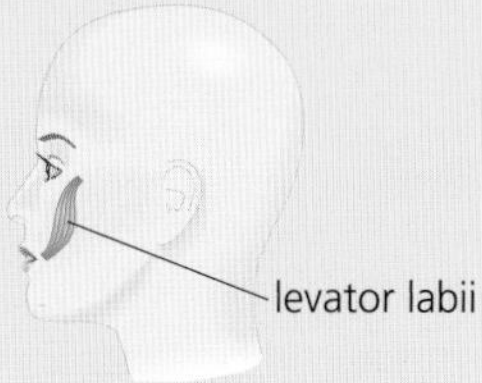	Distaste 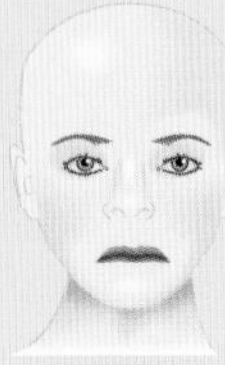	Surrounds the upper lip.	Raises and draws back the upper lips and nostrils.

Muscle	Expression	Location	Action
Depressor labii 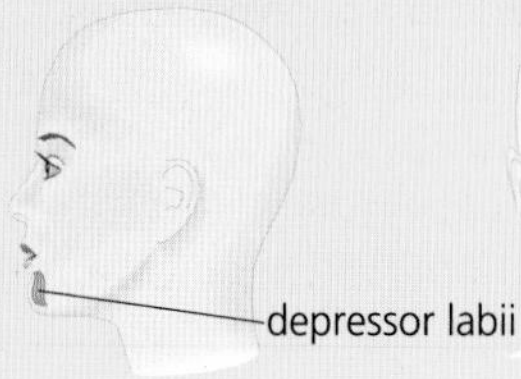	Sulking 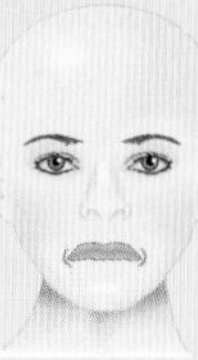	Surrounds the lower lip.	Pulls down the lower lip and draws it slightly to one side.
Orbicularis oris 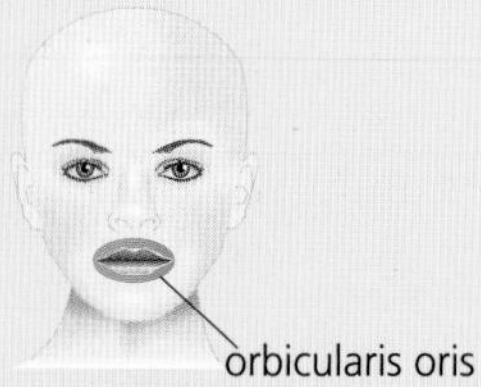	Pout, kiss, doubt 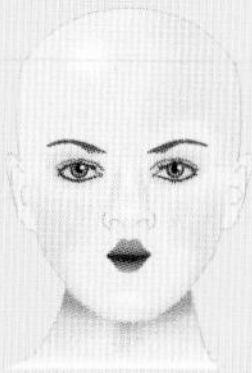	Surrounds the mouth.	Purses the lip (as in blowing), closes the mouth.
Triangularis 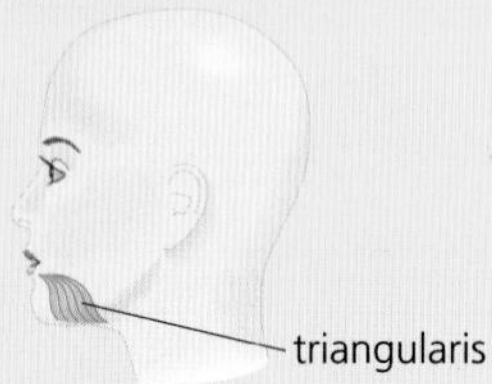	Sadness 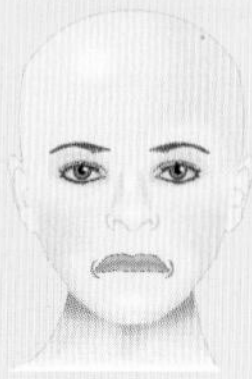	The corner of the lower lip extends over the chin.	Draws down the mouth's corners.
Mentalis 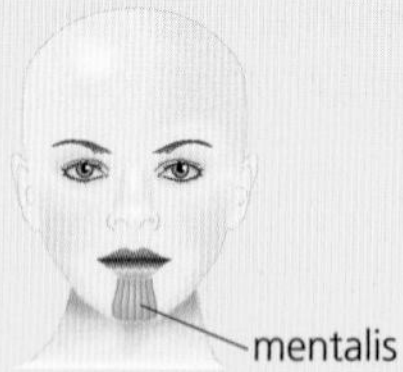	Doubt 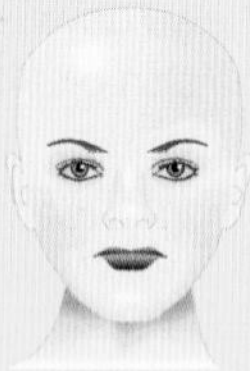	Covers the front of the chin.	Raises the lower lip, causing the chin to wrinkle.
Platysma 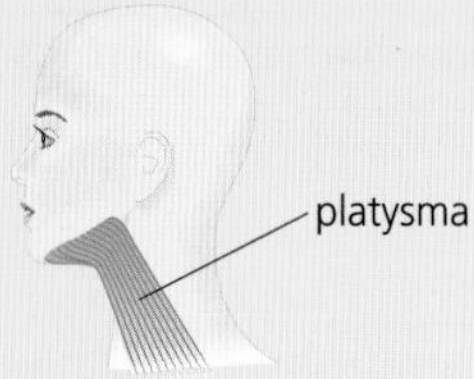	Fear, horror 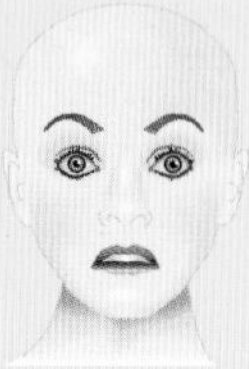	The sides of the neck and chin.	Draws the mouth's corners downwards and backwards.

depressor labii

orbicularis oris

triangularis

mentalis

platysma

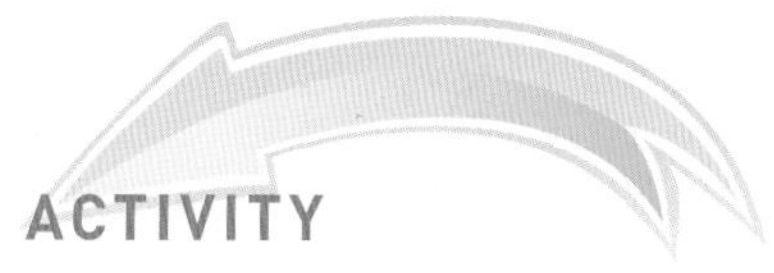

ACTIVITY

Facial expressions

In front of a mirror, move the muscles of your face to create the expressions that you might form each day.

What expressions can you make? Which part or parts of the face are moving? Which facial muscles do you think have contracted to create these expressions?

TOP TIP

Crow's feet

To avoid the premature formation of 'crow's feet':

- **avoid squinting in bright sunlight – wear sunglasses**
- **have your eyes tested regularly**
- **if you use a visual display unit, ensure that you take regular breaks, and have a protective filter screen to remove glare**

Muscles of mastication The muscles responsible for the movement of the lower jawbone (the **mandible**) when chewing are called the **muscles of mastication**.

Muscles of the upper body When massaging the shoulder area you will cover the following **muscles of the upper body**. You will also cover the trapezius muscle that makes up the majority of the upper back (see above).

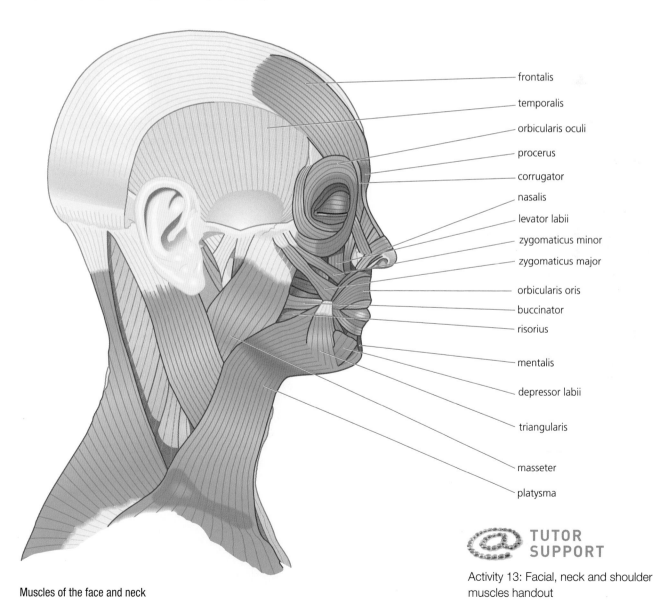

frontalis
temporalis
orbicularis oculi
procerus
corrugator
nasalis
levator labii
zygomaticus minor
zygomaticus major
orbicularis oris
buccinator
risorius
mentalis
depressor labii
triangularis
masseter
platysma

Muscles of the face and neck

TUTOR SUPPORT

Activity 13: Facial, neck and shoulder muscles handout

Muscle	Location	Action
Masseter	The cheek area: extends from the zygomatic bone to the mandible.	Clenches the teeth; raises the lower jaw and closes the mouth.
Temporalis	Extends from the temple region at the side of the head to the mandible.	Raises the jaw and draws it backwards, as in chewing.

Muscles that move the head

Muscle	Location	Action
Sterno-cleido-mastoid	Runs from the sternum to the clavicle bone and the temporal bone.	Flexes the neck; rotates and bows the head.
Trapezius	A large diamond or kite-shaped muscle, covering the back of the neck and the upper back. (Also a muscle of the upper-body).	Draws the head backwards and allows movement at the shoulder.
Occipitalis	Covers the back of the head.	Draws scalp backwards.

TOP TIP

An adult head weighs 5kg. Strong muscles of the neck and back are required to allow movement of the head.

TOP TIP

Muscles that move the head assist those of facial expression when communicating, e.g. nodding the head.

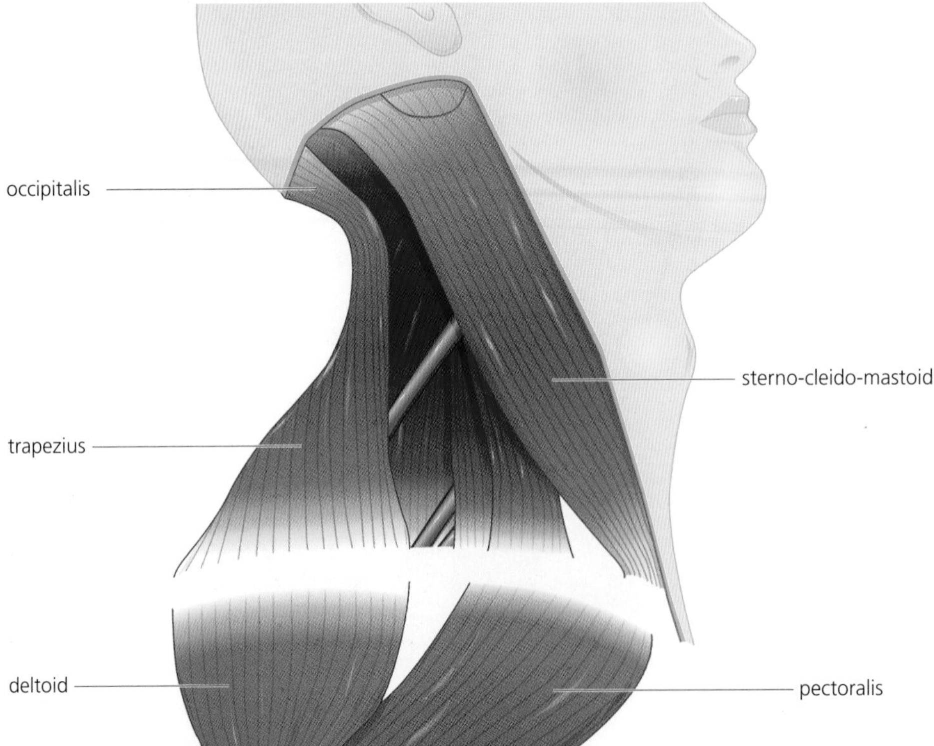

Muscles that move the head and muscles of the upper body

Muscle	Location	Action
Pectoralis major	The front of the chest.	Moves the arm towards the upper body.
Deltoid	A thick triangular muscle, covering the shoulder joint.	Takes the arm away from the side of the body.

The muscles of the hand and arm

The hand and fingers are moved primarily by muscles and tendons in the forearm. These muscles contract, pulling the tendons, and thereby move the fingers much as a puppet is moved by strings.

The **muscles of the hand and arm** that bend the wrist, drawing it towards the forearm, are **flexors**; other muscles, **extensors**, straighten the wrist and the hand.

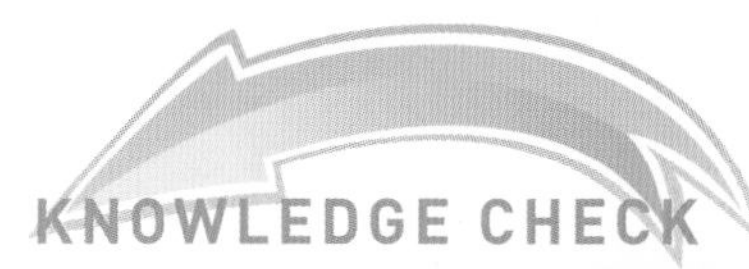

KNOWLEDGE CHECK

On the diagram of the muscles of the face, name muscles 1–6. What are the actions of these muscles?

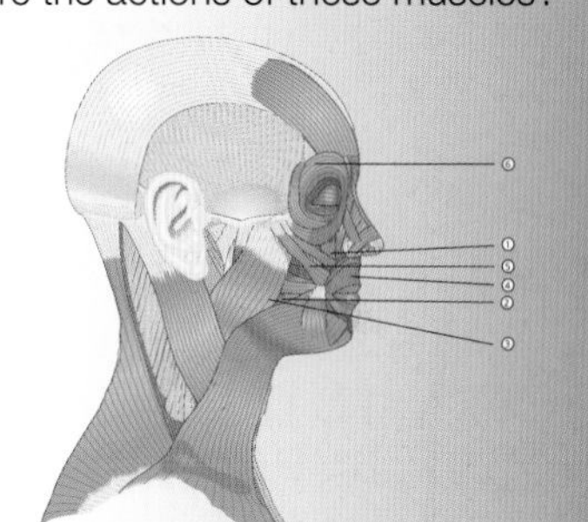

Need more time... refer to page 69 to help you.

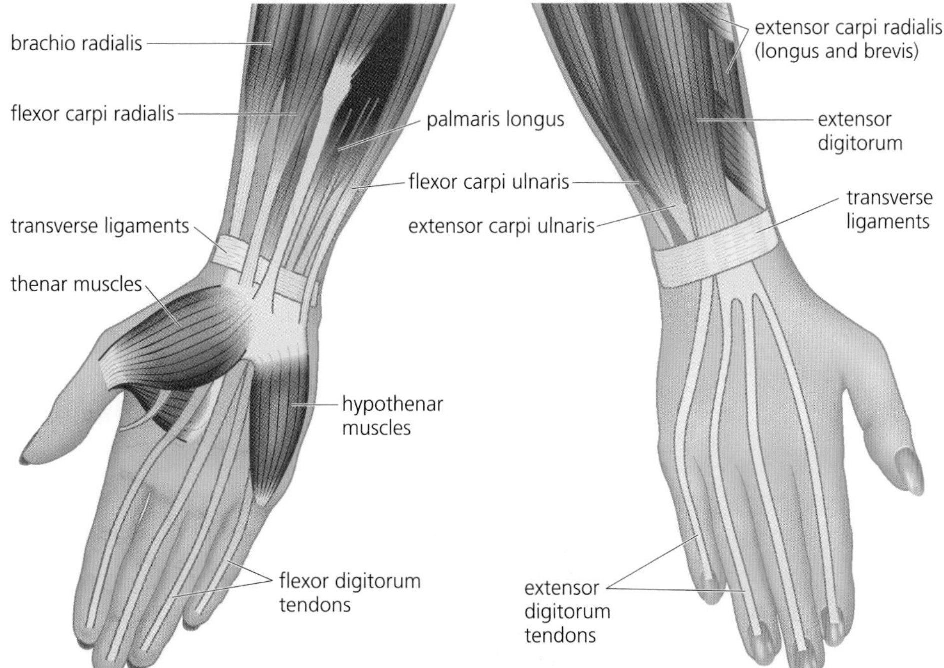

Muscles of the arm and hand

ACTIVITY

Observing the tendons

Tendons are made of strong connective tissue and attach muscle to bone. Hold your palm face upwards, with your sleeve pulled back so that you can see your forearm. Move the fingers individually towards the palm. Can you see the tendons moving?

Muscle	Location	Action
Brachio radialis	On the outer (thumb side) of the forearm.	Flexes arm at the elbow.
Flexor carpi radialis	Middle of the forearm.	Flexes and abducts the wrist.
Extensor carpi radialis (longus and brevis)	Thumb side of the forearm.	Extends and abducts the hand and wrist.

Muscle	Location	Action
Flexor carpi ulnaris	Front of the forearm.	Muscle that flexes and adducts the wrist joint in towards the body.
Extensor carpi ulnaris	Back of the forearm.	Extends and adducts the wrist.
Palmaris longus	Middle of the front of the forearm.	Flexes the wrist and tenses the palm of the hand.
Hypothenar muscle	In the palm of the hand, below the little finger.	Flexes the little finger and moves it outwards and inwards.
Thenar muscle	In the palm of the hand, below the thumb.	Flexes the thumb and moves it outwards and inwards.
Flexor digitorum tendons	Front of fingers.	Flexes the fingers when contracted.
Extensor digitorum tendons	Back of fingers.	Extends the fingers when contracted.

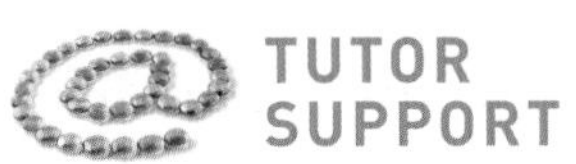

Activity 14: Muscles of the leg and foot handout

The muscles of the foot and lower leg

The **muscles of the foot** work together to help move the body when walking and running. In a similar way to the movement of the hand, the foot is moved primarily by **muscles in the lower leg**; these pull on tendons, which in turn move the feet and toes.

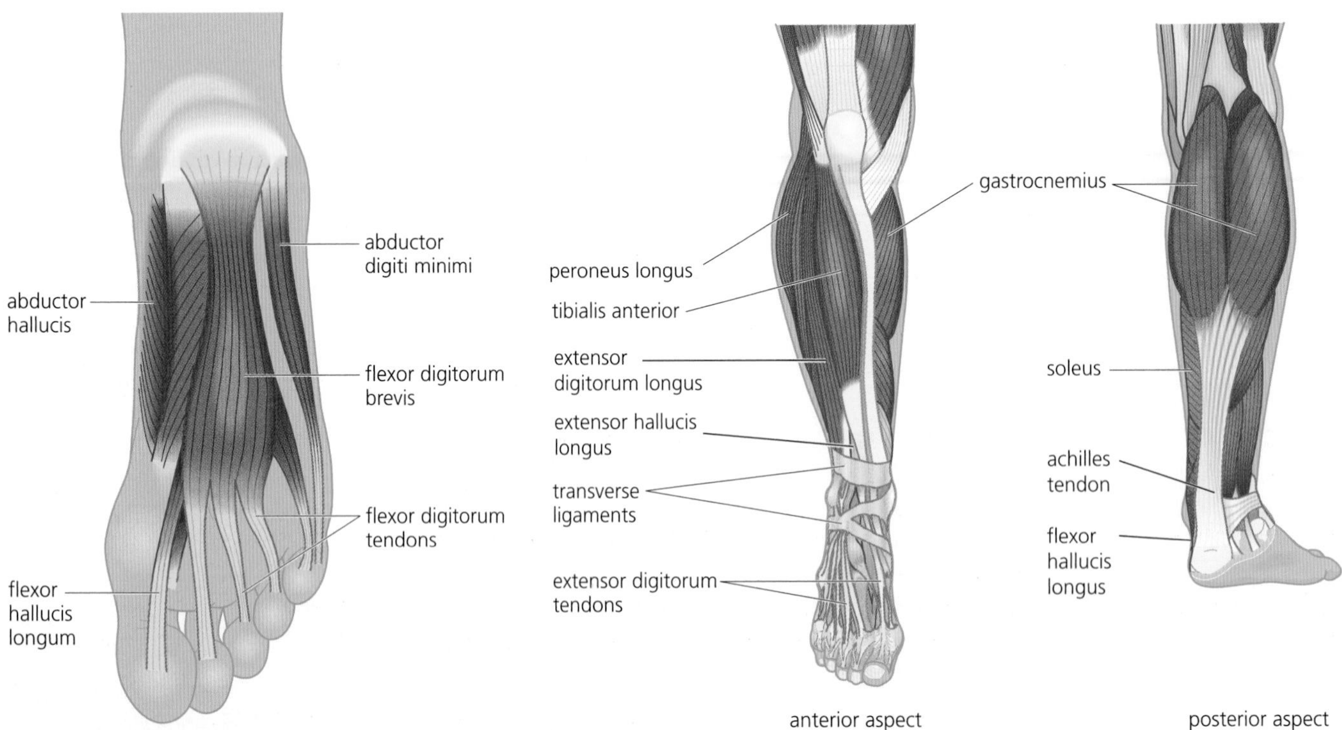

Muscles and tendons of the foot

Muscles of the lower leg

Muscles and tendons of the lower leg and foot

Muscle	Location	Action
Gastrocnemius	Calf of the leg, inserts through the Achilles tendon into the heel.	Flexes the lower leg; plantar flexes the foot (extends and points the toes down).
Tibialis anterior	Front of the lower leg.	Inverts the foot (turns sole inwards) dorsi flexes the foot (flexes and points the toes up); rotates foot outwards. Supports the medial longitudinal arch of the foot when running or walking.
Soleus	Calf of the leg, situated below the gastrocnemius muscle. Inserts through the Achilles tendon into the heel.	Plantar flexes the foot (flexes and points toes down). Assists forward motion when walking or running.
Peroneus longus	Lateral side of the lower leg.	Plantar flexes the foot and everts (turns sole outwards). Supports the foot arches.
Extensor digitorum longus	Lateral side of the front of the lower leg.	Dorsi flexes the foot up at the ankle and extends the toes.
Extensor hallucis longus	Arises from the middle front surface of the fibula, passing the transverse aspect of the foot and inserting into the big toe.	Extends the big toe.
Flexor digitorum longus	Back of the tibia in the lower leg and inserts into the distal four toes.	Plantar flexes foot downwards and inverts the foot. Helps the toes to grip. Supports the lateral longitudinal arch of the foot.
Flexor hallucis longus	Arises from the back of lower leg and inserts to the plantar aspect of the foot to the base of the big toe.	Flexes the big toe and pushes the foot off the ground when walking.
Achilles tendon	Attached to the soleus and gastrocnemius down to the heel.	Raises the foot when related muscle contracts.
Extensor digitorum tendons	Tops of toes.	Straightens the toes when related muscle contracts.
Flexor digitorum tendons	Underneath the toes.	Bends the toes when related muscle contracts.

The bones

When carrying out a massage to the face, head, shoulders, arms, hands legs and feet, you will feel below your hands the underlying bones. **Bone** is the hardest structure in the body: is made up of water; non-living (inorganic) material including calcium and phosphorus and living (organic) material such as the cells which form bones called **osteoblasts**. It protects the underlying structures, gives shape to the body and provides an attachment point for our muscles, thereby allowing movement. There are two main classifications of bone tissue, **compact** and **cancellous** (spongy). Bones are made up of both types of tissue which varies according to size and function.

Compact appears to have no visible spaces and is solid in structure making it strong and hardwearing. However, under a microscope it can be seen that it is supplied with blood and lymph vessels and nerves.

Name one muscle located in each of the following: the shoulder, arm and hand.

What are the group of muscles called that bend the wrist, drawing it towards the forearm?

Need more time... refer to page 71 to help you.

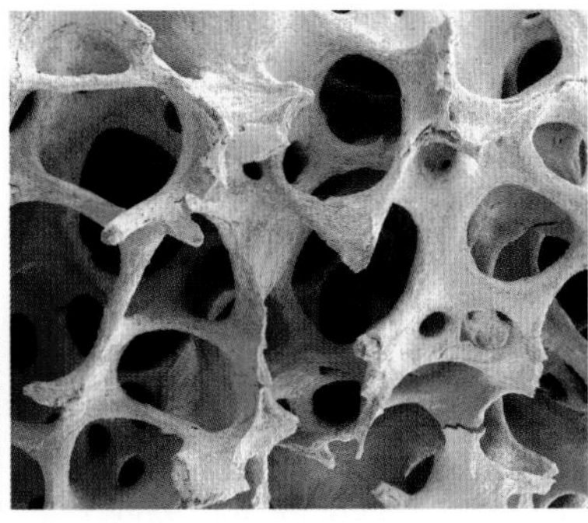

Bone tissue

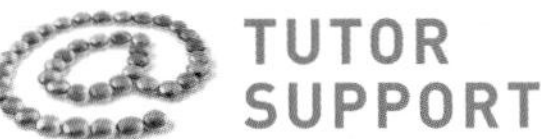

Activity 7: Label the bones of the neck, chest and shoulder

TOP TIP

Bone acts as a reservoir for important minerals such as calcium and phosphorus and also makes new cells for the blood in certain bones in tissue called bone marrow.

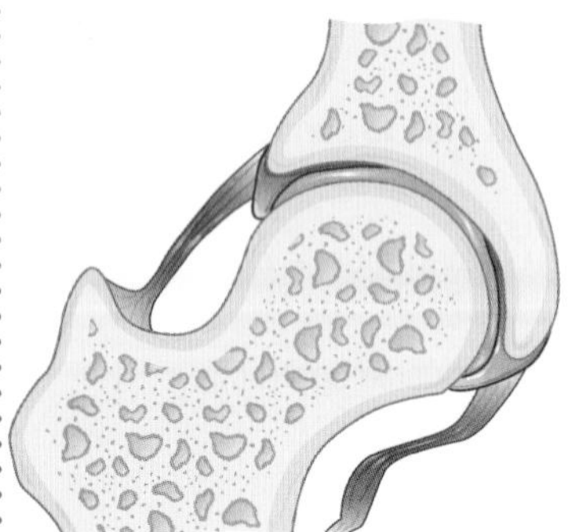

Ball and socket joint, as in the shoulder

Cancellous (spongy) has many spaces which contains red and yellow bone marrow. Red bone marrow produces new red blood cells and yellow bone marrow stores fat cells.

The skeleton is made up of many bones. The average skeleton has 206 bones. It forms a strong framework which supports the softer tissues, maintains the shape of the body and keeps the internal organs anchored in position. Muscles are attached to the bones which contract and relax allowing movement. Together with the muscles and joints, the skeleton allows movement. Many organs are surrounded by a protective cage of bone. Many of the blood cells are made in bone marrow (found inside the bones).

Bones have different shapes, accord to their function. Bones can be classified as: flat; short; irregular; long and sesamoid.

Each bone is connected to its neighbour by *connective tissue*, a structural tissue that supports, surrounds and links different parts of the body. Fibrous connective tissue is used for immovable joints such as those of the cranium. *Fibro-cartilage* is used for

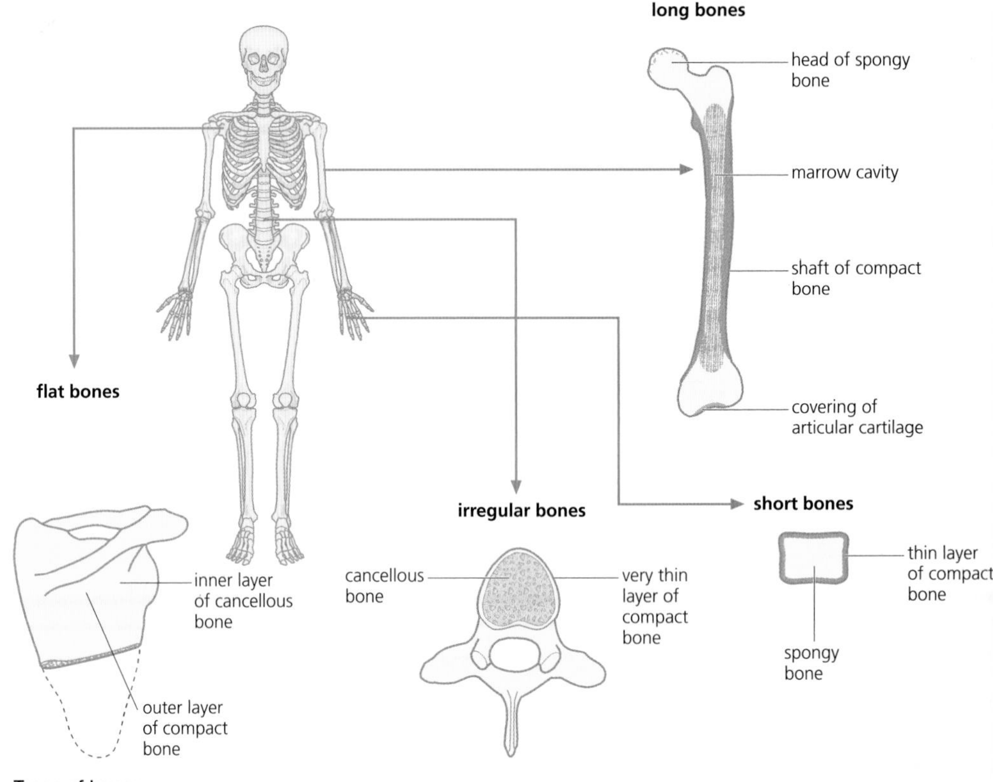

Types of bones

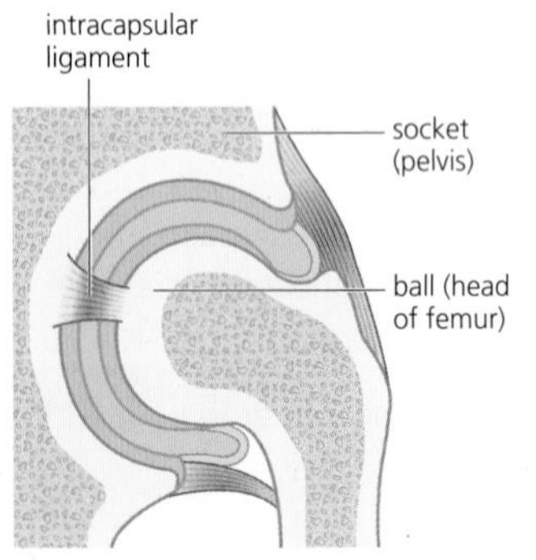

Hip

Shoulder

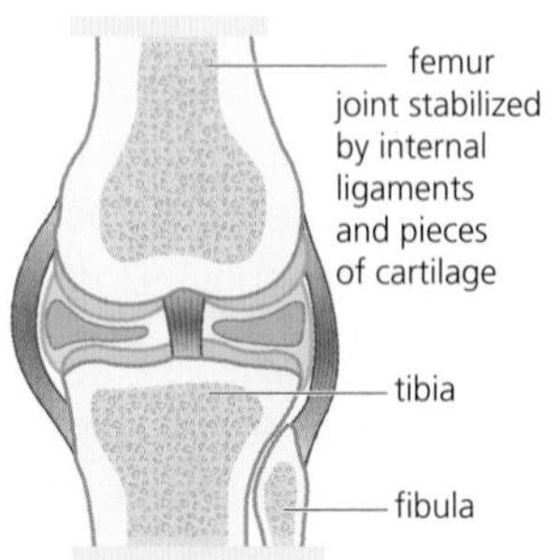

Knee

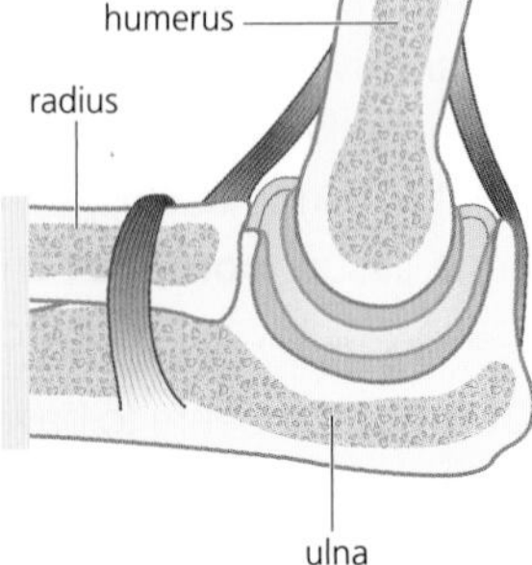

Elbow

semi-immovable joints such as those between the bones of the vertebrae. The most common joints – *synovial joints* – are freely moveable and are loosely held together by a form of connective tissue called a *ligament*.

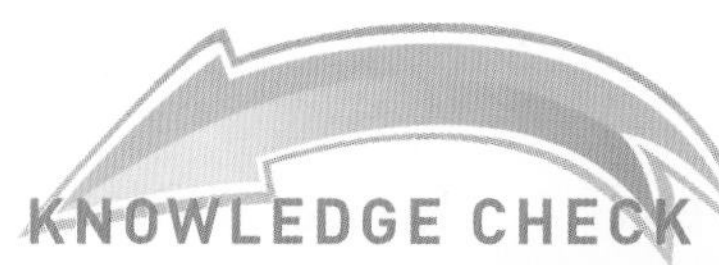

Name two muscles located in the foot and lower leg and their actions.

Need more time... refer to pages 72–73 to help you.

Bones of the head, neck, chest and shoulders

The bones which form the head are collectively known as the **skull**. The skull can be divided into two parts, the face and the cranium, which together are made up of 22 bones:

- the fourteen **facial bones** form the face
- the eight cranial bones form the rest of the head

As well as forming our facial features, the facial bones support other structures such as the eyes and the teeth. Some of these bones, such as the nasal bone, are made from **cartilage**, connective tissue, a softer tissue than bone.

The cranium surrounds and protects the brain. The bones are thin and slightly curved, and are held together by connective tissue. After childhood, the joints become immovable, and are called **sutures** appearing as wavy lines.

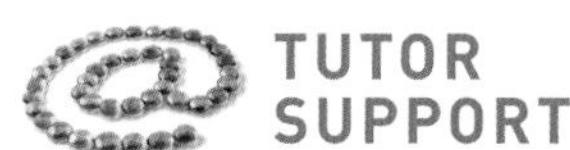

Activity 6: Label the bones of the face

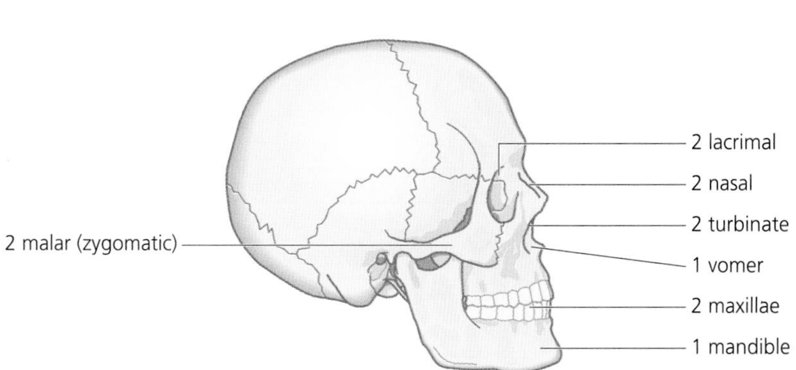

Bones of the face (14 in total)

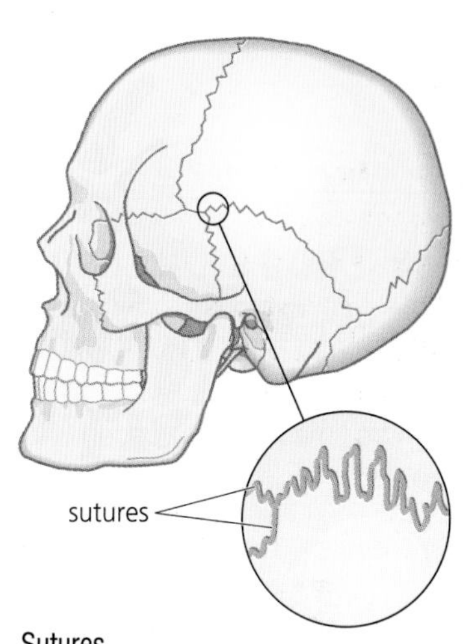

Sutures

Facial bones

Bone	Number	Location	Function
Nasal	2	The nose	Form the bridge of the nose.
Vomer	1	The nose	Forms the dividing bony wall of the nose.
Palatine	2	The nose	Form the floor and wall of the nose and the roof of the mouth.
Turbinate	2	The nose	Form the outer walls of the nose.
Lacrimal	2	The eye sockets	Form the inner walls of the eye sockets; contain a small groove for the tear duct.
Malar (zygomatic)	2	The cheek	Form the cheekbones.
Maxillae	2	The upper jaw	Fused together, to form the upper jaw, which holds the upper teeth.
Mandible	1	The lower jaw	The largest and strongest of the facial bones; holds the lower teeth.

Cranial bones

Bone	Number	Location	Function
Occipital	1	The lower back of the cranium	Contains a large hole called the *foramen magnum:* through this pass the spinal cord, the nerves and blood vessels.
Parietal	2	The sides of the cranium	Fused together to form the sides and top of the head (the 'crown').
Frontal	1	The forehead	Forms the forehead and the upper walls of the eye sockets.
Temporal	2	The sides of the head	Provide two muscle attachment points: the mastoid process and the zygomatic process.
Ethmoid	1	Between the eye sockets	Forms part of the nasal cavities.
Sphenoid	1	The base of the cranium, the back of the eye sockets	A bat-shaped bone that joins together all the bones of the cranium.

KNOWLEDGE CHECK

What are the basic functions of bone?

Need more time... refer to page 73 to help you.

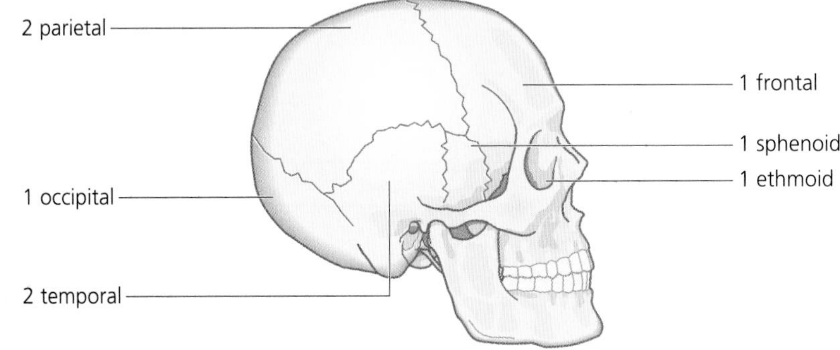

Bones of the cranium (8 in total)

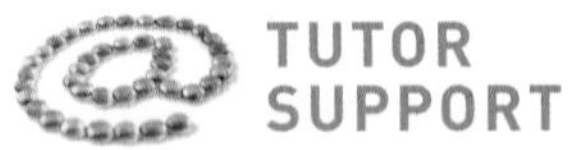

TUTOR SUPPORT

Activity 5: Label the bones of the cranium

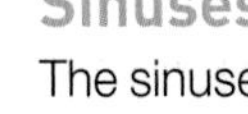

Sinuses

The sinuses are hollow spaces in the facial and cranial bones containing air and lined with a mucous membrane, producing mucus which drains into the nose and keeps the nasal cavities moist and traps bacteria and dirt. The mucous membrane is continuous with the nasal cavities. They can also get blocked by airborne allergens, e.g. pollen, air pollution and chronic drug misuse. They connect with the inside of the nasal cavity through small openings called ostia. The main sinuses are the:

- maxillary, in each cheekbone
- frontal, either side of the forehead, above the eyes
- sphenoid, between the upper part of the nose and between the eyes
- ethmoid, behind the bridge of the nose and between the eyes

The sinuses contain fibres that slow the flow of lymph fluid through them and which enables macrophages to ingest microorganisms that could lead to infection.

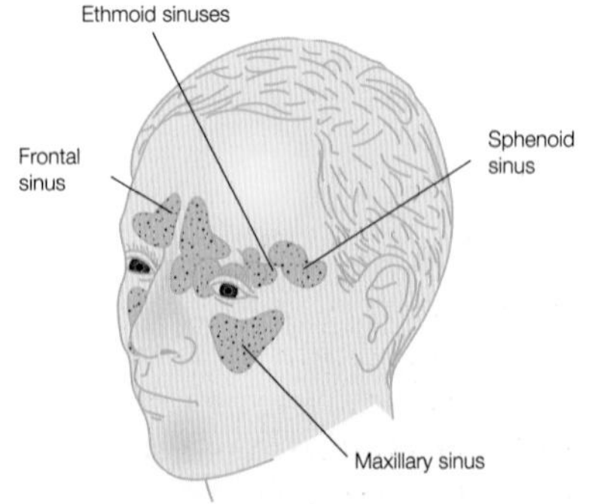

Sinuses

Bones of the torso

Bone	Number	Location	Function
Cervical vertebra	7	The neck.	These vertebrae form the top of the spinal column: the *atlas* is the first vertebra, which supports the skull; the *axis* is the second vertebra, which allows rotation of the head.
Thoracic vertebrae	12	Upper and middle back.	The rib cage joins to the thoracic vertebra and protects the body's vital organs, i.e. heart and lungs.
Hyoid	1	A U-shaped bone at the front of the neck.	Supports the tongue.
Clavicle	2	Slender long bones at the base of the neck.	Commonly called the *collar bones*, these form a joint with the sternum and the scapula bones, allowing movement at the shoulder.
Scapula	2	Triangular bones in the upper back.	Commonly called the *shoulder blades*, the scapulae provide attachment for muscles which move the arms. The **shoulder girdle**, which allows movement at the shoulder, is composed of the clavicles and the scapulae.
Humerus	2	The upper bones of the arms.	Form ball-and-socket joints with the scapulae: these joints allow movement in any direction.
Sternum	1	The breastbone.	Protects the inner organs; provides a surface for muscle attachment and supports muscle movement.

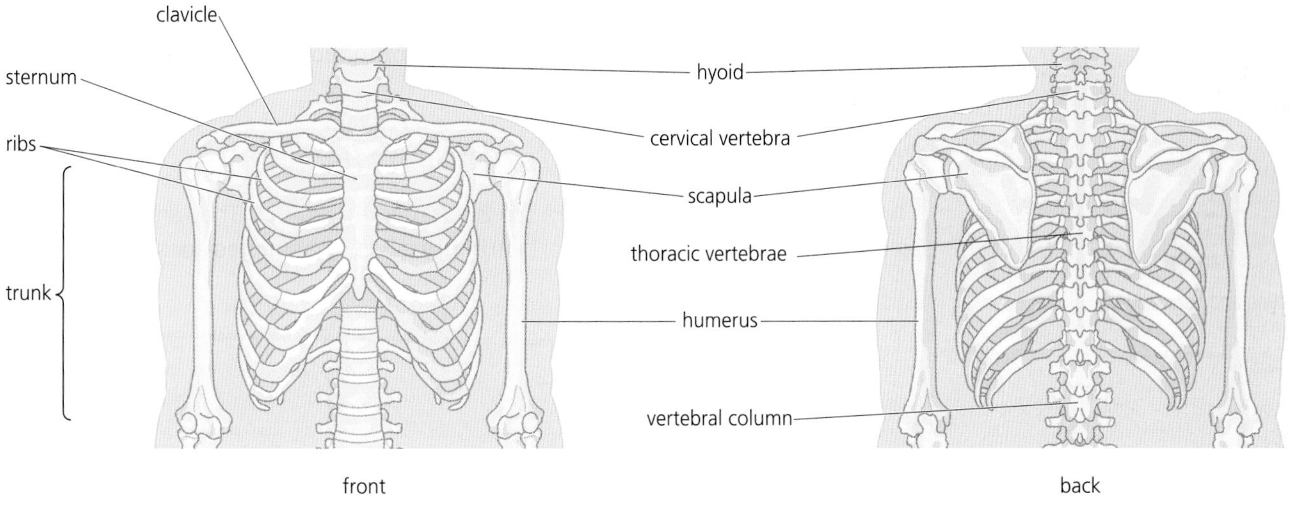

Bones of the torso

Bones of the hands and upper limbs (arms)

The bones of the hand There are 27 **bones of the hand**. The wrist consists of eight small **carpal** bones, which glide over one another to allow movement. This is called a **condyloid** or **gliding joint**.

There are then five **metacarpal** bones that make up the palm of the hand.

The fingers are made up of 14 individual bones called **phalanges** – two in the thumb, and three in each of the fingers.

The bones of the arm The **bones of the arm** are three long bones: the **humerus** is the bone of the upper arm, from the shoulder to the elbow; the **radius** and **ulna** lie side by side in the lower arm, from the elbow to the wrist.

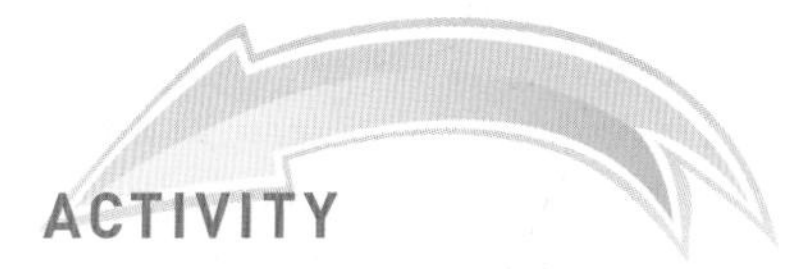

Identifying bones in the hand
Look very closely at your hand. Can you identify where the bones are? Try feeling the bones with your other hand. How many can you feel?

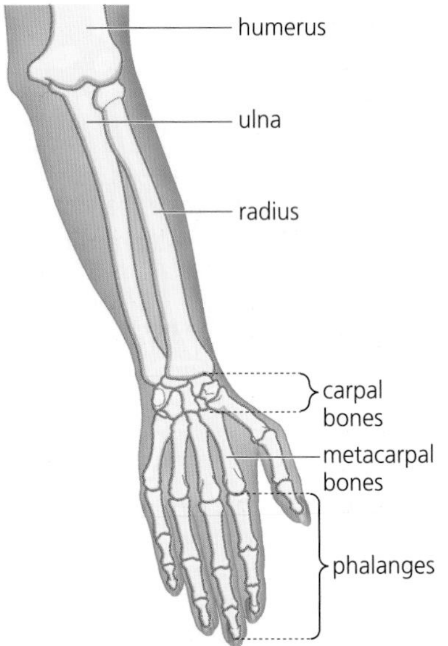

Bones of the arm and hand

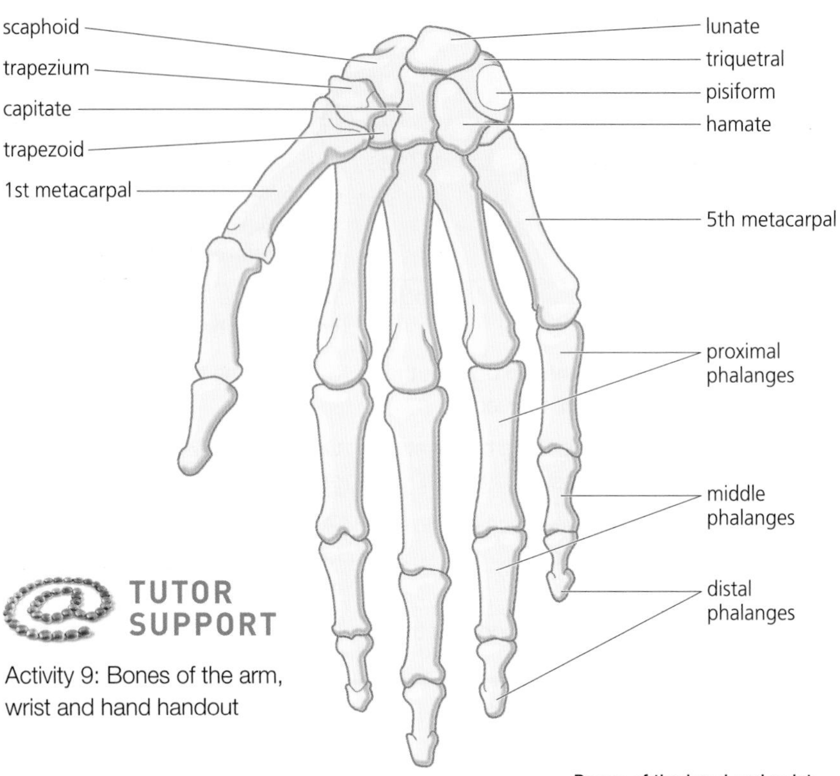

TUTOR SUPPORT

Activity 9: Bones of the arm, wrist and hand handout

Bones of the hand and wrist

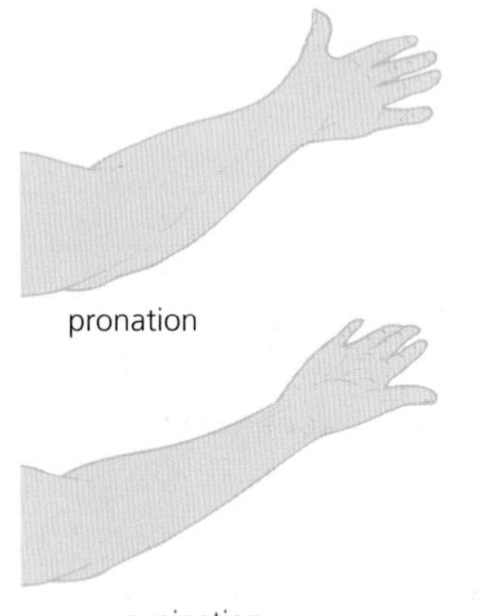

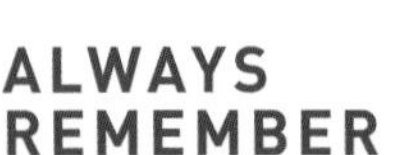

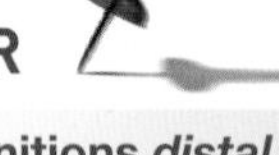

Pronation and supination

Having two bones in the lower arm makes it easier for your wrist to rotate. This movement that causes the palm to face downwards is called **pronation**; the movement that causes it to face upwards is called **supination**.

Bones of the foot and the lower limbs (legs)

The bones of the foot There are 26 **bones of the foot**. They are seven **tarsal** (ankle) bones, five **metatarsal** (ball of foot) bones, and 14 **phalanges** (toes). These bones

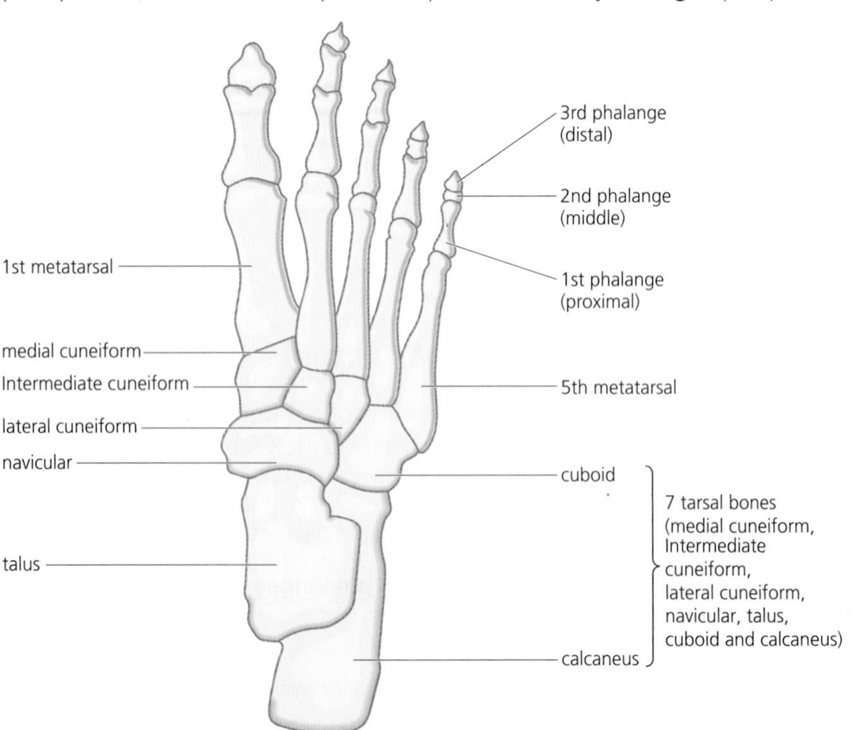

Bones of the foot

ALWAYS REMEMBER

Anatomical definitions *distal* and *proximal*

These are used to explain the location of anatomical structures.

Proximal: means nearest to

Distal: means furthest away

You can see on the diagram of the foot, the phalanx bones next to the metatarsal bones are referred to as proximal and the phalanx bones at the ends of the toes are referred to as distal.

Anatomical terminology descriptions are found on page 28.

fit together to form arches, which help to support the foot and to absorb the impact when we walk, run and jump.

The arches of the foot The **arches** of the foot are created by the formation of the bones and joints, and supported by ligaments. These arches support the weight of the body and help to preserve balance when we walk on even surfaces.

The longitudinal arch runs longitudinally from the calcaneus to the metatarsals. The arch on the inside aspect of the foot is the medial longitudinal arch, on the outside aspect it is the lateral longitudinal arch. The transverse arch lies perpendicular to this in the metatarsal area, as shown below.

TOP TIP

Arches

Footprints made by bare feet show that only part of the foot touches the ground. Weight transfers from the heel to the ball to the big toe when walking. Feet with reduced arches are referred to as 'flat feet', caused by weak ligaments and tendons.

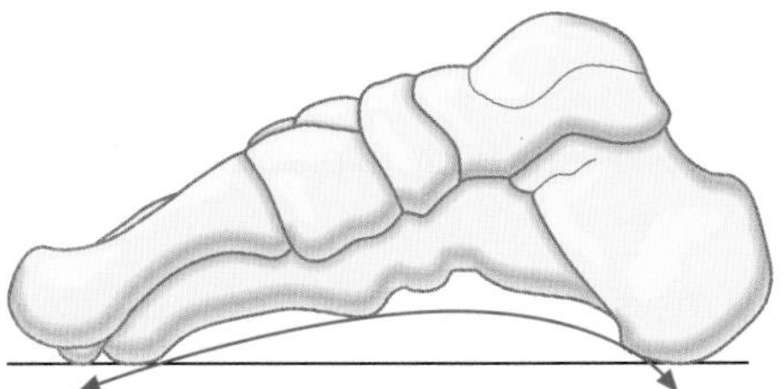

Medial Longitudinal Arch

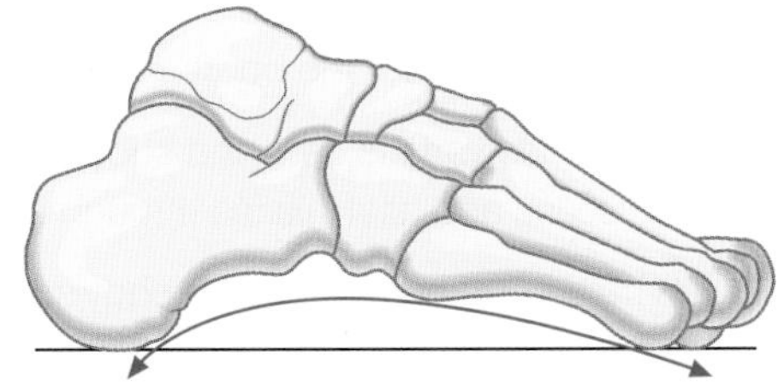

Lateral Longitudinal Arch

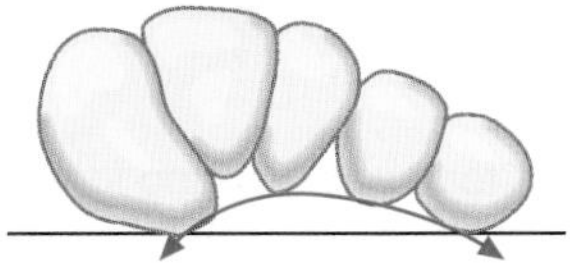

Transverse Arch

The bones of the leg The bones of the lower leg are two long bones, the **tibia** and the **fibula**. These bones have joints with the upper leg (at the knee) and with the foot (at the ankle). Having two bones in the lower leg – as with the forearm – allows a greater range of movement to be achieved at the ankle.

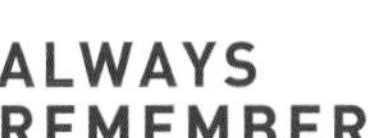

ALWAYS REMEMBER

Anatomical definitions

Medal: towards the midline (middle) of the body

Lateral: away from the median line (middle) line of the body. The outer side of the body.

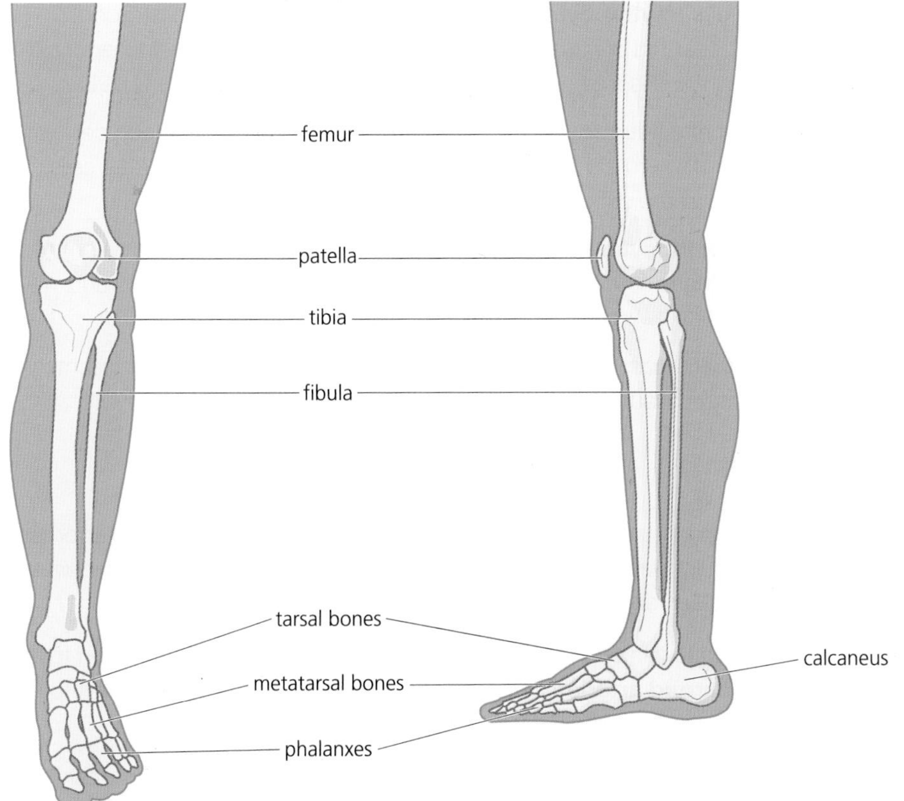

Bones of the lower leg

KNOWLEDGE CHECK

Name the bones that form the ankle.

Need more time... refer to page 78 to help you.

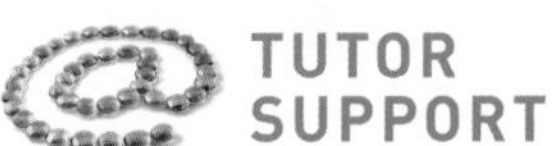

TUTOR SUPPORT

Activity 8: Bones of the leg, ankle and foot handout

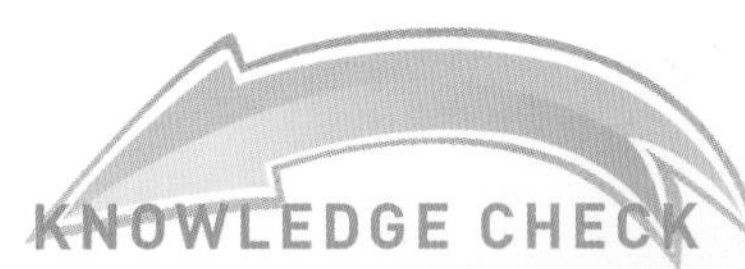

KNOWLEDGE CHECK

The wrist is made up of eight small carpal bones, which glide over one another to allow movement. Name them.

Need more time... refer to page 78 to help you.

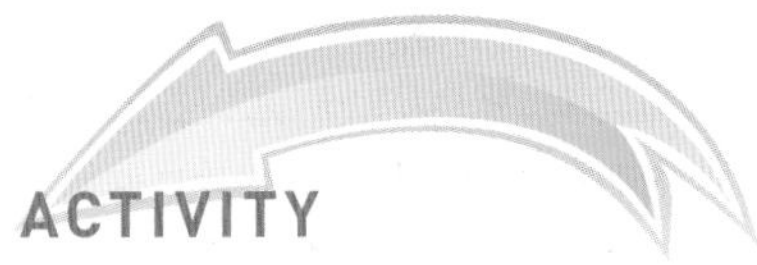

ACTIVITY

30 bones form each leg and foot, 60 in both! State where each bone can be found:

1 femur
1 patella
1 tibia
1 fibula
7 tarsal bones
5 metatarsal bones
14 phalanges

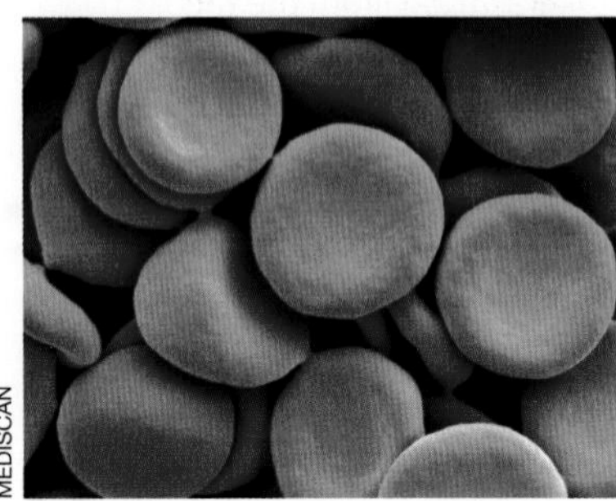

Blood cells

TOP TIP

Blood

Blood helps to maintain the body temperature at 36.8°C. Varying blood flow near to the skin's surface increases or diminishes heat loss.

The blood

Composition and function of blood

Blood is a collection of specialized cells suspended in a liquid called plasma supplying the needs of the body's cells keeping the body healthy. It is transported around the body by a network of vessels with a length of 90,000 miles.

Blood transports various substances around the body:

- It carries oxygen from our lungs, and nutrients from our digested food to the cells of the body supply energy – these allow the cells to develop and divide, and the muscles to function.
- It carries waste products and carbon dioxide from the cells and tissues away for elimination from the body.
- It carries various cells and substances which allow the body to prevent or fight disease and heal injuries through blood clotting.
- Transports hormones, the body's chemical messengers to their target tissue to cause a particular response.
- Helps to maintain the body temperature at 36.8°C: carrying blood flow near to the skin surface increases or diminishes heat loss.

The main constituents of blood

Blood consists of the following:

- **Plasma** This constitutes 50 per cent of blood and is a straw-coloured liquid: mainly water (90 per cent), with foods and carbon dioxide.
- **Red blood cells (erythrocytes)** These constitute 40–50 per cent of blood. These cells appear red because they contain **haemoglobin** a protein responsible for their colour. It is this that carries oxygen from the lungs to the body cells.
- **White blood cells (leucocytes)** There are several types of white blood cells. Their main role is to protect the body destroying foreign bodies and dead cells, and carrying away the debris (a process known as **phagocytosis**).
- **Platelets (thrombocytes)** When blood is exposed to air, as happens when the skin is injured, these cells bind together to form a clot. White blood cells and platelets constitute 1–2 per cent of blood.
- **Other chemicals** Hormones also are transported in the blood – 'chemical messengers' to target tissues.

Circulation

The circulation of blood is under the control of the **heart**, a powerful muscular organ, the size of a clenched fist, which pumps the blood around the body. The heart requires a constant supply of oxygen and energy from blood.

Blood leaving the heart is carried in large, elastic tubes called **arteries**. The blood to the head arrives via the **carotid arteries**, which are connected via other main arteries to the heart. There are two main carotid arteries, one on each side of the neck.

These arteries divide into smaller branches, the *internal carotid* and the *external carotid.* The **internal carotid artery** passes the temporal bone and enters the head, taking blood to the brain eyes, eyelids, forehead, nose and internal ears). The **external**

carotid artery stays outside the skull, and divides into branches which supply blood to various regions of the head, face and neck.

- the **occipital branch** supplies the back of the head and the scalp
- the **temporal branch** supplies the sides of the face, the head, the scalp and the skin. Some of its important branches are:
  - frontal: supplies the forehead
  - parietal: supplies the top and sides of the head
  - transverse: supplies the masseter muscle
  - middle temporal supplies the temples and the eyelids
  - anterior auricular: supplies the front part of the ear
- the **facial branch**, also known as the external maxillary artery, supplies the muscles and tissues of the face
- **posterior auricular branch** supplies the scalp, back and above the ear.

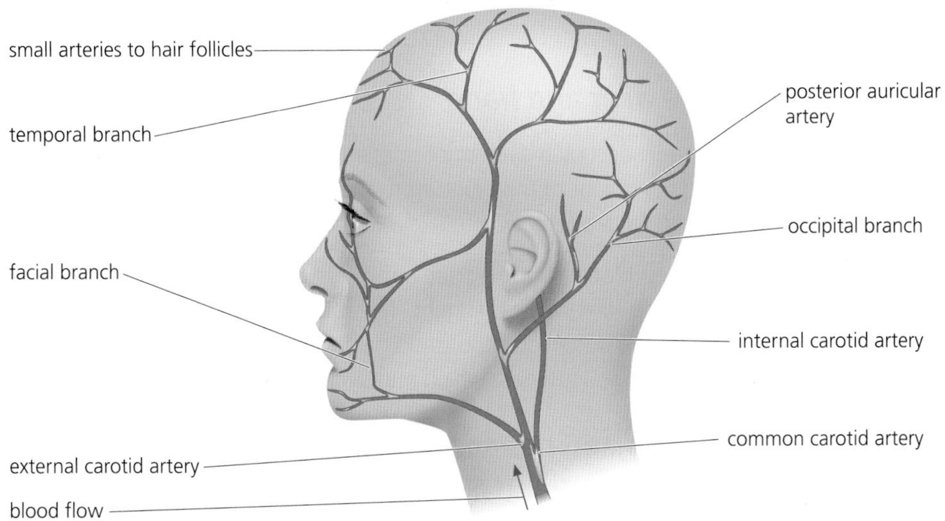

The blood supply to the head

These arteries also divide repeatedly, successive vessels becoming smaller and smaller until they form tiny blood **capillaries**. These vessels are just one cell thick, allowing substances carried in the blood to pass through them into the **tissue fluid** which bathes and nourishes the cells of the various body tissues.

The blood capillaries begin to join up again, forming first small vessels called **venules**, then larger vessels called **veins**. These return the blood to the heart.

Veins are less elastic than arteries, and are closer to the skin's surface. Along their course are **valves**, which prevent the backflow of blood.

The main veins are the external and internal jugular veins. The **internal jugular vein** and its main branch, the **facial vein**, carry blood from the face and head. The **external jugular vein** carries blood from the scalp and has two branches: the **occipital branch** and the **temporal branch**. The jugular veins join to enter the **subclavian vein**, which lies above the clavicle.

Blood returns to the heart, which pumps it to the lungs, where the red blood cells take on fresh oxygen, and where carbon dioxide is expelled from the blood. The blood returns to the heart, and begins its next journey round the body.

TOP TIP

Pulse rate

The pumping of the blood under pressure through the carotid arteries can be felt as a pulse in the neck. Press gently on the neck just inside the position of the sternomastoid muscle.

Pulse rate relates to the speed of the heartbeat. The strength of the pulse is affected by the pressure of the blood flow leaving the heart. The heart on average beats 70 times per minute.

Blood pressure increases during activity and decreases during rest.

Relaxing treatments such as facial massage lower blood pressure.

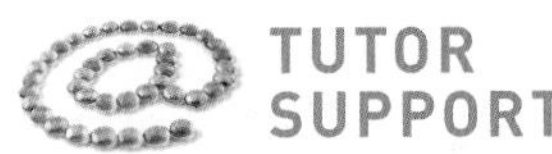

TUTOR SUPPORT

Activity 17: Label the blood supply to and from the head

KNOWLEDGE CHECK

What are the main constituents of blood?

Need more time... refer to page 80 to help you.

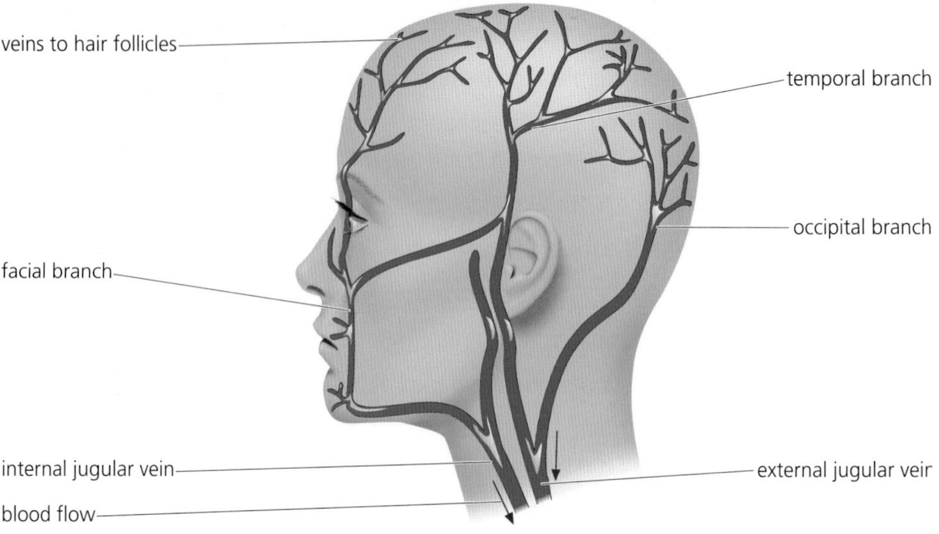

The blood supply from the head

The arteries of the arm and hand

The arm and hand are nourished by a system of arteries that carry oxygen-rich blood to the tissues. You can see the colour of the blood from the capillaries beneath the nail: it is these that give the nail bed its pink colour.

The brachial artery supplies blood to the upper arm. This branches into the ulnar and radial artery which supply the forearm and fingers. The radial and ulnar arteries are connected across the palm by the superficial and deep palmar arches. These arteries divide to form the metacarpal and digital arteries, which supply the palm and fingers.

The veins of the arms and hands Veins deliver deoxygenated blood back to the heart. Blood which has had oxygen removed appears blue. Veins often pass through muscles. Each time muscles contract, veins are squeezed and the blood is pushed along. Massage is particularly beneficial to help this process.

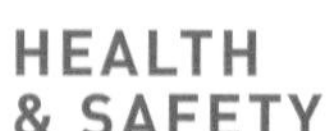

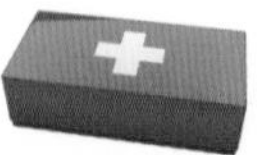

Capillaries

The strength and elasticity of the capillary walls can be damaged, for example by a blow to the tissues. Broken capillaries are capillaries whose elasticity is damaged and they remain constantly dilated with blood.

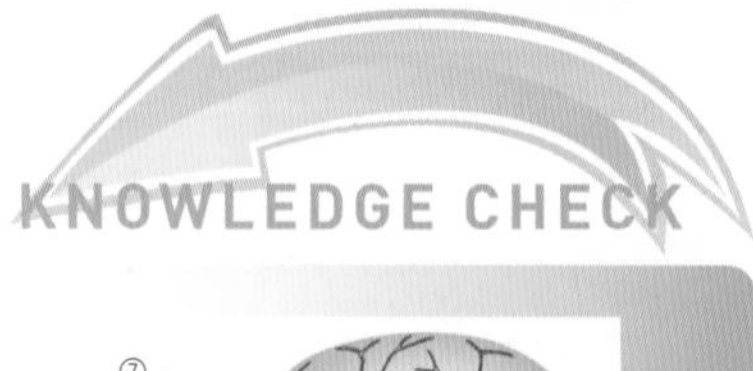

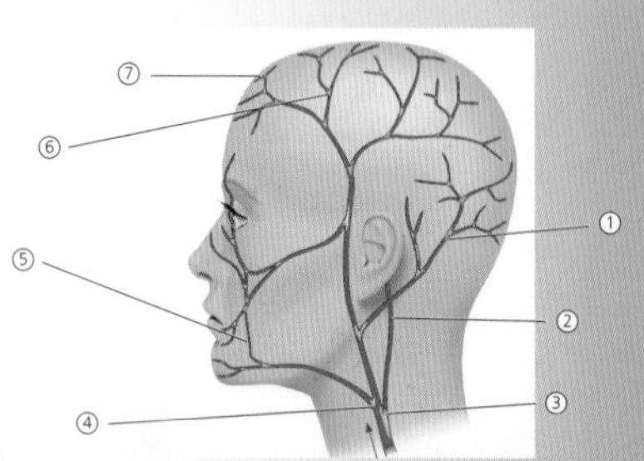

Blood supply to the head

Label the arterties that transport blood to the head.

Need more time... refer to page 81 to help you.

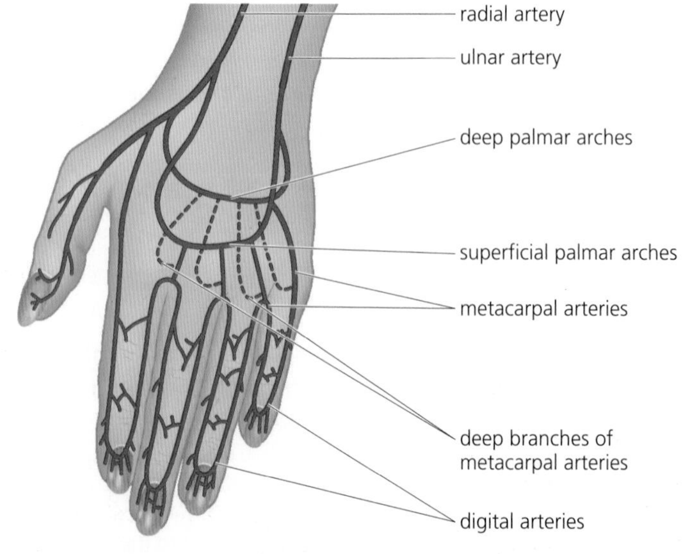

Arteries of the hand

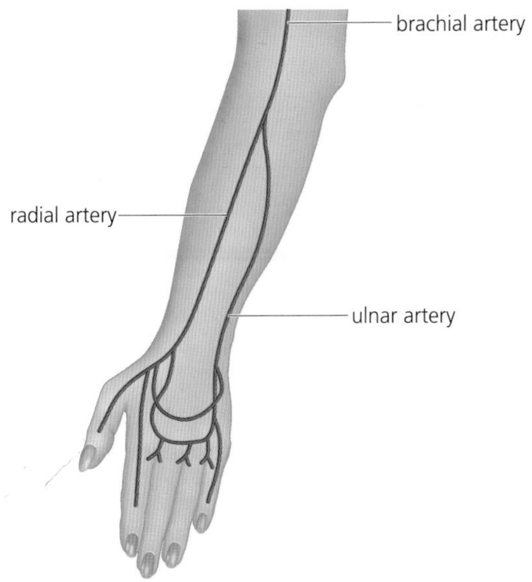

Arteries of the arm

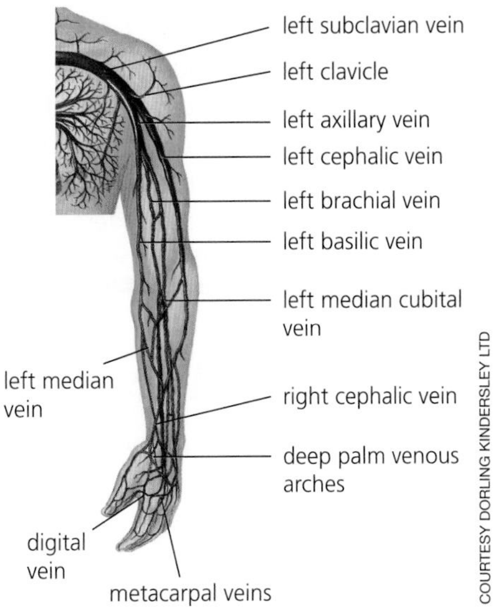

Veins of the arms and hands

Blood in the digital veins drains blood from the fingers. The palmar venous arches drains blood from the hands. The cephalic and basilic veins drain blood from the forearm.

The arteries of the foot and leg

The leg and feet are nourished by a system of arteries that carry oxygen rich blood to the tissues.

In the thigh the external iliac arteries carry blood into the femoral artery. Below the knee the femoral artery branches forming the posterior and anterior tibial artery.

The anterior and tibial artery supplies blood to the lower leg and foot. The peroneal artery branches off the posterior tibial artery. At the ankle the anterior tibial artery becomes the dorsalis pedis artery. The posterior tibial artery divides at the ankle to form the medial and lateral plantar arteries. The plantar and dorsalis pedis arteries supply the digital arteries of the toes.

When it is cold, and when the circulation is poor, insufficient blood reaches the feet and they feel cold. Severe circulation problems in the feet may lead to **chilblains**.

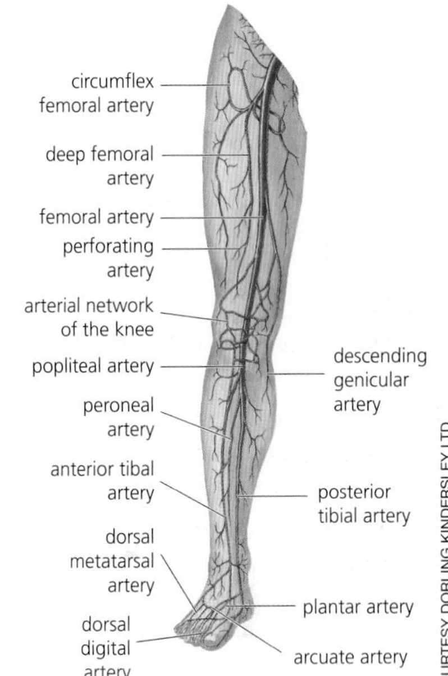

Arteries of the foot and leg

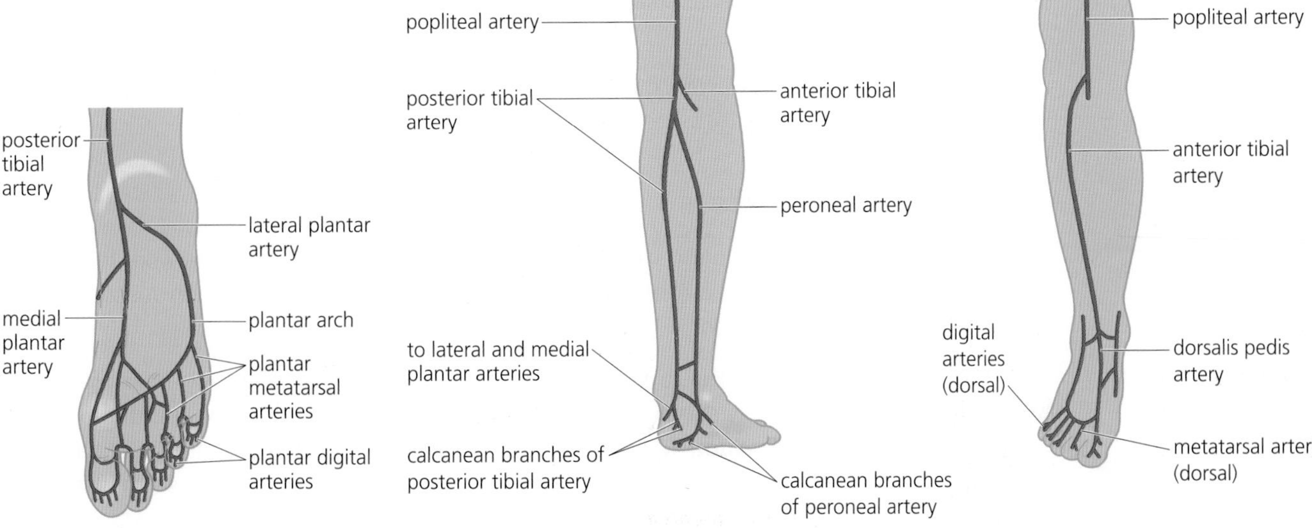

Arteries of the foot

Arteries of the lower leg

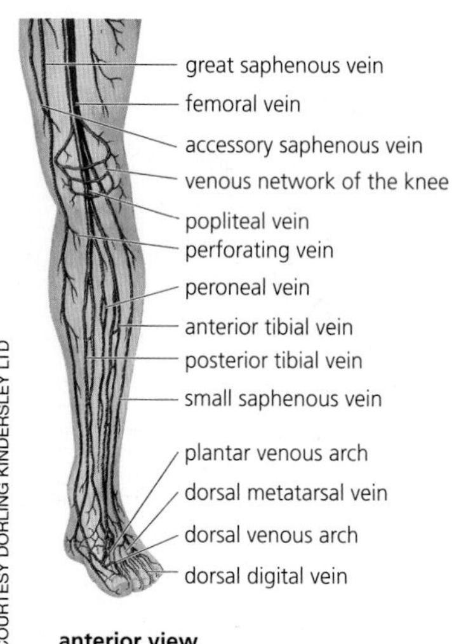

Veins of the foot and leg

The veins of the foot and leg The digital veins from the toes drain into the plantar and dorsal venous arch. The dorsalis pedis veins drain to the saphenous vein. The following deep veins drain the lower leg: the posterior tibial vein at the back of the leg and the peroneal vein, and the anterior tibial vein at the front of the leg. The deep tibial veins join to form the popliteal vein. Above the knee the popliteal vein continues up the back of the thigh as the femoral vein, which enters into the external iliac vein. The blood from the leg returns to the heart in the inferior vena cava.

How are arteries different to veins?

Need more time... refer to page 81 to help you.

The lymphatic system

The **lymphatic system** is closely connected to the blood system, and can be considered as supplementing it. Its primary function is defensive: to remove bacteria and foreign materials, thereby preventing infection. It also drains away excess fluids for elimination from the body.

The lymphatic system consists of the fluid **lymph**, the **lymph vessels** and the **lymph nodes** (or glands). You may have experienced swelling of the lymph nodes in the neck when you have been ill i.e. tonsilitis.

Unlike the blood circulation, the lymphatic system has no muscular pump equivalent to the heart. Instead, the lymph moves through the vessels and around the body because of movements such as contractions of large muscles. Contractions of the body muscles push the lymph through a series of one-way valves. Massage can play an important part in assisting this flow of lymph fluid, thereby encouraging the improved removal of the waste products transported in the lymph.

Lymph

Lymph is a straw-coloured fluid, derived from blood plasma, which has filtered through the walls of the capillaries. Lymph drains into a network of lymph capillaries and then into larger vessels known as lymphatics which contain special filters called nodes or glands. The composition of lymph is similar to that of blood, though less oxygen and fewer nutrients are available. In the spaces between the cells where there are no blood capillaries, lymph provides nourishment. It also carries **lymphocytes** (a type of white blood cell), which play an important role in the immune system. They can destroy dangerous cells and disease-causing bacteria and viruses directly before they return to the bloodstream.

Lymph travels only in one direction: from body tissues back towards the heart.

Lymph vessels

Lymph vessels often run very close to veins, forming an extensive network throughout the body. The lymph moves quite slowly, and the valves along the lymph vessels prevent backflow of the lymph.

The lymph vessels join to form larger lymph vessels, which eventually flow into one or other of two large lymphatic vessels: the **thoracic duct** (or **left lymphatic duct**) and the **right lymphatic duct**. The thoracic duct receives lymph from the left side of the head, neck, chest, abdomen and lower body; the right lymphatic duct receives lymph from the right side of the head and upper body.

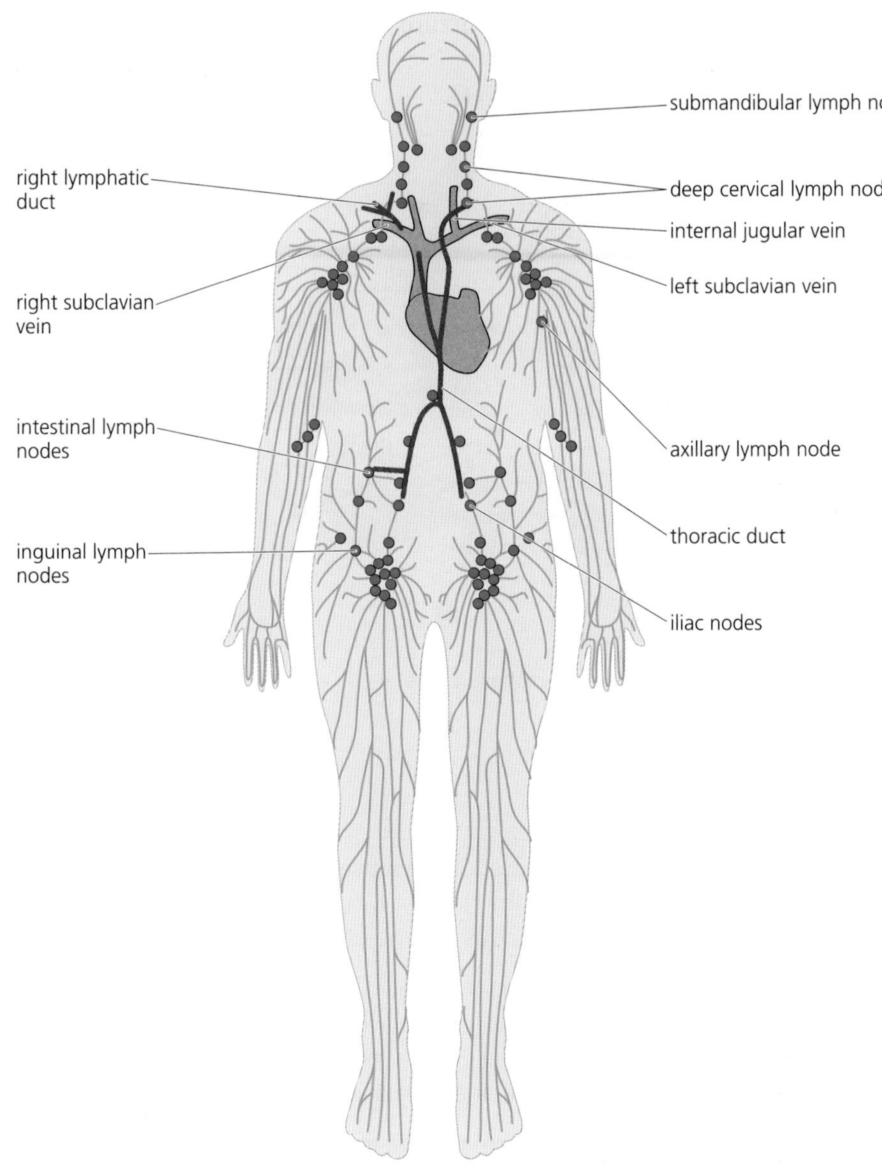

Lymph vessels and nodes (glands) in the body

These principal lymphatic vessels then empty their contents into a vein at the base of the neck, which in turn empties into the **vena cava**. The lymph is mixed into the venous blood as it is returned to the heart.

Lymph nodes

Lymph nodes or **glands** are tiny oval structures between 1mm and 25mm in length, made from lymphatic tissue encased in a fibrous capsule which filters the lymph, extracting poisons, pus and bacteria, and thus defending the body against infection by destroying harmful organisms. When we suffer an infection, the lymph nodes closest to the site of infection may swell up and become tender as the white cells attempt to destroy the germs. They are located along the routes of the principal lymphatic vessels. Lymph enters a node through an **afferent** vessel and leaves through an **efferent** vessel. **Lymphocytes** and macrophages, found in the lymph glands, are special cells which produce **antibodies** which enable us to resist invasion by microorganisms, preventing disease.

Lymph filters through at least one lymph node before returning to the bloodstream.

ALWAYS REMEMBER

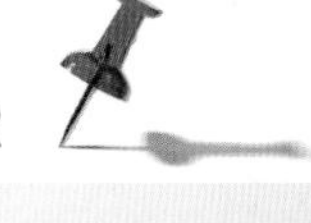

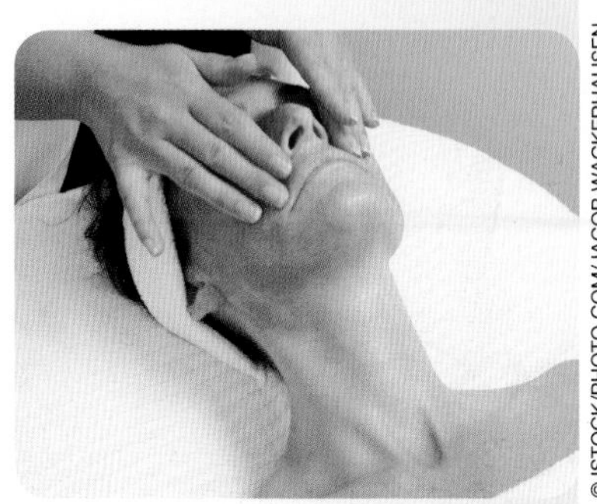

An effect of facial massage is to increase blood and lymphatic circulation in the area

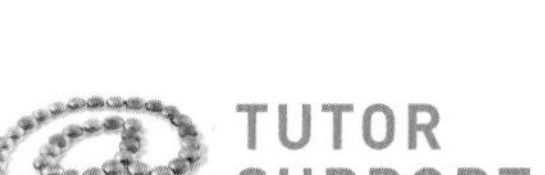

TUTOR SUPPORT

Activity 16: Label the lymph nodes of the body

KNOWLEDGE CHECK

What are the main constituents of lymph?

Need more time... refer to page 84 to help you.

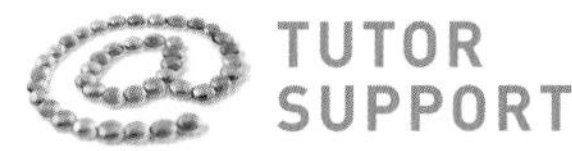

TUTOR SUPPORT

Activity 19: A&P wordsearch

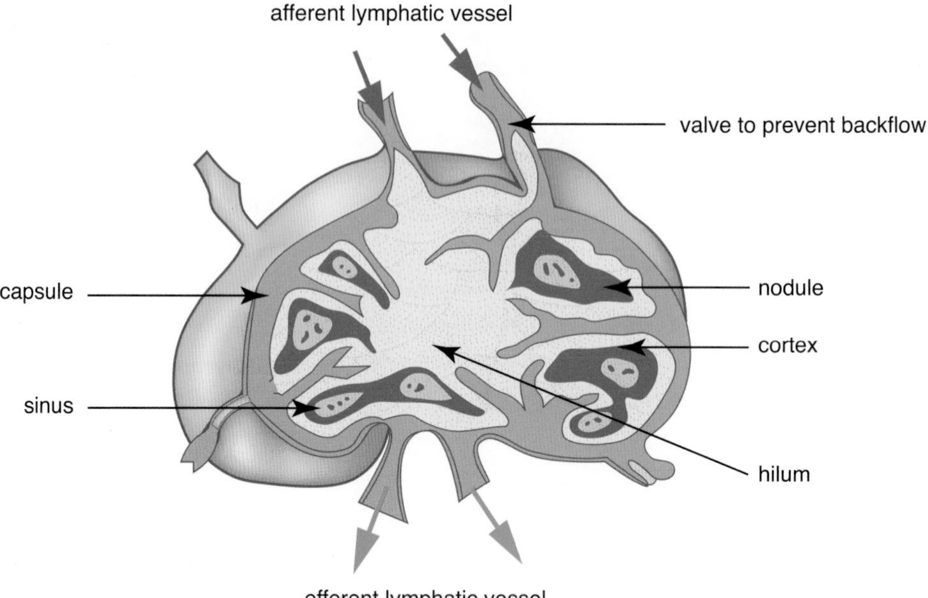

Lymph node

LEARNER SUPPORT

A&P mini crossword

When performing massage, the hands should be used when appropriate to apply pressure to direct the lymph towards the nearest lymph node: this encourages the speedy removal of waste products. Various groups of lymph nodes drain the lymph of the head and neck.

Lymph nodes of the head

- The buccal group drains the eyelids, the nose and the skin of the face.
- The mandibular group drains the chin, the lips, the nose and the cheeks.
- The **mastoid group** drains the skin of the ear and the temple area.
- The **occipital group** drains the back of the scalp and the upper neck.
- The **submental group** drains the chin and the lower lip.
- The **parotid group** drains the nose, eyelids and ears.

Lymph nodes of the neck

- The **superficial cervical group** drains the back of the head and the neck.
- The **lower deep cervical group** drains the back area of the scalp and the neck.

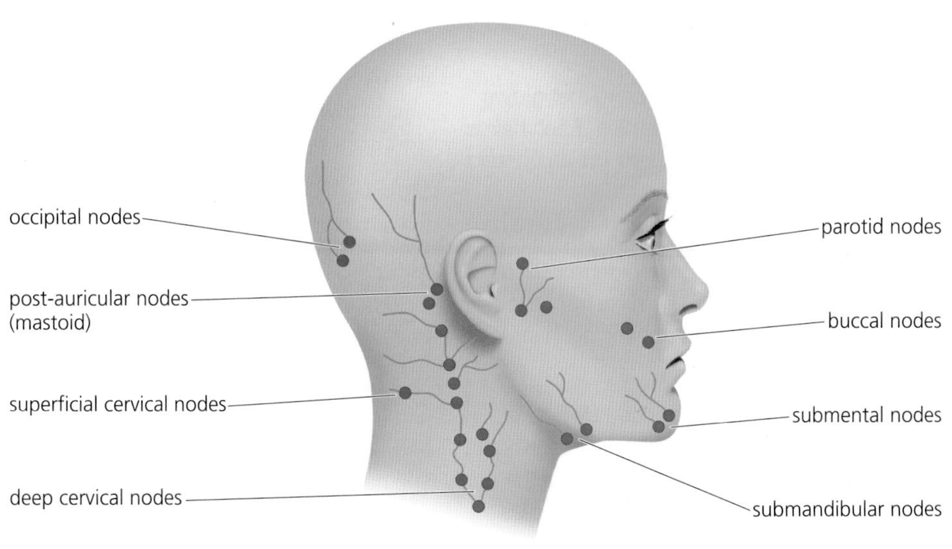

Lymph nodes of the head and neck

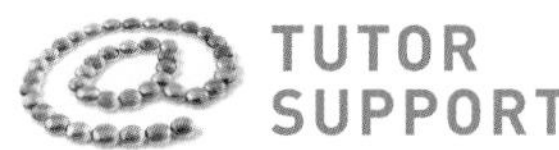

Activity 15: Label the lymph nodes of the head

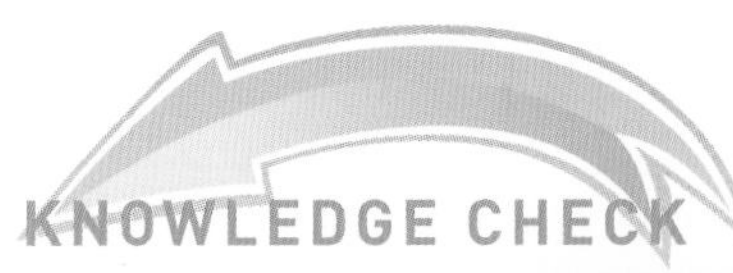

What are the functions of lymph nodes and glands?

Need more time... refer to page 85 to help you.

Lymph nodes of the chest and arms The nodes of the armpit area drain various regions of the arms and chest.

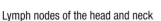

TOP TIP

Frontal–Temporal–Parietal–Occipital–Mandible (mandibular)–Cervical

Learn and remember these names of the main regions of the head and neck. Not only will this assist you in recalling the names and locations of the bones, it will also help you greatly with the names and locations of muscles, arteries, veins, nerves and lymph nodes.

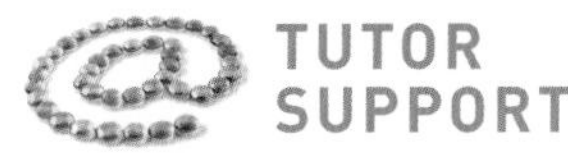

Activity 20: Multiple choice quiz

GLOSSARY OF KEY WORDS

Anagen the active growth stage of the hair growth cycle.

Apocrine gland sweat gland found in the armpit, nipple and groin area. Larger than the eccrine sweat gland and attached to the hair follicle. These sweat glands are controlled by hormones and become active at puberty.

Arrector pili muscle a small muscle attached to the hair follicle and base of the epidermis. When the muscle contracts (shortens) it causes the hair to stand upright in the hair follicle.

Blood nutritive liquid circulating through the blood vessels. It transports essential nutrients to the cells and removes waste products. It also transports other important substances such as oxygen and hormones.

Blood vessel transports blood through the body in either an artery or a vein. An artery transports blood away from the heart at high pressure, the vein returns blood to the heart at low pressure.

Bone the hardest structure in the body. A type of tissue that protects the underlying structures, gives shape to the body and provides an attachment point for muscles.

Bones of the chest connective tissue that protects the inner organs, and provides a surface for muscle attachment that allows movement and includes the sternum.

Bones of the foot and lower leg connective tissue that provides a surface for muscle attachment. These include in the foot the tarsals, metatarsal and phalanxes. In the lower leg the tibia and fibula.

Bones of the lower arm and hand connective tissue that provide a surface for muscle attachment. These include in the lower arm the radius and ulna. In the hand the carpals, metacarpals and phalanges.

Bones of the neck connective tissue that supports the skull and includes the cervical vertebrae.

Catagen the stage of the hair growth cycle where the hair becomes detached from its source of nourishment, the dermal papilla, and stops growing.

Cell basic units of life which specialize in carrying out particular functions in the body. Groups of cells which share function, shape, size or structure are called tissues. The human body consists of trillions of cells.

Circulatory system transports material around the body.

Collagen protein fibre found in the dermis of the skin that gives the skin its strength.

Cortex the thickest layer of the hair structure.

Cyclical pattern of growth the hair growth cycle, which can be divided into three phases: anagen, catagen and telegen.

Dermal papilla an organ that provides the hair with blood, necessary for hair growth.

Dermis the inner portion of skin situated underneath the epidermis.

Ear the external or outer part of the ear collects sound waves and directs these to the inner ear. This part of the ear that stands out at the side of the head is called the pinna, which comprizes of the helix and lobule.

Eccrine gland simple sweat producing gland responsive to heat, appearing as tiny tubes which are straight in the epidermis, and coiled in the dermis. Its function is to maintain the body temperature by sweating.

Elastin protein fibre found in the dermis of the skin which gives the skin its elasticity.

Epidermis the outer layer of the skin.

External ear structure funnels sound waves into the ear to enable hearing. It comprises the pinna, lobe, cartilage and cartilaginous tissue.

Facial bones connective tissue that forms the face and is an attachment point for muscles. Facial bones include the zygomatic, mandible, maxilla, nasal, vomer, turbinate, lacrimal and palatine.

Hair a long slender structure that grows out of, and is part of, the skin. Each hair is made up of dead skin cells, which contain the protein called keratin.

Hair follicle an appendage (structure) in the skin formed from epidermal tissue. Cells move up the hair follicle from the bottom (the hair bulb), changing in structure, to form the hair.

Keratin a protein produced by cells in the epidermis called keratinocytes. Keratin makes the skin tough and reduces the passage of substances into our bodies. Each hair and nail contains keratin.

Lymph a clear, straw-coloured liquid circulating in the lymph vessels and lymphatics of the body, filtered out of the blood plasma.

Lymphatic system closely connected to the blood system. Its primary function is defensive: to remove bacteria and foreign materials to prevent infection.

Lymph vessel referred to as lymphatics. They transport lymph from the tissues to the blood.

Melanin a pigment in the skin and hair that contributes to skin and hair colour.

Melanocytes cells that produce the skin pigment melanin that contributes to skin colour.

Muscle contractile tissue responsible for movement of the body.

Muscle tone the normal degree of tension in healthy muscle.

Muscles of facial expression muscles which when contracted, pull the facial skin in a particular way and create facial expressions. These include the frontalis, corrugators, temporalis, orbicularis oculi, levator labii, orbicularis oris, buccinators, risorius, mentalis, zygomaticus, masseter, depressor labii.

Muscles of the foot and lower leg the muscles of the foot work together to help move the body. The foot is moved by muscles in the lower leg which pull on tendons that attach the muscle to the bone.

Muscles of the lower arm and hand the hands and fingers are moved by muscles and tendons. The muscles that bend the wrist in towards the forearm are flexors; the extensors straighten the wrist and hand.

Muscles of the upper body these move the arm and include pectoralis and deltoid.

Muscles that move the neck these include sternocleido mastoid, platysma, trapezius.

Nail growth cells divide in the matrix and the nails grow forward over the nail bed until they reach the end of the finger. The nail cells harden as they grow through a process called keratinization.

Nail structure composed for protection the nail is made up of the following parts: nail plate, nail bed, matrix, cuticle, lunula, hyponychium, eponychium, nail wall, free edge, lateral nail fold.

Nail the structure on the end of each finger and toe formed from hard, horny, epidermal cells that protect the living nail bed of fingers and toes.

Nerve a collection of single neurones surrounded by a protective sheath through which impulses are transmitted between the brain or spinal cord and another part of the body.

Neurones nerve cells which make up nervous tissue.

Nervous system co-ordinates the activities of the body by responding to stimuli received by sense organs.

Pigment the skin's and hair's colour, called melanin. The amount of pigment varies for each client, resulting in different skin/hair colour.

Sebaceous gland a minute sac-like organ usually associated with the hair follicle. The cells of the gland decompose and produce the skin's natural oil sebum. Found all over the body, except for the soles of the feet and the palms of the hands.

Sebum the skin's natural oil, which keeps the skin supple.

Sensory nerve endings these nerves receive information and relay this to the brain. They are found near the skin's surface and respond to touch, pressure, temperature and pain.

(Hair) Shaft the part of the hair that can be seen above the skin's surface, extending from the hair follicle.

Shoulder girdle bones connective tissue that provides attachment for the muscles which move the arms, and includes the clavicle and scapula.

Skin appendages structures within the skin including sweat glands (that excrete sweat), hair follicles (that produce hair), sebaceous glands (produce the skin's natural oil, sebum) and nails (a horny substance that protects the ends of the fingers/toes).

Skin characteristics while looking at the skin type, the skin's additional characteristics may be seen. These include skin that may be sensitive, dehydrated, moist or oedematous (puffy).

Sweat gland or sudoriferous glands are composed of a specialized lining tissue called epithelial tissue. Their function is to control body temperature through the evaporation of sweat from the surface of the skin.

Skin type the different physiological functioning of each person's skin dictates their skin type. There are four main skin types: normal (balanced), dry (lacking in oil), oily (excessive oil) and combination (a mixture of two skin types, e.g. dry or oily).

Skull bones a type of connective tissue forming a hard structure. It surrounds and protects the brain and forms an attachment point for muscles. These include the occipital, frontal, parietal, temporal, sphenoid and ethmoid.

Subcutaneous layer a layer of fatty tissue situated below the epidermis and dermis.

Telogen the resting stage of the hair growth cycle, when the hair is finally shed.

Terminal hair deep-rooted, thick, coarse, pigmented hair found on the scalp, underarms, pubic region, eyelash and brow areas.

Tissues cells in the body which specialize in carrying out particular functions. These include epithelial, connective, muscular and nervous tissue.

Vellus hair fine, downy and soft hair – found on the face and body.

Vitamin D a fatty substance in the skin converted to vitamin D with UV light from the sun. Vitamin D circulates in the blood and, with the mineral salts calcium and phosphorus, helps the formation and maintenance of the health of the body's bones.

ASSESSMENT OF KNOWLEDGE AND UNDERSTANDING

You have now learnt about anatomy and physiology in the beauty therapy workplace. To test your level of knowledge, answer the following short questions. These will prepare you for your summative (final) assessment.

1. The tissue that contracts and moves the various parts of the body is:
   a. connective
   b. epithelial
   c. liquid
   d. muscular

2. The muscle attached to the lower surface of the heel and pulls the foot down is the:
   a. gastrocnemius
   b. soleus
   c. peroneus brevis
   d. peroneus logus

3. The flat bone that protects the inner organs located between the ribs on the anterior view of the body is the (sternum) bone.
   a. thorax
   b. scapula
   c. hyoid
   d. sternum

4. List the primary functions of the skeletal system:
   a. Give shape and support to the body
   b. Protect various internal organs
   c. Serve as attachments for muscles
   d. Help produce blood cells

5. Match the following bones of the face with its correct description:

1) nasal	a) largest and strongest facial forms the lower jawbone
2) zygomatic	b) form the cheekbones
3) maxillae	c) form the bridge of the nose
4) mandible	d) bones of the upper jaw

6. The system that is also referred to as the cardiovascular system and controls the steady circulation of the blood flow is:
   a. muscular
   b. skeletal
   c. circulatory
   d. nervous

7. The thick-walled, muscular, flexible tubes that carry oxygenated blood away from the heart are the:

a. capillaries
b. arteries
c. veins
d. vessels

8. The arteries that are located on either side of the neck and are the main sources of blood supply to the head, face and neck are the __________ arteries. The internal carotid artery enters the head and supplies blood to the _______________. The external carotid artery supplies blood through it branches to the outside of the skull _____________. The _______ and _______ arteries are the main blood supply for the arms and hands.

9. Label the parts of the nail.

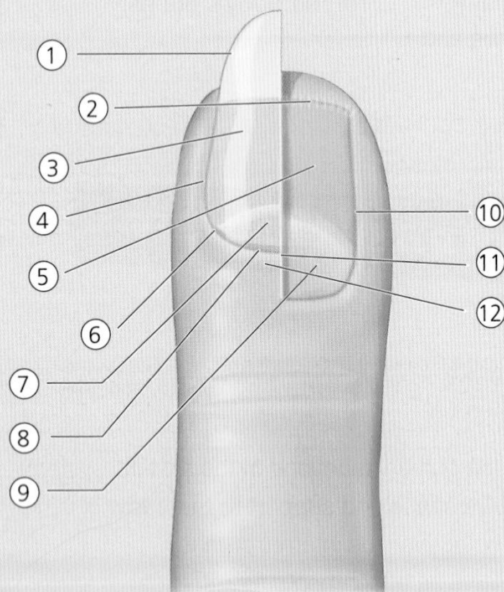

10. The growth of the nail plate is affected by what?

11. The appendages of the skin include:

a.
b.
c.
d.

12. The sebaceous or oil glands of the skin are connected to the what?

13. The reticular layer contains the following structures within its structure:

a.
b.
c.
d.
e.
f.

14. Label the cross-section of the hair follicle.

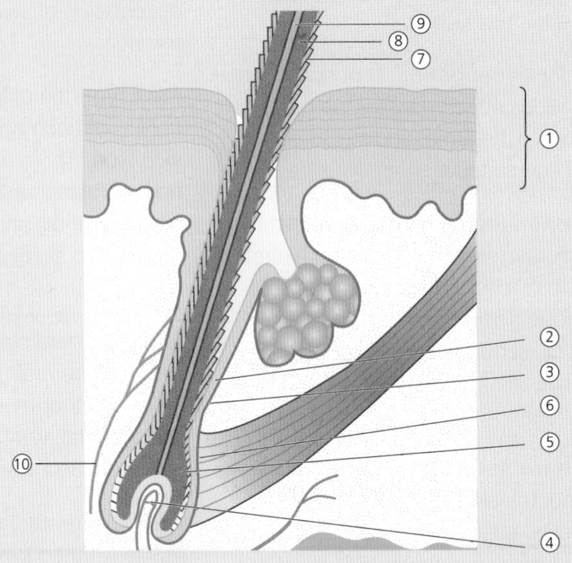

15. Match the following ear parts with its correct description:

1) helix	a) The part of the ear that stands out from the sides of the head
2) pinna	b) Made up of fibrous fatty tissue with no cartilage, it forms the lower part of the earlobe
3) lobule	c) Made up of cartilage tissue, it forms the upper part of the ear lobe

16. Label the lymph nodes of the head.

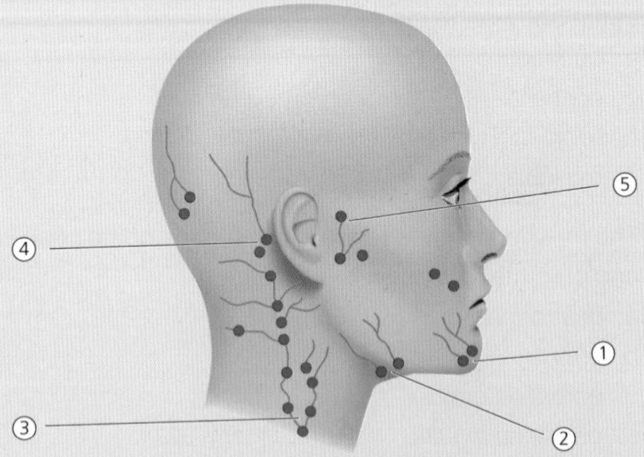

3 Health and Safety

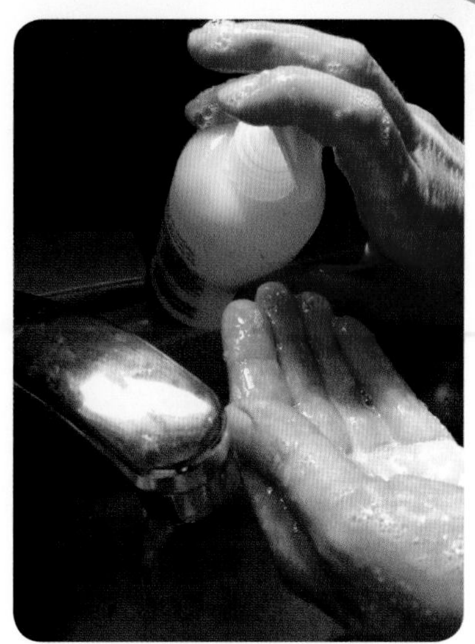

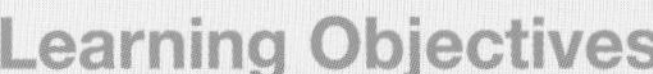

Learning Objectives

This chapter covers **VRQ Unit Follow health and safety practice in the salon.**

This unit is all about knowing what makes a safe working environment and how safe working practices are implemented to ensure the safety of yourself, clients and colleagues. The chapter covers health and safety, security and emergency duties and responsibilities for everyone in the workplace.

You will assessed whilst performing health and safety practice in the salon.

Health and safety practice should be considered at all times within all work areas.

There are **two** learning outcomes for this unit which you must achieve:

1 **Be able to maintain health, safety and security practices**

2 **Be able to follow emergency procedures**

From the range statement, you must show that you can:

- deal with **hazards** within own area of responsibility
- maintain appropriate level of **personal presentation**
- follow salon policy for **security**
- use required **personal protective equipment (PPE)**
- describe and dispose of all types of **salon waste**
- outline the main provisions of **health and safety legislation**
- state the **employers' and employees' health and safety responsibilities**
- state the **difference between a hazard and a risk**

(continued on the next page)

International hazard symbols

HSE

- describe the **methods used in the salon to ensure hygiene**
- identify named **emergency personnel**
- state the dangers of the incorrect **use of fire fighting equipment on different types of fires**
- describe **procedures for dealing with emergencies**

You must be able to show you have the necessary practical skills and underpinning knowledge to follow health and safety practice in the salon.

This unit is linked to the Beauty Therapy NOS **Unit G20.**

Outcome 1: Be able to maintain health, safety and security practices

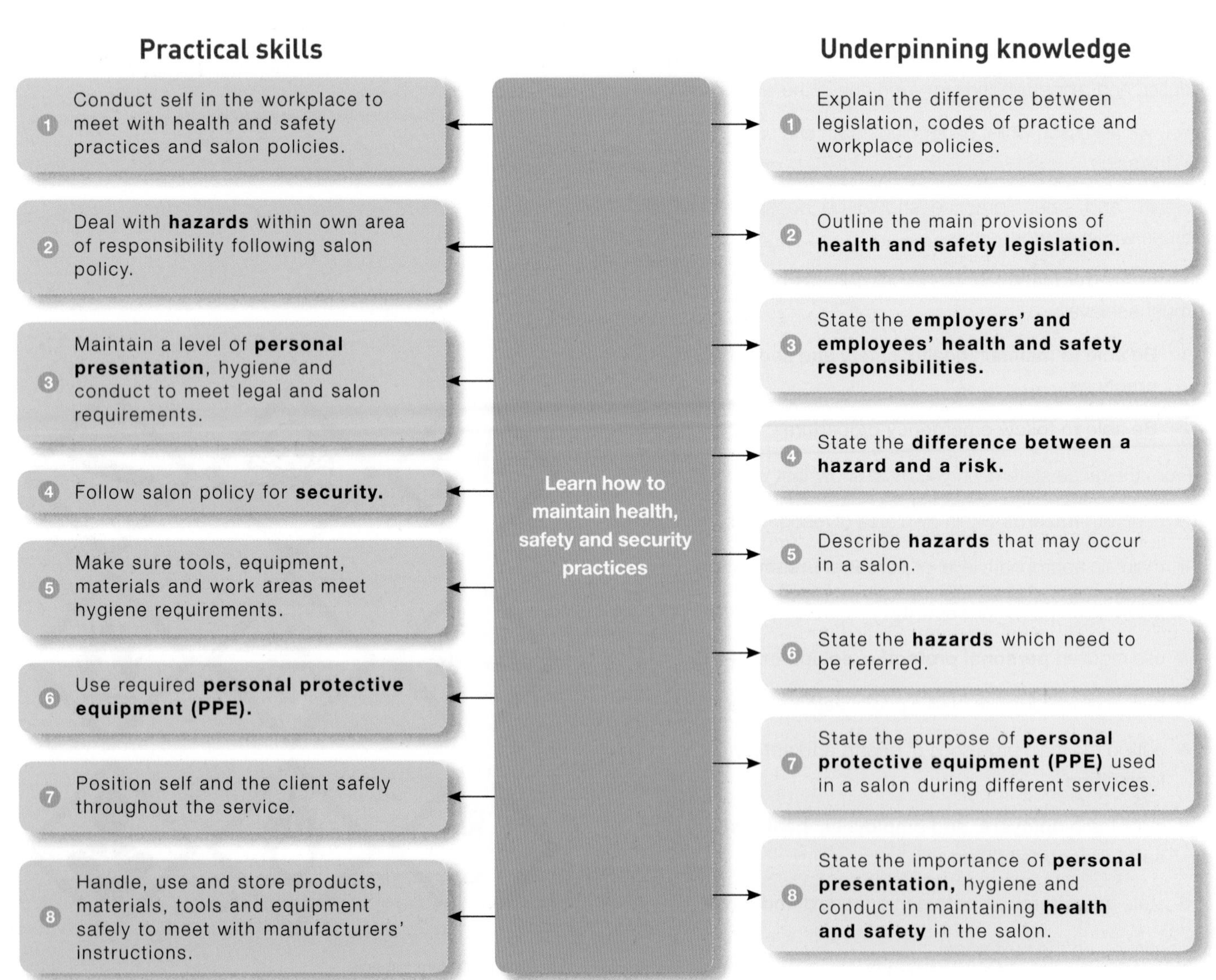

Practical skills
Underpinning knowledge
Learn how to maintain health, safety and security practices
1 Conduct self in the workplace to meet with health and safety practices and salon policies.
2 Deal with hazards within own area of responsibility following salon policy.
3 Maintain a level of personal presentation, hygiene and conduct to meet legal and salon requirements.
4 Follow salon policy for security.
5 Make sure tools, equipment, materials and work areas meet hygiene requirements.
6 Use required personal protective equipment (PPE).
7 Position self and the client safely throughout the service.
8 Handle, use and store products, materials, tools and equipment safely to meet with manufacturers' instructions.
1 Explain the difference between legislation, codes of practice and workplace policies.
2 Outline the main provisions of health and safety legislation.
3 State the employers' and employees' health and safety responsibilities.
4 State the difference between a hazard and a risk.
5 Describe hazards that may occur in a salon.
6 State the hazards which need to be referred.
7 State the purpose of personal protective equipment (PPE) used in a salon during different services.
8 State the importance of personal presentation, hygiene and conduct in maintaining health and safety in the salon.

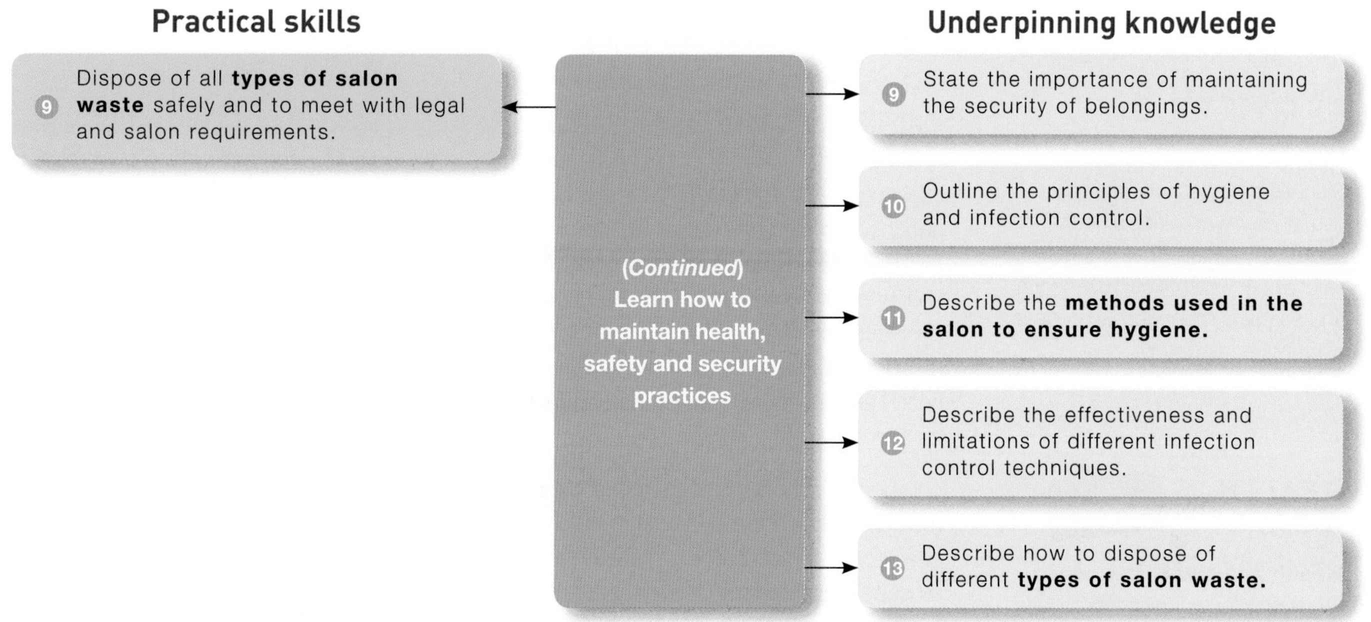

Practical skills
9 Dispose of all **types of salon waste** safely and to meet with legal and salon requirements.
(Continued) Learn how to maintain health, safety and security practices
Underpinning knowledge
9 State the importance of maintaining the security of belongings.
10 Outline the principles of hygiene and infection control.
11 Describe the **methods used in the salon to ensure hygiene.**
12 Describe the effectiveness and limitations of different infection control techniques.
13 Describe how to dispose of different **types of salon waste.**

Taking care of all in the workplace

When working in a service industry, you are legally required to provide a **safe, secure and hygienic environment**. This applies wherever you are working: in a hotel, a spa, a department store or a beauty salon. Even when operating a freelance beauty therapy service, you must pay careful attention when in clients' homes: it is essential to follow all health and safety guidelines, just as you would when working in a salon.

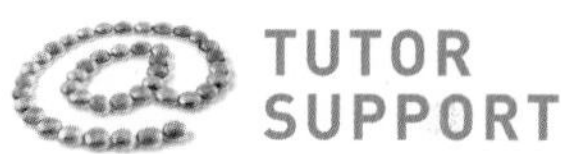

Activity 6: Health and safety wordsearch

Legal responsibilities

If you cause harm to your client, or put a client at **risk**, you will be held responsible and you will be liable for **prosecution**, with the possibility of being fined.

There is a good deal of **legislation** relating to health and safety. You will need to know the laws relating to your work role and you must be aware of your rights and responsibilities.

You will need an awareness and understanding of all of the following legislation:

Health and Safety at Work Act, Personal Protective Equipment at Work Regulations, Workplace (Health, Safety and Welfare) Regulations, Manual Handling Operations Regulations, Control of Substances, Hazardous to Health Regulations (COSHH), Provision and use of Work Equipment Regulations, Electricity at Work Regulations, Reporting injuries, Diseases and Dangerous Occurrences (RIDDOR), Fire Precautions Act, Health and Safety First Aid Regulations, Health and Safety (Display Screen Equipment) Regulations.

This chapter will outline the main provisions of health and safety legislation.

It is a good idea to obtain and read all relevant publications from your local Health and Safety Executive (HSE) offices. The HSE provides guidance and information on all aspects of health and safety legislation. Information can also be accessed online.

In addition, as the standards-setting body for beauty therapy, the hair and beauty industry authority Habia provide health and safety working guidelines and legislative requirements. **Codes of practice** are available from Habia, sharing best and mandatory working practice approved by both industry experts and health and safety advisors. Approved codes of practice are recognized by the HSE.

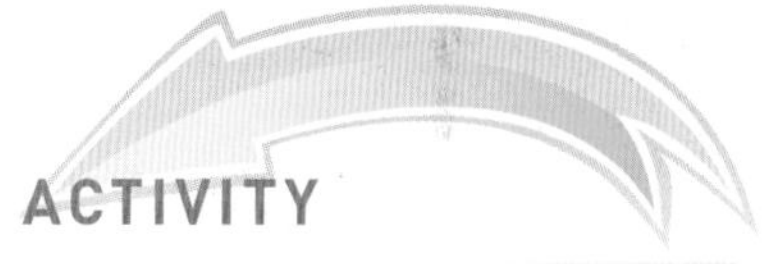

Keep up to date

Health and safety information is continually updated. Write to your local Health and Safety Executive (HSE) office (www.hse.gov.uk) or Local Authority Environmental Health Department, the bodies appointed to support and enforce health and safety law, to ask for a pack of relevant health and safety information. Legislation relevant to business operations can also be found in the Health and Safety pack for salons.

Visit www.habia.org to research current beauty therapy health and safety legislation and minimum requirements.

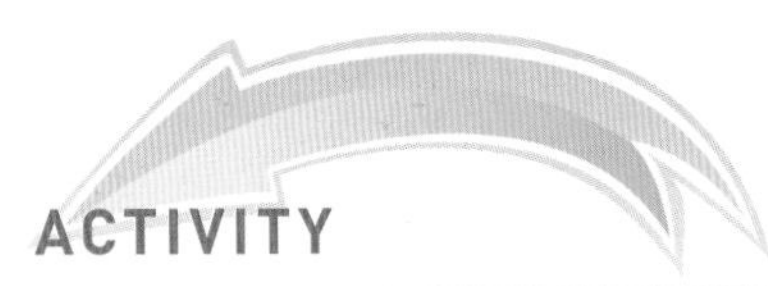

ACTIVITY

Health and safety rules
Discuss the rules which apply to you in your workplace's health and safety policy. The health and safety policy identifies how health and safety is managed: who does what, when and why.

HEALTH & SAFETY

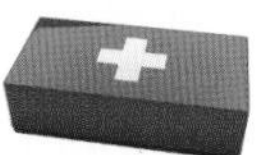

Health and safety law notice
Every employer is obliged by law to display a health and safety law poster in the workplace. This explains the responsibilities of employers and also employees, what action to take if a health and safety problem arises and employment rights. A leaflet is available called 'Your health and safety – a guide for workers'. Both poster and leaflets are available from the HSE.

HEALTH & SAFETY

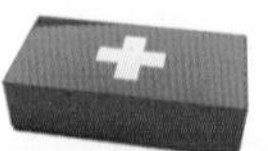

Lone workers
If you are self employed and work alone, consider your safety. Guidance is provided in the information 'Working alone: health and safety guidance on the risks of lone working', INDG73 (rev2).

Health and safety legislation

The Health and Safety at Work Act (1974) (HASAWA) The **Health and Safety at Work Act (1974)** is continually reviewed and is the main piece of legislation affecting health and safety issues. It was developed from experience gained over 150 years and incorporates any earlier legislation, including the Offices, Shops and Railway Premises Act (1963) and the Fire Precautions Act (1971). It lays down the minimum standards of health, safety and welfare required in each area of the workplace. For example, it requires business premises and equipment to be safe and in good repair. It is the employer's legal responsibility to implement the Act and to ensure, so far as is reasonably practicable, the health and safety at work of the people for whom they are responsible and those who may be affected by the work they do. This will include clients and any visitors to the workplace.

The Local Authority Environmental Health Department appoints inspectors called Environmental Health Officers (EHOs) to enforce health and safety law by visiting the workplace to check compliance is being met with all relevant health and safety legislation. Your business must be registered with the relevant enforcing authority. Workplace Contract Officers (WCOs) are available to provide advice and guidance and gather relevant data in relation to health and safety of your business.

The Health and Safety (Information for Employees) Regulations (1989) (HSIER) were amended in April 2009. Employers are required to provide information relating to health, safety and welfare in the workplace by displaying a copy of the approved health and safety poster or providing a copy of the leaflet.

Each employer of more than five employees must formulate a written **health and safety policy** for their business. Habia have resources providing guidance on creating a written policy. The health and safety policy identifies how health and safety is managed for that business, who does what, when and why. The policy must be issued and discussed with each employee at induction and should outline the health and safety responsibilities they should undertake. It should also include items such as:

- details of the storage of chemical substances
- details of the stock cupboard or dispensary
- details and records of the checks made by a qualified electrician on specialist electrical equipment
- names and addresses of key holders
- escape routes and emergency evacuation procedures
- whom to report emergencies and significant risks to.

The health and safety policy should be reviewed regularly to ensure it continues to meet all relevant legislation guidelines including any updates. Health and safety training should also be carried out regularly and recorded. Regular health and safety checks should be made and procedures reviewed to ensure that safety is being satisfactorily maintained.

Hazards and risks

Employees must always cooperate with their employer to provide a safe, secure and healthy workplace. As soon as an employee observes a **hazard** (anything that has potential to cause harm) this must be reported to the relevant responsible person so that the problem can be put right. Risk is the likelihood of a hazard's potential being realized. Hazards include:

- obstructions to corridors, stairways and fire exits (an obstruction is anything that blocks the traffic route in the salon work environment)
- spillages and breakages
- trailing wires
- faulty electrical equipment.

You should use your initiative and deal with low risk hazards within your responsibility, following workplace policy and legal requirements.

If there are fewer than five employees, appropriate health and safety arrangements and procedures should be in place. In 1992, European Union (EU) directives updated the legislation on health and safety management. Current legislation (at the time of writing) is outlined below.

The Health and Safety at Work Act covers many other smaller regulations also which are discussed.

Health and safety rules and regulations and examples of compliance to be displayed include:

- fire evacuation procedures
- public liability insurance certificate
- Health and Safety (Information for Employees) Regulations (1989) poster, updated April 2009 (the previous poster can continue to be displayed until 2014).
- health and safety policy (dependent upon employee numbers)
- risk assessment records and guidance.

HEALTH & SAFETY 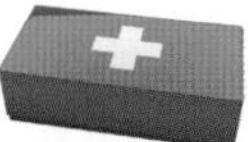

Non-smoking legislation
An example of the need to be responsive to safe working conditions and practices is the non-smoking legislation in the workplace, introduced 1 July 2007.

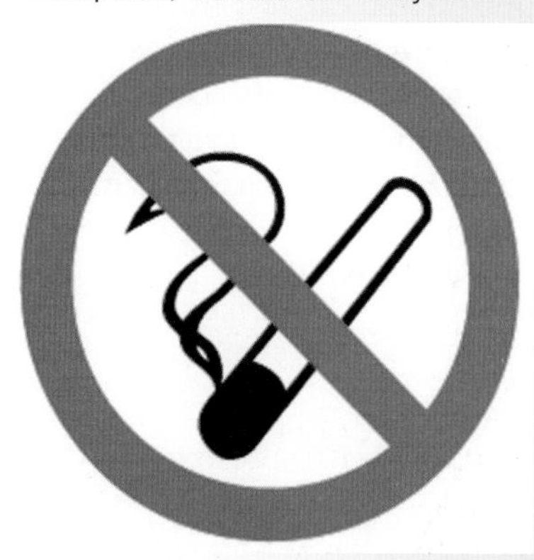

No smoking sign

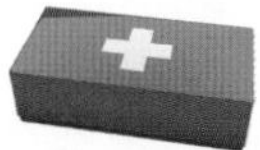

TUTOR SUPPORT

Activity 2: Accident report form

HEALTH & SAFETY 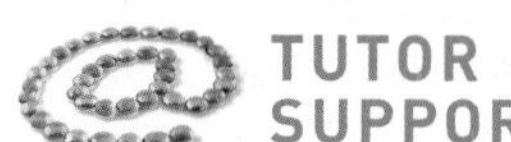

Five steps to risk assessment
This is an HSE publication providing guidance on risk assessment.

Inspection and registration of premises

Inspectors from the HSE or your local authority enforce the health and safety laws. They visit the workplace to ensure compliance with government legislation.

If the inspector identifies any hazards, it is the responsibility of the employer to remove the hazard within a designated period of time. The inspector issues an **improvement notice**. Failure to comply with the notice will lead to prosecution. The inspector also has the authority to close a business or stop a particular activity until they are satisfied that all potential danger to employees and public has been removed. A closure involves the issuing of a **prohibition notice**.

Certain services carried out in beauty therapy, such as ear piercing, pose additional risk because they might produce blood and body tissue fluid. Inspection of the premises is necessary before such services can be offered to the public. The inspector will visit to make sure that the guidelines listed in the Local Government (Miscellaneous Provisions) Act (1982) relating to this area are being complied with in terms of levels of hygiene and training. Good infection control systems are essential and the working environment must be suitable. When the inspector is satisfied, a certificate of registration will be awarded.

The Personal Protective Equipment (PPE) at Work Regulations (2002) The Personal Protective Equipment (PPE) at Work Regulations (1992) require employers to identify – through a **risk assessment** – those activities or processes which require special protective clothing or equipment to be worn. This clothing and equipment must then be made available, and must be suitable and in adequate

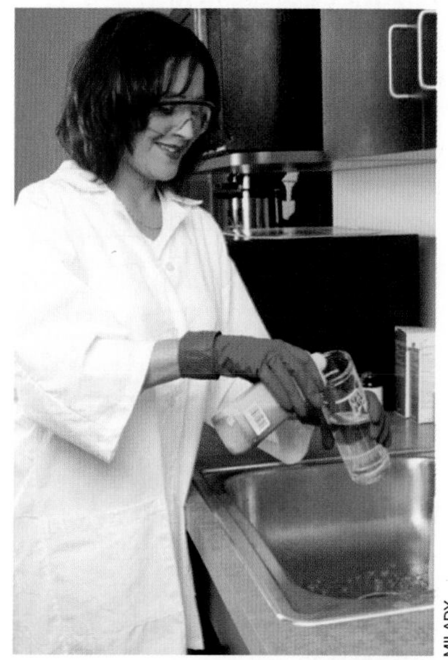

MILADY

PPE for handling chemicals

HEALTH & SAFETY

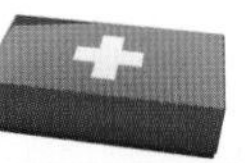

Protective equipment: gloves
If you are to come into contact with body tissue fluids or with chemicals, wear protective disposable surgical gloves. Latex gloves can cause allergic reactions and in some cases the development of asthma, and are not recommended.
An alternative glove that provides adequate protection from contamination should be used, e.g. nitrile or PVC formulation.

KNOWLEDGE CHECK

What is a hazard?

What is a risk?

Need more time... refer to pages 94–95 to help you.

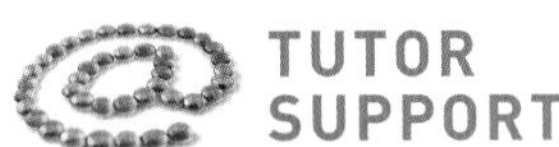

TUTOR SUPPORT

Activity 3: Risk assessment form

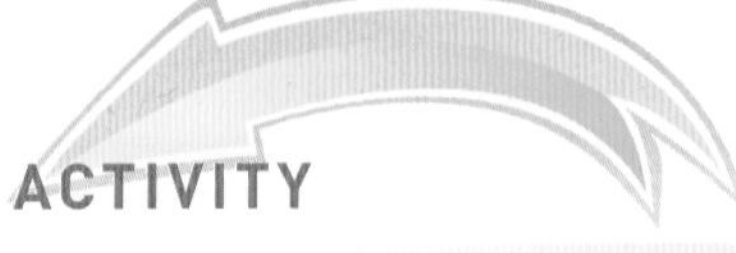

ACTIVITY

PPE Risk assessment
Carry out your own risk assessment on risks of cross-infection by contamination. List the potentially hazardous substances that you may be required to handle. What protective clothing should be available?

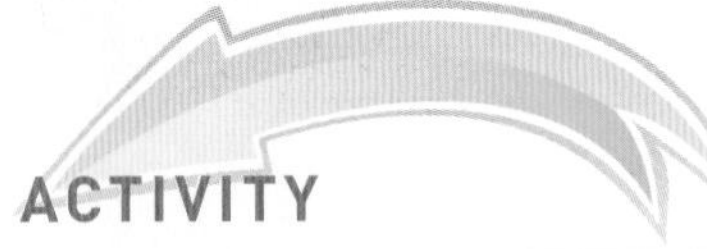

ACTIVITY

Moving objects in the salon
What equipment or objects may you be required to move in the salon? Think of three examples and how best they should be lifted and handled.

supplies. PPE includes aprons, gloves and particle masks. Employees must wear the protective clothing and use the protective equipment provided, and make employers aware of any shortage so that supplies can be maintained.

Training should be provided on the correct use and application of PPE and its use should be monitored. If not used the reason should be investigated as this becomes a risk.

You should use PPE to protect yourself against potentially hazardous substances such as:

- disinfectants – can cause chemical irritation to the skin
- body tissue fluids – direct contact can lead to skin infections and disease
- other harmful products and materials, such as the fumes and dust created during the application of artificial nails.

PPE should be 'CE' marked, which means it complies with the Personal Protective Equipment at Work Regulations 1992 and satisfies basic safety requirements.

The Workplace (Health, Safety and Welfare) Regulations (1992)

The **Workplace (Health, Safety and Welfare) Regulations (1992)** cover a broad range of basic health, safety and welfare issues and require all that work to maintain a safe, healthy and secure working environment. These regulations aim to ensure the workplace meets the health, safety and welfare needs of all the employees, including those with disabilities, and accessibility should be made where practicable. A 'disabled person' is defined in the Equality Act (2010). The regulations include legal requirements in relation to the following aspects of the working environment:

- maintenance of the workplace and equipment
- ventilation to ensure the air is changed regularly and fumes or strong smells are removed. Fresh air should be drawn from outside the workplace.
- working temperature
- lighting adequate to enable people to move safely and perform tasks competently
- cleanliness of furniture, equipment, furnishing and fittings and correct handling and disposal of **waste** materials
- safe salon layout, dimensions adequate for traffic flow (pedestrian traffic) and nature of the work
- safety protection against falls and falling objects, objects should be stored safely
- windows, doors, gates and walls should be safe and fit for purpose
- safe floor and traffic routes
- escalators and moving walkways should operate safely and have appropriate safety mechanisms
- sanitary conveniences for all staff and clients should be suitable and sufficient
- washing facilities of hot and cold running water should be available with soap and a means of drying hands
- drinking water: adequate supply
- facilities for changing and storage of clothing should be adequate and secure
- facilities for staff to rest and eat meals should be suitable
- fire exits and fire fighting equipment.

Manual Handling Operations Regulations (1992) The **Manual Handling Operations Regulations (1992)** apply in all occupations where manual lifting occurs, the aim being to prevent skeletal and muscular disorders and repetitive strain disorders due to poor working practice. The employer is required to carry out a risk assessment of all activities undertaken which involve manual lifting. Risk assessment records must be available for audit when required.

The risk assessment should provide evidence that the following have been considered:

- risk of injury
- the manual movement involved in performing the activity
- the physical constraint the load incurs
- the environmental constraints imposed by the workplace
- workers' individual capabilities
- action taken to minimize potential risks.

Manual lifting and handling Always take care of yourself when moving goods around the salon. Assess the risk. Do not struggle or be impatient: get someone else to help. When **lifting**, reduce the risk; lift from the knees, not the back. When **carrying**, balance weights evenly in both hands and carry the heaviest part nearest to your body.

Provision and Use of Work Equipment Regulations (PUWER) (1998) The **Provision and Use of Work Equipment Regulations (PUWER) (1998)** lay down the important health and safety controls on the provision and use of work equipment. They state the duties for employers and for users, including the self-employed. The regulations affect both old and new equipment. They identify the requirements in selecting suitable equipment and in maintaining it. They also discuss the information provided by equipment manufacturers, and instruction and training in the safe use of equipment. Specific regulations address the dangers and potential risks of injury that could occur during operation of the equipment. Suitable safety measures must be in place, including protective devices and warning signage as appropriate.

Health and Safety (Display Screen Equipment) Regulations (1992) The **Health and Safety (Display Screen Equipment) Regulations (1992)** cover the use of display screen equipment and computer screens. They specify acceptable levels of radiation emissions from the screen and identify correct posture, seating position, permitted working heights and rest periods. Employers have a responsibility to comply with this regulation to ensure the welfare of their employees in avoiding the potential risks of eyestrain, mental stress and muscle fatigue.

ALWAYS REMEMBER

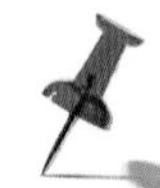

Temperature and lighting

The salon temperature should be a minimum of 16°C within one hour of employees arriving for work. The salon should be well ventilated, or carbon dioxide levels will increase, which can cause nausea. Many substances used in the salon can become hazardous without adequate ventilation. If the working environment is too warm this can cause heat stress, a condition that is recognized by the HSE. Lighting should be adequate to ensure that services can be carried out safely and competently, with the minimum risk of accident.

BEST PRACTICE

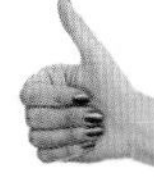

Broken goods

When you unpack a delivery, make sure the product packaging is undamaged, to avoid possible personal injury from broken goods.

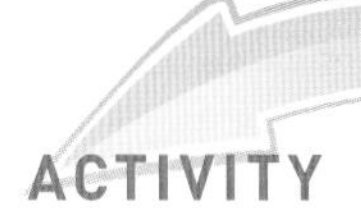

ACTIVITY

European directives

The Workplace (Health, Safety and Welfare) Regulations were implemented following a European Union directive on minimum safety and health requirements for the workplace.

1. Obtain a copy of the *Workplace (Health & Safety & Welfare) Regulations 1992* (available online at www.hse.gov.uk).
2. Look through the publication, and make notes on any information relevant to you in the workplace.

KNOWLEDGE CHECK

What is PPE? What is it used for?

Need more time... refer to pages 95–96 to help you.

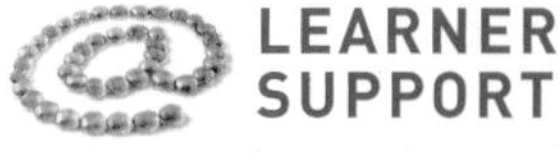

LEARNER SUPPORT

Health & safety fill-in-the-blanks

HEALTH & SAFETY

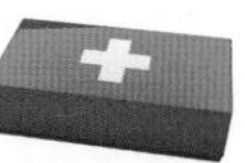

COSHH assessment

All hazardous substances must be identified when completing the risk assessment. This includes cleaning agents such as a wax equipment cleaner.

High-risk products should, where possible, be replaced with lower risk products.

COSHH assessments should be reviewed on a regular basis and updated to include any new products.

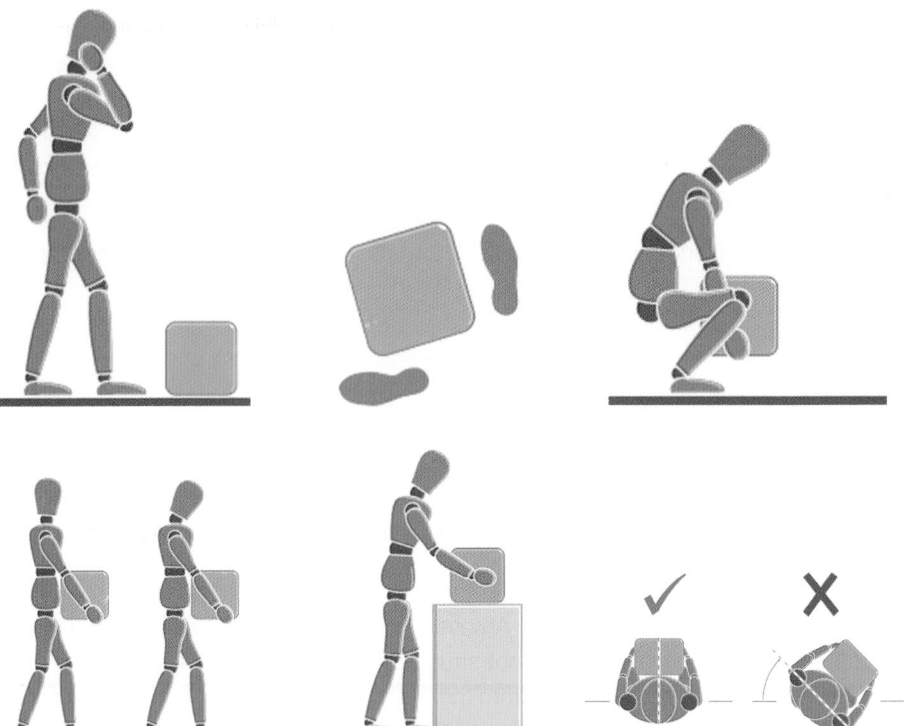

Best practice for manual handling

ACTIVITY

Identifying electrical hazards

Make a list of potential electrical hazards in the workplace, e.g. damaged plugs. Who should these be reported to?

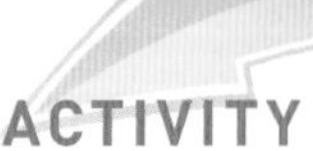

ACTIVITY

COSHH assessment

Carry out a COSHH assessment on selected treatment products used in the salon. Consider nail treatments, waxing and facial and eye treatments.

TOP TIP

COSHH essential information for beauticians is available on the HSE website in a section called, COSHH and your industry. How does COSHH affect you?

Control of Substances Hazardous to Health (COSHH) Regulations (2002) The **Control of Substances Hazardous to Health (COSHH) Regulations (2002)** were designed to make employers consider the substances used in their workplace and assess the possible risks to health. Many substances that seem quite harmless can prove to be hazardous if used or stored incorrectly. A hazardous substance is anything that can harm your health. All cosmetic products must comply with the Cosmetic Products (Safety) Regulations (2008). This legislation requires that cosmetics and toiletries are safe in their formulation and safe for use for their intended purpose.

Employers are responsible for assessing the risks from hazardous substances and controlling exposure to them to prevent ill health. Any hazardous substances identified must be formally recorded in writing. Safety precaution procedures should then be implemented and training given to employees to ensure that the procedures are understood and will be followed correctly. Employers must control substances that can harm employees' health.

Hazardous substances are identified by the use of known symbols, examples of which are shown below. Any substance in the workplace that is hazardous to health must be identified on the packaging and stored and handled correctly.

Hazardous substances can enter the body via the:

- eyes
- skin
- nose (**inhalation – breathing in**)
- mouth (**ingestion – swallowing**)

Each beauty product supplier is legally required to make guidelines available on how materials should be used and stored. These are called material safety data sheets (MSDSs) and will be supplied on request.

REACH (2007) **REACH 2007** is a European Union Regulation concerning the:

Registration

Evaluation

Authorization; and restriction of

CHemicals.

It operates alongside COSHH and is designed to improve the information provided by chemical manufacturers through the provision of adequate safety data sheets.

Electricity at Work Regulations (1989) The **Electricity at Work Regulations (1989)** state that every piece of electrical equipment in the workplace must be tested every 12 months by a qualified electrician. This is called portable appliance testing or (PAT). A written record of testing must be retained and made available for inspection. A list of all salon electrical equipment should be available with its unique serial number and date of purchase/disposal.

In addition to annual testing, a trained member of staff should regularly check all electrical equipment for safety. This is recommended every three months. Report to your supervisor if you see any of these potential hazards:

- exposed wires in flexes
- cracked plugs or broken sockets
- worn cables
- overloaded sockets

Although it is the employer's responsibility to ensure all equipment is safe to use, it is also the responsibility of the employee to check that equipment is safe before use, and never to use it if it is faulty. This complies with the requirements of public liability insurance. Failure to do so could lead to an accident which would be considered negligent.

Any pieces of equipment that appear faulty must be checked immediately and, if necessary, repaired before use. If faulty they must be labelled to ensure that they are not used by accident.

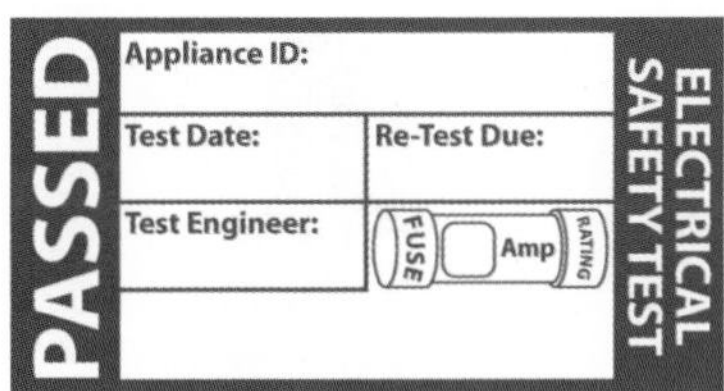

PAT test sticker

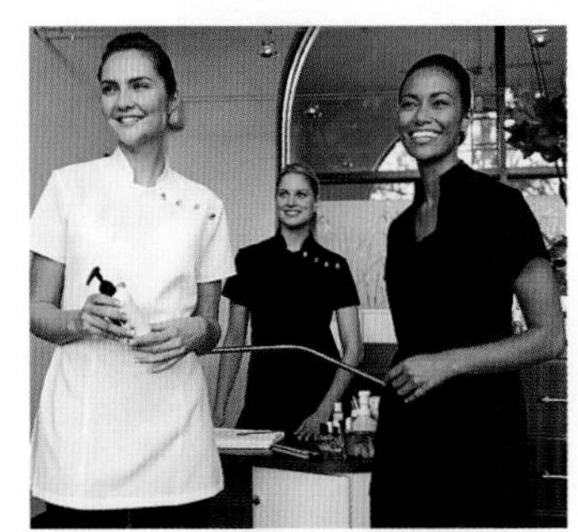

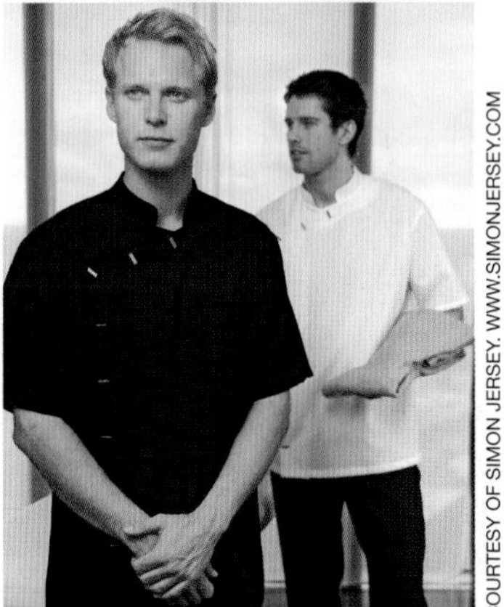

Personal presentation should project a professional image

Personal health, hygiene and presentation

Your appearance enables the client to make an initial judgment about both you and the salon, so make sure that you create the correct impression! Employees in the workplace should always reflect the desired image of the profession that they work in. This is discussed in more detail in Chapter 1 Introduction.

ACTIVITY

Personal appearance

1. Collect pictures from various suppliers of overalls. Select those that you feel would be most practical for a Level 2 beauty therapist, make-up artist or receptionist. Briefly describe why you feel these are the most suitable.
2. Design various hairstyles, or collect pictures from magazines, to show how the hair could be smartly worn by a beauty therapist with medium-length to long hair.

Ethics

Beauty therapy has a **code of ethics**. This is a code of **behaviour** and expected standards for the professional beauty therapist to follow, which will uphold the reputation of the industry and ensure best working practice for the safety of the industry and members of the public. Beauty therapy professional bodies produce **Industry Codes of Practice** for their members. A business may have its own code of practice. Although not a legal requirement, this code may be used in criminal proceedings as evidence of improper practice.

Lifestyle

A beauty therapist requires stamina and energy. To achieve this you need to eat a healthy, well-balanced diet, drink an adequate amount of water, take regular exercise and have adequate sleep.

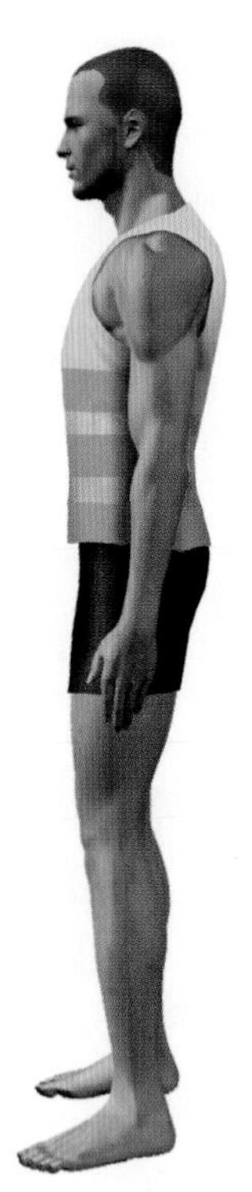
Good standing posture

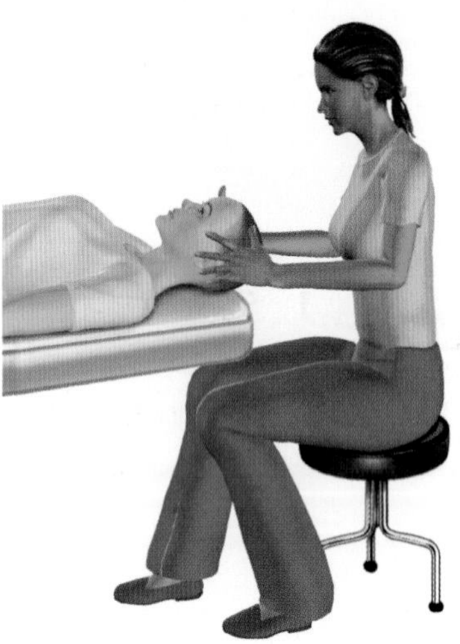
Good sitting posture

HEALTH & SAFETY

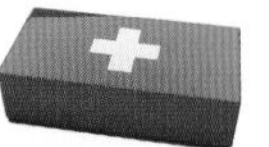

Repetitive strain injury (RSI)
If you do not follow correct postural positional requirements when performing services, muscle and ligaments may become overstretched and over-used resulting in repetitive strain injury (RSI). This may result in you being unable to work in the short term, and potentially long term in the occupation.

Posture

Posture is the way you hold yourself when standing, sitting and walking. *Correct* posture enables you to work longer without becoming tired, it prevents muscle fatigue, repetitive strain injury (RSI) and stiff joints, and it also improves your appearance.

Good standing posture If you are standing with good posture, you will have your:

- head up, centrally balanced
- shoulders slightly back, and relaxed
- chest up and out
- abdomen flat
- hips level
- fingertips level
- bottom in
- knees level
- feet slightly apart and weight evenly distributed.

Good sitting posture To have good sitting posture, sit on a suitable chair or stool with a good back support and:

- sit with the lower back pressed against the chair back
- keep the chest up and the shoulders back
- distribute the body weight evenly along the thighs
- keep the feet together, and flat on the floor
- do not slouch, or sit on the edge of your seat.

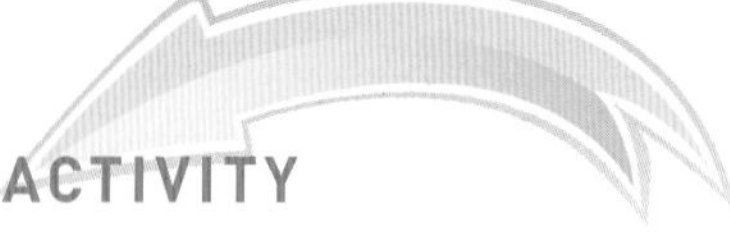

ACTIVITY

The importance of posture

1. Which services will be performed sitting, and which standing?
2. In what way do you feel your services would be affected if you were not sitting or standing correctly?

Personal hygiene

It is vital that you have a high standard of personal **hygiene**. You are going to be working in close proximity with people.

Bodily cleanliness is achieved through daily showering or bathing. This removes the stale sweat, dirt and bacteria which cause body odour. An antiperspirant or deodorant may be applied to the underarm area to reduce perspiration and thus the smell of sweat. Clean underwear should be worn each day.

Hands Your hands and everything you touch are covered with germs. Although most are harmless, some can cause ill health or disease. Wash your hands regularly, especially after you have been to the toilet and before eating food. You must also wash your hands before and after treating each client, and during a service if necessary. Washing the hands before treating a client minimizes the risk of cross-infection and presents to the client a hygienic, professional, caring image. Disinfecting hand gel may also be applied to the clean hands before services are delivered.

Step by step: How to wash your hands

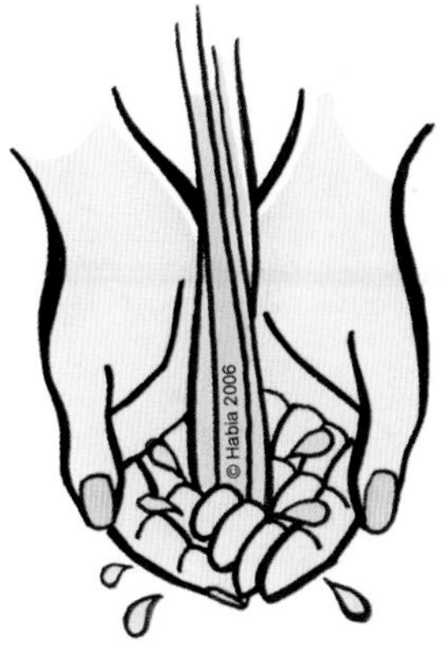

1 Wet your hands, wrists and forearms thoroughly using running water

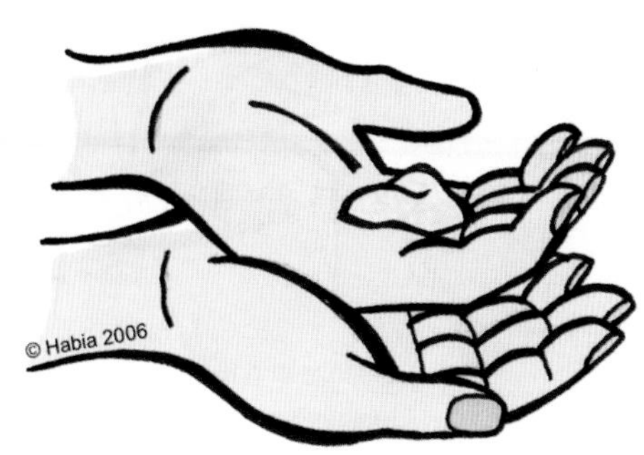

2 Apply around 3ml to 5ml of liquid soap

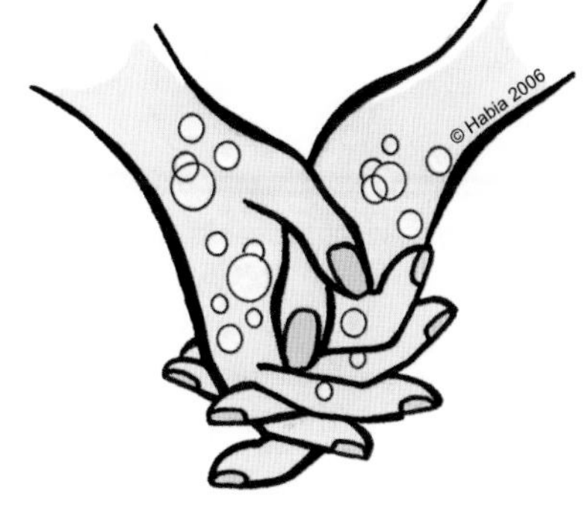

3 Start the lathering process, rubbing palm to palm

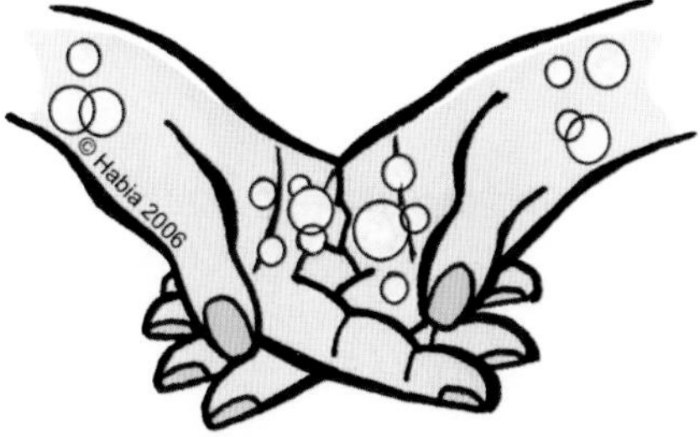

4 Interlock fingers and rub, ensuring a good lather

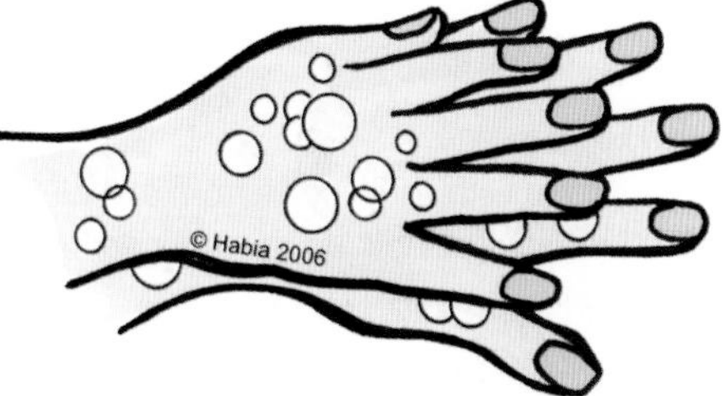

5 Rub right hand over back of left, then left over right hand

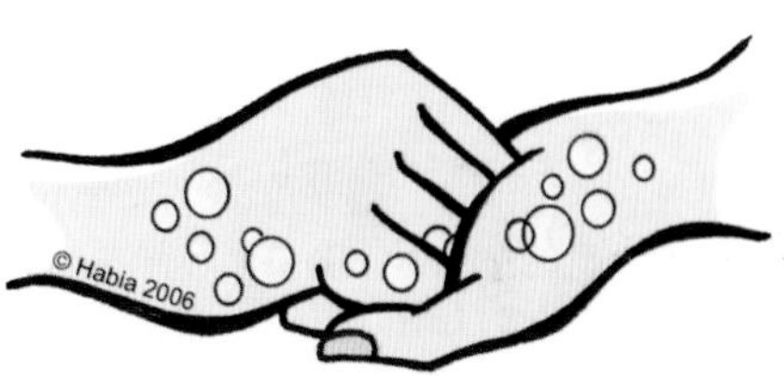

6 Rub with fingers locked in palm of hand ensuring fingertips are cleaned

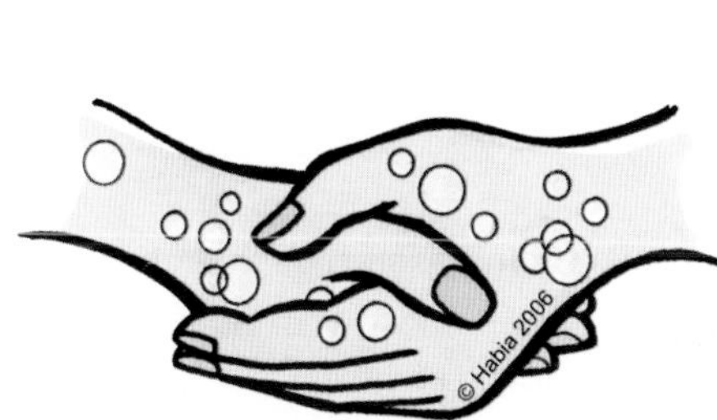

7 Lock thumbs and rotate hands

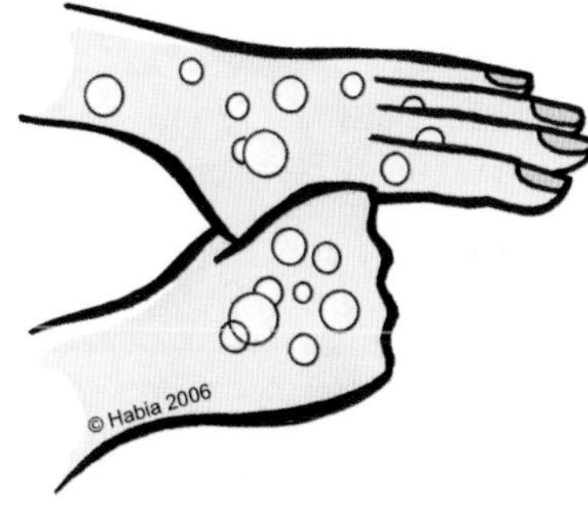

8 Grasp thumb with hand and rotate, repeat with opposite thumb

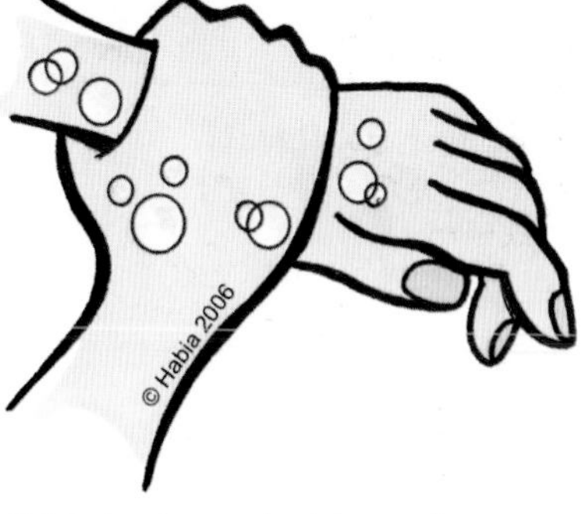

9 Rotate hand around wrist, repeat on opposite wrist

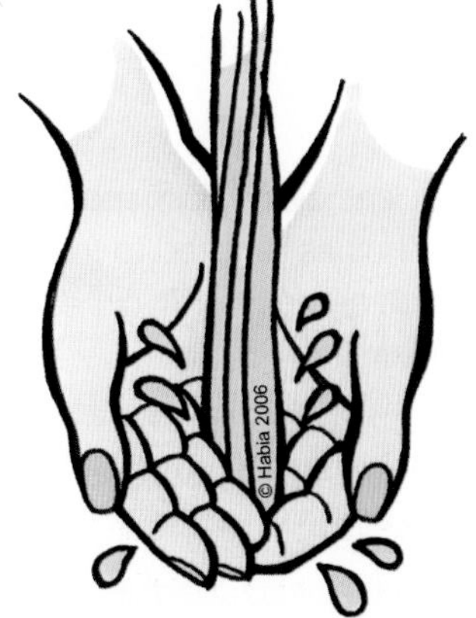

10 Rinse hands and wrists thoroughly using running water

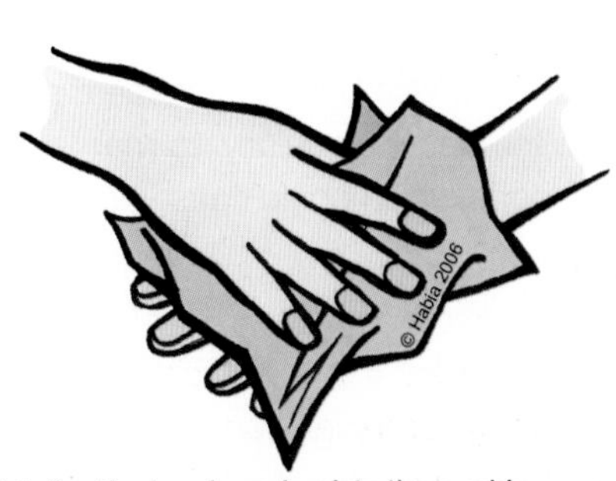

11 Dry the hands and wrists thoroughly

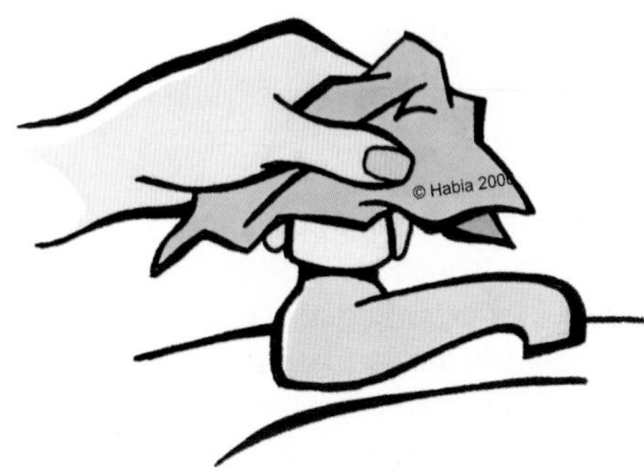

12 Turn off the tap using a paper towel

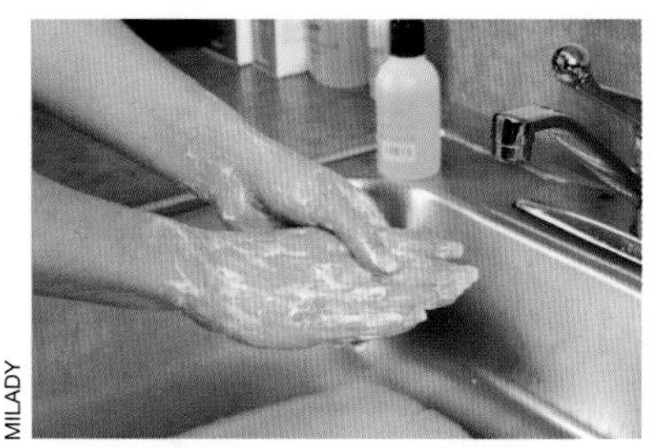

Personal hygiene for the hands

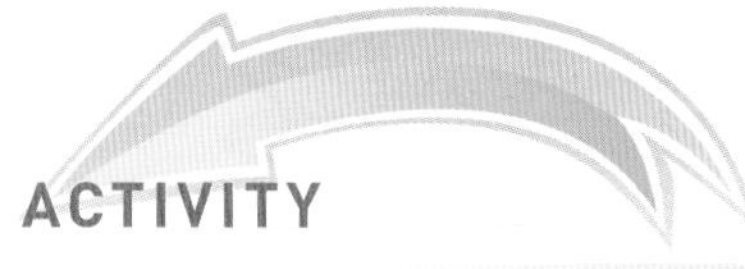

ACTIVITY

Hand hygiene
What further occasions can you think of when it will be necessary to wash your hands when treating a client?

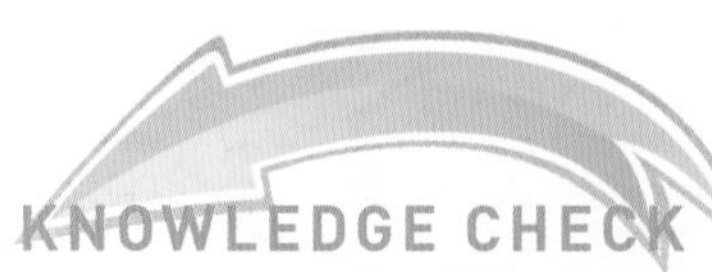

KNOWLEDGE CHECK

Why is good posture important?

Need more time... refer to page 100 to help you.

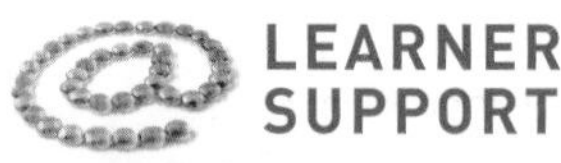

LEARNER SUPPORT

Health & safety true or false?

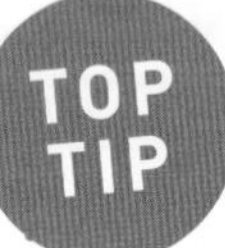

TOP TIP

Fresh breath
When working, avoid eating strong-smelling highly spiced food.

HEALTH & SAFETY

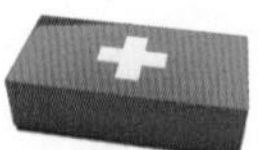

Long hair
If long hair is not taken away from the face, the tendency will be to move the hair away from the face repeatedly with the hands, and this in turn will require that the hands be washed repeatedly.

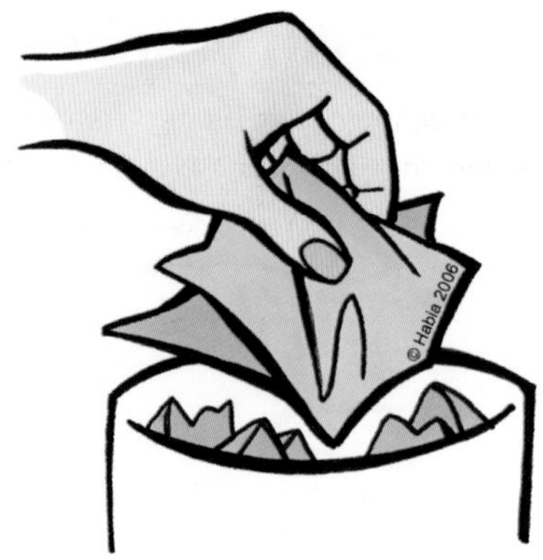

13 Dispose of paper towel without touching any part of the waste bin

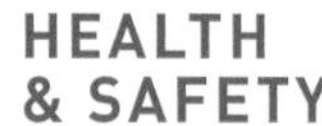
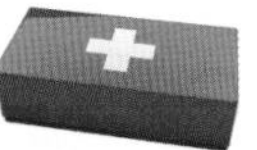

HEALTH & SAFETY

Soap and towels
Wash your hands with liquid soap from a sealed dispenser. This should take 10–20 seconds. Don't refill disposable soap dispensers when empty: if you do they will become a breeding ground for bacteria.

Disposable paper towels or warm-air hand dryers should be used to thoroughly dry the hands.

Protecting yourself
You will be wise to have the relevant inoculations, including those against tetanus and hepatitis, to protect yourself against ill health and even death.

Protecting the client
If you have any cuts or abrasions on your hands, cover them with a clean dressing to minimize the risk of secondary infection. Disposable gloves may be worn for additional protection.

Certain skin disorders are contagious. Therapists suffering from any such disorder must not work, but must seek medical advice immediately.

Face masks may be worn when working in close proximity to the client.

Feet Keep your feet fresh and healthy by washing them daily and then drying them thoroughly, especially between the toes to avoid foot disorders developing such as athlete's foot. Deodorizing foot powder may then be applied.

Oral hygiene Avoid bad breath by brushing your teeth at least twice daily and flossing the teeth frequently. Use breath fresheners and mouthwashes as required to freshen your breath. Visit the dentist regularly, to maintain healthy teeth and gums. Avoid eating strong flavoured foods which could cause offence in close proximity.

Hair Your hair should be clean and tidy. Have your hair cut regularly to maintain its appearance, and shampoo and condition your hair as often as needed.

If your hair is long, wear it off the face and taken to the crown of the head. Medium-length hair should be clipped back, away from the face, to prevent it falling forwards.

Hygiene and infection control in the workplace

Infections Effective hygiene and infection control is necessary in the salon to prevent *cross-infection* and *secondary infection.* Infection can occur through poor practice, such as the use of tools that are not sterile. Reusable (as opposed to disposable) tools and equipment become contaminated – infected with skin and nail debris. An infection can be recognized by red and inflamed skin, or the presence of pus. All staff must be trained in and carry out effective decontamination procedures to remove and/or destroy the contamination.

Cross-infection occurs because some microorganisms are contagious – they may be transferred through personal contact or by contact with an infected tool that has not been disinfected or sterilized. Cross-infection can occur through blood contamination and skin or nail infections.

Secondary infection can occur as a result of injury to the client during the service or, if the client already has an open wound bacteria can penetrate the skin and cause infection. **Sterilization** and disinfection procedures (below) are used to minimize or destroy the harmful microorganisms which could cause infection – **bacteria**, **viruses** and **fungi**.

Infectious diseases that are contagious **contra-indicate** beauty service: they require medical attention. People with certain other skin disorders, even though these are not contagious, should likewise not be treated by the beauty therapist, as treatment might lead to secondary infection.

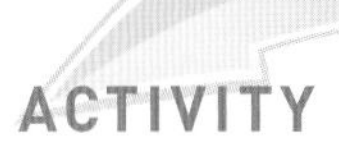

ACTIVITY

Avoiding cross-infection

1. List the different ways in which infection can be transferred in the salon.
2. How can you avoid cross-infection in the workplace?

Sterilization and disinfection **Sterilization** is the total destruction of all living micro-organisms from metal tools and equipment. **Disinfection** is the destruction of most living micro-organisms from non-metal tools, equipment and work areas. Disinfection aims to reduce the level of micro-organisms to a level that will not lead to infection. Sterilization and disinfection techniques practised in the beauty salon involve the use of ***physical*** agents such as radiation and heat and ***chemical*** agents such as antiseptics and disinfectants. Sterilization and disinfection procedures must be performed between each client.

HEALTH & SAFETY

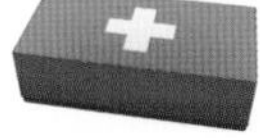

UV lamps
Ultra-violet light is dangerous, especially to the eyes. The lamp must be switched off before opening the cabinet. A record must be kept of usage, as the effectiveness of the lamp decreases with use.

Radiation – a quartz mercury-vapour lamp can be used as the source for ultra-violet (UV) light, which minimizes harmful micro-organisms. However, UV light has limited effectiveness and cannot be relied upon for complete sterilization. A UV cabinet is a good place to store previously sterilized objects.

The UV lamp must be contained within a closed cabinet. This cabinet is an ideal place for storing sterilized objects.

Heat – dry and moist heat can both be used for sterilization. One method is to use a dry **hot-air oven**. This is similar to a small oven and heats to 150–180°C. It is seldom used in the salon.

Water is boiled in an **autoclave** (similar to a pressure cooker): because of the increased pressure, the water reaches a temperature of 121–134°C. Autoclaving is the most effective method and highly recommended for sterilizing objects in the salon.

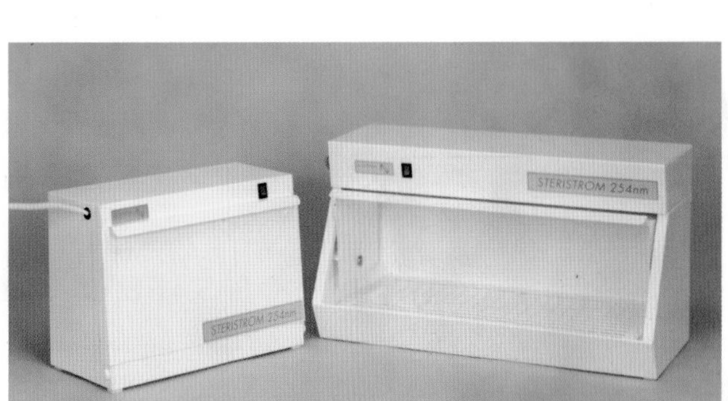

An ultra-violet light cabinet

Disinfectants and antiseptics If an object *cannot* be sterilized, it should be placed in a chemical **disinfectant** solution. A disinfectant destroys most micro-organisms, but not all. Hypochlorite is a disinfectant – bleach is an example of a hypochlorite. Hypochlorite is suitable for cleaning work surfaces but is particularly corrosive and unsuitable for use with metals – use as

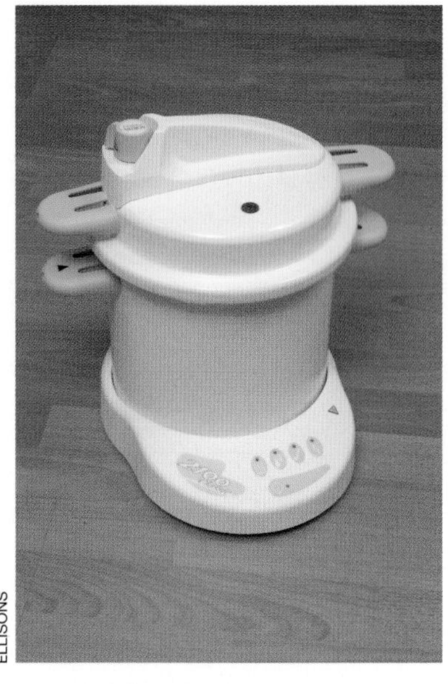

ELLISONS

An automatic medical autoclave

HEALTH & SAFETY

Using an autoclave

- The autoclave should only be used by those trained to do so.
- Not all objects can safely be placed in the autoclave. Before using this method, check whether the items you wish to sterilize can withstand this heating process.
- All objects should be cleaned, using an effective cleaning agent, e.g. surgical spirit, to remove surface dirt and debris before placing in the autoclave.
- To avoid damaging the autoclave, always use distilled de-ionized water.
- To avoid rusting, metal objects placed in the sterilizing unit must be of good-quality stainless steel.
- Never overload the autoclave. Follow manufacturer's instructions in its use.

directed by the manufacturer. Ammonium compound disinfectants such as 'Barbicide' can be used with metal and plastic items. Alcohol-impregnated wipes are a popular way to clean the skin using a disinfectant such as isopropyl alcohol.

An **antiseptic** prevents the multiplication of micro-organisms. It has a limited action and does not kill all micro-organisms.

All sterilization/disinfection techniques must be carried out safely and effectively following the manufacturer's instructions for correct use:

1. Select the appropriate method of sterilization or disinfectant for the object. ***Always*** follow the manufacturer's guidelines on the use of the sterilizing or disinfecting unit or agent.
2. Always clean the object in clean water and a detergent, such as liquid soap, to remove dirt, debris and grease. This is often referred to as sanitization in the salon. (Dirt left on the object might prevent effective sterilization or disinfection.)
3. Dry it thoroughly with a clean, disposable paper towel.
4. Sterilize or disinfect the object, allowing sufficient time for the process to be completed. Contact with all surfaces of the object must be made.
5. Following disinfection/sterilization handle the objects with clean tongs or protective gloves. Place objects that have been sterilized or disinfected in a clean, covered container, ideally labelled. After 24 hours the object will be clean but not disinfected.

Keep several sets of the tools you use regularly, so that you can carry out effective sterilization and disinfection.

HEALTH & SAFETY

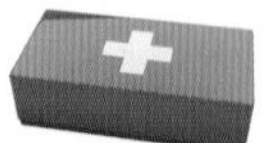

Aseptic conditions

This is the situation you should try to ensure occurs in the workplace by eliminating bacteria. All treatment procedures must be aseptic, i.e. wearing PPE, hand hygiene, correct methods of waste disposal etc.

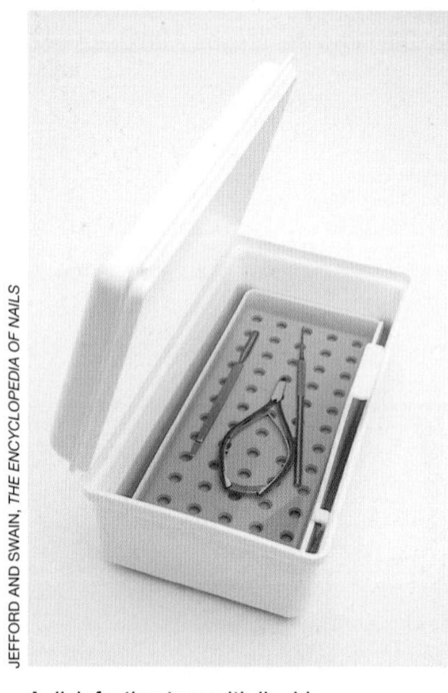

JEFFORD AND SWAIN, *THE ENCYCLOPEDIA OF NAILS*

A disinfection tray with liquid

HEALTH & SAFETY

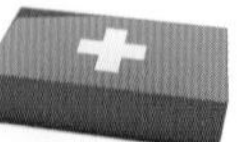

Using disinfectant

Disinfectant solutions should be changed as necessary to ensure their effectiveness. After removing the object from the disinfectant, rinse it in clean water to remove traces of the solution. (These might otherwise cause an allergic reaction on the client's skin.)

HEALTH & SAFETY 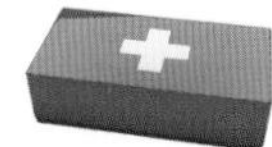

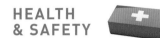

Damaged equipment
Any equipment in poor repair must be repaired or disposed of. Such equipment may be dangerous and may harbour germs.

Using chemical agents
Always wear protective gloves when using cleaning materials to prevent drying and irritation of the skin, which could lead to the skin disorder dermatitis.

ALWAYS REMEMBER 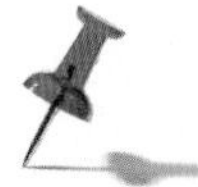

Before sterilization, surgical spirit applied with clean cotton wool may be used to remove debris from small objects.

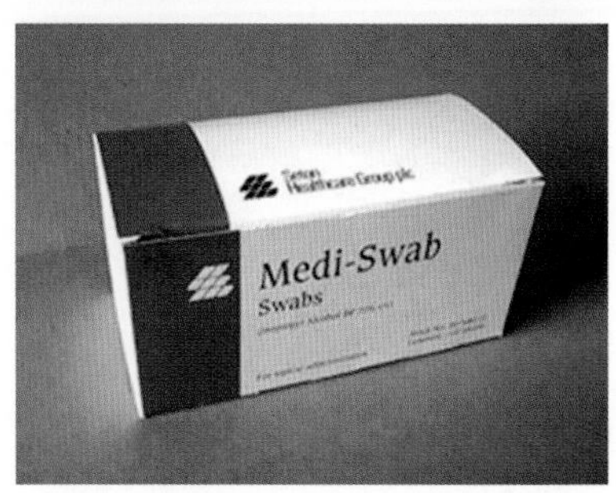

ELLISONS

Medi-swabs (sterile isopropyl tissues)

Workplace policies Each workplace should have its own workplace policy to identify hygiene rules.

- *Health and safety* Follow the health and safety policies for the workplace.
- *Personal hygiene* Maintain a high standard of personal hygiene. Wash your hands with a detergent containing **chlorhexidine gluconate**, which protects against a wide range of bacteria. The addition of isopropyl alcohol provides a stronger hand disinfectant, removing surface bacteria and fungi.
- *Cuts on the hands* Always cover any cuts on your hands with a protective dressing.
- *Cross-infection* Take great care to avoid cross-infection in the salon. *Never* treat a client who has a contagious skin disease or disorder, or any other contra-indication. Refer the client tactfully to their GP.
- *Use hygienic tools* Never use an implement unless it has been effectively sterilized or disinfected as appropriate.
- *Disposable applicators* Wherever possible use disposable applicators, also referred to as 'single use' tools.
- *Working surfaces* Disinfect all working surfaces (such as trolleys and couches) with a chlorine preparation, diluted to the manufacturer's instructions. Cover all working surfaces with clean, disposable paper tissue.
- *Gowns and towels* Clean gowns and towels must be provided for each client. Towels should be laundered at a temperate of 60°C.
- *Laundry* Dirty laundry should be placed in a covered container.
- *Waste* including clinical waste and non-contaminated waste, must be disposed of following the COSHH procedures and guidelines provided by the local authority and training by the employer. For contaminated waste comply with the Controlled Waste Regulations (1992). Put waste in a suitable container lined with a disposable waste bag. A yellow '**sharps**' **container** or heavy duty yellow bag, should be available for clinical waste contaminated with blood or tissue fluid. Protective gloves should be worn to avoid risk of contamination.
- *Eating and drinking* Never eat or drink in the service area of the salon. Not only is it unprofessional, but harmful chemicals may also be ingested.
- *Drugs and alcohol* Never carry out services in the workplace under the influence of drugs or alcohol. Your competence will be affected putting yourself, clients and possibly colleagues at risk. Any accident as a result would be termed negligent and you would be liable.

TOP TIP

HSE advice on cleaning
Advice on cleaning work surfaces and equipment can be found on the COSHH Essentials website:
www.coshh-essentials.org.uk.

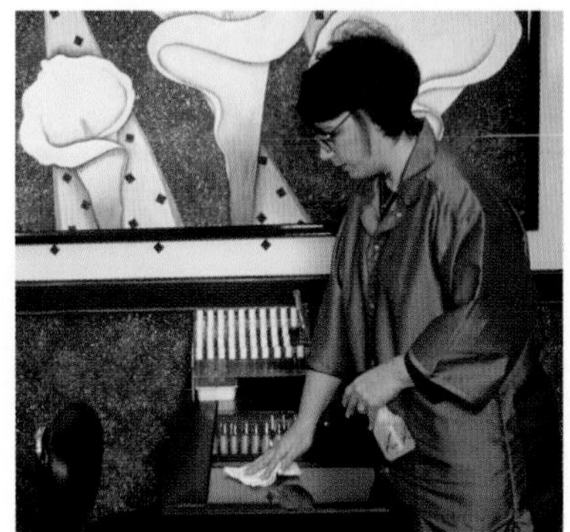

MILADY

Disinfecting work surfaces

HEALTH & SAFETY 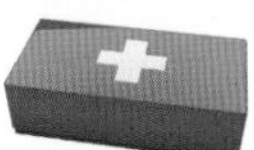

Cuts on the hands
Open, uncovered cuts provide an easy entry for harmful bacteria, and may therefore lead to infection. Always cover cuts.

HEALTH & SAFETY 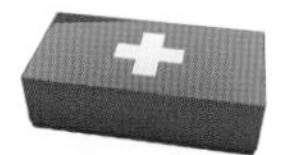

Misuse of Drugs Act (1971)
This Act categorizes drugs into classes and details the penalties for those caught possessing them. Therefore, you are acting illegally.

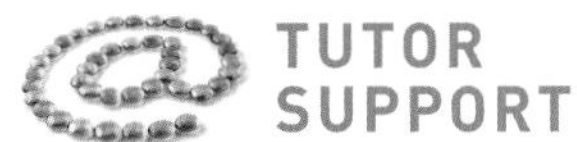

TUTOR SUPPORT

Activity 5: Workplace policies task

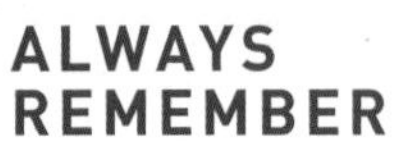 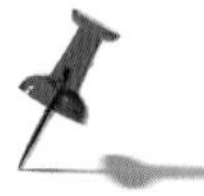

ALWAYS REMEMBER

Security procedures should be:

- current
- fit for purpose
- implemented
- performed by a designated person.

Ensure that your behaviour at work is in accordance with your workplace policies and doesn't endanger yourself or others.

Salon security

HEALTH & SAFETY 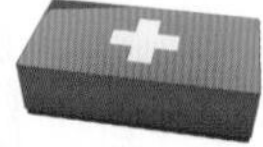

Security
A Crime Prevention Officer can complete a security check and provide advice on effective ways of securing the business premises.
Some businesses used closed circuit television (CCTV).

It is important that adequate precautions are taken to secure the premises against theft (during business hours) and burglary (outside business hours). Insurance companies will not insure a business where there are inadequate security measures. Staff must be trained in all aspects of security with procedures. Updates should be discussed at staff meetings. All staff at induction should be made aware of the consequences of theft. Theft is often referred to as gross misconduct and may lead to dismissal and prosecution.

The employer should have a formal policy and procedures to ensure the security of:

- people and possessions
- premises
- tools and equipment
- stock
- cash and equivalents.

Security concerns should be taken into consideration at all times. Systems should be in place to monitor till transactions, stock and personal possessions, including client and staff belongings.

- Personal possessions – secure areas such as lockers should be available to staff for storing personal possessions while they are at work. If a service requires the removal of clothing and/or jewellery, the client's possessions should be given to the client for safe keeping or kept within view of the client. It is customary to display a notice disclaiming responsibility in the event of theft.
- Stock – areas vulnerable to theft, such as the retail area, should be designed so as to be in full view of staff. Only authorized staff should handle and have access to stock. Expensive equipment may be locked away when not in use. Regular and random stock checks will show up any missing stock.
- Cash and equivalents – only authorized staff should handle money. Security systems should be in place so that all errors are traceable. There should be a salon policy to deal with fraudulent monetary transactions. In accordance with the Data Protection Act (1998), confidental information about staff or clients must only be recorded and stored if consent has been given. Records must be stored in a secure area.

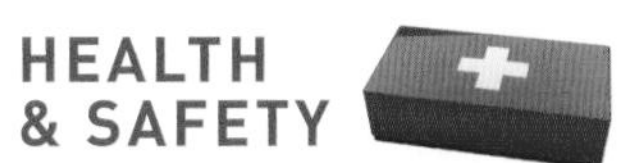
HEALTH
& SAFETY

Fire!

If there is a fire, never use a lift. A fire quickly becomes out of control. You do not have very long to act!

Fire drill notices should be visible to show people to the emergency exit route.

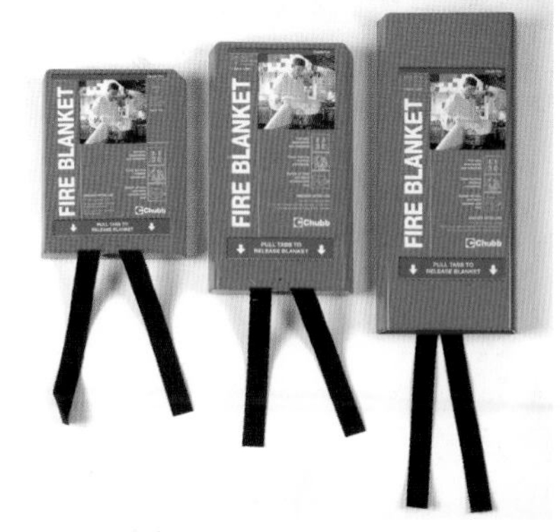
FIRE BLANKET
FIRE BLANKET
FIRE BLANKET

Fire blankets

Fire-fighting equipment Fire-fighting equipment must be available, located in a specified area. The equipment includes fire extinguishers, blankets, sand buckets and water hoses. Fire-fighting equipment should be used only when the cause of the fire has been identified – using the ***wrong*** fire extinguisher could make the fire worse.

Fire classifications include class A, B and C. Symbols are used to identify these classifications and choice of fire extinguisher as shown below.

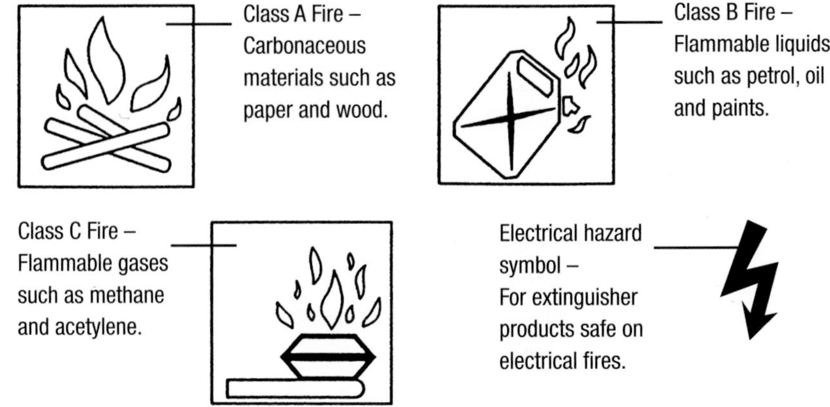
Class A Fire –
Carbonaceous materials such as paper and wood.
Class B Fire –
Flammable liquids such as petrol, oil and paints.
Class C Fire –
Flammable gases such as methane and acetylene.
Electrical hazard symbol –
For extinguisher products safe on electrical fires.

Fire extinguisher symbols

Class D Fires involve metals.

Never use fire-fighting equipment unless you are trained in its use.

Fire extinguishers Fire extinguishers are available to tackle different types of fire. These should be located in a set place known to all employees. It is important that these are checked and maintained as required.

Fire blankets are used to smother a small, localized fire or if a person's clothing is on fire. **Sand** is used to soak up liquids if these are the source of the fire and to smother the fire. **Water hoses** are used to extinguish large fires caused by paper materials and the like – buckets of water can be used to extinguish a small fire. *Remember turn off the electricity at the mains first!*

Never put yourself at risk – fires can spread quickly. Leave the building at once if in danger and raise the alarm by telephoning the emergency services on the emergency telephone numbers, **999** or **112**.

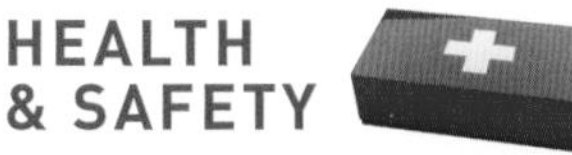
HEALTH
& SAFETY

Fire exits

Fire-exit doors must be clearly marked, remain unlocked during working hours and be free from obstruction.

ALWAYS REMEMBER

Fire extinguishers

Label colour and symbols indicate the use of particular fire extinguishers. Make sure you know the meaning of each of the colours and symbols.

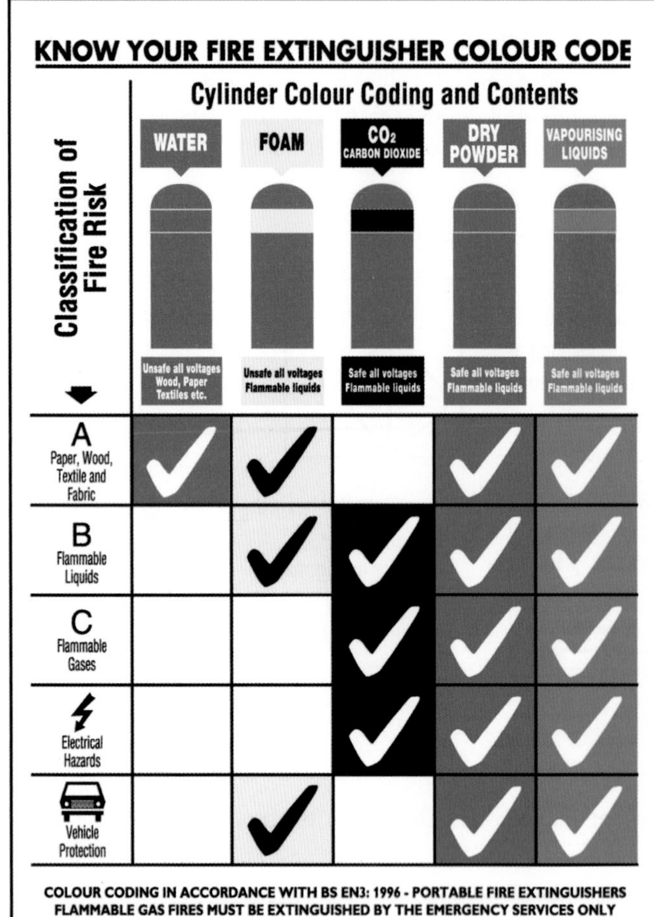

KNOW YOUR FIRE EXTINGUISHER COLOUR CODE
Cylinder Colour Coding and Contents
Classification of Fire Risk
WATER
FOAM
CO_2 CARBON DIOXIDE
DRY POWDER
VAPOURISING LIQUIDS
Unsafe all voltages Wood, Paper Textiles etc.
Unsafe all voltages Flammable liquids
Safe all voltages Flammable liquids
Safe all voltages Flammable liquids
Safe all voltages Flammable liquids
A Paper, Wood, Textile and Fabric
B Flammable Liquids
C Flammable Gases
Electrical Hazards
Vehicle Protection
COLOUR CODING IN ACCORDANCE WITH BS EN3: 1996 - PORTABLE FIRE EXTINGUISHERS
FLAMMABLE GAS FIRES MUST BE EXTINGUISHED BY THE EMERGENCY SERVICES ONLY

Fire extinguisher label colour code

Cause of fire and choice of fire extinguisher

Cause	Extinguisher type	Label colour code
Electrical fire	Carbon dioxide (CO_2) extinguisher	Black
Solid material fire (paper, wood, etc.)	Water extinguisher	Red
Flammable liquid	Foam extinguisher	Cream/yellow
Electrical fire	Dry-powder extinguisher	Blue
Flammable metal fire	Vapourizing liquid	Green

KNOWLEDGE CHECK

Which set of regulations determines fire safety in the workplace?

Need more time... refer to page 110 to help you.

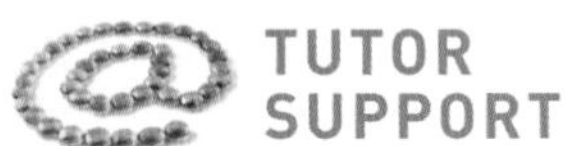

TUTOR SUPPORT

Activity 1: Firefighting equipment handout

Other emergencies

Other possible emergencies that could occur relate to fumes and flooding. Learn where the water and gas stopcocks are located. In the event of a gas leak or a flood, the stopcocks should be switched off and the appropriate emergency service contacted.

In the event of a bomb alert staff must be trained in the appropriate emergency procedures. This will involve recognition of a suspect package, how to deal with a bomb threat, evacuation of staff and clients and contacting the emergency services. Your local Crime Prevention Officer (CPO) will advise on bomb security.

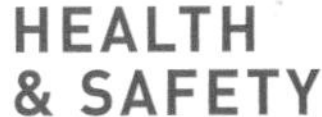

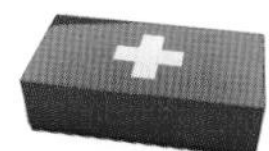

Using fire extinguishers
The vapours emitted when using vapourizing liquid extinguishers 'starve' a fire of oxygen. They are therefore dangerous when used in confined spaces, as people need oxygen too!

ACTIVITY

Health and Safety awareness
Where can you find the following in your workplace:

1. Fire extinguisher(s)?
2. Information sheets stating how products should be stored/used. MSDS (Material Safety Data Sheets)?
3. Health and safety workplace information?
4. First aid kit?
5. Sterilization/disinfection equipment?
6. Personal protective equipment (PPE)?
7. The fire exit/s?
8. Accident book?
9. Sharps box and waste bags for contaminated waste?

Environmentally friendly working practices Reflect on how you work, use and dispose of products within your work. Are you always environmentally friendly? Consider the following changes:

- use biodegradable packaging for disposal of non-contaminated waste
- for hospitality drinks rather than use disposable plastic cups revert back to cups and glasses that can be washed
- dispose of chemicals safely, not down the sinks
- use wooden spatulas from sustainable wood sources
- use recycled consumable materials where possible, e.g. bed-roll, tissues and cleaning products
- use light bulbs that minimize energy use
- switch off lights in rooms not being used and also equipment when not in use – if safe to do so

- turn down the heating thermostat rather than opening windows (this will save money too)
- buy in bulk, reducing trips to the wholesaler, and buy locally
- recycle your waste and packaging where possible, use colour-coded waste bags that are of course made from recycled materials
- recycle used printer cartridges
- some beauty companies will provide a free product on the return of a used product packaging.

Small steps can make a big difference.

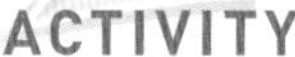

ACTIVITY

Noise levels

Assess the noise level at your workplace. Are there any intrusive noise levels preventing normal communication, e.g. do voices need to be raised?

Control of Noise at Work Regulations (2005) Loud noise can damage hearing. Noise is measured in decibels (db) and have different kinds of weighting. A-weighting is sometimes written as 'dB(A)', which is average noise level. C-weighting is 'dB(C)' – noise which is at its highest point, e.g. explosives.

As an employer a safe working environment should be provided with noise levels kept within safe levels. This does not include low-level noise. As in all **workplace practices**, noise levels can be classified as a risk. If a risk is identified, action should be taken to correct it. This could be a PPE hearing protection. Information, instruction and training must be provided and must be is monitored.

Insurance

Insurance must cover all activities in the workplace. **Public Liability Insurance** protects employers and employees against the consequences of death or injury to a third party while on the premises. Professional indemnity insurance extends public liability insurance to cover named employees against claims.

Product and **treatment liability insurance** is usually included with your public liability insurance but this should be checked with the insurance company. Product liability insurance covers you for risks which might occur as a result of the products you are using and/ or selling.

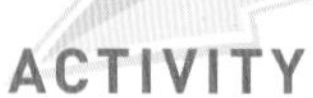

ACTIVITY

Causes of fires

Can you think of several potential causes of fire in the salon? How could each of these be prevented?

It is a legal requirement under the **Employer's Liability (Compulsory Insurance) Act (1969)** that every employer must have **employer's liability insurance**. This provides financial compensation to an employee should they be injured as a result of an accident in the workplace. A current employee/public liability insurance certificate notice must be displayed in a prominent place indicating that a policy of insurance has been obtained.

ALWAYS REMEMBER

To avoid potential hazards and risks in the workplace you should:

- be aware of the workplace health and safety policy and your responsibility in its implementation
- ensure your personal presentation and conduct at work meets health and safety and legislative requirements in accordance with workplace policies
- follow the most recent workplace policies for your job role and manufacturers' instructions for the safe use of resources
- follow the latest health and safety legislation related to your work
- know who is responsible for health and safety in your workplace. Pass on any suggestions for reducing health and safety risks within your job role
- report or deal immediately with any risk which could be a hazard, complying with workplace policies and legal requirements
- be aware of first aid arrangements in the event of an accident or illness
- know the workplace fire evacuation advice and procedure
- ensure your working practice minimizes the possible spread of infection or disease.

Why is it important to have insurance?

Need more time... refer to page 114 to help you.

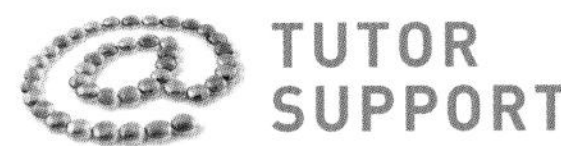

Activity 7: H&S multiple choice questions

GLOSSARY OF KEY WORDS

Accident book a written record of any accident in the workplace. Incidents in the accident book should be reviewed to see where improvements to safe working practice could be made.

Accident form a detailed report form to be completed following any accident in the workplace.

Antiseptic a chemical agent that prevents the multiplication of microorganisms. It has limited action and does not kill all microorganisms.

Aseptic The methods used to eliminate bacteria when performing treatment procedures from British standards. See also terms relating to disinfectants.

Autoclave an effective method of sterilization, suitable for small metal objects and beauty therapy tools. Water is boiled under increased pressure and reaches temperatures of 121–134°C.

Bacteria minute, single-celled organisms of various shapes. Large numbers live on the skin's surface and are not harmful (they are non-pathogenic); others, however, are harmful (pathogenic) and can cause disease.

Behaviour this refers to how we conduct ourselves in the workplace. It is important to be polite and friendly at all times, work cooperatively with others and conform with all workplace policies and procedures.

Contra-indication a problematic symptom that indicates the service may not proceed.

Control of risk the means by which risks identified are removed or reduced to acceptable levels.

Control of Substances Hazardous to Health (COSHH) (2002) these regulations require employers to identify hazardous substances used in the workplace and state how they should be correctly stored and handled.

Controlled Waste Regulations (1992) categorizes waste types. The local authority provides advice on how to dispose of waste types in compliance with the law.

Cosmetic Products (Safety) Regulations (2008) part of consumer protection legislation that requires that cosmetics and toiletries are safe in their formulation and are safe for use for their intended purpose as a cosmetic and comply with labelling requirements.

Cross-infection the transfer of contagious micro-organisms.

Disinfectant a chemical agent that destroys most micro-organisms.

Electricity at Work Regulations (1989) these regulations state that electrical equipment in the workplace should be tested every 12 months, by a qualified electrician. The employer must keep records of the equipment tested and the date it was checked.

Employers' Liability (Compulsory Insurance) Act (1969) this provides financial compensation to an employee should they be injured as a result of an accident in the workplace. A certificate indicating that a policy of insurance has been purchased should be displayed.

Environmental conditions this includes heating, lighting, ventilation and general comfort requirements for the workplace or service.

Fire Precautions Act (1971) legislation that states that all staff must be familiar with, and trained in fire, and emergency evacuation procedures for their workplace.

Fungus (fungi) microorganisms that can cause fungal diseases of the skin and feed off the waste products of the skin. They are found on the skin's surface or they can attack deeper tissues.

Hazard a hazard is something with potential to cause harm.

Health and Safety at Work Act (1974) legislation that lays down the minimum standards of health safety and welfare requirements in all workplaces.

Health and Safety (Display Screen Equipment) Regulations (1992) these regulations cover the use of visual display units (VDUs) and computer screens. They specify acceptable levels of radiation emissions from the screen and identify correct posture, seating position, permitted working heights and rest periods.

Health and Safety (First Aid) Regulations (1981) legislation that states that workplaces must have appropriate and adequate first aid provision.

Health and safety policy each employer of more than five employees must have a written health and safety policy issued to their employees outlining their health and safety responsibilities.

Hygiene requirements the expected standards as required by law, industry codes of practice or written procedures specified by the workplace.

Industry Code of Practice a set of guidelines written by the industry to provide a framework for good practice and minimum standards.

Infection the communication of disease from one body to another. An infection is the colonization of a host organism by parasite species. If a client has an infection, do not treat the client.

Infestation a condition where animal parasites live off and invade a host.

Legislation laws affecting the beauty therapy business relating to products and services, the business premises and environmental conditions, working practices and those employed.

Local Government (Miscellaneous Provisions) Act (1982) legislation that requires that salons offering any form of skin piercing be registered with the local health authority. This registration includes both the operators who will be carrying out the service and the salon premises where the service will be carried out.

Management of Health and Safety at Work Regulations (1999) this legislation provides the employer with an approved code of practice for maintaining a safe, secure working environment.

Manual Handling Operations Regulations (1992) legislation that requires the employer to carry out a risk assessment of all activities undertaken which involve manual handling (lifting and moving objects).

Personal Protective Equipment (PPE) at Work Regulations (1992) this legislation requires employers to identify through risk assessment those activities that require special protective equipment to be worn.

Posture the position of the body, which varies from person to person. Good posture is when the body is in alignment. Correct posture enables you to work longer without becoming tired; it prevents muscle fatigue and stiff joints.

Provision and Use of Work Equipment Regulations (PUWER) (1998) this regulation lays down important health and safety controls on the provision and use of equipment.

Public liability insurance protects employers and employees against the consequences of death or injury to a third party while on the premises.

Regulatory Reform (Fire Safety) Order (2005) this legislation requires that the employer or designated 'responsible person' must carry out a risk assessment for the premises in relation to fire evacuation practice and procedures.

Reporting of Injuries, Diseases and Dangerous Occurrences Regulations (RIDDOR) (1995) these regulations require the employer to notify the local enforcement officer in writing, in cases where employees or trainees suffer personal injury at work.

Responsible persons in health and safety, this term is used to mean the person or persons at work to whom you should report any issues, problems or hazards. This could be a supervisor, line manager or your employer.

Risk the likelihood of a hazard's potential being recognized.

Secondary infection bacterial penetration into the skin, causing infection.

Skin allergy if the skin is sensitive to a particular substance, an allergic skin reaction will occur. This is recognized by irritation, swelling and inflammation.

Sterilization the total destruction of all micro-organisms in metal tools and equipment.

Viruses the smallest living bodies, too small to see under an ordinary microscope. Viruses invade healthy body cells and multiply within the cell. Eventually the cell walls break down and the virus particles are freed to attack further cells.

Waste items, substances and materials requiring disposal following a service. Waste must be disposed of safely and in accordance with legal and salon requirements.

Workplace (Health Safety and Welfare) Regulations (1992) these regulations provide the employer with an approved code of practice for maintaining a safe, secure working environment.

Workplace policies the documentation prepared by your employer on the procedures to be followed in your workplace. Examples are your employer's safety policy statement, or general health and safety statements and written safety procedures covering aspects of the workplace that should be drawn to the employees' (and other persons') attention, pricing policies and customer service policies.

Workplace practices any activities, procedures, use of materials or equipment and working techniques used in carrying out your job. Lifting techniques and maintaining good posture whilst working are also included.

ASSESSMENT OF KNOWLEDGE AND UNDERSTANDING

You have now learnt about health and safety in the beauty therapy workplace. To test your level of knowledge, answer the following short questions. These will prepare you for your summative (final) assessment.

1. Cleaning agents that are formulated for use on skin are:
   a. disinfectants
   b. antiseptics
   c. sterilizers
   d. sanitizers
2. The hygiene control method of sterilization:
   a. is the destruction of most living organisms
   b. is the cleaning method using a disinfectant cleaning agent
   c. is the total destruction of all living micro-organisms
   d. uses ultra-violet light (UVL) to minimize harmful micro-organisms
3. What is a disinfectant?
   a. a chemical solution that destroys most micro-organisms
   b. a solution that prevent the multiplication of micro-organisms
   c. a type of distilled water to avoid damaging the autoclave
   d. a physical agent that destroys most micro-organisms
4. How often should the beauty therapist wash their hands?
   a. after each service to prevent cross-infection
   b. before each service to prevent secondary infection
   c. after eating to maintain personal hygiene
   d. regularly to prevent cross-infection
5. If a towel accidentally dropped onto the floor, what should you do with it?
   a. pick it up, fold it and replace on the work surface to prevent somebody tripping over it
   b. place it in the laundry bin for washing
   c. use it to dry your hands on after washing rather than use it on a client
   d. use it when cleaning to dry the work surfaces before washing
6. What do the Control of Substances Hazardous to Health (COSHH) regulations regulate for health and safety?
   a. those activities or processes that require special protective clothing or equipment to be worn
   b. substances used in the work place that may cause a risk to health
   c. the provision and use of work equipment
   d. the clinical disposal of contaminated waste
7. When completing a client's record card, you recognize that the client has a contra-indication as the client has an infectious skin disorder. Identify this from the list below:
   a. eczema
   b. bruising
   c. verruca
   d. lentigo
8. Which fire fighting equipment should be used on an electrical fire?
   a. water extinguisher
   b. vaporizing liquid
   c. foam extinguisher
   d. carbon dioxide (CO_2) extinguisher
9. What is a fire drill?
   a. fire detection equipment
   b. testing the fire alarm system to comply with health and safety procedures
   c. a notice to show people to the emergency exit route
   d. practice of the fire evacuation procedure
10. A risk is:
    a. anything that has the potential to cause harm
    b. the likelihood of potential harm from a hazard happening
11. Clients' records should be stored securely in accordance with the
    a. Data Protection Act
    b. Provision and Use of Work Equipment Regulations
    c. Health and Safety at Work Act
    d. Health and Safety (Display Screen Equipment) Regulations
12. If an accident occurs in the workplace:
    a. you should provide immediate assistance
    b. you would report this to the Health and Safety Executive (HSE) Incident contact centre
    c. record the details immediately on the accident report form and enter it into the accident book
    d. you would inform the member of staff with a HSE approved basic first aid qualification

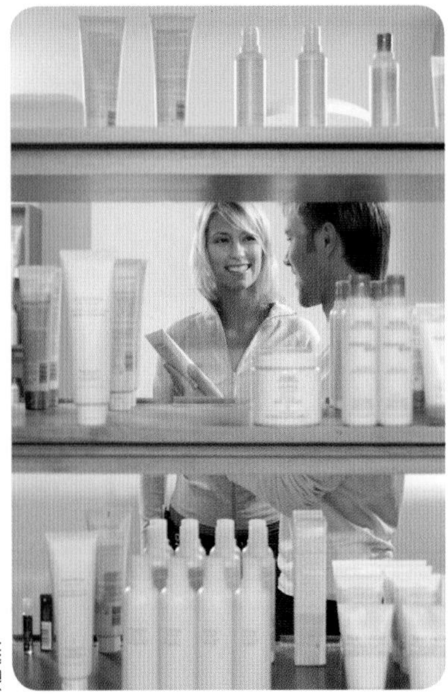
ALAMY

4 Selling Skills

Learning Objectives

This chapter covers **VRQ Unit Promote products and services to clients in a salon**. The salon benefits from maintaining client interest through awareness of the different services that are available to meet their on-going needs. Businesses must continuously launch new or improved products and services to be able to survive in a competitive environment. However, it is also important for a business, even one without local competitors, to encourage its clients to try new services or products to maximize overall service results.

This unit is all about your need to keep pace with new developments in the beauty workplace and educate and inform your clients about them. Clients expect more and more from their beauty treatments and related products; their awareness of what is available will give them greater choice to meet their needs.

There is **one** learning outcome for this unit which you must achieve:

1 Be able to promote products and services to the client

From the range statement, you must show that you can:

- use appropriate **communication and consultation techniques**
- promote **services and/or products** to clients
- provide accurate and relevant information on the **features and benefits** of services/products
- maintain a high level of **personal presentation**
- demonstrate the **stages of the sales process**

(continued on the next page)

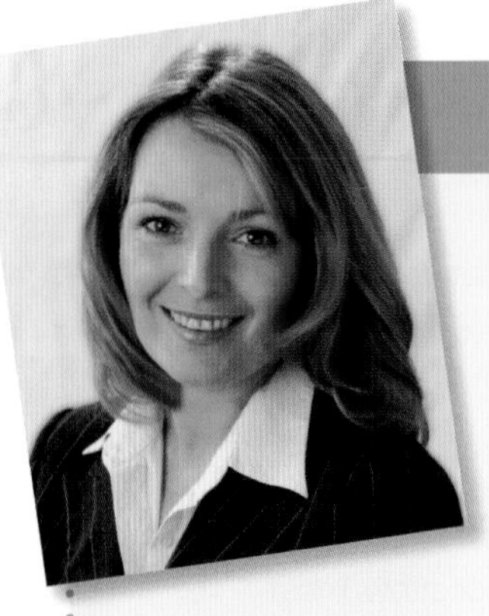

ROLE MODEL

Ruth Langley

Salon owner and beauty therapist
Pink Orchid Hair and Beauty Salon

“Ruth began her beauty therapy career in 1985 by renting a tiny room inside a hair salon. After five years she opened Pink Orchid, which now employs 18 hair and beauty therapists. The salon has won many regional and national awards.

Her main responsibilities are ensuring the continual growth and success of the salon, training the teams and ensuring each client receives the very best service and customer care.

Ruth works as a sales consultant for Habia and wrote their Selling Skills course. She is the author of the book *Beautiful Selling* which was written to help and encourage therapists everywhere to sell. Ruth says that she is very proud of the book and the wonderful feedback which she has received.

- comply with relevant **legislation**
- deal with different **methods of payment**

You must be able to show you have the necessary practical skills and underpinning knowledge to promote products and services to clients.

This unit is linked to the Beauty Therapy NOS **Unit G18**.

TOP TIP

Client refreshments

Healthy light refreshments may be promoted as an additional retail opportunity.

The importance of product or service promotion

When clients select a beauty therapy service or product they do so for one or a number of reasons. This may be:

- to improve their appearance, e.g. an eyelash tint or manicure
- for a special occasion, e.g. make-up application
- for therapeutic reasons, to receive a quality professional service in tranquil surroundings, e.g. a de-stress facial massage
- for aspirational reasons, e.g. to imitate the appeal of an advertising campaign
- to seek professional guidance on what would best suit their needs, e.g. skincare advice
- for performance, the product or service has guaranteed results
- to maintain the benefits of a particular service they have received before, e.g. repeat booking for leg waxing service
- for social reasons, they enjoy visiting the salon as much as receiving the service
- to give a friend a service or product as a gift, e.g. a **gift voucher**

Whatever the reason, you want the client to feel pleased with their choice, enjoy their experience and inform others of their satisfaction – thus promoting the business.

Retail sales are of considerable importance to the beauty salon business: they are a straightforward way of increasing income without too much extra time and effort. Beauty therapy services are time-consuming and labour-intensive; selling a product in addition to providing the service will immediately increase profitability. Importantly it can also benefit and support the client to achieve their treatment aim. For example, if the client receives a manicure and has weak, flaking nails recommend a specialized nail service and a strengthening retail product.

Clients need to be given on-going information about further products and services available. This will help maintain their interest and awareness of salon services and overall satisfaction with the salon. In Chapter 5 we look at the importance of creating an initial positive impression to the client. A high level of personal presentation, including personal hygiene, is very important and will encourage the client to initially engage with

TOP TIP

Seeking selling opportunities

The client's skincare preparations need to alter throughout the different seasons. As such, the client should be advised on products that are most suitable to maintain skin health and appearance. This gives you the opportunity to promote additional products and maintain client interest.

ACTIVITY

Express services

Increasingly clients are requiring a fast service often received in their lunch break. Examples include express artificial lashes for that unexpected special occasion. Find out what other services may be offered as an express service.

HEALTH & SAFETY

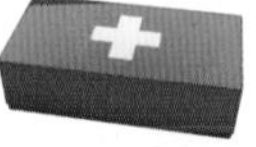

Contra-indications

If the client has a contra-indication to a service they wish to receive, recommend they seek their GP's approval first. You may require written evidence of this.

Give good advice

You have a duty to provide your clients with good home-care advice and help them to buy. Do your best to make the buying process easy and enjoyable for the client.

Ruth Langley

you. You must inspire confidence. Staff knowledge of products and services is vital to ensure personal effectiveness and helps in gaining client loyalty.

If you have got it right the client will maintain their loyalty to you and this helps the business to grow. For example, a facial service might take one hour and cost the client £40. You might then sell the client a moisturiser costing £40, of which £10 might be clear profit. Supposing that you sold eight products each day each yielding £10 profit. That would be a profit of £80 per day or £400 per week, or £1,600 each month and thus, £19,200 profit over the whole year: a significant sum.

Outcome 1: Promote products and services to clients in a salon

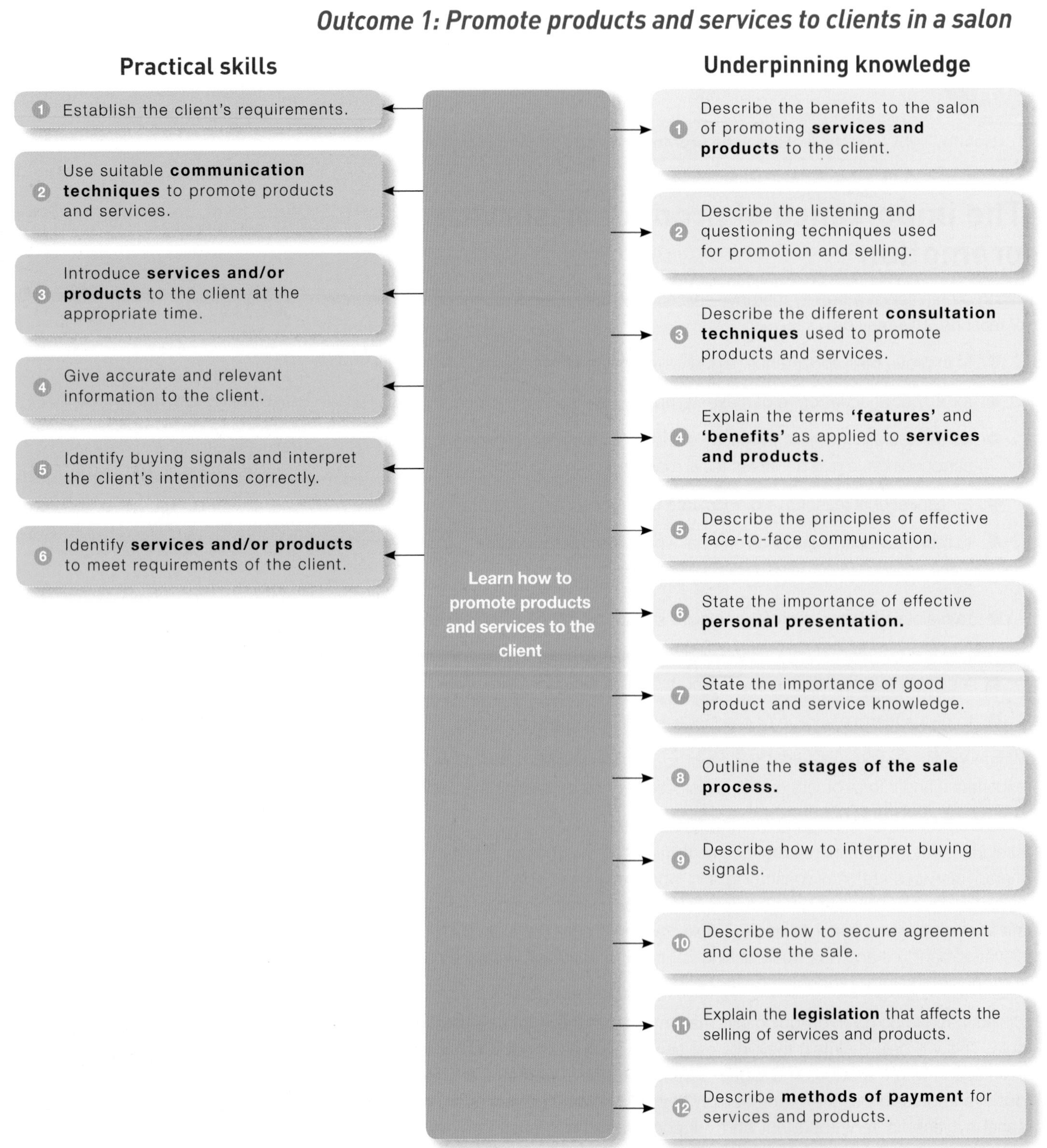

Practical skills
1 Establish the client's requirements.
2 Use suitable **communication techniques** to promote products and services.
3 Introduce **services and/or products** to the client at the appropriate time.
4 Give accurate and relevant information to the client.
5 Identify buying signals and interpret the client's intentions correctly.
6 Identify **services and/or products** to meet requirements of the client.
Learn how to promote products and services to the client
Underpinning knowledge
1 Describe the benefits to the salon of promoting **services and products** to the client.
2 Describe the listening and questioning techniques used for promotion and selling.
3 Describe the different **consultation techniques** used to promote products and services.
4 Explain the terms **'features'** and **'benefits'** as applied to **services and products**.
5 Describe the principles of effective face-to-face communication.
6 State the importance of effective **personal presentation.**
7 State the importance of good product and service knowledge.
8 Outline the **stages of the sale process.**
9 Describe how to interpret buying signals.
10 Describe how to secure agreement and close the sale.
11 Explain the **legislation** that affects the selling of services and products.
12 Describe **methods of payment** for services and products.

When promoting products or services, find out first about the client's needs and expectations. This will help you identify appropriate services or products for them. Carry out a **consultation** – an assessment of the clients' needs. This will use your questioning and listening skills. Consider the following.

- What is the client's main priority? What would they like to achieve? This information will guide you on selecting and advising them of the most suitable product or service.
- Is a skin sensitivity test necessary before the service? Ensure there will be sufficient time to carry out any necessary tests when promoting a service.
- Is the client allergic to any particular substance, contact with which should be avoided?
- Does the client have a skin disorder or nail disease which might contra-indicate use of a particular product? Contra-actions to products must always be noted on your salon records and the appropriate action to take explained to the client.
- Is the client planning to use the product over a skin disorder, e.g. eczema? If so, is this safe?
- Find out what services the client has received before. Were they satisfied or disappointed in any way with them? If so, find out why.
- How much is the client used to spending on products? Ask about what they are presently using: this will give you an idea of the types of product they have experience with using, and the sort of prices they are used to paying.

Bearing in mind the client's needs, you can now guide them to the most suitable service or product. This is where your expertise and knowledge are so important: you can describe fully and accurately the features and benefits of the services and products you can offer.

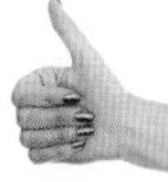

BEST PRACTICE

Testers for products
Encourage your client to try the product testers. You can also take the opportunity to apply the product, explaining its special qualities, to show it at its best effect to suit the client.

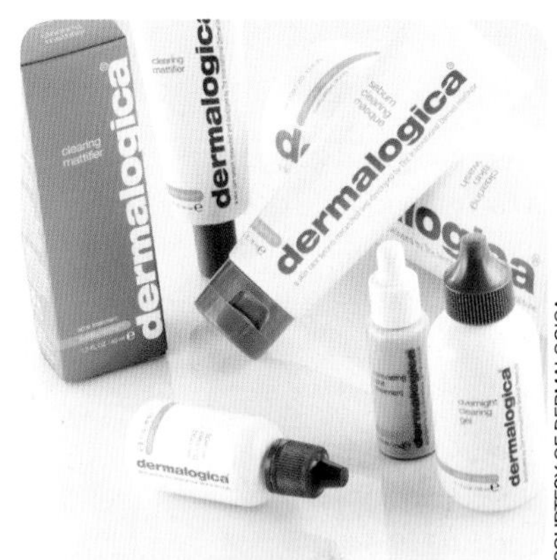

COURTESY OF DERMALOGICA

Skincare retail products

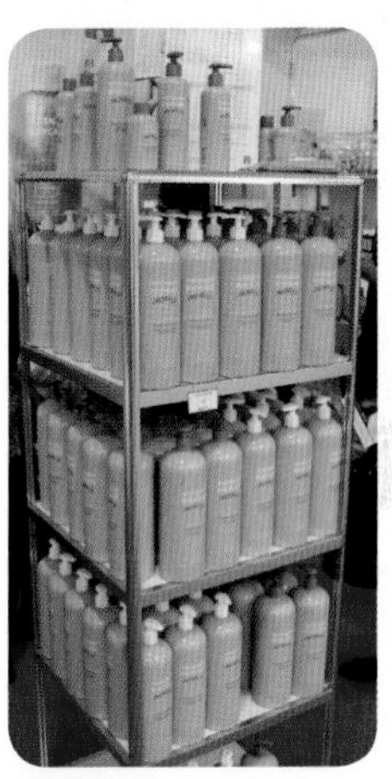

Retail product display

Features and benefits

This can be repeated again later to help the client make a purchase decision when there maybe several items to consider.

A **feature** is the uniqueness or individuality of a product or service, e.g. new technology used in the ingredient formulation of a product or the design technology of a piece of equipment.

A **benefit** is the gain to be made by the client from using the product or service.

Selling products

The products themselves must be presented to the client in such a way that they seem both attractive and desirable: the presentation should further encourage the client to purchase them. The packaging and the product should be clean and in good condition, and **testers**/samples to take away should be available wherever possible so that the client can try the product before purchasing it.

The final choice of product is with the client, of course, but often the client will ask for a recommendation, for example if they cannot decide between two possibilities. It is in these circumstances that your ability to answer technical questions fully, from a complete knowledge of the product, will help in closing the sale. Speaking with confidence and authority on the one product that will particularly suit the client's requirements may well persuade them to buy it.

TOP TIP

Features and benefits
A *feature* is the product's specialist ingredients and the effects they can achieve.

A *benefit* is what the client can expect from buying the product.

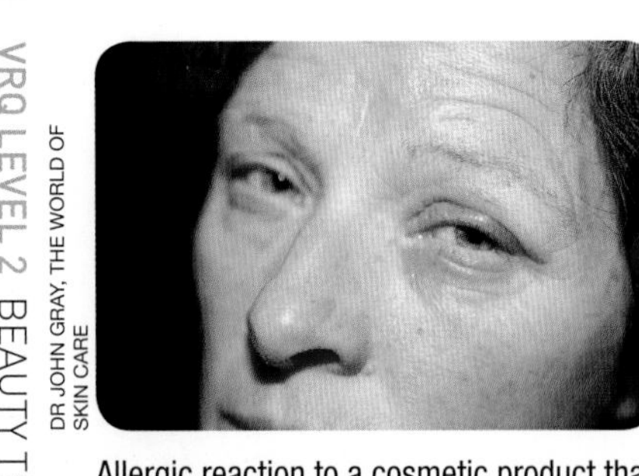

Allergic reaction to a cosmetic product that has affected the eyes

Product suitability

If the client has not used the product or received the service before there is always a possibility of an allergic reaction.

If the client does not know what an **allergic reaction** is – or how to recognize an allergy – it is important that you describe it to them (red, itchy, flaking and even swollen skin). If they experience this, which is termed professionally as a contra-action, they should contact you immediately or, in the case of product intolerance, stop applying the product the client suspects is producing it.

ACTIVITY

Features and benefits
Discuss and write down the features and benefits of a product or service sold in your training establishment.

HEALTH & SAFETY

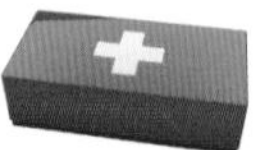

Skin sensitivity tests
If the client has not tried a product before, or if there is doubt as to how their skin will react, a skin patch test must be carried out.

1. Select either the inner elbow or the area behind the ear. The skin here is thinner, more sensitive and less tolerant.
2. Make sure the skin is clean.
3. Apply a little of the product to the skin, using a clean applicator.
4. Leave the area alone for 24 hours.
5. If there is no reaction (referred to as a negative reaction) after 24 hours, the client is not allergic to the product: they can go ahead and use it. If there has been any itching, soreness, erythema, or swelling in the area where the product has been applied, the client is allergic to it and should not use it (referred to as a positive reaction).

> **Know your clients' needs**
> The products that you recommend must be the right choice for your clients and deliver the results they require.
>
> **Ruth Langley**

Techniques in selling

The first rule of selling is *know your products*. This applies to all retail products and to all salon services.

KNOWLEDGE CHECK

Why are retail sales important to the beauty business?

Need more time... refer to pages 119–120 to help you.

Staff training

It is important that everybody is knowledgeable and able to answer the client's questions – this also includes the receptionist, who is often the first and last person the client comes into contact within a salon. In conversation, especially during quieter periods, they have opportunities to discuss products and services informally.

Often product companies provide training either at the business or at another venue. This is a great opportunity to update your knowledge and skills, which you will be able to share enthusiastically with your clientele. Often certificates to prove training are issued and these should be professionally displayed in the salon.

If not all staff can participate it is important that new information is passed on to them to make them effective in their jobs. Team meetings are a good opportunity to discuss salon policy and new products and promotions.

Information on products and services must be supplied for clients to read, and **displays** should be set up to gain attention. Be aware of your **competitors** and their current advertising displays and campaigns.

ACTIVITY

Updating your knowledge
It is recommended that you update your skills and knowledge annually, referred to as **continuous professional development (CPD)**. This allows you to be aware of current products, services and trends. Keep a record or log of all the different training activities you have been on.

If your business has a website, ensure it is kept updated. It is a great resource for keeping clients updated and details of sharing product/service promotions. If you have the software facility, clients may be able to purchase products or services online also.

Personal presentation is very important when promoting and selling products and services. Your appearance should instill confidence in the client and be a positive advertisement for the products and services you are selling. Refer to Chapter 3 Health and Safety for more information.

ALWAYS REMEMBER

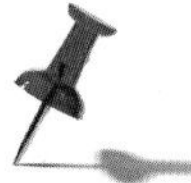

Consumer protection legislation

Legally you are required to comply with legislation including the **Prices Act (1974)** and the **Trade Descriptions Acts (1968 and 1972)**. These Acts prohibit false descriptions and prices of goods and services by the business. You must ensure accuracy of all media information provided in relation to products and services.

Methods of promoting products and services

When promoting products and services it is good to raise client interest and awareness by considering the following.

- Eye-catching promotional material (usually provided by the product supplier): displays in the window will encourage new clients! This should be changed regularly to maintain interest.
- Updated salon literature discussing benefits and costs of products and services may be provided.
- A promotional launch event, where clients can enjoy a social event and perhaps book services or buy products at discounted prices, may be held.
- Promotional packages may be presented at reduced cost or limited edition products can be purchased.
- Sample products may be given following a service for the client to try at home.
- Products to enhance the service may be promoted, e.g. specially formulated mascara to wear with individual false lashes. Always spot and make use of a selling opportunity without being 'too pushy'. Which may be off putting to the client.
- If you have a website you may wish to promote products and services on your homepage. Special offers may be featured and you may have the facility for clients to book online.
- Special events or occasions: e.g. if the client is going on holiday, recommend travel-size products.
- Remember your personal appearance is important and affects how we are viewed by others. It is important to look like you have made an effort with your appearance and this will reflect that you have pride in your work, products and services. If promoting a particular service or product such as nails – your nails should look great!

TOP TIP

Promotional launch events

Promotions are an ideal opportunity to establish your new product line with special offers.

Clients may have the opportunity to:

- purchase products at a special discounted rate
- purchase products with complimentary gifts
- receive complimentary samples

Clearly signpost these offers at different areas of the salon, e.g. reception and service rooms, using professional marketing materials. Provide the opportunity for the client to try the products.

Know your products and services **Product usage** must be discussed with clients, as necessary, and advice given on which product and service will best suit each of them. The only way to be able to do this is to memorize the complete range: all your products and services, including for example which skin types or treatment conditions each is for, what the active ingredients are, when and how each should be used, and its cost. Any questions asked must be answered with authority and confidence. Clients expect the staff in a beauty salon to be professionals, able to provide expert advice.

- Speak with confidence and enthusiasm.
- Avoid confusing technical words.
- Explain the features and benefits and personalize these, matching them to the needs of each client.

Always give accurate and relevant information to the client. If the client requests advice on products or services that are outside of your responsibility, refer them to the relevant

TOP TIP

Product knowledge

Use the products yourself. It is always good to be able to speak from experience and shows your confidence in them. You will also be able to give tips on how best to use them.

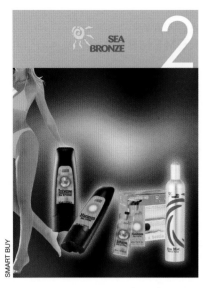

SMART BUY

A promotional poster for self-tanning products

colleague who has the expertise. You may have information literature you are able to provide to your client to find out more that will prevent possible loss of a sale, so pass it on.

Information to read The **information** available to clients can start from the salon window display. Use the **window adverts** if supplied with product ranges, and include information that advertises the salon's services.

Promotional **posters** are supplied with good-quality product and service ranges, and most suppliers provide **information leaflets** for clients. Use the posters and display leaflets in the reception area; clients can then help themselves, and read about the products and their benefits. This will generate questions – and sales.

Product and retail displays Two types of display can be used in the beauty salon. In the first, the display is there simply to be looked at, and seen as part of the decor. It should be attractive and artistically arranged, and can use dummy containers. It is not meant to be touched or sold from, so it can be behind glass or in a window display.

On the other hand, in the second, products are there to be sold. In this case products must be attractive but also accessible. The display should include testers so that clients can freely smell and touch. Each product must be clearly priced, and small signs placed beside the products or on the edge of the shelves to describe the unique selling points of each product.

This sort of active display must always be in the part of the salon where most people will see and walk past it -- the area of 'highest traffic'. A large proportion of cosmetic and perfume sales are **impulse buys**. It is no accident that perfumery departments are beside the main entrances to department stores, or right beside access points such as escalators.

Product displays must also feature in the beauty treatment service area. As the beauty therapist uses the products, they can discuss and recommend them for the client. If displays are there to see and to take from, the sale can be closed even before the client returns to reception. Although in theory clients can of course change their minds between the service area and actually paying, in practice once they have the product in their hands they will go on to buy it.

Most small salons will design and create their own displays using the counter **display packs** provided by the product companies. Some larger businesses will have a professional **window dresser** to regularly change the window displays for the best effect.

Be a great salesperson Believe in yourself. You have the potential to become a great salesperson. Most sales are lost because they were never asked for.

Ruth Langley

ACTIVITY

Learning the product range
Learn about and memorize the product range sold in the training establishment you attend. Once you have learnt about the range, memorize the cost of the products.

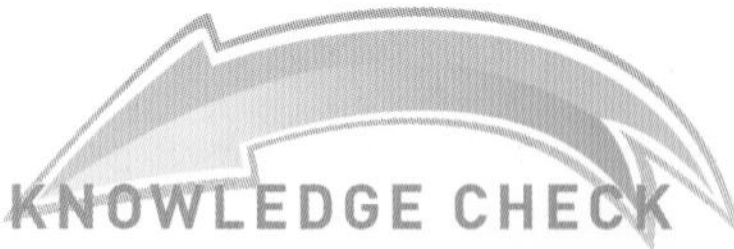

KNOWLEDGE CHECK

How do you think speaking with confidence and authority about a product will influence the client to buy?

Need more time... refer to pages 122–123 to help you.

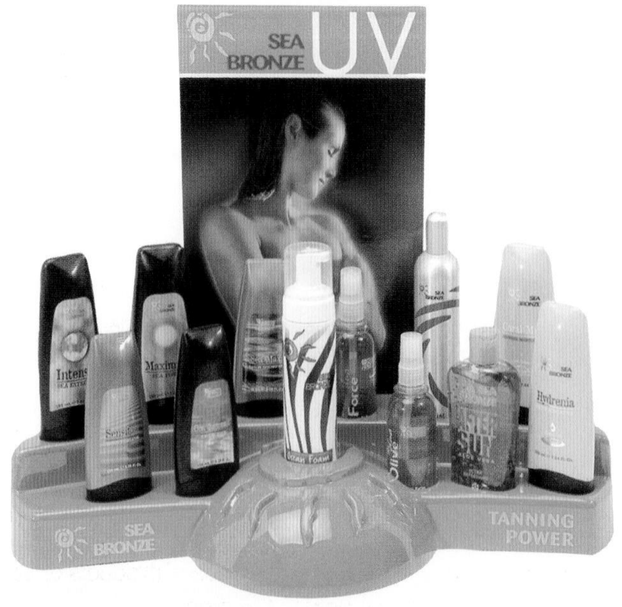

SMART BUY

Promotional product display for self-tanning products

Displays should always be well stocked, with smart undamaged packaging. Eye-level displays are best and ideally should be accessible. Change the display regularly according to the **promotion**, for example UV skin protection products in summer.

Displays must be checked and cleaned regularly – in busy salons this will usually mean daily. A window display will need to be dusted, straightened, and looked at from outside to make sure that it looks its best. The display from which products are being sold will also need to be dusted, perhaps wiped over (if testers have dripped), and straightened up. Testers need to be checked to make sure they are not sticky and spilt, and that no one has left dirty fingerprints on them.

HEALTH & SAFETY

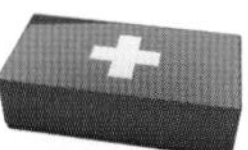

Maintaining hygiene and preventing cross-infection
To prevent contamination, spatulas must be used so customers do not put their fingers into the pots either when testing or during home use. You may also like to sell spatulas for clients to use at home.

The range of products

It is not enough to stock just a few items and expect clients to fit in with the range you carry: different ranges must be available for each skin type, and a number of specialist products – such as eye gel, skin serums or creams – that will suit all skin types. Make-up and nail polish should be attractive to all ages and types of customer. Sales must not be lost because of a lack of product range.

Information provided to the client should be accurate and not false or misleading. Legal action could follow in the case of non-compliance with consumer protection **legislation**.

ACTIVITY

Collecting information
Collect information leaflets from local beauty salons and beauty product counters in department stores. Is this literature attractive? Will the presentation encourage sales?

Email wholesalers and product companies for information about the display packs they supply with their products.

Look at websites also. What are the features of a good business website?

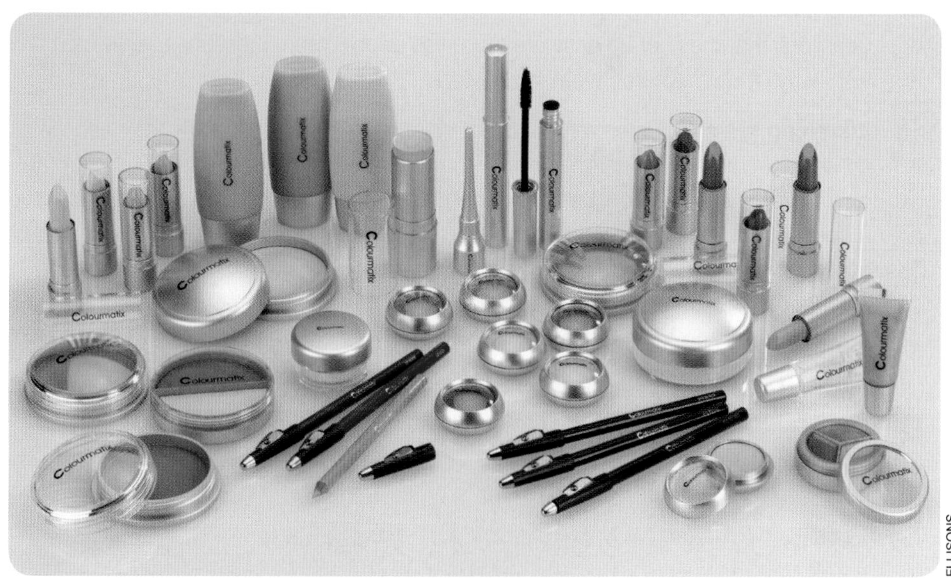

A cosmetic product range

Knowing when to promote the product or service

Choose the most appropriate time to inform the client about **additional products and services**. Present information on the product or service at a pace relevant to the client's knowledge and experience. If the information is new this may be slower and detailed. If the client is receiving a service this may be at the consultation, when discussing the service objectives, during service delivery when you have the opportunity to recommend and share advice, or when discussing aftercare. Here you will be able to reinforce the importance of further products and services to enhance the service benefits gained. Establish the clients requirements. This may be further use of products or services that the client has used before or of those that are new to the client.

ACTIVITY

Product and service promotion
Think of different services or products that your workplace offers that are not as popular as they once were. Consider a promotion you could offer to gain client interest. How would this promotion be presented?

Using good communication techniques

Good communication with clients, both verbal and non-verbal, is important. Establish a rapport with your client and give your attention fully to the client above any other tasks. Use your client's name: this increases their sense of self-importance and value.

- At all times remain polite, friendly and respect the client's individual opinions and preference. Never be critical; this may lose a sale.
- A client may be already considering purchasing a product or service and the type of questions they ask will signal this. The most common question is 'How much is it?'
- Make eye contact, observe the client's **body language**: are they interested in what you are telling them? If the client is interested, they will agree with you and their body language will be relaxed yet attentive. There are many customer types: those that are decisive, indecisive, chatty, quiet, opinionated, awkward and disbelieving. This should be considered in your approach: it is important that the client gains confidence in you and ultimately your products or service. This will be secured through your appearance, communication, style and manner.
- **Questions** must be accurate and detailed. You are the expert: show your knowledge. Do not ask the client what sort of skin they have – they are not the expert, and will probably give the wrong answer. Instead, ask more detailed questions, such as 'Does your skin feel tight?' (which may indicate dryness), or 'Do you have spots in a particular area?' (which may indicate an oily area). Use open questions. These are questions that may not be answered with yes or no. Open questions usually start with 'why,' 'how,' 'when,' 'what' and 'which'.
- **Listening** is a skill. Listen to your client; this will help you to identify their service or product needs. Always listen carefully to the answers your client gives: do not talk over their answer or interrupt. Only when they have finished talking should you give a considered, informed reply. Summarize simply and repeat what you they have said to show you understand – this is called reflective listening. You may need to ask another question, or you may be able straightaway to direct them to the best product or service for their needs based upon your conversation.
- Ensure that the client receives adequate attention whilst providing them with the products that they have agreed to purchase. Present the products to them and explain any specific requirements in their use in order that they gain maximum benefit from their use.
- Allow time for the client to think about the purchase.
- In the case of a service, make an appointment and provide the client with an appointment card and relevant literature relating to the service. If the client has made a decision to receive a service or purchase a product, you may find there is a delay in its availability. Ensure any delay is minimal. Do not be tempted to offer unsuitable alternatives, which are not as suited to the client's needs or service requirements. Inform the client honestly and realistically of their availability. In the case of a product you may be able to give the client a sample to use until the product is available.
- Ensure that the client has sufficient information to make a confident selection in their service or product choice.
- Give the client opportunity to ask questions and answer these confidently.
- Questions may lead to the opportunity to increase the sale of more products or services.

BEST PRACTICE

Create your own selling opportunity

- If the client is having a manicure and has weak nails, you could recommend a course of nail services and an appropriate nail strengthener.
- If the client is going away on holiday tell them about the special 'holiday package promotion'.
- If the client is having an eyelash tint, tell them how quick and simple an eyebrow wax is and the difference it can make!

TOP TIP

Always pay careful attention to your client and their responses. Remember: question, listen, answer:

- ***Question*** **your client as to their needs.**
- ***Listen*** **to the answer.**
- ***Answer*** **with the relevant information.**

TOP TIP

Competitions and free gifts are a popular incentive for clients to purchase products. Make your client aware of any promotions.

- Ensure the environment is conducive to the client feeling comfortable to ask questions.
- If a sale is achieved, be positive – smile, this will help to make the client feel they have made a good decision.
- Ask the client if there is anything else they need when closing the sale on the product. Confirm the size of product the client wishes to purchase, explaining any financial benefit to their selection.
- Explain any policies that relates to the sale of the services/products, e.g. the salon's policy on the return/exchange of products or when a gift voucher expires.
- Be appreciative, and thank the client when they are about to leave even if an enquiry has not resulted in a purchase.
- Record all sales on the client's record card. This is a useful reference point for the therapist and client to refer back to.

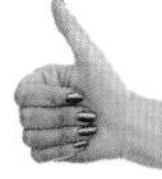

BEST PRACTICE

Packaging
Gift bags and a wrapping provide a thoughtful customer care service. If packaging carries the salon name and contact details this may generate future business.

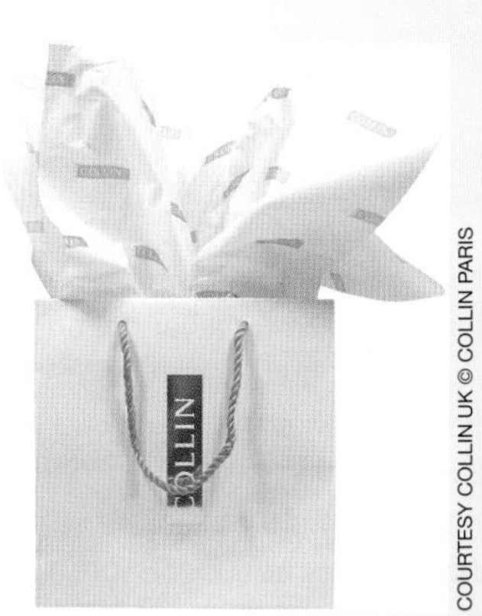

COURTESY COLLIN UK © COLLIN PARIS

Client suitability

If the client is not interested, they will probably not engage with you, and will appear disinterested in what you are saying. If this occurs go back to the beginning and suggest alternatives to attempt to regain their interest, but avoid pressuring the client. Following discussion about a product or service, you may feel that the client is unsuitable. Tactfully explain to the client why this is. If it is for medical reasons, ask them to seek permission from their GP before the product or service is provided. The expectations of some clients may be unrealistic. If this is the case, patiently and diplomatically explain why and aim to agree to a realistic service programme. Remember your legal duty under the **Health and Safety at Work Act (1974)** to take reasonable care to avoid harm to yourself or others.

Methods of payment for products and services

When the sale of products/services is closed and the client is satisfied, the final stage is payment. There are different methods of payment including cash, cheque, credit card, debit card and vouchers. These are discussed in more detail in Chapter 6 Salon Reception.

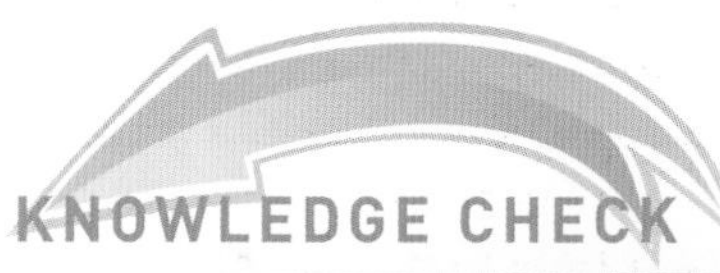

KNOWLEDGE CHECK

How can you interpret buying signals?

Need more time... refer to page 126 to help you.

Promotion

Promotions are another way of informing your clients about products or services that are available. They are also a great way of gaining interest in a product or service from a wider audience.

General benefits of a promotion

- Clients may take the opportunity of using a product or service because it is on offer at a reduced cost. If they do not like it, it is less of a costly mistake.
- A service or product on promotion may cost less and therefore be accessible to a wider client base.
- Limited editions or offers are a way of gaining client interest as the product or service may not be available or on offer at a later date.
- The enthusiasm of some clients will motivate others to purchase.

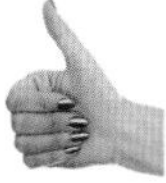

BEST PRACTICE

Effective stock control
It is important that you try to always have the range of retail stock available so effective **stock-keeping** is important. It is disappointing for the client if they are unable to purchase a retail item and this could potentially result in the loss of a sale – especially if they source an alternative elsewhere.

Demonstration

Demonstrating to an audience needs particularly careful planning if the demonstration is to achieve the maximum benefit. Everything required must be available, and all the relevant literature to be given out to the audience or clients.

Consider all possibilities in your planning. What type of demonstration is required? Will you be working on one client, to demonstrate and sell a product, or demonstrating to a group? Is a range of products or services to be demonstrated, or just one item?

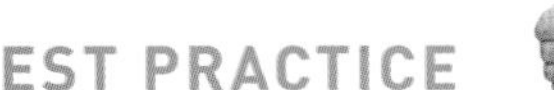

BEST PRACTICE

Promotion

All staff should be aware of any promotions that their business is offering so that they can build on a client's initial interest in a product or service and turn it into a sale. Always know about your products and services.

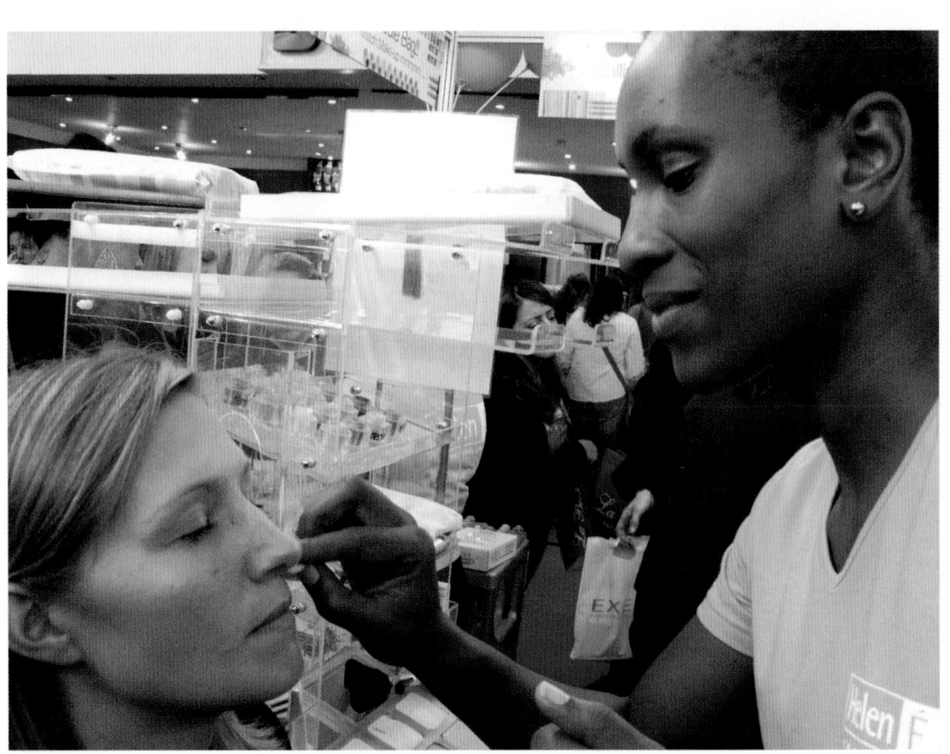

Trade demonstration

TOP TIP

Demonstrations

An effective demonstration will always create sales. Have the product ready to sell, or give out vouchers to encourage clients to purchase the product or service at a discounted rate.

Single client Demonstrations may be used to discuss facial skincare, make-up application and strip lash extension and removal techniques. When demonstrating on a client, have a mirror in front of them so that you can explain as you go along and the client can watch. They can then see the benefit of the product and learn how to use it at the same time. This is a simple but effective way to sell products.

A group The presentation should include an introduction to the demonstrator and the product, the demonstration itself, and a conclusion with thanks to the audience and model. Written **promotional material** can be placed on the seats before the audience arrives, or handed out at an appropriate point during the demonstration; **samples** can be handed around the audience to try while being discussed.

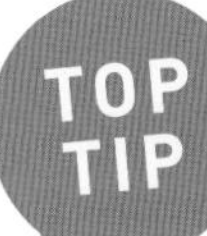

Visual promotional resources

You may wish to have the demonstration professionally recorded. This may then be used as a video on your website (if available) or in reception to capture clients' interest and generate questions from those who did not attend.

KNOWLEDGE CHECK

Describe three different methods of payment that may be used for products and services.

Need more time... refer to page 127 to help you.

The demonstration itself must be clear, simple and not too long. The audience *must* be able to see what is being done and hear the commentary. Maximize the impact of the demonstration by giving the audience the opportunity to buy the product immediately.

If this is not possible – because the demonstration is in another room, away from the products or at another venue, not the salon business premises – ensure that members of the audience leave with a **voucher** to exchange for the product. This should offer some incentive, such as a **discount**, to encourage potential buyers to make the effort to come to the salon and buy. Never sell the features and benefits to potential customers, creating the desire for the product, without also giving them the chance to buy it.

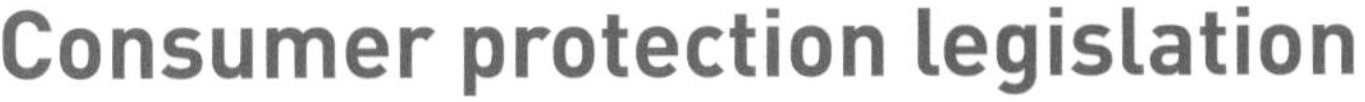

Consumer protection legislation

The salon has a legal obligation to implement and/or abide by the following legislation, designed to protect the rights of clients.

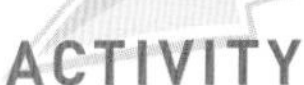

ACTIVITY

Siting of product displays

In your nearest large town, go into the big department stores and note where the cosmetic and perfumery department displays are situated. Research and list why this is a good place to site these products.

Consumer Safety Act (1978)

The **Consumer Safety Act (1978)** aims to reduce risk to consumers from potentially dangerous products. It outlines the minimum safety standards to be met. Amendments to this Act includes the **Consumer Protection Act 1987**.

Consumer Protection Act (1987)

The **Consumer Protection Act (1987)** follows European Union (EU) directives to protect the customer from unsafe, defective services and products that do not reach safety standards. It is important, therefore, to only use reputable products, purchased from a reliable source and that adequate information is provided to the client on their correct use. All staff should be trained in using products and maintaining them so they are in consistently good condition. It also covers misleading price indications about goods or services available from a business. Up-to-date prices for products and services must be available. Local authorities are responsible for protecting consumers. Trading Standards or Consumer Protection Departments check that trading standards and laws are adhered to and investigate any complaint. This Act makes provisions with respect to the liability of persons for the damage caused by defective products. If proven at fault and an offence has occurred the business may face legal action. For more information visit www.ico.gov.uk.

Prices Act (1974)

The **Prices Act (1974)** states that the price of products or services has to be displayed in order to prevent the buyer being misguided.

Trade Descriptions Acts (1968 and 1972)

The **Trade Descriptions Acts (1968 and 1972)** prohibit the use of false descriptions of goods and services provided by a business. Products must be clearly labelled. When retailing, the information supplied both in written and verbal form must always be accurate. The supplier must not:

- supply misleading information
- describe products falsely
- make false statements.

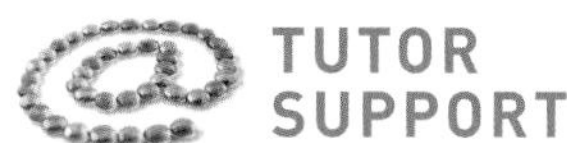

TUTOR SUPPORT

Activity 2: Product and retail display project

In addition they must not:

- make false comparisons between past and present services
- offer products at what is said to be a 'reduced' price, unless they have previously been on sale at the full price quoted for a 28-day minimum
- make misleading price comparisons.

The Acts also require accurate information to be included in advertisements.

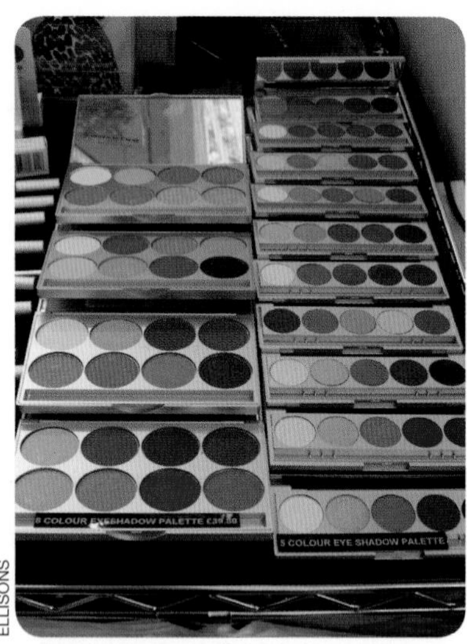

A range of eye cosmetics for make-up services

Resale Prices Acts (1964 and 1976)

Under the provisions of the **Resale Prices Acts (1964 and 1976)** the manufacturer can supply a recommended retail price (MRRP), but the seller is not obliged to sell at the recommended price.

Sale and Supply of Goods Act (1994)

This Act amended the previous Sale of Goods Act (1979) but the customers' rights as outlined in 1979 remain unchanged. The **Sale and Supply of Goods Act (1994)** provides that goods must be as described, of satisfactory quality including fit for their intended purpose, in appearance and finish, free from minor defects and safe and durable. The Act also covers the conditions under which customers can return goods. It is the responsibility of the retailer to correct a problem where the goods are not as described. This may be by refund, credit note, repair or replacement.

Cosmetic Products (Safety) Regulations (2004)

The **Cosmetic Products (Safety) Regulations (2004)** consolidates earlier regulations and incorporates current European Union directives. Part of consumer protection legislation, it requires that cosmetics and toiletries are safe in their formulation and are safe for use for their intended purpose as a cosmetic and comply with labelling requirements.

KNOWLEDGE CHECK

Clients have consumer rights. Why is it important to give accurate information about products or services?

Need more time... refer to page 129 to help you.

Data Protection Act (DPA) (1998)

The **Data Protection Act (1998)** applies to any business that uses computers or paper-based systems to store information about its clients and staff.

Through **communication** with your client it is necessary to ask clients a series of questions before the service plan can be finalized. Client details are recorded on the client record card. This information is confidential and should be stored in a secure area. The client should understand the reason behind the questions asked of them and how the information will be used. Confidential information on staff or clients should only be made available to persons to whom consent has been given.

Clients who have given information need to know how it will be used; otherwise they have a right to withhold it. Information stored must be accurate and up to date. It is necessary to register with the Data Protection Registrar, who will place the business on a public register of data users. A code of practice is provided, which must be complied with. For more information visit www.ico.gov.uk.

Consumer Protection Act (1987)

This Act follows European laws to protect the customer from unsafe, defective services and products that do not reach safety standards. It also covers misleading price indications about goods or services available from a business.

Consumer Protection (Distance Selling) Regulations (2000)

These regulations, as amended by the Consumer Protection (Distance Selling) (Amendment) Regulations (2005) are derived from a European Union directive and cover the supply of goods/services made between suppliers, acting in a commercial capacity, and consumers. They are concerned with purchases made where there is no face-to-face contact, that is, by telephone, fax, internet, digital television or mail order, including catalogue shopping.

Consumers must receive clear information on goods or services, including delivery arrangements and payment, suppliers' details and consumers' cancellation rights, which should be made available in writing. The consumer also has a seven working-day cool-off period where they may cancel their purchase. The point at which the right to cancel services is reached is detailed in the 2005 amendment to the 2000 Regulations.

KNOWLEDGE CHECK

Name three pieces of legislation/regulations relating to the way products or services are delivered to clients which protect legal rights.

Need more time... refer to pages 130–131 to help you.

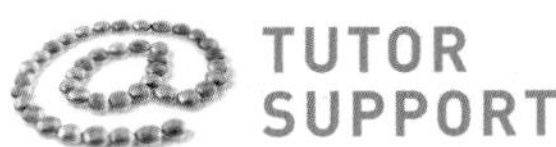

TUTOR SUPPORT

Activity 1: Customer rights task

GLOSSARY OF KEY WORDS

Additional products and services products and services offered by your salon that a client may receive or purchase to enhance their service benefits.

Benefit the gain to be made from using a product or service.

Body language communication involving the body.

Code of practice the expected standards and behaviour for the professional beauty therapist to follow, which will uphold the reputation of the industry and ensure best working practice for the industry and protect members of the public. Beauty therapy professional bodies produce codes of practice for their members. A business may have its own code of practice.

Communication the exchange of information and the establishment of understanding between people.

Consumer Protection Act (1987) this Act follows European Union directives to protect the customer from unsafe, defective services and products that do not reach safety standards.

Consumer Protection (Distance Selling) Regulations (2000) these Regulations, as amended by the Consumer Protection (Distance Selling) (Amendment) Regulations (2005), are derived from a European Union directive and cover the supply of goods/services made between suppliers acting in a commercial capacity and consumers. They are concerned with purchases made by telephone, fax, internet, digital television and mail order.

Consumer Safety Act (1978) this Act aims to reduce risks to consumers from potentially dangerous products.

Cosmetic Products (Safety) Regulations (2004) part of consumer protection legislation that requires cosmetics and toiletries be safe in their formulation and safe for use for their intended purpose as a cosmetic and comply with labelling requirements.

Data Protection Act (1998) legislation designed to protect client privacy and confidentiality.

Feature a unique or defining characteristic of a product or service.

Gift voucher a pre-payment method for beauty therapy services or retail sales.

Legislation laws affecting the workplace in relation to services, systems and procedures, the premises, employers and employees.

Prices Act (1974) this Act states that the price of products has to be displayed in order to prevent the buyer being misguided.

Promotion ways of communicating products or services to clients to increase sales.

Resale Prices Acts (1964 and 1976) this Act states that the manufacturer can supply a recommended price (MRRP), but the seller is not obliged to sell at the recommended price.

Retail the selling of goods e.g. products for clients to use at home.

Sale and Supply of Goods Act (1994) goods must be as described, of merchantable quality and fit for their intended purpose.

Stock-keeping maintenance of stock levels to anticipate needs. Stock records note how much stock has been used and when a new order is needed. This may be achieved using a manual or computerized system.

Trade Descriptions Acts (1968 and 1972) legislation that states that, when selling products, both written and verbal information should be accurate.

ASSESSMENT OF KNOWLEDGE AND UNDERSTANDING

You have now learnt about selling skills in the beauty therapy workplace. To test your level of knowledge, answer the following short questions. These will prepare you for your summative (final) assessment.

1. Which piece of consumer legislation states that goods must be as described, of merchantable quality and fit for their intended purpose?
   a. Disability Discrimination Act (1996)
   b. Sales and Supply of Goods Act (1994)
   c. Resale Prices Acts (1964 and 1976)
   d. Trade Descriptions Acts (1968 and 1972).
2. The feature of a product or service is described as:
   a. the individuality of a product or service
   b. the gain to be made from using a product or service.
3. Body language is important when selling, and is also known as:
   a. non-verbal communication
   b. non-verbal questioning techniques
   c. observation techniques
   d. eye contact.
4. To provide accurate information to the client when making recommendations you should:
   a. write down information about the products/services that you are recommending
   b. use technical words
   c. explain the features and benefits of all products/services
   d. ask the client if they have any questions.
5. Client record keeping is important as it helps you:
   a. remember recommendations made on a previous salon visit
   b. refer to previous products/services used when recommending other suitable products/services
   c. provide advice in the instance of a contra-action to product/service
   d. all of the above.
6. When selling, it is important to:
   a. recommend products/services based upon your client's needs
   b. use effective questioning techniques to find out the client's needs
   c. explain the features and benefits of the products/services
   d. all of the above.
7. Before most clients will purchase products/services from you they must:
   a. have received a beauty service previously
   b. have confidence in you
   c. observe that your salon is busy
   d. have a specific treatment requirement.
8. If a client is undecided on what product to use:
   a. advise them to go away and do some research
   b. recommend that they purchase all the products/services recommended
   c. suggest they to go away and think about it
   d. guide the client as to the most suitable choice following your consultation.
9. When are the client's needs identified when promoting products and services?
   a. following the consultation
   b. following service aftercare
   c. after skin analysis
   d. when demonstrating the products/services.

5 Client Care and Communication

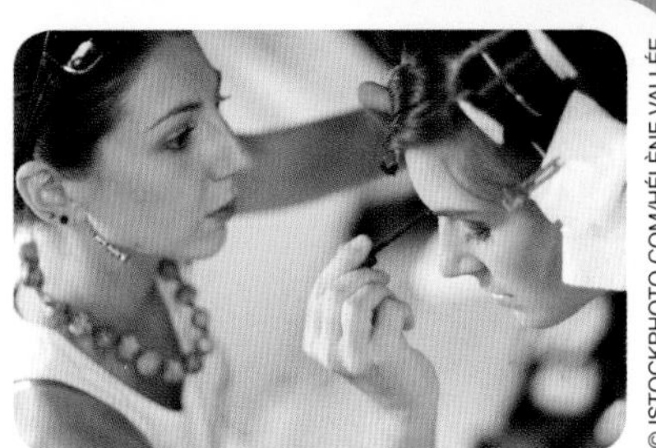

Learning Objectives

This chapter covers **VRQ Unit 203 Client care and communication in beauty related industries.**

This unit is all about taking personal responsibility to improve your communication and performance at work. This also includes ensuring positive, professional relationships are established with clients, colleagues and the team of people you work with, to contribute to the effectiveness and ultimately the success of the business. You will develop your communication skills to perform effectively in a range of situations and salon based activities. These include handling enquiries; selling; appropriately dealing with difficult situations and carrying out client consultations to identify the most appropriate service and/or product.

There are **two** learning outcomes for this unit which you must achieve:

1 Be able to communicate with clients

2 Be able to provide client care

From the range statement, you must show that you can:

- use **communication and consultation techniques**
- provide **clear advice and recommendations**
- comply with all related **legislation**
- refer a complaint to the **relevant person**

You must be able to show you have the necessary practical skills and underpinning knowledge to communicate with clients and provide client care.

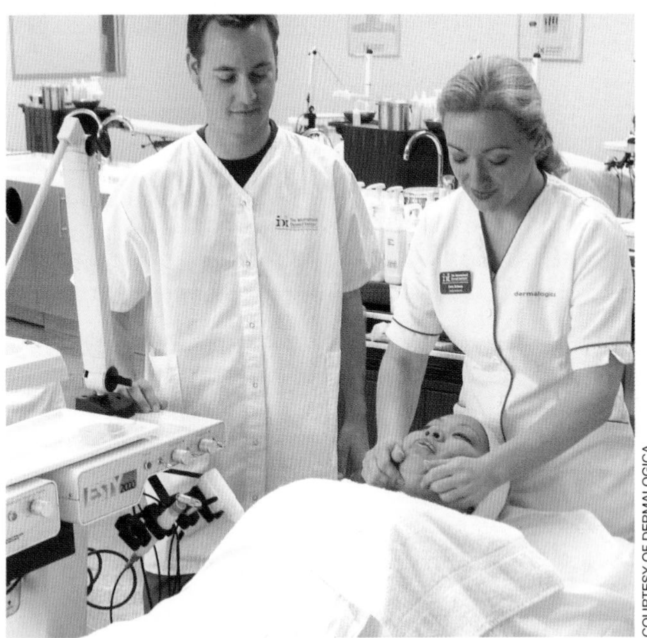

Beauty therapists demonstrating their client care skills

Client relationships

Outcome 1: Be able to communicate with clients

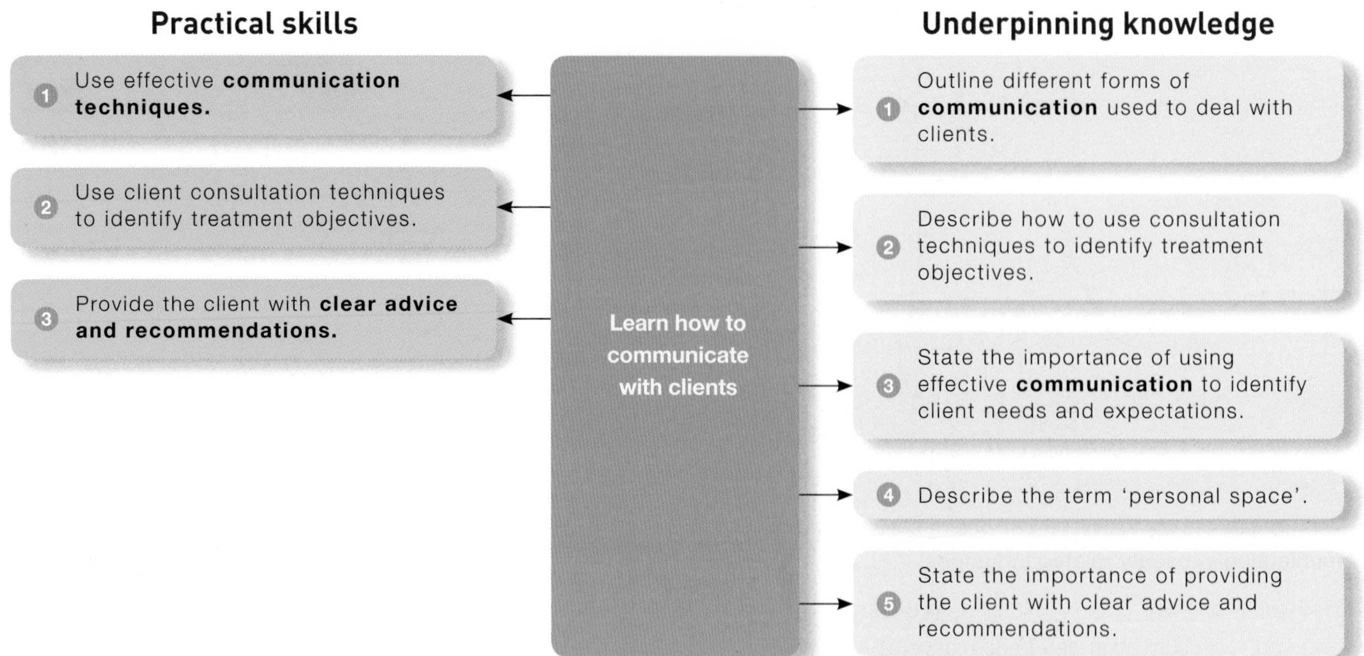

Practical skills
Underpinning knowledge
1 Use effective **communication techniques.**
2 Use client consultation techniques to identify treatment objectives.
3 Provide the client with **clear advice and recommendations.**
Learn how to communicate with clients
1 Outline different forms of **communication** used to deal with clients.
2 Describe how to use consultation techniques to identify treatment objectives.
3 State the importance of using effective **communication** to identify client needs and expectations.
4 Describe the term 'personal space'.
5 State the importance of providing the client with clear advice and recommendations.

For any beauty therapy business, to be a success requires the commitment of each employed individual to ensure quality at all levels and in all services.

For this to occur it is important both that you are effective in your job role and that you develop and maintain positive working relationships with your colleagues and clients which will create the right work environment.

Good working relationships in the workplace are essential. Each employee, whatever their job role, is valuable as part of the team in ensuring the success of the business. All staff at **induction** should be told of the goals of the business, and their role in achieving them. The induction should take place as soon as you start work, or progress into a new job role. Its aim is to provide you with general and essential information such as a description of the work environment facilities, health and safety, security, the staffing structure, roles and responsibilities of colleagues in the organization and how they relate to your welfare. For example who to report to if you require advice in area outside of your responsibility or you have a concern. The induction should leave you more confident about the expectations required from you and how you will be supported. Relevant responsibilities should be clearly defined in a **job description**.

Your training establishment will have certain salon service standards with regard to the expected standard of **behaviour** and appearance to perform successfully in the job role. These are often referred to as **codes of conduct**.

General beauty therapy codes of conduct

- Have a smart, professional appearance at all times and follow the expected dress code – it creates an impression of the quality standard that can be expected.
- Always have high standards of personal hygiene.
- Never eat, drink or chew gum in front of the client.

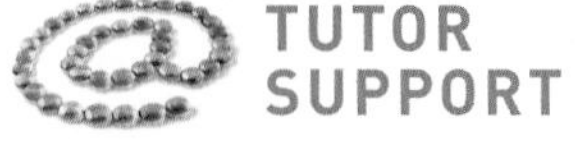

Activity 1: Code of conduct poster

- Ensure that you follow your health and safety responsibilities, never putting yourself or anybody else at risk through your actions.
- Communicate clearly and positively, both verbally and non-verbally.
- Be polite and courteous at all times to both clients and colleagues.
- Never lose your temper, or swear in front of a client.
- Avoid controversial and personal topics of conversation.
- If you are unable to give the client information they need, quickly find somebody suitably qualified to assist.
- If there are any personal issues among staff or towards a client, do not let these show in front of the client. Settle the grievances (reasons for complaint) as soon as possible, to avoid job satisfaction and productivity being affected.

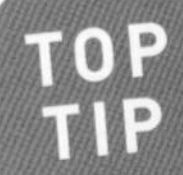

Image

A professional image creates confidence in clients, who learn to trust that they will be treated in a certain way – professionally and with respect.

Client care

Many organizations have a **customer care statement**, which outlines the standards of service customers can expect.

Clients want to enjoy their visits to the beauty salon and they are paying for a service. It is important that during each visit they are made to feel relaxed and comfortable and their needs are met. Good communication helps achieve this. It is the exchange of information between two people or groups of people that is effectively understood.

Remember that each client has a different personality and different service needs, requiring an individual service approach.

A client can be made to feel intimidated, uncomfortable or ignored – and this can happen without your saying anything! Even without speaking you communicate with your eyes, your face and your body, transmitting some of your feelings. This is called **non-verbal communication**. How you look and how you behave in front of your clients is important.

ACTIVITY

Client care

Find out whether your organization has a customer care statement. If so, how well do you do in providing that level of client care? Monitor yourself against the statement, and ask colleagues for feedback.

Positive relationships with clients

On meeting a client, always smile, make eye contact and greet her cheerfully – however bad your own day is! As you communicate you can:

- promote yourself, and gain the client's confidence in your professionalism and technical expertise
- develop a professional relationship with the client
- establish the client's needs
- promote services

Verbal communication occurs when you talk directly to another person, either face to face or over the telephone. Always speak clearly and precisely, and avoid slang. It is important to be a good listener: this will help you identify the client's service requirements and understand their personality. You can then guide the conversation appropriately.

ACTIVITY

Telephone calls

A telephone call is often the first contact the client has with the salon and is an important method of communication.

- How should the phone be answered?
- What should you confirm if the client requires an eyelash tint?
- What action would you take if there was not sufficient time for the appointment at the time requested?
- How would you handle a complaint about a service?

Conversing with a client

Having developed a professional relationship with your client, centre the conversation on them, so that they feel special. Avoid interrupting the client while they are speaking, listen carefully and be patient.

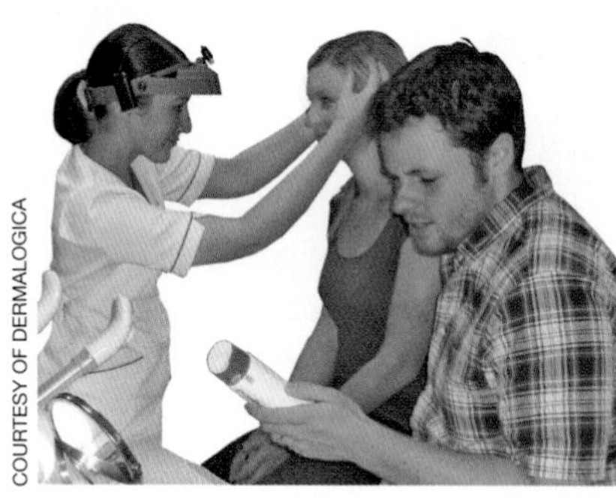
COURTESY OF DERMALOGICA

Client consultation

Listening skills When you listen, give the person all your attention, the other person then knows you are listening. You must ensure that you *hear* what the other person is saying and you *understand* what they are saying. Then you will be able to *respond* appropriately to what they have said or asked. Do not be afraid of silence, allow the other person to think and consider when listening.

A nervous client may need to be reassured. Gain their confidence by being pleasant and cheerful without chattering constantly. When asking questions, don't interrogate your client. Never talk down to them, and avoid technical jargon – instead, use commonly understood words.

Questioning skills Asking questions allows you to find out information you need to know and learn more to make a decision. Ask open questions; those that encourage the other person to talk and cannot be answered with *yes* or *no* (these are called closed questions). Open questions start with 'how,' 'why,' 'what,' 'when,' and 'which.' Probing questions can used and are necessary when you need to gain further detail or information. These may ask for precise detail, e.g. 'How long exactly do you want to wear your false lashes for?'

Certain technical information may not appear complicated, but if for example a client has bought several skincare products it is important that they know how to use them safely and efficiently. Always check tactfully with the client to ensure that they have fully understood the information provided.

Avoid all controversial topics, such as sex, religion and politics! When a relationship has been established, value it but be discreet – clients will often share confidences with you. Never pass judgment, and ensure that you deserve clients' trust by maintaining confidentiality.

TOP TIP

Conversation topics

Make notes on the client's record card of topics that interest them. You can introduce these topics in conversation next time the client receives a service, and they will be pleased that you have taken the trouble to remember.

Responding appropriately

It may be that the client requests information that you are unable to help with or which lies outside your responsibility. If this occurs politely inform them that you are not able or qualified to deal with their request but will get somebody else to assist. Always indicate how long this will take if it will not be immediately.

Keeping your client informed is reassuring and important to avoid dissatisfaction with the service provided.

TOP TIP

Client confusion

If a client is confused about the information you have given them, identify which part is confusing.

Repeat the information clearly and logically to clarify your instructions, checking for understanding.

Always allow time for clients to consider your response and provide further explanation as necessary.

Confirm the client's understanding with them and ensure that they are now clear and satisfied.

Non-verbal communication

Non-verbal communication is also referred to as **body language**. Interpreting body language is an important skill: learn to notice how the client is behaving, including their voice, their eyes, their body and their arm and hand movements. An instinctive 'feel' for customers' behaviour can be developed with experience.

Noticing client behaviour will help you to recognize the client's different needs and expectations. You must be able to adapt to these.

When approaching potential customers in a situation, such as a client who shows an interest in a product on a retail display, be aware that conflicting signals may be given. For example, a person may smile and nod as if interested but may, in fact, not be. On the other hand, if the customer makes the first approach then they obviously have an active interest already.

Initially the customer may be formal and may even have a stiff body posture and a reserved manner. As they become more interested, however, their posture will relax: they may begin to lean forward. It will become obvious at this stage that they are interested, and they then will go on to nod and agree, and to listen actively.

You must use your own body language to good effect. You must be relaxed but attentive, and listen actively – nodding and shaking your head, and smiling in agreement. Use relaxed, gentle hand movements: do not twitch or turn away from the customer.

If the customer is not agreeing with you, or is not interested, they may look bored, tap their fingers, fiddle with their shopping, look away, or even look at their watch. If these signs are evident, go back to the beginning and try to find out why they are not interested. This is important when selling. Perhaps they do not want the product you have recommended? Or perhaps it is too expensive? Suggest alternatives and see whether you can get their interest again.

When the customer has decided to buy, smile – help them to feel that they have made an excellent decision. They should leave feeling proud to have purchased the product.

TOP TIP

Using the correct title

It is important that a client is greeted appropriately according to their expectations.

Never use a client's first name unless invited to do so.

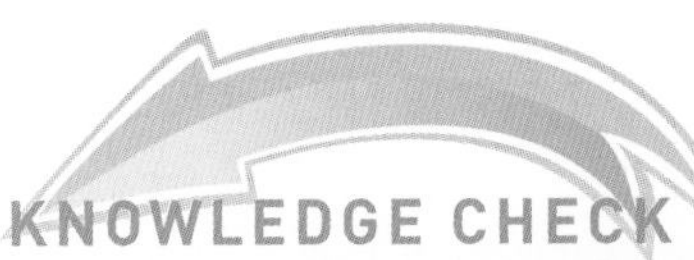

Define communication.

Need more time... refer to pages 135–137 to help you.

Consultation techniques

When you carry out a consultation you use all your communication techniques, both verbal and non-verbal, to correctly identify their treatment objectives. Through the consultation process you assess the needs of the client and identify their service/product needs.

It is necessary to ask the client a series of questions before the service plan/product can be finalized. This should ideally be carried out in a private area to maintain client confidentiality and the details recorded on the client **record card**. Remember at all times to ensure that the client feels comfortable, ensure that there is sufficient space between yourself and them. This is especially important when communicating with a client you have never met before. If the client feels uncomfortable they may feel you have invaded their **personal space**. Personal space is the space around a person that they sees as theirs. Intrusion of this can make them feel uncomfortable. A common reaction will be that they will move away from you, put up a personal barrier by folding their arms, avoiding eye contact. Ensure that you explain fully the consultation techniques in order that the client feels comfortable. Avoid touching the client unnecessarily, again as this is an invasion of their personal space. Always observe and read your client's body language.

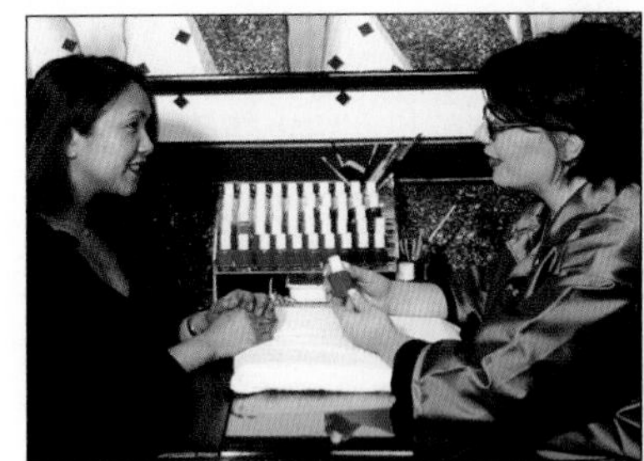

Personal space. There is sufficient space between the client and nail technician and good eye contact, showing the client is comfortable.

Open questions helps you find out the information you need to recommend a product or service to meet the clients needs. Use visual aids to aid understanding if necessary. An example may be the use of 'before and after' images to show the benefit of using a nail treatment product.

The information recorded on the record card is confidential and should be stored in a secure area following client service. This is enforced through the Data Protection Act (1998).

The client should understand the reason behind the questions asked and feel comfortable when answering them. As such, they should be asked in a sensitive and supportive manner. Avoid technical terms, choosing commonly understood words to ensure client understanding. Ask 'open' questions, which will encourage the client to give more than a one word response of 'yes' or 'no' and will help you to make informed decisions based on the information provided.

If, after the consultation, you are unsure of the client's suitability for service, tactfully explain to the client why this is and ask them to seek permission from their GP if relevant before the service is given. Some clients' expectations may be unrealistic. If this is the case, tactfully explain why and aim to agree to a realistic service programme.

Designing an effective service plan includes:

- completion of the client record card
- checking for client suitability to services
- providing clear advice and recommendations
- design and explanation of a suitable, realistic service plan
- agreeing the service plan with the client.

Outcome 2: Be able to provide client care

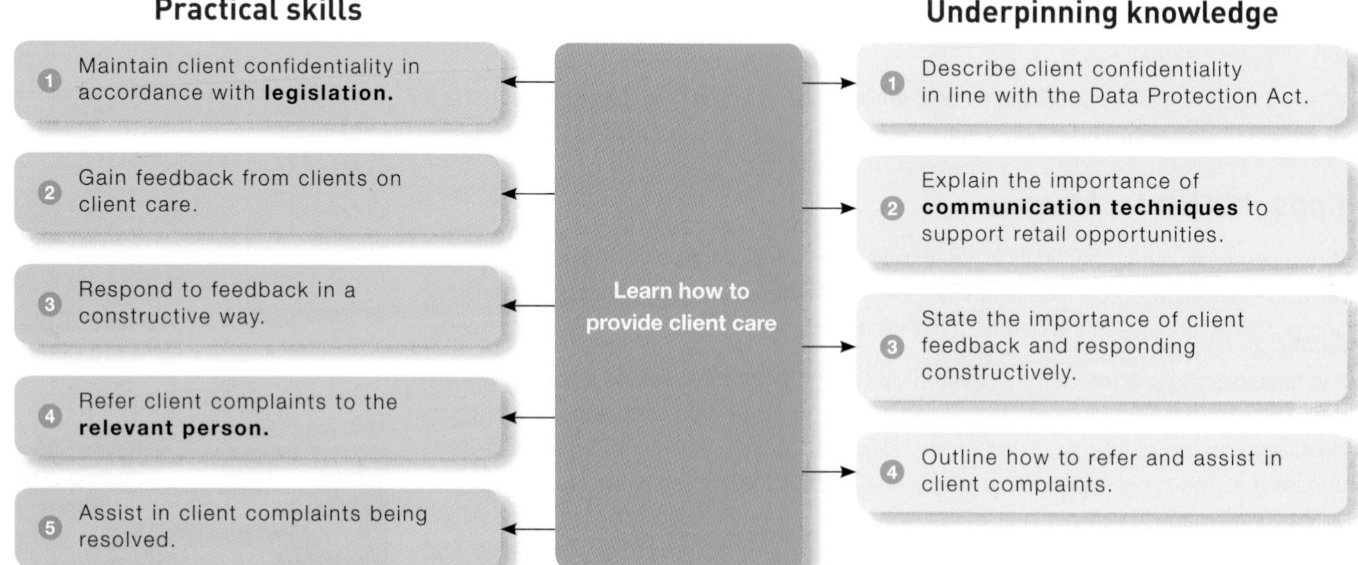

Practical skills
1 Maintain client confidentiality in accordance with **legislation.**
2 Gain feedback from clients on client care.
3 Respond to feedback in a constructive way.
4 Refer client complaints to the **relevant person.**
5 Assist in client complaints being resolved.
Learn how to provide client care
Underpinning knowledge
1 Describe client confidentiality in line with the Data Protection Act.
2 Explain the importance of **communication techniques** to support retail opportunities.
3 State the importance of client feedback and responding constructively.
4 Outline how to refer and assist in client complaints.

Complaints

Sometimes clients are unhappy with an aspect of the service received or a product they purchased.

ACTIVITY

Handling customer complaints
The client shown is unhappy about how long she has been waiting. What action would you take? List five other complaints that might be made by a client. How would you handle each situation to ensure a positive outcome?

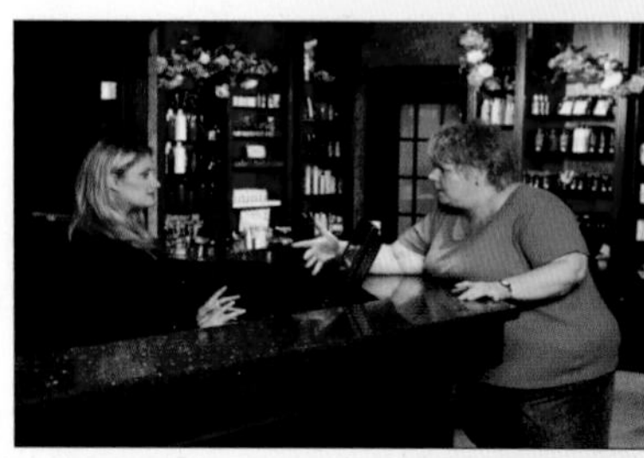

Avoiding client dissatisfaction

Some dissatisfied clients will voice their dissatisfaction; others will remain silent and simply not return to the salon. This situation can often be prevented through good customer care and effective communication.

- Always ensure that the client has a thorough consultation before any new service. This should be carried out by a colleague with the appropriate technical expertise.
- Regularly check the client's satisfaction. If there is any concern that you cannot handle, inform the **relevant person** of this immediately.
- Inform the client of any disruption to service – do not leave them wondering what the problem may be. Politely inform them of the situation, for example 'I'm sorry but we are running ten minutes late – are you able to wait?' If your salon has the facilities, you may offer them a drink.
- Inconvenience caused by disruption to service can usually be compensated in some way. It is important to resolve problems and keep clients satisfied.

Customer care is vital: clients provide the salon's income and your wages. The success of the business depends upon satisfied clients.

Complaints procedure

Unfortunately problems do sometimes arise in which the client cannot be appeased or satisfied. Many complaints are easily resolved but require a procedure to deal with them. A **complaints procedure** is a formal, standardized approach adopted by the organization to handle any complaints. It should also be used to handle complaints of discrimination.

Whatever the procedure for handling a complaint, all employees should be familiar with it. You should play your part when aware of a client complaint in ensuring that it is quickly resolved.

Clients should be advised of the standard complaint procedure and if not able to be dealt with immediately, they should be left with confidence knowing how it is to be dealt with, and how and when they will be contacted with an update or outcome.

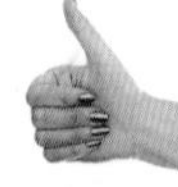

BEST PRACTICE

Handling and monitoring complaints

A complaint from a dissatisfied client gives us the opportunity to put things right and turn a negative into a positive!

Complaints received should be logged, however minor, and reviewed at team meetings. There may be patterns to the complaints which if not fixed could affect long-term customer satisfaction.

KNOWLEDGE CHECK

What are listening skills? Why are they important when ascertaining the client's needs?

Need more time... refer to page 136 to help you.

Dealing with client dissatisfaction or complaint

If a client is dissatisfied they may appear angry and complain or they may say nothing. However they react, remember that a dissatisfied client is bad for business.

You may be required to deal with a dissatisfied client.

- Stay calm and listen to the client's complaint.
- If you are unable to handle it refer it as quickly as possible to somebody who can. Inform the client of your actions at all times. (It is important that you know the limits of your authority when handling a complaint.) Inform the relevant person. This may be the manager, receptionist or senior therapist depending upon the nature of the complaint.
- Establish the facts and take appropriate action as laid down in your client complaints procedure.
- Always aim to repair the relationship, although at times this may not be possible.
- Not all clients are always genuine in their complaint – establish the facts and tactfully advise the client of the outcome.
- Always remain courteous, professional and create a positive impression.

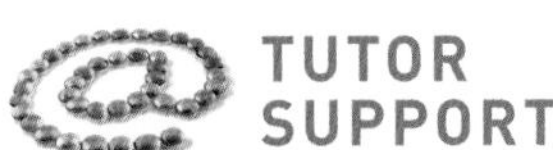

TUTOR SUPPORT

Activity 3: Communicating to clients

Legal requirements

The salon has a legal obligation to implement legislation designed to protect clients' rights. The relevant legislation is discussed below.

Health and safety Following the consultation you may feel that the client is unsuitable for service. Explain tactfully why this is and ask them to seek permission from their GP before the service is given. Some clients may have unrealistic expectations. If this is the case, tactfully explain why and aim to agree to a realistic service programme.

Remember your legal duty under the **Health and Safety at Work Act (1974)** to take reasonable care to avoid harm to yourself and others. Refer to Chapter 3 Health and Safety for more information.

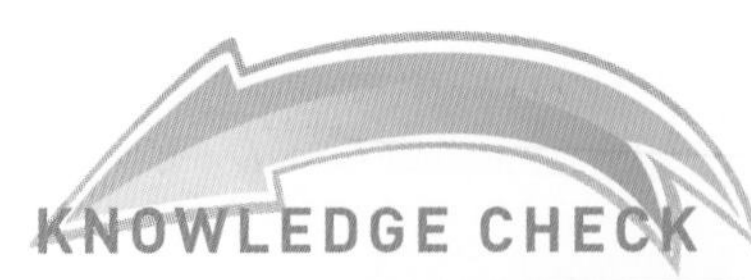

KNOWLEDGE CHECK

How can you interpret non-verbal communication when identifying retail opportunities?

Need more time... refer to page 136 to help you.

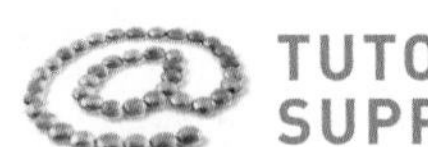

TUTOR SUPPORT

Activity 2: Evaluating client care project

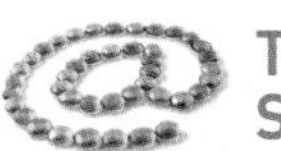

TUTOR SUPPORT

Activity 4: Which Act? handout

KNOWLEDGE CHECK

If a client was dissatisfied or had a complaint with a product or services how could you assist in resolving this?

Need more time... refer to page 139 to help you.

TOP TIP

Opportunities to improve technical skills and knowledge

Use your time effectively in the workplace; observe colleagues if you are not busy, ask questions, make opportunities to improve your knowledge and experience.

ACTIVITY

In your organization do you know:

- Who to report a client complaint to?
- Who you would refer to if information requested was outside of your area of responsibility?

ALWAYS REMEMBER

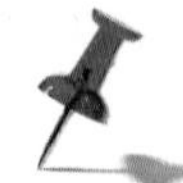

Legislation

Important legislation relating to communication and supply of products/services includes:

- Data Protection Act
- Sale and Supply of Goods Act
- Consumer Protections Act
- Trade Descriptions Act

You need to be able to describe the importance of each piece of legislation, see page 130 for more information.

Data Protection Act (1998) Before treating your client it is necessary to ask them a series of questions so that a service plan can be finalized.

Client details are recorded on the client record card. This information is confidential and should be stored in a secure area. The client should understand the reason behind the questions asked of them.

Confidential information on staff or clients should only be made available to persons to whom consent has been given.

Consumer protection legislation This is legislation designed to protect the client from harm for products/services and protects their rights when purchasing products/services. Refer to page 123 to find out more.

Improving your performance

In order to develop personally and to improve your skills professionally, it is important to set yourself targets against which you can measure your achievement.

To an employer it is important that you are *consistent*. You must always perform your skills to the highest standard, and present and promote a positive image of the industry and the organization in which you are employed and which you represent.

Developing your communication and client care skills

There will be many opportunities to develop your communication and client care skills and experience, including:

- Active participation in training and development activities.
- Watching and talking to colleagues who have more advanced qualifications or experience.
- Using time effectively, and by practising – all skills take time to master: the more you practise, the more skilled and confident you will become.

Communicate effectively as part of a team

There can be no place in a customer care industry for poor working relationships. A great portion of your time is spent in the workplace alongside your colleagues, and if the environment becomes stressful this will affect your effectiveness. It will also be apparent to clients, and relationships between staff members should not trouble them. Disputes must be resolved immediately.

When handling a dispute:

- Your behaviour can affect others for the worse or the better, remember 'behaviour breeds behaviour'. Stay calm and the other person will become calm, become angry and so will the other person.
- Do not be defensive, this is a negative behaviour.
- Behave appropriately for the workplace, remembering your salon 'codes of conduct': there may be clients in the work environment.
- Explain your case clearly and what your issues are. Avoid repeating yourself.
- Listen to the other person's case without interrupting.
- Suggest ideas to resolve the dispute. What outcomes do you need?
- Agree a solution, negotiate, including the other person's ideas also.
- Agree mutually to move forward.

If the dispute cannot be resolved report this to a senior colleague who has the responsibility to deal such personnel issues.

Personnel problems may occur if there are ineffective communication systems.

It is important that you understand the salon's **staffing structure**. You need to know who is responsible for what, and who you should approach in various circumstances.

KNOWLEDGE CHECK

What is the purpose of the client consultation?

Need more time... refer to page 137 to help you.

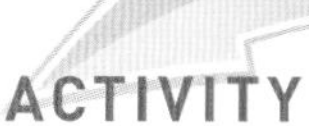

ACTIVITY

Dealing with the unexpected
How would you deal with the unexpected situations listed opposite? With colleagues, discuss your experiences and record your ideas.

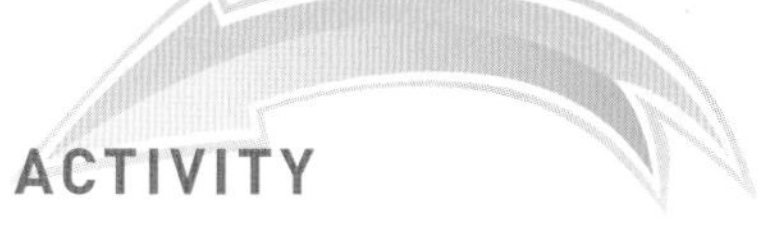

ACTIVITY

How good are we?
A questionnaire may be useful in monitoring client satisfaction. Questionnaires can be anonymous, and collected at a central point.

Ask questions that are important to the team and the business. Collate the findings and use them to evaluate effectiveness and identify areas requiring development. Simple changes can make all the difference!

Working under pressure

Sometimes you will be extremely busy and you may be feeling tired and weary. This is not the client's problem! Remain cheerful, courteous and helpful. You should also use your initiative in helping others, for example by preparing a colleague's work area when you are free and they are busy.

You must be able to cope with the unexpected such as:

- clients arriving late for appointments
- clients' services overrunning the allocated service times
- double bookings, with two clients requiring service at the same time
- the arrival of unscheduled clients
- changes to the bookings

With effective **teamwork** such situations can usually be overcome.

Gaining client feedback

In the service industry feedback from clients is important when measuring levels of service and satisfaction. It enables you to evaluate marketing methods, salon image and service.

Client feedback can be gathered in a variety of ways, both formally and informally.

- Client questionnaires can be used at random to evaluate performance, for example following a promotion. The results should be analyzed and appropriate action taken to improve areas of weakness, build on strengths and investigate potential areas of development.
- Simply asking the client if they have enjoyed or been satisfied with the service received is another method of service evaluation.

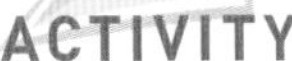

ACTIVITY

Evaluating customer care

Visit a local salon. Beforehand, think of questions you would like to ask in relation to services offered. Then evaluate the customer care and services you received. Were the staff:

- friendly?
- dressed smartly?
- knowledgeable?
- efficient and eager to assist you?
- helpful?

If you answered 'no' to any of these questions, discuss your reasons with your colleagues. What have you learnt from this experience?

GLOSSARY OF KEY WORDS

Assistance providing help or support.

Behaviour this refers to how we conduct ourselves in the workplace. It is important to be polite and friendly at all times, work cooperatively with others and conform with all workplace policies and procedures.

Body language communication involving the body.

Code of conduct workplace service standards with regard to appearance and behaviour while in the working environment.

Complaints procedure a formal, standardized approach adopted by the organization to handle any complaints.

Customer care statement defined customer service standards that are expected.

Induction an introductory activity delivered when you start or progress into a new job role. Its aim is to provide you with general and essential information related to the work environment, welfare and your job roles and responsibilities.

Job description written details of a person's specific work role, duties and responsibilities.

Limits of your own authority the extent of your responsibility as determined by your own job description and workplace policies.

Personal space the space around a person that they see as theirs. Invasion of this can make them feel uncomfortable.

Relevant person the person (or persons) at work to whom you should report any issues which are not within the limits of your own authority, e.g. manager, receptionist, senior therapist/nail technician, so they can resolve the problem.

Teamwork supportive work by a team.

Verbal communication occurs when you talk directly to another person either face to face or over the telephone.

Workplace policies this covers the documentation prepared by your employer on the procedures to be followed in your workplace. Examples are your employer's safety policy statement, or general health and safety statements and written safety procedures covering aspects of the workplace that should be drawn to the employees' (and other persons') attention, pricing policies and customer service policies.

ASSESSMENT OF KNOWLEDGE AND UNDERSTANDING

You have now learnt about client care and communication in the beauty therapy workplace. To test your level of knowledge, answer the following short questions. These will prepare you for your summative (final) assessment.

1. The first time you meet a client you should be:
   a. polite, friendly, aloof
   b. polite, friendly, chatty
   c. friendly, inviting, distant
   d. casual, friendly, distant.
2. The client consultation is the most import any part of any service.
   a. true
   b. false
3. When a scheduling mix-up occurs, you should:
   a. not admit that you or anyone in the salon made a mistake
   b. argue with the client who wrote the appointment down wrong
   c. be polite and never argue to see which one of you is correct
   d. blame the salon receptionist and call the manager.
4. Which of the following ways are appropriate ways of dealing with unhappy clients?
   a. Find out why the client is unhappy.
   b. Do not change what the client dislikes until their next visit.
   c. Tactfully explain the reasons why you cannot make changes.
   d. Argue with the client to inform them of your opinion.
   e. Call on the advice of the relevant person to help.
5. The legislation designed to protect client privacy and confidentiality is:
   a. Data Protection Act
   b. Workplace Regulations
   c. Health and Safety at Work Act
   d. Provision and use of Work Equipment Regulations.
6. Non-verbal communication is:
   a. communicating using the telephone
   b. communicating using body gestures
   c. completion of the client record card
   d. the tone of voice used when talking to the client.
7. Personal space is:
   a. the space around a person that they see as theirs
   b. the appointment space booked for each client
   c. where the client's details are recorded
   d. where the client can store their personal belongings.
8. A consultation should be provided:
   a. at every service
   b. if the client is new to you
   c. each time the client receives a different service
   d. at every other appointment.
9. The consultation uses the following:
   a. verbal communication
   b. non-verbal communication
   c. listening techniques
   d. verbal and non-verbal communication.
10. Verbal questioning techniques at consultation used to find out your clients need use:
    a. open questions
    b. closed questions
    c. a record card to tick the correct answer to a question
    d. a list of set questions that the client provides short answers to.

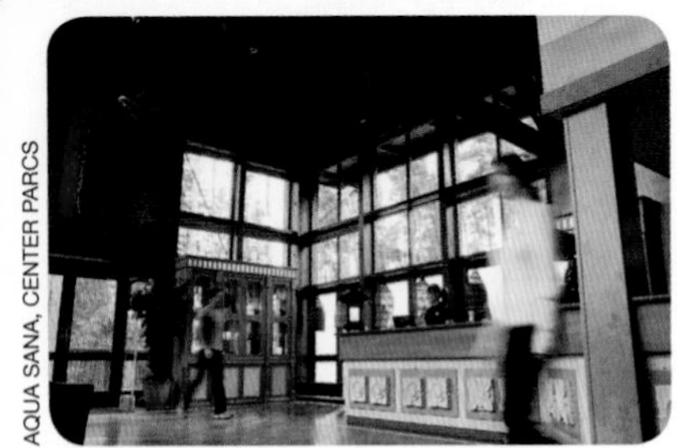

AQUA SANA, CENTER PARCS

6 Salon Reception

Learning Objectives

This chapter covers **VRQ Unit 216 Salon reception duties**. It explains how to carry out the important reception skills of welcoming and receiving people entering the beauty therapy work area, handling enquiries, making appointments, dealing with client payments and generally maintaining the appearance of the reception area. Dealing with people in a polite, efficient manner while questioning them to find out what they require forms an important part of this unit.

There are **three** learning outcomes for this unit which you must achieve:

1 **Be able to carry out reception duties**

2 **Be able to book appointments**

3 **Be able to deal with payments**

From the range statement, you must show that you can:

- deal with a variety of enquiries through a **variety of techniques**
- **communicate and behave** in an appropriate and professional manner
- identify the **nature of the enquiry**
- observe all **legislation** when handling client details
- deal with the different **methods of payment**
- deal with all types of payment **problems**

You must be able to show you have the necessary practical skills and underpinning knowledge to fulfil salon reception duties.

This unit is linked to the Beauty Therapy NOS **Unit G4**.

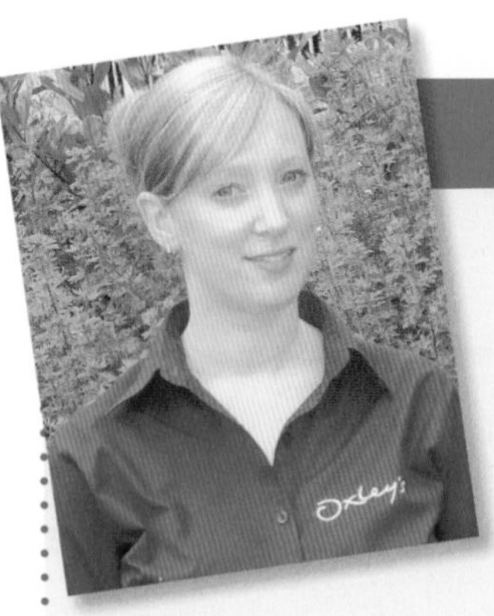

ROLE MODEL

Sally-Anne Braithwaite

Sally-Anne Braithwaite
Front of House Manager
Oxley's at Ambleside
Blue Fish Spa

"My current job role as front of house manager includes all sorts of responsibilities such as running reception, meeting and greeting customers, product sales and helping with marketing and accounts.

When I first started the job in October 2006 I was new to the beauty industry and had to learn all aspects of the job as I went along. I was trained up to have a good knowledge of all the treatments we have to offer, which I feel is a very important part of my role. Now I am part of a great team and have a very rewarding and enjoyable job.

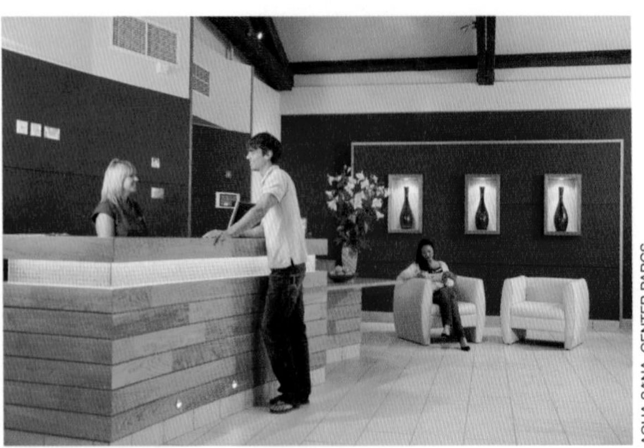

AQUA SANA, CENTER PARCS

Spa reception

Reception introduction

Reception is a client's first and also final impression of the business, whether this is on the telephone or in person when they visit. It is becoming increasingly more popular to book appointments online. If your salon has an online facility this must be handled smoothly and efficiently. Clients observe the quality of service, making judgments through every contact they have with the business. It is important that the attitude of the **receptionist** and their response to any query is knowledgeable and extremely helpful. The reception area must be kept clean and tidy at all times. First impressions count, so ensure that the client gets the *right* impression!

Clients need to feel valued. Good **interpersonal skills** are essential in a receptionist. Interpersonal skills are behaviours – everything you say and do. Clients will reach conclusions based upon your behaviour. Always:

- act positively and confidently
- speak clearly
- be friendly, and smile
- look at the client and maintain eye contact
- use good listening skills
- be interested in everything that is going on around the reception area
- give each client individual attention and respect.

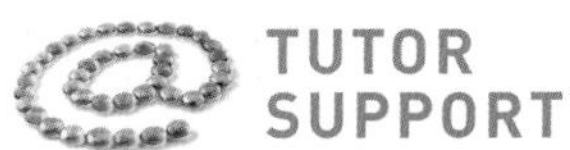

Activity 1: Requirements for reception area tasks

TOP TIP

Cleanliness

An attractive heavy-duty foot mat at the entrance to reception will protect the main floor covering from becoming marked. This may be embossed with the salon logo. Keep the entrance clean and smart at all times and reduce possible accidents from slipping on wet flooring.

Outcome 1: Be able to carry out reception duties

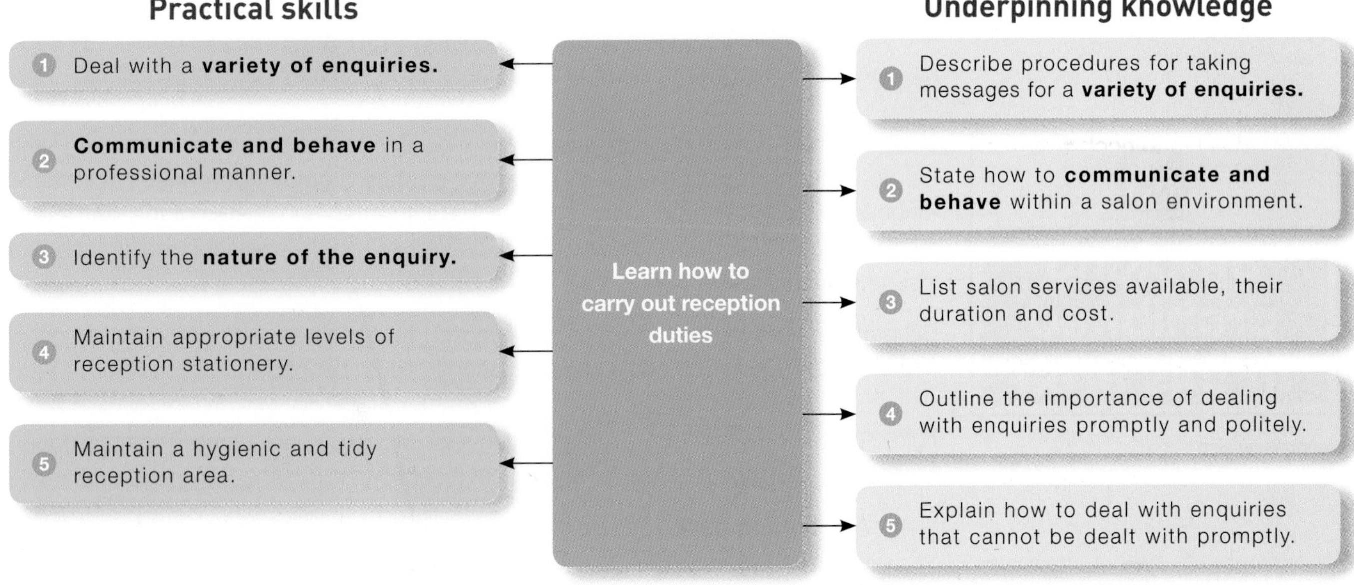

Practical skills
1 Deal with a variety of enquiries.
2 Communicate and behave in a professional manner.
3 Identify the nature of the enquiry.
4 Maintain appropriate levels of reception stationery.
5 Maintain a hygienic and tidy reception area.
Learn how to carry out reception duties
Underpinning knowledge
1 Describe procedures for taking messages for a variety of enquiries.
2 State how to communicate and behave within a salon environment.
3 List salon services available, their duration and cost.
4 Outline the importance of dealing with enquiries promptly and politely.
5 Explain how to deal with enquiries that cannot be dealt with promptly.

ACTIVITY

Magazines

What magazines do you think would be appropriate for the beauty salon? Consider your clientele.

TOP TIP

DVD promotion presentation

Facilities in reception may be used to promote salon services. Many suitable DVDs are available from beauty manufacturers and suppliers.

Reception area

Location Reception is usually situated at the front of a beauty salon; in a large department store, reception may be a cosmetic counter. It should be clean, tidy and inviting.

With a salon, the advantage of having reception at the front is that the window can be used to attract and capture the attention and interest of potential clients. Clients who are waiting in reception, however, may seek privacy, so the window should be attractively curtained and the seating should be situated away from the view of the main window if possible.

Size The entrance to reception should be large enough for wheelchair access. There should be adequate seating, and an area in which to hang clients' coats and wet umbrellas. If the entrance floor becomes wet for any reason, all necessary action should be taken immediately to avoid slippage.

HEALTH & SAFETY

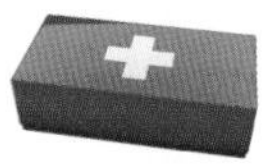

Disability Discrimination Act (DDA) (2005) – wheelchair access

The Disability Discrimination Act (2005) is a piece of legislation that promotes civil rights for disabled people and protects disabled people from discrimination. Your business provides an everyday service that those with disabilities have a right to get access to. It is important every effort is made to comply with this legislation and the appointment of reception and access design should take this into account.

It may be that small services, such as manicures, are carried out at reception. These services can then be seen by others, and may attract further clients.

Hospitality is important and shows the salon's commitment to client care. If the client arrives early or their service is likely to be delayed, offer magazines or refreshments such as coffee or water. Clients may also like refreshments following their service for example while waiting for their nail polish to dry or while waiting between different services. It is also a pleasant gesture to have boiled sweets on reception for the client to take.

Magazines should be stored in an area of the reception. They should be collected as necessary and returned to this area. Magazines should be renewed regularly and disposed of if in poor condition.

Smoking It is illegal to smoke on enclosed or partially enclosed business premises and you are required by law to display a mandatory sign stating this. Out of courtesy if you have an area where clients are able to smoke outside you may inform them of this.

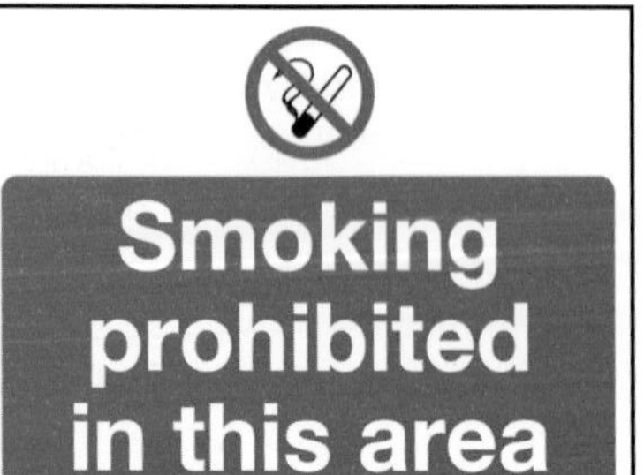

No smoking sign

Decoration The reception area should be decorated tastefully in keeping with the décor in the rest of the salon. Attractive posters promoting proprietary cosmetic ranges/services may be displayed on the walls. Framed certificates of the staff's professional qualifications can be displayed, as well as health-legislation registration and insurance certificates.

Decorative plants or fresh flowers displayed on reception are attractive. Avoid heavily fragranced flowers which could cause irritation to some people.

Reception resources The reception area should be uncluttered. The main equipment and furnishings required for an efficient reception include the following:

- **A *reception desk*** The size of the desk will depend on the size of the salon; some salons may have several receptionists. The desk should include shelves and drawers; some have an in-built lockable cash or security drawer. The desk should be at a convenient height for the client to write a **cheque**, note down the appointment time, etc. It should also be large enough to house the **appointment** book or computer (or both). Consider clients who may be in a wheelchair – the desk must be accessible to them so you can communicate effectively with them and handle their payments.
- **A *comfortable chair*** The receptionist's chair should provide adequate back support and be the correct height for working at a computer screen.

HEALTH & SAFETY

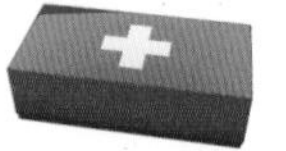

Ventilation

Ensure that the air is fresh and the room adequately ventilated to remove any smells created from services such as nail services performed in the reception area.

- **A *computer*** Computers can be used to store data about clients, to book appointment schedules, handle electronic communication (e.g. email), to carry out automatic stock control, and to record business details such as accounts and marketing information. They can also be programmed to recommend specific services on the basis of personal data about the client! Space should be provided for a printer if required. A shredder is useful to dispose of confidential information when necessary.
- **A *calculator*** This is used for simple financial calculations, especially if the salon does not have a computer.
- ***Stationery*** This should include price lists, gift vouchers, appointment cards and a receipt pad. Keep a supply available in line with your salon policy.
- **A *notepad*** This is for taking notes and recording **messages**.
- ***Address and telephone contact details*** All frequently used telephone numbers should be available in an electronic or non-electronic format.
- ***Sales-related equipment*** Items such as till rolls, credit card equipment and a cash book if used.
- **A *telephone and an answering machine*** The answering machine allows clients to notify you, even when the salon is closed, of an appointment request, or an unavoidable change or cancellation. You can then re-schedule appointments as quickly as possible. If you are working on your own, the answering machine avoids interruptions during a service, yet without losing custom.
- **A *fax machine*** This may be available at reception. The fax is capable of transmitting text and image via a telephone line to another fax machine. This is useful when information needs to be passed on quickly.
- ***Record cards*** Record cards are confidential cards that record the personal details of each client registered at the salon. They should be kept in alphabetical order in a filing cabinet or a card-index box, and should be ready for collection by the therapist when treating new or existing clients. See the general beauty therapy units of this book for complete unit-specific examples of record cards. Each card records:
  - the client's name, address and telephone number
  - any medical details
  - any contra-indications (such as allergies and contra-actions)
  - results and dates of any skin tests carried out
  - service aims and outcomes
  - a base on which to plan future services
  - services received, products used and merchandise purchased

  These records may be updated by the receptionist at a later stage following the client's service if a central electronic database is used for this purpose.
- **Pens, pencils and a rubber** Make sure these stay at the desk!
- **A display cabinet** This may be used to store proprietary skincare and cosmetic products, and any other merchandise sold by the salon.
- **Waste bin** A covered, lined waste bin may be provided at the reception area. Ensure this is emptied regularly following salon policy.

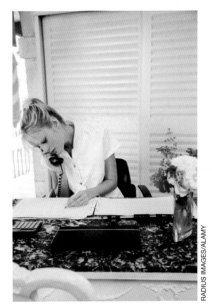

RADIUS IMAGES/ALAMY

A receptionist booking an appointment

Employability skills
Someone who is well presented, willing to learn, adaptable and a confident communicator makes a good impression.

Sally-Anne Braithwaite

HEALTH & SAFETY 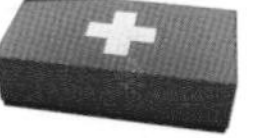

Eating and drinking
The receptionist and other employees should not eat or drink at reception.

ALWAYS REMEMBER 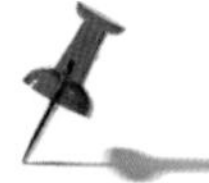

Data Protection Act (1998)
Client records
The record card records confidential information about your client. Ensure that how client information is stored and used complies with the Data Protection Act (1998).

A sample client record card

BEAUTY WORKS	
Date	Beauty therapist name
Client name	Date of birth
Address	Postcode
Evening phone number	Daytime phone number
Name of doctor	Doctor's address and phone number
Related medical history (Conditions that may restrict or prohibit service application.)	
Are you taking any medication (especially antibiotics, steroids, the pill, etc.)?	

CONTRA-INDICATIONS REQUIRING MEDICAL REFERRAL	
(Preventing facial service application)	
☐	bacterial infection (e.g. impetigo)
☐	fungal infection (e.g. tinea corporis)
☐	viral infection (e.g. herpes simplex)
☐	eye infections (e.g. conjunctivitis)

CONTRA-INDICATIONS WHICH RESTRICT SERVICE	
(Service may require adaption)	
☐	cuts and abrasions
☐	recent scar tissue
☐	skin allergies
☐	styes
☐	bruising and swelling
☐	eczema
☐	vitiligo
☐	hyper keratosis

Data Protection Act (DPA) (1998)

The **Data Protection Act (1998)** was passed by Parliament to control the way information is handled and to give legal rights to people who have information stored about them. With more and more organizations using computers to store and process personal data, access to confidential information has become increasingly possible.

This legislation is designed to protect the client's privacy and confidentiality. It is necessary to ask the client questions before the service plan can be finalized. The relevant information gathered on the client is confidential and should be stored in a safe and secure area following client service, whether on a computer or organized paper filing system. Inform the client that their personal details are being stored and will only be accessed by those individuals who are authorized to do so. Remember also, do not provide confidential information over the telephone or in email correspondence.

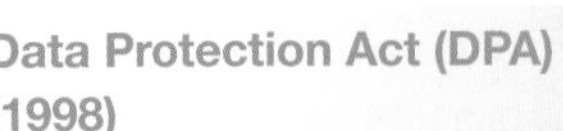

Data Protection Act (DPA) (1998)

To keep up to date and be aware of the full legislation requirements for the DPA visit www.hmso.gov.uk.

TOP TIP

Client attention at reception

It is important to give the right amount of attention to all clients according to their specific requirements, to ensure client satisfaction. This must always be considered in a busy situation where a client may be kept waiting. Always acknowledge their arrival.

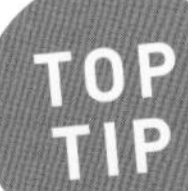

Business cards

Visitors to the salon may leave a business card, stating the name of the company, and the representative's name, address and telephone number. These cards should be filed by the receptionist for future reference. At a convenient time, store these electronically for ease of reference in the future.

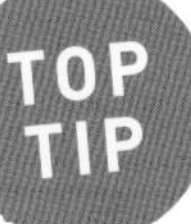

Price lists

Some salons' price lists are in booklet form, detailing the services offered and explaining their benefits. Ensure adequate supply is available at the reception area. Your prices should be kept updated if shown on a website.

Receptionists' duties

Receptionists should have a smart appearance and be able to communicate effectively and professionally, creating the right impression.

The receptionist's duties include:

- maintaining the reception and product displays
- looking after clients and visitors on arrival and departure
- answering telephone calls
- dealing with **enquiries** face-to-face, by telephone, fax or possibly email
- scheduling appointments
- dealing with complaints and compliments
- telling the appropriate therapist that a client or visitor has arrived
- assisting with retail sales

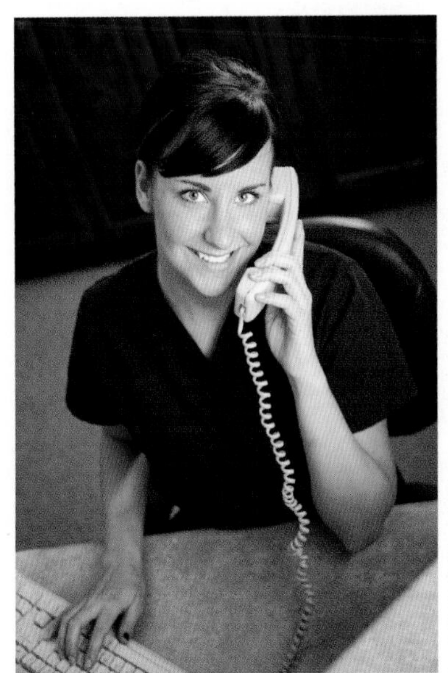

ISTOCKPHOTO/©RICH LEGG

A receptionist

TOP TIP

Electronic mail (email)
Email is a popular method of telecommunication. If your salon has an email address this should be provided to your clients. Also, collect your clients' email addresses as an alternative method of communicating if preferred.

HEALTH & SAFETY

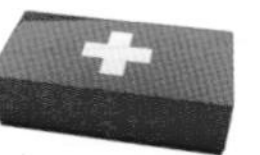

Contact numbers
Just in case a client should become ill while in the salon, a contact number should be recorded on the client's card.

- operating the payment point and handling payments
- filing client records (increasingly this is performed electronically).

The receptionist should know:

- the name of each member of staff, their role and their area of responsibility
- who to refer enquiries to that cannot be dealt with
- the salon's hours of opening, and the days and times when each beauty therapist is available
- the range of services or products offered by the salon, their duration and their cost
- any booking service restrictions such as skin testing requirements
- who to refer different types of enquiries to
- the person in your salon to whom you should refer reception problems
- any current discounts and special offers that the salon is promoting
- the benefits of each service and each retail product
- the approximate time taken to complete each service
- how to schedule follow-up services

TOP TIP

Useful contact numbers
It is useful to have the contact details of other service providers that a client may ask for that you could personally recommend. Examples include local taxi companies, hairdressers and florists. You may work collaboratively with these businesses, displaying their business cards.

TOP TIP

Opportunities for promoting products and services
Within your area of training and responsibility, bring to the attention of clients waiting in the reception area any new products, services or promotions.

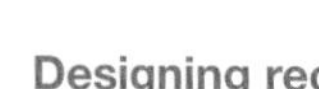

ACTIVITY

Designing record card/salon service menu
Design a record card to be used to record the client's service details. Alternatively, you could design a salon service menu, explaining the different services available and their costs. Be creative, and include a business name you may wish to use in the future.

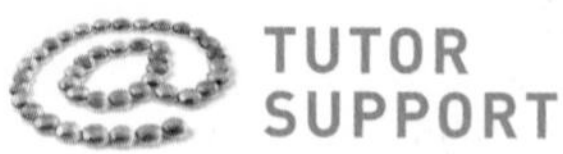

TUTOR SUPPORT

Activity 2: Record cards task

Skin sensitivity (patch) tests Before clients receive certain services, it may be necessary to carry out **skin sensitivity tests** to test skin sensitivity. The skin sensitivity test is often carried out at reception, and the receptionist or NVQ/SVQ Level 1 therapist will be able to perform the test once they have been trained. Every client should undergo a skin test before a permanent tinting service to the eyelashes or eyebrows. Further tests may be necessary, depending on the sensitivity of the client, before services such as those for artificial eyelashes or wax depilation. Refer to the relevant chapters to familiarize yourself with the test required.

As a reception duty it may be your responsibility to check that the necessary test has been received on client arrival following the salon policy for this.

The importance of good communication

As discussed previously clients make quality judgments based on their contact with the business. Effective **communication** is important to the success of the business. This may be **verbal communication**, that is face-to-face, over the telephone or written communication – including email – and remember **non-verbal communication** – we speak through our bodies' gestures. Conclusions about how we see other people are based on their behaviour both spoken and unspoken.

Always remember the **diversity** or range of people you will come into contact with. Diversity includes:

- personality
- beliefs and attitudes
- age
- religion, morality
- background and culture.

Diversity should be considered in communication, respond to any enquiry and allow time for the client to respond. Consider if you feel you have dealt with their enquiry adequately. It is important that a client is listened to and responded to appropriately.

Communication should always suit the situation. In all situations you should speak slowly and clearly, avoid rushing the conversation even in busy trading situations. Avoid confusing the client in your communication by avoiding the use of technical terminology unless this is something they are familiar with. Avoid slang words and informal phrases such as 'hang on a minute'. Your tone of voice is important; you should always sound calm, cheerful, helpful, knowledgeable and professional. Your voice and manner should inspire confidence and trust.

Adopting good posture will also positively affect your speech and professional appearance. You will sound and look more energized.

Non-verbal communication This is often referred to as **body language** and is how we communicate using our face, body movements and gestures.

Often we do this unconsciously and our body language may contradict what we are actually saying. It is an important skill to be able to interpret body language and the mood of clients. Observing clients' behaviour will help you to recognize their needs and expectations. Your body language should also show you to be attentive; examples include nodding your head and smiling in agreement.

Asking questions It is important to ask verbal questions to ensure, for example, that you are confident and understand what the client has asked you, do not be embarrassed to do this. It will ensure you give an appropriate answer, make the correct decision and that client satisfaction will be achieved. You may ask 'open' or 'closed' questions. Always ask open questions if you need more information as these questions cannot be answered with 'yes' or 'no'. Open questions start with 'what', 'when', 'who' and 'why' etc. Closed questions are used when you need to confirm something quickly. These are answered 'yes' or 'no'.

ACTIVITY

Planning a reception area
Design a reception area, to scale, appropriate to a small or large beauty salon. Discuss the choice of wall and floor coverings, furnishings and equipment, and give the reasons for their selection and the image you want to create. Consider clients' comfort, and health and safety.

To help you plan this you may refer to a specialist beauty therapy equipment suppliers' brochure or online information.

Customer service
"A friendly and helpful approach is the key to good customer service."
Sally-Anne Braithwaite

HEALTH & SAFETY

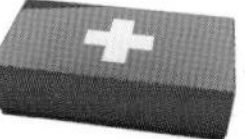

Cleaning
In a large salon a cleaner may be employed to maintain the hygiene of the reception area. In a smaller salon this may be the responsibility of the receptionist, assistant therapist or a junior therapist. Reception must be maintained to a high standard at all times. Use quieter periods for this purpose and to check stock levels, etc.

TOP TIP

Eye contact
In some cultures eye contact is considered to be disturbing or inappropriate. Always consider client diversity.

BEST PRACTICE 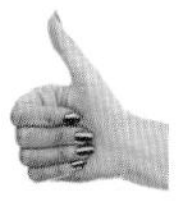

Client care
If you are engaged on the telephone when a client arrives, look up and acknowledge their presence. This is positive body language and an example of good interpersonal skills, which makes the client feel welcome.

HEALTH & SAFETY 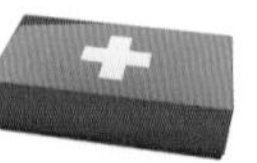

Fire drill
As the receptionist you should be familiar with the emergency procedure in case of fire.

ACTIVITY

Reception
Pair up with a colleague and share your experiences of a well managed and a badly managed reception.

TOP TIP

Do's and don'ts
List *five* important do's and *five* don'ts for the receptionist. Think also of things that *should not* be discussed at reception.

TOP TIP

Clients matter most
Don't regard the phone ringing as an interruption. Always remember that clients matter – it is they ensure the success of your business!

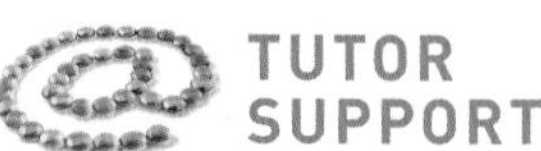 TUTOR SUPPORT

Activity 9: Telephone technique task

BEST PRACTICE 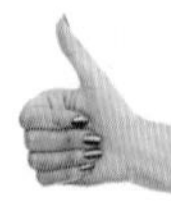

Name badges
It is a good idea for the receptionist to wear a badge indicating their name and position.

Telephone calls: communication

A good telephone technique can gain clients; a poor technique can lose them. Here are some guidelines for good technique:

- ***Answer quickly*** On average, a person may be willing to wait up to nine rings: try to respond to the call within six rings.
- ***Build a rapport*** Do this by introducing yourself when you answer the telephone.
- ***Be prepared*** Have information and writing materials ready to hand in the event you need to write down a message or record an instruction. It should not normally be necessary to leave the caller waiting while you find something.
- ***Be welcoming and attentive*** Speak clearly without mumbling, at the right speed. Pronounce your words clearly, and vary your tone. Sound interested, and never abrupt.

ACTIVITY

Listening to yourself
A pleasant speaking voice is an asset. Do you think you could improve your speech or manner?

Record your voice as you answer a telephone enquiry, then play it back. How did you sound? This is how others hear you!

Helping clients
Recognize the needs of each individual client and work to build a rapport with them. Show a genuine interest in them and their lifestyle, family and hobbies, etc. and your customer will come to trust you and listen to your recommendations.

Sally-Anne Braithwaite

TOP TIP

Telephone services
Telephone directories, codebooks and guides to charges provide a great deal of useful information. Read them carefully to make yourself familiar with the telephone services that are available.

Remember: the caller may be a new client ringing several salons, and their decision whether to visit your salon may depend on your attitude and the way you respond to their call.

Here are some more ideas about good telephone technique:

- ***Smile*** – this will help you put across a warm, friendly response to the caller.
- ***Alter the pitch of your voice*** as you speak, to create interest.
- ***As you answer give the standard greeting for the salon*** – for example: 'Good morning, Visage Beauty Salon, Susan speaking. How may I help you?'
- ***Listen attentively*** to the caller's questions or requests. You will be speaking to a variety of clients: you must respond appropriately and helpfully to each.
- ***Evaluate the information*** given by the caller, and be sure to respond to what they have said or asked.
- ***Use the client's name*** if you know it; this personalizes the call.
- ***In your mind summarize the main requests from the call***. Ask for further information if you need it.
- ***If you have an enquiry that you cannot deal with yourself*** refer to the relevant person promptly for assistance. Tell the client what you are doing.
- ***At the end*** repeat the main points of the conversation clearly to check that you and the client have understood each other.
- ***Close the call pleasantly*** – for example, 'Thank you for calling, Mrs Smith. Goodbye.'

If you receive a business call, or a call from a person seeking employment, always take the caller's name and telephone number. Your supervisor can then deal with the call as soon as they are free to do so.

Transferring calls

If you transfer a telephone call to another extension, explain to the caller what you are doing and thank them for waiting. If the extension to which you have transferred the call is not answered within nine rings, apologize and explain to the caller that you will ask the person concerned to ring back as soon as possible. Take the caller's name and telephone number and offer to take a message. Always make sure the person gets the message.

Taking messages

Messages should be recorded neatly on a memorandum ('memo') pad. Each message should record:

- who the message is for
- who the message was from
- the date and the time the message was received
- accurate details of the message including the reason for the call, details of information requested or to be passed on
- the telephone number or address of the caller
- the signature of the person who took the message.

ACTIVITY

Open and closed questions

Think of an open question you could ask a client to check their suitability for leg waxing, when making a waxing appointment.

Think of a closed question you may ask to confirm client satisfaction with their service that day.

ACTIVITY

Non-verbal communication

In conversation you give signals through your behaviour that tell others whether you are listening or not.

1 What do you think the following signals indicate:
   - a smile?
   - head tilted, and resting on one hand?
   - frowning?
   - eyes semi-closed?
   - head nodding?
   - fidgeting?
2 Can you think of further facial or body signals that indicate your mood?

ACTIVITY

Communicating with clients

Listen to experienced receptionists and notice how they communicate with clients.

TOP TIP

Personal calls
Check the salon's policy on personal calls. Usually they are permitted only in emergencies. This is so that staff are not distracted from clients, and to keep the telephone free for clients to make appointments.

When taking a message, listen actively and attentively. Repeat the details you have recorded so that the caller can check that you've got it right. Pass the message directly to the correct person as soon as possible. The message should be received in time to be acted upon.

A memo

TELEPHONE MESSAGE RECEIVED			
To	Angela	Date	10.7.10
From	Jenny Heron	Time	9.30 am
Number	273451	Taken by	Sandra
Please ring Jenny Heron regarding her appointment on Saturday			

ACTIVITY

What do you need to know?
Think of different questions that you might be asked as a receptionist. Then ask an experienced receptionist what the most common requests are.

Listening skills

It is important to listen closely to what people are saying to you in your role to ensure you correctly identify the purpose of any enquiry in order to choose the correct response when dealing with it.

Listening skills include:

- being focused on the other person, paying them your full attention
- ensuring that your facial expressions show your interest
- not interrupting the other person speaking
- using positive body language to show your interest; maintain eye contact; nod your head and lean forward
- observing the other person's body language, reading what it is telling you while you listen
- summarizing what the other person has said to confirm understanding
- asking further questions as necessary if unsure in order to give the right response
- asking a client to rephrase what you have said in their own words if they appear confused.

TOP TIP

A client who has received a poor response to their telephone call may tell others about it.

How to deal with a dissatisfied client or complaint

Occasionally a client may be dissatisfied and wish to complain. The receptionist is usually the first contact with the client (either face to face or through telephone contact) and may have to deal with dissatisfied, angry or awkward customers. Considerable skill is needed if you are to deal constructively with a potentially damaging situation.

If your business has a procedure for handling complaints this should be followed. Procedures are useful as these can be audited to identify emerging problems that may require correction. If ignored these problems could be harmful to the business.

Never become angry or awkward yourself. Always remain courteous and diplomatic, and communicate confidently and politely.

1 Listen to the client as they describe their problems, without making judgments. Do not make excuses for yourself or for colleagues. Do not interrupt.

TOP TIP

If the salon uses a cordless phone or a mobile phone, keep it in a central location where it can easily be found when it rings. After each call, be sure to return the phone to its usual location.

2 Ask questions to check that you have the full background details. Summarize the client's concerns to confirm this.

3 If possible, agree on a course of action, offering a solution if you can. Check that the client has agreed to the proposed course of action. It may be necessary to consult the salon supervisor before proposing a solution to the client: if you're not sure, always check first.

4 Log the complaint: the date, the time, the client's name, the nature of the complaint and the course of action agreed.

5 There should also be a system for handling compliments. Again it is good to see those aspects of the business that are particularly successful. This can also be rewarding and motivational for staff to hear. Such compliments can be used in marketing materials.

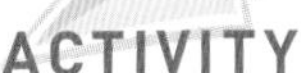

ACTIVITY

Finding the right approach
What telephone manner should you adopt when dealing with people who are:

- angry
- talkative
- nervous?

BEST PRACTICE

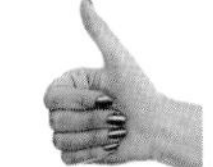

Taking messages
It is important to interpret the mood of a client leaving a message. If they have are making a complaint listen to their complaint, ensure you have the key facts and where possible provide a time that somebody will get back to them. Never become angry or defensive yourself. If skilled, you should be able to calm and provide reassurance to the complainant.

Appointments

Outcome 2: Be able to book appointments

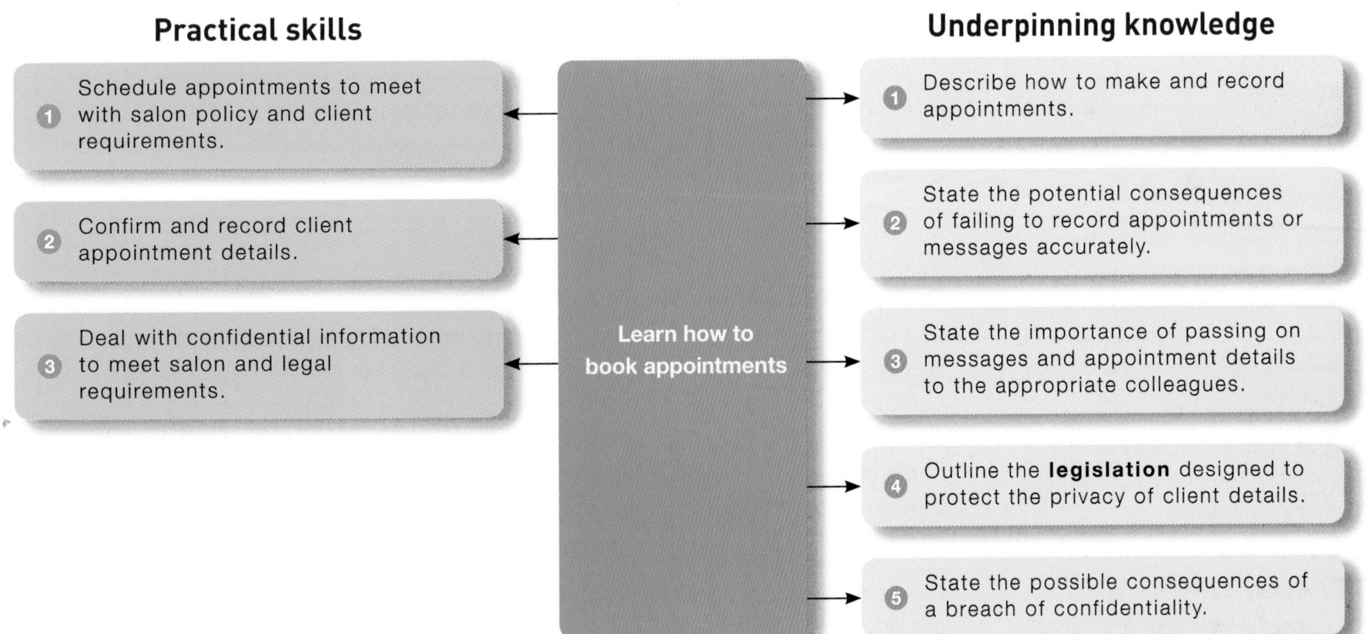

Practical skills
1 Schedule appointments to meet with salon policy and client requirements.
2 Confirm and record client appointment details.
3 Deal with confidential information to meet salon and legal requirements.
Learn how to book appointments
Underpinning knowledge
1 Describe how to make and record appointments.
2 State the potential consequences of failing to record appointments or messages accurately.
3 State the importance of passing on messages and appointment details to the appropriate colleagues.
4 Outline the legislation designed to protect the privacy of client details.
5 State the possible consequences of a breach of confidentiality.

Making correct entries in the **appointment book** or salon **computer** is one of the most important duties of the receptionist. The way you handle client records and the information held on them must conform with the Data Protection Act (see page 130). Always handle confidential information in line with both salon policies and legal requirements. Failure to do so is unprofessional and also breaks the law. If the Data Protection

ALWAYS REMEMBER

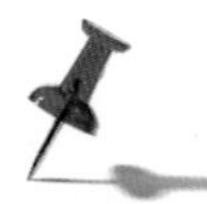

Behaviour breeds behaviour
If you behave calmly, the client will become less angry. If you become angry, the client will become even angrier!

Your behaviour can effect the other person for the worse or the better.

Act is not complied with the client may have the legal right to take action. All staff have a responsibility to maintain client confidentiality at all times.

As receptionist you must familiarize yourself with the salon's appointment system, column headings, service times and any abbreviations used.

Each therapist will usually have their name at the head of a column. Entries in columns must not be reallocated without the consent of the therapist or supervisor, unless they are absent.

Bookings

When a client calls to make an appointment, record the client's name and the service they want. Allow adequate time to carry out the required service (as indicated in the following chapters). Take the client's telephone number or other contact details in case the therapist falls ill or is unable to keep the appointment for some other reason. If the client requests a particular therapist, be sure to enter the client's name in the correct column.

In addition, software enabling online appointment booking and scheduling is becoming more popular. This is accessed through the business website and clients can book appointments and view the business's information (services offered, specials offers, etc.) at any time. The business can make the final decision to accept or reject the appointment. As receptionist this may be your responsibility.

TOP TIP

Gaining client satisfaction

Occasionally you will have to disappoint a client such as when cancelling their appointment or explaining they cannot proceed with a service for reasons of health and safety. This you should be able to do without offending or upsetting the client. Consider your tone of voice, how you are going to present the information and what alternative options there may be. Through your words and tone you should be able to demonstrate genuine empathy and resolve to recover the situation.

ACTIVITY

Reception role play
With colleagues, act out the following situations, which may occur when working as a receptionist. You may wish to video the role plays for review and discussion later.

1 A client arrives very late for an appointment but insists that she be treated.
2 A client questions the bill.
3 A client comes in to complain about a service given previously (choose a particular service).

Alternatively you may choose to do this as a written activity with a discussion of your answers.

Finally the hours of the day are recorded along the left-hand side of the appointment page, divided into 15-minute intervals. You must know how long each service takes so that you can allow sufficient time for the therapist to carry out the service in a safe, competent, professional manner. If you don't allow sufficient time, the therapist will run late, and this will affect all later appointments. On the other hand, if you allow too much time, the therapist's time will be wasted and the salon's earnings will be less than they could be. Suggested times to be allowed for each service are given in the service chapters.

Ensure that you regularly check scheduled appointments and plan ahead where you can see any potential problem – put a strategy in place to rectify it. This may involve asking others to help you.

Confirm the name of the therapist who will be carrying out the service, the date and the time.

Finally, confirm or estimate the cost of the service to the client.

Service	*Abbreviation*	*Service time allowed**
Cleanse and make-up: day	C/M/up day	30 mins
special occasion	C/M/up special	45 mins
Eyebrow shaping	E/B reshape or trim	15 mins
Eyebrow tint	EBT	10 mins
Eyelash tint	ELT	20 mins
Manicure	Man	45 mins
Pedicure	Ped	50 mins
Leg wax: half	½ leg wax	30 mins
three-quarter	¾ leg wax	30–40 mins
full	Full leg wax	50 mins
Bikini wax	B/wax	15 mins
Underarm wax	U/arm wax	15 mins
Arm wax	F/arm wax	30 mins
Facial wax	F/wax	10–15 mins
Eyebrow wax	E/B wax	15 mins
Threading	EB/Thread	10–15 mins
	F/Thread	10–15 mins
Ear pierce	E/P	15 mins
Facial	F	60 mins
Artificial eye lashes strip/individual flare	F/Lash	10–20 mins
Artificial nails: full set	N/ext F/S	120 mins
nail maintenance	N/Infill	90 mins
removal	N/rem	60 mins
Natural nail overlays	N/O'lays	75 mins
Nail art	N/art	30 mins
Manual tan-full body	Man/tan	60 mins

*Service time does not include preparation for service and consultation.

Services are usually recorded in an abbreviated form. All those who use the appointment page must be familiar with these abbreviations.

If an appointment book is used, write each entry neatly and accurately. It is preferable to write in pencil: appointments can be amended by erasing and rewriting, keeping the book clean and clear.

Electronic appointment booking systems, if used, allow you to read the appointment schedule and add or edit appointments immediately.

HEALTH & SAFETY

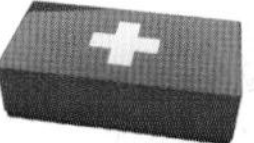

Health and Safety (Display Screen Equipment) Regulations (1992)

These regulations cover the use of visual display units and computer screens. They specify acceptable levels of radiation emissions from the screen, and identify correct posture, seating position, permitted working heights and rest periods.

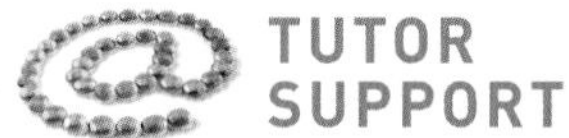

Activity 3: Treatment list task

TOP TIP

Software business management features

The software which can be used for booking and scheduling appointments often has the benefits of stock control and ordering, managing client data, and issuing gift cards.

TOP TIP

Appointment reminder

Some software can email or text your clients an appointment reminder directly to their mobile phone.

Teamwork

"A good team member has the ability to listen and communicate well, respect their colleagues and be able to get their point across in the appropriate manner.

Sally-Anne Braithwaite

DAY SATURDAY DATE 15th JANUARY

THERAPIST	JAYNE	SUE	LIZ
9.00	Mrs Young	DNA	
9.15	1/2 leg wax	Jenny Newley	
9.30	Carol Kreen	ELT/EBT	
9.45	Full leg wax	EB trim	
10.00	B /Wax		
10.15		Sandra Smith	Fiona Smith
10.30	Ms Lord E/B wax	C / M / up	C / M / up
10.45			Strip / lash
11.00		Mrs Jones	
11.15		U/arm wax	
11.30		F/arm wax	Carol Brown
11.45			E/P
12.00			
12.15			
12.30	Nina Farrel		
12.45	Man		
1.00	Ped		
1.15		Sue Uip E/P	
1.30	1/2 leg wax	T Scott	
1.45		3/4 leg wax	
2.00	Karen Davies	U/arm wax	
2.15	Facial		
2.30			
2.45			Pat king
3.00			C / M / up (C)
3.15	Anno Wood		Man
3.30	Man		
3.45	E/B Reshape		
4.00			

TOP TIP

Service time allowed

Dependent upon the manufacturers' guidelines and the service needs of the client including any procedure modifications required, the service times may take less or more time.

Appointment cards may be offered to the client, to confirm the client's appointment. The card should record the service, the date, the day and the time. The therapist's name may also be recorded.

When the client arrives for their service, draw a line or checkmark through their name to indicate that they have arrived.

If the client cancels, indicate this on the appointment page *immediately*, usually with a large C, placed through the booking. This enables another client to take the appointment.

If a client fails to arrive, the abbreviation DNA ('did not arrive') is usually written over the booking. The client's telephone number should then be used to see if a re-booking is required.

Use the relevant recording icon if using an online appointment booking system.

Some salons will have a policy to charge for a missed appointment.

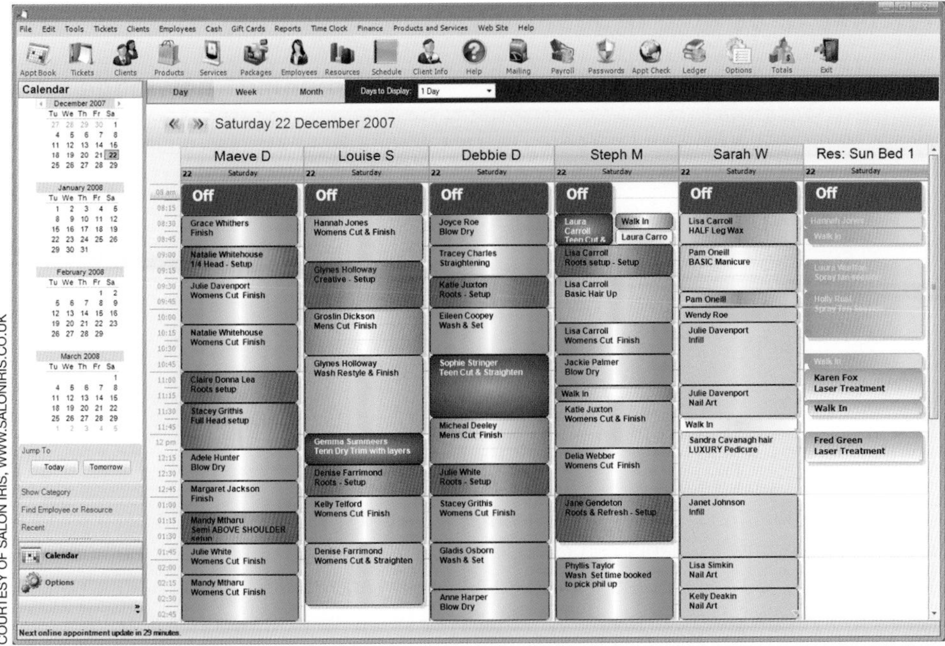

COURTESY OF SALON IRIS, WWW.SALONIRIS.CO.UK

Online appointments page

Dealing with appointment problems

You are often required to use your initiative in helping colleagues and clients and be able to cope with the unexpected such as:

- clients arriving late for appointments
- double-bookings, with two clients requiring service at the same time
- the arrival of unscheduled clients
- staff absence with a column of appointments!

Effective teamwork can usually overcome any of these situations. Inform your colleague/supervisor of the problem and, dependent upon your experience, state what action needs to be taken or ask them to support you in identifying a solution. You must always:

- aim to accommodate clients
- not disadvantage or compromise any clients in terms of quality of service
- keep the client informed of what action is being taken
- state how long any delay to service will be and if this is unsuitable offer an alternative future appointment
- use your excellent communication skills!

ACTIVITY

How would you deal with the following reception problems:

- a client arriving late for a service
- a double-booking
- the arrival of an unscheduled client?

ALWAYS REMEMBER

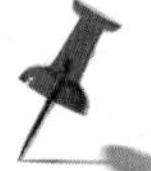

Appointments can usually be made up to six weeks in advance. Often clients will book their next appointment while still at the salon. How far ahead the receptionist is able to book appointments will vary from salon to salon.

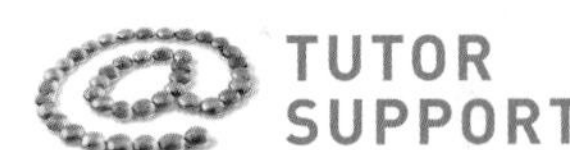

Activity 8: Reception book scheduling task

Using initiative

If you see something that needs to be done, do it without having to be asked. If you think a procedure could be done better or more efficiently, don't be afraid to suggest it to your employer.

Sally-Anne Braithwaite

Outcome 3: Be able to deal with payments

Learn how to deal with payments

Practical skills

1. Calculate service costs accurately.
2. Deal with payments for services and/or products to meet with salon policy.
3. Follow security procedures when handling payments.

Underpinning knowledge

1. State how to process different **methods of payment.**
2. Describe how to deal with **problems** that may occur with payments.
3. Explain how to keep payments safe and secure.

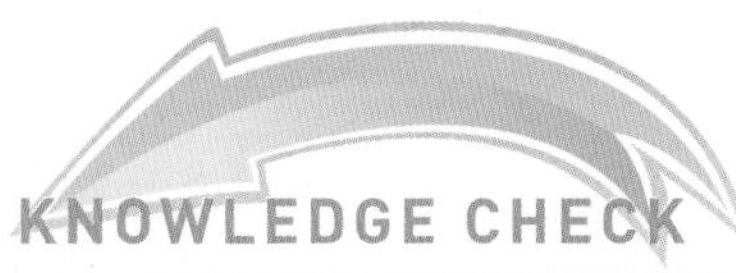

When taking messages what is the important information you should record?

Need more time... refer to page 153 to help you.

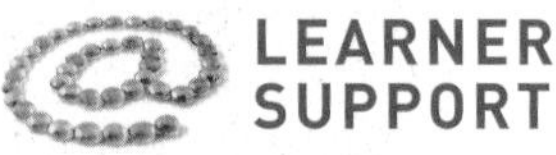

Reception mini crossword

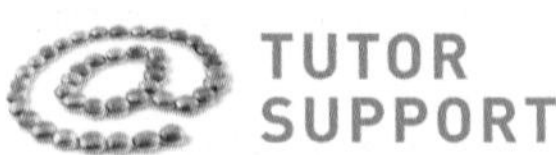

Activity 4: Handling payments handout

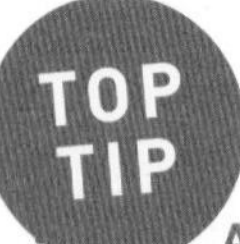

Advertisement vouchers
Sometimes the salon may publish other offers, such as a discount on producing a newspaper advertisement for the salon or a website voucher. The advertisement voucher is a form of payment, and must be collected.

Every beauty therapy or cosmetic business will have a policy for handling cash and for handling the payment. Clients can choose from a wide range of payment methods. It's important that you handle each payment efficiently and correctly. Not all businesses accept every **method of payment** so this should be checked in your training.

It is important that you have received training and are confident to take payment in the client's preferred method, which may be cash or cash equivalent (e.g., **gift voucher**), cheque or payment card.

Before processing payment confirm what it is the client is paying for, i.e. the services received and/or the products to be purchased. Confirm the price; ask how they would like to pay. Gaining client confirmation will reduce **discrepancies** later. Always check for any defects in products as you process a sale, e.g. breakage or leakage. If you are responsible for stock control when a product is found to be defective a replacement product is required.

The payment point

Kinds of payment points

Manual tills With **manual tills** a lockable drawer or box is used to store cash: this may form part of the reception desk. Each transaction must be recorded by hand.

At the end of the working day, record the total cash register in a book, to ensure that accurate accounts are kept. Records of petty cash, small amounts of monies used for expenditures, e.g. milk for clients' coffee, must also be kept so that the final totals will balance.

Automatic tills **Electrical automatic tills** use codes, one for each kind of service or retail sale. These are identified by keys on the till. Using these with each transaction makes it possible to analyze the salon's business each day or each week.

With each sale during the day a receipt is given to the client; the total is also recorded on the till's **audit roll**.

Automatic tills also provide **subtotals** of the amounts taken: these can be cross-checked against the amount in the till, to determine the daily takings:

- The X reading provides subtotals throughout the day, as required.
- The Z reading provides the overall figures at the end of the day.

Computerized tills **Computerized tills** provide the same facilities as automatic tills, with additional features to help with the business, record-keeping, including client service cards and stock records.

Both electronic and computerized tills help calculate the client's bill for you, including change to be given.

Equipment and materials required

- ***Calculator*** This is useful in totalling large amounts of money or when using a manual till.
- ***Credit card equipment*** If your business is authorized to accept credit cards you may use either an *imprinter* or *electronic terminal*. An imprinter is a manual system whereby the client's credit card is placed on a self-carbonating voucher within the machine and a manual sliding mechanism imprints the details of the card upon the voucher. If this system is used you require a supply of vouchers. Alternatively, where an electronic payment system is used a special till roll which provides a printout for yourself and a copy for the client is required.
- ***Cash float*** At the start of each day you need a small sum of money comprising coins and perhaps a few notes, to provide change: this is called the **float**. (At the end of the day there will be money surplus to the float: if no mistakes have been made, this should match the takings.)
- ***Till roll*** This records the sales and provides a receipt. Keep a spare to hand. If you're using a manual cash drawer, you'll need a **receipt book**.
- ***Audit roll*** The retailer's copy of the till roll.
- ***Cash book*** This is a record of income and expenditure, for a manual till.
- ***Other stationery*** A date stamp and a salon name stamp (for cheques), pens, pencils and an eraser, and a container to hold these.

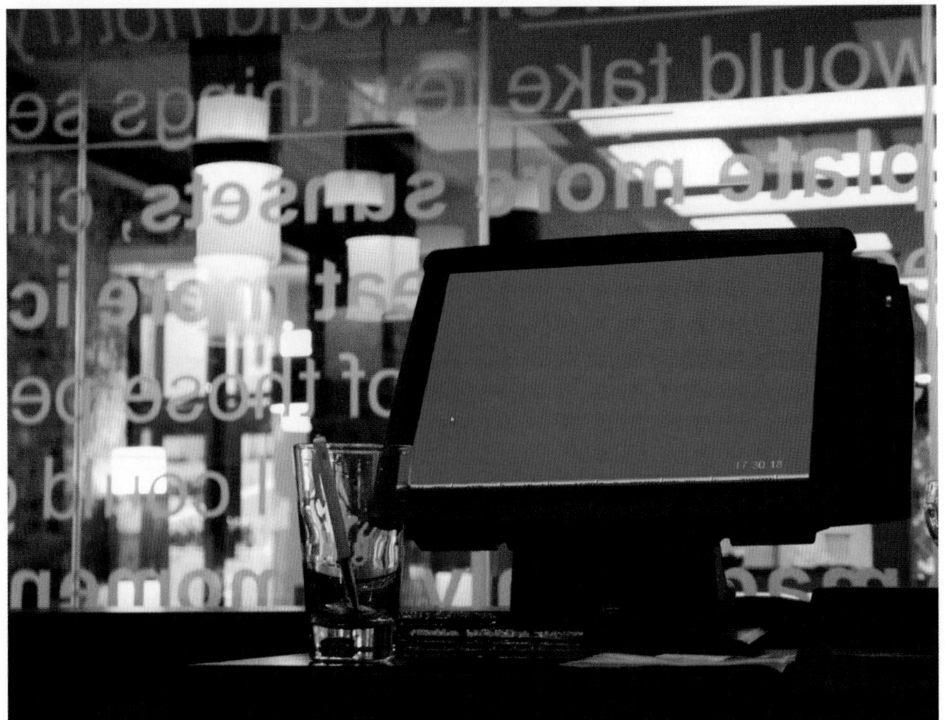

Computerized till

ALWAYS REMEMBER

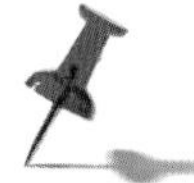

Sale and Supply of Goods Act (1994)

You have a duty to comply with the responsibilities of this Act, ensuring all products sold are of merchantable quality. They must 'conform to contract'. This means fit for purpose and of satisfactory quality.

KNOWLEDGE CHECK

What is the importance of passing on messages?

Need more time... refer to page 154 to help you.

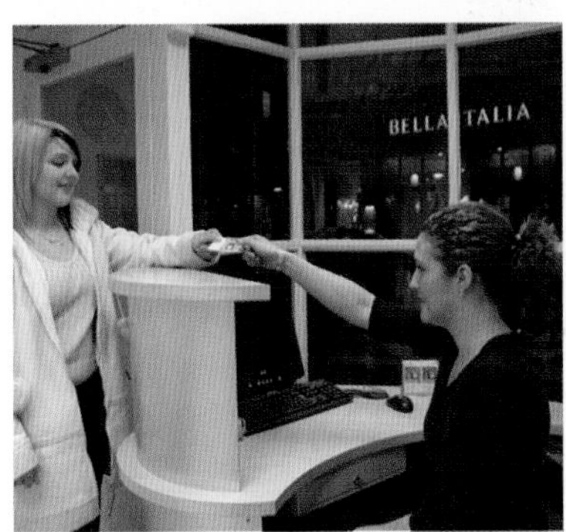

Receptionist returning the card to the client

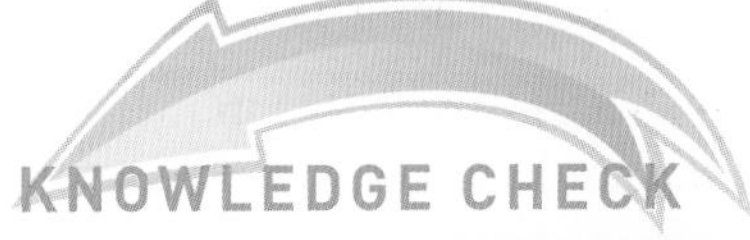

KNOWLEDGE CHECK

What are the common systems used in salons to make appointments?

Need more time... refer to page 158 to help you.

BEST PRACTICE

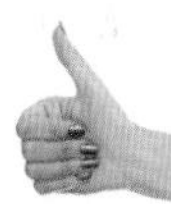

Tills

If there is too little change in the till, inform the relevant person. Running out of change would disrupt service and spoil the impression clients receive.

ACTIVITY

Fraud
Find out about your salon's policy in the case of fraudulent monetary transactions, using either cash or cards. What actions should you take?

KNOWLEDGE CHECK

Why is it important to inspect the quality of goods before payment is processed?

Need more time... refer to page 160 to help you.

TOP TIP

Forgeries

Hold notes to the light to check for forgeries. You should be able to see the watermark (picture of the Queen's head), the continuous metal strip that runs through the note and a hologram decal in the mid-left section of the note.

An ultra-violet detector machine may also be used to check for forgeries.

The police will often provide a list of forged bank note numbers to businesses to be aware of.

TOP TIP

Cheques

Most cheques may only be valid for six months from the date on the cheque – however this is at the discretion of the bank.

Security at the payment point

Having placed money in the cash drawer and collected change as required, always close the cash drawer firmly – never leave it open. Do not leave the key in the drawer, or lying about reception unattended.

Some members of staff will be appointed to authorize cheques and credit card payments; one of these should initial each cheque.

Errors may occur when handling cheques or when operating an electronic or computerized payment point. Don't panic! If you can't correct the error yourself, seek assistance – but don't leave the cash drawer unattended and open.

Be aware of stolen cards and forged notes and coins. Check at every payment transaction and follow the salon policy if presented. Remember that this must be handled sensitively as the client may not know they are in receipt of a cash forgery.

You may periodically be informed of cards that are invalid, on a credit card warning list from the service provider. If you receive a card that is on a credit card warning list, politely detain the customer, hold onto the card, and contact your supervisor, who will implement the salon's procedure. If the card is unsigned, do not allow the cardholder to sign the card unless you first get authorization from the credit card company's service provider. (The service provider's telephone number should be kept near the telephone.)

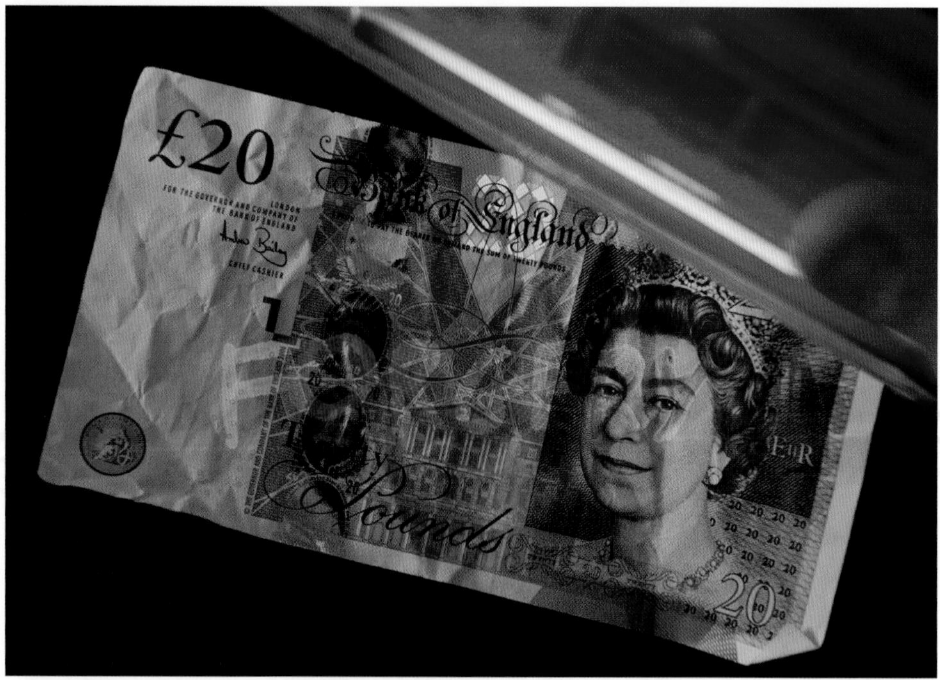

Forged note detector

Methods of payment

Cash When receiving payment by **cash**, follow this sequence:

1. Accurately total the charge for the services/products received. Inform the client of the amount to be paid.
2. Check that the money offered is **legal tender** – that is, money you will be able to pay into your bank. (Your salon will probably not accept foreign currency, for example.)

3 Place the customer's money on the till ledge until you have given change, or at least state to the customer verbally the sum of money that they have given you.

4 Aloud, count the change as you give it to the client. This will help avoid payment disputes.

5 Thank the client, and give them a receipt.

6 If a client disputes the change given as too little, ask how much money they are missing. Inform the client that when the takings are cashed at the end of the day if there is a surplus and it matches that amount they will be reimbursed. Ensure that you have the client's details so that you can inform them of the outcome the next day. Always follow your salon policy.

What security measures may be in place at the payment point?

Need more time... refer to page 162 to help you.

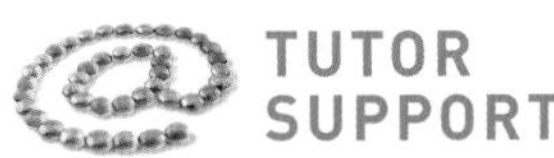

Activity 5: Cheque payment handout

Cheques **Cheques** are an alternative form of payment, and must be accompanied by a **cheque guarantee card**. This proves identity and guarantees the spending limit, usually £100. The debit card is usually the same card as the cheque guarantee card. Your salon may be willing to accept cheques for larger amounts if the client can show some other identification, such as a driving licence, but you must always check first with your supervisor.

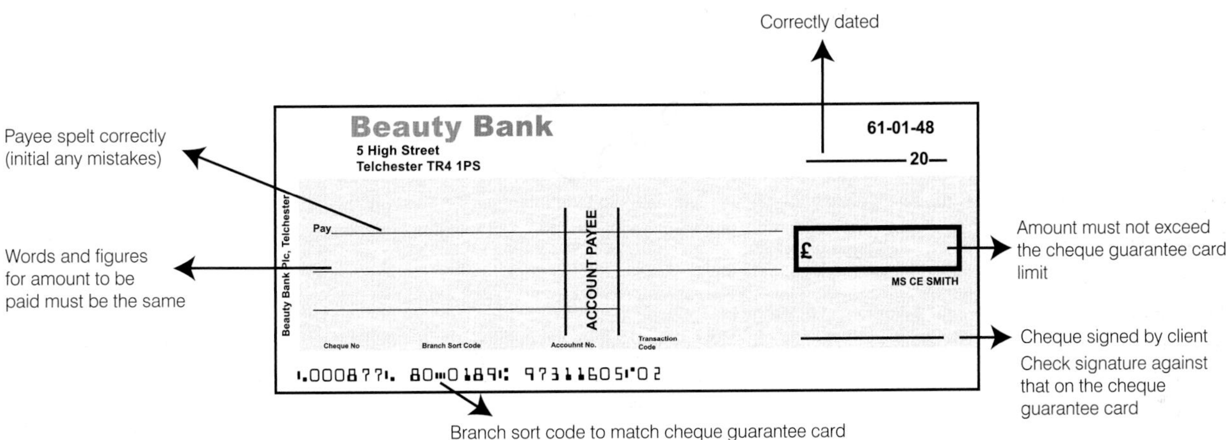

A cheque

Some businesses are no longer accepting cheques as it is becoming more costly to accept as a form of payment.

When receiving payment by cheque, follow this sequence of checks:

1 The cheque must be correctly dated.

2 The cheque must be made payable to the salon (you may have a salon stamp for this).

3 The words and figures written on the cheque must match those in the box.

4 Any errors or alterations must have been initialled by the client.

5 The signature on the back of the cheque guarantee card must match that on the cheque – compare these as the customer writes their signature on the cheque.

6 The bank's 'sort code' numbers on the cheque must match those on the cheque guarantee card.

7 The date on the cheque guarantee card must be valid.

TOP TIP

Card non-authorization

If a card is declined when processing, it may be requested that the card is retained. Refer this to the designated responsible person without causing embarrassment to the client following salon policy.

8 The value on the cheque must not exceed the cheque guarantee card limit.

9 The cheque card number must be recorded on the back of the cheque.

10 The cheque must be signed by the client.

Debit cards **Debit cards** include Switch/Maestro and Solo. The card authorizes immediate debit of the cash amount from the client's account and is an alternative to writing a cheque. (This card may also be a cheque guarantee card.) You cannot perform this kind of transaction unless your salon has an electronic terminal. This processes payment automatically through a telephone connection (chip and PIN). The card processing company applies a fixed fee for each transaction made. Duplicated receipts are produced following authorization; one copy is given to the client, the other kept by the salon. If there is a connection problem a manual imprinter is used as an alternative, details of the sale are written on the voucher which is signed by the client. The client is then given one copy of the sales voucher; a copy is sent to the debit card company; the third copy is kept by the salon.

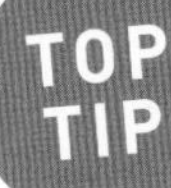

TOP TIP

Security

When paying for goods with a debit or credit card the client will need to enter their PIN (personal identity number). This is usually entered into an electronic handheld device, but in some cases they may have to sign.

Debit and credit cards can also be used to make payments by phone or over the internet. In this case the client will need to provide certain details that are printed on their card.

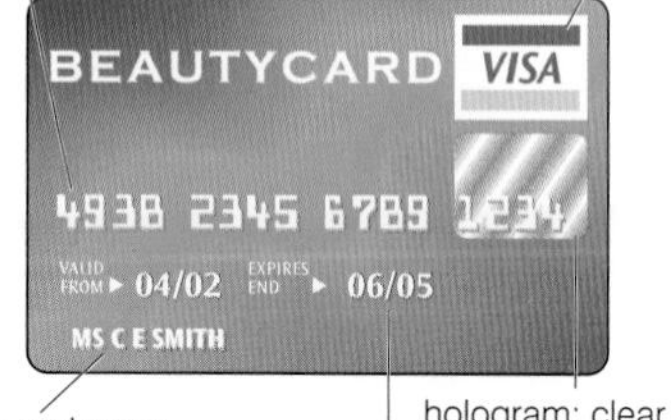
embossed account number should be valid – not on a credit card company's warning list
card logo
BEAUTYCARD
VISA
4938 2345 6789 1234
VALID FROM ▸ 04/02
EXPIRES END ▸ 06/05
MS C E SMITH
sex and name should fit your client
hologram: clear sharp image
valid to (expiry) date

Credit card checks

Credit cards **Credit cards** can be used only if your business has an arrangement with the relevant credit card company. In this case the company will give the salon a credit limit (a **ceiling**), the maximum amount that may be accepted with the card. Any amount greater than this must be individually authorized by the credit card company. (This is done by telephone at the time of transaction.)

Credit cards allow the client to 'buy goods now and pay later' with interest paid each month on the outstanding balance if not paid off in full.

Electronic payment systems An electronic computerized terminal may be used for payment by both credit and debit cards.

1 Check that the terminal display is in 'SALE' mode.

2 Confirm that a sale is to be made by pressing the YES button.

3 The terminal will request that you swipe the card. Do this, ensuring that the magnetic strip passes over the reader head and that you retain the card in your hand. In some cases the magnetic strip cannot be read by the swipe card reader: in this situation you will have to key the complete card number into the terminal manually. This does not necessarily mean that there is any reason for suspicion, but do look carefully at it for any signs that the card has been tampered with.

4 When prompted, use the 'AMOUNT' button on the keypad to input the purchases and total them. (If you make a mistake, you can clear the figures using the CLEAR button.)

KNOWLEDGE CHECK

What should you check when receiving payments by cheque?

Need more time... refer to page 163 to help you.

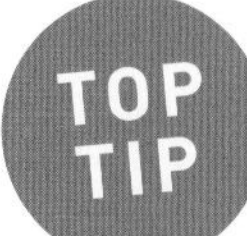

Cards

If cards are accepted as a method of payment, those that are accepted by the business will usually be displayed at the payment point.

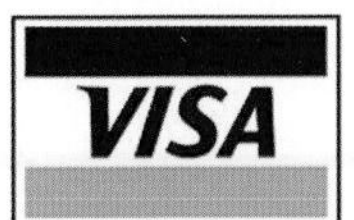

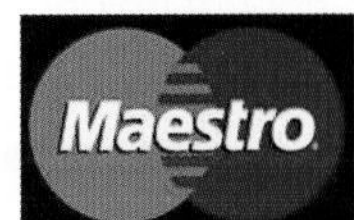

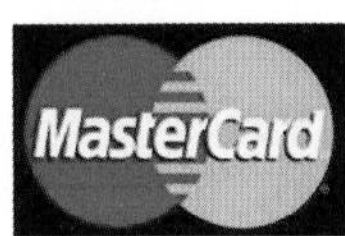

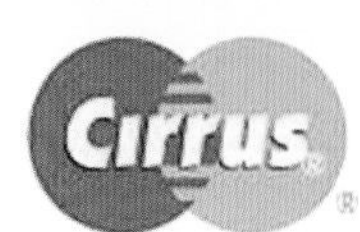

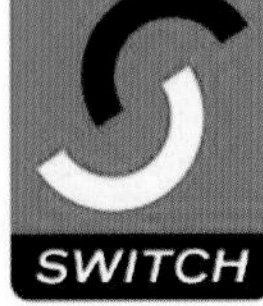

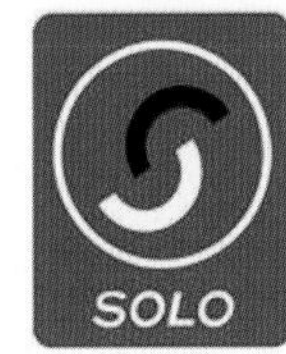

Types of credit and debit card

5 Press ENTER, which will automatically connect the terminal to the credit card company. A message will indicate first 'DIALLING', and then 'CONNECTION MADE'.

6 Customer details are accessed automatically. After a few moments you should receive one of two messages. If the payment is authorized you will see 'AUTH CODE', and a code number will be printed on the receipt with the other purchase details. If the transaction is declined, you will see 'CARD NOT ACCEPTED'.

7 While holding the card, check the details and tear off the two-part receipt and ask the cardholder to sign in ballpoint pen, in the space provided. Alternatively the 'chip and PIN' system may be used, where the client enters their personal identity number instead of signing their name. The transaction will be declined if the PIN is incorrect.

8 Where a signature is used, check the signature matches the signature on the card, and give the customer the top, signed copy, with the card.

9 Place the copies in the till. One copy is for the debit/credit card company, the other for your records.

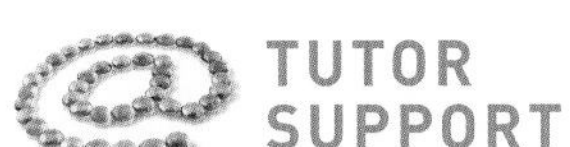

Activity 6: Credit and debit card payment handout

When receiving payment by debit or credit card, check these points:

1 The card logo for a credit card is at the upper right-hand corner on the front of the card. For a debit card, it should be at the lower right-hand corner of the card.

2 The hologram should have a clear, sharp image and be in the centre right of the card.

3 The date on the card must be valid: if it is out of date ask for another form of payment.

4 The sex (Ms, Miss, Mrs, Mr) and the name of the customer must fit your client.

5 The cardholder's signature on the reverse of the card must match the name on the front of the card.

6 The cardholder's card number should be embossed and across the width on the front of the card.

7 The cardholder's card number must not be one of those on the credit card company's warning list.

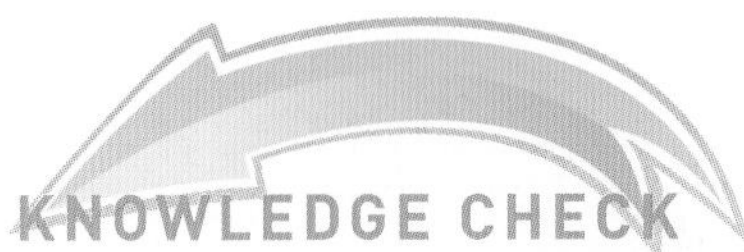

If you make an error when operating the payment point, why must you report this?

Need more time... refer to page 162 to help you.

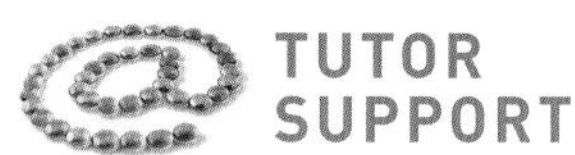

Activity 7: Reception area Wordsearch

Travellers' cheques **Travellers' cheques** are pre-printed fixed-amount cheques. They may be acceptable, provided they are in particular currencies (usually sterling). Such cheques must be compared with the client's passport for validity. Also available are travellers' cheque cards.

Charge cards Some businesses accept **charge cards** such as American Express. These differ from credit cards in that the account holder must repay to the card company the complete amount spent each month. They are considered a more convenient alternative to cash.

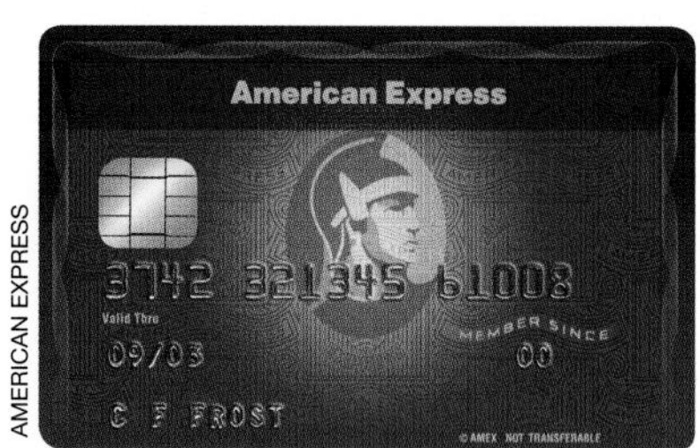

AMERICAN EXPRESS

A charge card

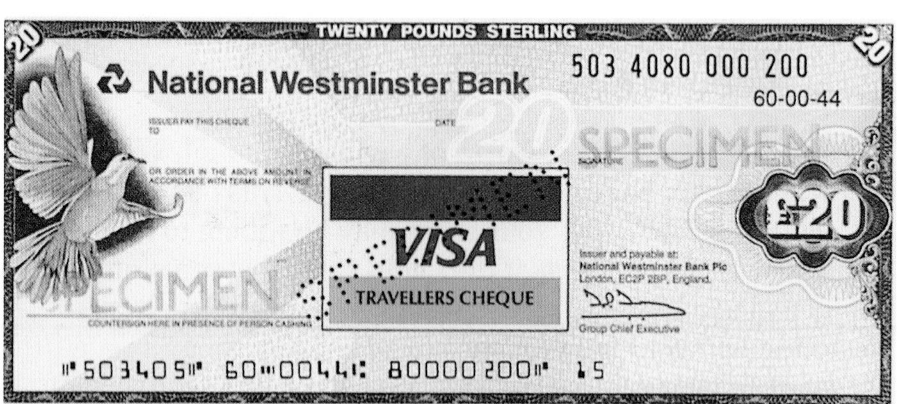

A travellers' cheque

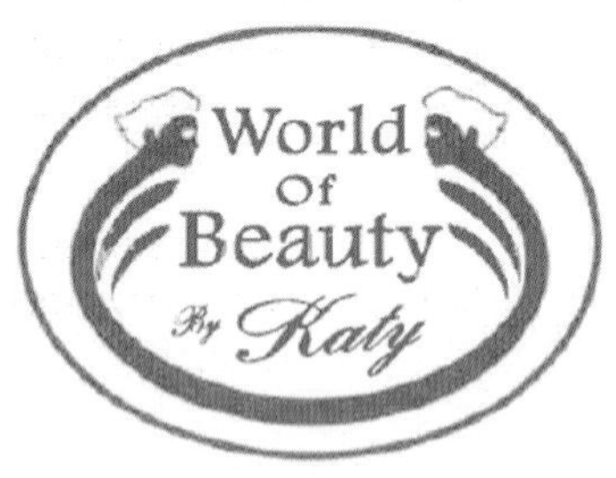

Amount or Treatment
for the value of

SAMPLE

Valid to

WORLD OF BEAUTY by KATY
88 Park Road
Crouch End, London N8 8JQ

COURTESY OF THE WORLD OF BEAUTY BY KATY, LONDON

A gift voucher

Gift vouchers Gift vouchers are purchased from the salon as pre-payments for beauty therapy services or retail sales. Check the following:

- There is usually a specific time period in which gift vouchers must be used. Check to see if this is the case and if they are still valid.
- Check the value of the voucher, and remember to request another form of payment if the cost of the service is higher than the voucher.

It is important that all financial transactions are handled competently. However busy you are always follow the guidelines for handling each method of payment.

If you are ever unsure when handling a financial transaction or make a mistake, inform your supervisor immediately. It may be that you have to be discreet when doing this, for example if a client has handed you a forged bank note! This will also enable a specific financial discrepancy to be justified.

GLOSSARY OF KEY WORDS

Appointment an arrangement made for a client to receive a service on a particular date and time.

Body language communication involving the body.

Charge card an alternative form of payment where the complete amount of credit spent must be repaid by the card-holder each month to the card company.

Cheque an alternative form of payment to that of using cash. A cheque must be accompanied by a cheque guarantee card.

Communication the exchange of information and the establishment of understanding between people.

Credit card an alternative form of payment to that of using cash. These cards are held by those who have a credit account, where there is a pre-arranged borrowing limit. These can only be used if your business has an arrangement to deal with the relevant credit card company.

Data Protection Act (1998) legislation designed to protect client privacy and confidentiality.

Debit card alternative method of payment where the card authorizes immediate debit of the cash amount from the client's account.

Discrepancy a disagreement over amounts of money, etc. This is referred to in instances where a client disagrees with what they are being asked to pay or the amount of change received.

Enquiries questions presented by clients or business contacts to find out more information.

Gift voucher a pre-payment method for beauty therapy services or retail sales.

Health and Safety (Display Screen Equipment) Regulations (1992) these regulations cover the use of visual display units (VDUs) and computer screens. They specify acceptable levels of radiation emissions from the screen and identify correct working posture, seating position, permitted working heights and rest periods.

Hospitality this covers welcoming the client, being helpful and offering refreshments and magazines, and ensuring the client is comfortable while at reception.

Messages communication of information to another person in written, electronic or verbal form.

Method of payment different forms of payment that may be accepted to pay for a product or service including cash, cash equivalents, cheque and payment cards.

Non-verbal communication communicating using body language, i.e. using your eyes, face and body to transmit your feelings.

Reception the area where clients are received.

Receptionist person responsible for maintaining the reception area, scheduling appointments and handling payments.

Record cards confidential cards recording the personal details of each client registered at the business. This information may be stored electronically on the salon's computer.

Sale and Supply of Goods Act (1994) goods must be as described, of merchantable, satisfactory quality and fit for their intended purpose.

Salon services covers all the services offered in your workplace.

Skin sensitivity patch test method used to assess skin tolerance/sensitivity to a particular substance or service.

Travellers' cheques alternative form of payment used when travelling abroad and must be compared with the client's passport.

Verbal communication occurs when you talk directly to another person, either face to face or over the telephone.

ASSESSMENT OF KNOWLEDGE AND UNDERSTANDING

You have now learnt about salon reception in the beauty therapy workplace.

To test your level of knowledge, answer the following short questions. These will prepare you for your summative (final) assessment.

1. When a scheduling mix-up occurs, you should:
   a. not admit that you or anyone in the salon made a mistake.
   b. argue with the client about who wrote the appointment down wrong.
   c. be polite and never argue the point of which one of you is correct.
   d. blame the salon receptionist and call the manager.
2. How long should you allow when making an appointment for the following services?

   Match the service to the correct service timing:

Eyebrow tint	20 mins
Manicure	60 mins
Facial	45 mins
Individual flare lashes	10 mins

3. The reception area should always be:
   a. clean and tidy.
   b. clean and noisy.
   c. comfortable and messy.
   d. dirty and quiet.
4. Which important functions does the receptionist handle?
   a. booking appointments
   b. dealing with a variety of enquiries
   c. operating the payment point and handling payments
   d. all of the above
5. If a client disputed the change given as too little following payment what could you do?
6. Which of the following types of card is a debit card?
   a. gift voucher
   b. Switch/Maestro
   c. American Express card
   d. loyalty card
7. What are the important details to take and record when taking a message?
8. What is the legislation designed to protect the privacy of the client's details?
9. What may be the consequence of non-compliance with privacy legislation?
10. If you were presented with a fraudulent credit card what action should you take?

7 Facial Skincare

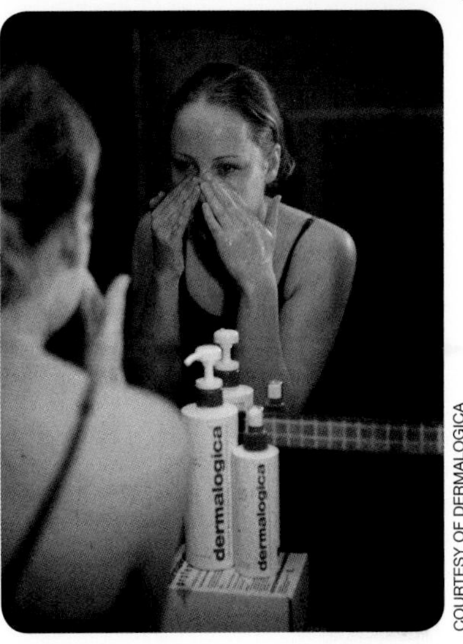

COURTESY OF DERMALOGICA

Learning Objectives

This chapter covers **VRQ Unit 204 Provide facial skincare**.

This unit is all about improving and maintaining your client's facial skin condition. A facial includes the application of facial products, use of associated equipment and facial massage techniques adapted to suit your client's skin type and condition.

There are **two** learning outcomes for this unit which you must achieve competently:

1 Be able to prepare for facial skincare treatments

2 Be able to provide facial skincare treatments

From the range statement, you must show you can:

- use **consultation techniques** to identify the treatment **objectives**
- use **products, tools and equipment** as appropriate
- treat all **skin types and conditions**
- ensure the **environmental conditions** are suitable
- complete a consultation and skin analysis to identify any **contra-indications**
- **communicate and behave** in an appropriate and professional manner
- follow all **health and safety working practices**
- provide relevant **aftercare and contra-action advice**

You must be able to show you have the necessary practical skills and underpinning knowledge to provide facial skincare.

This unit is linked to the Beauty Therapy NOS **Unit B4**.

ROLE MODEL

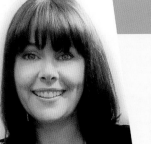

Sally Penford

Education Manager, UK and Ireland
The International Dermal Institute

"As Education Manager for the International Dermal Institute, I am responsible for training and development of a highly specialized team of lecturers, along with overall operations of eight training centres across UK and Ireland.

I studied at the London College of Fashion and achieved a Higher National Diploma in Beauty Therapy. From this I gained extensive experience in spas and industry consultancy and went on to run my own skin centre. It was 15 years ago that I joined the International Dermal Institute, the world's largest and most influential postgraduate education centre for professional skin therapists.

I share my knowledge in various ways such as traditional lecturing and more recently, through contemporary media methods, such as Twitter. As skincare treatments evolve, it is important to keep up with new advances.

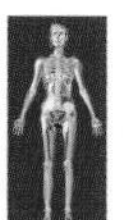

Essential anatomy and physiology knowledge for this unit is identified on the checklist in Chapter 2, page 27.

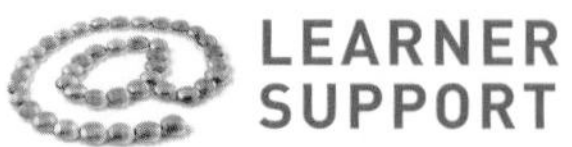

Health multiple choice quiz

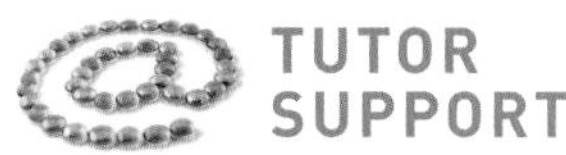

Activity 4: Healthy living task

Basics of skincare

If the skin is to function efficiently the skin must be cared for both internally and externally. Our **lifestyle** – the way we care about ourselves – affects the condition and appearance of the skin.

Healthy eating

Internally, a nutritionally balanced diet is vital to the health and appearance of the skin. A number of skin allergies and disorders are in part the result of poor nutrition, caused by a poorly balanced diet, including highly processed food, alcohol and lack of essential nutrients.

Foods contain the chemical substances we need for health and growth, the **nutrients**: a healthy diet contains all the essential nutrients. The nutrients are carried to the skin in the blood, where they nourish the cells in the processes of growth and repair.

A balanced diet prevents malnutrition (undernourishment) and vitamin/mineral deficiencies. The following food triangle diagram illustrates the different food groups. The daily recommended amounts to be consumed are:

Fats/oils	1 serving*
Fruit	2–4 servings
Milk and yoghurt	2–3 servings
Proteins	2–3 servings
Starch	6–11 servings
Sugar	1 serving*
Vegetables	3–5 servings

*use scarcely

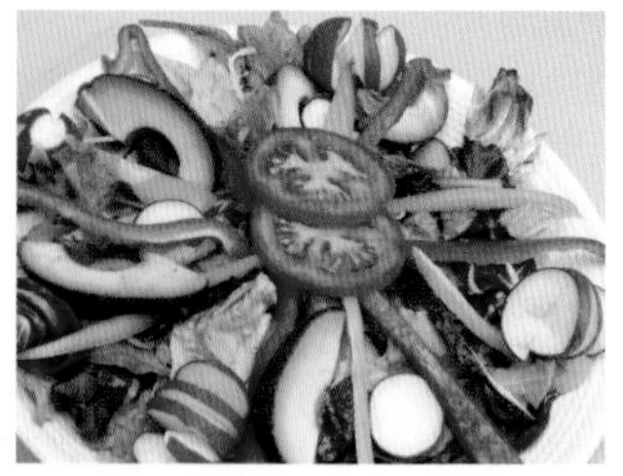

A traffic light system of food package labelling shows information on the nutritional content of foods to inform healthy food choice.

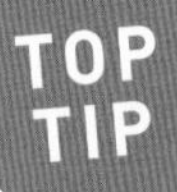

Five a day rule

Eat at least the recommended five servings of fruit and fresh vegetables every day. These foods provide vital vitamins and minerals that keep the skin healthy. A serving is:

- **1 small glass of pure fruit juice**
- **3 heaped tablespoons of fruit salad**
- **4 heaped tablespoons of vegetables**
- **1 medium fruit (an orange); 2 small fruits (plums)**
- **1 dessert bowl of salad**

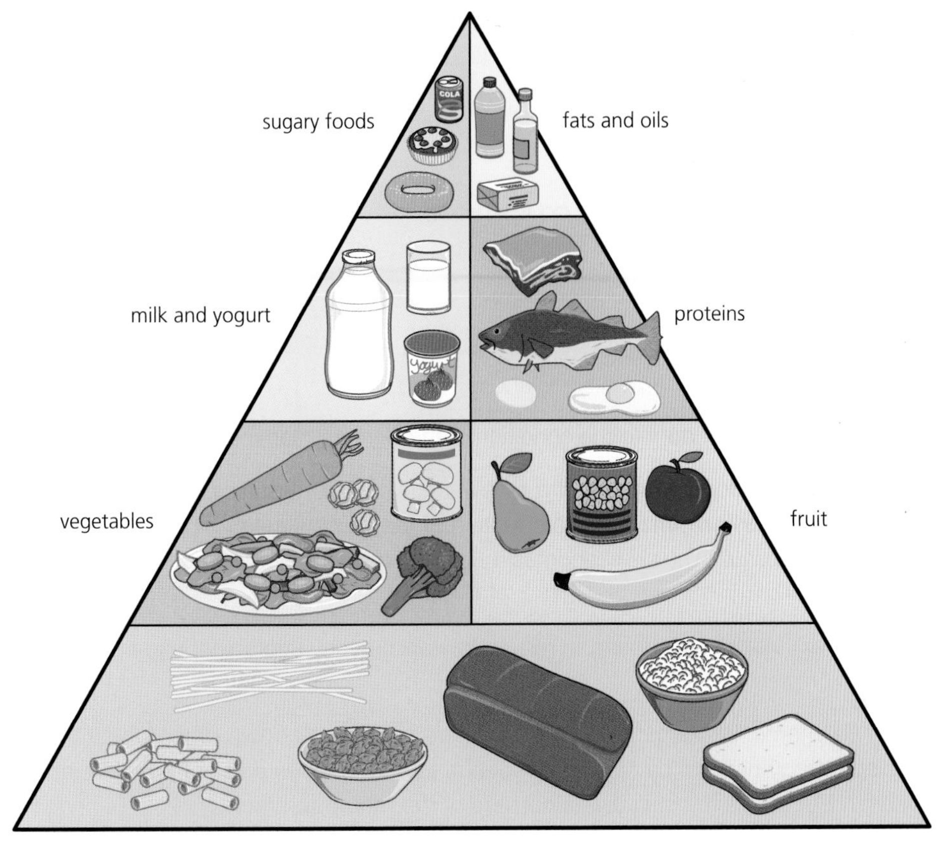

Chart for a balanced diet

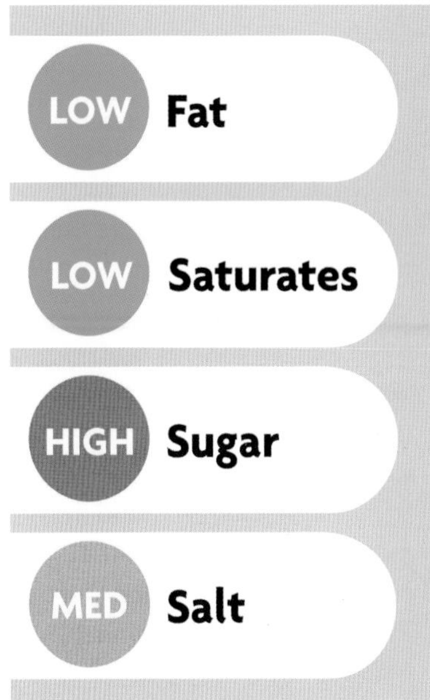

Traffic light system food label

There are six principal groups of nutrients:

Carbohydrates Carbohydrates provide energy quickly. They are either simple sugars or starches that the body can turn into simple sugars.

Food sources: Carbohydrates are found in fruit, vegetables, milk, grains, sugar and honey.

Fats Fats provide a concentrated source of energy, and are also used in carrying certain vitamins (see below) around the body. Fat is stored in the body around organs and muscles and under the skin. However, if too much fat is deposited under the skin, the elastic fibres there may be damaged by the expansion of the adipose tissue. Fat is also used in the formation of sebum, the skin's natural lubricant.

Food sources: Although this is not always evident, fats are present in almost all foods, from plants and from animals.

Proteins Proteins provide material for the growth and repair of body tissue, and are also a source of energy. Severe protein deficiency in children gives the skin a yellowish appearance, known as **jaundice**.

Food sources: Proteins are found in meat, fish, eggs, dairy products, grains and nuts.

Minerals Minerals provide materials for growth and repair and for regulation of the body processes. The major minerals are calcium, iron, phosphorus, sulphur, sodium,

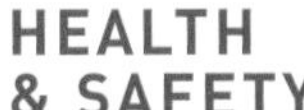
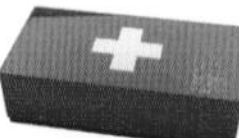

HEALTH & SAFETY

Vegan diets

Proteins are composed of many smaller units called *amino acids*. Animal protein sources contain all the amino acids essential to health. A *vegetarian* consuming dairy food will likewise obtain all the essential amino acids. A *vegan*, however, must be careful to eat an adequate quantity and variety of vegetables and other foods, in order to be sure that they receive all the amino acids they need.

Vegans must take vitamin B_{12} as a vitamin supplement as this vitamin occurs naturally only in animal-derived foods.

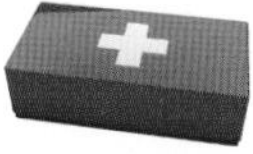

HEALTH & SAFETY

Special diets

Warn your clients about the danger of very low-fat, low-carbohydrate or low-protein diets: these can deprive the body of the nutrients it needs for growth, repair and energy.

TOP TIP

Antioxidant foods

As we know, antioxidants are essential to maintain the health of the skin, fighting the damaging effects of free radicals in your body. Vitamins A, C and E and the mineral selenium all have good antioxidant properties. These can be found in significant amounts in the following foods: blueberries, kale, strawberries, spinach, avocado and broccoli.

ACTIVITY

How do each of the following vitamins benefit the skin's appearance and its function: A, B, C and E?

HEALTH & SAFETY

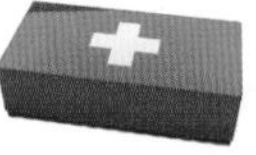

Weight loss

If you lose weight too quickly, your skin will sag and wrinkle. A healthy weight loss plan should be followed, drinking the recommended amount of water to stay hydrated.

HEALTH & SAFETY

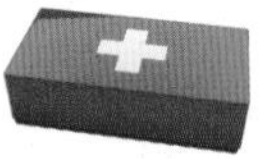

Effects of dehydration

Adequate water consumption means that we avoid being dehydrated, which can lead to symptoms such as headaches, tiredness and loss of concentration.

In hot weather or following active physical exercise more water must be consumed.

potassium, chlorine and magnesium. Of these, the most important to the skin is iron. A pale, dry skin may indicate **anaemia**, caused by a shortage of iron.

Food sources: Fruit and vegetables; iron is found in liver, egg yolks and green vegetables.

Vitamins Vitamins regulate the body's processes and contribute to its resistance to disease. Vitamins are divided into two groups, according to whether they are soluble in water or in fat:

- the fat-soluble vitamins are A, D, E and K
- the water-soluble vitamins are B and C

The vitamins most important to the condition of the skin are vitamins A, B_2, B_3, C and E.

Vitamin A Essential for the growth and renewal of skin cells. Insufficient vitamin A in the diet leads to **hyperkeratinization** (production of too much keratin). This causes blockages in the skin tissue. The skin becomes rough and dry, and eye disorders such as styes may occur.

Food sources: Vitamin A is found in red, yellow and green vegetables, and in egg yolk, butter and cheese.

Vitamin B_2 Vitamin B_2 (also called **riboflavin**) helps to break down other foodstuffs, releasing energy needed by cells to desquamate and function efficiently. A deficiency of vitamin B_2 causes the skin at the corners of the mouth to crack.

Food sources: Vitamin B_2 is found in brewer's yeast, milk products, leafy vegetables, liver and whole grains.

Vitamin B_3 Vitamin B_3 (also called **niacin**) has the same function as vitamin B_2, but is also vital in the maintenance of the tissues of the skin.

Food sources: Vitamin B_3 is found in meat, brewer's yeast, nuts and seeds.

Vitamin C Vitamin C (also called **ascorbic acid**) maintains healthy skin and is important for the production of collagen, providing tone and elasticity. A lack of vitamin C causes the capillaries to become fragile, and haemorrhages of the skin, such as bruising, may occur. Severe deficiency results in **scurvy**.

Food sources: Vitamin C is found in fruit and vegetables.

Vitamin E Vitamin E is found in most foods. It is an antioxidant and helps prevent premature skin ageing. It helps to rehydrate the skin, calms inflammation, helps healing and maintains healthy skin.

Food sources: Vitamin E is found in most foods. The richest sources are vegetable oils, cereal products, eggs and meat.

Water Water forms about two-thirds of the body's weight, and is an important component both inside and outside the body cells. Water is essential for the body's growth and maintenance. It helps remove waste from the body through urine and sweat and regulates temperature. Water must be regularly replaced through the diet. At least one and a half litres of water should be drunk every day, to avoid dehydration of the body and the skin. Aim to drink 6–8 medium glasses daily.

Food sources: Water is also a constituent of many foods, including fruits and vegetables.

Fibre Fibre is not broken down into nutrients, but it is very important for effective digestion.

Food sources: Fibre is found in fruit, vegetables and cereals.

Lifestyle threats to the skin

Internal

Alcohol Alcohol deprives the body of its vitamin reserves, especially vitamins B and C, which are necessary for a healthy skin. Alcohol also tends to dehydrate the body, including the skin. Skin conditions such as acne rosacea, eczema and psoriasis are often aggravated by the consumption of alcohol.

Caffeine Coffee, tea, cocoa and soft fizzy drinks contain a mild stimulant drug called **caffeine**. In moderate doses, such as two or three cups of coffee per day, caffeine is safe. If you drink too much, however, caffeine can cause nervousness, interfere with digestion, block the absorption of vitamins and minerals, dehydrate and spoil the appearance of the skin, stimulating skin ageing.

Drugs Drugs are chemical substances that affect the way our body performs. When they enter the body they are transported throughout the body in the blood. Recreational drugs are taken because they cause a particular effect or sensation which may feel good initially. Long term, they are harmful and addictive. Most affect blood pressure and heart rate. Stimulants, for example, can cause sweating, shaking and headaches. Heroin, in the class of painkillers called *narcotics*, ravages the skin, causing chronic dryness and premature ageing.

Smoking Smoking interferes with cell respiration and slows down the circulation. This makes it harder for nutrients and oxygen to reach the skin cells and for waste products to be eliminated. Cigarette smoking also releases a chemical that destroys vitamin C. This interferes with the production of collagen, and thereby contributes to premature wrinkling. Nicotine is a **toxic** substance – a poison!

Medication Certain medicines taken by mouth can cause skin dehydration, **oedema** – swelling of the tissues – (this may for example be caused by steroids) or irregular skin pigmentation (sometimes caused by the contraceptive pill). During the initial **consultation** with the client, find out whether they are taking any medication – and take this into account in your diagnosis and **treatment plan**.

Stress Stress is shown in the face as tension lines where the facial muscles are tight. Because blood and lymph cannot circulate properly, this causes a sluggish skin condition and poor facial nutrition. A person suffering from stress usually experiences disturbed sleep or sleeplessness (**insomnia**). Lack of sleep causes the skin to become dull and puffy, especially the tissue beneath the eyes, where dark circles also appear. Too *much* sleep can also cause the facial tissue to become puffy – because the circulation is less active, body fluids collect in the tissues.

If someone is suffering from stress, they may drink more tea, coffee or alcohol, or smoke more cigarettes: this too damages the skin.

Stress and anxiety are often the underlying cause of certain skin disorders. Some skin conditions, such as boils and styes, appear at times of stress; others, such as psoriasis and eczema, may become much worse. At the consultation, try to determine whether the client is suffering from stress: if they are, make sure that the salon treatments promote relaxation.

HEALTH & SAFETY

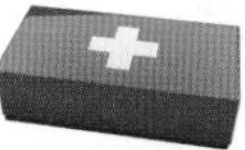

Alcohol intake

Alcohol intake is measured in units — one unit is one centilitre of pure alcohol and is equivalent to:

- 1 single measure of spirits
- 1/2 pint lager, beer or cider
- 1 small glass of wine.

A maximum of three units a day are recommended for men and a maximum of two units for women. It is increasingly recommended to have two alcohol-free days per week.

TOP TIP

Caffeine

Advise your clients to replace tea with herbal infusions and to drink decaffeinated coffee (in moderation) rather than regular coffee.

Caffeine is a diuretic, causing increased urination and loss of water leading to dehydration.

HEALTH & SAFETY

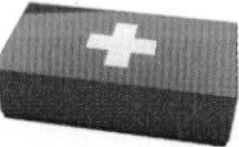

Smoking

Smoking depletes the body of vital nutrients, preventing their absorption.

ACTIVITY

Causes of stress

1. Can you think of everyday situations that may trigger stress?
2. How do you react physically when put in a stressful situation?
3. How can you create a relaxing environment in the salon?

TOP TIP

Retail opportunity

Some cosmetic companies offer bath preparations that aid relaxation by the inhalation of aromatic ingredients. These ingredients, combined with the warm water, may help a client who has difficulty in sleeping.

TOP TIP

UV light

UVB is most intense between 11 a.m. and 3 p.m., when the sun is at its highest. Advise clients to avoid the sun between these times.

HEALTH & SAFETY

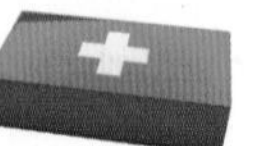

Cold sores

A client who suffers from cold sores (herpes simplex) should avoid excessive exposure to UV light as it can stimulate production of the sores.

ACTIVITY

The effects of UV

To see evidence of the damaging effects of ultra-violet on the skin, compare the skin on the back of your hands to skin on parts of the body that are not normally covered.

TOP TIP

Hyperpigmentation

Hyperpigmentation marks caused by repeated exposure to UV light eventually remain, even without the exposure to UV. Some clients dislike such marks, and you could advise them on camouflage make-up and daily application of a sun block skincare product.

External

As well as looking after the skin from the *inside*, by diet, it needs care from the *outside* – it must be kept clean, and it must be nourished.

With normal physiological functioning, the skin becomes oily, and sweat is deposited on its surface. The skin's natural oil (**sebum**) can easily build up and block the natural openings, the hair **follicles** and **pores**: this may lead to infection. Facial cosmetics too affect the health of the skin; if not regularly removed, they may cause congestion. Skincare treatments help to maintain and improve the functioning of the skin.

Ultra-violet light Although recently ultra-violet (UV) has been identified as a hazard to skin, it also has some *positive* effects. One of these is its ability to stimulate the production of **vitamin D**, which is absorbed into the bloodstream and nourishes and helps to maintain bone tissue. Second, UV light activates the pigment **melanin** in the skin, and thereby creates a **tan**. Many people feel better when they have a tan, as it gives a healthy appearance.

Ultra-violet light is divided into different bands. The most important to skin tanning are UVA and UVB. **UVA** stimulates the melanin in the skin to produce a rapid tan, which does not last very long. UVA penetrates deep into the dermis where it can cause premature ageing of the skin. **Free radicals** – highly reactive molecules which cause skin cells to degenerate – are also formed. These molecules disrupt production of collagen and elastin, the fibres that give skin its strength and elasticity. Reduced elasticity leads to wrinkling.

UVB stimulates the production of vitamin D. Melanin activation by UVB produces a longer-lasting tan than that produced by UVA. UVB is partially absorbed by the atmosphere – it has a shorter wavelength than UVA – and only 10 per cent reaches the dermis. UVB causes thickening of the stratum corneum layer, which reflects ultra-violet away from the skin's surface. UVB causes **sunburn**: the skin becomes red as the cells are damaged, and the skin may blister. UVB is also implicated in skin cancers, especially malignant melanoma.

The relaxing, warming effect of the sun is caused by the **infra-red (IR)** light. This penetrates the skin to the subcutaneous layer and is thought to speed skin ageing and possibly to cause a cancer called squamous cell carcinoma. The tan is actually a sign of skin damage, therefore, and both UV and IR probably contribute to photo-ageing – the premature ageing of the skin by light.

Although black skin has a high melanin content, which absorbs more ultraviolet and allows less to reach the dermis, it is not fully protected against the UV and still requires additional protection.

Chemical skin protection, or sunscreens, are designed to absorb ultra-violet light (UVA and UVB), reducing the rate of skin ageing in all skin types. Various sunscreens are available, classified by number according to their sun-protection factor (SPF). This is the amount of protection that the sunscreen gives you from the sun. A SPF of at least 15 is recommended in winter and 30 in summer. The application of the sunscreen extends your natural skin protection, allowing you to stay in the sun for longer without burning. For example, if normally you can be in the sun for 10 minutes before the skin begins to go red, a sunscreen with an SPF of 10 will allow you 10 × 10 minutes' (i.e. 100 minutes') safe exposure in the sun. Always check the expiry date of sunscreens, they only have a shelf life of 2–3 years.

Artificial UV light produced by sun beds, used for cosmetic skin tanning, also causes premature ageing. Most sun beds use concentrated UVA, which causes dermal tissue damage resulting in lines and wrinkles.

It may take years to see the effects of the dermal damage caused by unprotected UV exposure, but once they have occurred the effects are irreversible. UVA rays are present all year round, so to prevent premature ageing, cosmetic preparations containing sunscreens should be worn at all times.

Climate Sebum, the skin's natural grease, provides an oily protective film over the surface of the skin that reduces evaporation. Despite this, unprotected exposure of the skin to the environment allows evaporation from the epidermis which results in a dry, dehydrated skin condition.

The climate has several effects on the skin:

- ***Sebum production*** When the skin is exposed to the cold, less sebum is produced. The skin has reduced protection, allowing moisture to evaporate.
- ***Perspiration*** In very hot weather more moisture is lost as **perspiration**: perspiration increases to cool the skin and regulate the body's temperature.
- ***Humidity*** Moisture loss from the skin is also affected by the **humidity** (water content) of the surrounding air. In hot, dry weather humidity will be low, so water loss will be high. In temperate, damp conditions humidity will be high, so water loss will be low.
- ***Extremes of temperature*** Alternating heat and cold often leads to the formation of **broken capillaries**. These appear as fine red lines on Caucasian skin, and as discolouration on black skin.
- ***Stratum corneum*** The cells of the stratum corneum multiply with repeated unprotected exposure to the climate, as the body's natural defence.

The damaging effects caused by the climate can be reduced by using protective skincare preparations such as moisturisers. These spread a layer of oil over the skin's surface, reducing evaporation.

HEALTH & SAFETY

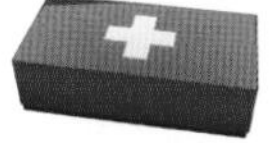

Ashiness
A black skin can sometimes appear ashen, with patches of skin becoming grey and flaky. This is caused by sudden changes in temperature combined with low humidity, which can cause the skin to lose moisture. Moisturisers help in alleviating this problem.

Environmental stress and pollution Further causes of moisture loss include harsh alkaline chemicals such as detergents and soaps – which remove sebum from the skin's surface – and air conditioning and central heating.

Environmental **pollutants** such as lead, mercury, cadmium and aluminium can accumulate in the body. One result is the formation of dangerous chemicals that attack proteins in the cells. Such pollutants find their way into food through polluted waters, rain and dust. To protect the body, always wash vegetables thoroughly, and eat a diet rich in vitamins C and E.

Air pollution, involving carbon from smoke, chemical discharges from factories, and fumes from car exhausts, should be removed from the skin by effective cleansing. Absorption of these pollutants is reduced by the application of **moisturiser**: this forms a barrier over the skin's surface.

HEALTH & SAFETY

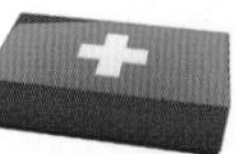

Sunbathing
Never wear perfume, cosmetic products or deodorants when sunbathing, either in natural sunlight or in artificially produced (sun-canopy) ultra-violet. The chemicals in these products can sensitize the skin, causing an allergic skin reaction.

Ultra-violet can penetrate water to a depth of one metre, so even when swimming you need to wear a sunscreen. Special waterproof products are designed for this purpose.

BEST PRACTICE

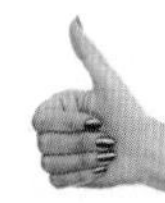

To acquire a tan without the damaging effects of the sun or sun beds, your client can use a *fake tanning* preparation. This treatment is becoming popular in the beauty therapist's salon.

ALWAYS REMEMBER

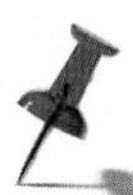

At the consultation, ask the client their occupation: this will guide you as to their likely skincare requirements. The client who works outdoors, for example, will have different treatment needs from the one who works indoors.

ACTIVITY

Geographical variations
Consider the effects of climate on the skin. Name four different geographical locations, and state the humidity level and climate you would expect at each location.

Think of the probable effects on the skin. What treatments by a beauty therapist might be needed in each country?

TOP TIP

Dry skin in winter

Central heating creates an environment with humidity similar to that of the desert. Unless you use a moisturiser, the loss of moisture from the skin will cause a dry, dehydrated skin condition.

HEALTH & SAFETY

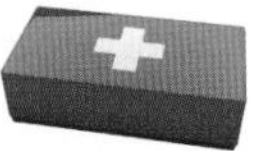

Effects of water loss

Water loss can sometimes be sufficient to disrupt living cells in the skin to the extent that some actually die. This results in skin irritation and reddening.

ACTIVITY

Environmental factors

It is important that you are aware of all the factors that can affect the health of a client's skin: this knowledge allows you to assess each client's treatment needs. Summarize the different factors you have learnt about.

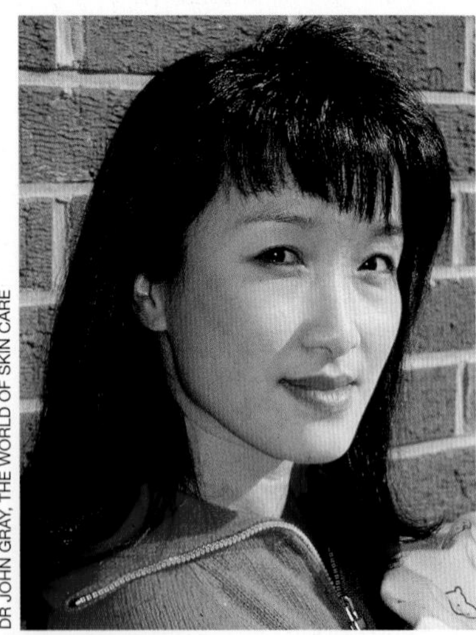

DR JOHN GRAY, THE WORLD OF SKIN CARE

Normal skin

Skincare treatments

The beauty therapist has the professional expertise to help each client improve the appearance and condition of their skin by the application of appropriate skincare treatments and products. The facial skin treatments you may offer include:

- consultation and skin analysis
- skin cleansing
- exfoliation
- manual **massage** of the face, neck and shoulders
- the application of face **masks**

The beauty therapist cannot change the underlying skin type, which is genetically determined, but they can keep the physiological characteristics of each skin type in check.

Skin types

The basic structure of the skin does not vary from person to person, but the physiological functioning of its different features does; it is this that gives us **skin types**, recognized by specific visible characteristics.

The first and most important part of a **facial** treatment is the correct diagnosis of the skin type. This is carried out at the beginning of each facial treatment. The beauty therapist must choose the correct skincare products and facial treatment for the client's skin type. This assessment is called a **skin analysis**.

Basic types

There are four main skin types:

- normal
- dry
- oily
- combination

Normal skin Normal skin is often referred to as **balanced**, the water and oil content is constant, it is neither too oily nor too dry. Because when young this skin type seldom has any problems, such as blemishes, it is often neglected. Neglect causes the skin to become dry, especially around the eyes, cheeks and neck, where the skin is thinner.

HEALTH & SAFETY

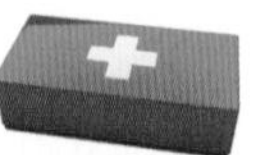

Air pollution

There are many components to air pollution. Car exhaust fumes, for example, release nitrogen oxide and volatile organic compounds. These react with sunlight to form ozone, a highly reactive form of oxygen. This can penetrate deep inside the skin and damage the cells' DNA (their main component), which can lead to skin cancer. Also, accelerated skin ageing is caused by free radical damage caused by unstable molecules, which affect the skin's elasticity. Moisturisers containing antioxidants are essential and should be recommended to neutralize free radicals or repel them from the skin before skin damage is caused.

A normal skin type in adults is very rare. It has these characteristics:

- the pore size is small or medium
- the moisture content is good
- the skin texture is smooth and even, neither too thick nor too thin
- the colour is healthy (because of good blood circulation)
- the skin elasticity is good, when young
- the skin feels firm to the touch
- the skin pigmentation is even-coloured
- the skin is usually free from blemishes

Dry skin Dry skin is lacking in either sebum or moisture, or both. Because sebum limits moisture loss by evaporation from the skin, skin with insufficient sebum rapidly loses moisture. The resulting dry skin is often described as **dehydrated**.

Dry skin has these characteristics:

- the pores are small and tight
- the moisture content is poor
- the skin texture is coarse and thin, with patches of visibly flaking skin
- there is a tendency towards sensitivity (broken capillaries often accompany this skin type)
- premature ageing is common, resulting in the appearance of fine lines leading to deeper wrinkles, seen especially around the eyes, mouth and neck
- skin pigmentation may be uneven, and disorders such as ephelides (freckles) usually accompany this skin type
- milia are often found around the cheek and eye area

Oily skin In oily skin the sebaceous glands become very active at puberty, when stimulated by the male hormone **androgen**. An increase in sebum production often causes the appearance of skin blemishes. Sebaceous gland activity begins to decrease when the person is in their twenties.

Oily skin has these characteristics:

- the pores are enlarged
- the moisture content is high
- the skin is coarse and thick
- the skin is sallow in colour, as a result of the excess sebum production, dead skin cells become embedded in the sebum, and the skin has sluggish blood and lymph circulation
- the **skin tone** is good, due to the protective effect of the sebum
- the skin is prone to shininess, due to excess sebum production
- there may be uneven pigmentation
- certain skin disorders may be apparent – comedones, pustules, papules, milia or sebaceous cysts

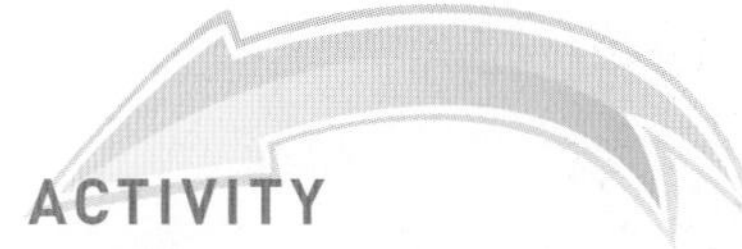

ACTIVITY

Recognizing skin types and conditions

Refer to the illustration below. What skin characteristics conditions would you expect to see in each of the numbered areas if performing a skin analysis on a:

- dry skin type?
- oily skin type?
- combination skin type?

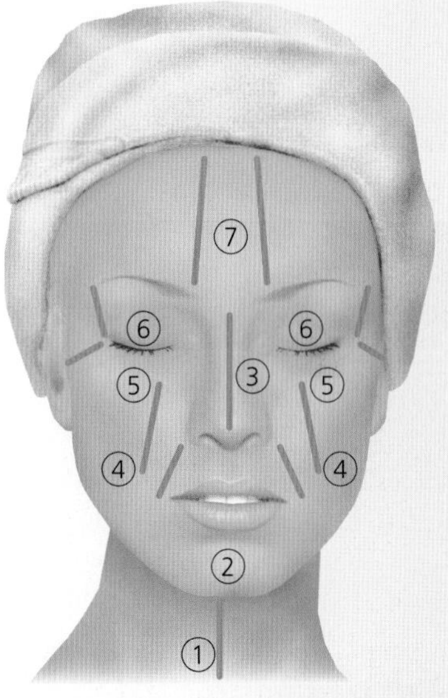

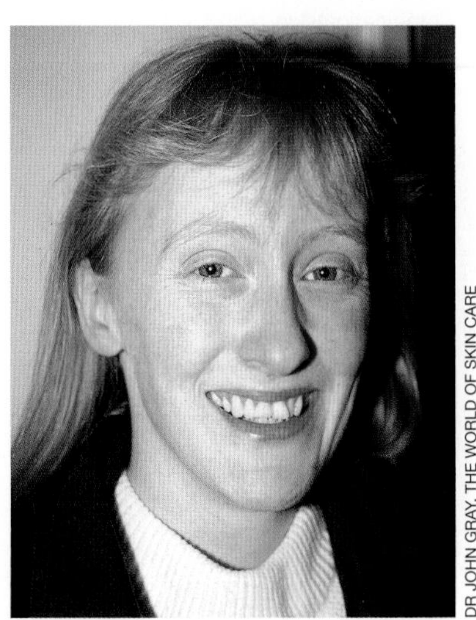

Dry skin

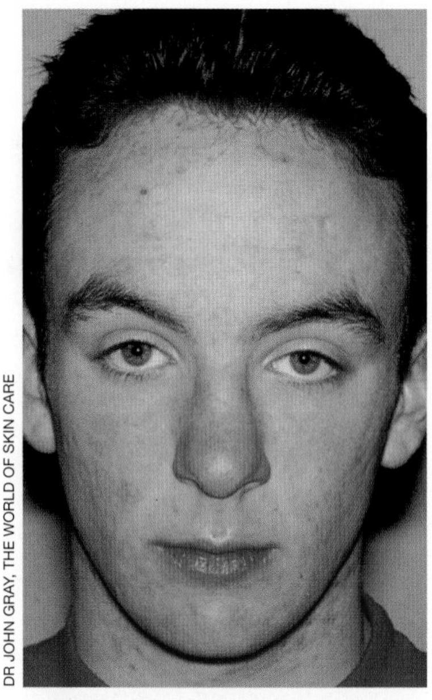

Oily skin

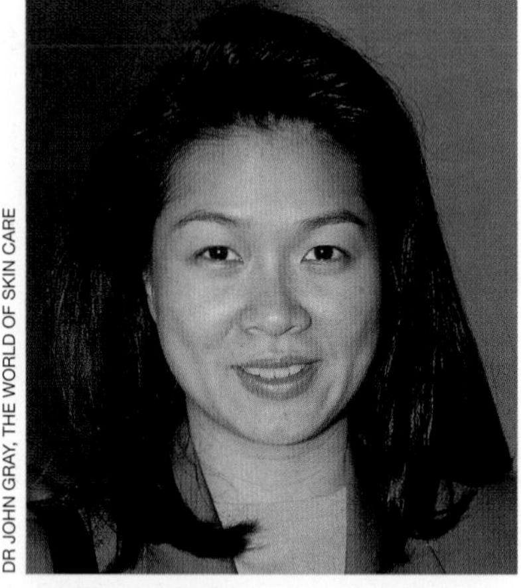

Combination skin

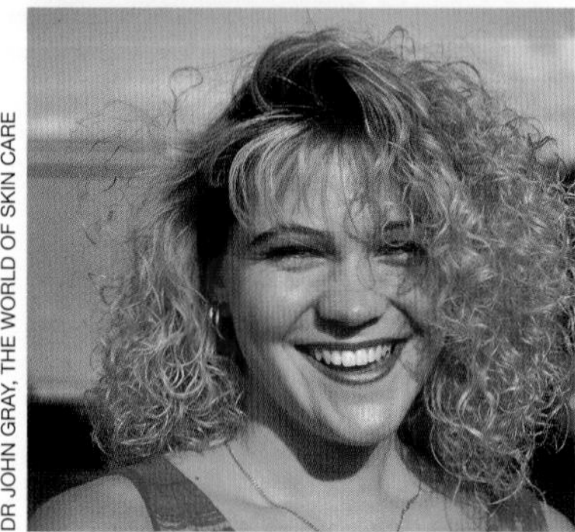

Sensitive skin

BEST PRACTICE

Dehydrated skin

Encourage clients, especially those with dehydrated skin, to drink six to eight glasses of water a day to replenish the moisture in the body.

Acne vulgaris and **seborrhoea** are skin disorders that occur when the skin becomes excessively oily due to the influence of hormones. Treatment of these skin disorders should be carried out to control and reduce sebum flow.

Combination skin Combination skin is partly oily and partly dry. The oily parts are generally the chin, nose and forehead, known as the **T-zone**. The upper cheeks may show signs of oiliness, but the rest of the face and neck area is usually dry.

Combination skin is the most common skin type. It has these characteristics:

- the pores in the T-zone are enlarged, while in the cheek area they are small to medium
- the moisture content is high in the oily areas, but poor in the dry areas
- the skin is coarse and thick in the oily areas, but thin in the dry areas
- the skin is sallow in the oily areas, but shows sensitivity and high colour in the dry areas
- the skin tone is good in the oily areas, but poor in the dry areas
- there is uneven pigmentation, usually seen as ephelides and lentigines
- there may be blemishes such as pustules and comedones on the oily skin at the T-zone
- milia and broken capillaries may appear in the dry areas, commonly on the cheeks and near the eyes

Additional skin conditions

While looking closely at the skin, further **skin characteristics** may become obvious. The skin may be:

- sensitive
- dehydrated
- moist
- oedematous (puffy)

Sensitive skin Sensitive skin usually accompanies a dry skin type, but not always. The characteristics of sensitive skin are these:

- the skin may show high colouring as it is easily irritated
- there are usually broken capillaries in the cheek area
- the skin feels warm to the touch
- there is superficial flaking of the skin
- the skin may show high colouring and tightness after skin cleansing, if it is sensitive to pressure

In black skin, instead of the redness shown by Caucasian skin, irritation shows up as a darker patch.

Allergic skin Allergic skin is irritated by external **allergens**, including chemicals in some cosmetics. The allergens inflame the skin and may damage its protective function. At the consultation, always try to discover whether the client has any allergies, and if so, to what.

The allergies of most concern to the beauty therapist are those caused by substances applied to the skin. The therapist must be aware of such substances and avoid their use. Contact with an allergen, especially if repeated, may cause skin disorders such as eczema or dermatitis (see pages 40–53, where skin diseases and disorders are dealt with in more detail).

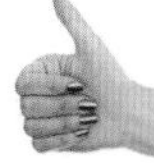

BEST PRACTICE

Oedematous skin

While completing the record card you may be able to recognize aspects of your client's lifestyle that probably contribute to the oedematous skin. If so, you can advise the client accordingly.

Dehydrated skin Dehydrated skin is skin that has lost water from the skin tissues. The condition can affect any skin type, but most commonly accompanies dry or combination skin types. The problem may be related to the client's general health. If they have recently been ill with a fever, for example, the skin will have lost fluid through sweating. If they are taking medication, this too may cause dehydration, as may drastic dieting. In many cases the dehydration is caused by working in an environment with a low humidity, or in one that is air-conditioned. You must try to discover the cause, and provide both corrective treatment and advice.

The characteristics of dehydrated skin are as follows:

- the skin has a fine orange-peel effect, caused by its lack of moisture
- there is superficial flaking
- fine, superficial lines are evident on the skin
- broken capillaries are common

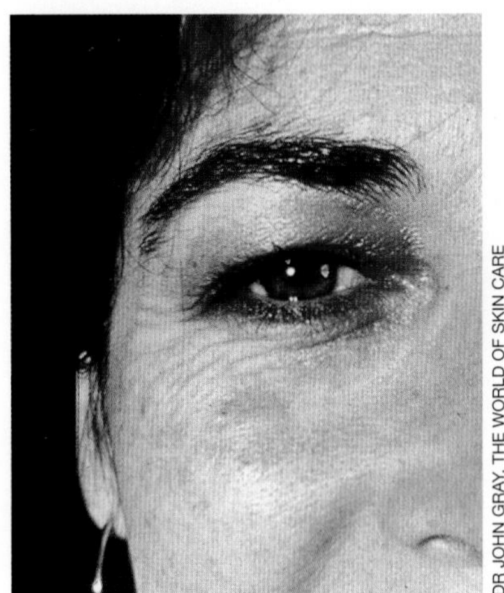

DR JOHN GRAY, THE WORLD OF SKIN CARE

Dehydrated skin

Moist skin Moist skin appears moist and feels damp: this is due to the over-secretion of sweat. The beauty therapist cannot correct this skin condition, which is often caused by some internal physiological disturbance such as a hormonal or metabolic imbalance.

Advise the client to use lightweight cleansing preparations. The client should avoid skin-toning preparations with a high alcohol content; these would stimulate the skin, causing yet further perspiration and skin sensitivity. They should avoid highly spiced food, and be aware that alcoholic or hot drinks will cause dilation of the skin capillaries, thereby increasing the skin's temperature.

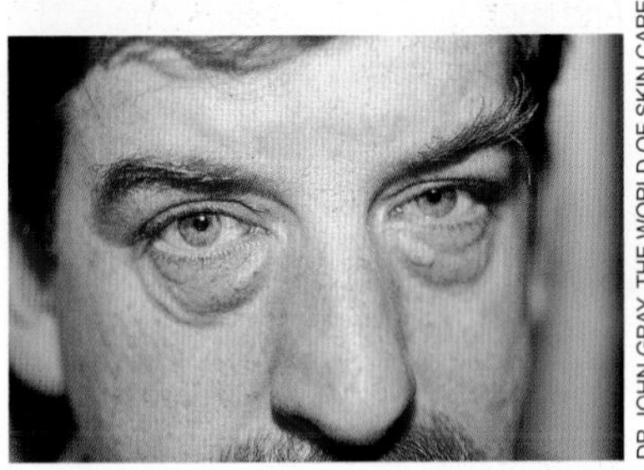

DR JOHN GRAY, THE WORLD OF SKIN CARE

Puffy skin

Oedematous (puffy) skin Oedematous skin is, and appears, swollen and puffy: this is because the tissues are retaining excess water. The condition may be caused by a medical disorder, or may be a side-effect of medication. Hot weather can cause temporary swelling of the tissues, as can local injury to the tissues. Poor blood circulation and lymphatic flow may cause puffy skin, too; this is often seen around the eyes. In this case the condition may benefit from gentle massage around the eye area. Tissue-fluid retention in the facial skin may be caused by an incorrect diet, such as one that includes too much salt or the drinking of too much alcohol, tea or coffee and insufficient water.

Unless you are quite sure about the cause of the oedema, always seek permission from your client's doctor before treating the skin.

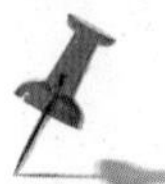

ALWAYS REMEMBER

Sensitive skin

Use hypoallergenic products – these do not contain any of the known common skin sensitizers such as perfume that can cause skin irritation.

Skin that is sensitive may also be allergic to certain substances such as adhesives that may be used in false lash application.

Recommend avoiding lifestyle factors that can make sensitive skin worse. These include alcohol, smoking, poor diet and stress.

The sex of the client

Men have a more acidic skin surface than females and the stratum corneum is thicker on males than females. However, males have coarse facial hair and shaving daily removes cells of the stratum corneum before they are ready to desquamate naturally. This can sensitize and dry the skin, especially if aftershave lotions with a high alcohol content are directly applied. A moisturiser should be applied to protect the skin.

The collagen content of the skin is different in men and women. Collagen and sebum production falls in menopausal women causing skin ageing. Skin does not appear to age

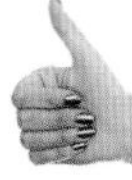

BEST PRACTICE

Male facials
Recommend that the male client shaves before a facial treatment. This will soften the skin and facilitate skin cleansing.

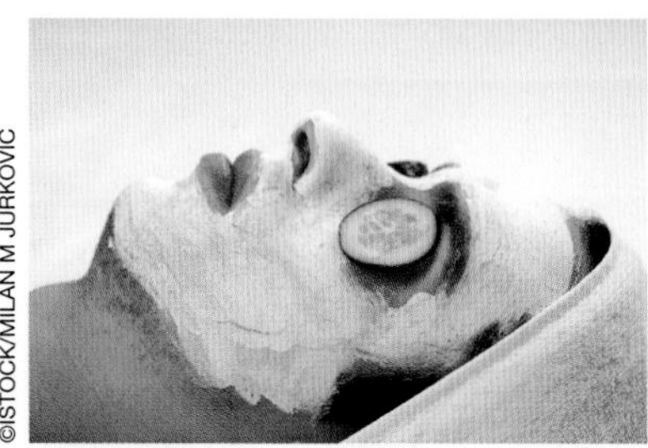

Male facial

ALWAYS REMEMBER

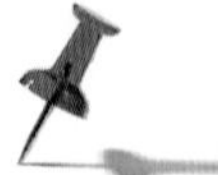

Skin tone
To test skin tone, gently lift the skin at the cheeks between two fingers and then let go. If the skin tone is good, the skin will spring back to its original shape.

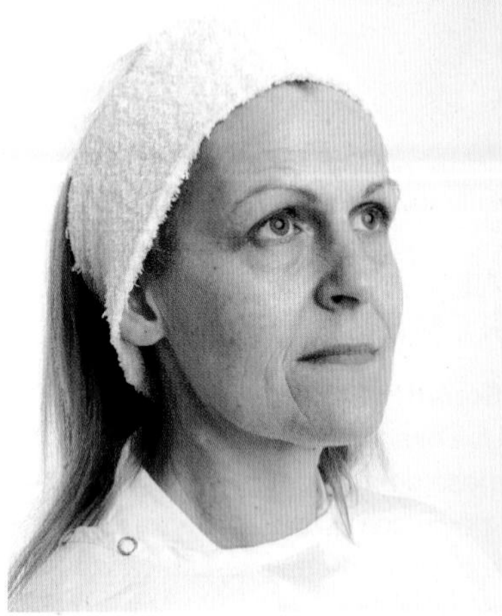

Mature skin

as quickly in males as females because collagen, elastin and sebum production remain constant. The skin of males typically feels firmer.

The main reason males choose to have a facial is for relaxation, to improve the appearance of the skin, and increasingly for the anti-ageing benefits.

The age of the skin

Having identified the skin type, the beauty therapist must classify the age of the skin. This can vary between people of different race because of evolution which may delay the visible signs of ageing due to differences in sebaceous gland and melanin activity in skin.

Often the age of a client will relate to skin problems that are evident. A young client, for example, may have skin blemishes such as comedones, pustules and papules. These disorders are caused by over-activity of the sebaceous gland at puberty, when the body is developing its secondary sexual characteristics. It is at this time that acne vulgaris is most likely to occur, due to the hormonal imbalance. The skin of clients aged over 25 years, however, is generally termed **mature skin**.

The beauty therapist should also consider the client's skin tone and **muscle tone** in relation to their age. A young skin will probably have good skin tone, and the skin will be supple and elastic. This is because the collagen and elastin fibres in the skin are strong. Poor skin tone, on the other hand, is recognized by the appearance of facial lines and wrinkles.

A healthy young skin will also have good muscle tone, and the facial contours will appear firm. With poor muscle tone, the muscles becomes slack and loose.

Poor lifestyle choices and general health will also affect how quickly our skin shows visible signs of ageing.

Mature skin The change in appearance of women's skin during ageing is closely related to the altered production of the hormones oestrogen, progesterone and androgen at the menopause.

Mature skin has the following characteristics:

- The skin becomes dry, as the sebaceous and sudoriferous glands become less active.
- The skin loses its elasticity as the elastin fibres harden, and wrinkles appear due to the cross-linking and hardening of collagen fibres.
- The epidermis grows more slowly and the skin appears thinner, becoming almost transparent in some areas such as around the eyes, where small veins and capillaries show through the skin.
- Broken capillaries appear, especially on the cheek area and around the nose.
- The facial contours become slack as muscle tone is reduced.
- The underlying bone structure becomes more obvious, as the fatty layer and the supportive tissue beneath the skin grow thinner.
- Blood circulation becomes poor, which interferes with skin nutrition, and the skin may appear sallow.
- Due to the decrease in metabolic rate, waste products are not removed so quickly, and this leads to puffiness of the skin.
- Patches of irregular pigmentation appear on the surface of the skin, such as lentigines and chloasmata.

The skin may also exhibit the following skin conditions, although these are not truly *characteristic* of an ageing skin:

- Dermal naevi may be enlarged.
- Seborrhoeic warts may appear on the epidermal layer of the skin.
- Verruca filliformis warts may increase in number.
- Hair growth on the upper lip or chin, or both, may become darker or coarser, due to hormonal imbalance in the body.
- Dark circles and puffiness may occur under the eyes.

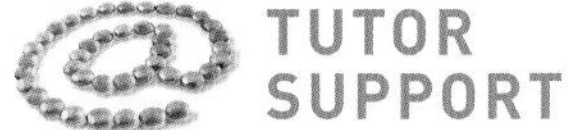

Activity 1: Consultation sheet task

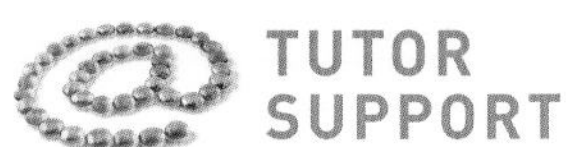

Activity 2: Skin analysis handout

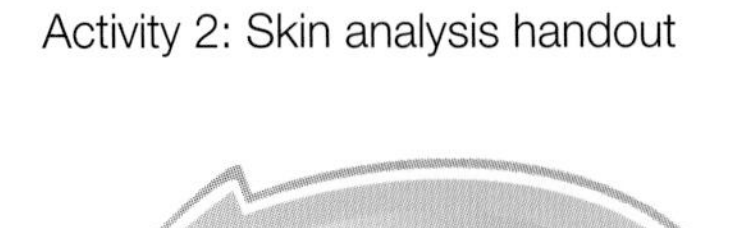

KNOWLEDGE CHECK

How do you identify a client's skin type?

Need more time... refer to pages 176–178 to help you.

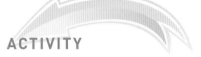

ACTIVITY

The ageing process

Cut out photographs from magazines or newspapers showing men and women of different cultures and various ages.

1 Can you identify the visible characteristics of ageing?
2 Does ageing occur at the same rate in men and women and in different cultures?
3 Discuss your findings with your colleagues and tutor.

HEALTH & SAFETY

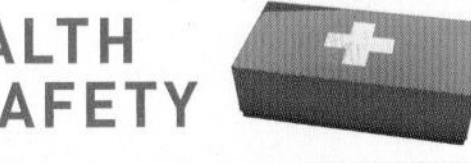

UV light and ageing

The ageing process is accelerated when the skin is regularly exposed to ultra-violet light.

Differences in skin

Although there is no difference between skin functions such as sweat and sebaceous gland activity in white and black skin, the amount of pigment, called *melanin*, varies, resulting in different skin and hair colour.

There are two forms of the melanin pigment: *eumelanin*, produced in black and brown skin colours, and *phaeomelanin*, found in lighter skins. Both forms of pigment can be present together but the amount of each can vary.

People who originate from hot countries and are nearer the equator have more melanin and a darker skin pigment. This is because the UV is very intense and the skin requires more protection. Those who originate from cooler countries have less melanin and a lighter skin pigment. The pigmentation of the skin is the result of millions of years of evolution.

TOP TIP

Skin appearance

As the surface of the skin reflects light and shows the skin colour, the therapist's aim is for the skin surface to be smooth and healthy. This is achieved by the removal of dead skin cells and ensuring it is adequately moisturised.

African-Caribbean The skin colour is dark and ranges in tone to almost black. This is because it has more melanin, which absorbs ultra-violet (UV) light. As black skin is exposed to UV light it becomes darker and darker.

Care must be taken when dealing with blemishes on darker skins as scars may occur as the skin heals. The scars may become keloids, scarring that becomes enlarged and projects above the skin's surface. Even minor scratches may result in keloid formation.

Hyperpigmentation (uneven patches of skin tone which are darker than the surrounding skin) may also occur with exposure to UV light. It is more common in darker skinned people due to increased melanin. Hyperpigmentation most commonly occurs following skin inflammation, such as acne vulgaris. Keloids may become hyperpigmented if exposed to the sun in the early stages of their formation.

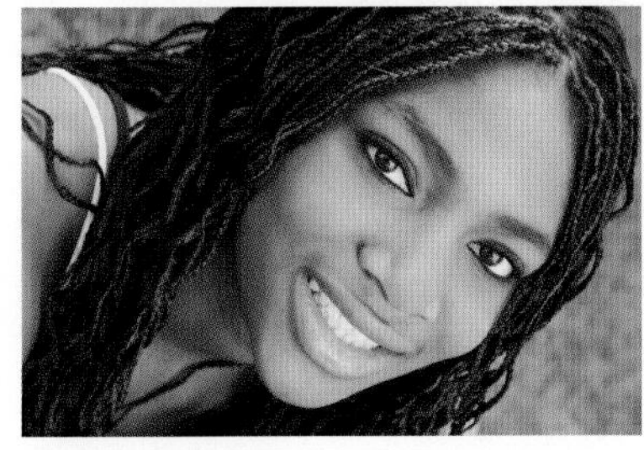

African-Caribbean skin

ALWAYS REMEMBER

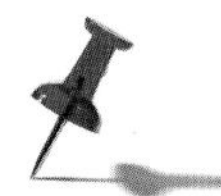

Skin and UV light defence

Very dark skin offers up to 30 times more protection against the sun than lighter skin.

ALWAYS REMEMBER

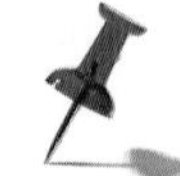

Hyperpigmentation and **hypopigmentation** can affect the skin of any race.

Chloasma or 'liver spots' are an example of hyperpigmentation and are commonly seen as dark brown marks on the backs of the hands. These occur as a result of skin damage caused by sun damage, skin trauma or hormonal imbalance.

Freckles or ephelides are another example of hyperpigmentation. These become darker when the skin is exposed to the sun.

Prescription creams containing hydroquinone bleach and laser treatment may be used to lighten the skin. However, care must be taken using hydroquinone bleach on black and Asian skin as hypopigmentation and skin allergy can occur.

Increasing in popularity are botanical brightners which include the professional application of an exfoliant to remove the pigmented surface cells and serum.

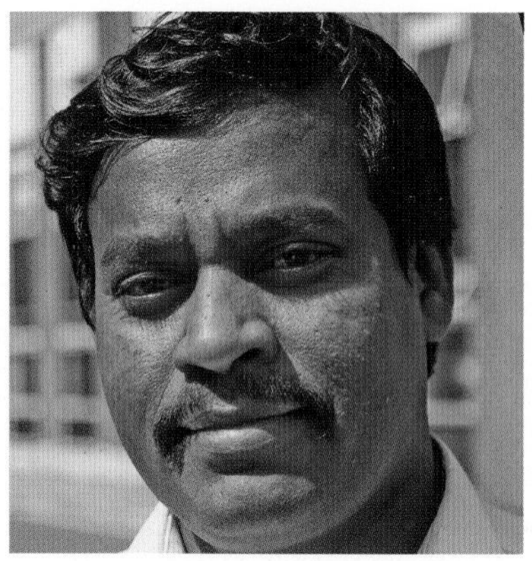

Asian skin

Vitiligo (a type of hypopigmentation or loss of skin pigment) is a considerable problem when it occurs in dark skin, as it is very obvious. Cosmetics may be applied as a corrective technique.

Male African-Caribbean clients may have a tendency towards *pseudo folliculitis*, an inflammatory skin disorder. This occurs as the hair is coarse and curly and has a tendency as it grows out of the skin to curl back and re-enter it, becoming ingrown. This foreign object in the skin becomes irritated and inflamed. Hyperpigmentation may also accompany this condition.

Dermatosis papulosis nigra, also called flesh moles, can occur. These are brown or black hyperpigmented markings, resembling moles, usually seen on the cheeks. Their cause is unknown but they are sometimes found to be hereditary. They also occur more frequently in women than men.

Hair colour is dark brown to black.

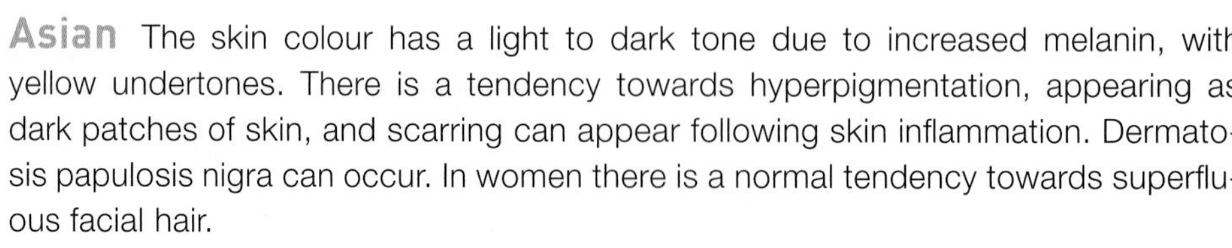

Asian The skin colour has a light to dark tone due to increased melanin, with yellow undertones. There is a tendency towards hyperpigmentation, appearing as dark patches of skin, and scarring can appear following skin inflammation. Dermatosis papulosis nigra can occur. In women there is a normal tendency towards superfluous facial hair.

Hair colour is dark brown to black.

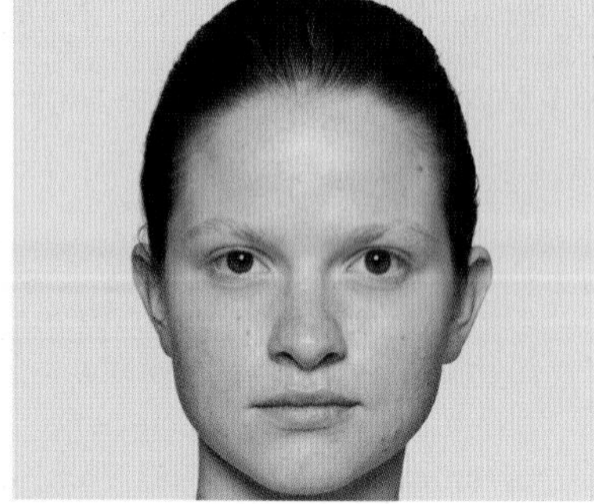

Caucasian skin

Caucasian The skin colour is pink. This skin has less melanin and so less defence in the presence of UV light; sun damage results in skin burning and premature ageing. Caucasian skin has a tendency to show freckles (ephelides), as a result of uneven melanin distribution in the skin.

Hair colour is usually fair, red or brown.

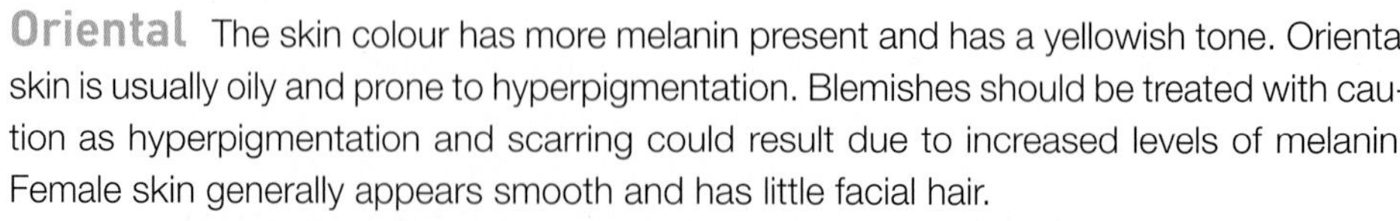

Oriental The skin colour has more melanin present and has a yellowish tone. Oriental skin is usually oily and prone to hyperpigmentation. Blemishes should be treated with caution as hyperpigmentation and scarring could result due to increased levels of melanin. Female skin generally appears smooth and has little facial hair.

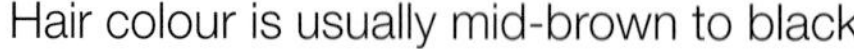

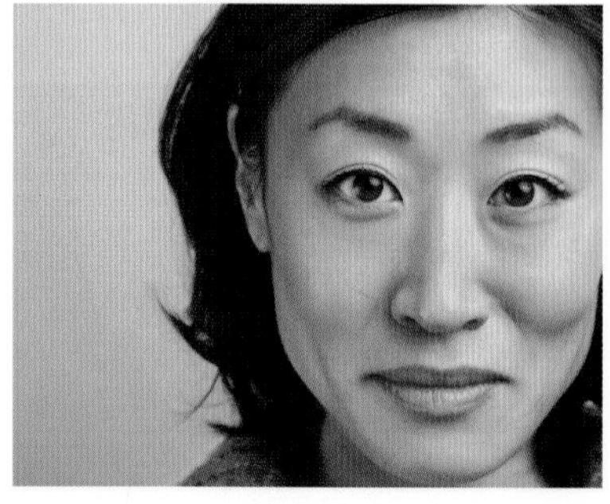

Oriental skin

Hair colour is usually mid-brown to black.

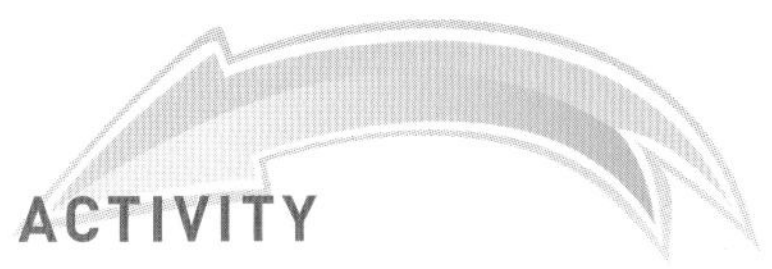

ACTIVITY

Which countries do people with the skin types listed below originate from:

- Caucasian?
- Oriental?
- Asian?
- African-Caribbean?

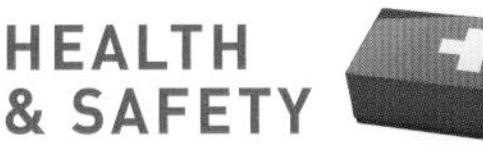
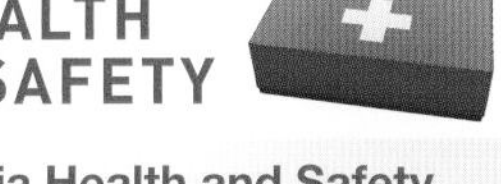

HEALTH & SAFETY

Habia Health and Safety *Hygiene for Hairdressers and Beauty Therapists* booklet is available as a download from www.habia.org providing practical advice on how to avoid infection in the workplace.

Outcome 1: Be able to prepare for facial skincare treatments

Learn how to prepare for facial skincare treatments

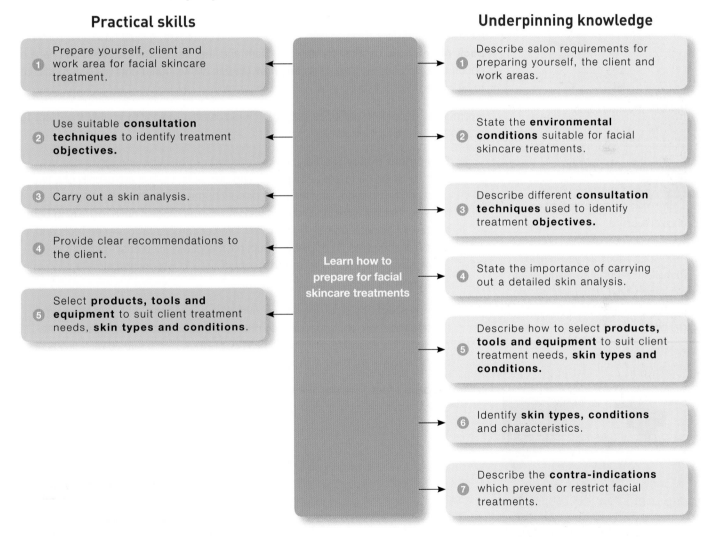

Practical skills

1. Prepare yourself, client and work area for facial skincare treatment.
2. Use suitable **consultation techniques** to identify treatment **objectives.**
3. Carry out a skin analysis.
4. Provide clear recommendations to the client.
5. Select **products, tools and equipment** to suit client treatment needs, **skin types and conditions**.

Underpinning knowledge

1. Describe salon requirements for preparing yourself, the client and work areas.
2. State the **environmental conditions** suitable for facial skincare treatments.
3. Describe different **consultation techniques** used to identify treatment **objectives.**
4. State the importance of carrying out a detailed skin analysis.
5. Describe how to select **products, tools and equipment** to suit client treatment needs, **skin types and conditions.**
6. Identify **skin types, conditions** and characteristics.
7. Describe the **contra-indications** which prevent or restrict facial treatments.

Chapter 3 Health and Safety covers general legal hygiene and safety practice which you legally have to carry out. You will learn about further specific health and safety.

Remember to always:

- Give due consideration to general health and safety legislation throughout the treatment.

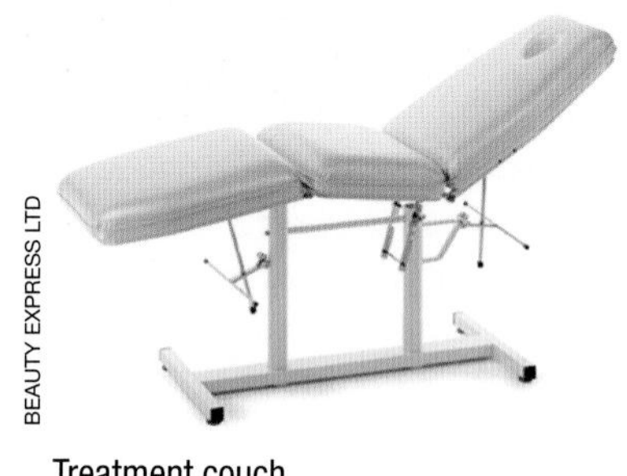
BEAUTY EXPRESS LTD

Treatment couch

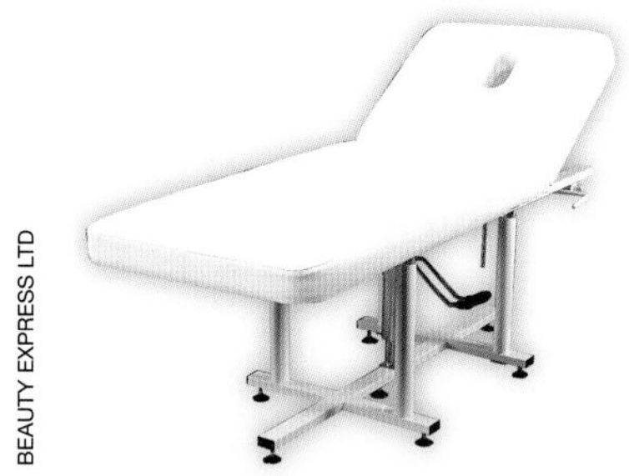
BEAUTY EXPRESS LTD

Hydraulic treatment couch

Be thorough Creating a unique, personalized experience is essential. Think about how you can go the extra mile, and what extra special touches you can add to make it an out-of-this world treatment every time. Your client will see excellent results, and you'll never get bored!

Sally Penford

- Implement any hygiene, health and safety requirements as identified in the unit practical skills and underpinning knowledge.
- Follow industry hygiene, health and safety practices throughout the treatment application. Refer to the Habia website to keep up to date with current health and safety practice.
- Dispose of any waste materials safely and correctly.

Preparing the work area

Consideration should be given to the positioning of **equipment** for ease and safety of use.

Each facial work area should have the following basic equipment: a **treatment couch or beauty chair.** The couch or chair should be covered with easy-to-clean upholstery; it must withstand daily cleaning with warm water and detergent. It must have an adjustable **back rest**, for the comfort of both the client and the therapist. If possible, purchase a couch that also has an adjustable **leg rest**, as this allows treatments such as pedicure to be carried out.

Hydraulic couches are useful as they can be adjusted in height to enable the client to position herself on the couch with ease.

- **Equipment trolley** The equipment trolley should be large enough to accommodate all the necessary equipment and products; trolleys are usually of a two- or three-shelf design. Like the chair or couch, the trolley should be made of a material that will withstand regular cleaning. Some models have restraining bars to prevent objects sliding off the trolley. Drawers are useful in storing tools and small consumables. The trolley should have securely fixed easy-glide castors. Some salons may use a large surface work area to display and store equipment and products.
- **Beauty stool** The stool should be covered in a fabric similar to that covering the treatment couch. It may or may not have a back rest; in some designs the back rest is removable. For the comfort of the therapist, it should be adjustable in height; to allow mobility, it should be mounted on castors.
- **Step-up stool** To assist clients as necessary to position themselves on the couch, have available a step-up stool.

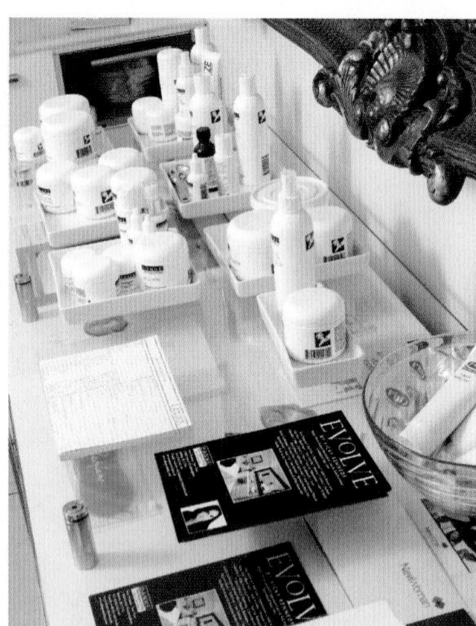

A prepared and organized work area

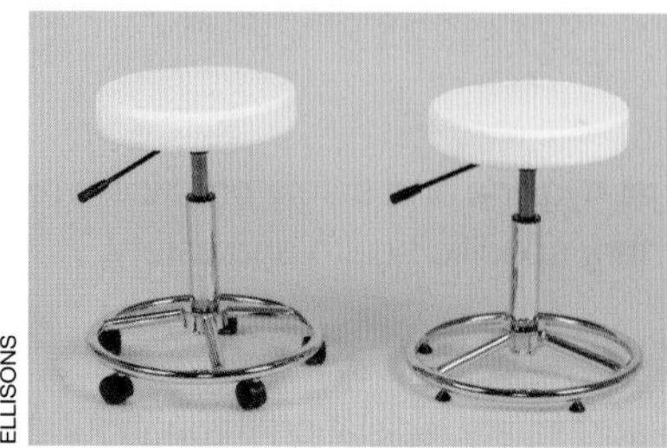
ELLISONS

Beauty stools

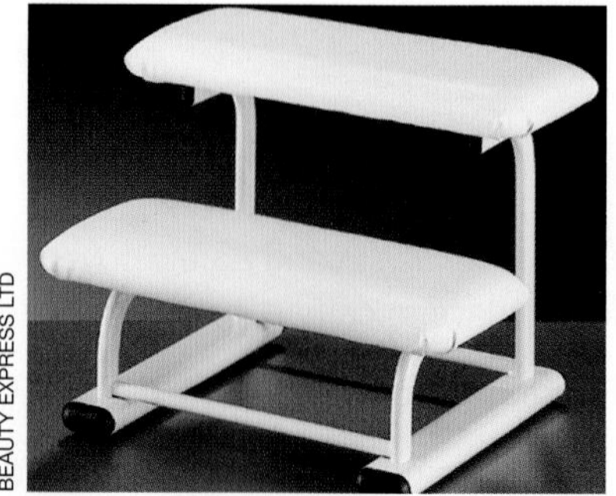
BEAUTY EXPRESS LTD

Step-up stool

- **Magnifying lamp** The magnifying lamp is available in three models: floor-standing, wall-mounted and trolley-mounted.
- **Covered waste bin** A covered waste bin should be placed unobtrusively within easy each. It should be lined with a disposable bin-liner. You should also have a 'sharps' box for the disposal of contaminated equipment.

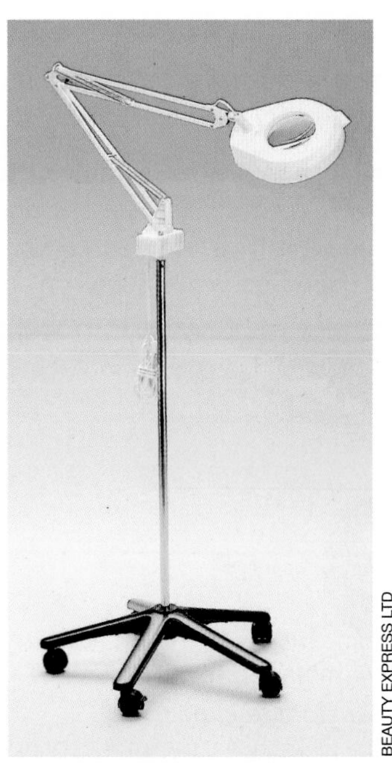
BEAUTY EXPRESS LTD

Magnifying lamp

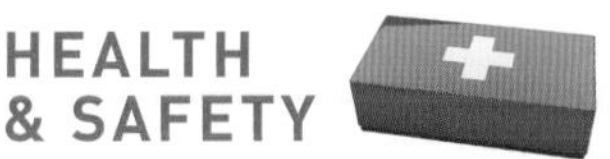

HEALTH & SAFETY

The couch and chair
The couch should be wiped over with a disinfectant solution after each client, and should be cleaned thoroughly with hot water and detergent at the end of each day. If protected with a towelling couch cover this must be protected with a covering that is replaced after each client, i.e. large towel or disposable paper.

Arrangements for the collection and disposal of contaminated waste should be made with your local environmental health office.

The following equipment guidelines describe the basic products, tools and equipment for all facial treatments. Further products, tools and equipment relevant to specific facial treatments are discusses later in the chapter.

PRODUCTS, TOOLS AND EQUIPMENT

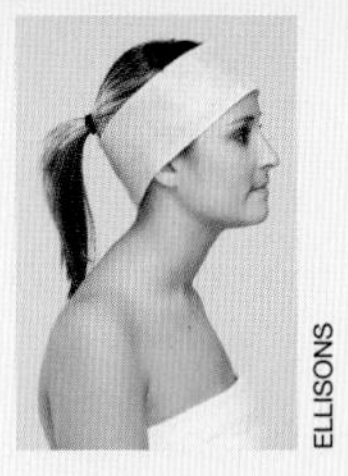
ELLISONS

Headband
A clean headband should be provided for each client. Use either a material headband or disposable. Disposable are useful as they can be discarded after the treatment

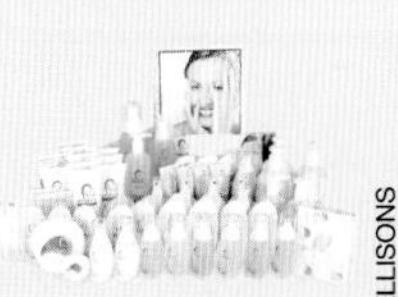
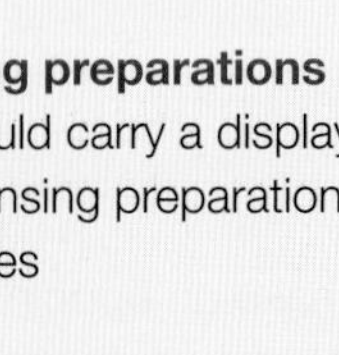
ELLISONS

Skin-cleansing preparations
The trolley should carry a display of facial skin-cleansing preparations to suit all skin types

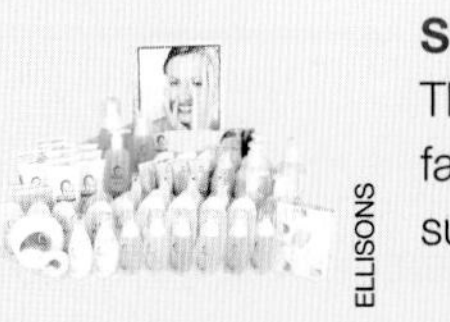
ELLISONS

Cotton wool
There should be a plentiful supply of both damp and dry cotton wool, sufficient for the treatment to be carried out. Dry cotton wool should be stored in a covered container; damp cotton wool is usually placed in a clean bowl

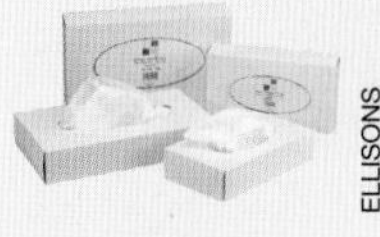
ELLISONS

Tissues
Facial tissues should be large and of a high quality. They should be stored in a covered container

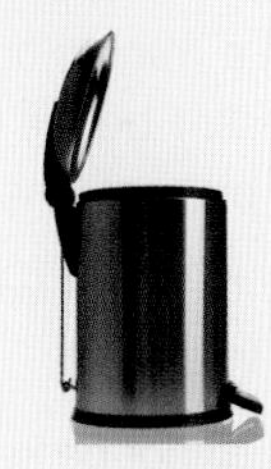

Waste bin
A covered container for waste may be placed on the bottom shelf of the trolley or it can be put into the waste bin at once

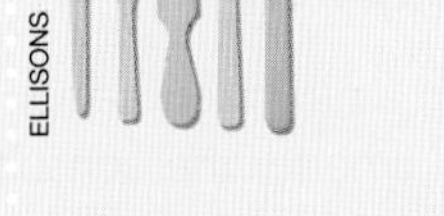
ELLISONS

Spatulas
Several clean spatulas (preferably disposable) should be provided for each client. One should be used in tucking any stray hair beneath the headband. Others will be used in removing products from their containers

YOU WILL ALSO NEED:

Towel drapes There should be a large towel to cover the client's body, and a small hand towel to drape across the client's chest and shoulders

Trolley The surface of each shelf can be protected with a sheet of 500mm disposable bedroll

Bowls To store damp and dry cotton wool

Steamer Use to warm the skin for cleansing and skin stimulation, e.g. facial steamer (vapour unit)

Towel A clean towel should be placed on the trolley for the therapist to wipe their hands on as necessary

Gown A clean gown should be provided for each client as necessary

Facial sponges, facial mitts or towels Used to remove facial products from the skin during treatment. They are particularly useful when working on a male client where cotton wool would collect on coarse facial hair

Mirror A clean hand mirror should be available for use in consulting with the client before during and after their treatment

Container for jewellery A container may be provided in which the client can place their jewellery if they need to remove it prior to treatment – follow your salon procedures in respect of client possessions

TOP TIP

Towel racks

Wall-mounted towel racks save storage space.

TOP TIP

Cotton wool

It is bad practice to leave the client in order to fetch more cotton wool. It is also bad practice to prepare too much and be wasteful!

Pre-shaped cotton wool discs are ideal for facial treatments. Alternatively, cut high-quality cotton wool into squares (6cm × 6cm).

HEALTH & SAFETY

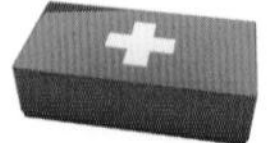

Containers

Bottles and other containers should be clean and clearly labelled.

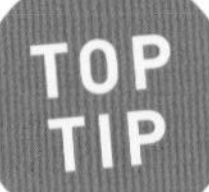

On arrival

When the client arrives for the treatment, generally the **record card** is completed. Record the client's personal details, such as their name and address. Check that there are no contra-indications to facial treatment.

If a client is a **minor**, under the age of 16 years of age, it is necessary to obtain signed written consent before treatment is carried out. It is also necessary that the parent or guardian is present when the treatment is given.

The beauty therapist will add further information to the record card at the consultation and during treatment.

Clients should not be kept waiting on arrival for their appointment. It is important that the work area is ready to proceed. The work area should always be maintained in a condition suitable for further treatments.

KNOWLEDGE CHECK

What environmental conditions should be considered when setting up the facial work area?

Need more time... refer to pages 95–96 – The Workplace (Health, Safety and Welfare) Regulations (1992) to help you.

Reception

When a new client telephones to make an appointment for a treatment, always allocate extra time for the consultation beforehand. Explain to the client how long they should allow for the appointment. For example, if a client is seeking a basic skin cleansing and mask treatment, allow 30 minutes; if they are a new client allow 45 minutes so that there is time for the consultation and filling in the record card. If it is necessary to remove facial blockages and to carry out other specialized treatments, allow 45 minutes to one hour. For a full facial treatment, allow one hour.

ALWAYS REMEMBER

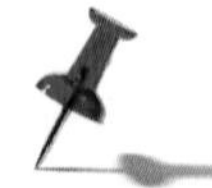

Compliance with the Data Protection Act (1998)

Ensure all client records are stored securely, with only those staff who have the client's permission having access to them.

HEALTH & SAFETY

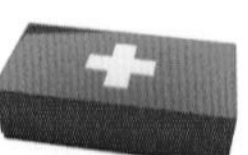

Poor health

If the client is in poor health, or is taking medication that affects their skin condition, it may not be possible to treat them until the medical condition has been treated by their general practitioner.

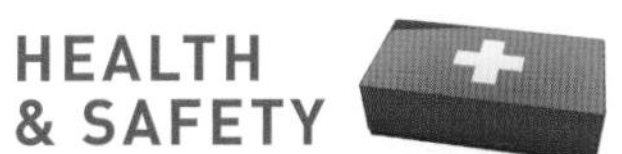

HEALTH & SAFETY

Consultation check

Check if a client has received any specialist electrical facials such as micro-dermabrasion or chemical peels. These treatments involve removing the surface epidermal cells from the skin, which may cause it to be sensitive. Ensure that you check at the consultation if the client has been receiving any specialized treatments for the facial skin, and if so what and when. Seek guidance as necessary from a senior therapist as to client suitability.

Depending on the facial treatment to be carried out, the client may need to remove some clothing. Offer them a **gown** to wear for modesty. Privacy must be maintained at all times.

Before carrying out *any* facial treatments, the beauty therapist must consult with the client to determine their treatment needs. **Consultation** is a service that should be offered separately: there should be no pressure on the client to book a treatment following the consultation. Excellent communication skills should be used at consultation to ensure your judgements on the needs of the client are correct.

The consultation

In the privacy of the facial treatment work area, carry out the consultation. This takes place when the client first meets the therapist and again whenever a new treatment is to be carried out.

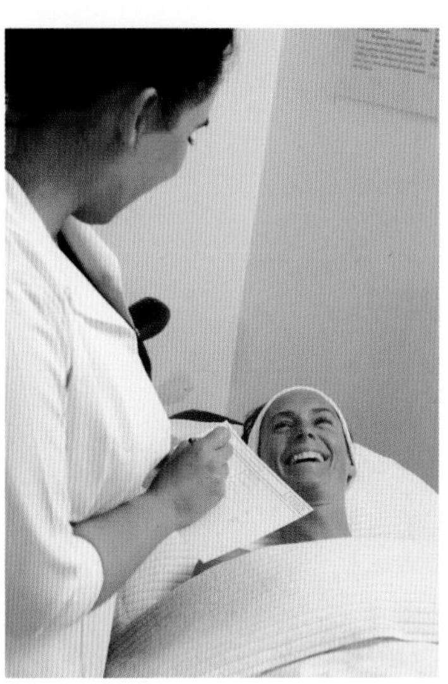

Confirming details following the consultation

The consultation is the time when the beauty therapist can assess whether the client is actually suited to treatment. The therapist must look for contra-indications, and must give no treatment if there are any – this is to safeguard the therapist, the client and, in the case of a client with a contagious skin disorder, other clients who would be at risk of cross-infection. Remember you are not qualified to diagnose a contra-indication. Refer the client to their GP without causing unnecessary cause for concern. Further information on specific skin diseases and disorders can be found on pages 40–53.

ALWAYS REMEMBER

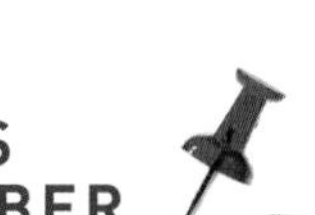

Treatment modification

Examples of facial treatment modification include:

- altering the pressure or choice of manipulations during massage to suit the client's skin and muscle tone
- altering the distance and application of steam heat to take into account skin sensitivity. The more sensitive the skin the greater the distance from the skin.

Be empathetic

Being able to 'connect' with your client is invaluable as a therapist. Try to see the world through the other person's eyes, think about how they might feel and adapt your communication as necessary. For instance, if it is their first ever skin treatment, are they shy or embarrassed? How can you help them to feel more at ease?

Sally Penford

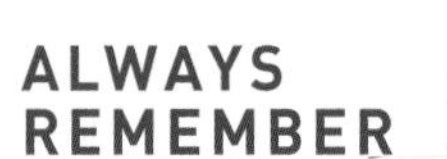
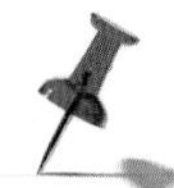

ALWAYS REMEMBER

Never make assumptions about what the client can afford. Usually the client will indicate to you what they are prepared to spend.

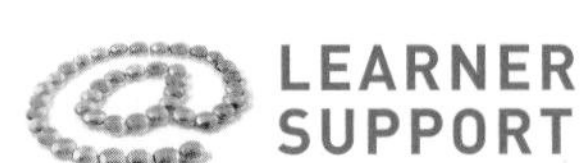

LEARNER SUPPORT

Facial skincare: match the statements

Ask the client specific questions about their present skincare routine and their general health and lifestyle. Listen carefully to their responses to guide you in your assessment.

The beauty therapist's knowledge of facial treatments and advice on skincare will instil confidence in the client. Explain what is involved with the treatment, how long it takes and the aftercare that is recommended. This will demonstrate your professional knowledge and expertise.

The client is likely to ask which is the most suitable product for them, and you must advise them as to which would best meet their needs.

Make the client aware of the cost of the individual treatment – or treatment programme, if necessary – so that they can decide whether or not to undertake the financial commitment involved.

Invite the client to ask questions during the consultation. Visual aids may be used to explain aspects of the treatment. You could demonstrate some of the products e.g. an exfoliation product, directly on your own skin or theirs usually the back of the hand. Marketing literature may also be available to refer to. By the end, they should understand fully what the proposed treatment involves.

The client may receive the treatment immediately, following the consultation, or go away to consider the proposals.

During the consultation, details are noted on the client's record card. You can fill this in as you speak to them, without diverting your attention away from them.

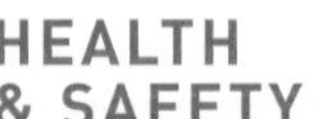
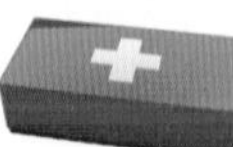

HEALTH & SAFETY

Herpes simplex (cold sore)

A small skin lesion due to herpes simplex may initially appear to be simply a pustule with a scab. At the consultation, always check whether the client knows if they suffer from any skin disease or disorder.

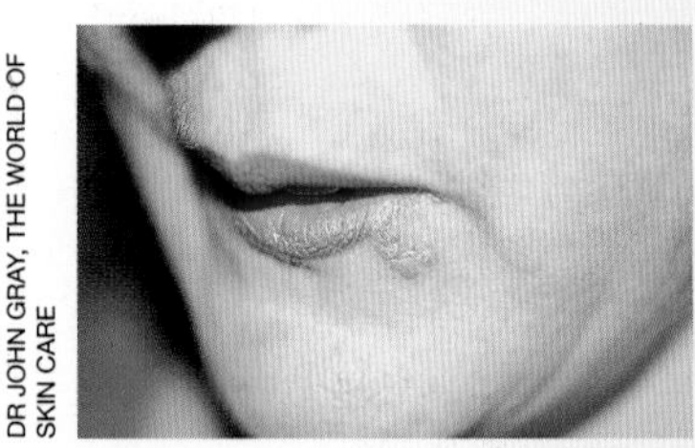

DR JOHN GRAY, THE WORLD OF SKIN CARE

Herpes simplex

ACTIVITY

Recognizing contra-indications

Think of six skin disorders and six skin diseases. List them in a chart.

Briefly describe how you would recognize each skin condition. Why would it be inappropriate to treat each?

Contra-indications

The consultation and skin analysis will draw your attention to any contra-indications or conditions that may that require special care and attention.

Remember that not all contra-indications are visible. Refer to the checklist of contra-indications on the client's record card.

The following contra-indications are relevant to *all* facial treatments:

- ***skin disorder***, such as active acne vulgaris (unless medical approval has been sought and given)
- ***skin disease***, such as impetigo

A sample client record card

Date	Beauty therapist	
Client name	Date of birth (identifying client age group)	
Home address	Postcode	
Email address	Landline	Mobile phone number
Name of doctor	Doctor's address and phone number	
Related medical history (conditions that may restrict or prohibit treatment application)		
Are you taking any medication? (this may affect the appearance of the skin or skin sensitivity)		

CONTRA-INDICATIONS REQUIRING MEDICAL REFERRAL
(preventing facial treatment application)

- ☐ bacterial infection (e.g. impetigo)
- ☐ viral infection (e.g. herpes simplex)
- ☐ fungal infection (e.g. tinea corporis)
- ☐ parasitic infection (e.g. pediculosis and scabies)
- ☐ eye infections (e.g. conjunctivitis)
- ☐ severe eczema
- ☐ systemic medical condition
- ☐ severe skin condition
- ☐ during chemotherapy or radiotherapy treatment

CONTRA-INDICATIONS WHICH RESTRICT TREATMENT
(treatment may require adaptation)

- ☐ cuts and abrasions
- ☐ recent scar tissue
- ☐ skin allergies
- ☐ styes
- ☐ bruising and swelling
- ☐ vitiligo
- ☐ hyperkeratosis
- ☐ diabetes
- ☐ undiagnosed lumps, bumps and swellings
- ☐ high or low blood pressure
- ☐ skin disorders
- ☐ epilepsy
- ☐ broken bones

SKIN TYPE

- ☐ oily
- ☐ combination
- ☐ normal
- ☐ dry

SKIN CONDITION

- ☐ sensitive
- ☐ mature
- ☐ dehydrated

FACIAL PRODUCTS

- ☐ cleanser
- ☐ toner
- ☐ eye cleanser
- ☐ exfoliant
- ☐ mask – setting
- ☐ mask – non-setting
- ☐ massage medium
- ☐ moisturiser
- ☐ specialist skin products (e.g. eye cream/gel)

MASSAGE MEDIUMS

- ☐ oil
- ☐ cream

SKIN CONDITION CHARACTERISTICS

- ☐ broken capillaries
- ☐ pustules
- ☐ open pores
- ☐ hypopigmentation
- ☐ keloids
- ☐ pseudo folliculitis
- ☐ milia
- ☐ comedones
- ☐ papules
- ☐ hyperpigmentation
- ☐ dermatitis papulosa nigra
- ☐ ingrowing hairs
- ☐ hyperkeratosis

Following skin analysis, identify on the illustration below skin condition characteristics found and in which numbered area they appear.

EQUIPMENT AND MATERIALS

- ☐ magnifying light
- ☐ consumables
- ☐ skin warming devices
- ☐ facial steamer

MASSAGE TECHNIQUES

- ☐ effleurage
- ☐ tapotement
- ☐ petrissage
- ☐ frictions
- ☐ vibrations

Beauty therapist signature (for reference)

Client signature (confirmation of details)

A sample client record card (continued)

TREATMENT ADVICE
Full facial treatment – this treatment will take 60 minutes (1 hour).

TREATMENT PLAN
Record relevant details of your treatment and advice provided for future reference.
Ensure the client's records are up-to-date, accurate and fully completed following treatment. Non-compliance may invalidate insurance.

DURING
Find out:
- what products the client is currently using to cleanse and care for the skin of the face and neck
- how regularly the products are used
- satisfaction with their current skincare routine – what they are pleased with and what they don't like

Explain:
- how the products used should be applied and removed by the client

Note:
- any adverse (unwanted) skin reaction, if any occurs

AFTER
Record:
- specific areas treated
- any modification to treatment application that has occurred, e.g. less pressure applied over the cheek area when working on a sensitive skin with broken capillaries in the area.
- what products have been used in the facial treatment
- the effectiveness of treatment – did you achieve what you set out to do?
- any samples provided (review their success at the next appointment)

Advise on:
- product application and removal in order to gain maximum benefit from product use
- use of make-up following facial treatment
- recommended time intervals between treatments
- the importance of a course of treatment to improve the skin condition

RETAIL OPPORTUNITIES
Advise on:
- progression of the treatment plan for future appointments
- products that would be suitable for the client to use at home to care for their skin
- recommendations for further facial treatments
- further products or treatments that you have recommended that the client may or may not have received before

Note:
- any purchase made by the client

EVALUATION
Record:
- comments on the client's satisfaction with the treatment
- how you will progress the treatment to maintain and advance the treatment results in the future

HEALTH AND SAFETY
Advise on:
- avoidance of activities or product application that may cause a contra-action
- appropriate action necessary to be taken in the event of an unwanted skin reaction

- ***bruising*** in the area
- ***haemorrhage***, if recent – wait until the condition has healed
- ***operation*** in the area, if recent – wait for six months
- ***fracture***, if recent – wait for six months
- ***furuncle*** (boil)
- ***inflammation or swelling*** of the skin
- ***scar tissue,*** if recent – wait for six months
- ***sebaceous cyst***
- ***eye disorder***, such as conjunctivitis

Certain contra-indications restrict treatment; that is, the treatment may have to be adapted or delayed until the contra-indication has gone. For example, if eczema is present but the skin is not broken, the treatment can proceed but the area should be avoided as much as possible.

If the client has an allergy to an ingredient in the cosmetic preparations used, treatment cannot proceed until an alternative, non-allergenic product suited to the client is obtained. If the client has a stye, treatment cannot proceed. However, when the eye disorder has gone treatment may be carried out. These are referred to on pages 40–53, where skin diseases and disorders are illustrated and discussed.

Be attentive

When talking with your client give them your undivided attention. Even if you have only ten minutes to give. By being truly present when engaging in interpersonal communication, such as product sampling, you will add value and worth over and above your competitors.

Sally Penford

Following the consultation, the client's answers will indicate to the therapist what is required, and what is achievable, from a skincare programme.

When finalizing the most suitable treatment plan:

- explain what is involved in each treatment, how long it takes, and what aftercare and home care are required (if relevant)
- assess how much the client is willing to spend, and design a treatment programme within their budget

This allows the client to:

- discover what the beauty therapist can offer to meet their needs
- ask questions, and receive honest professional advice concerning the most appropriate choice of skincare treatment
- decide how much they are willing to spend

The beauty therapist should ensure that the client fully understands and is realistic about what the proposed treatment involves and what can be achieved.

KNOWLEDGE CHECK

Describe the different communication skills that you would need to use when performing a client consultation.

Need more time... refer to pages 187–188 to help you.

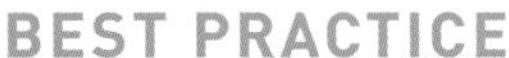

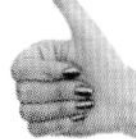

BEST PRACTICE

Client care

Always give clear instructions to your client. This will help to ensure that they are not embarrassed or uncomfortable at any time.

Headbands

Check that the headband is comfortable. A tight headband will cause tension and eventually a headache.

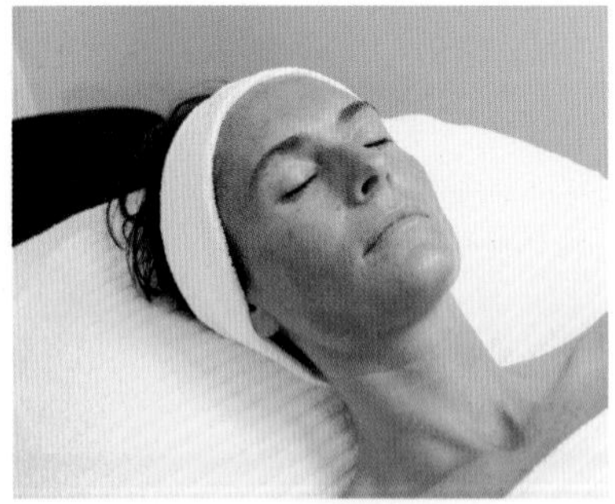

Client prepared and positioned for treatment

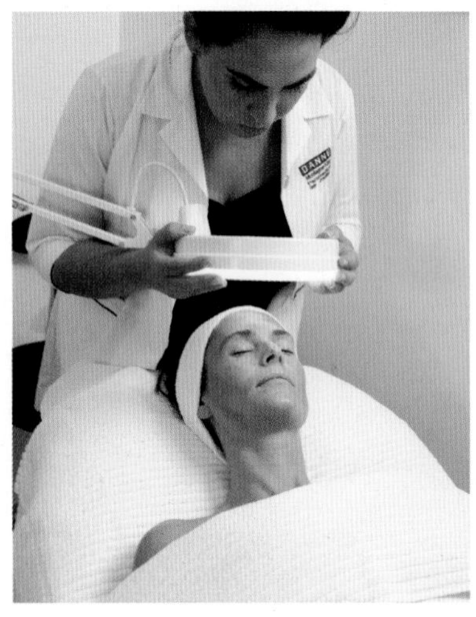

Skin analysis

ACTIVITY

Answering questions

You should be able to answer honestly, competently and tactfully any questions related to the beauty treatments you offer. Below are examples of the questions you may be asked at consultation.

- 'I have always used soap and water upon my face. Is this a satisfactory way to cleanse my face?'
- 'Why do I need to use a separate night cream as well as a day moisturiser?'
- 'How often should I have a facial?'
- 'I have extremely oily skin. Why do I need to wear a moisturiser?'
- 'What can I do to treat these fine lines around my eyes?'

What answers would you give? Think of further questions you might be asked with regard to skincare. A senior beauty therapist will be able to advise you.

Be a receptive communicator

Employers often ask for a range of skills, however often two skills come from the opposite end of the spectrum. Which do you have your strength in? For example, communication in writing versus communicating face to face, or following rules versus thinking creatively. One skill will be your natural preference but by developing the opposite skill you will be more appealing to potential employers.

Sally Penford

When the treatment plan has been agreed, prepare and position the client for treatment.

1. Position the client on the couch. Ensure the client is comfortable and relaxed. Cover the client with the clean, large bath towel or alternative suitable covering. If necessary, drape a small hand towel across their shoulders. Some salons offer a quilt cover to keep the client warm and relaxed.
2. If facial, neck and shoulder massage is to be given, ask the client politely to remove their arms from their bra straps in preparation: this avoids disturbance later. All jewellery should be removed from the client in the treatment area and contact lenses may need to be removed to avoid eye irritation.
3. Fasten a clean headband around the client's hairline. Position the headband so that it does not cover the skin of the face. If using an facial steamer cover the hair to stop it getting damp.
4. After preparing the client, wash your hands: this demonstrates to the client your concern to work hygienically.

The skin should than be cleansed prior to completing a more detailed skin analysis where you can correctly diagnose the skin type and condition.

Choice of products selected will be decided upon from the information you have gained so far.

All **facial products** and equipment should be used with due regard to health and safety following manufacturers' instructions.

Outcome 2: Be able to provide facial skincare treatments

Learn how to provide facial skincare treatments

Practical skills

1. **Communicate and behave** in a professional manner.
2. Follow **health and safety working practices.**
3. Position yourself and client correctly throughout the treatment.
4. Use **products, tools, equipment and techniques** to suit clients treatment needs, **skin type and condition.**
5. Complete the treatment to the satisfaction of the client.
6. Record the results of the treatment.
7. Provide suitable **aftercare advice.**

Underpinning knowledge

1. State how to **communicate and behave** in a professional manner.
2. Describe **health and safety working practices.**
3. State the importance of positioning yourself and the client correctly throughout the treatment.
4. State the importance of using **products, tools, equipment and techniques** to suit clients treatment needs, **skin type and conditions.**
5. Describe how treatments can be adapted to suit client treatment needs, **skin type and condition.**
6. State the **contra-actions** that may occur during and following treatments and how to respond.
7. State the importance of completing the treatment to the satisfaction of the client.
8. State the importance of completing treatment records.
9. State the **aftercare advice** that should be provided.
10. Describe the structure and functions of the skin.
11. Describe diseases and disorders of the skin.
12. Explain how natural ageing, lifestyle and environmental factors affect the condition of the skin and muscle tone.
13. State the position and action of the muscles of the head, neck and shoulders.
14. State the names and position of the bones of the head, neck and shoulders.
15. Describe the structure and function of the blood and lymphatic system for the head, neck and shoulders.

ALWAYS REMEMBER

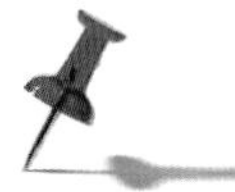

Seasonal changes
Seasonal changes affect the skin. You may need to alter the client's basic skincare routine through the year.

HEALTH & SAFETY

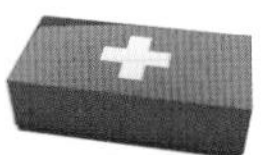

Sensitive skin
When treating sensitive skin, choose a cleansing product that does not contain common known allergens such as mineral oil, alcohol or lanolin. Such products are usually referred to as *hypoallergenic* or *dermatologically tested*.

Cleansing

Skin cleansing is essential in promoting and maintaining a healthy skin. There are various cleansing preparations to choose from; basically their action is the same in each case:

- to gently exfoliate dead skin cells from the stratum corneum, exposing younger, fresher cells and improving the skin's appearance
- to remove make-up (if worn), dirt and pollutants from the skin's surface, reducing the possibility of blemishes and skin irritation
- to remove excess sweat and sebum from the skin's surface, reducing congestion of the skin and the subsequent formation of comedones and pustules
- to prepare the skin for further treatments

Be positive

Having a positive attitude will not only help you to continually improve yourself, it will also rub off on your fellow team members. Show your initiative with suggestions and ideas that make moves towards the goals of your skin centre. Don't be scared to get creative and think outside of the box with new ideas for treatments, promotions or events.

Sally Penford

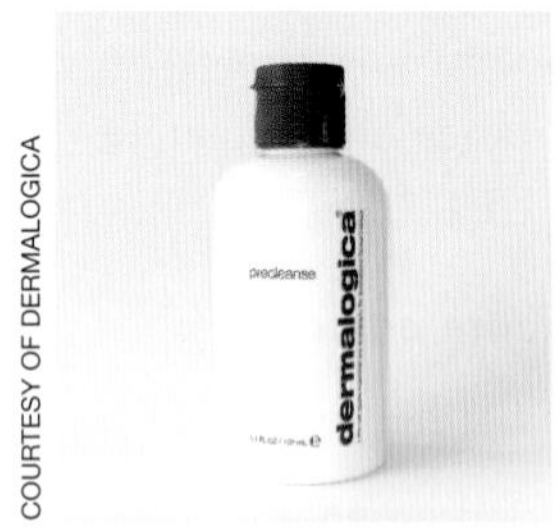

COURTESY OF DERMALOGICA

Cleansing preparation cream

Cleansing preparations

A **cleanser** is required that will remove both oil-soluble and water-soluble substances without drying the skin. Oil is capable of dissolving grease; water will dissolve other substances. Usually, therefore, a cleanser is a combination of both oil and water.

Oil and water do not combine: if you simply mix the two together they separate again, with the oil floating on the top of the water. If the two substances are shaken together vigorously, however, one substance will break up and become suspended in the other. The result is known as an **emulsion**.

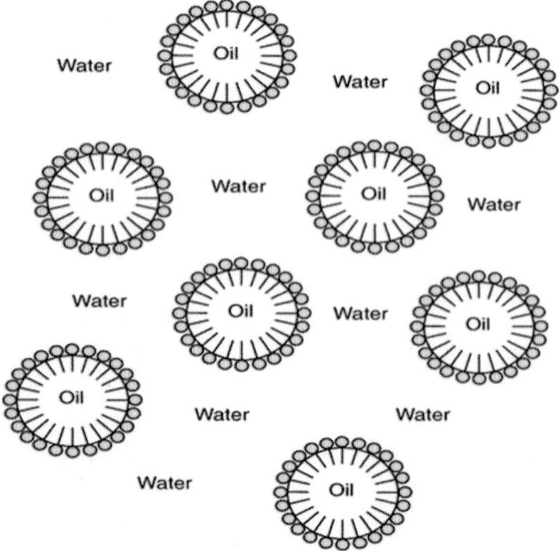

Oil-in-water emulsion

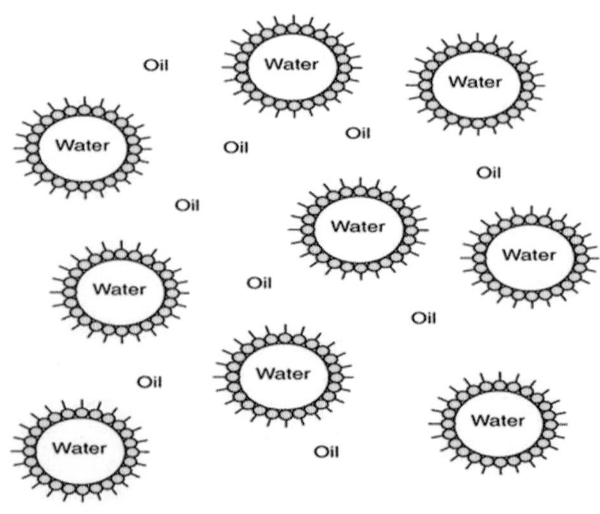

Water-in-oil emulsion

Emulsions are used in many cosmetic preparations. They are either:

- **oil-in-water** (O/W) – minute droplets of oil, surrounded by water
- **water-in-oil** (W/O) – minute droplets of water, surrounded by oil

To give the emulsion stability, and to stop it separating out again, an **emulsifier** is added.

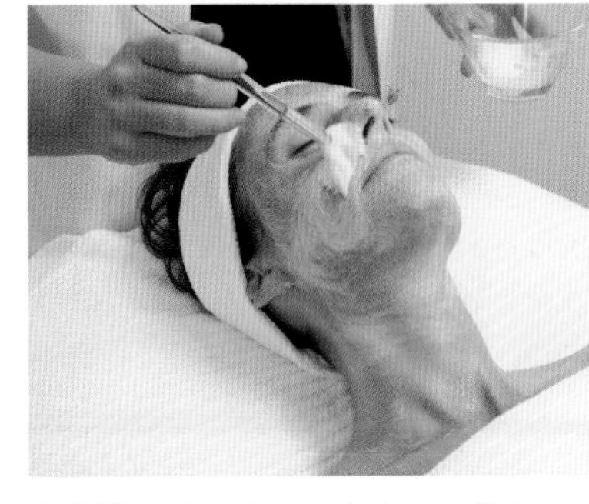

Facial foaming cleanser being applied

Various cleansing preparations are available to the beauty therapist, with formulations designed to suit the different skin types. They include:

- cleansing milks
- cleansing creams
- cleansing balms
- cleansing lotions
- facial gel or foaming cleansers
- cleansing bars
- eye make-up removers

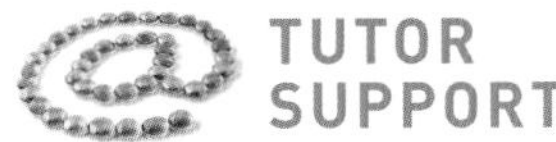

TUTOR SUPPORT

Activity 3: Facial products handout

Whichever cleanser is chosen, it should have the following qualities:

- it should cleanse the skin effectively, without causing irritation
- it should remove all traces of make-up and grease
- it should feel pleasant to use
- it should be easy to remove from the skin
- ideally, it should be pH-balanced

ACTIVITY

Acidic or alkaline?

To discover whether a liquid product is acidic or alkaline, carry out a simple test using litmus paper. Litmus changes colour according to the pH:

- litmus paper turns *blue* if an *alkali* is present
- litmus paper turns *red* if an *acid* is present

Test the pH of various cleansing preparations.

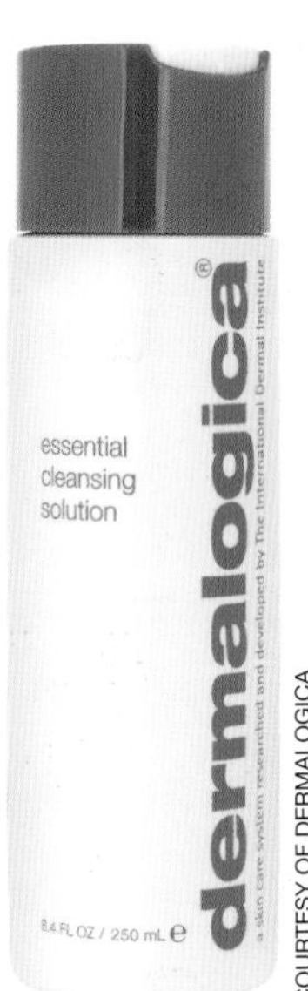

COURTESY OF DERMALOGICA

Cleansing lotion

The pH scale The **pH scale** is used to measure the **acidity** or **alkalinity** of a substance. Using a numbered scale of 1–14, acids have a pH less than 7; alkalis have a pH greater than 7. Substances with a pH of 7 are **neutral**.

The skin is naturally slightly acidic: it has an **acid mantle**. Alkalis strip the skin of its protective film of sebum, making it feel dry and taut. To avoid skin irritation it is preferable to use a product that matches the acid mantle, a product whose pH is 5.5–5.6.

Cleansing milks **Cleansing milks** are usually oil-in-water emulsions, with a relatively high proportion of water to oil, making the milk quite fluid and light in its consistency.

Cleansing milks have these specific treatment uses:

- treating normal to dry skin that is prone to sensitivity
- treating sensitive skin

Cleansing creams **Cleansing creams** have a relatively high proportion of oil to water, making the emulsion thicker and richer in its consistency than cleansing milks. The high oil content allows the product to be massaged over the skin surface without dragging the tissues. The cream is also more effective in removing grease and oil-based make-up from the skin.

Cleansing creams have these specific treatment uses:

- removing facial cosmetics
- treating by deep cleansing massage
- treating very dry skin

Cleansing balms **Cleansing balms** are usually light weight cleansers which quickly transform from a solid balm to a fluid. They moisturise and improve the texture of the skin while cleansing.

Cleansing balms have these specific treatment uses:

- moisturising, non-drying effect
- improvement of skin texture
- suitable for all skin types except oily

Cleansing lotions **Cleansing lotions** are solutions of detergents in water. They do not usually contain oil, and are therefore unsuitable for the removal of facial cosmetics.

Cleansing lotions have these specific treatment uses:

- cleansing a normal to combination skin type
- treating oily skin (where a high oil content could aggravate the skin, causing yet further sebum production)

Medicated ingredients may be included in a cleansing formulation: these are only suitable for oily, congested, pustular skin types.

Be different

What makes you stand out from the crowd? As well as a good all-round basic knowledge, try to offer something that no other skin therapist in your area offers. There are plenty of postgraduate training facilities to help you progress, so step outside of the treatment room and learn something new!

Sally Penford

TOP TIP

Dry skin

If a client has very dry skin, advise them to avoid them use of tap water on the face – tap water contains salts and chlorine, which can dry the skin.

Male skin

Cleansing rinse-off formulations are very popular with male clients.

The use of a soft nylon bristle face brush is beneficial to use with a facial foaming cleanser or bar to prevent ingrowing hairs forming.

If the client has a mature, normal or combination skin, a cleansing lotion may not be effective because of the reduced oil content. A mature skin benefits from oil content to compensate for reduced sebum production.

Facial gel or foaming cleansers **Facial gel or foaming cleansers** usually contain a mild detergent which foams when mixed with water. Additional ingredients are selected for the treatment of different skin types. These cleansers are quick to use and afford a suitable alternative for the client who likes to cleanse their face with soap and water. If the client wears an oil-based make-up, advise them to use a cleansing cream first to remove make-up thoroughly before using this cleanser.

Facial foaming cleansers have a general application:

- treating most skin types except very dry or sensitive skin
- particularly suitable for oily and combination skin due to their formulation which effectively removes sebum without drying the skin

Cleansing bars Although it is efficient as a cleanser, **soap** is usually considered unsuitable for use on the skin. It has an alkaline pH, which disturbs the skin's natural acidic pH balance. Soap strips the skin of its protective acid mantle, leaving insoluble salts on the skin's surface. The skin may be left feeling itchy, taut and sensitive.

Cleansing bars are a milder alternative to soap, and are specially formulated to match the skin's acidic pH of 5.5–5.6. They are less likely to dry out the skin.

Cleansing bars have this specific application:

- treating oily to normal skin that is not sensitive

Eye make-up remover Eye tissue is a lot finer than the skin on the rest of the face. It readily puffs if aggravated by oil-based cleansing preparations, and becomes very dry if harsh cleansing preparations are used.

To remove make-up from this area, use an **eye make-up remover.** This product cleanses the eyelid and lashes, gently emulsifying the make-up. It also conditions the delicate skin. Formulated as a lotion or a gel, it is designed to remove either water-based or oil-based products (or both) from the eye area.

Oily eye make-up removers have these specific treatment uses:

- treating clients who wear waterproof mascara
- removing wax or oil-based eye shadow

Non-oily eye make-up removers have these applications:

- treating clients with sensitive skin around the eyes
- treating clients who wear contact lenses
- treating clients who wear individual false eyelashes

Cleansing treatment

There are two manual processes involved in the cleansing routine: *the superficial cleanse* and the *deep cleanse*.

The superficial cleanse uses lightweight cleansing preparations to emulsify surface make-up, dirt and grease. This is followed by the more thorough deep cleanse, in which a heavier cleansing cream is applied to the face. The high percentage of oil contained in

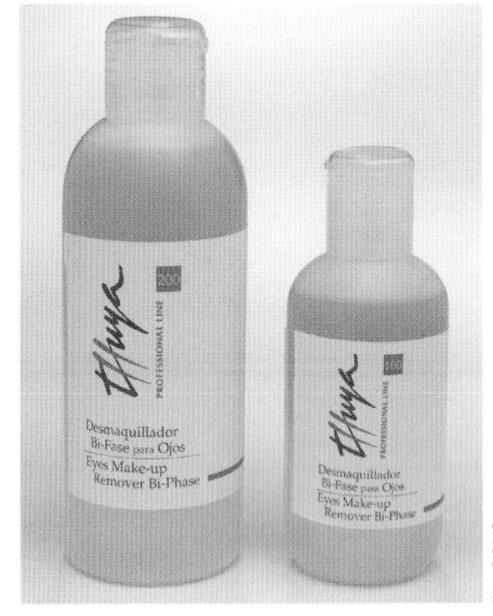

Eye make-up remover

TOP TIP

Eye treatments

Many eye make-up removers are also eye treatments. If your workplace uses a commercial product in this way apply it to the dampened eye pads used during mask treatment. This may also assist your retail sales, as the client may wish to buy some for home use.

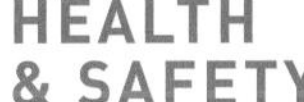

HEALTH & SAFETY

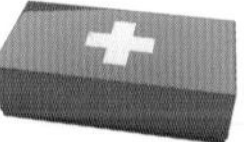

Eye care

Never apply pressure over the eyeball when cleansing the eye area.

The ring finger is always used in the eye area when applying products as it provides the least pressure.

HEALTH & SAFETY

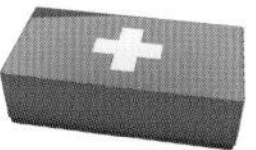

Hygiene

Never use the reverse side of the cotton wool pad – this is unhygienic.

Never use the same piece of cotton wool to cleanse both eyes, use a separate piece for each eye to avoid cross-infection.

TOP TIP

Removing artificial lashes

If the client is wearing semi-permanent false eyelashes avoid the application of high oil content eye make-up removal skincare preparations. These will weaken the adhesive that secures the artificial lashes. Take general care.

the cream formulation allows the cream to be massaged over the skin's surface without evaporation of the product.

ALWAYS REMEMBER

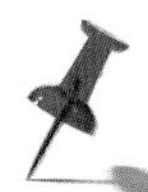

Unlike the muscles of the body, which attach to bones, most of the facial muscles are attached to the facial skin itself. You should therefore avoid stretching the skin unnecessarily – if you do, you may also stretch the facial muscles and contribute to premature ageing.

Step-by-step: Superficial cleansing

Each part of the face requires a special technique in the application and removal of the cleansing product. The face is usually cleansed in the following order:

- the eye tissue and lashes
- the lips
- the neck, chin, cheeks and forehead

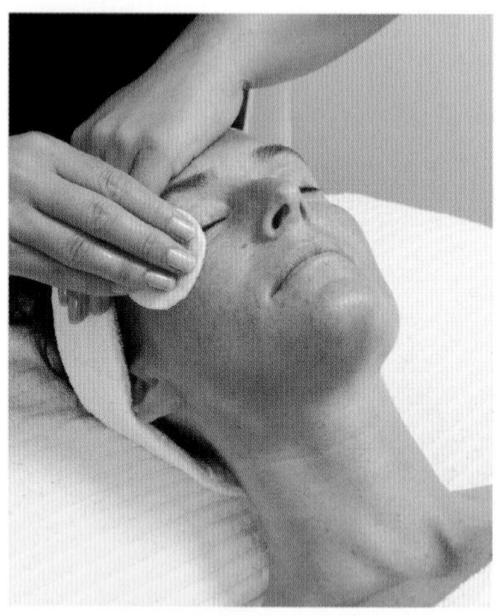

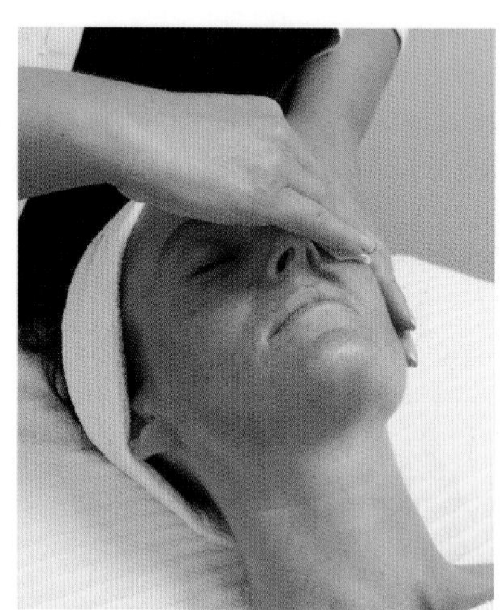

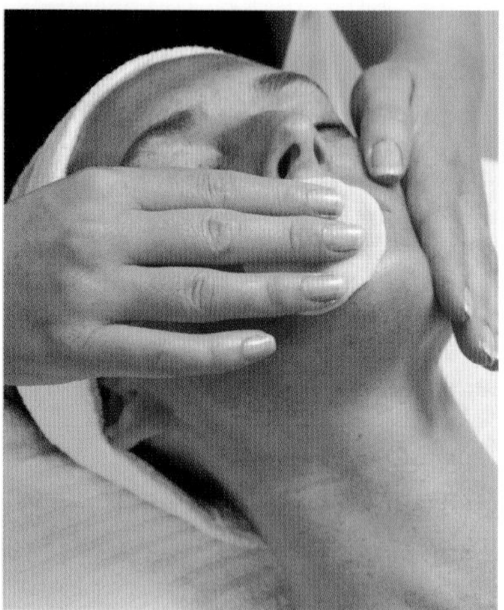

1 Wash your hands.

Gloves may be worn if a male client has coarse facial hair that may cause skin irritation to the hands. Ensure that the client's contact lenses are removed if worn.

2 Cleanse the eye area, using a suitable eye make-up remover. If the client is not wearing make-up this product has been formulated for use around the eye area and can still be used. Each eye is cleansed separately. Your non-working hand lifts and supports the eye tissue while the working hand applies the eye make-up remover.

If eye make-up remover is used, this is applied directly to a clean piece of cotton wool. Stroke down the length of the eyelashes, from base to points. Next, cleanse the eye tissue in a sweeping circle, outwards across the upper eyelid, circling beneath the lower lashes towards the nose. Repeat, regularly changing the cotton wool until the eye area and the cotton wool show clean.

Sometimes a cleansing milk is used to remove eye make-up. In this case, apply a little of the product to the back of one hand. The ring finger is then used to apply the cleansing milk to the lashes.

Use damp cotton wool to remove the emulsified product.

Repeat the cleansing process until the eye area is clean.

3 Cleanse the lips, preferably with a cleansing milk or lotion (as this readily emulsifies the oils or waxes contained in lipstick if worn).

Apply a little of the product to the back of your non-working hand. Support the left side of the client's mouth with this hand. With the working hand, apply the product in small circular movements across the upper lip, from left to right; and then across the lower lip, from right to left.

Remove the cleanser from the lips. Support the corner of the mouth; using a clean damp piece of cotton wool wipe across the lips.

Repeat the cleansing process as necessary, until the lips and the cotton wool show clean. A cotton bud may be used to clean directly under the lower eyelashes.

4 Select a cleansing product to suit your client's skin type.

Place the product into one hand – sufficient to cover the face and neck – and to massage gently over the surface of the skin. Massage the surface of the hands together when using a milk, cream or balm: this warms the product (so that it isn't cold on the client's skin) and distributes it over your hands.

Clasp the fingers together at the base of the neck, and unlink them as you move up the neck.

Clasp the fingers together again at the chin, drawing the fingers outwards to the angle of the jawbone.

Stroke up the face, towards the forehead, with your fingertips pointing downwards and your palms in contact with the skin.

Using a series of light circular movements with your fingertips, gently massage the product into the skin, beginning at the base of the neck and finishing at the forehead.

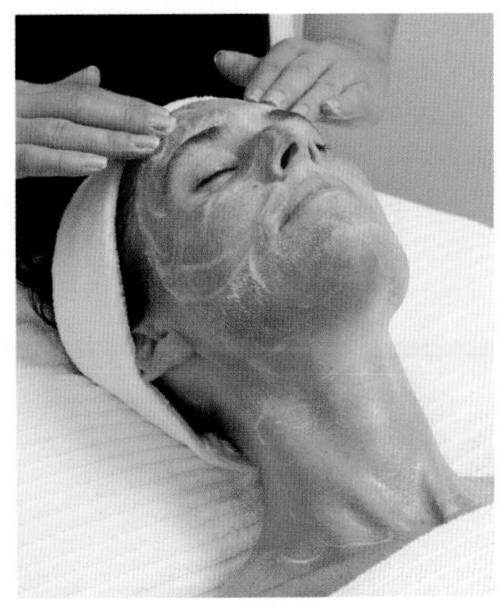

Superficial cleanse

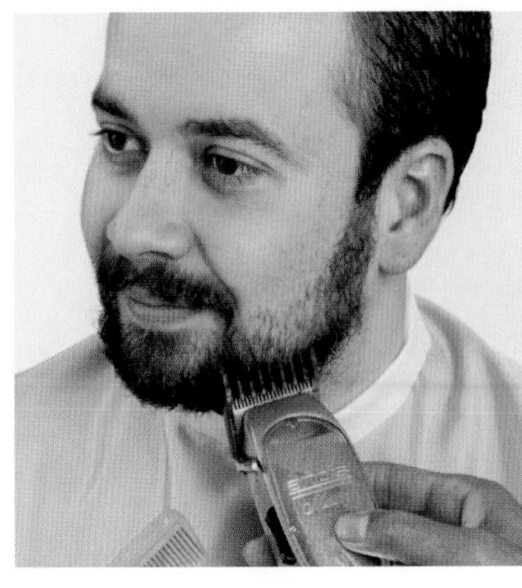

For male clients most movements for the beard and moustache area should follow the hair growth patterns

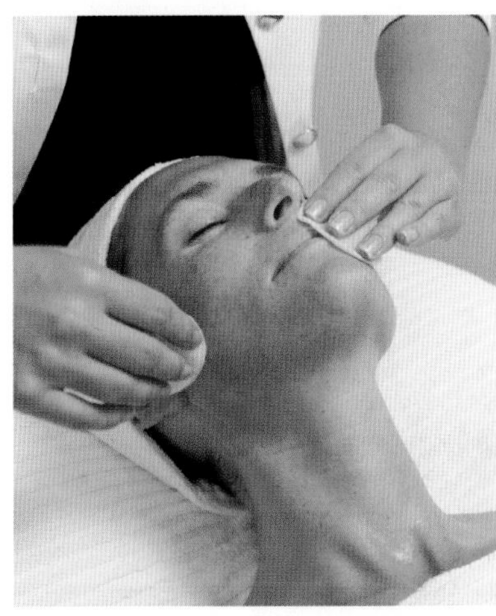

Removal of cleansing product with damp cotton wool

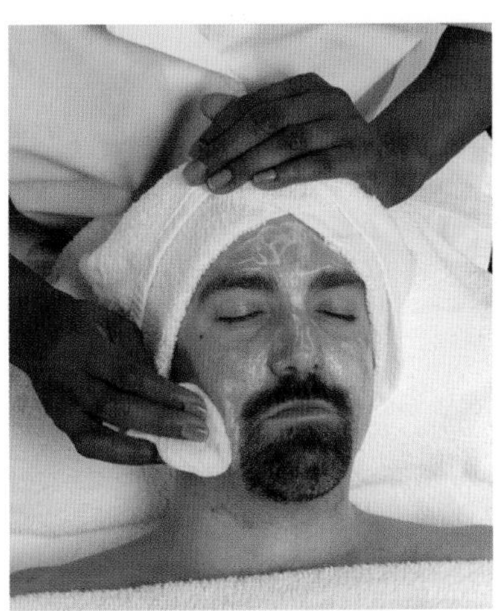

Removal of cleansing product with damp cotton wool

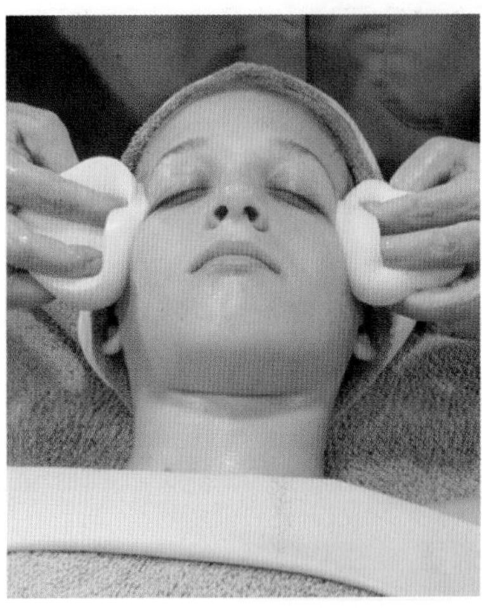

Removal of cleansing product with damp sponges

5 Remove the cleanser thoroughly with clean damp cotton wool, facial sponges or facial mitts simultaneously stroking over the skin surface, upwards and outwards. Repeat this process as necessary, using clean cotton wool, if used. each time. Facial sponges and mitts will require regular rinsing with clean, warm water.

TOP TIP

Make-up removal

If there is any make-up left at the base of the lower lashes after eye cleansing, this may be removed with a cotton bud or a thin piece of damp, clean cotton wool. Ask the client to look upwards, support the eye tissue with the other hand and gently draw the cotton wool along the base of the lower lashes, towards the nose.

If the client is wearing facial make-up, it is usual to perform the superficial cleanse twice to ensure all cosmetics are effectively removed.

HEALTH & SAFETY

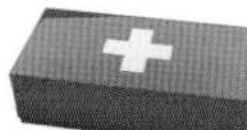

Careful cleansing

When cleansing, be careful that cleanser does not enter the eyes or mouth. When cleansing around the nose, avoid restricting the client's nostrils.

HEALTH & SAFETY

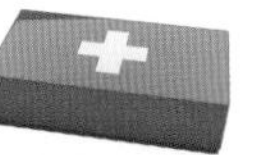

Safe pressure

Reduce pressure when working over the *hyoid bone* at the throat and bony prominences such as the *zygomatic bone* (the cheekbone) and the *frontal bone* (the forehead).

Pressure must always be *upwards* and *outwards*, to avoid stretching the tissues.

Step-by-step: Deep cleansing

The deep cleanse involves a series of massage manipulations which reinforce the cleansing achieved with the cleansing product. Blood circulation is increased to the area; this has a warming effect on the skin, which relaxes the skin's natural openings, the hair follicles and pores. This aids the absorption of cleanser into the hair follicles and pores, where it can dissolve make-up if worn, sebum and skin debris.

There are various deep-cleansing sequences; all are acceptable if carried out in a safe, hygienic manner, and all can achieve the desired outcomes. Here is one sequence for deep cleansing.

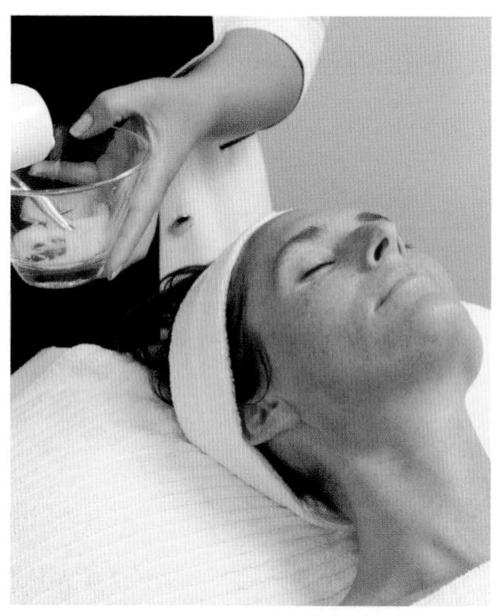

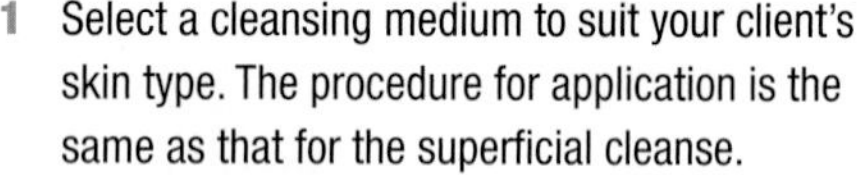

1 Select a cleansing medium to suit your client's skin type. The procedure for application is the same as that for the superficial cleanse.

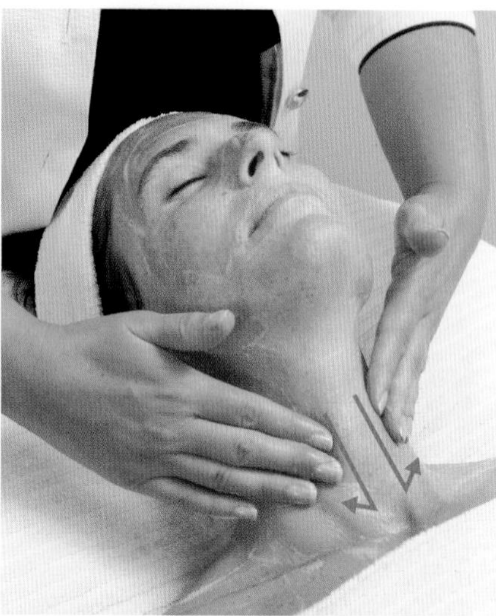

2 Stroke up either side of the neck, using your fingertips. At the chin, draw the fingers outwards to the angle of the jaw, and lightly stroke back down the neck to the starting position.

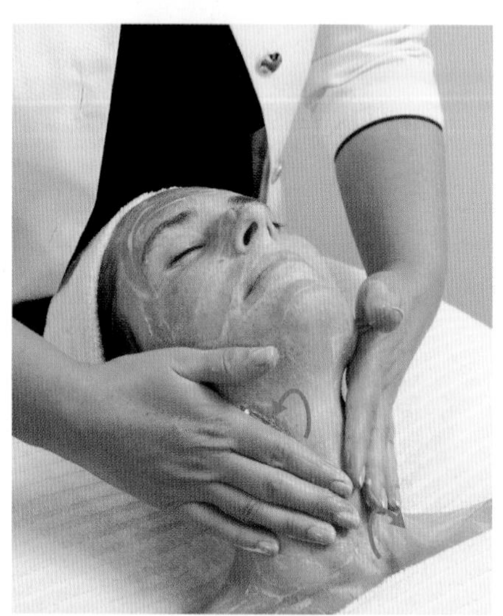

3 Apply small circular manipulations over the skin of the neck.

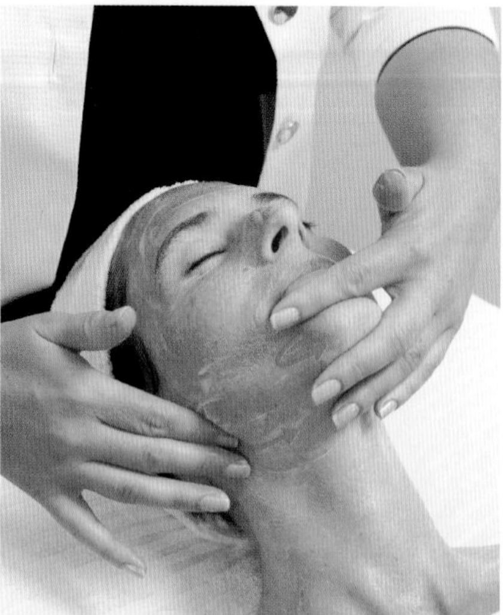

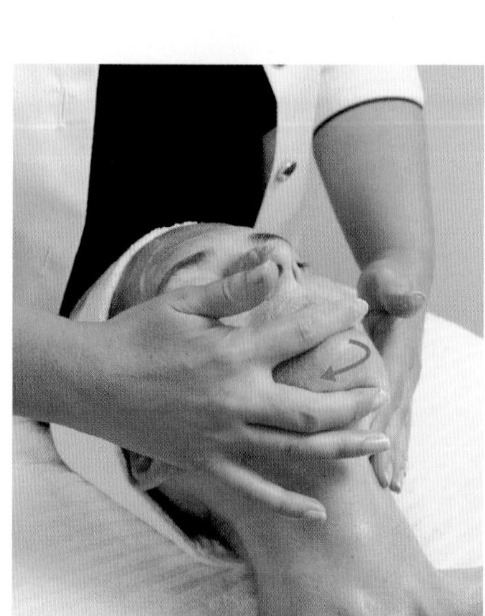

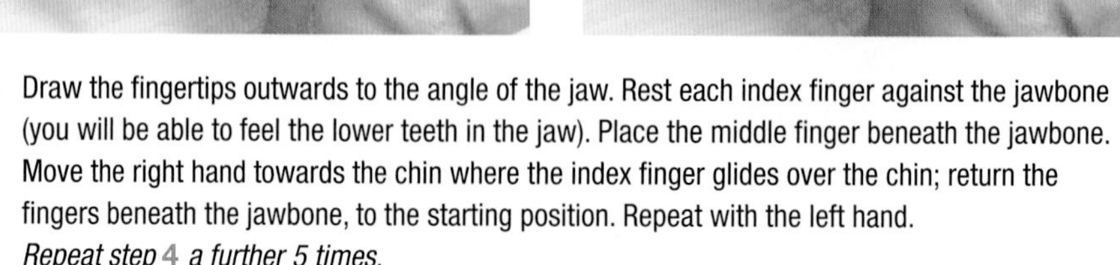

4 Draw the fingertips outwards to the angle of the jaw. Rest each index finger against the jawbone (you will be able to feel the lower teeth in the jaw). Place the middle finger beneath the jawbone. Move the right hand towards the chin where the index finger glides over the chin; return the fingers beneath the jawbone, to the starting position. Repeat with the left hand.
Repeat step 4 a further 5 times.

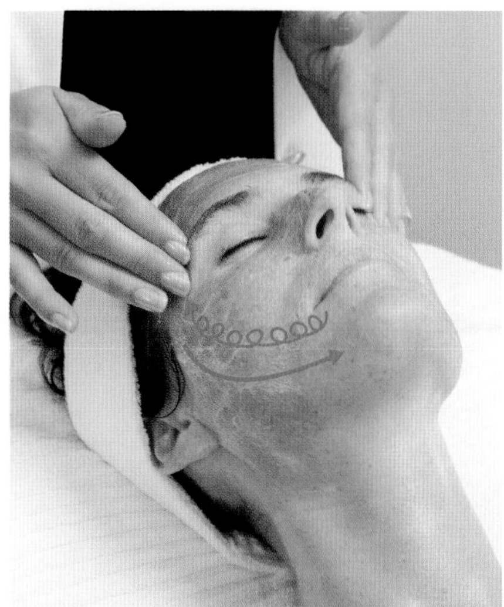

5 Apply small circular manipulations, commencing at the chin working up towards the nose, and finishing at the temples. Slide the fingers from the temples back to the chin.

Repeat step 5 a further 5 times.

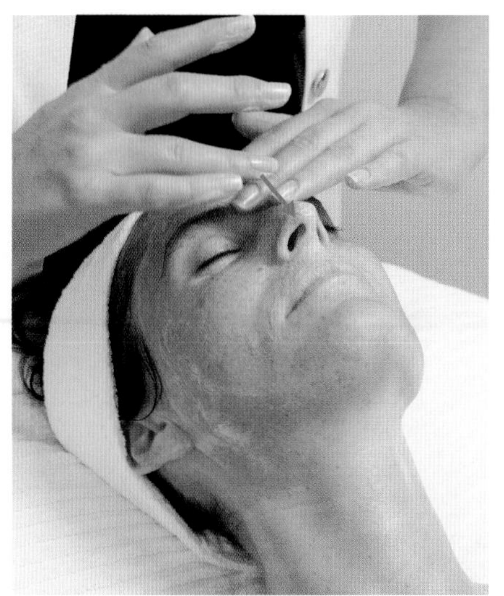

6 Position the ring finger of the right hand at the bridge of the nose. Perform a running movement, sliding the ring, middle and index fingers off the end of the nose. Repeat immediately with the left hand.

Repeat step 6 a further 5 times with each hand.

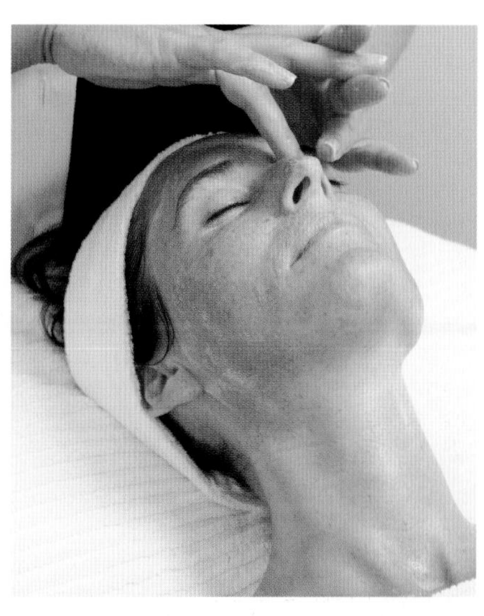

7 With the ring fingers, trace a circle around the eye orbits. Begin at the inner corner of the upper brow bone; slide to the outer corners of the brow bone, around and under the eyes, and return to the starting position.

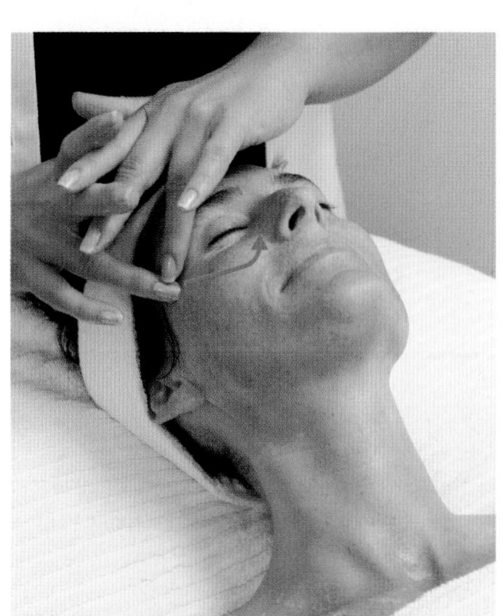

Repeat step 7 a further 5 times.

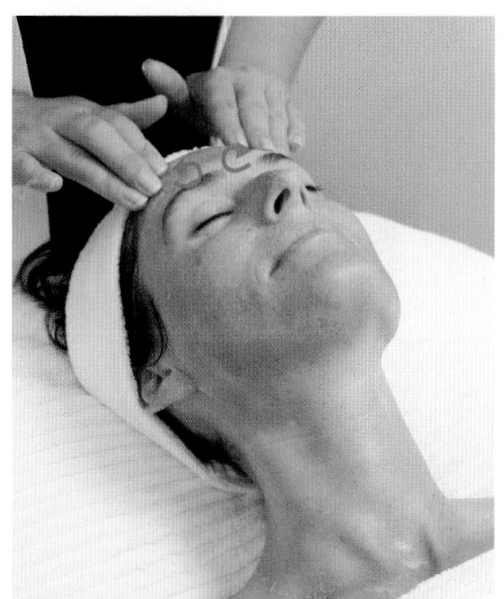

8 Using both hands, apply small circular manipulations across the forehead. *Repeat step 8 a further 5 times.*

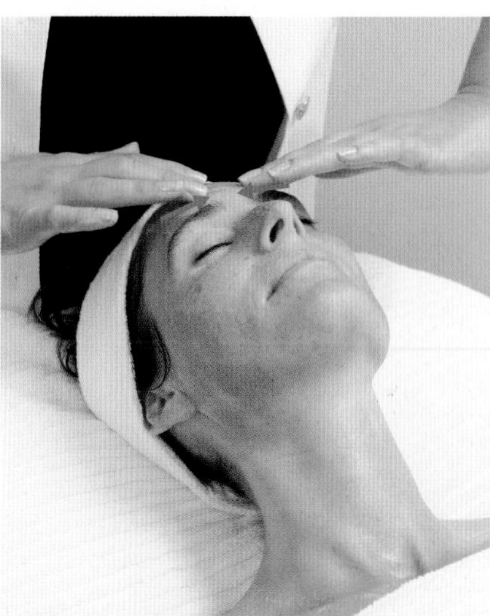

9 Open the index and middle fingers of each hand and perform a cross-cross stroking movement over the forehead.

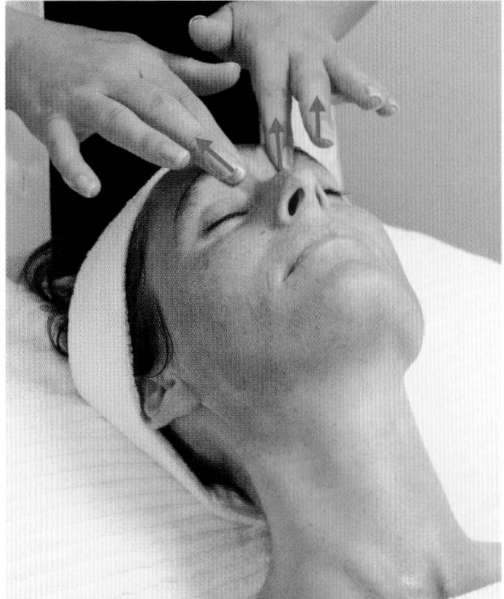

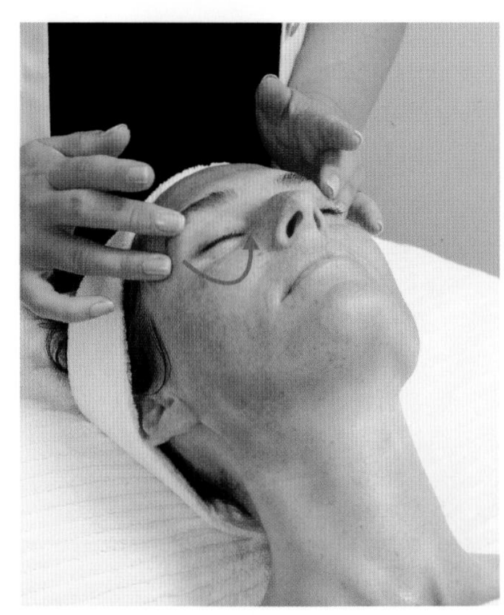

10 Slide the index finger upwards slightly, lifting the inner eyebrow. Lift the centre of the eyebrow with the middle finger. Finally, lift the outer corner of the eyebrow with the ring finger. Slide the ring fingers around the outer corner and beneath the eye orbit.
Repeat step 10 a further 5 times.

TOP TIP

Brow cleansing
Check that the brow hair and the skin beneath the chin are free of grease: it is easy to overlook some cleansing product in these areas.

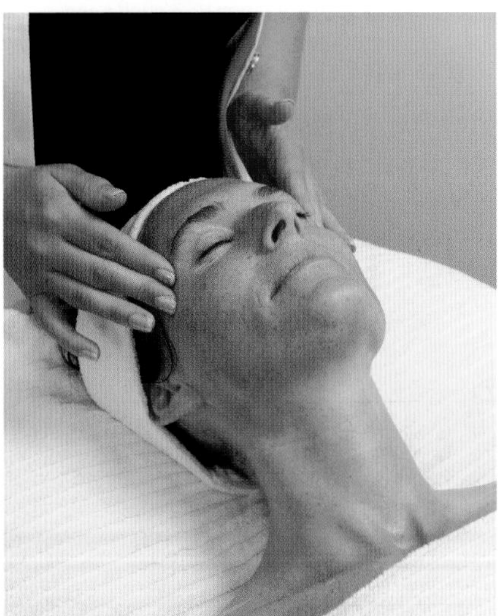

11 With the finger pads of each hand, apply slight pressure at the temples. This indicates to the client that the cleansing sequence is complete.

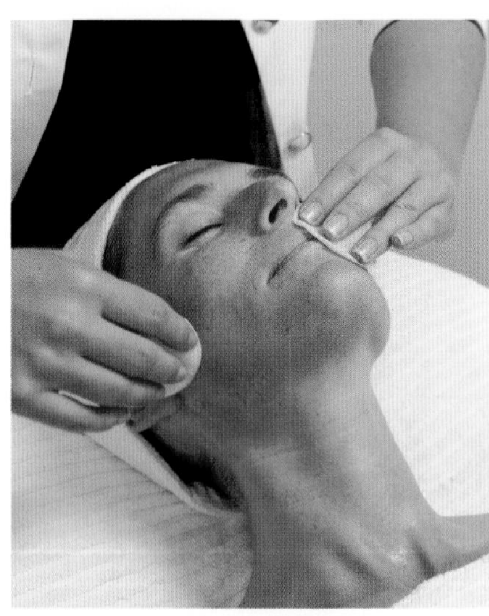

12 Remove the cleansing cream from the skin, using damp cotton wool, facial sponges or facial mitts.

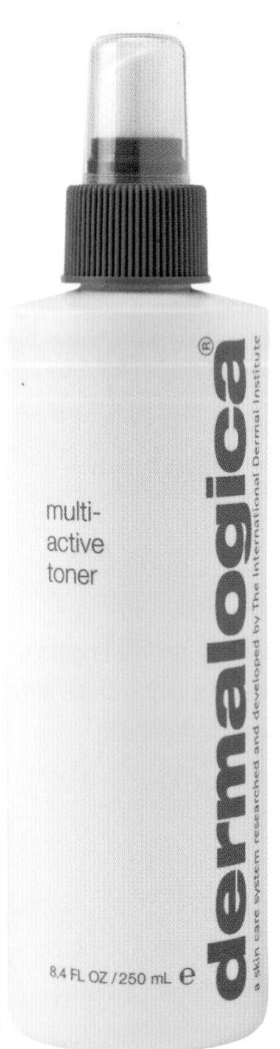

COURTESY OF DERMALOGICA

Toning lotion

Toning

After the skin has been cleansed it is then toned with an appropriate toning lotion.

Toning preparations

Toning lotions remove from the skin all traces of cleanser, grease and skincare preparations. The toning lotion's main action is as follows:

- It produces a cooling effect on the skin when the water or alcohol in the toner evaporates from the skin's surface. (When a liquid evaporates it changes to a gas, which takes energy. In the case of toner, the energy is taken from the skin, which therefore feels cooler.)

- It creates a tightening effect on the skin, because of a chemical within the toner called an astringent. This causes the pores to close, thereby reducing the flow of sebum and sweat onto the skin's surface.
- It helps to restore the acidic pH balance of the skin. Milder skin toners have a pH 4.5–4.6; stronger astringents disturb the pH more severely, and may cause skin irritation and sensitivity.

There are three main types of toning lotions, the main difference being the amounts of alcohol they contain. They include:

- bracers and fresheners
- tonics
- astringents

Skin bracers and fresheners **Skin bracers** and **skin fresheners** are the mildest toning lotions: they contain little or no alcohol. They consist mainly of purified water, with floral extracts such as **rose water** for a mild toning effect.

Skin bracers and fresheners are recommended for:

- dry, delicate skin
- sensitive skin
- mature skin

Skin tonics **Skin tonics** are slightly stronger toning lotions. Many contain a little of some astringent agent such as orange flower water.

Skin toners are recommended for:

- normal skin

Astringents **Astringents** are the strongest toning lotions; they have a high proportion of alcohol which can be very drying. They may contain antiseptic ingredients such as witch hazel or tea tree oil; these are for use on blemished skin, to reduce the growth of bacteria and promote skin healing. Strong astringents can cause the skin to become dry and irritated if there is any skin sensitivity – so care must be taken.

Astringents are recommended for:

- oily skin with no skin sensitivity
- mild acne in young skin

Toning lotions which are suitable for oily skin are becoming increasingly available and rely upon their botanical formulations to control sebum flow and promote skin healing.

Application

Toning lotion may be applied in several ways. Whichever method you choose, it should leave the skin thoroughly clean and free of grease.

The most popular method of application is to apply the toner directly to two pieces of clean damp cotton wool, which are wiped gently upwards and outwards over the neck and face.

TOP TIP

Toning lotions

All **toning lotions have some astringent effect on the skin, but those that contain a relatively high alcohol content are actually marketed as astringents.**

Do not use toning lotions that contain more than 20 per cent alcohol on dry skin – they may cause skin irritation.

Avoid the excessive use of astringent on oily skin – the astringent will make the skin dry, and it will then produce more sebum.

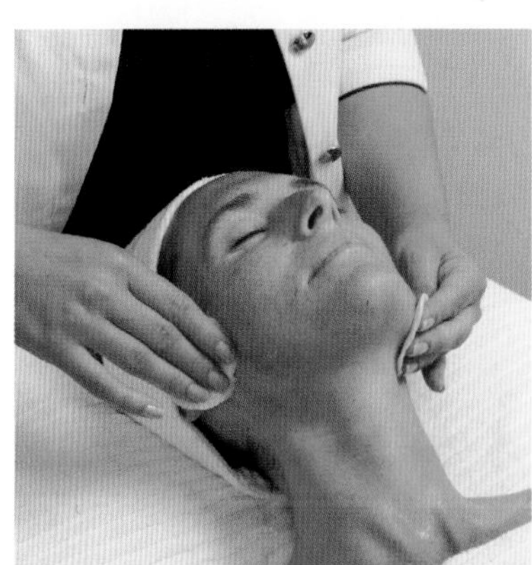

Toning

TOP TIP

Combination skin

When applying toning lotion to a combination skin, you may need to apply different toning lotions to treat separate skin conditions.

For home use, advise the client to apply toning lotion using dampened cotton wool: this is more economical.

TOP TIP

Client care

Before facial application it is a good idea to spray the mist onto the back of the client's hand: this helps them to relax.

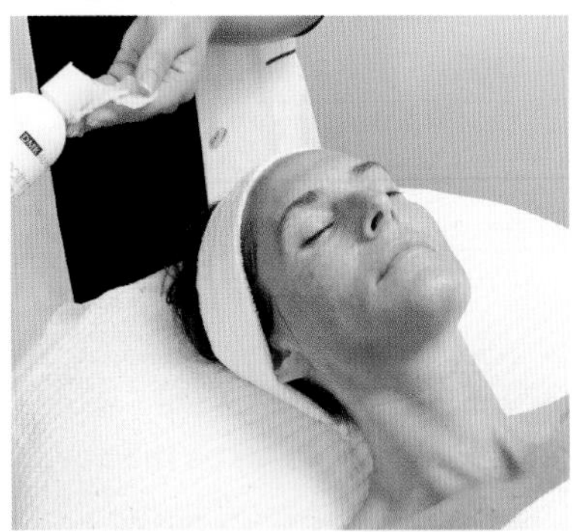
Application of toning lotion

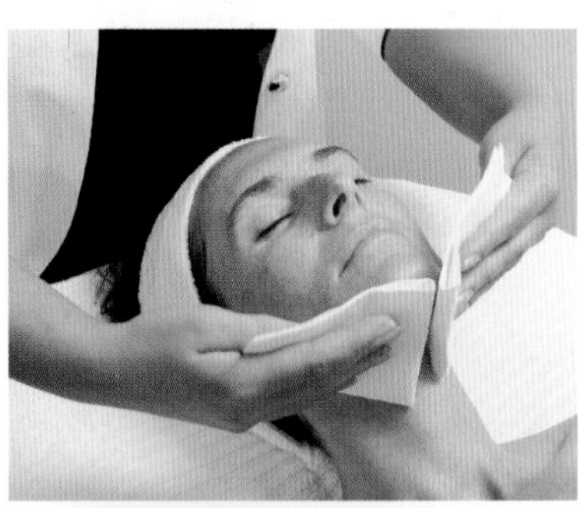

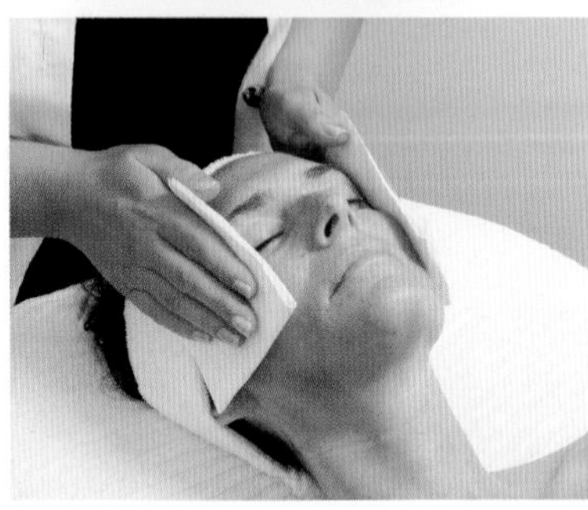
Blotting the skin

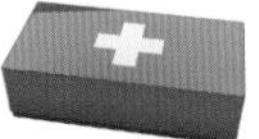
HEALTH & SAFETY

Client comfort

To avoid claustrophobia and discomfort, tell the client before you start how and why facial blotting is carried out.

Alternatively, the toner may be applied under pressure as a fine spray, using a vaporizer. This produces a fine mist of the toning lotion over the skin. If using this method, always protect the eye tissue with cotton wool pads and hold the vaporizer about 30cm from the skin, directing the spray across the skin in a sweeping movement. This is preferable when treating a male client, where the cotton wool application technique would be unsuitable.

To produce a stimulating effect, the toning lotion can be applied to dampened cotton wool: hold this firmly at one corner, and gently tap it over the skin.

Blotting the skin

After applying toning lotion, immediately blot the skin dry with a soft facial tissue to prevent the toner evaporating from the skin's surface (which would stimulate the skin). Alternatively you can make a small tear in the centre of a large facial tissue for the client's nose. Place the tissue over their face and neck, and mould it into position to absorb excess moisture. Alternatively, blot over the face with large facial tissues as shown.

When skin is thoroughly cleansed and toned a thorough skin analysis can occur using a magnifying lamp. If the client is sensitive to light protect the client's eyes with damp cotton wool pads. The skin's surface will be magnified enabling you to comment further and note any characteristics of skin type and skin conditions requiring attention. Record these on a record card.

Moisturising

The skin depends on water to keep it soft, supple and resilient. Two-thirds of our body is composed of water and the skin is an important reservoir, containing about 20 per cent of the body's total water content. Most of the fluid is in the lower layers of the dermis, but it circulates to the top layer of the epidermis, where it evaporates.

The skin protects its water content in these ways:

- sebum keeps the skin lubricated, and reduces water loss from skin
- the skin cells have **natural moisturising factors** (**NMFs**), a complex mix of substances which are able to fix moisture inside the cells
- a cement of fats (lipids) between the skin cells forms a watertight barrier

The natural moisture level is constantly being disturbed. The application of a cosmetic **moisturiser** helps to maintain the natural oil and moisture balance by locking moisture into the tissues, offering protection and hydration.

The basic formulation of a moisturiser is oil and water to make an oil-in-water emulsion. The water content helps to return lost moisture to the surface layers; the oil content prevents moisture loss from the surface of the skin. Often a **humectant**, such as **glycerine** or **sorbitol**, is included: this attracts moisture to the skin from the surrounding air and stops the moisturiser from drying out. If a humectant is included, less oil is used in the formulation: this results in a lighter cream.

Moisturiser also has the following benefits:

- it protects the skin from external damage caused by the environment
- it softens the skin and relieves skin tautness and sensitivity

- it plumps the skin tissue with moisture, which minimizes the appearance of fine lines
- it provides a barrier between the skin and make-up cosmetics
- it may contain additional ingredients which improve the condition of the skin (such as vitamin E, which has a humectant action and is an excellent skin conditioner)
- it may contain ultra-violet filters, which protect the skin against the age-accelerating sunlight.

Moisturisers are available for wear during the day or the night. These are available in different formulations, to treat all skin types and conditions.

Moisturisers are applied at the final stage of the facial when the skin is clean and toned, providing a protective barrier.

TOP TIP

Tinted moisturisers

If your client likes a natural look for the day, they may wish to wear a moisturiser that is tinted; this gives the skin a healthy appearance.

Antioxidant moisturisers

Antioxidant moisturisers protect against free-radical damage from UV exposure, cigarette smoke, pollution and stress.

Moisturisers for daytime use

Moisturising lotions **Moisturising lotions** contain up to 85–90 per cent water and 10–15 per cent oil. They have a light, liquid formulation, and are ideal for use under make-up.

Moisturising lotions have these specific applications:

- oily skin
- young combination skin
- dehydrated skin
- normal skin

Moisturising creams **Moisturising creams** contain up to 70–85 per cent water and 15–30 per cent oil. They have a thicker consistency, and cannot be poured.

Moisturising creams have these specific applications:

- mature skin
- dry skin

HEALTH & SAFETY 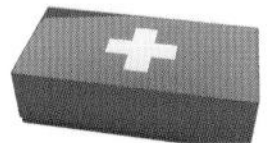

Allergies

Hypoallergenic moisturisers are available for clients with sensitive skin. These are screened from all common sensitizing ingredients, such as lanolin and perfume, and they also have soothing properties.

ALWAYS REMEMBER 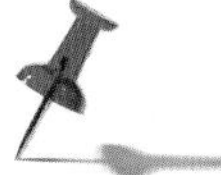

Oily skin

Even oily skin requires a moisturiser. This skin can become dehydrated by the over-use of harsh cleansers and astringents.

HEALTH & SAFETY 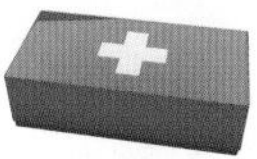

UV light

Even on an overcast day, as much as 80 per cent of the sun's age-accelerating UVA can penetrate the skin.

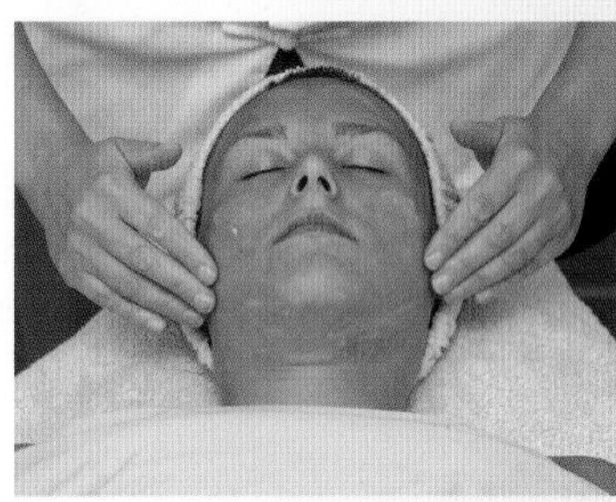

Apply sun protection

TOP TIP

Moisturising creams

Some clients dislike heavier cream, feeling that it is too heavy for their skin. Offer them a suitable moisturising lotion alternative.

COURTESY OF DERMALOGICA

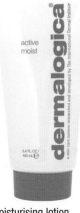

Moisturising lotion

Step-by-step: Applying how to apply moisturiser

Moisturiser is applied after the final application of toning lotion. If the moisturiser is being applied before make-up, use a light formulation so that it does not interfere with the adherence of the foundation.

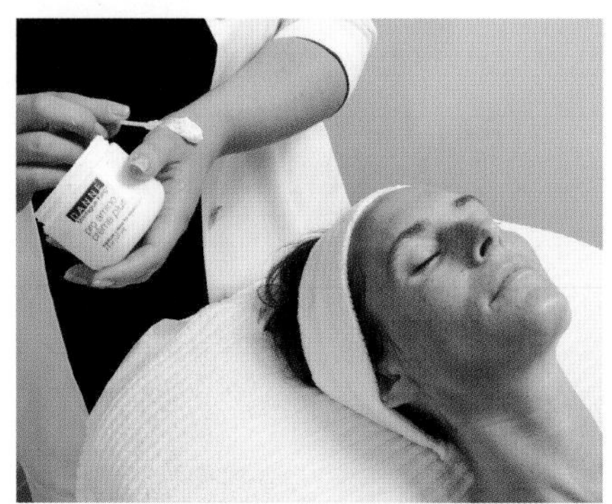

1 Remove some moisturiser from the jar, using a disposable spatula or disinfected plastic spatula. Place it on the back of the non-working hand, then take it on the fingertips of your working hand.

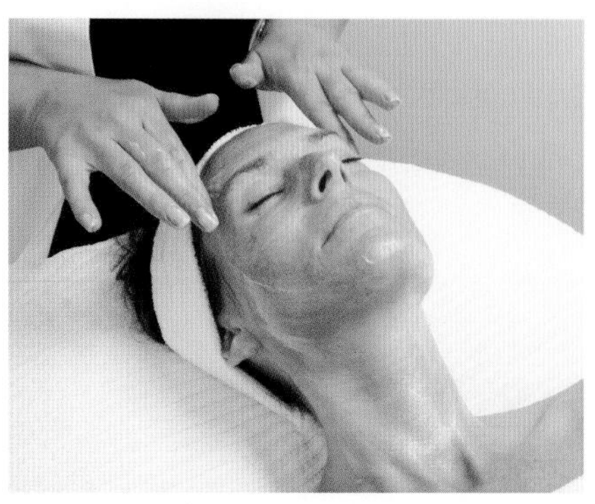

2 Apply the moisturiser in small dots to the neck, chin, cheeks, nose and forehead. Quickly and evenly spread it in a fine film over the face, using light upward and outward stroking movements.

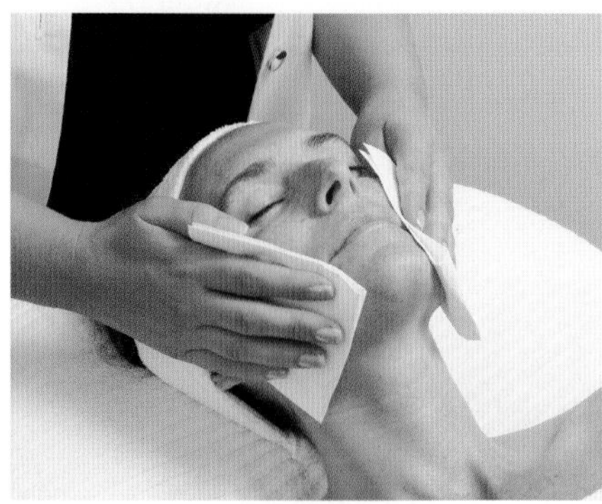

3 Blot excess moisturiser from the skin using a facial tissue.

BEST PRACTICE

If the moisturiser is very fluid, apply it directly to the fingertips of the non-working hand – it would run if applied to the back of the hand.

Moisturisers for night-time use

Moisturisers are applied to the skin in the evening, after the skin has been cleansed, toned and blotted dry.

An emulsion **night cream** with a higher proportion of oil is the most effective for application in the evening: by this time the surrounding air is dry and warm, which encourages water loss from the skin; the oil seals the surface of the skin, preventing this water loss.

A small amount of **wax** (such as beeswax) may be included in the formulation: this improves the *slip* of the product, making it easier to apply and helping its skin-conditioning effect.

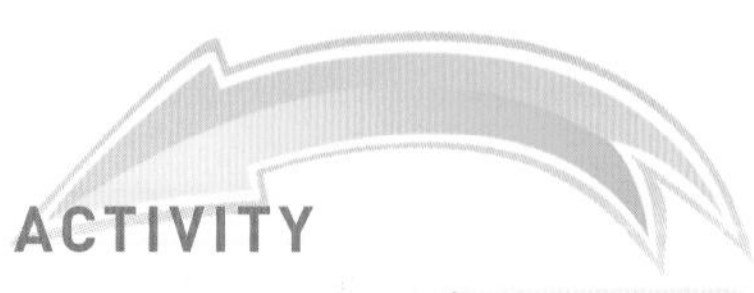

ACTIVITY

Moisturisers

Collect information on different moisturisers from various skincare suppliers. You could visit local beauty salons, retail stores or beauty wholesale suppliers, or write to professional skincare companies.

Specialist skin treatment products

In addition to basic skincare products, **specialist skincare treatment products** are available to target improvement for specific facial areas.

Neck creams The neck can become dry as it is exposed to the weather, often without the protection of a moisturiser. As a client ages, the collagen molecules in the dermis become increasingly cross-linked; they are then unable to retain the same volume of water, and the skin loses its plump appearance.

The formulation for a **neck cream** is similar to that for a night cream; it also contains various skin conditioning supplements, such as collagen or vitamin E, which help maintain moisture in the stratum corneum.

Encourage your client to include the neck in their cleansing routine, applying facial moisturiser to the neck during the day and either a night cream or specially formulated throat cream in the evening. Recommend that they always apply the throat cream gently in an upward and outward direction, using their fingertips.

BEST PRACTICE

Weight loss

Advise the client against losing weight quickly, especially when older – the neck tissue can look loose and very wrinkled as the underlying fat is lost.

To improve the appearance of the neck, good posture is important. If the client is round-shouldered the head often drops forwards, putting strain on the muscles of the neck. This causes tension in the muscles, which become tight and painful. Correct the client's posture, and advise them to massage the neck when applying the throat cream to relieve tension.

Eye creams The eye tissue is very thin and readily becomes very dry, emphasizing fine lines and wrinkles (**crow's feet**). Special care must be taken when applying products near this area: it contains a large number of **mast cells**, the cells that respond to contact with an irritant by causing an allergic reaction.

Eye cream is a fine cream formulated specifically for application to the eye area. A small quantity of the product is applied to the eye tissue using the ring finger of one hand, gently stroking around the eye, inwards and towards the nose. Support the eye tissue with the other hand. Do not apply the product too near to the inner eyelid or you will cause irritation to the eye.

Eye gel **Eye gel** is usually applied in the morning; it has a cooling, soothing, slightly astringent effect. (This is caused partly by the evaporation of the water in the gel, and partly by the inclusion of plant extracts such as **cornflower** or **camomile**.)

Eye gel is recommended for all clients, but especially for those suffering with slightly puffy eye tissue. It may also be applied following a facial treatment, to normalize the pH of the skin.

Eye gel may be applied with a light tapping motion, using the pads of the fingers. This will mildly stimulate the lymphatic circulation in the area and help to reduce any slight swelling.

Ampoule treatment **Serums** are chemicals used to revitalize the skin. They are supplied in **ampoules**, sealed glass or plastic phials which prevent the content from evaporating and losing their effectiveness. Serums are usually applied for 7–28 days as a skin tonic course for the treatment of different skin types and conditions.

Blemished skincare preparations Professional products are available for the client to apply specifically to blemishes such as pustules and papules. Benzoyl peroxide is an example of a product ingredient that dries and promotes healing of skin blemishes. The skincare aims to purify the skin while keeping it hydrated.

After cleansing the skin thoroughly the skin is exfoliated.

Exfoliation

The natural physical process of losing dead skin cells from the stratum corneum layer of the epidermis is called **desquamation**. **Exfoliation** is a salon technique used to accelerate this process. It is normally carried out after the skin has been cleansed and toned, and before further facial treatments.

Exfoliation has the following benefits:

- dead skin cells, grease and debris are removed from the surface of the skin
- fresh new cells are exposed, improving the appearance of the skin
- skin preparations such as moisturising lotions are more easily absorbed

TOP TIP

Specialist lip products

Products designed to firm the skin around the lips and reduce visible lines are becoming popular. The result aims to smooth and firm and even 'plump' the lip line, reducing the appearance of visible lines caused by lifestyle factors such as smoking and stress.

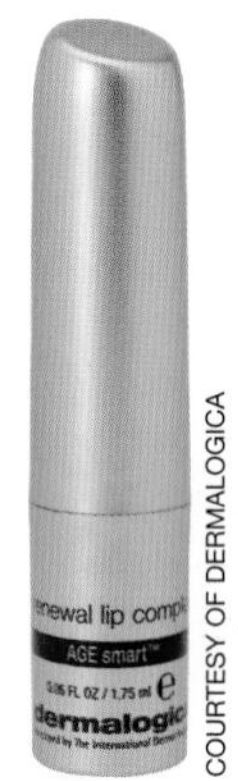

COURTESY OF DERMALOGICA

Specialist lip product

ACTIVITY

Eye conditions

Think of different *non-medical* conditions affecting the skin around the eye for which a client might seek your advice. Discuss with colleagues the possible cause of these conditions, and what you could recommend to improve the appearance in each case.

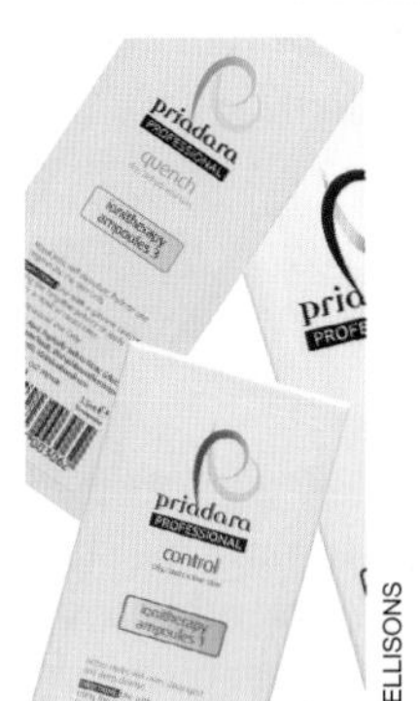

ELLISONS

Ampoule products

- the blood circulation in the area is mildly stimulated, bringing more oxygen and nutrients to the skin cells and improving the skin colour
- hyperpigmentation is improved in appearance by the removal of the pigmented surface skin cells

ACTIVITY

Exfoliants

Apply an exfoliant to the back of your own – or a colleague's – hand or arm. Compare the appearance and the feeling of the skin before and after application.

This technique produces a particularly marked effect on black skin, as it reduces the greyish appearance of the skin. (This is due to the skin having a thicker stratum corneum.)

TOP TIP

Male skin

A man who shaves exfoliates every day, as shaving removes the top layer of skin. You can recommend that he also uses a cosmetic exfoliating product on areas such as the nose and forehead. If a male client suffers from pseudo folliculitis recommend an electric shave rather than a wet shave which tends to make this disorder worse.

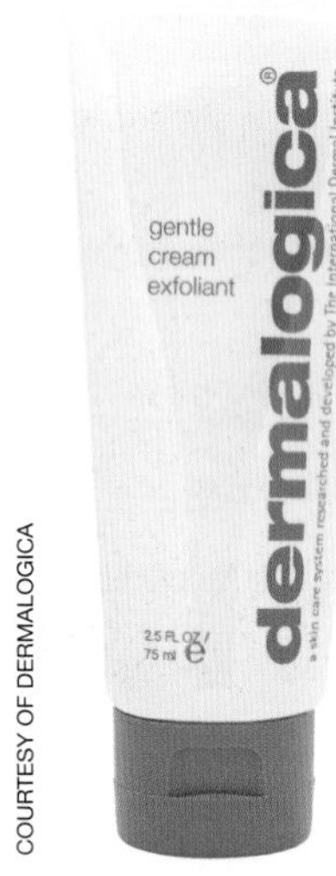

COURTESY OF DERMALOGICA

Exfoliator product

TOP TIP

Steaming

Steaming before exfoliation softens the outer skin cells, making them easier to remove. This is particularly beneficial when treating a male client.

HEALTH & SAFETY 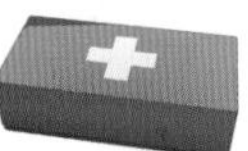

Exfoliants

Avoid exfoliating products that contain sharp grains of nut shells: these can scrape, split and damage the epidermis. Before purchasing, test the exfoliating product on the back of your own hand to feel its action.

Contra-indications

Exfoliation is beneficial for most skin types; however, avoid application if the client has the following:

- highly sensitive skin
- a vascular skin disorder such as telangiectases or damaged broken veins in the area of treatment application
- pustular, blemished skin

Exfoliants

Various **exfoliants** are available; they may be of chemical or vegetable origin. Alternatively, mechanical exfoliation may be used.

Biochemical skin peel **Natural acids** (alpha-hydroxy acids – AHAs), derived from fruits, sugar cane and milk, are applied to the skin as a face mask. The natural acids dissolve dead surface cells and stimulate circulation in the underlying skin. These masks are available to suit all skin types.

AHAs may be combined with enzymes derived from fruits such as papaya (papain) to help remove surface dead skin to achieve maximum effect.

When you apply this type of face mask, warn the client that there will be a stinging sensation and then a tightening effect as the mask sets.

Pore grains **Pore grains** are the most popular exfoliants: a base of cream or liquid containing tiny spheres of polished plastic or crushed nuts is gently massaged over the skin's surface.

Clay exfoliants Gentler **clay exfoliants** have a clay base which is applied like a face mask. As it dries, the clay absorbs dead skin cells and sebum. The mask is then gently stroked away, using the pads of the fingers. A mask style exfoliant is more suitable for a blemished skin accompanying an oily skin type.

Mechanical exfoliation **Mechanical exfoliation**, or 'facial brushing', softens and cleanses the skin. Dead skin cells and excess sebum are removed as the soft hair bristles rotate over the skin's surface. The rotary action also increases the cleansing action of exfoliation.

If steam is applied before mechanical exfoliation, this will soften the dead skin cells, and **skin peeling cream** may be applied: together these will maximize the result of exfoliation.

Be careful to avoid over-stimulation, and over-exfoliation resulting in sensitizing the skin's surface, or disturbing the skin's natural protective qualities. Permanent sensitization could result from incorrect exfoliation techniques or over-exfoliation.

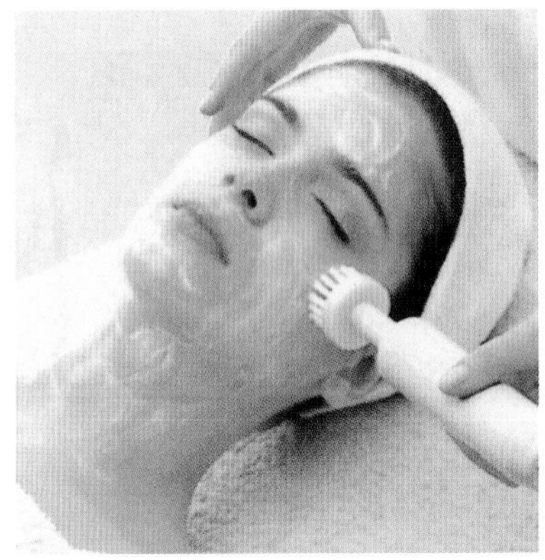

Mechanical exfoliation

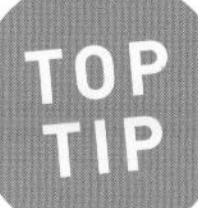

TOP TIP

Exfoliation

Exfoliation should be strongly recommended for the mature client. The removal of the surface dead cells has a rejuvenating effect on the skin's appearance.

Teenagers regenerate external skin cells every 14 days. This increases to 30–40 days as a client reaches their forties.

Step-by-step: Exfoliation treatment

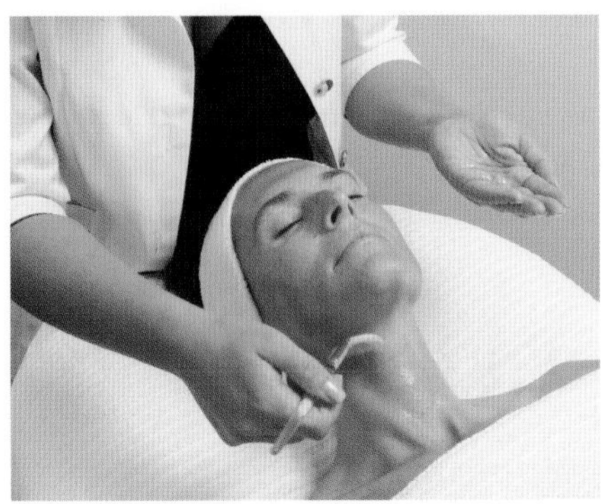

Exfoliant lotion is applied to a dry, sensitive skin type.

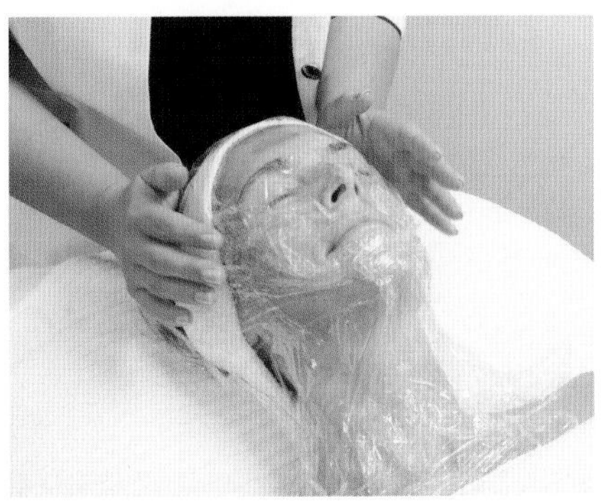

Plastic film is placed over the exfoliant to speed up the action of the exfoliant lotion.

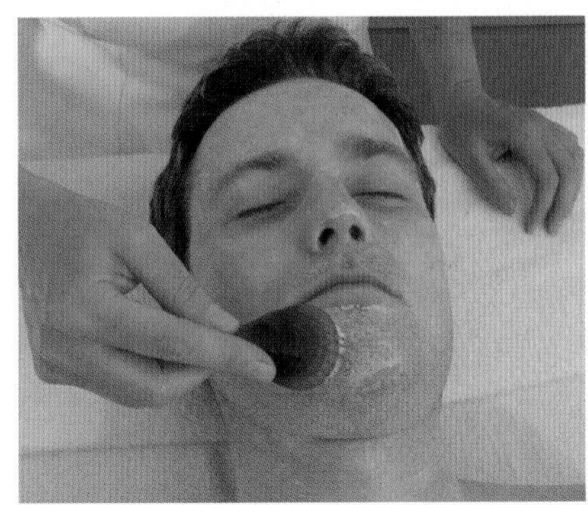

Mechanical exfoliation with pore grains.

1 Facial exfoliant is applied to the skin following cleansing and steaming to warm and soften the skin. The exfoliant containing hydroxy acids is applied, which removes dead skin cells and stimulates skin renewal. Warn the client a mild stinging sensation may be experienced, but will disappear quickly upon removal.

2 A soft facial brush may be used in a rotary action to further enhance the effectiveness of the exfoliant to remove areas of dead skin and sebum. This is particularly beneficial when working on a male client to loosen dead skin and debris surrounding coarse facial hair. A client may purchase the brush to use as part of their home care programme.

ALWAYS REMEMBER

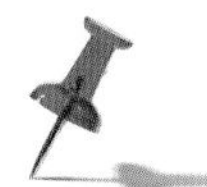

Body exfoliants

Point out to clients that exfoliants designed for use on the *body* are unsuitable for use on the *face* – their action is not as gentle and their ingredients unsuitable unless specifically designed for dual use.

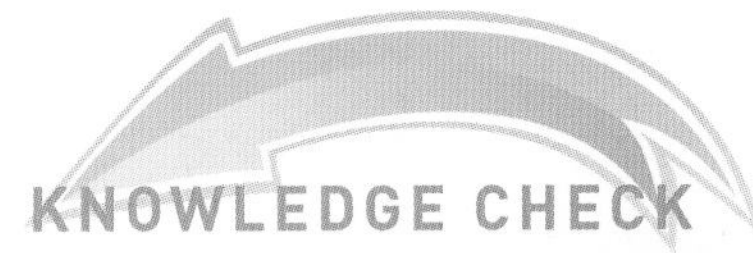

KNOWLEDGE CHECK

What is the purpose of an exfoliant?

Need more time... refer to pages 208–209 to help you.

Advice on home use

The client can be advised to use exfoliants at home as a specialized cleansing treatment after normal cleansing and toning. Exfoliants should be applied once a week for all skin types except oily, for which it may be applied twice a week.

Advise the client to massage the product gently over the skin using their fingertips. Application should always be upwards and outwards. The application and removal technique will differ according to the exfoliant product type.

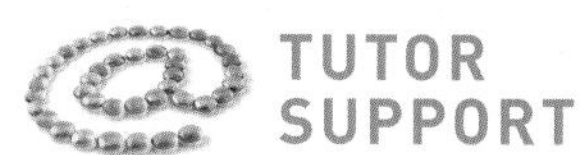
TUTOR SUPPORT

Activity 5: Comparing exfoliant treatments task

HEALTH & SAFETY 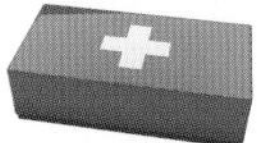

Exfoliants

- Tell the client how the skin should look after exfoliation treatment. The skin's colour should be *slightly* heightened; but too vigorous a massage application may cause the formation of broken capillaries.
- Tell the client to avoid contact with the delicate eye tissue.
- A client with a pustular skin should not use exfoliant products – they would probably cause discomfort, and any lesions present might burst.

BEST PRACTICE 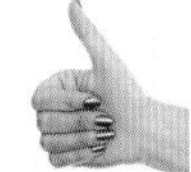

Heat the water in the vapour unit in advance of its application. This usually takes about 12 minutes. This will avoid an unnecessary delay in the facial routine waiting for the water to heat! Ensure that the couch is correctly positioned before treatment when using steam, to allow the vapour unit to be positioned at the correct distance from the client's skin.

HEALTH & SAFETY 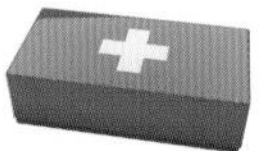

Vapour application

Keep the vapour directed away from the client's face until a visible jet of steam can be seen. To avoid skin sensitization, consider carefully where to position the steam so as to ensure even heat distribution.

TOP TIP

Retail opportunity

To encourage sales of this skincare product, demonstrate the product on the back of one of the client's hands. They will be amazed when they compare the appearance of their hands.

After application, any product residue should be thoroughly rinsed from the face using clean, tepid water. The client may then apply a face mask or tone the skin and apply a nourishing skin moisturiser.

A UV sun block should be used to protect the skin to avoid skin damage.

Following the exfoliation technique applied to suit your client's skin type a suitable skin warming technique is used relevant to the client's needs.

Warming the skin

A **steam treatment** is the ideal means of producing the required warming effect on the skin to achieve both cleansing and stimulation. Skin warming is often incorporated into a facial treatment after the manual cleansing, so as to stimulate the skin and make it more receptive to subsequent treatments.

The effects are these:

- the pores are opened
- locally the blood circulation and the lymphatic circulation are stimulated
- the surface cells of the epidermis are softened, which helps desquamation
- sebaceous gland activity is improved, which benefits a dry mature skin type
- skin colour is improved

Steam is provided by an electric **vapour unit**. In this, distilled water is heated electrically until it boils to create steam.

The resulting steam is applied as a fine mist over the facial area. As the steam settles upon the skin, it is absorbed by the surface epidermal cells. These cells are softened and can be gently loosened with an exfoliation treatment.

HEALTH & SAFETY 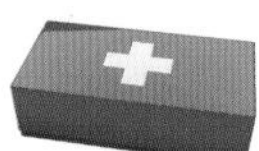

Safe use and care of the vapour unit

- Always follow manufacturer's instructions on correct usage. Have the unit tested annually by a qualified electrician to ensure its safety in compliance with the Electricity at Work Regulations (1989).
- Always use distilled water to avoid lime scale build-up in the heating element.
- Never fill the water vessel past the recommended level or 'spitting' could occur, where hot droplets of water are ejected and could burn the client's skin.
- Never use the equipment if the water vessel is below the recommended level or the heating element could be damaged. Most units have a cut-out feature so that the machine switches off if this occurs.
- Never leave the lead trailing across an area where somebody could trip and fall.

Contra-indications Although the treatment is suitable for most clients, do not use steam if you discover that the client has any of the following:

- ***Respiratory problems***, such as asthma or a cold.
- ***Vascular skin disorders*** – these would be aggravated by the heating action and increased blood circulation.
- ***Claustrophobia*** – fear of enclosure or confined space.
- ***Excessively dilated capillaries***.
- ***Skin with reduced sensitivity***.
- ***Diabetes***, unless the client's GP has given permission.
- ***Rosacea*** – a vascular skin disorder, where excess sebum production combined with a chronic inflammatory condition is caused by dilation of the blood capillaries. The skin becomes coarse, the pores enlarge, and the cheek and nose become inflamed.
- ***Dilated capillaries***, where capillaries near the surface of the skin are permanently dilated.

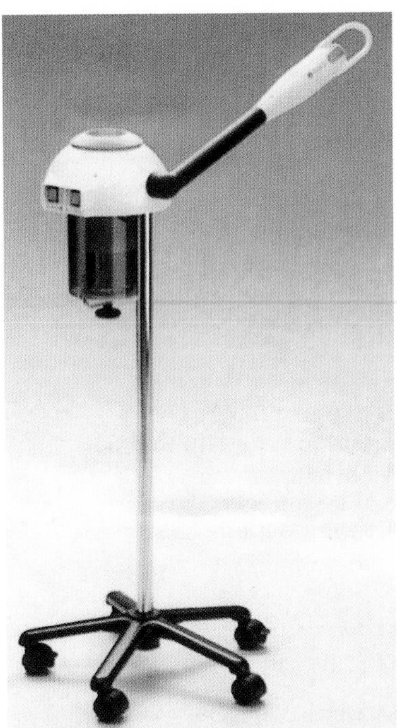
BEAUTY EXPRESS LTD

A vapour unit

HEALTH & SAFETY 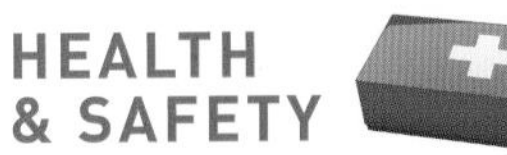

Steam application

Oily skin will tolerate a shorter application distance and a longer application time. For sensitive skin, increase the application distance and reduce the time. What are the manufacturer's guidelines for your equipment? Remember that these are only *guidelines* – observe the skin's reaction and check that the client is comfortable.

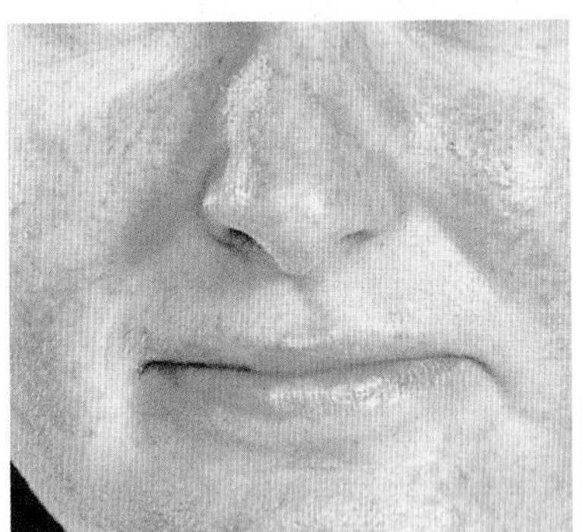
DR M H BECK

Rosacea

Explain to the client:

- how long the treatment is to be applied for
- the sensations that will be experienced
- the physical effect on the skin

The duration of the application and the distance differ according to the skin type.

The client should be positioned in a semi-reclined position for facial application.

Before applying steam, protect the client's eyes with damp cotton wool. Areas of delicate skin should be protected with damp cotton wool and if necessary a barrier cream.

The distance between the vapour outlet and the client's skin to be treated should be approximately 30–35cm. The application time will depend on the treatment effect and the type of skin that is being treated. Generally allow:

- 10 minutes for the face
- 15 minutes for the body

Ensure that an even flow of steam covers all the area being treated; reposition as necessary.

If you are using ozone, this is applied following the steam application for the final few minutes, as directed by the manufacturer. The steam will change in appearance to a bluish-white cloud.

After applying steam vapour, blot the skin dry with a soft facial tissue and proceed to remove any blockages.

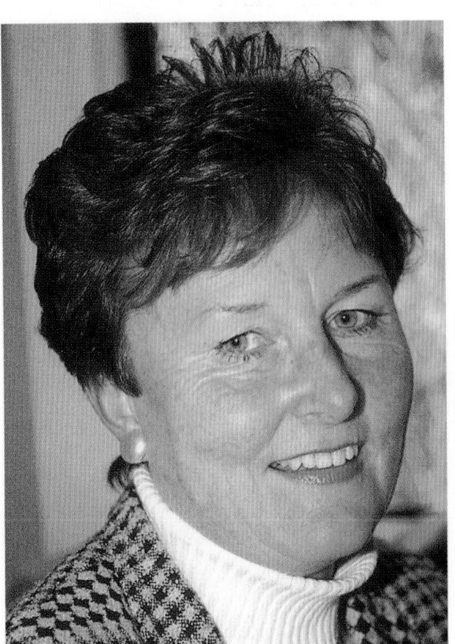
DR JOHN GRAY, THE WORLD OF SKIN CARE

Dilated capillaries

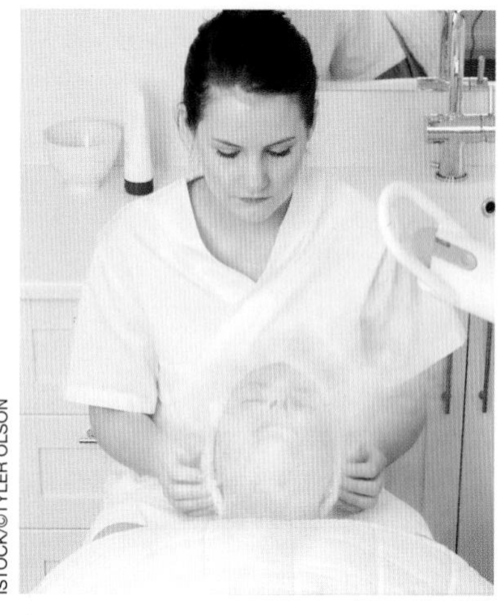
ISTOCK/©TYLER OLSON

Applying steam to the face

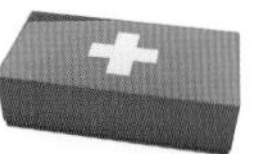
HEALTH & SAFETY

Ozone
Most vapour units produce ozone when the oxygen in the steam is passed over a high-intensity quartz mercury arc tube. Ozone is thought to be beneficial in the treatment of blemished skin, as it kills many bacteria, but it may also be carcinogenic (liable to cause cancer) if inhaled. Use a vapour unit only in a well-ventilated room, and only for short periods of time.

At the end of the treatment, turn off the machine and unplug it. Check that you have tidied away the trailing lead so that there is no risk of it causing an accident.

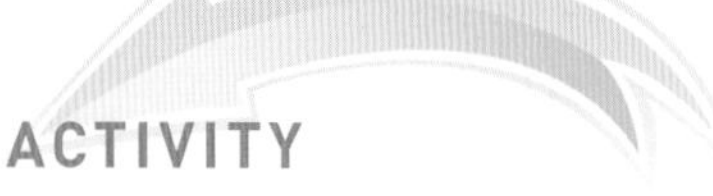
ACTIVITY

Vapour units
Collect literature on different vapour units. Compare their efficiencies and features. Which would be the best buy? Consider:

- Is the unit transportable, for marketing demonstrations?
- Is it height-adjustable, to suit the height of the treatment couch?
- Is it easy to clean?
- If floor-standing, does it move easily?
- Does it allow the addition of aromatic oils?
- Does it havesafety features to prevent overheating or the vessel running dry?

Contra-actions

Contra-actions to facial steaming include the following:

- *over-stimulation of the skin*, caused by incorrect application distance and duration of the steam
- *scalding*, caused by spitting from a faulty steam jet or by the vessel being over-filled
- *discomfort*, caused by the steam being too near the skin, leading to breathing difficulties, or by the treatment being applied for too long

After facial steaming, blot the skin dry with a soft facial tissue and proceed to remove any skin blockages – termed *extraction*.

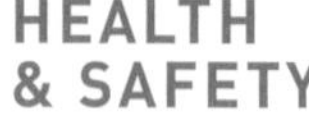
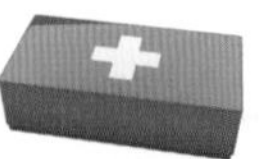
HEALTH & SAFETY

Treatment programme
If the client suffers from severe congestion, do not attempt to carry out all the removals in one session. This would sensitize the skin, making it appear very red, and would be most uncomfortable for the client. Instead they should visit the salon weekly for you to clear the skin gradually as part of an overall treatment programme.

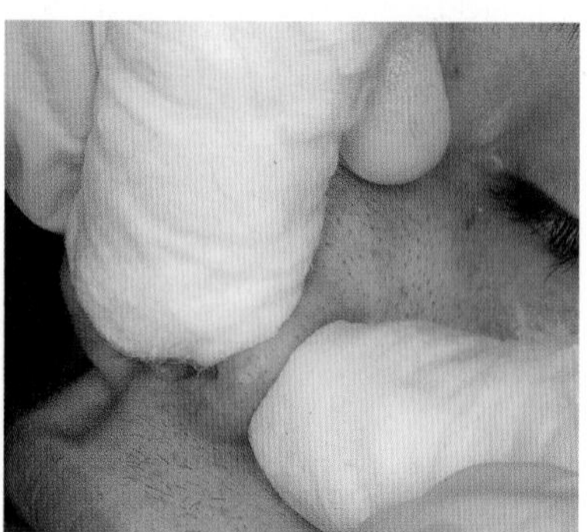
Comedone extraction

Removing skin blockages

After the skin has been cleansed, you may wish to remove minor skin blemishes such as comedones (blackheads). As discussed, it is preferable to warm up the skin tissues first; this softens the skin and relaxes the openings of the skin that are blocked. Milia (whitehead) extraction pierces the skin and therefore additional advanced training will be required in order to perform this treatment.

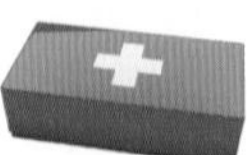
HEALTH & SAFETY

Skin blockages
Do not attempt to remove larger skin blockages such as sebaceous cysts – these should be treated by a general practitioner.

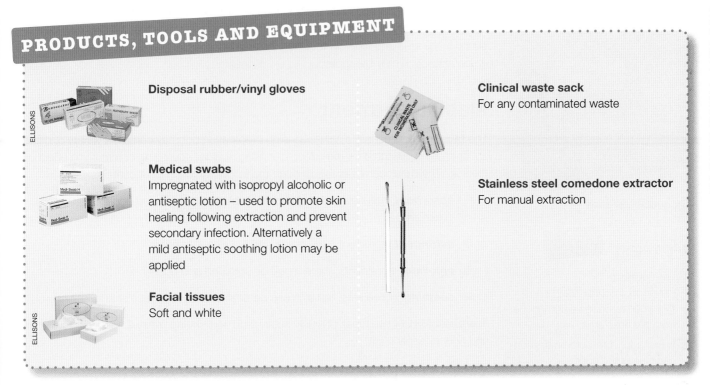

PRODUCTS, TOOLS AND EQUIPMENT

Disposal rubber/vinyl gloves

ELLISONS

Medical swabs
Impregnated with isopropyl alcoholic or antiseptic lotion – used to promote skin healing following extraction and prevent secondary infection. Alternatively a mild antiseptic soothing lotion may be applied

Facial tissues
Soft and white

ELLISONS

Clinical waste sack
For any contaminated waste

Stainless steel comedone extractor
For manual extraction

Sterilization and disinfection

All contaminated waste material from this treatment (such as facial tissues and gloves) should be disposed of in an identified waste container, as directed by your local health authority.

After use the stainless steel comedone extractor should be cleaned with an alcohol preparation and then sterilized in an autoclave.

Wear disposable gloves while carrying out the treatment.

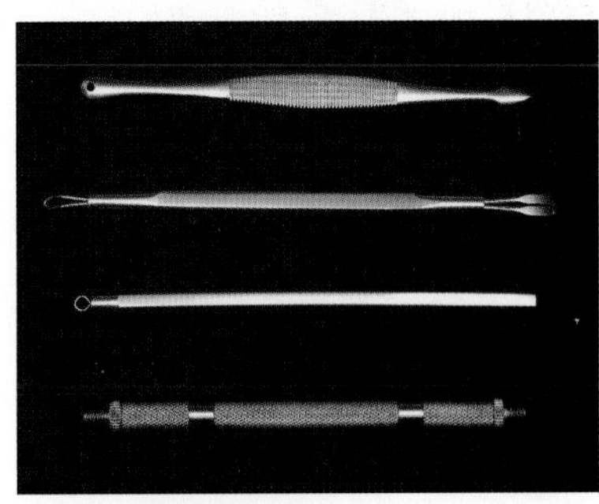

Comedone extractors

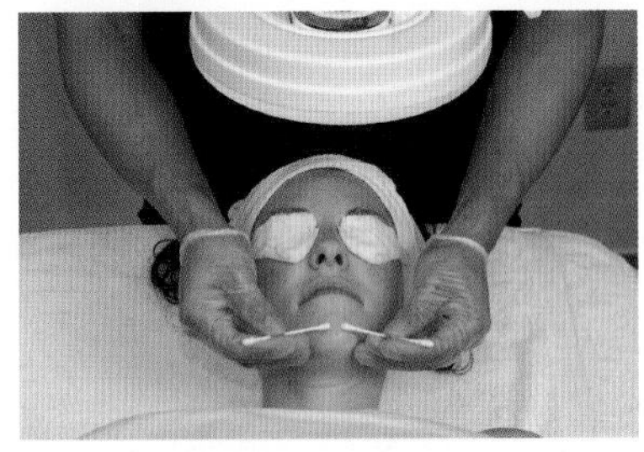

Using cotton buds on sensitive skin to remove blockages

Comedone removal For **comedone removal** the loop end of the extractor tool is used to apply gentle pressure around the comedone. The comedone should leave the skin, apparent as a plug. You may need to apply gentle pressure with your fingers at the sides of the comedone to ensure that it is effectively removed; when doing this, wrap a tissue around the pads of the index fingers.

Contra-actions:

- Skin bruising could occur if too much pressure is applied.
- Capillary damage could result if too much force is used when squeezing the comedone. The surrounding blood capillaries can rupture, causing permanent skin damage.

A mild antiseptic soothing lotion or medical swab maybe applied after extraction which will help the skin to heal.

Contra-action If extraction resulted in tissue damage resulting in blood loss, a medical swab should be applied to the area. The contaminated waste should be disposed of as

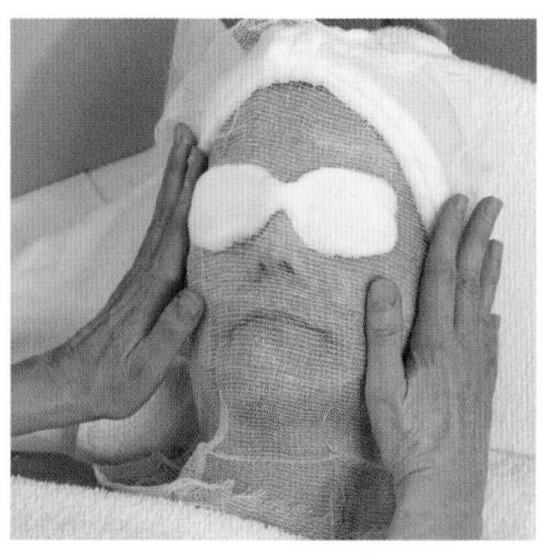
Gauze mask application

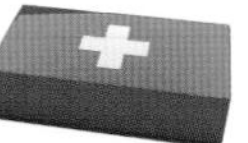
HEALTH & SAFETY

Client comfort

- Never obstruct the client's nostrils when removing a comedone from the nose area.
- Never apply pressure on the soft cartilage of the nose.

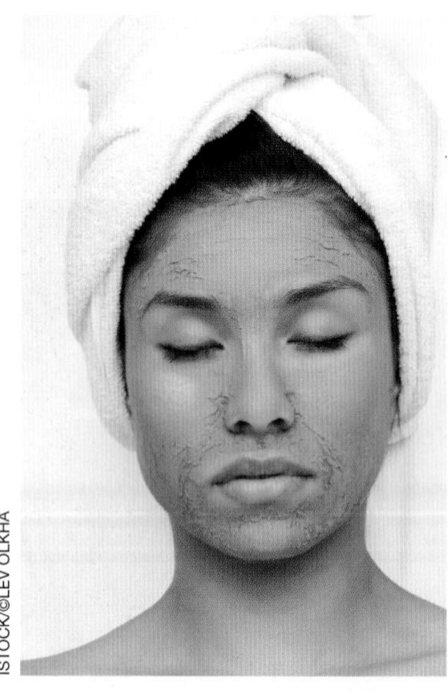
ISTOCK/©LEV OLKHA

A setting face mask

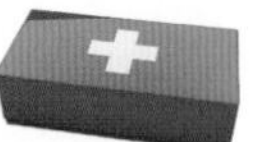
HEALTH & SAFETY

Avoiding infection

Clay mask ingredients must always be made from sterilized materials, because of the danger from tetanus spores.

Ensure that *all* contents of the skin blockage are removed, or infection may occur.

directed by your local authority. The area should then be avoided by the beauty therapist to prevent secondary infection. Inform the client following extraction that the skin may be reddened in the area and to avoid touching the area unnecessarily until the redness subsides. A soothing lotion may be applied.

Mask treatment

The **face mask** is usually a skin-cleansing preparation but may contain a variety of different ingredients selected for their deep cleansing, toning, nourishing or refreshing effect on the skin. The mask achieves this through the following actions. If it contains:

- ***absorbent*** materials, dead skin cells, sebum and debris will adhere to it when it is removed
- ***astringent*** ingredients, the pores and the skin will tighten
- ***emollient*** ingredients, the skin will be softened and nourished
- ***soothing*** ingredients, the skin can be desensitized to reduce skin irritation

There are basically two types of mask: setting and non-setting. You will need to know when and how to apply each.

Setting masks

Setting masks are applied in a thin layer over the skin and then allowed to dry. The mask need not necessarily set solid – a solid mask can become uncomfortable, and be difficult to remove especially if the client has a sensitive skin condition.

Setting masks come in these varieties:

- clay masks
- peel-off masks – including gel, polyvinyl acetate (PVA) and paraffin wax
- thermal masks

Clay masks The **clay mask** absorbs sebum and debris from the skin surface, leaving it cleansed. It can also stimulate or soothe the skin, according to the ingredients chosen. Various clay powders are available – select from these according to the physiological effects you require:

- ***Calamine*** A light pink powder which soothes surface blood capillaries. For sensitive or delicate skin.
- ***Magnesium carbonate*** A very light, white powder which creates a temporary astringent and toning effect. For open pores on dry and normal skins.
- ***Kaolin*** A cream-coloured powder which has a very stimulating effect on the skin's surface capillaries, thereby helping the skin to remove impurities and waste products. For congested, oily skin.
- ***Fuller's earth*** A green, heavy clay powder. It has a very stimulating effect, such that the skin will show slight reddening. It also produces a whitening, brightening effect. For oily skin with a sluggish circulation. Due to its strong effect, it is not suitable for a client with sensitive skin.
- ***Flowers of sulphur*** A light, yellow clay powder, which has a drying action on pustules and papules. Applied only to specific blemishes (pustules).

To activate these masks it is necessary to add a liquid – an **active lotion** – which turns the powder to a liquid paste. Active lotions are selected according to the skin type of the client and the mask to be used; they reinforce the action of the mask. Examples are:

- ***Rose water and orange-flower water*** These are very popular; they have a very mild stimulating and toning effect.
- ***Witch-hazel*** This has a soothing effect on blemished skin; it is also an astringent and natural antiseptic and is suitable for use on oily skin.
- ***Distilled water*** This is used on highly sensitive skin.
- ***Almond oil*** This is mildly stimulating. Because it is an oil, it does not allow the mask to dry: it is therefore recommended for highly sensitive skin or dehydrated skin.
- ***Glycerol*** A humectant, which prevents the mask drying and is suitable for dry mature skin.

Clay masks have the disadvantage when treating a black skin in that they tend on removal to leave streaks of white residue. Choose a mask that does not have this effect.

The mask should be kept in place for about 10–15 minutes.

Peel-off masks **Peel-off masks** may be made from gel, polyvinyl acetete (PVA) or paraffin wax. Because perspiration cannot escape from the skin's surface, moisture is forced into the stratum corneum. The mask also insulates the skin, causing an increase in temperature.

The **gel mask** is either a suspension of biological ingredients, such as starches, gums or gelatine, or a mixture of synthetic non-biological resin ingredients. The mask is applied over the skin; on contact with the skin it begins to dry. When dry it is peeled off the face in one piece. Depending on the biological ingredients added, the gel mask can be used to treat all skin types. (If the client has excessive facial hair, such as at the sides of the face, this mask may cause discomfort on removal. To avoid this place a lubricant under the mask, or use a different sort of mask.)

Peel-off masks contain a synthetic resin emulsion such as **polyvinyl acetate** (PVA) resin and are used to tighten the skin temporarily, and are suitable for mature skin; they can also be used with dry skin. Algae may be used as an ingredient which causes rapid setting.

The **paraffin-wax mask** is stimulating in its action. The paraffin wax is blended with petroleum jelly or acetyl alcohol which improve its spreading properties. The wax is heated to approximately 37°C and is then applied to the skin as a liquid. It sets on contact, so speed is essential if the mask is to be effective. The wax mask is loosened at the sides and removed in one piece after 15–20 minutes. The paraffin-wax mask is suitable for dry skin. Because of its stimulating action, it is unsuitable for oily skin or highly sensitive skin.

Thermal masks The **thermal mask** contains various minerals. The ingredients are mixed and applied to the face and neck, avoiding the mouth and eye tissue. The mask warms on contact with the skin: this causes the pores to enlarge, thereby cleansing the skin. As the mask cools it sets, and the pores constrict slightly. The mask is removed from the face in one piece. Thermal masks have a stimulating, cleansing action, suitable for a normal skin or for a congested, oily skin with open pores.

ALWAYS REMEMBER

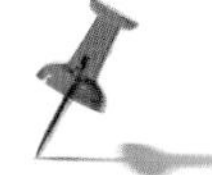

Face packs

The term *face pack* is sometimes used instead of face mask: a face pack does not set, but remains soft; a face mask sets and becomes firm.

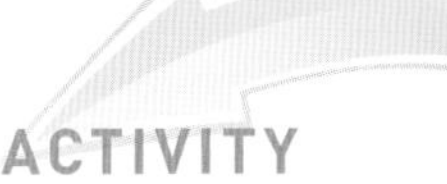

ACTIVITY

Choosing clay face masks

Which clay powder and which active lotion would you mix for clients with the following skin types:

1. A mature, sensitive skin type.
2. A young, normal skin type.
3. A combination skin type: cheeks, neck area dry; forehead, nose and chin area oily.

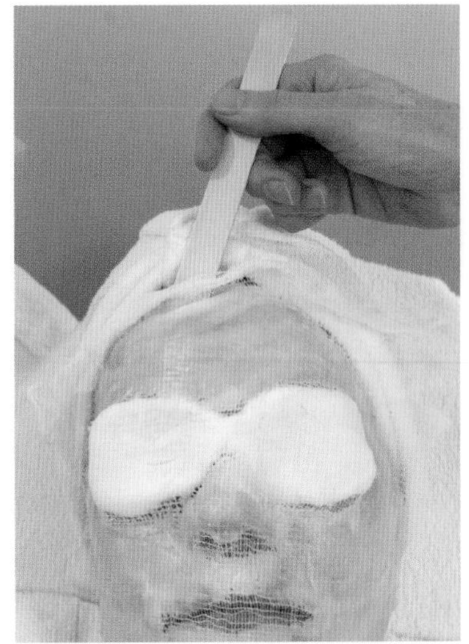

Removal of paraffin-wax mask – gently loosen the mask from the face with a wooden spatula

HEALTH & SAFETY

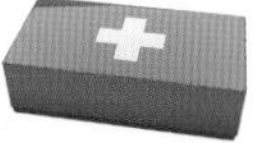

Contra-indications

Do not use thermal masks on a client with a circulatory disorder or one who has lost tactile sensation.

HEALTH & SAFETY

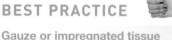

Client comfort
If a client is particularly nervous, choose an effective non-setting mask. Some clients feel claustrophobic when wearing a setting mask.

HEALTH & SAFETY

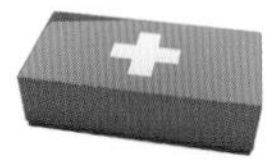

Client comfort
Before applying the wax to the client's skin always test the temperature of the wax on your own inner wrist.

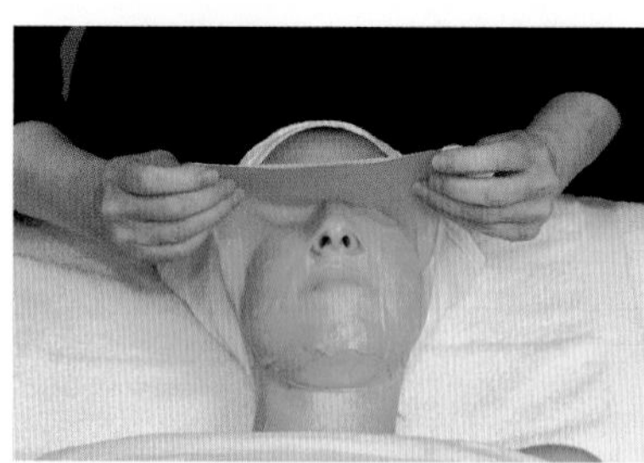

Japanese silk cream mask

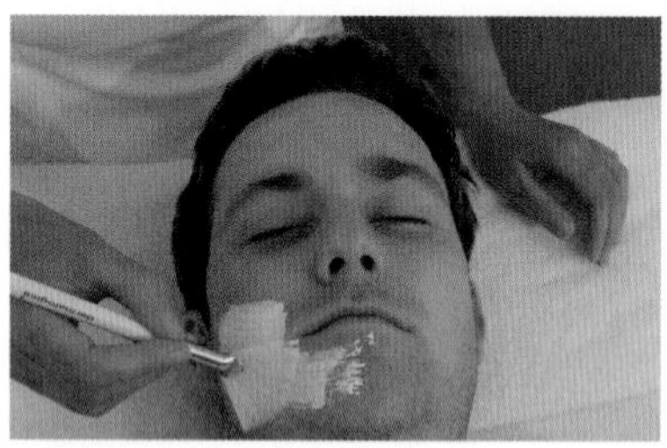

Applying a cream face mask

Non-setting masks

Some **non-setting masks** stay soft on application; others become firm, but they do not tighten like a setting mask. For this reason they do not tone the skin as effectively as setting masks. Non-setting masks include:

- warm oil
- natural masks – fruit, plant and herbal
- cream

Warm-oil masks A plant oil, typically **olive oil** or **almond oil**, is warmed and then applied to the skin. It softens the skin and helps to restore the skin's natural moisture balance. Warm-oil masks are recommended for mature skin and dry or dehydrated skin.

Gauze masks A **gauze mask** is cut to cover the face and neck, with holes for the eyes, nostrils and lips, e.g. Japanese silk cream mask. This is then soaked in warm oil. A dampened cotton wool eye pad is placed over each eye. The gauze is then placed over the face and neck. It is usually left in place for 10–20 minutes.

Impregnated tissue masks These are placed over the skin and have been impregnated or saturated in active ingredients to achieve specific treatment results e.g. collagen to hydrate and rejuvinate the skin.

Natural masks **Natural masks** are made from natural ingredients rich in vitamins and minerals. Fresh **fruit** and **vegetables** have a mildly astringent and stimulating effect. Usually the fruit is crushed to a pulp and placed between layers of gauze, which are laid over the face.

Honey is used for its toning, tightening, antiseptic and hydrating effect. **Egg white** has a tightening effect and is said to clear impurities from the skin. **Avocados** have a nourishing effect; **bananas** soften the skin, and are used for sensitive skins.

Cream masks **Cream masks** are pre-prepared for you. They have a softening and moisturising effect on the skin. Each mask contains various biological extracts or chemical substances to treat different skin types or conditions. Instructions will be provided with the mask, stating how the product is to be used professionally.

BEST PRACTICE

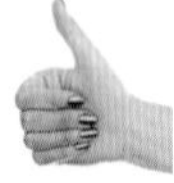

Gauze or impregnated tissue masks
Ensure that you position the gauze or tissue correctly so that the nose and eye holes are properly placed.

HEALTH & SAFETY

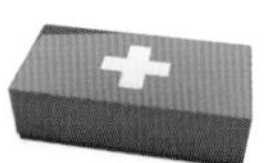

Allergies
When using biological masks, always check first whether the client has any food allergies. Avoid contact with any known allergen.

HEALTH & SAFETY

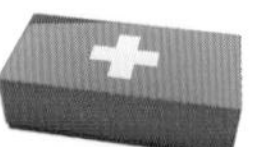

Natural masks
Because natural masks are prepared from natural foods, they must be prepared *immediately* before use – they very quickly deteriorate.

These masks are popular in the beauty salon: they often complement a particular facial treatment range used by the salon, and they are available for retail sale to clients.

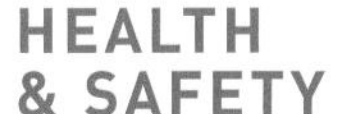

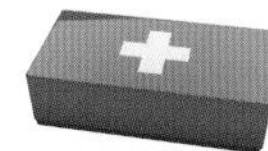

Acidic fruit

Lemon and grapefruit are generally considered too acidic for use on the face.

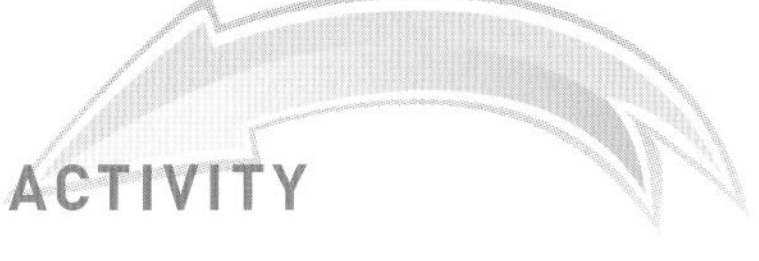

Creating natural masks

Create some masks, listing the ingredients to suit each of the following skin types:

- dry
- oily
- mature, with superficial wrinkling
- sensitive

If possible, arrange to carry out one of the masks on a suitable client. Evaluate the natural face mask. Consider: cost, preparation, application, removal and effectiveness. Remember to ask your client for *their* opinion!

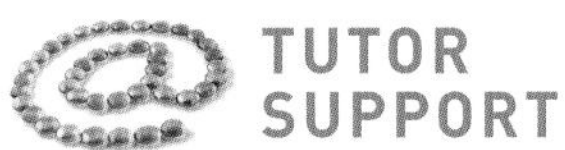

Activity 6: Face masks handout

Contra-indications

The contra-indications to general skincare apply also to face mask application. In addition, observe the following:

- ***Allergies*** Check whether your client knows if they have allergies. If so, avoid all contact with known allergens.
- ***Claustrophobia*** Do not use a setting mask on a particularly nervous client. Some clients feel claustrophobic under its tightening effect.
- ***Sensitive skins*** Do not use stimulating masks on clients with highly sensitive skin.

PRODUCTS, TOOLS AND EQUIPMENT

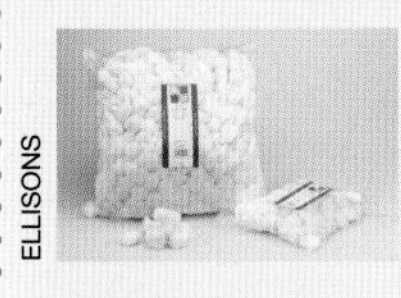

ELLISONS

Clean, dampened and clean, dry cotton wool
With sit-up and lie-down positions and an easy-to-clean surface

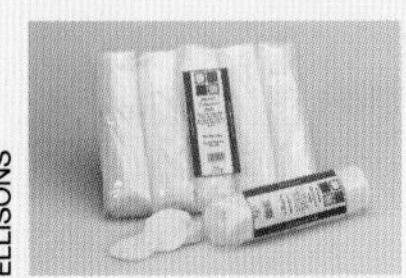

ELLISONS

Cotton wool eye pads
(2) Pre-shaped, round and dampened

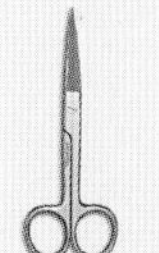

Scissors
To cut cotton wool eye pads (if cotton wool discs are not used)

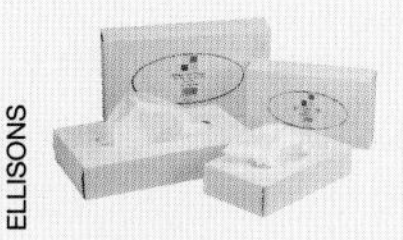

ELLISONS

Facial tissues (white)
To blot the skin dry after applying toner following mask removal

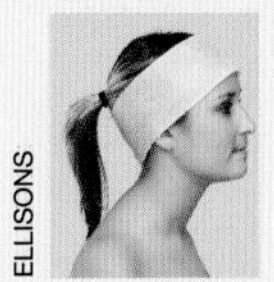

ELLISONS

Protective headband (clean)

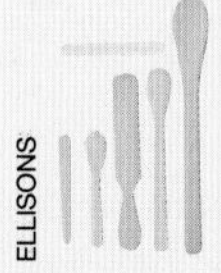

ELLISONS

Clean spatulas (several)
To mix individual masks (if required) and to remove products from containers

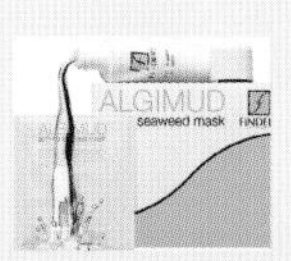

Face-mask ingredients

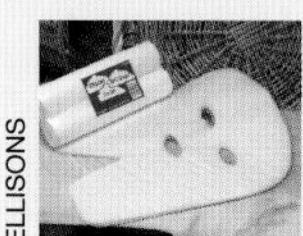
ELLISONS

Gauze
Used in applying certain masks

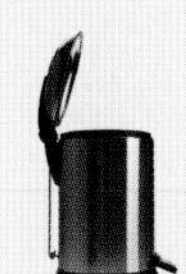

Waste bin (covered and lined)
For waste consumables

YOU WILL ALSO NEED:

Disposable tissue roll Such as bedroll

Towels (2) Freshly laundered for each client

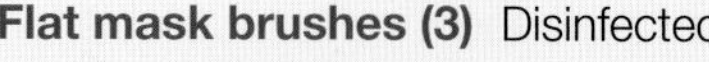

Flat mask brushes (3) Disinfected

Trolley To display all facial treatment products to be used in the facial treatment

Client's record card To record all the details relevant to the client's treatment

Facial toning lotions (a selection) To suit various types of skin

Sterilized mask-removal sponges (2) or facial mitts/ towels For use when removing the mask using clean warm water

Large bowl To hold warm water during removal of the mask

Lukewarm water If required for mask removal

Moisturisers (a range) To suit different skin types for use after mask removal

Hand mirror (clean) To show the client their skin following the facial treatment

BEST PRACTICE

Place a clean facial tissue under the edge of the headband at the forehead, so that it overlaps the headband. This will protect the headband from staining.

Don't mix the mask with the mask brush – if you do, the solid contents will tend to collect in the bristles, the mask won't be mixed effectively, and the brush won't spread the mask evenly.

Sterilization and disinfection After applying the mask, clean the mask brush thoroughly in warm water and detergent. Next, place it in a chemical disinfecting agent; rinse it in clean water; allow it to dry; and then store it in the ultra-violet cabinet.

If you use sponges to remove the mask, place them in warm water and detergent. After rinsing them in clean water, place them ready for disinfection in an autoclave. (With repeated disinfection, sponges will begin to break up.)

Thermal mitts should be washed at a temperature of 60°C.

A large high-quality cotton wool disc may be purchased to use in mask removal.

ALWAYS REMEMBER

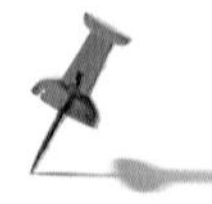

Brushes
When purchasing mask brushes, note that a plastic-handled brush is preferable to one with a painted wooden handle – the painted one would be likely to peel on immersion in water, which spoils the professional image!

Preparing the work area Check that you have all the materials you need to carry out the treatment. You may like to place a paper roll at the head of the couch, underneath the client's head, to collect any mask residue on mask removal.

The head of the couch should be flat or slightly elevated. Don't have it in a semi-reclined position during the mask application, as some masks are liquid in consistency and may run into the client's eyes and behind their neck.

HEALTH & SAFETY

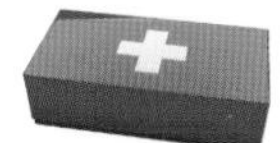

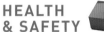

Client comfort

It is important to check that your client is comfortable while the mask is on their face. (They will suffer discomfort if their skin is intolerant to a particular mask.)

HEALTH & SAFETY

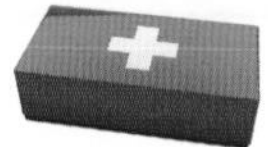

Maintaining hygiene

You need several mask brushes and mask sponges to allow effective disinfection of the tools, and so that you can provide freshly disinfected tools for each client.

Preparing the client For maximum effect, the mask must be applied on a clean, grease-free surface. If the mask application follows a facial massage, ensure that the **massage medium** has been thoroughly removed.

Select the appropriate mask ingredients to treat the skin type and the facial conditions that require attention.

How to apply and remove the mask The mask is usually applied as the *final* facial treatment, because of its cleansing, refining and soothing effects upon the skin. The methods of preparation, application and removal are different for the various face mask types, so the guidelines below are a general outline of effective treatment technique.

1 Having determined the client's treatment requirements, select the appropriate mask ingredients. If you use a commercial mask, always read the manufacturer's instructions first.

2 Discuss the treatment procedure with the client, explain:

- what the mask will feel like on application
- what sensation, if any, they will experience
- how long the mask will be left on the skin

Generally the mask will be left in place for 10–20 minutes, but the exact time depends on the client's skin type, the type of mask, the effect required and the manufacturer's instructions.

3 Prepare the mask ingredients for application.

ALWAYS REMEMBER

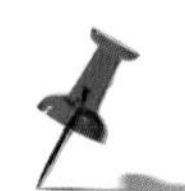

Ensure that you have plenty of dampened cotton wool – it is used to apply toner to the skin before mask application, to remove the mask or mask residue left on the skin, and to apply toner to the skin after mask removal.

Ideally, buy cotton wool discs to use for the eye pads. This will reduce preparation time and ensure an evenly shaped protective shield for the eye area.

ALWAYS REMEMBER

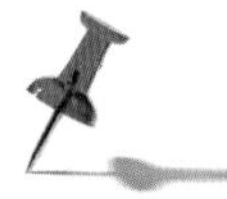

Paraffin wax
If you are using paraffin wax, remember to heat it in advance.

HEALTH & SAFETY

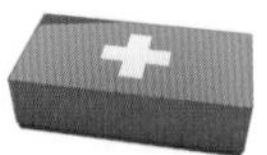

Allergies
When using a commercial mask, try to find out *exactly* what it contains, so that you don't apply a sensitizing ingredient to an allergic skin type.

Setting masks
When using a setting mask, ensure that the mask is evenly applied or it will dry unevenly.

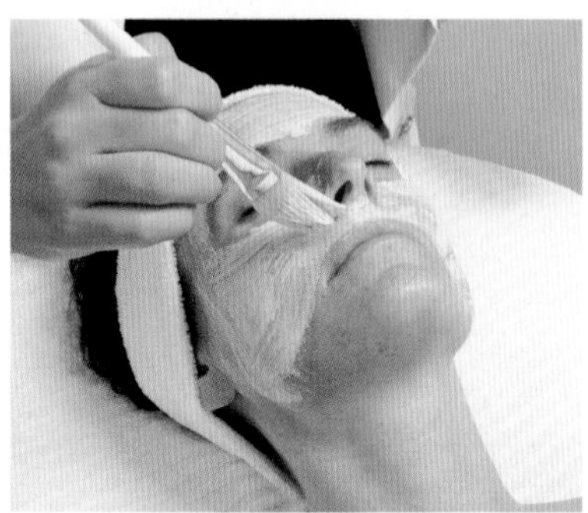

Applying a mask with a brush

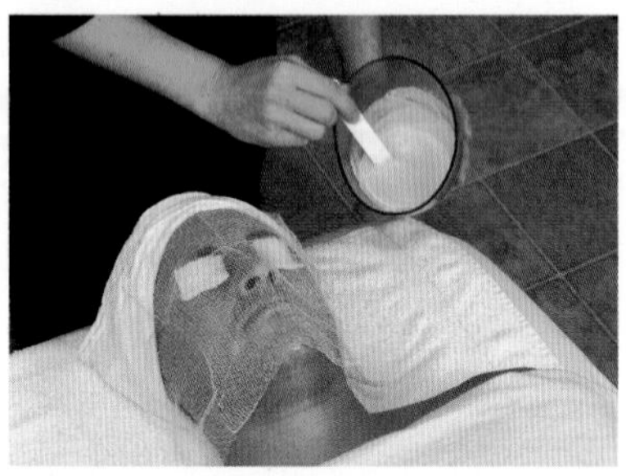

Mask application over gauze

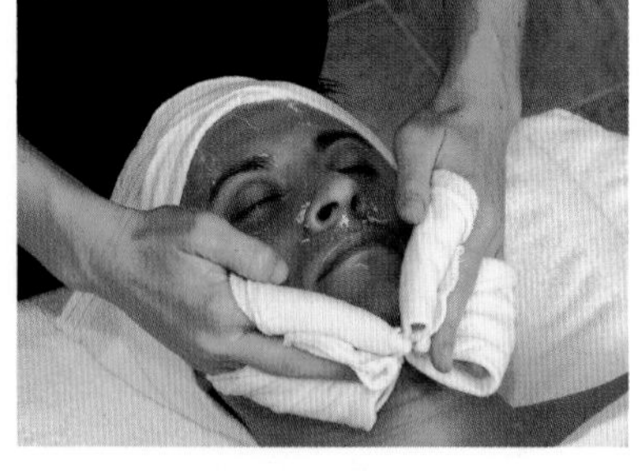

Removing the mask with damp towels

4. Using the sterilized mask brush or spatula, begin to apply the mask. The usual sequence of mask application is neck, chin, cheeks, nose and forehead.

   If you are using more than one mask to treat different skin conditions, apply the one that will need to be on longest first to achieve maximum benefit.

   Apply the mask quickly and evenly so that it has maximum effect on the whole face. Don't apply it too thickly; as well as making mask removal difficult, this is wasteful as only the part that is in contact with the skin has any effect.

   Keep the mask clear of the nostrils, the lips, the eyebrows and the hairline.

5. To relax the client, apply cotton wool eye pads dampened with clean water.
6. Leave the mask for the recommended time or according to the effect required. Take account also of the sensitivity of the skin and your client's comfort.
7. Wash your hands.
8. When the mask is ready for removal, remove the eye pads.

   Explain to the client that you are going to remove the mask. Briefly describe the process, according to whether this is a setting or a non-setting mask.

   Remove the mask using an appropriate technique, e.g. mask removal sponges. Some beauty salons use a warm towel method in which towels are steamed to make them hot and damp and then they wrapped around the face and then used to gently wipe away the mask.

9. When the mask has been completely removed, apply the appropriate toning lotion using dampened cotton wool. Blot the skin dry with a facial tissue.
10. Apply an appropriate moisturiser to the skin.
11. Remove the headband and tidy the client's hair.
12. With a mirror, show the client their skin. Evaluate the treatment.
13. Record the results on their record card.

Contra-actions Before you apply the mask, explain to the client what the action of the mask will feel like on the skin. This will enable them to identify any undesirable skin reaction, evident to them as skin irritation – a burning sensation.

Ask the client initially whether they are comfortable: this will give them the opportunity to tell you if they are experiencing any discomfort. Should there be a contra-action to the mask, remove the mask immediately and apply a soothing skincare product.

If on removal of the mask you can see that there has been an unwanted skin reaction (that is, if you see inflammation), apply a soothing skincare product. In either case, note the skin reaction on the record card, and choose a different mask next time.

Advice on home use The client may be given a sample of the face mask for use at home. Explain to them the procedure for application and removal, so that they achieve maximum benefit from the mask. Encourage them to purchase a suitable mask for their skin type and condition to apply at home once or twice a week, depending on their skin type, to dislodge dead skin cells and to cleanse and stimulate the skin. The suitability of the mask must be reviewed periodically dependent upon the client's skin needs and environmental and lifestyle factors.

Advise the client not to apply the mask directly before a special occasion, in case it causes blemishes, as sometimes happens.

The skin should be toned and moisturised after removing the mask.

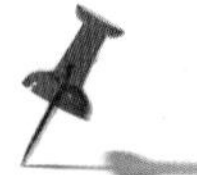

ALWAYS REMEMBER

Mask removal
When using water to remove a mask you may need to renew the water as you work to ensure effective removal.

Facial massage

Manual massage is the external manipulation, using the hands, of the soft tissues of the face, neck and upper chest. Massage can improve the appearance of the skin and promote a sensation of stimulation or relaxation.

Each massage performed is adapted to the client's physiological and psychological needs. The skin's physiological needs are observed during the skin analysis; the client's psychological needs are usually discovered during the consultation.

The benefits of the facial massage include the following:

- Dead epidermal cells are loosened and shed. This improves the appearance of the skin, exposing fresh, younger cells.
- The muscles receive an improved supply of oxygenated blood, essential for cell growth. The tone and strength of the muscles are improved, firming the facial contour.
- The increased blood circulation in the area warms the tissues. This induces a feeling of relaxation, which is particularly beneficial when treating tense muscles.
- As the blood capillaries dilate and bring blood to the skin's surface, the skin colour improves.
- The lymphatic circulation and the venous blood circulation increase. These changes speed up the removal of waste products and toxins, and tend therefore to purify the skin. The removal of excess lymph improves the appearance of a puffy oedematous skin (provided that this does not require medical treatment).
- The increased temperature of the skin relaxes the pores and follicles. This aids the absorption of the massage product, which in turn softens the skin.
- Sensory nerves can be soothed or stimulated, depending on the massage manipulations selected.
- Massage stimulates the sebaceous and sudoriferous glands and increases the production of sebum and sweat. This increase helps to maintain the skin's natural oil and moisture balance.

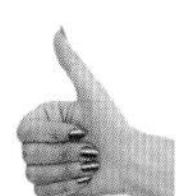

BEST PRACTICE

While the mask is on the face you can tidy the working area and collect together the materials required for mask removal. Do not disturb the client, who will be relaxing at this time. A hand massage may also be offered.

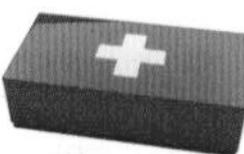

HEALTH & SAFETY

Peel-off masks
When using a peel-off mask, make sure that the border of the mask is thick enough – if it isn't, it will be difficult to remove and the client may experience discomfort.

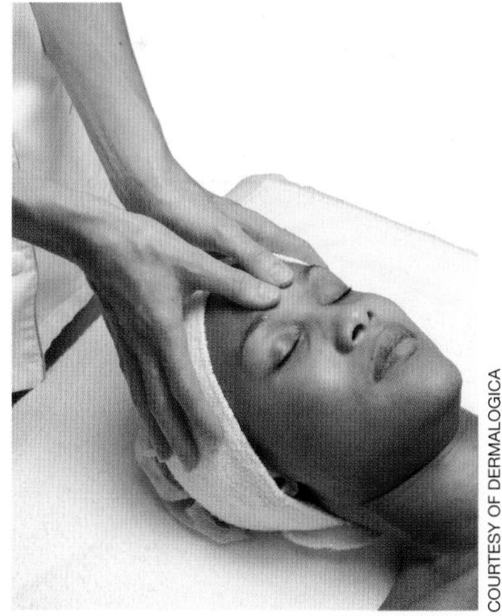

Facial massage

Reception

Facial massage is carried out as required, usually once every four to six weeks. Before the facial massage is given, the skin is cleansed; afterwards it is usual to apply a face mask, which absorbs any excess massage medium from the skin or can enhance further the skin nourishing effect of the treatment.

When booking a client for this treatment, allow one hour. The facial massage itself should take approximately 20 minutes, but this may vary according to the client's skin type.

Warn the client that the skin may appear slightly red and blotchy after the treatment, due to the increase in blood circulation to the area: this reaction will normally subside after four to six hours. If it does not the client should be advised to contact the salon for further guidance.

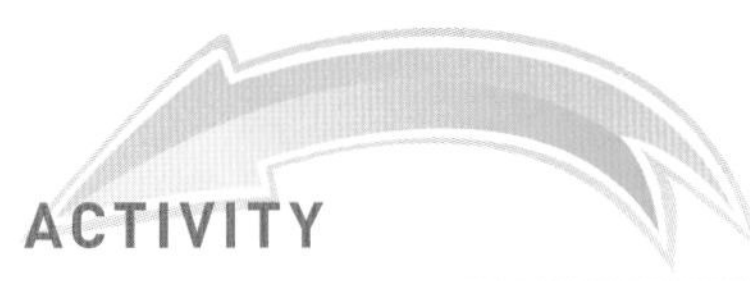

ACTIVITY

Planning a massage
How will observations from the skin analysis and the client consultation influence the facial massage treatment?

ALWAYS REMEMBER

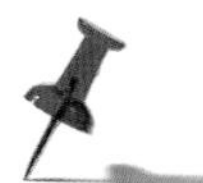

Client care
The headband can spoil the hair, and the massage medium may enter the hairline. Recommend that the client does not style their hair directly before the facial treatment.

BEST PRACTICE

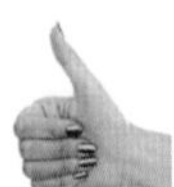

Neck and shoulders
Pressure may be increased when working on larger muscles in the neck or shoulders, especially if the client has tension in this area.

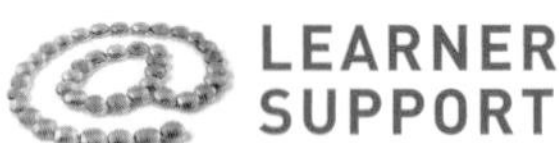

LEARNER SUPPORT

Facial skincare: mini crossword

Because of the stimulating effect on the skin recommend to the client that they receive this treatment when they do not have to apply any cosmetic products directly afterwards.

Sometimes the skin develops small blemishes after facial massage; this is due to its cleansing action. If the client is preparing for a special occasion, therefore, such as a wedding, make the appointment for at least five days in advance.

Massage manipulations

The facial massage is based on a series of classic massage movements, each with different effects. There are four basic groups of massage movements:

- effleurage
- petrissage
- percussion (also known as tapotement)
- vibrations

The therapist can adapt the way each of these movements is applied, according to the needs of the client. Either the *speed of application* or the *depth of pressure* can be altered.

Effleurage **Effleurage** is a stroking movement, used to begin the massage, as a link manipulation, and to complete the massage sequence. This manipulation is light, has an even pressure, and is applied in a rhythmical, continuous manner to induce relaxation.

The pressure of application varies according to the underlying structures and the tissue type, but it must *never* be unduly heavy.

Effleurage has these effects:

- desquamation is increased
- arterial blood circulation is increased, bringing fresh nutrients to the area
- venous circulation is improved, aiding the removal of congestion from the veins
- lymphatic circulation is increased, improving the absorption of waste products
- the underlying muscle fibres are relaxed

Uses in treatment: to relax tight, contracted muscles.

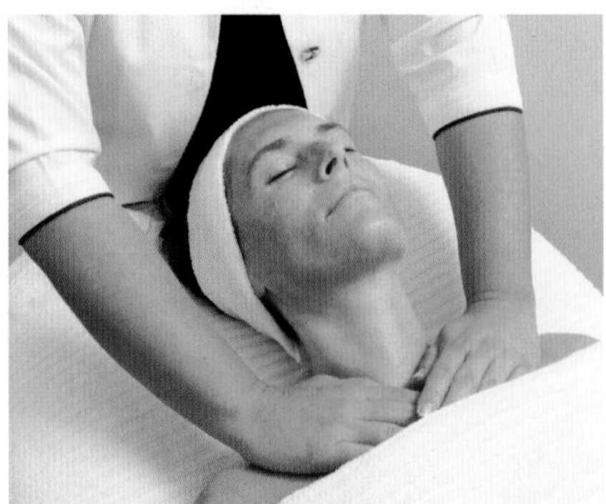

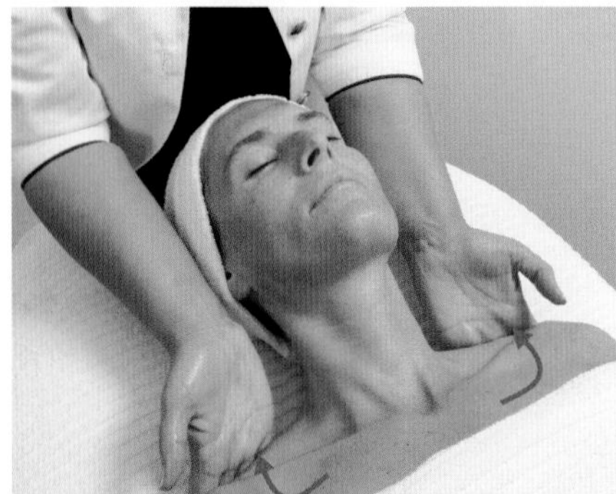

Effleurage

Petrissage **Petrissage** involves a series of movements in which the tissues are lifted away from the underlying structures and compressed. Pressure is intermittent, and should be light yet firm.

Petrissage has these effects:

- improvement of muscle tone, through the compression and relaxation of muscle fibres
- improvement in blood and lymph circulation, as the application of pressure causes the vessels to empty and fill
- increased activity of the sebaceous gland, due to the stimulation

Movements include picking up, kneading, knuckling, pinching, rolling frictions and scissoring.

Uses in treatment: to stimulate a sluggish circulation; to increase sebaceous gland and sudoriferous gland activity when treating a dry skin condition.

BEST PRACTICE

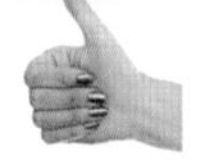

Stimulation
When a stimulating massage is required, incorporate more petrissage and tapotement into the massage sequence.

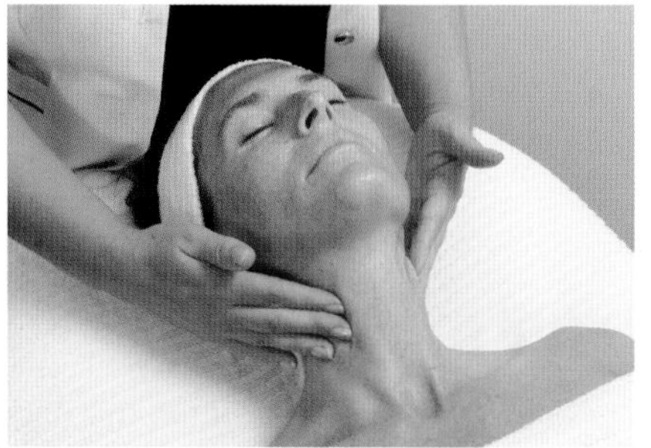

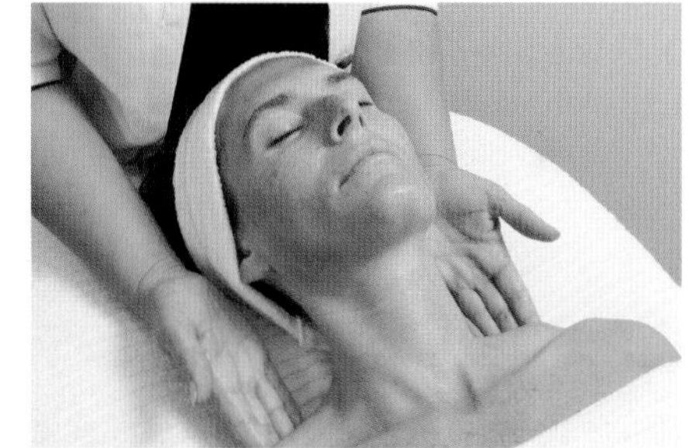

Petrissage

Percussion Percussion, also known as **tapotement**, is performed in a brisk, stimulating manner. Rhythm is important as the fingers are continually breaking contact with the skin; irritation could occur if the movement were performed incorrectly

Percussion has these effects:

- a fast vascular reaction because of the skin's nervous response to the stimulus – this reaction, **erythema**, has a stimulating effect
- increased blood supply, which nourishes the tissues
- improvement in muscle and skin tone in the area

Movements include clapping and tapping. In facial massage, only light tapping should be used.

Uses in treatment: to tone areas of loose, crepey skin around the jaw or eyes.

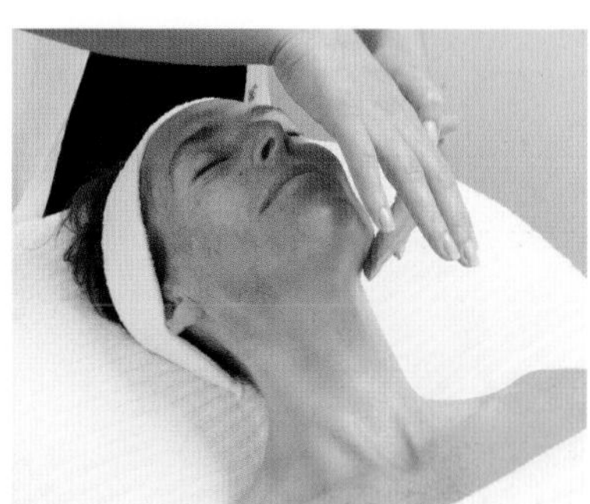

Percussion

Vibrations **Vibrations** are applied on the nerve centre. They are produced by a rapid contraction and relaxation of the muscles of the therapist's arm, resulting in a fine trembling movement.

Vibration has these effects:

- stimulation of the nerves, inducing a feeling of wellbeing
- gentle stimulation of the skin

Movements include *static* vibrations, in which the pads of the fingers are placed on the nerve, and the vibratory effect created by the therapist's arms and hands is applied in one position; and *running* vibrations, in which the vibratory effect is applied along a nerve path.

Uses in treatment: to stimulate a sensitive skin in order to improve the skin's functioning without irritating the surface blood capillaries.

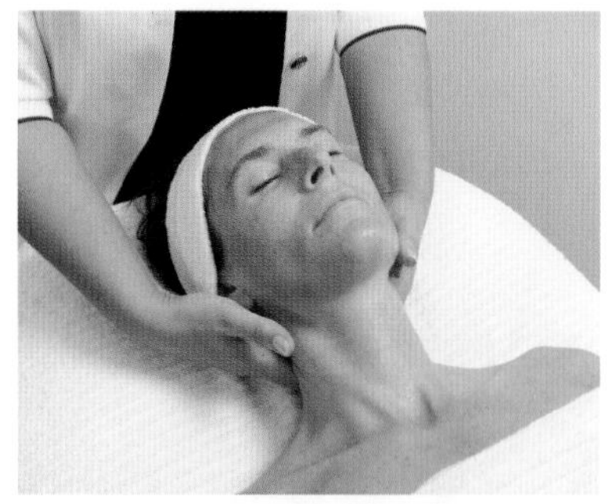

Vibrations

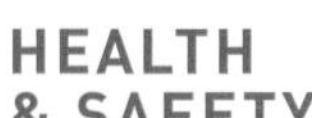

HEALTH & SAFETY

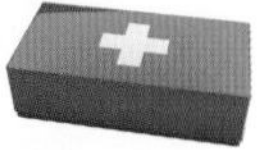

Contra-indications
Do not apply percussion over highly sensitive or vascular skin conditions to avoid excessively increasing blood circulation in the area and over-stimulating the skin.

TOP TIP

Posture

It is important to maintain good posture during facial massage. If you slouch, you will experience muscle fatigue and long-term postural problems!

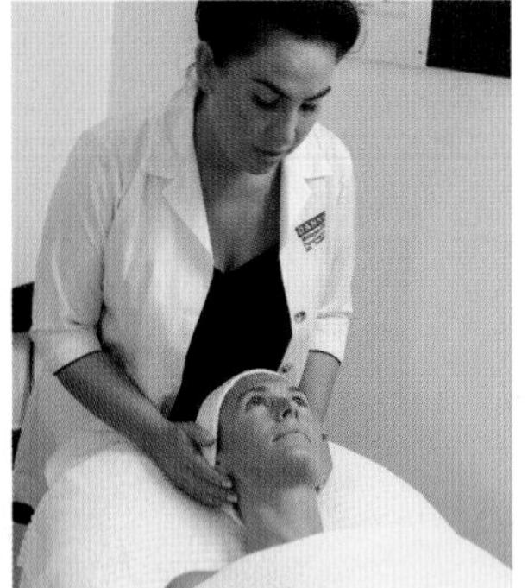

Beauty therapist working position

Equipment and materials

The massage is carried out using a **massage medium** that acts as a lubricant. A massage cream or oil may be used; these are slightly penetrating, and soften the skin. Choose a product that contains ingredients to suit the client's skin type and the age of the skin.

Whichever product you choose, it should provide sufficient slip while allowing you to control the massage movements.

ACTIVITY

Choosing a massage medium

Compare two professional skincare ranges. Look at:

- the choice of facial-massage preparations
- the ingredients used in their formulation, and the effects claimed

Step-by-step: Massage treatment

There are many different massage sequences, but each uses one or all of the massage manipulations discussed above. What follows is a basic sequence for facial massage.

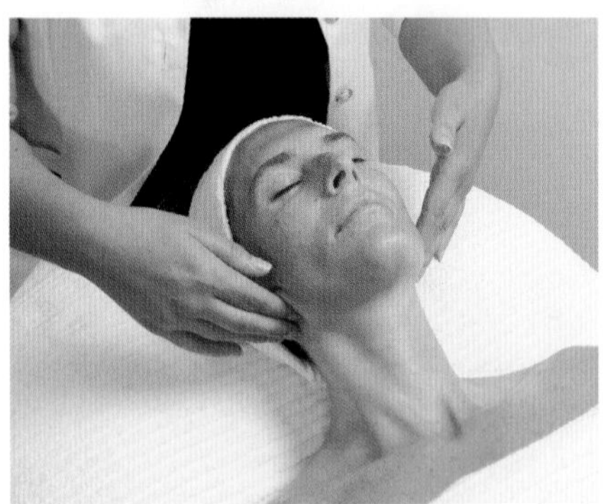

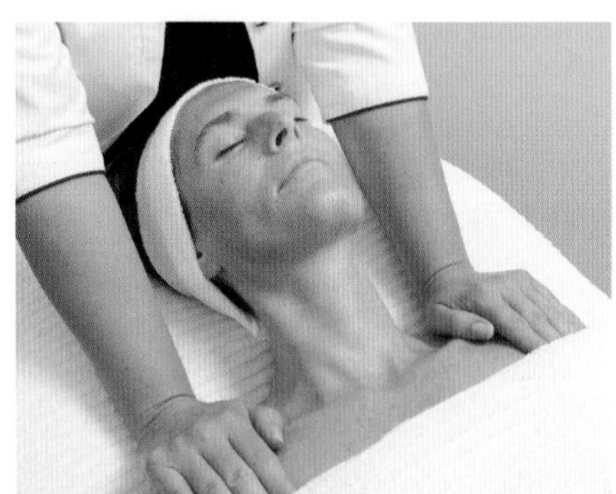

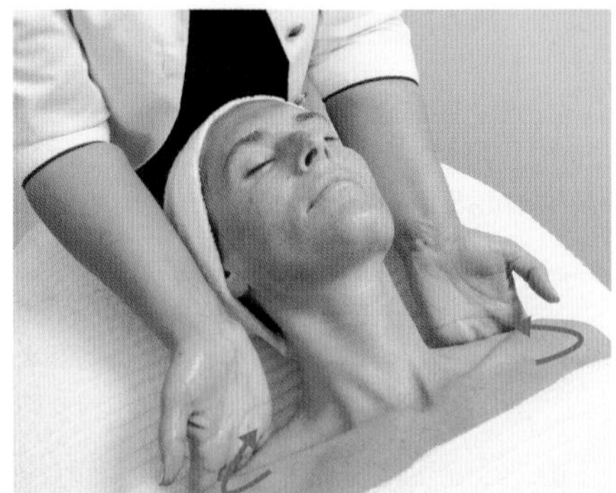

1 **Effleurage to the neck and shoulders** Slide the hands down the neck, across the pectoral muscles around the deltoid muscle, and across the trapezius muscle. Slide the hands up the back of the neck to the base of the skull.

Repeat step 1 a further 5 times.

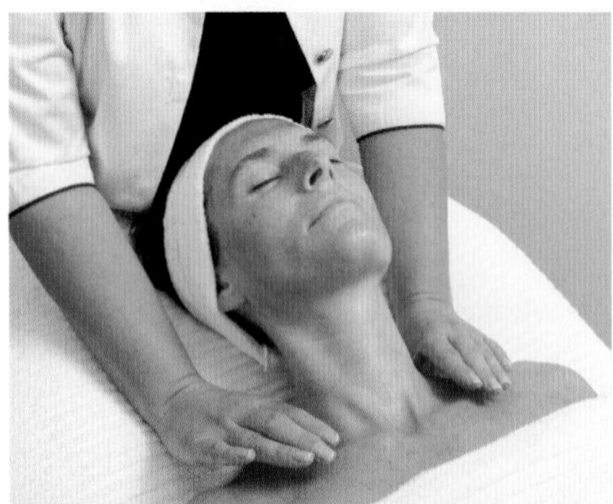

2 **Thumb kneading to the shoulders** Using the pad of both thumbs, make small circles (frictions) along the trapezius muscle, working towards the spinal vertebrae.

Apply each movement 3 times; then repeat the sequence (step 2) a further 2 times.

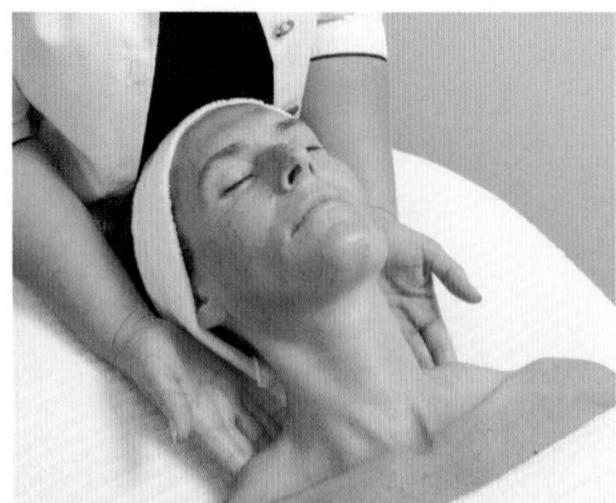

3 **Finger kneading to the shoulders** Position the fingers of each hand behind the deltoid, and make large rotary movements along the trapezius.

Apply each rotary movement 3 times; repeat the sequence (step 3) a further 2 times.

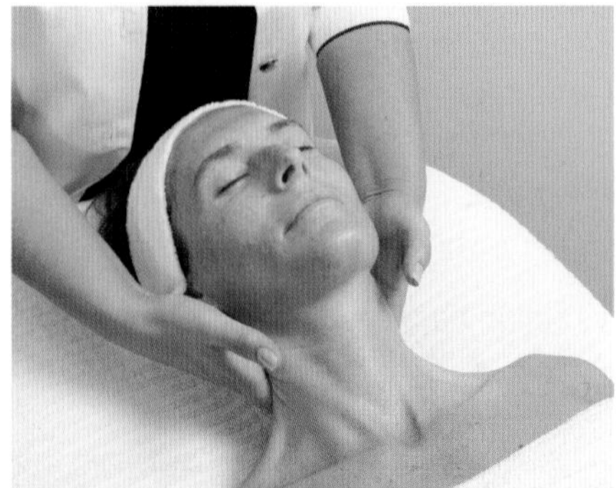

4 **Vibrations** Place the hands, cupped, at the base of the neck: perform running vibrations up the neck to the occipital bone.

Repeat step 4 a further 6 times.

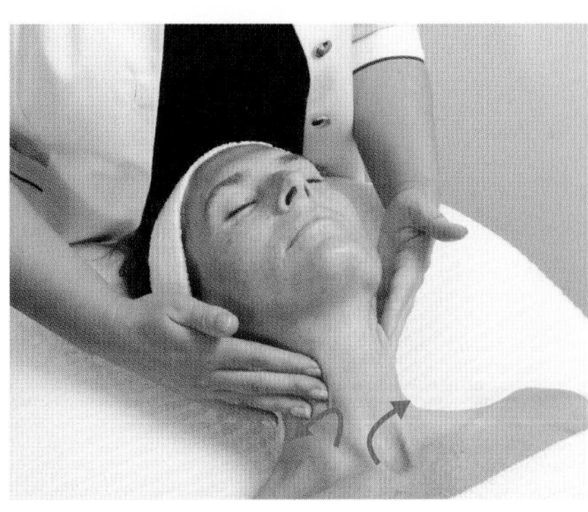

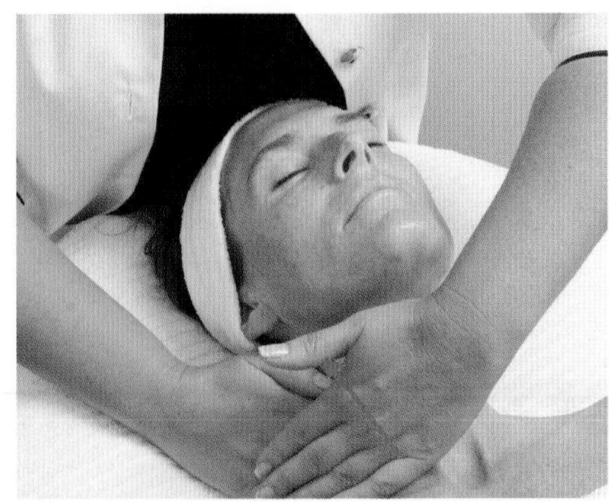

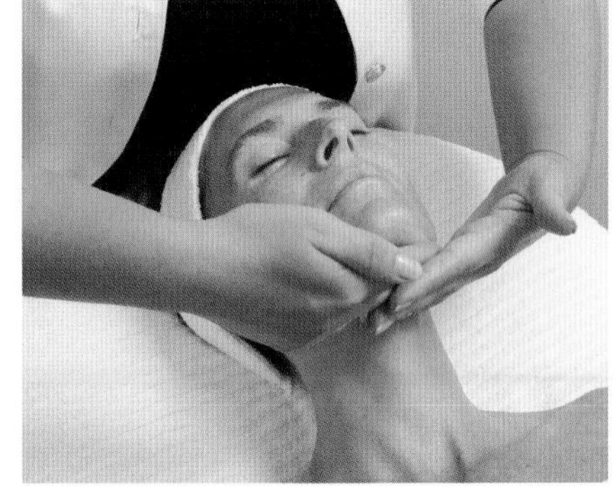

5 **Circular massage to the neck** Perform small circular movements over the platysma and the sternomastoid muscle at the neck.

6 **Hands cupped to the neck** Cup your hands together. Place the hands at the left side of the neck, above the clavicle. Slide the hands up the side of the neck, across the jaw line, and down the right side of the neck; then reverse.

Repeat step 6 a further 2 times.

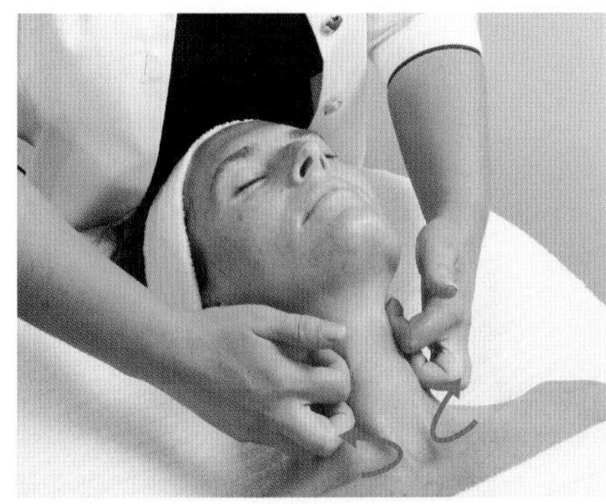

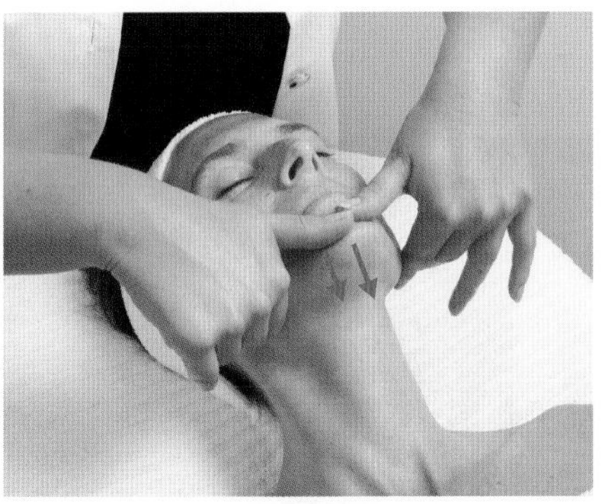

7 **Knuckling to the neck** Make a loose fist: rotate the knuckles up and down the neck area.

Repeat step 7 to cover, a further 2 times.

8 **Up and under** Place the thumbs on the centre of the chin, and the index and middle fingers under the mandible. Slide the thumbs firmly over the chin. Bring the index finger onto the chin, and place the middle finger under the mandible forming a V shape. Slide along the jaw line to the ear. Replace the index finger with the thumb, and return along the jaw to the chin.

Repeat step 8 a further 5 times.

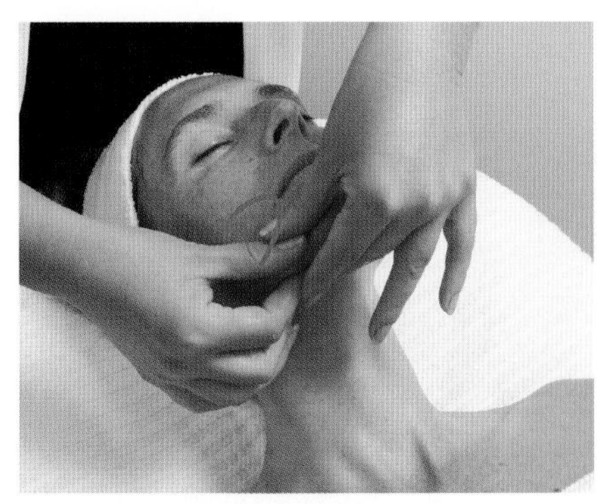

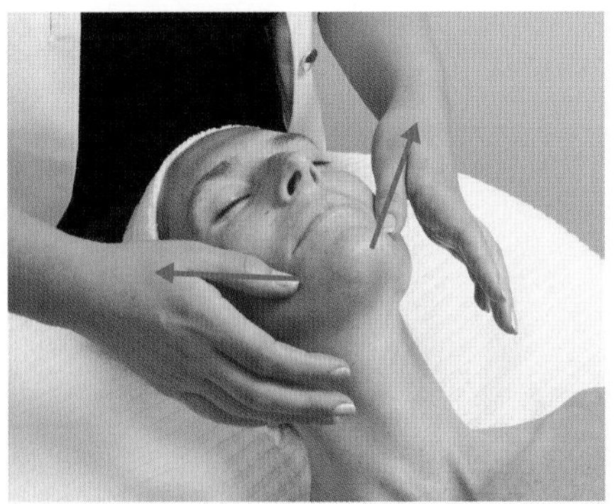

9 **Circling to the mandible** Place the thumbs one above the other on the chin, and proceed with circular kneading along the jaw line towards the ear. Reverse and repeat.

Repeat step 9 a further 2 times.

10 **Flick-ups** Place the thumbs at the corners of the mouth. Lift the orbicularis oris muscle, with a flicking action of the thumbs.

Repeat step 10 a further 5 times.

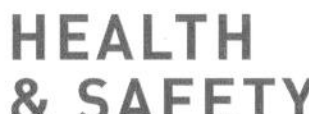

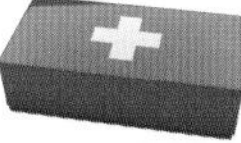

HEALTH & SAFETY

The trachea

Never apply pressure when working on the neck over the trachea area, which could cause discomfort.

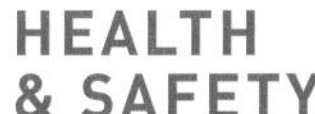

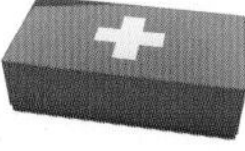

HEALTH & SAFETY

Sensitive skin

Do not use knuckling on sensitive skin to avoid over-stimulation.

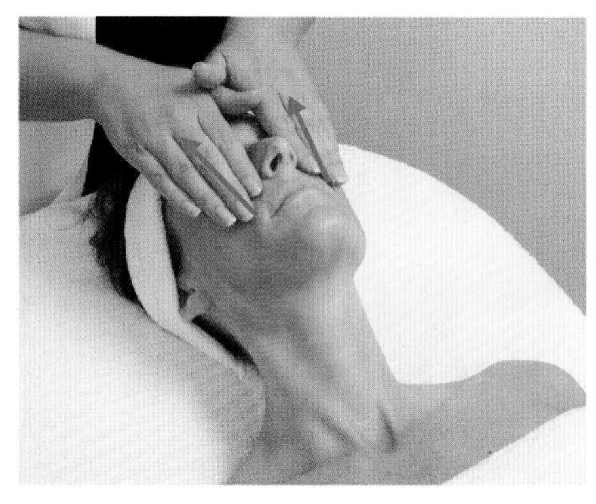

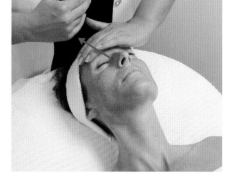

11 Half face brace Clasp the fingers under the chin; turn the hands so that the fingers point towards the sternum. Unclasp, and slide the hands up the face towards the forehead.

Repeat step 11 a further 2 times.

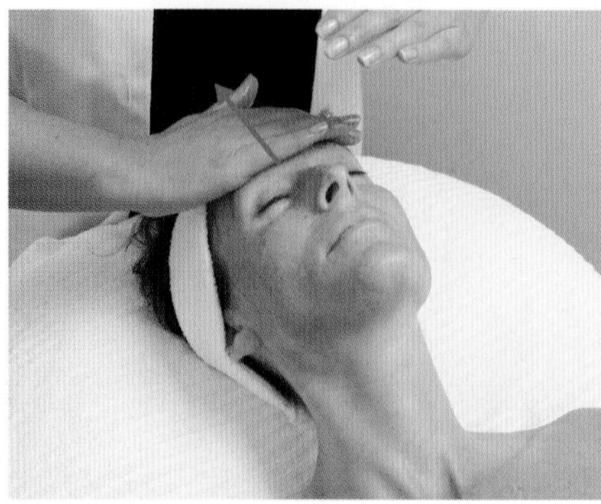

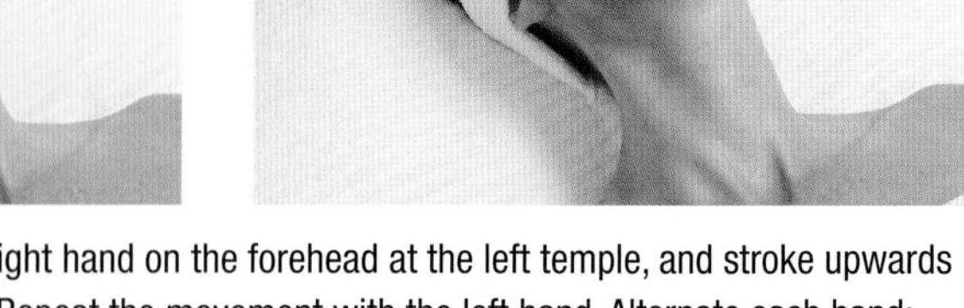

12 Lifting the eyebrows Place the right hand on the forehead at the left temple, and stroke upwards from the eyebrow to the hairline. Repeat the movement with the left hand. Alternate each hand; repeat the movement across the forehead.

Repeat step 12 a further 2 times.

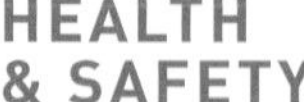

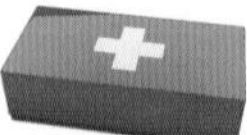

HEALTH & SAFETY

Massage manipulation 'flick-ups': the lips

Do not flick the lips. Position the thumbs 5mm from the corner of the mouth to avoid this.

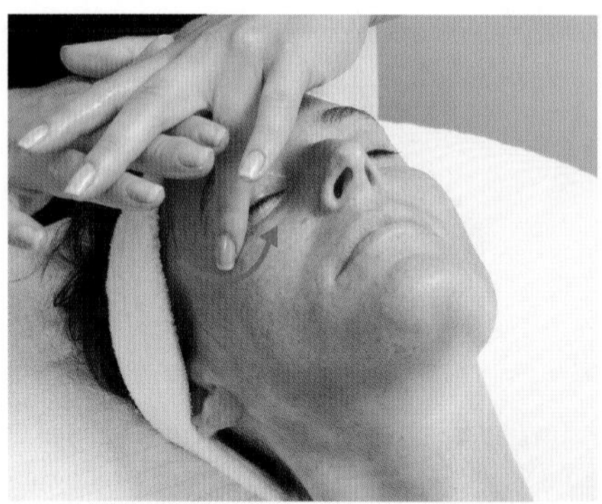

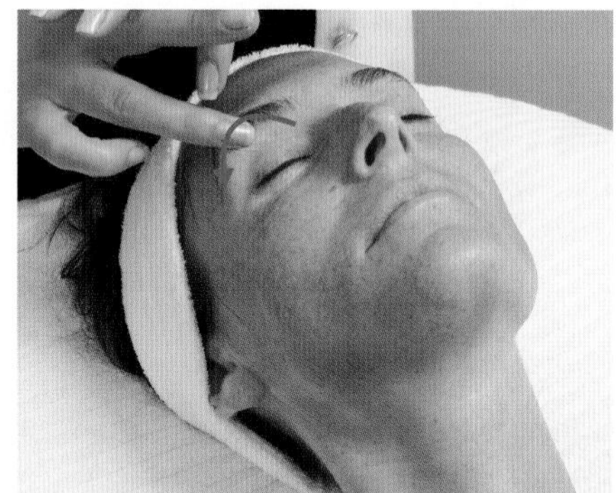

13 Inner and outer eye circles Using the ring finger, *gently* draw 3 outer circles and 3 inner circles on each eye, following the fibre direction of the orbicularis oculi muscle.

Repeat step 13 a further 2 times.

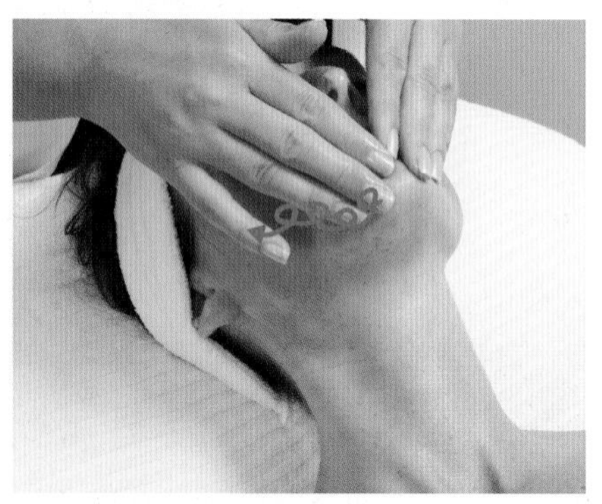

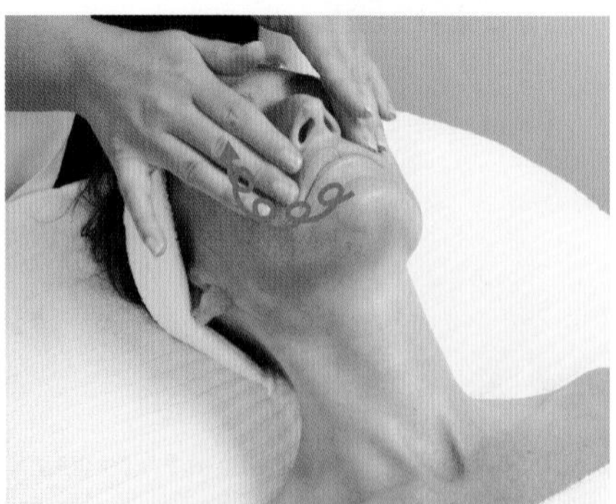

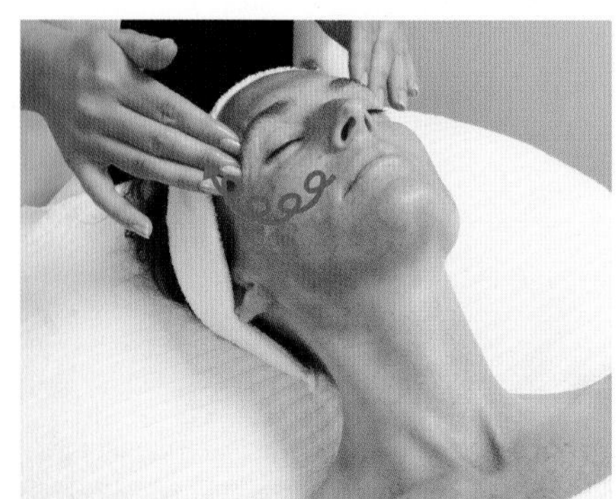

15 Circling to the chin, the nose and the temples Apply circular kneading to the chin, the nose and the temples. Return to the starting position.

Repeat step 15 a further 2 times.

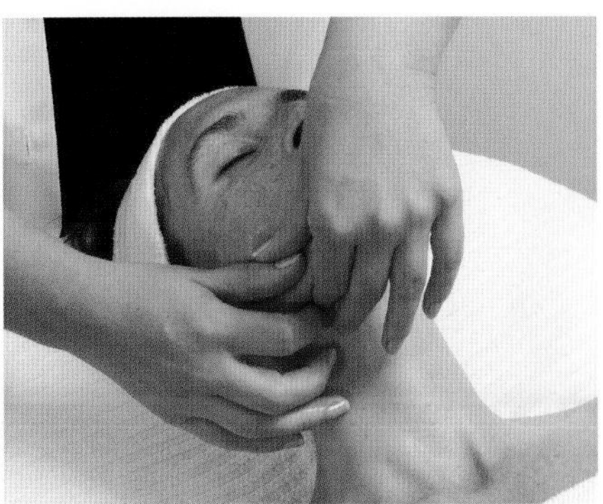

16 Thumb kneading under the cheeks Place the thumbs under the zygomatic bones. Carry out a circular kneading over the muscles in the cheek area.

Repeat step 16 a further 5 times.

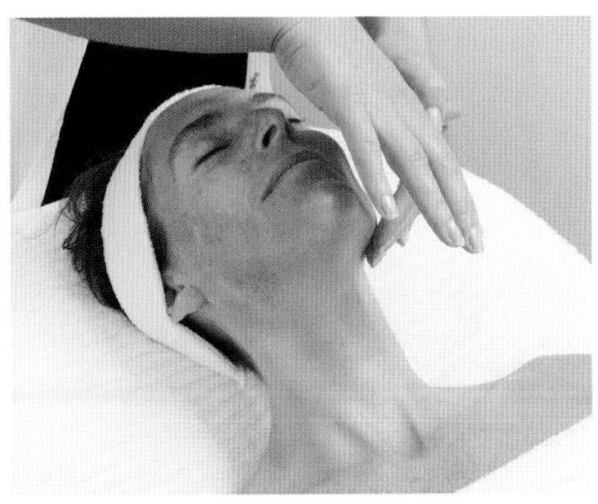

17 Tapping under the mandible Tap the tissue under the mandible, using the fingers of both hands. Work from the left side of the jaw to the right; then reverse.

Repeat step 17 a further 5 times.

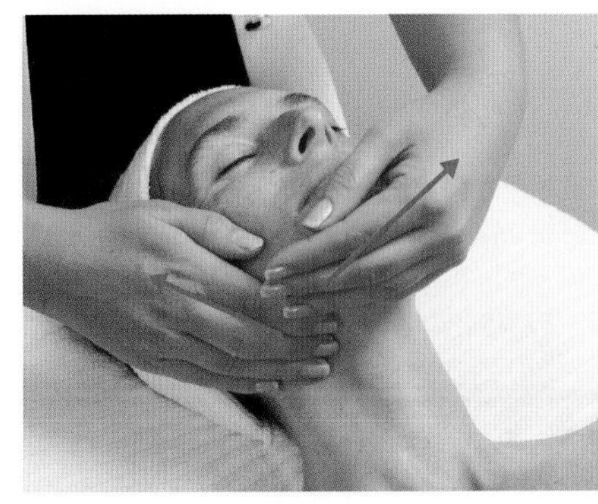

18 Lifting the masseter Cup the hands. Using the hands alternately, lift the masseter muscle.

Repeat step 18 a further 5 times.

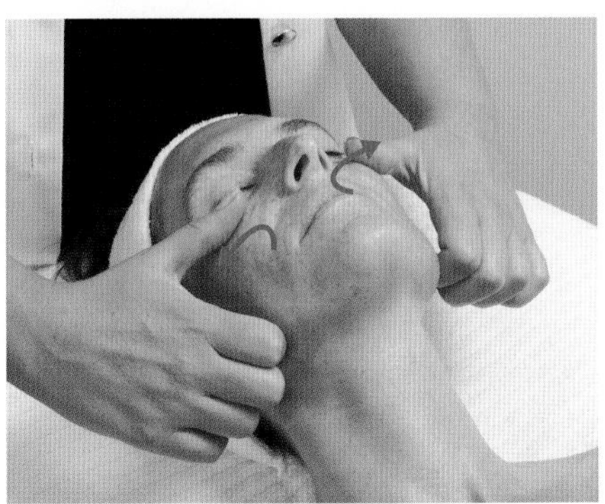

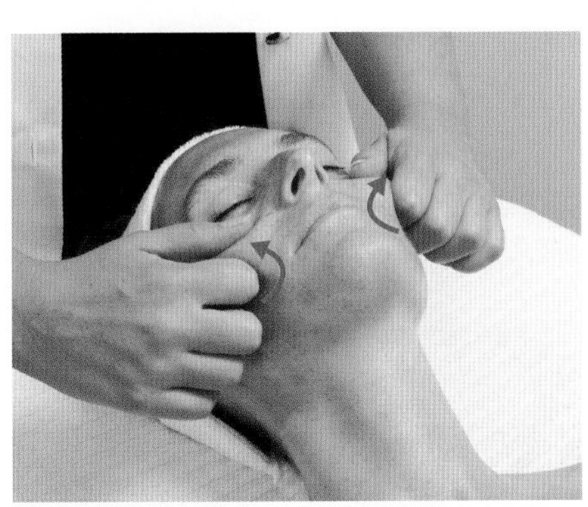

19 Rolling and pinching Using a deep rolling movement, draw the muscles of the cheek area towards the thumb in a rolling and pinching movement.

Repeat step 19 a further 5 times.

HEALTH & SAFETY

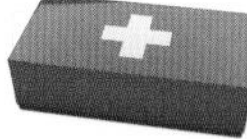

Sensitive skin

Avoid the use of tapotement over areas of sensitivity.

ALWAYS REMEMBER

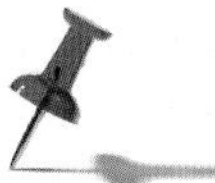

Massage medium

If the skin appears to drag during massage, stop and apply more massage medium. If you keep going you may cause skin irritation or discomfort.

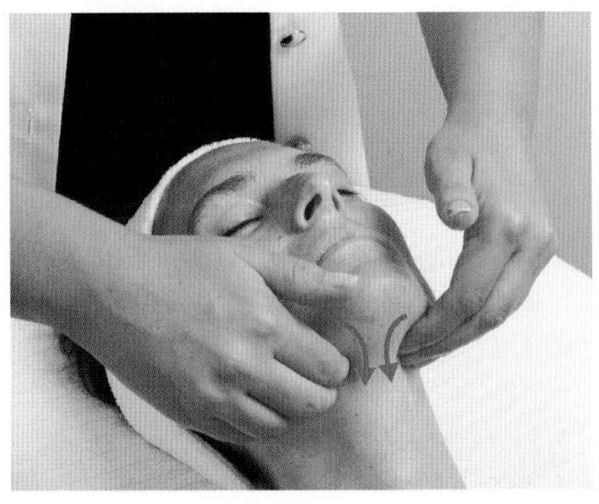

20 Lifting the mandible Place the pads of the fingers underneath the mandible and pivot diagonally. Lifting the tissues work towards the ear.

Repeat step 20 a further 2 times.

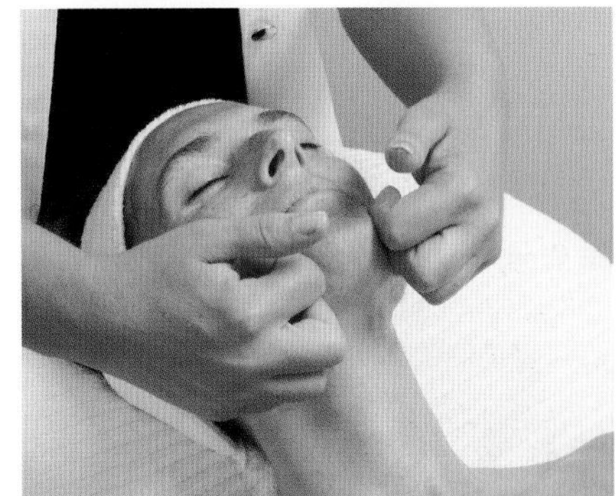

21 Knuckling along the jaw line Knuckle along the jaw line and over the cheek area.

Repeat step 21 a further 2 times.

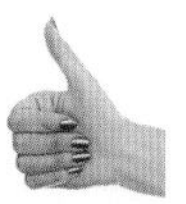

BEST PRACTICE

During the facial massage, the client's face should relax. If there are evident signs of tension, such as vertical furrows between the eyebrows, check that the client is warm and comfortable.

ACTIVITY

Hand and wrist mobility exercises

Devise ten exercises to increase the strength and mobility of your hands and wrists.

ACTIVITY

Massage at home

Design a simple massage routine that a client could be taught to use at home.

Which type of manipulation is involved in each movement in your sequence? What effect do you wish to achieve by incorporating it?

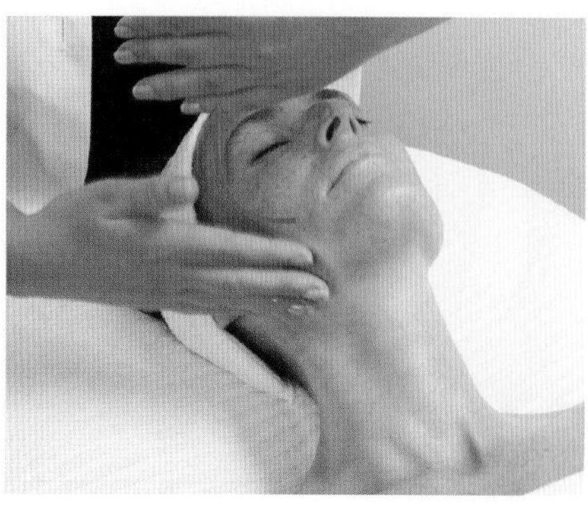

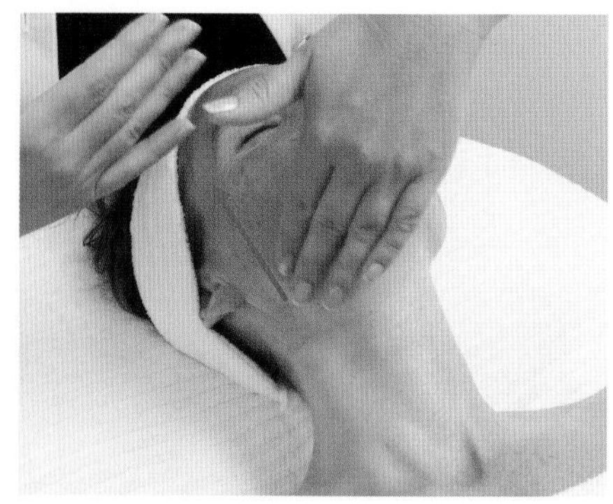

22 Upwards tapping on the face Using both hands, gently slap along the jaw line from ear to ear, lifting the muscles.

Repeat step 22 a further 5 times.

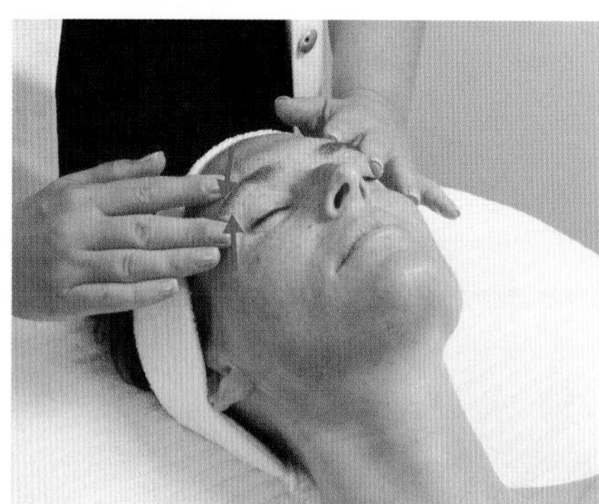

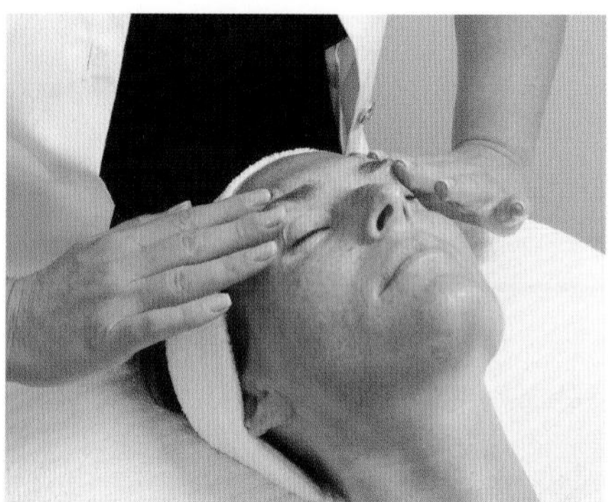

24 Scissor movement to the forehead Open the index and middle fingers to make a V shape at the outer corner of each eyebrow. Open and close the fingers in a scissor action towards the inner eyebrow.

Repeat step 24 a further 2 times.

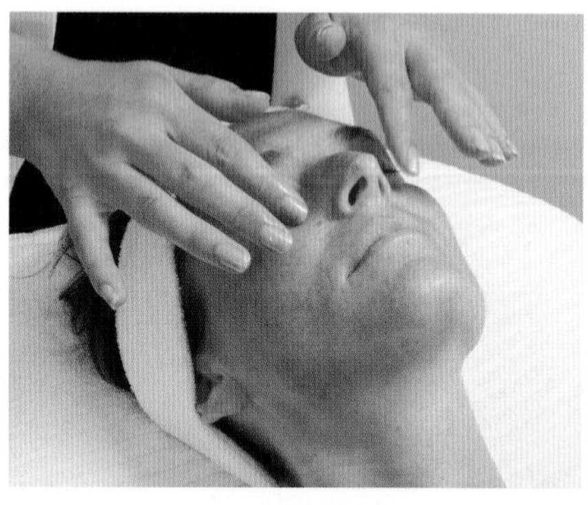

25 Tapotement movement around the eyes Using the pads of the fingers, tap gently around the eye area.

Repeat step 25 a further 2 times.

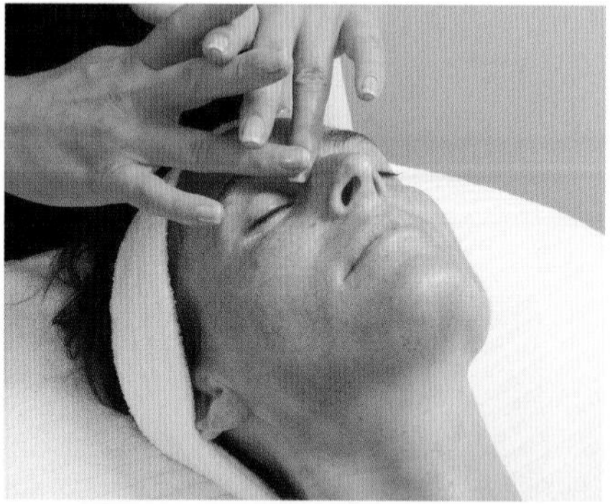

26 Eye circling *Repeat step 13, a further 3 times.*

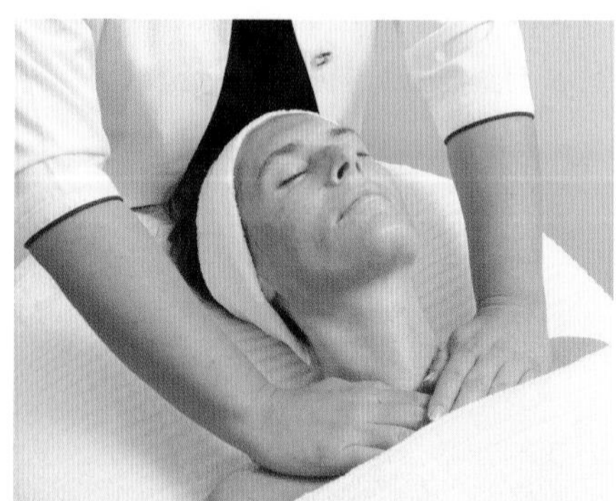

27 Apply effleurage to the neck and shoulders to complete the massage service.

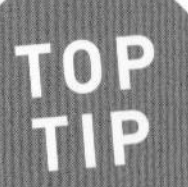

TOP TIP

Practise

When learning the facial massage you need to practise. Practise the movements on a Styrofoam® head block with facial features, or mannequin head as used in hairdressing, to perfect the manipulations. If these are unavailable, practise each manipulation on your knee – this will increase the agility and strength of your fingers and wrists.

After the massage

After the facial massage, remove the massage medium thoroughly using clean, damp cotton wool, facial mitts or towels. Check thoroughly that all product has been removed.

Apply toner to remove any traces of massage medium, leaving the skin grease-free. Finally, blot the skin dry.

You may then proceed with further skin treatments, such as a face mask, or simply apply an appropriate moisturiser to conclude the treatment.

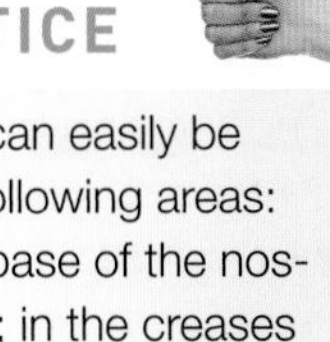

BEST PRACTICE

Massage medium can easily be overlooked in the following areas: the eyebrows; the base of the nostrils; under the chin; in the creases of the neck; behind the ear and on the shoulders. Ensure all massage medium is thoroughly removed.

Advice on home care

Encourage your client to use massage movements when applying emollient skincare products. Show them how to perform such movements correctly.

Facial exercises may be given to the client to practise at home. These should be carried out at least four times per week.

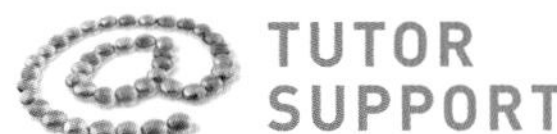

TUTOR SUPPORT

Activity 7: Facial treatment wordsearch

Specialist facial treatments

Specialist treatments should be offered to your client when there is a specific need or if they feel they would like to benefit from such a treatment. Specialist training in these advanced techniques is usually offered by the main product companies.

ACTIVITY

What products may you recommend a client uses as part of their home care routine?

Need more time... refer to page 209 to help you.

Aftercare

Aftercare and advice is discussed throughout the chapter in relation to each of the facial treatment procedures.

At the conclusion of your facial treatment ensure that you have covered the following in your **aftercare advice**:

- checked that the treatment has been completed to the satisfaction of the client
- explained what products have been used in the facial treatment and why
- advised what products would be suitable for the client to use at home, a basic home care routine, to gain maximum benefit from the treatment
- advised on product application and removal, again in order to gain maximum benefit from their use
- provided contra-action advice, i.e., action to be taken in the event of an unwanted skin reaction for contra-actions (including severe erythema, swelling, allergic reactions to products and tissue damage resulting in blood loss)
- suggested lifestyle changes that may improve the overall condition and appearance of the skin, e.g. the importance of a healthy regular diet and adequate water consumption (refer to pages 170–173 for guidance on caring for and avoiding threats to the skin)
- discussed the use of make-up following treatment (only eye and lip make-up should be worn directly after a facial treatment; allow up to eight hours before make-up application to avoid congestion of the stimulated, cleansed skin)
- explained the recommended time intervals between treatments

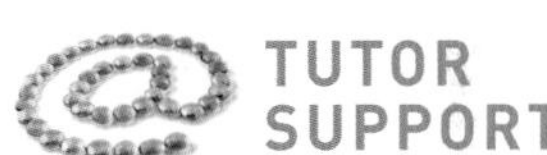

TUTOR SUPPORT

Activity 9: Multiple choice quiz

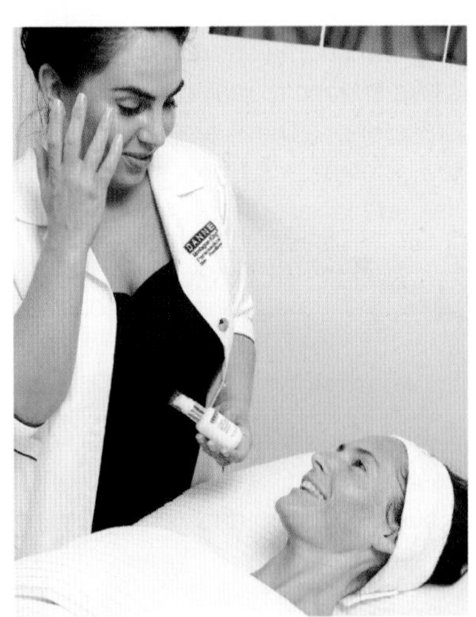

Home care routine advice

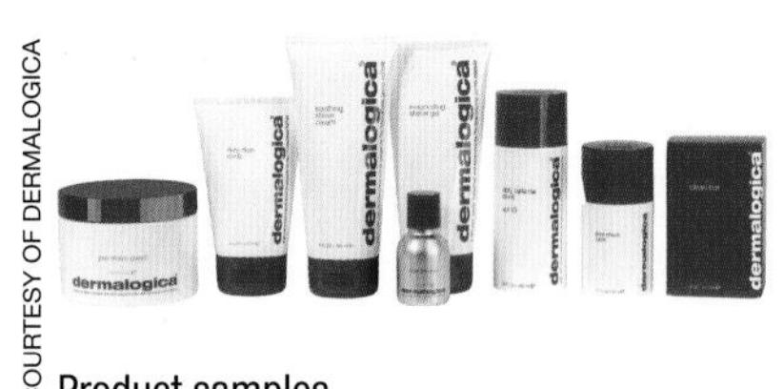

COURTESY OF DERMALOGICA

Product samples

- provided guidance on what further treatments you would recommend to maintain or improve further the facial skin condition in written form or verbal form
- discussed if product samples are to be provided, when and how they are to be used
- provided the opportunity for the client to ask any further questions

Update and record all details on the client record card, including products purchased. You can discuss their effectiveness at the next facial treatment.

Take the client to the reception to book their next appointment if required.

GLOSSARY OF KEY WORDS

Acid mantle the combination of sweat and sebum on the skin's surface, creating an acid film. The acid mantle is protective and discourages the growth of bacteria and fungi. The pH scale is used to measure the acidity or alkalinity of a substance using a numbered scale. The skin's pH is acid at 5.5–5.6.

Aftercare advice recommended advice given to the client following treatment to continue and enhance the benefits of the treatment.

Antioxidant properties of some foods that maintain the health of the skin, fighting the damaging effects of free radicals (unstable molecules which can cause skin cells to degenerate) in the body. Antioxidant ingredients are increasingly being included in skincare preparations to neutralize free radicals or repel them from the skin.

Cleanser a skincare preparation that removes dead skin cells, excess sweat and sebum, make-up and dirt from the skin's surface to maintain a healthy skin complexion. These are formulated to treat the different skin types, skin characteristics and facial areas.

Comedone removal facial techniques used to extract comedones (blackheads) from the skin. A small tool called a comedone extractor is used for this purpose.

Consultation assessment of client's needs using different assessment techniques, including questioning and natural observation.

Contra-action an unwanted reaction occurring during or after treatment application.

Contra-indication a problematic symptom which indicates that the treatment may not proceed or may restrict treatment application. Contra-indications identified for facial treatments are discussed in more detail in Chapter 2.

Effleurage a stroking massage manipulation used to begin the massage, as a link manipulation, and to complete the massage sequence. Applied in a rhythmic, continuous manner, it induces relaxation.

Equipment tools used within a facial to enhance the effects and application of facial products and procedures e.g. magnifying light and skin warming devices.

Erythema reddening of the skin caused by increased blood circulation to the area.

Exfoliant a treatment used to remove excess dead skin cells from the surface of the skin, which has a skin cleansing, cell rejuvenating action. This process can be achieved using a specialized cosmetic, or mechanically by using facial equipment where a brush is rotated over the skin's surface.

Facial a treatment to improve the appearance, condition and functioning of the skin and underlying structures.

Facial products skincare used with a facial treatment which have specific benefits to care for and improve the function and appearance of the skin.

Hyperpigmentation increased pigment production.

Hypopigmentation loss of pigmentation.

Mask a skin-cleansing treatment preparation applied to the skin, which may contain different ingredients. It can have a deep cleansing, toning, nourishing or refreshing effect. It may be applied to the face, hands and feet.

Massage manipulation of the soft tissues of the body, producing heat and stimulating the muscular, circulatory and nervous systems.

Massage manipulations movements which are selected and applied according to the desired effect, and which may be stimulating, relaxing or toning. Massage manipulations include effleurage, petrissage, percussion (also known as tapotement) and vibrations.

Massage medium a skincare product which acts as a lubricant to allow sufficient slip over the skin's, surface while performing facial massage.

Minor a person classed as a child who requires by law to have a guardian or parent present.

Moisturiser a skincare preparation whose formulation of oil and water helps maintain the skin's natural moisture by locking moisture into the skin, offering protection and hydration. The formulation is selected to suit the skin type, facial characteristics and facial area.

Molecule an arrangement of two or more atoms to create specific chemical compound.

Muscle tone the normal degree of tension in healthy muscle.

Necessary action the action taken to deal safely with a contra-action or contra-indication.

Nutrition the nourishment derived from food, required for the body's growth, energy, repair and production.

Oedema extra fluid in an area, causing swelling.

Petrissage a massage manipulation in which the tissues are lifted away from the underlying structures and compressed. Petrissage improves muscle tone by the compression and relaxation of the muscle fibres.

pH scale a scale from 0–14 used to measure the level of acidity or alkalinity of a substance. In the range of 0–6.9, the lower the pH value, the greater the acidity; 1 being the most acidic. In the range 7+, the greater the pH value, the greater the alkalinity; 14 being the most alkaline. A pH of 7 is neutral, meaning it is neither acid nor alkaline.

Pigment the skin's and hair's colour, called melanin. The amount of pigment varies for each client, resulting in different skin/hair colour.

Skin analysis assessment of the client's skin type and condition.

Skin characteristics while looking at the skin type, the skin's additional characteristics may be seen. These include skin that may be sensitive, dehydrated, moist or oedematous (puffy).

Skin condition while looking at the skin type, additional characteristics may be seen that indicate its condition. These include skin that may be sensitive, dehydrated or mature.

Skin tone the strength and elasticity of the skin.

Skin type the different physiological functioning of each person's skin dictates their skin type. There are four main skin types normal (balanced), dry (lacking in oil), oily (excessive oil) and combination (a mixture of two skin types, e.g., dry and oily).

Specialist skincare treatment products additional skincare preparations available to target improvement. These products include eye gels, throat creams and ampoule treatments.

Steam treatment a warming effect created by boiling water, which is then vaporized and used on the skin to achieve both cleansing and stimulation.

Tapotement also known as percussion. A massage manipulation that is used for its general toning and stimulating effect.

Toning lotion a skincare preparation formulated to treat the different skin types and facial characteristics. It is applied to remove all traces of cleanser from the skin. It produces a cooling effect on the skin and has a skin-tightening effect.

Treatment plan after the consultation, suitable treatment objectives are established to treat the client's conditions and needs.

Vapour unit an electrical appliance that heats water to produce steam which is applied to the skin of the face and neck, to warm, cleanse and stimulate the skin.

Vibrations massage manipulations applied on the nerve centre. They stimulate the nerves to induce a feeling of wellbeing and to provide gentle stimulation of the skin.

ASSESSMENT OF KNOWLEDGE AND UNDERSTANDING

You have now learnt how to provide facial skincare in the beauty therapy workplace. To test your level of knowledge and understanding, answer the following short questions. These will prepare you for your summative (final) assessment.

1. The massage manipulation shows finger stroking around the eye. Which muscle of the face is this being specifically applied to?
   a. occipital muscle

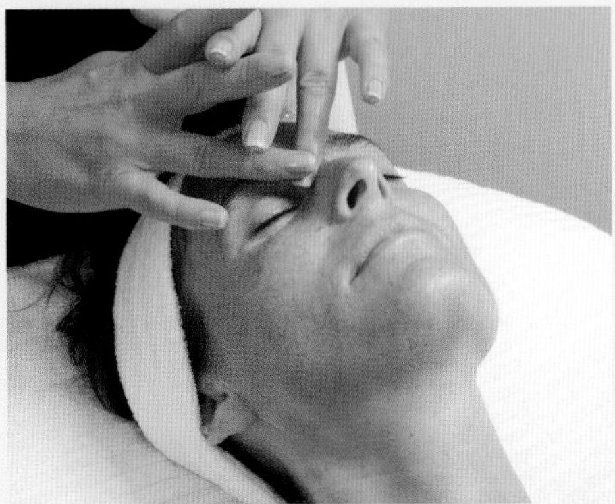

   b. orbicularis oris muscle
   c. orbicularis occuli muscle
   d. zygomaticus muscle.

2. An oily skin type has increased sebum production caused by over-activity of the:
   a. suderiferous gland
   b. lymph gland
   c. sebaceous gland
   d. sweat gland.

3. The following skin condition will restrict facial skincare treatment:
   a. severe psoriasis
   b. allergic skin
   c. sunburn
   d. impetigo.

4. The mask type most suitable of cleansing and absorbing dead skin cells and surface skin debris is:
   a. setting mask
   b. non-setting mask.

5. An exfoliant improves the appearance of the outer surface layer of the skin, which this is the:
   a. stratum granulosum
   b. stratum germinativum
   c. papillary layer
   d. stratum corneum.

6. Which massage manipulation can be incorporated to produce a quick erythema of the skin?
   a. effleurage
   b. vibrations
   c. tapotement
   d. petrissage.

7. The bone identified is the:
   a. frontal
   b. parietal
   c. ethmoid
   d. occipital.

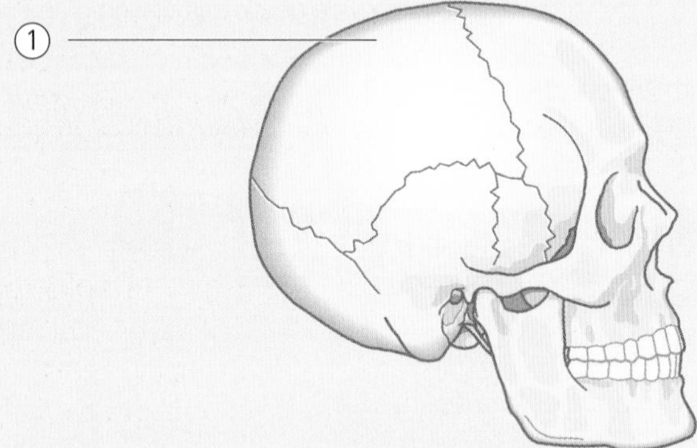

8. The lymph nodes identified are the:
   a. submental nodes
   b. submandibular nodes
   c. occipital nodes
   d. parotid nodes.

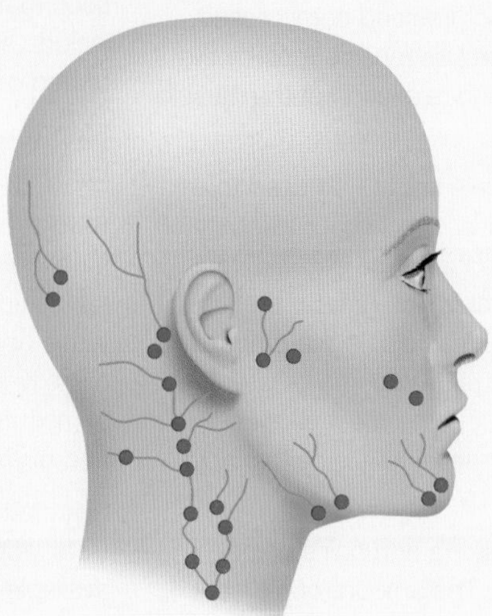

9. The following skin condition type may often contra-indicate facial steaming:
   a. oily skin type
   b. sensitive skin
   c. dehydrated skin
   d. mature skin.

10. Aftercare advice should be provided:
    a. the first time the client receives the facial treatment
    b. following every facial treatment.

8 Eyelash and Brow Treatments

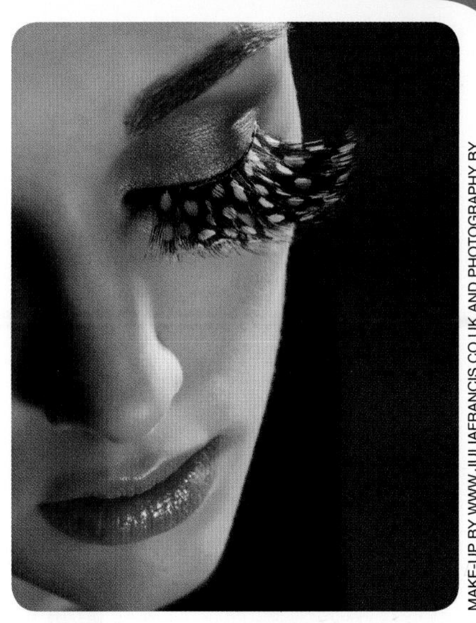

MAKE-UP BY WWW.JULIAFRANCIS.CO.UK AND PHOTOGRAPHY BY WWW.PETEWEBB.COM

Learning Objectives

This chapter covers **VRQ Provide eyelash and brow treatments.**

This unit is about how to enhance and emphasize the appearance of the client's eyebrows and eyelashes using the practical skills of brow shaping, lash and brow tinting and application of artificial lashes. This chapter also covers **VRQ Unit Shaping and colouring eyebrows** and **VRQ Unit Provide eyelash perming**, an eyelash treatment that permanently curls the eyelashes. The treatment application will be selected and performed to meet the outcomes required. Learning outcomes and range statements for **Shaping and colouring eyebrows** and **Provide eyelash perming** can be found in your qualification handbook.

There are **two** learning outcomes for this unit which you must achieve:

1 Be able to prepare for eyelash and eyebrow treatments

2 Be able to provide eyelash and eyebrow treatments

From the range statement, you must show you can:

- understand the different **eyelash and eyebrow treatments**
- use **consultation techniques** to identify the treatment **objectives**
- conduct skin sensivity **tests** as appropriate and understand the results
- use the **products, tools, equipment and techniques** required

(continued on the next page)

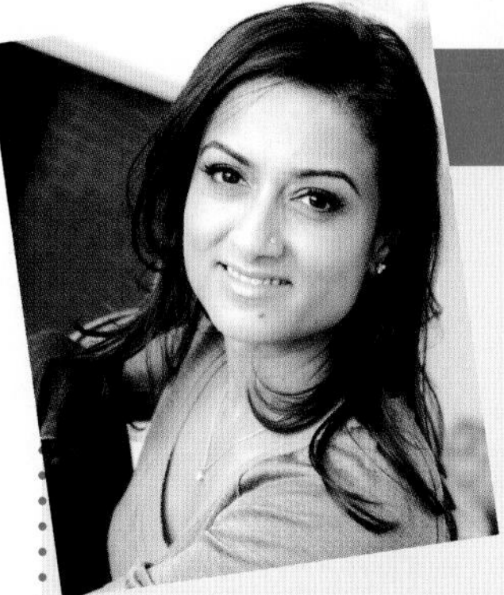

ROLE MODEL

Shavata Singh

Brand Director
Shavata UK (encompassing Shavata Brow Studio and Lash Lounge by Shavata)

“Eyebrows have always been a passion of mine. The entire process of creating the perfect arch fascinates me and I am constantly thinking of new ways to make this previously daunting beauty task simpler for my clients. This passion is one of the reasons I founded my first Brow Studio at the Urban Retreat, Harrods. This Brow Studio was my perfect solution for men and women who needed a quick, efficient, effective treatment, that takes just minutes and can transform your look. Shavata Brow Studios and Lash Lounges are now available in selected stores across the UK to help meet the demands of our clients and I have also developed my own range of fabulous products, which can help you to create the perfect brow in-between your studio appointments.

- ensure the **environmental conditions** are suitable
- identify **contra-indications** that prevent or restrict treatment
- **communicate and behave** in a professional manner
- follow all **health and safety working practices**
- identify **normal reaction of the skin** and **contra-actions**
- provide relevant **aftercare advice**

You must be able to show that you have the necessary practical skills and underpinning knowledge to provide eyelash and eyebrow treatments.

These units are linked to the Beauty Therapy NOS **Units B15** and **B5**.

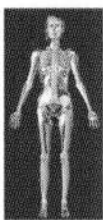

Essential anatomy and physiology knowledge for this unit is identified on the checklist on page 27.

Eyelash and brow treatments

The eyebrows and eyelashes protect the eye from moisture and dust as well as define the appearance of the eyes and enhance the facial features. Eyebrows can be shaped and tinted and eyelashes can be tinted and permed. Artificial eyelashes can also be attached to the natural lashes to further enhance the appearance of the eyes.

Outcome 1: Be able to prepare for eyelash and brow treatments

Learn how to prepare for eyelash and eyebrow treatments

Practical skills

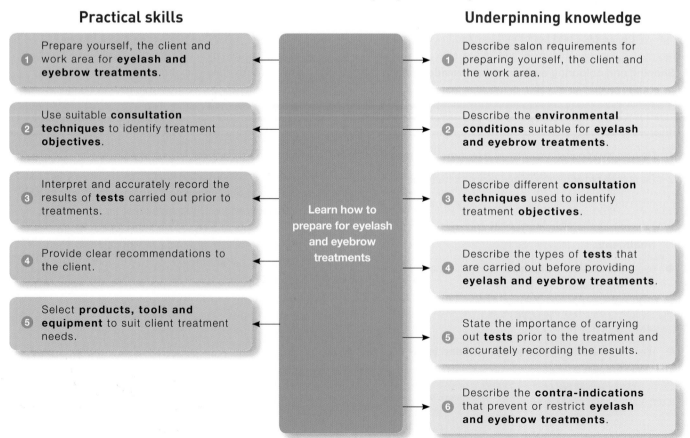

1. Prepare yourself, the client and work area for **eyelash and eyebrow treatments**.
2. Use suitable **consultation techniques** to identify treatment **objectives**.
3. Interpret and accurately record the results of **tests** carried out prior to treatments.
4. Provide clear recommendations to the client.
5. Select **products, tools and equipment** to suit client treatment needs.

Underpinning knowledge

1. Describe salon requirements for preparing yourself, the client and the work area.
2. Describe the **environmental conditions** suitable for **eyelash and eyebrow treatments**.
3. Describe different **consultation techniques** used to identify treatment **objectives**.
4. Describe the types of **tests** that are carried out before providing **eyelash and eyebrow treatments**.
5. State the importance of carrying out **tests** prior to the treatment and accurately recording the results.
6. Describe the **contra-indications** that prevent or restrict **eyelash and eyebrow treatments**.

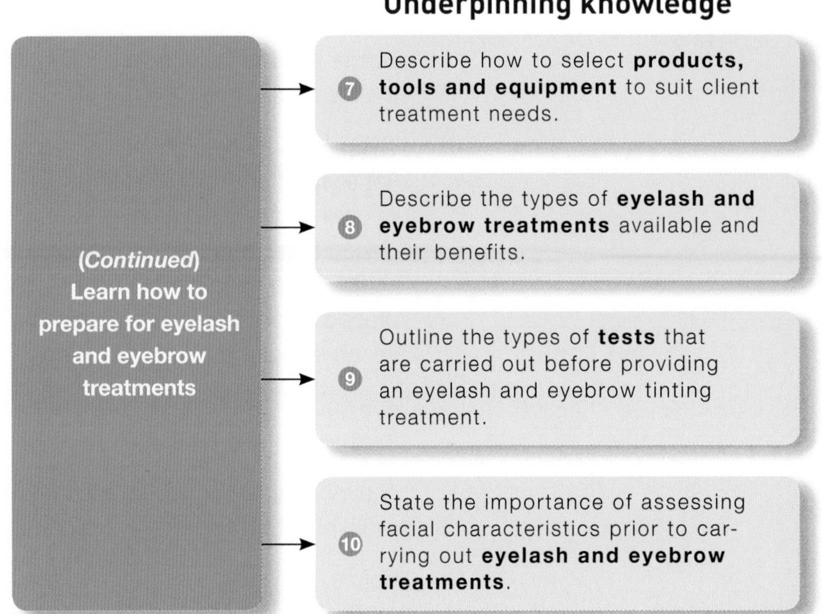

Underpinning knowledge
(Continued) Learn how to prepare for eyelash and eyebrow treatments
7 Describe how to select products, tools and equipment to suit client treatment needs.
8 Describe the types of eyelash and eyebrow treatments available and their benefits.
9 Outline the types of tests that are carried out before providing an eyelash and eyebrow tinting treatment.
10 State the importance of assessing facial characteristics prior to carrying out eyelash and eyebrow treatments.

HEALTH & SAFETY

Maintaining hygiene
Several pairs of tweezers must be purchased (perhaps five), due to the length of time required for sterilization. Buy good-quality stainless steel tweezers: cheaper metals rust after repeated sterilization. Disposable mascara wands are ideal for brushing the hairs during brow shaping.

TOP TIP

Tweezers
When purchasing tweezers, make sure that the ends meet accurately so they will grasp the hair effectively.

Eyebrow hair removal

The eyebrows, situated above the bony eye orbits of the face, help to protect the eyes from moisture and dust, and to cushion the skin from physical injury. Misshapen bushy brows give an untidy appearance to the face, but when correctly shaped, the brows give balance to the facial features and enhance the eyes – the most expressive feature of the face. Eyebrow hair removal can be carried out with temporary or permanent hair removal. Permanent methods include the advanced treatments of electrolysis and intense pulsed light (IPL). Temporary methods include threading (see Chapter 9) and waxing (see Chapter 15). This section will cover the removal of eyebrow hair with tweezers.

Eyebrow shaping is offered in the salon as either an **eyebrow reshape** or **eyebrow maintenance** – the former involves removing eyebrow hair to create a new shape, the latter involves removing only a few stray hairs in order to maintain the existing shape.

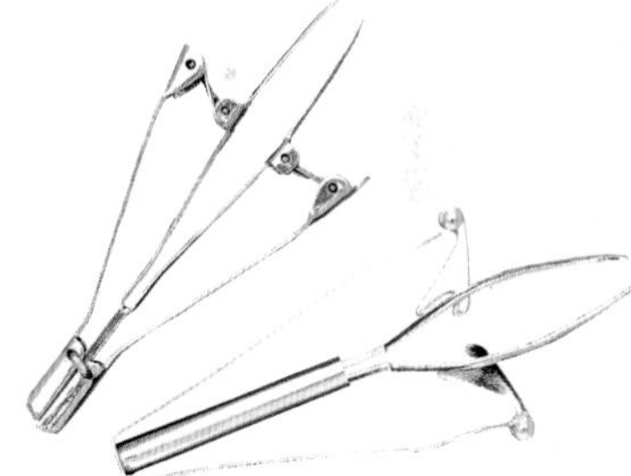
Automatic tweezers

Tweezers

There are two sorts of tweezers used to shape the eyebrows. **Automatic tweezers** are designed to remove the bulk of excess hair; they have a spring-loaded action. **Manual tweezers** are used to remove stray hairs, and to accentuate the brow shape where more accurate care is required. They are available with various ends including slant, claw and pointed; which you use is a matter of personal preference, but slanted ends are generally considered to be the best for eyebrow shaping.

Although many beauty therapists may complete an eyebrow shaping using only one of these – automatic or manual tweezers – it is important to be skilled in the use of both these tools.

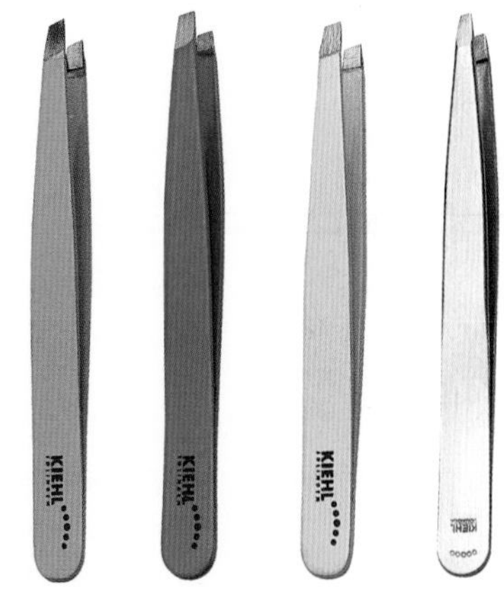
ELLISONS
Manual tweezers

Preparing the work area

Before the client is shown through to the work area, it should be checked to ensure that the area is clean and tidy.

The plastic-covered couch or chair should be clean, having been thoroughly washed with hot soapy water, or wiped thoroughly with a professional disinfectant cleaner. The couch or chair should be protected with a long strip of disposable paper bedroll which may be placed to cover a freshly laundered sheet or bath towel. A small towel should be placed neatly at the head of the couch — for hygiene and protection during service. This will be draped across the client's chest. The tissue will need changing and the towels should be freshly laundered for each client.

The couch should be positioned flat and the chair should be slightly elevated when performing the treatment.

The work area should be adequately lit to ensure that service can be given safely, but avoid bright lighting that could cause eye irritation.

Before beginning the eyebrow shaping treatment, check that you have the necessary products, tools and equipment to hand and that they meet the legal hygiene and industry requirements for eye treatments.

PRODUCTS, TOOLS AND EQUIPMENT

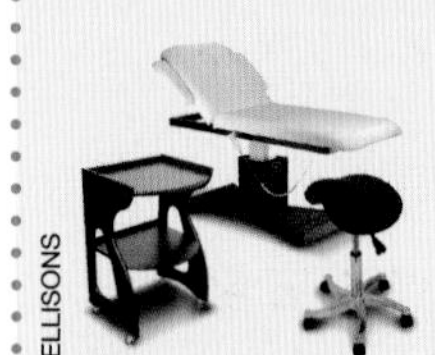

Couch or chair
With sit-up and lie-down positions and an easy-to-clean surface

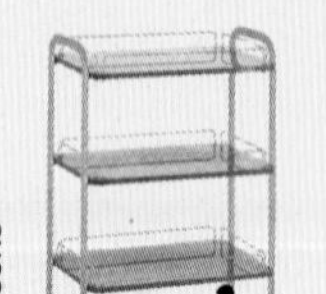

Trolley
On which to place everything

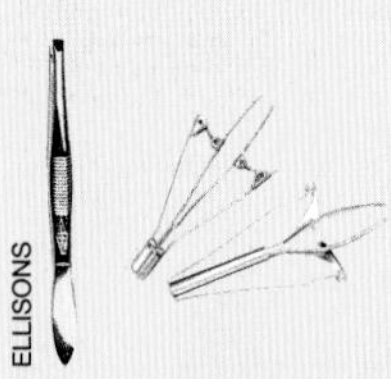
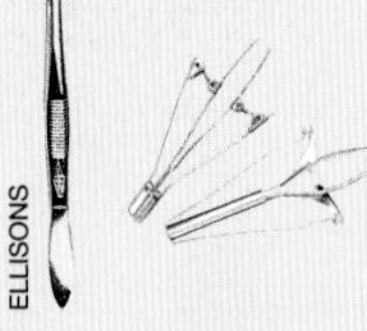

Tweezers (sterilized)
Both automatic and manual

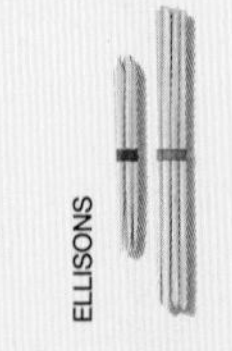

Orange sticks
To measure the length and arch of eyebrow when planning hair removal

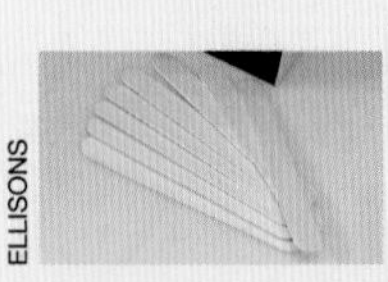

Disposable spatulas
To hygienically remove product from containers

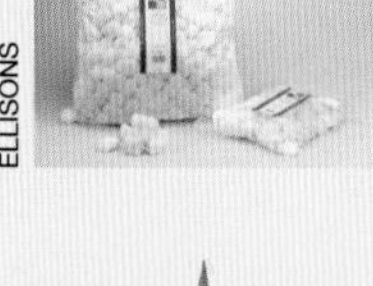

Dry and damp cotton wool
To apply cleansing and soothing agents – and to collect hair removed during service

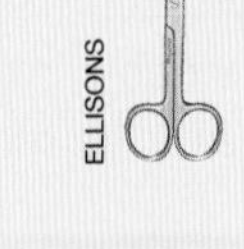

Scissors (stainless steel)
For trimming long hairs

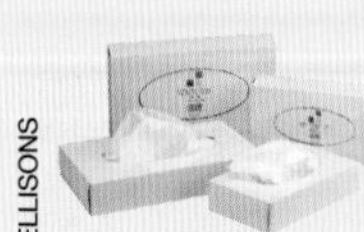

Facial tissues (white)
For blotting the skin dry in the area

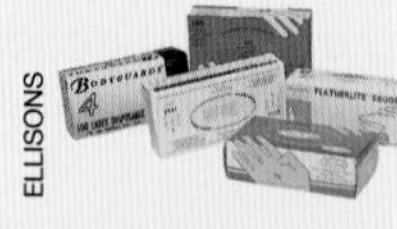

Disposable non-latex (synthetic), powder-free gloves
May be worn to prevent cross-infection

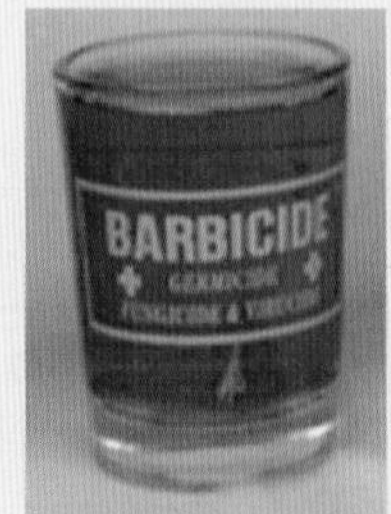

Disinfectant solution
To store small stainless steel sterilized tools

YOU WILL ALSO NEED:

Disposable tissue couch roll Placed over the couch cover before each treatment for reasons of hygiene

Towels (2) (medium sized) For draping over the client and placing over the top of the couch or chair

Eyebrow pencil Used to mark the skin when measuring brow length

Eyebrow brush or disposable brushes To comb through the brow hair during and following service

Headband (clean) To keep hair away from the brow shaping area

Pencil sharpener (stainless steel) Suitable for use in the autoclave, used to sharpen the eyebrow pencil

Skin disinfectant To cleanse and disinfect the client's skin

Cleansing lotion Used to remove facial make-up from the eye area

Soothing lotion or gel With soothing, healing and antiseptic properties, suitable for use on the skin of the face, e.g. witch hazel liquid/gel

Hand mirror (clean) Used when discussing the brow shaping requirements and to show the client the finished result

Client record card To record confidential details of each client registered at the salon including the clients personal details, products used and details of the service

Light magnifier (cold) To magnify the area to ensure all hairs have been removed

Disinfectant For cleaning tweezers and scissors before sterilization

Waste container This should be a lined metal bin with a lid

Sterilization and disinfection for eyebrow shaping

Sterilize tweezers at an appropriate time during the working day. Ensure that you always have sterile tweezers ready for use with each client. After they have been sterilized in the autoclave, the tweezers should be stored in the ultra-violet cabinet.

If used, an eyebrow brush should be cleaned in warm, soapy water or brush cleaner following use and, when dry, placed in the ultra-violet cabinet. Disposable brushes are effective as they can be thrown away immediately after use.

A fresh disinfectant solution may be used to store a spare pair of tweezers while carrying out an eyebrow service. This solution is usually dispensed into a small container stored on the trolley. (Spare tweezers are necessary in case you should accidentally drop the other tweezers during the service.) After the eyebrow shaping service, tweezers must be replaced and resterilized. Following sterilization store tweezers in a clean covered container.

Disposable gloves may be worn for protection avoiding cross-infection during the eyebrow shaping service – the therapist may come into contact with tissue fluids from the client's skin.

As the waste from the service may contain body fluids and pose a health threat, it must be collected and disposed of carefully, in accordance with the local authority Environmental Health Department.

During an eyebrow shaping treatment when would you select the use of:

- automatic tweezers?
- manual tweezers?

Need more time... refer to page 235 to help you.

Permanent eyelash and eyebrow tinting

The hair of the eyelashes and eyebrows protects the eyes from moisture and dust, but the lashes and brows also give definition to the eye. Many clients, especially those with fair lashes and brows, feel that without the use of eye cosmetics their eyes lack this definition.

Further definition of the brow and lash hair can be created if a permanent dye is applied to them. Most clients will benefit from eyelash and eyebrow tinting because the tips and the bases of these hairs are usually lighter than the body of the hairs, causing the hairs to appear shorter than they actually are. Tinting the length of the lash or brow hair makes it appear longer and bolder, yet the effect created looks natural.

TOP TIP

Blue tint

When a client requests a blue eyelash tint, make clear that this will not produce an 'electric blue' fashion colour.

HEALTH & SAFETY

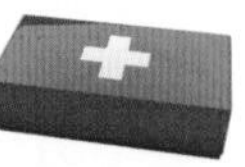

Peroxide strength

Do not use a higher strength than 10-volume or 3% hydrogen peroxide. If you do, skin irritation or minor skin burning may occur.

HEALTH & SAFETY

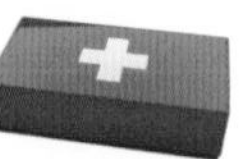

Permanent tinting

Always use a tint that is permitted for use under EU regulations and complies with the Cosmetic Products (Safety) Regulations 2003. If you use any other tint your insurance may be invalid.

HEALTH & SAFETY

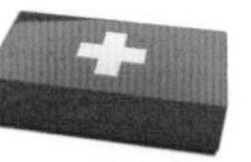

Storage

Permanent tint should be stored in a cool, dark area to avoid heat which would affect the quality and effectiveness of the product.

Always check MSDS sheets to ensure correct storage of products.

ALWAYS REMEMBER

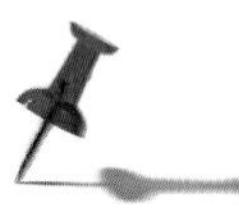

Peroxide

Replace the cap of the hydrogen peroxide container *immediately* after use, or the peroxide will lose its strength.

Because the skin around the eye area is very thin and sensitive, dyes designed for permanently tinting the hair in this area have been specially formulated to avoid any eye or tissue reactions. ***The application of any other dye materials in this area is dangerous and may even lead to blindness***.

Permanent tints are available in different forms, including jelly, liquid and cream tints. The most popular and acceptable permanent tinting product is the cream tint: this is thicker, so it does not run into the eye and it is easy to control during mixing, application and removal.

Several colours of permanent tint are available, including brown, grey, blue and black.

If the shade you want is not available, you can vary the shade of available tints by leaving the dye on the hair for different lengths of time, or by mixing different colours together. For example, to produce a navy blue colour; leave the tint to process for three to five minutes. If left to process for ten minutes, the same tint will produce a raven blue-black colour.

The development of colour

Two products are essential for the permanent tinting service:

- professional **eyelash** or **eyebrow tint**
- **hydrogen peroxide (H_2O_2)**

The tint contains small molecules of permanent dye called **toluenediamine**. These need to be 'activated' before their colouring effect becomes permanent: this is achieved by the addition of hydrogen peroxide. The peroxide is said to **develop** the colour of the tint.

Chemically, hydrogen peroxide is an **oxidant**, a chemical that contains available oxygen atoms and encourages certain chemical reactions – in this case, tinting.

The hydrogen peroxide container will state either its volume or its percentage strength. To activate the tint and for safe use around the eye area, a 3% or 10-volume strength peroxide is used.

When you add the hydrogen peroxide to the tint, the small dye molecules together form large molecules, which remain trapped in the **cortex** of the hair. The hair is thus permanently coloured, but in time, as it continues to grow, the new hair will show the natural colour.

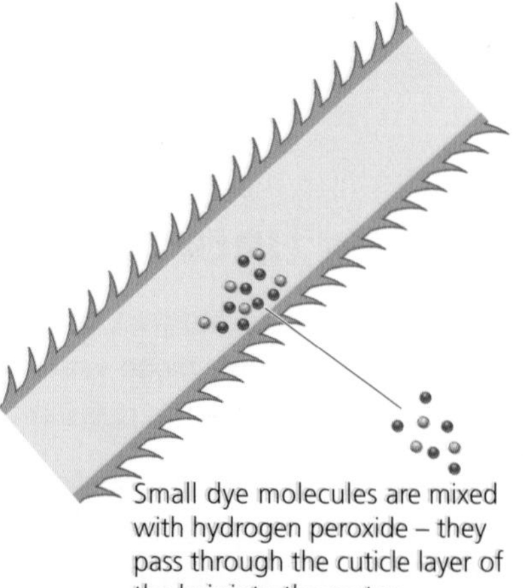

Small dye molecules are mixed with hydrogen peroxide – they pass through the cuticle layer of the hair into the cortex
Small dye molecules swell and join together, becoming permanently trapped in the cortex of the hair

Permanent hair colouring

Preparing the work area

Before the client is shown through to the work area, it should be checked to ensure that the area is clean and tidy.

Clean and protect the couch or chair as for the eyebrow-shaping service. The couch should be flat and the chair should be slightly elevated.

The work area should be adequately lit to ensure that service can be given, safely, but avoid bright lighting that could cause eye irritation.

Before beginning the tinting treatment, check that you have the necessary products, tools and equipment to hand and that they meet the legal hygiene and industry requirements for eye treatments.

PRODUCTS, TOOLS AND EQUIPMENT

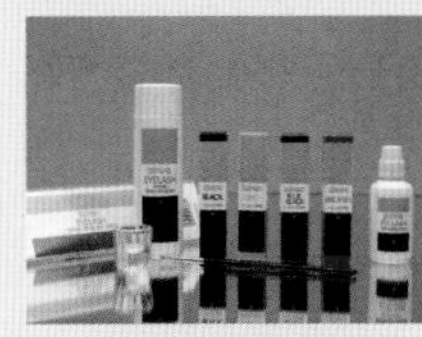

Coloured tints (a selection) Jelly, liquid or cream, select from blue, black, brown or grey (used as is or mixed to the appropriate colour desired)

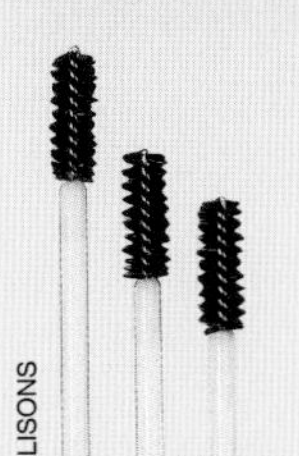

Disposable brushes To comb through the lash/brow hair following service

YOU WILL ALSO NEED:

Couch or chair With sit-up and lie-down positions and an easy-to-clean surface

Trolley On which to place everything

Towels (2) (medium-sized) Freshly laundered for each client

Headband (clean) To keep hair away from the brow and eye area and protect long hair or bleached hair from the tint

Cleansing lotion Used to remove facial make-up and the skin's natural oils and debris from the eye area

Eye make-up remover (non-oily) To cleanse the eye area before service application

Hydrogen peroxide (10-volume/3%)

Petroleum jelly To protect the skin and prevent skin staining

Brush To apply the tint

Damp cotton wool For cleansing the eye area and for lash and brow tint removal and to soothe the area following eyelash tinting

Eye shields (commercial) To prevent skin staining during eyelash tinting

Facial tissues (white) For blotting the eye area dry

Disposable spatulas For removing the petroleum jelly from its container

Disposable non-latex (synthetic), powder-free gloves To be worn if allergic to permanent tint products

Non-metallic bowl For mixing the permanent tint (note that some metals cause immediate release of the oxygen from the hydrogen peroxide, causing ineffective processing of the tint)

Skin stain remover To remove any accidental staining

Bowl (clean) To hold dampened cotton wool

Waste container This should be a lined metal bin with a lid

Hand mirror (clean) To show the client the finished results

Client record card To record confidential details of each client registered at the salon including the client's personal details, products used and details of the service.

KNOWLEDGE CHECK

What are the names of the two active ingredients used in permanent tinting?

Need more time... refer to page 238 to help you.

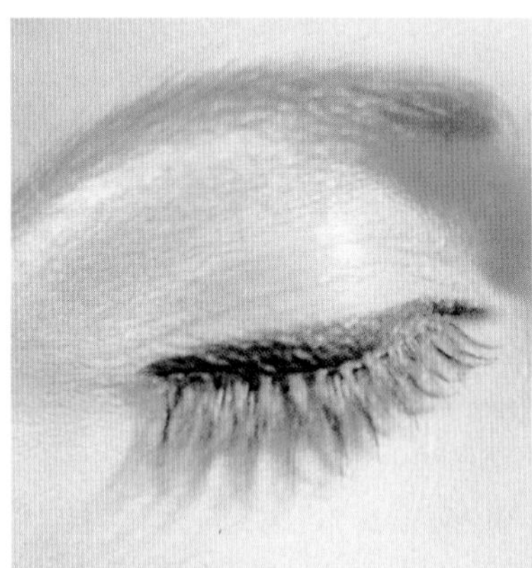

False eyelashes

Sterilization and disinfection for eyelash and brow tinting

Hygiene must be maintained in a number of ways:

- It is best practice to use disposable applicator brushes for the application of the petroleum jelly and the permanent tint because it is impossible to disinfect brushes effectively. If using a non-disposable brush applicator this should be placed in the ultraviolet cabinet after cleaning. Clean brushes should be stored in a clean, covered container.
- Dispense products from containers using disposable or disinfected plastic spatulas.

HEALTH & SAFETY

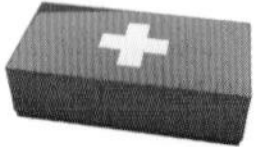

Applicator brushes

Because it is impossible to sterilize applicator brushes effectively, use disposable brushes for the application of petroleum jelly and permanent tint.

ACTIVITY

Choosing lash and brow colours

Which colour do you think would be most suitable for the eyelashes and eyebrows of the following clients:

- dark hair
- fair hair
- red hair
- white/grey hair
- elderly client?

ALWAYS REMEMBER

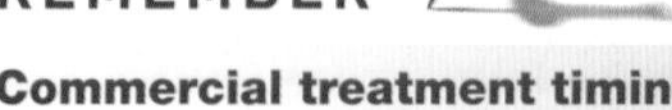

Commercial treatment timing

For artificial lash application, allow 20 minutes.

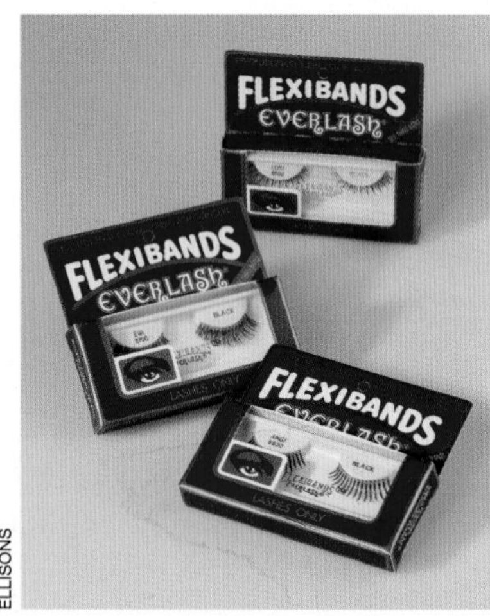

ELLISONS

Strip lashes

Artificial eyelashes

Artificial (false) eyelashes are made from small threads of nylon fibre or real hair. They are attached to the client's natural lash hair imitating natural eyelashes and making the lashes appear longer and thicker, and thereby drawing attention to the eye. There are two main types: **semi-permanent strip lashes** and **individual flare lashes**.

Artificial lashes are applied for the following reasons:

- to create shape and depth in the eye area, when completing corrective eye make-up
- simply to add definition to the eye area
- to enhance evening or fantasy make-up
- to provide thick long lashes for photographic make-up
- to provide an alternative eyelash-enhancing effect for a client who is allergic to mascara

Strip lashes Artificial **strip lashes** are designed to be worn for a short period, either for a day or an evening. They are attached to the natural eyelashes with a soft, weak adhesive. After removal the strip must be cleaned before re-application.

Individual flare lashes Artificial individual flare lashes are attached to the natural lashes with a strong adhesive. They may be worn for approximately four to six weeks, and are therefore known as **semi-permanent lashes**.

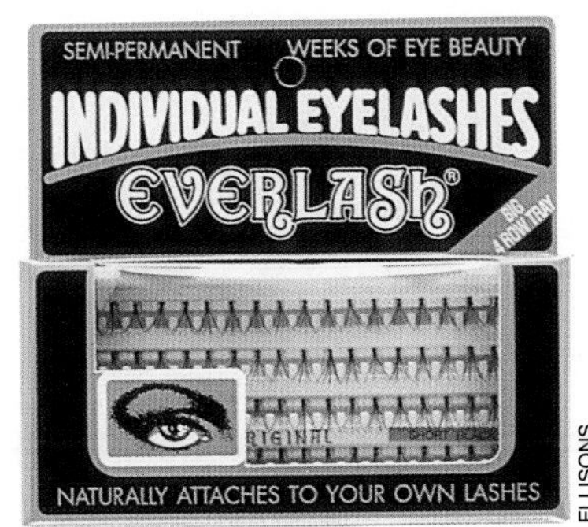

Individual flare lashes

Preparing the work area

Before the client is shown through to the work area, check the area is clean and tidy. The plastic-covered couch or chair should be clean, having been thoroughly washed with hot, soapy water or wiped thoroughly with a professional disinfectant cleaner. The couch or chair should be protected with a long strip of disposable-paper bedroll, placed to cover a freshly laundered sheet or bath towel. A small towel should be placed neatly at the head of the couch, ready to be draped across the client's chest for protection during treatment. The tissue will need changing and the towels will need to be laundered for each client.

The couch or chair should be in a slightly elevated position, to give the optimum position for the beauty therapist when applying the artificial lashes. In this position, too, the client will not be staring into the overhead light (which might cause the eyes to water).

Before beginning the artificial eyelash application, check that you have the necessary products, tools and equipment to hand and that they meet the legal, hygiene and industry requirements for eye treatments.

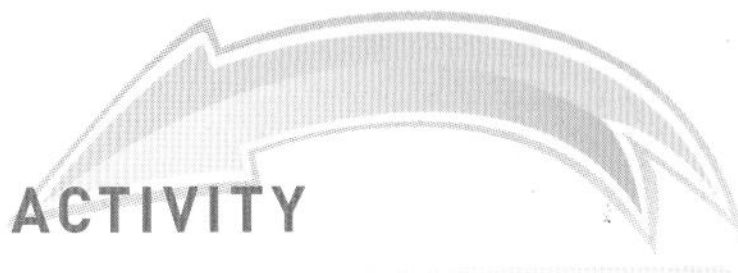

ACTIVITY

Position of client
Can you think of further disadvantages of having the client lying flat when applying artificial lashes?

PRODUCTS, TOOLS AND EQUIPMENT

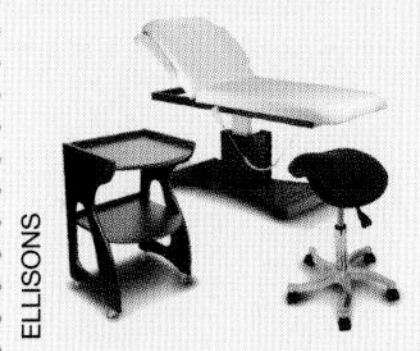

Couch or chair
With sit-up and lie-down positions and an easy-to-clean surface

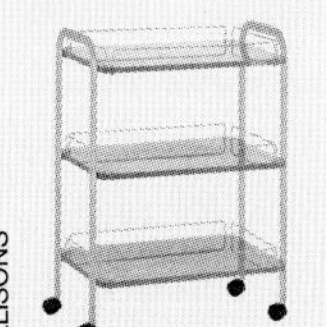

Trolley
On which to place everything

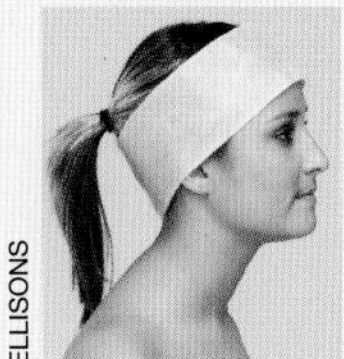

Headband (clean)
To to keep hair away from the treatment area
A large clip may be used if the hair been styled

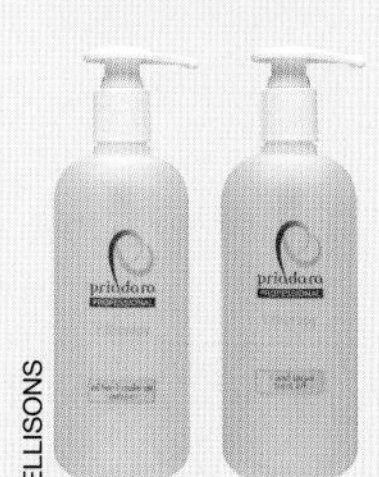

Eye make-up remover (non-oily)
To remove make-up and general skin debris and natural oils from the area

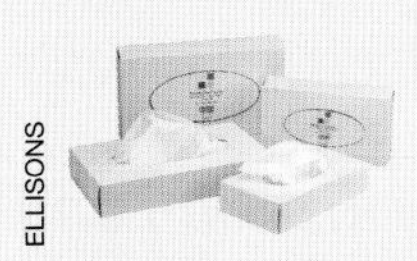

Facial tissues (white)
For blotting the eyelashes dry

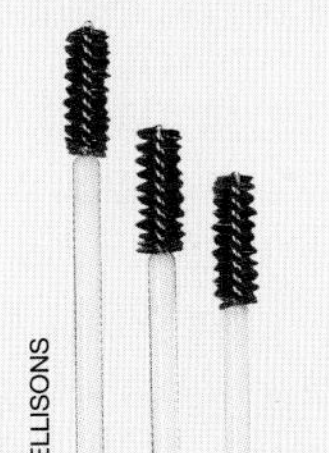

Disposable mascara brush
To brush through the lashes after cleansing and before lash application

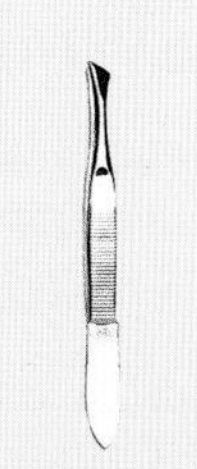

Manual tweezers (2 pairs) (sterilized)
To hold and place the artificial lash in position. Special tweezers are available, designed specifically to assist in attaching individual eyelashes

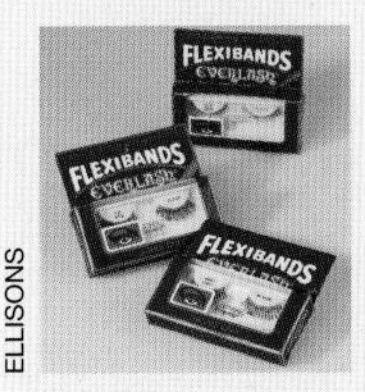

Strip eyelash lengths (a selection)
In a choice of colours

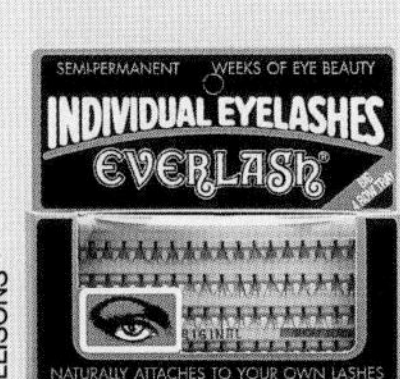

Individual flare eyelash lengths (a selection)
In a choice of colours

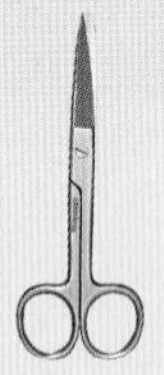

Sterilised scissors (1 pair)
Used for trimming the length of strip lashes

YOU WILL ALSO NEED:

Solvent To soften and dissolve the adhesive when removing artificial lashes

Towels (2) (medium-sized) Freshly laundered for each client

Disposable tissue roll To be placed over the couch cover before each treatment for hygiene reasons

Cleansing lotion Used to remove facial make-up from the eye area

Damp cotton wool For removing cleansing product from the eye area and protect the skin during individual flare lash removal

Cotton wool buds To apply solvent when removing individual flare lashes

Surgical spirit For wiping the points of the tweezers to remove adhesive

Plastic palette (disinfected) On which to place the artificial lashes prior to application (if preferred)

Disinfected dish (small) Lined with foil, in which to place the eyelash adhesive during individual flare lash application

Hand mirror (clean) To show the client the finished result

Client record card Confidential card recording details of each client registered at the salon to record the clients personal details, products used and details of the service.

Waste container Should be a lined metal bin with a lid

HEALTH & SAFETY

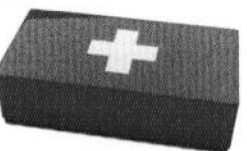

Cleaning

In order that you can effectively clean the dish containing the eyelash adhesive after the treatment, you need to line the dish with a disposable lining

Sterilization and disinfection for artificial eyelashes

Hygiene must be maintained in a number of ways:

- When preparing to apply artificial *strip* lashes, clean the surface of the palette onto which you will stick the lashes (if used) once you have removed them from their packet. Use disinfectant, applied with clean cotton wool for this purpose. The palette may be stored in the ultra-violet light cabinet until ready for use. *Individual* flare lashes come in a special 'contoured' package: you can hold this securely while removing individual flare lashes, so the lashes can be kept hygienically until required.
- Always have a spare pair of tweezers available during application of the individual or strip artificial lashes. Should you accidentally drop the tweezers with which you are working, you will need a clean, sterile pair available.
- Scissors, used to trim strip lashes, should be sterilized before use.
- Dispense products like artificial lash adhesive hygeinically from containers.

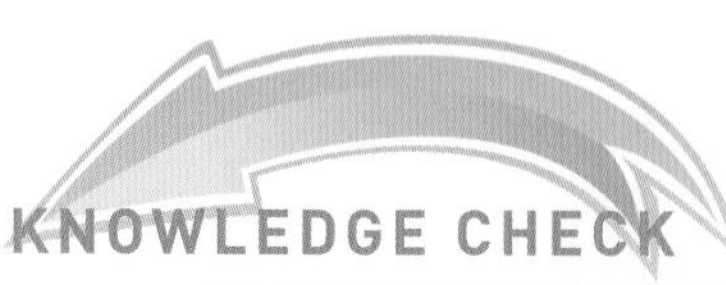

KNOWLEDGE CHECK

What is the difference between strip lashes and individual flare lashes?

Need more time... refer to pages 240–241 to help you.

Eyelash perming

Eyelash perming is the process of permanently curling the lashes, which enhances the appearance of the eyes. The lashes immediately appear longer, which suits most clients. The treatment also suits:

- short, sparse lashes, to make them appear longer and denser
- downward-slanting eyes, as the eyes appear lifted when the outer lashes are curled
- special occasions and holidays
- clients who are unable to wear eye make-up at work
- clients who want a natural effect to enhance the eyes

The effect lasts as long as the hair growth cycle of the eyelashes.

Chemical process of eyelash perming

Hair maintains its shape and strength by chemical cross bonds in the cortex (the thickest layer of the hair) called **disulphide bonds** (two sulphur bonds joined together). In the perm **processing** stage, these bonds must be broken to alter the shape of the hair. When the perm solution is applied to the hair, the chemical cross bonds are broken by the addition of hydrogen and the hair is softened. The hair then assumes the shape of the rod that it is curled around.

This shape is made permanent by the application of the fixing/neutralizing lotion. This stops the action of the perm lotion. This stage is called the **neutralizing** stage, where the chemical cross bonds in the cortex are reformed by adding oxygen (known as oxidation) and removing the hydrogen. This stage is completed before the rods are removed. On removal of the rods, the eyelash hair assumes its new shape.

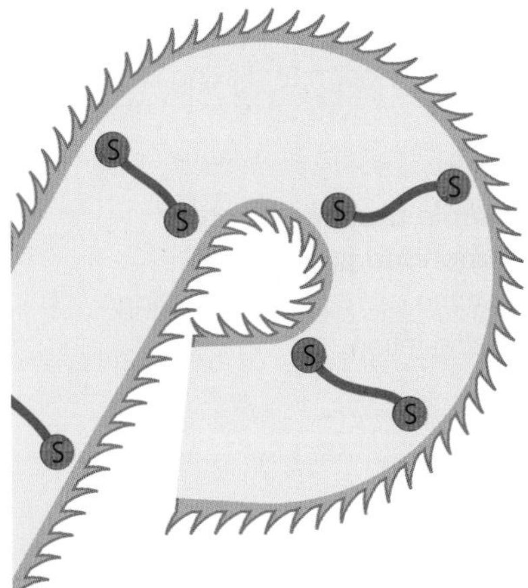

Disulphide bonds

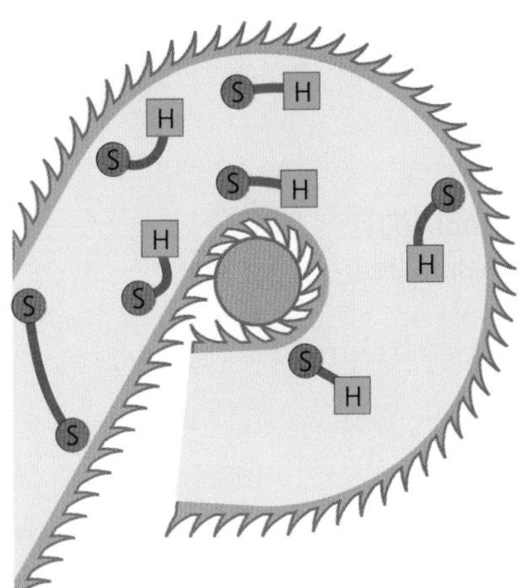

Processing stage: Breaking existing disulphide bonds by the addition of hydrogen

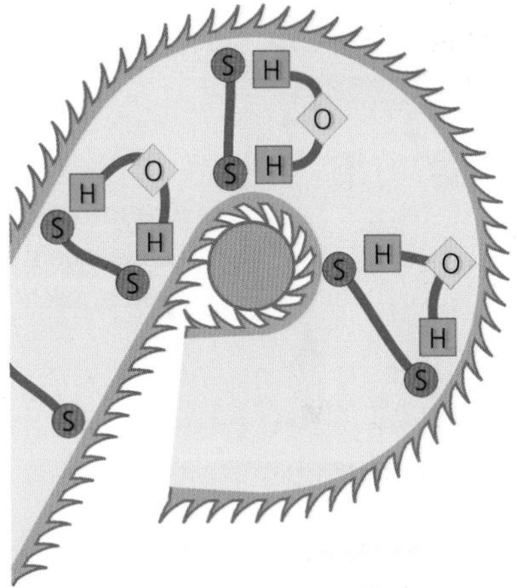

Neutralizing stage Oxidation: Forming new disulphide bonds

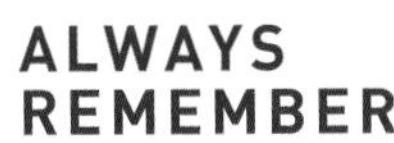

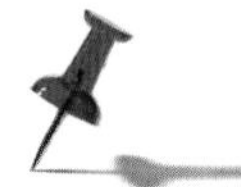

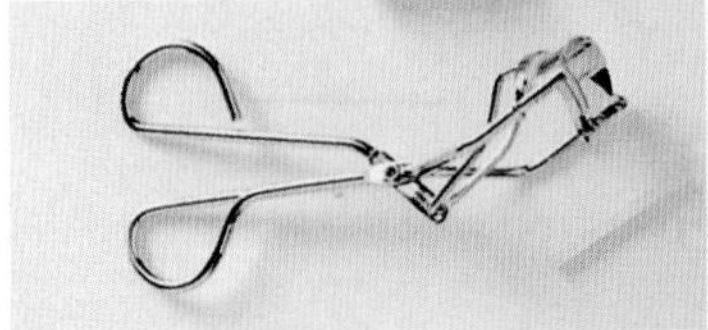

Mechanical eyelash curlers

Eyelash curling

Repeated mechanical eyelash curling is time-consuming and can weaken the lashes, causing breakage of the natural lash. Permanent curling is the ideal alternative.

HEALTH & SAFETY

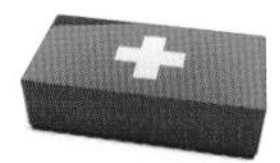

Storage

Store the perm solution in a well-ventilated area, away from direct sources of heat and light. If a spillage occurs, wear gloves while you clean it up, and increase ventilation in the area.

Preparing the work area Before the client is shown through to the work area, it should be checked to ensure the area is clean and tidy. Clean and protect the couch or chair as for an eyebrow-shaping treatment. The couch or chair should be flat or slightly elevated.

The work area should be adequately lit to ensure that the treatment can be given safely, but avoid bright lighting, which might cause eye irritation.

Before beginning the eyelash perming service check that you have the necessary products tools and equipment to hand and that they meet the legal, hygiene and industry requirements for eye treatment services.

PRODUCTS, TOOLS AND EQUIPMENT

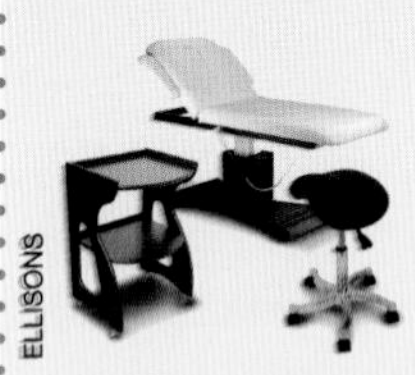

ELLISONS

Couch or chair
With sit-up and lie-down positions and an easy-to-clean surface

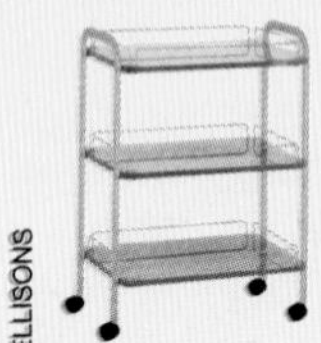

ELLISONS

Trolley
On which to place everything

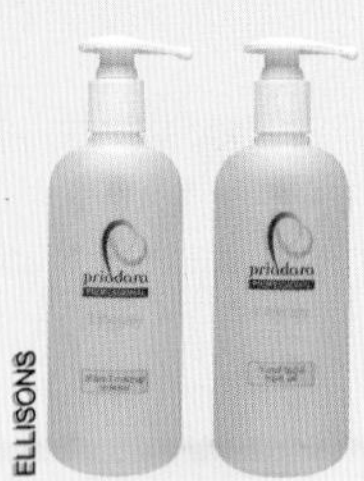

ELLISONS

Eye make-up remover (non-oily)
To cleanse the eye area before treatment application

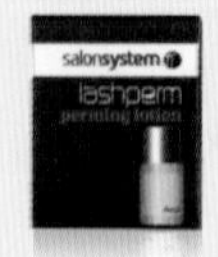

Mild perm solution (usually 6% thioglycollate)
Especially designed for use in the eye area, it is this solution that curls the lash into the desired new shape

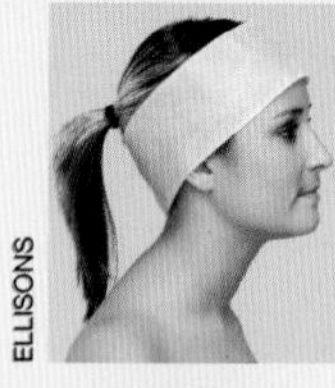

ELLISONS

Headband (clean)
To protect the hair

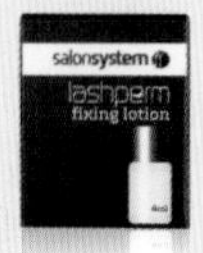

Fixing/neutralizing lotion (sodium bromate)
To make the new curl permanent

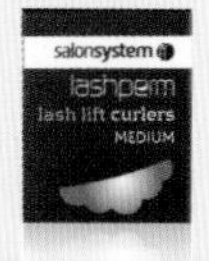

Eyelash curlers (a selection of different sizes)
Small curlers are used for fine hair, larger curlers for thicker hair

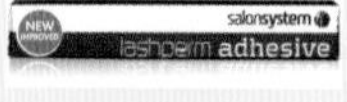

Eyelash adhesive
To secure the lashes to the curlers

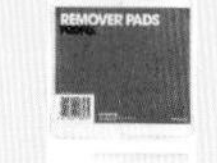

Lint-free pads
To remove the perm and fixing lotion

SALON SYSTEM

Disposable brushes or other recommended applicators
To apply the perm lotion and fixing/neutralizing lotion

YOU WILL ALSO NEED:

Hand mirror To show the client the results

Towels (medium-sized) Freshly laundered for each client

Bowls (2, clean) To hold damp cotton wool or lint-free pads

Timer To accurately time the curling and fixing processes

Waste container This should be a lined metal bin with a lid

Disposable wooden sticks or other recommended applicators To secure the natural lashes to the curlers

Damp cotton wool For cleansing the eye area and to remove excess products

Moisturising agent To facilitate removal of the curlers

Client record card To record confidential details of each client registered at the salon including the client's personal details, products used and details of the service

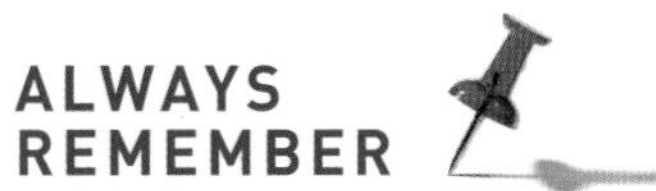

ALWAYS REMEMBER

Gel lotions

Perm lotions for the eye area are usually of *gel* formulation: this makes the lotion easy to control. Bear this in mind when selecting this product. The bottles are small to reduce the risk of oxidation, which would make the lotion ineffective.

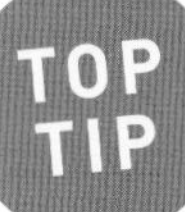

TOP TIP

Lash conditioning

A specialized conditioning agent may be applied to the lashes. This would be professionally applied as part of the perming service to rehydrate the lashes.

Sterilization and disinfection for eyelash perming

Ideally, applicators used for the perming chemical agents should be disposable. Alternatively, several brushes must be available to allow effective disinfection between clients.

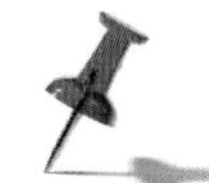

ALWAYS REMEMBER

Permanent brow colouring

By permanently tinting brow hair before shaping, you will colour any finer lighter hairs, which will then form part of the brow.

Eyebrow shaping consultation

Reception

When making an appointment it is usual to allow 15 minutes for an eyebrow shaping service.

It is wise to have a designated time between services so that there is no confusion between the two services; a trim or a maintenance service and a reshape. For example, under two weeks could be regarded as a maintenance, and over two weeks as a reshape.

If the client has thick, heavy brows, or if they do not have their brows shaped regularly, they should be encouraged to have them shaped gradually over a period of treatments, until the desired shape is achieved. This will allow the client to become accustomed to the new shape and will minimize any discomfort.

Eyebrow shaping may be carried out as an independent service, or combined with other services such as permanent tinting of the brows. In the latter case, the brows should be tinted before shaping, to avoid the tint coming into contact with the open follicle and perhaps causing an allergic reaction.

Before brow-shaping service commences, carry out a **consultation**. Discuss the shape and the effect that might be achieved. Consider such factors as age, the natural shape of

BEST PRACTICE

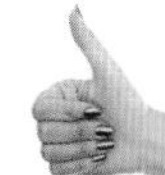

Positive promotion

While the client is having their eyebrows shaped, you have an ideal opportunity to discuss further possible services, such as an eyebrow tint.

Communication

At the consultation, identify any peculiarities such as bald patches or scarring in the brow area to avoid any confusion or concern later.

the brow, and fashion. It is important that you fully understand what the client's requirements because you will be temporarily removing the hair. Ensure that the client agrees the amount of brow hair to be removed and the shape to be achieved.

Remember for all eye services, that if a client is under the age of 16, it is necessary to obtain parent/guardian permission for the service. They will also have to be present when the service is received.

Contra-indications

When a client attends for an eyebrow shaping treatment, the therapist should always check that there are no **contra-indications** that might prevent the treatment.

If, while completing the record card or on visual inspection of the skin, the client is found to have any of the following in the eye area, eyebrow shaping treatment must not be carried out:

- ***hypersensitive skin*** – the skin could become excessively red and swollen
- ***any eye disorder***, such as those described in the chart below
- ***inflammation or swelling***– the cause may be medical
- ***skin disease***
- ***skin disorder***, such as severe psoriasis or eczema
- ***bruising*** – client discomfort could be caused and the condition made worse
- ***cuts or abrasions*** – secondary infection could occur
- ***scar tissue under six months old*** – the skin lacks elasticity

The following chart will help you to identify some eye disorders that contra-indicate eyebrow shaping treatment and also tinting eyebrows and lashes, artificial eyelash application, threading and eyelash perming.

Name	Description	Name	Description
Conjunctivitis or pink eye (WELLCOME)	Infectious bacterial infection. Inflammation of the mucous membrane that covers the eye and lines the eyelid. The skin of the inner conjunctiva of the eye becomes inflamed, the eye becomes very red, itchy and sore, and pus may exude from the eye area.	Watery eye or epiphora (WELLCOME)	The eye over-secretes tears, which would normally drain into the nasal cavity.
Stye or hordeola (WELLCOME)	Infectious bacterial infection. Infection of the sebaceous glands of the eyelash hair follides. Small lumps appear on the inner rim of the eyelid containing pus.	Blepharitis (WELLCOME)	Inflammation of the eyelid caused by infection or an allergic reaction.

Name	Description	Name	Description
Cyst © CHRISTOPH HER-MANN/ALAMY	Localized pocket of sebum, which forms in the hair follicle or under the sebaceous glands in the skin. Semi-globular in shape, either raised or flat, and hard or soft. The cysts are the same colour as skin, or red if bacterial infection occurs. A cyst appearing on the upper eyelid is known as a chalazion or meibomian cyst.	**Benign (non-malignant) tumor** WELLCOME	Harmless skin-coloured growths. They may appear as a 'thread' of skin on the eyelids growing between the eyelashes. Chemical services such as tinting and perming should be avoided to avoid skin irritation. Refer the client to their GP.

If you are unsure about the safety of proceeding with service – for example, if there is an undiagnosed lump in the area – ask your client to seek medical approval first. Remember you are not qualified to diagnose a contra-indication. Refer the client to their GP without causing unnecessary cause for concern.

Discuss possible contra-actions that may occur during or after the eyebrow shaping service with your client at consultation.

Contra-actions

Severe erythema is considered to be a **contra-action** to the service: it is recognized as a marked reddening of the skin seen over the whole area or specifically around one damaged follicle. It is usually accompanied by minor swelling of the area. If this occurs the beauty therapist must try to reduce the redness by applying a cool compress and soothing antiseptic lotion or cream to the area. In extreme cases it may be necessary to apply ice. Record details of any contra-action on the client's record card.

If the reddening reduces in response to your corrective action, you may decide in future to remove only a few stray hairs at each eyebrow-shaping service, to minimize the risk of this reaction recurring.

If you accidentally pinch the skin with the tweezers and break the skin, apply a suitable soothing, antiseptic lotion for the skin, whilst wearing gloves. Inform the client not to touch the area and recommend the further application of a suitable antiseptic lotion. The main aim is to avoid secondary infection. All details of action taken must be recorded on the client record card.

Dispose of any contaminated waste according to the local environmental health regulations.

HEALTH & SAFETY

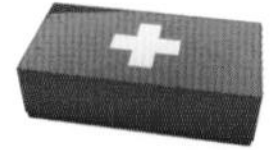

Contra-action: using ice
To maintain hygiene, place the ice cube in a new small freezer food bag. Dispose of the bag hygienically after use.

Discuss possible contra-actions that may occur during or after the eyebrow shaping service with your client at consultation.

KNOWLEDGE CHECK

Why is it important to have a thorough consultation before you commence the eyebrow shaping treatment?

Need more time... refer to pages 245–247 to help you.

Believe in the product

Believe in what you are selling: if you do not like the products it will be very hard to convince someone else that they should have them.

Be confident when selling and use the products yourself.

Shavata Singh

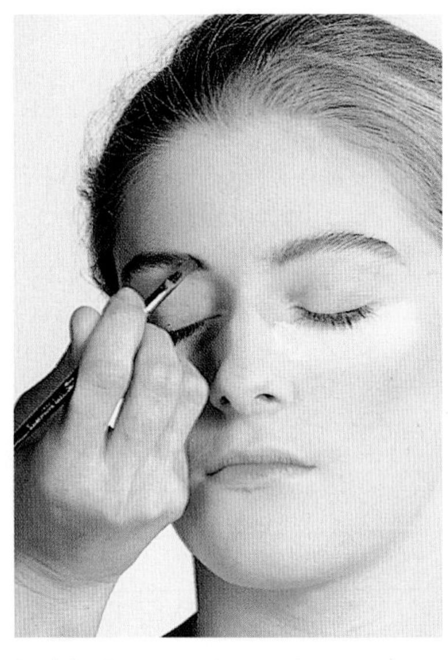

Applying temporary brow colour

Planning the service: factors to be considered

Before shaping the brows you must consider the following factors.

The natural shape of the brow The natural brow follows the line of the eye socket. This varies greatly between clients, and affects what is achievable.

If the client has been shaping their own brows, it may be necessary to let them grow for a short period before shaping them professionally. If the brows are very thin or very thick, it may take several sessions before the desired shape is achieved.

If the brows have been plucked over a long period of time, they may not grow back successfully; this should be discussed with the client. In such instances, temporary eyebrow pencil or matt powder eye shadow may be used to achieve the desired effect. Temporary brow colour is useful to apply when growing hairs into a new brow shape, to create a defined brow shape.

Fashion Each season sees new fashion trends, which also affect eye make-up and eyebrow shapes. This should be considered before using any form of permanent hair removal to shape the brows.

TOP TIP

Temporary brow colour

A sharpened eyebrow pencil may be used to simulate brow hairs – apply feathery strokes using the pencil point. To create a natural effect, two different pencil colours may be used, for example brown and grey.

TOP TIP

Male eyebrow shaping

Men may require a result that emphasizes their natural brow shape. This generally requires removing hair as shown below:

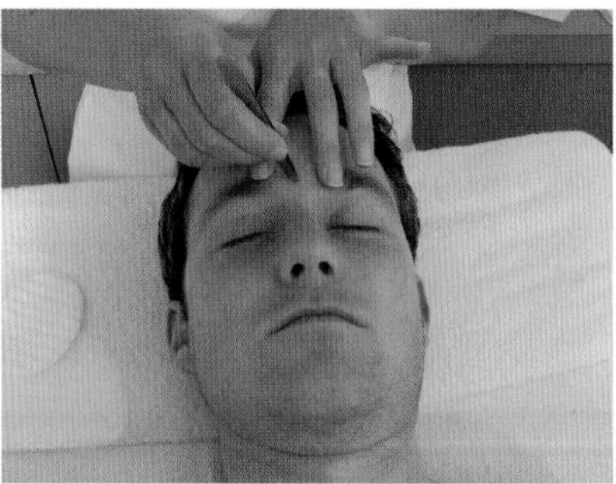

From the area between the brows where the brow hairs may meet. If this brow hair is not removed it can give the client a stern look.

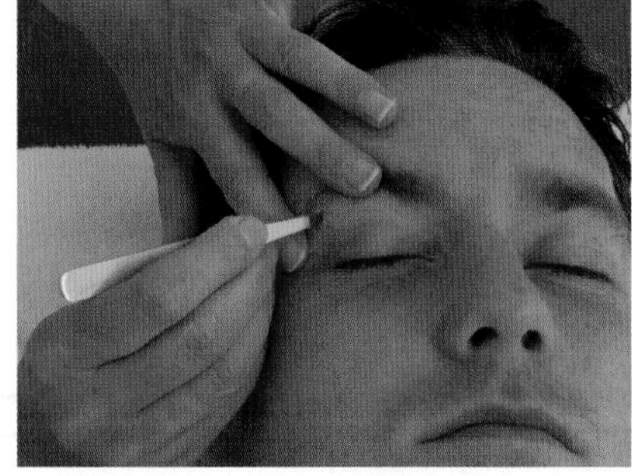

Underneath the lower outer brow which will open up the eye area. If this brow hair is not removed it can create a hooded effect to the eyelid.

Practise excellent customer service

- Promote great grooming.
- Be passionate about eyebrows.
- A successful beauty therapist will have a natural talent with people.
- Stay level-headed.
- Be precise!

Shavata Singh

The age of the client The brow hair of older clients may include a few coarse, long, discoloured white or grey hairs. These may be removed provided that this does not alter the brow line or leave bald patches.

In general, thick eyebrows make the client look older, by creating a hooded appearance; and thin eyebrows will make the client look severe. Ideally the brows should therefore be shaped to a medium thickness.

The natural growth pattern The shape and effect that the client requests may be made impossible by the pattern of the natural growth of the hair, which is genetically determined. When shaping the brows of the Oriental client, for example, you will notice that the eyebrow hair grows in a downward direction. To create an arch it may be necessary to trim the hairs, using a small, sterile pair of sharp nail scissors. Alternatively, you may remove the outer eyebrow length and use a cosmetic pencil to create a new brow-line. Use your professional judgement to advise the client.

Choosing an eyebrow shape

The eyebrows should be in balance with the rest of the facial features: the right brow shape for each client will depend on the client's facial proportions and natural brow shape.

There is no single ideal brow shape; different brow shapes are shown below.

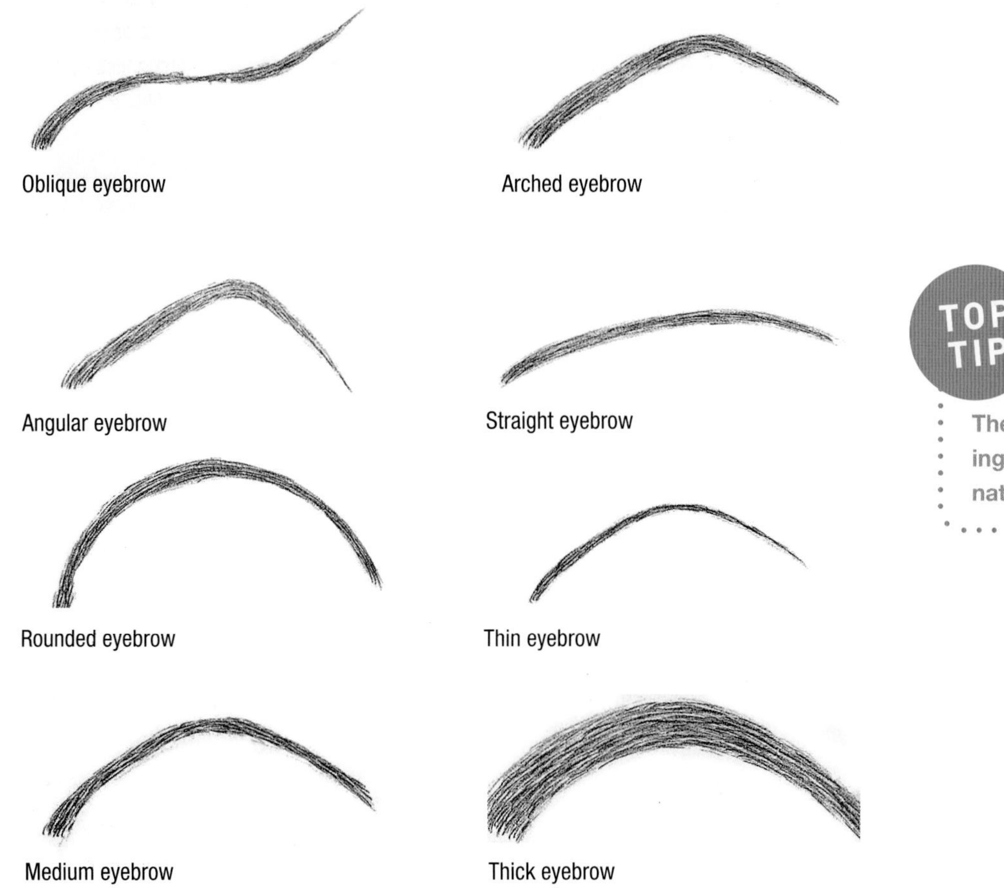

TOP TIP

False eyebrows

These are ideal for disguising any bald areas in the natural eyebrow hair.

What is achievable? Obviously not all of these brow shapes are achievable for every client, but the skilful application to the eyebrows of temporary cosmetic colour can create the illusion of the desired brow shape.

The quantity of brow hair removed during shaping produces a thin, medium or thick final shape, as illustrated. Other approaches, too, may be used:

- ***Semi-permanent make-up***, also referred to as micro-pigmentation, can be used to add colour permanently to the brows, for example to disguise a bald patch.
- ***Hair transplants*** are available for the client with sparse eyebrows.
- ***False individual eyebrow hairs*** are applied in the same way as individual false eyelashes.

Ideally, the distance between the two eyebrows should be the width of one eye. If this is not the case, the illusion may be created by removing hairs or by applying temporary brow colour to create this effect.

TOP TIP

Semi-permanent make-up

Suspended pigment particles in a liquid base are inserted into the outer skin using a disposable needle. Many of the popular dyes are based on plant extracts.

The effect gradually fades, lasting up to three years.

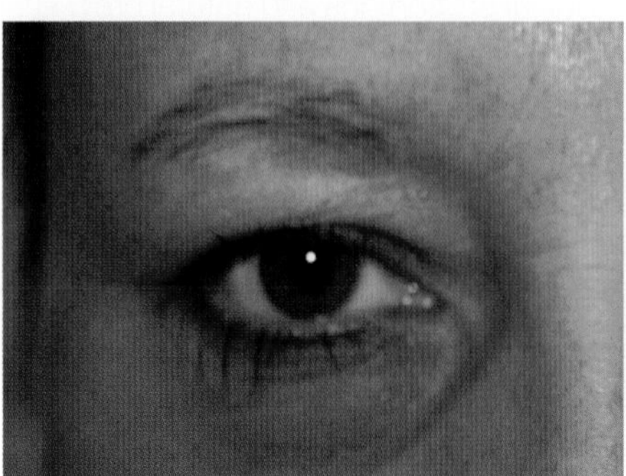

Before

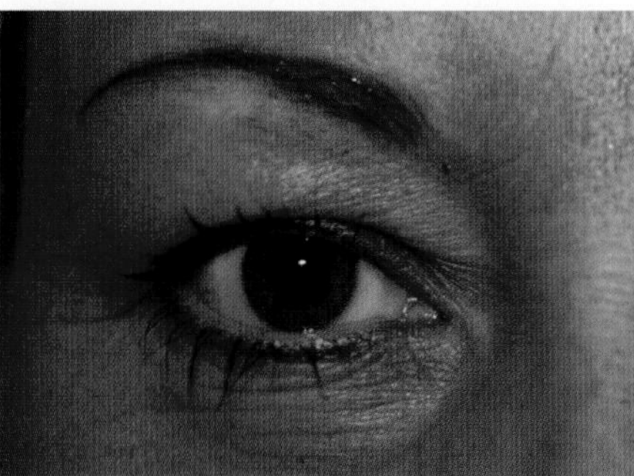

After

Wide-set eyes can be made to appear closer together by extending the brow-line beyond the inside corner of the eye; close-set eyes can be made to look further apart by widening the distance between them.

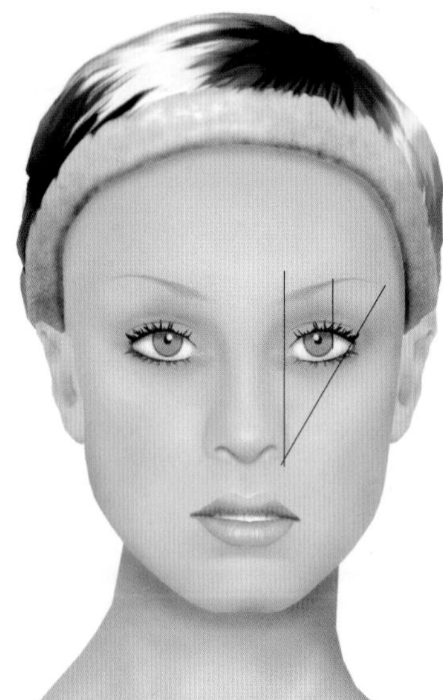

Measuring the eyebrow

How to measure the eyebrows to decide length

In order to determine the correct length of the client's eyebrows, there are three main guidelines:

1. Place an orange stick or spatula beside the nose and the inside corner of the eye. This is usually in line with the tear duct. Any hairs that grow between the eyes and beyond this point should be removed. If the client has a very broad nose, however, this guide is inappropriate: tweezing would commence near the middle of the brow. In this instance, use the tear duct at the inside corner of the eye as a guide (as per image).
2. Place an orange stick or spatula in a line from the base of the nose (to the side of the nostril) to the outer corner of the eye. Any hairs that grow beyond this point should be removed.
3. Place an orange stick or spatula in a vertical line from the centre of the eyelid. This is where the highest point of the arch should be.

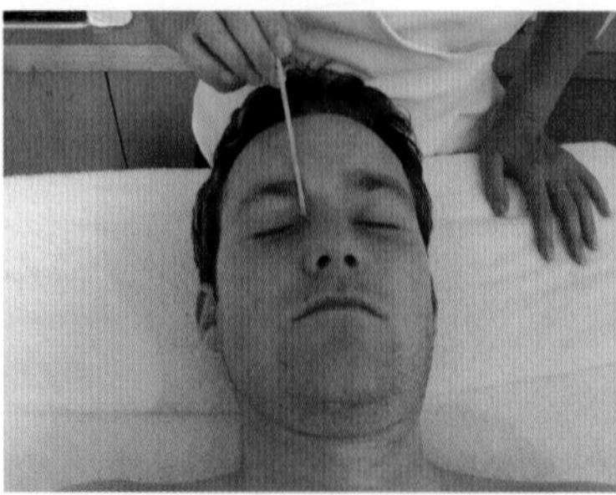

Measuring the eyebrow: the inner corner of the eye

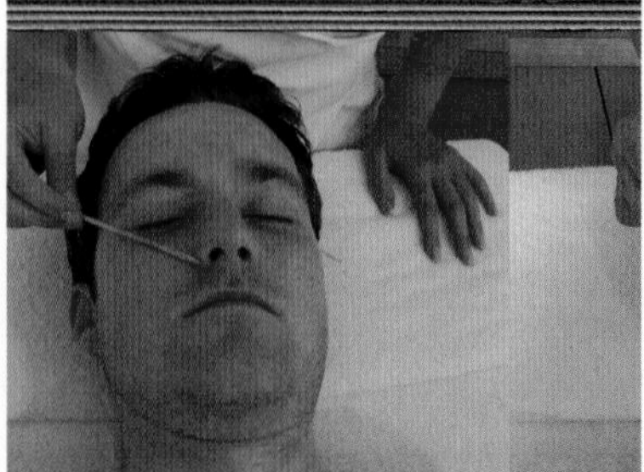

Measuring the eyebrow: the outer corner of the eye

Initially these guidelines will be needed to ensure that the correct length and brow shape are achieved, but the experienced therapist will recognize the corrective work to be carried out without the need for measuring.

ACTIVITY

Correcting brow shapes

You cannot change the bone structure of the facial features without cosmetic surgery, but brow shaping can create the illusion of improved facial balance and proportion. Discuss why each of the brow shapes below would complement the accompanying face shape.

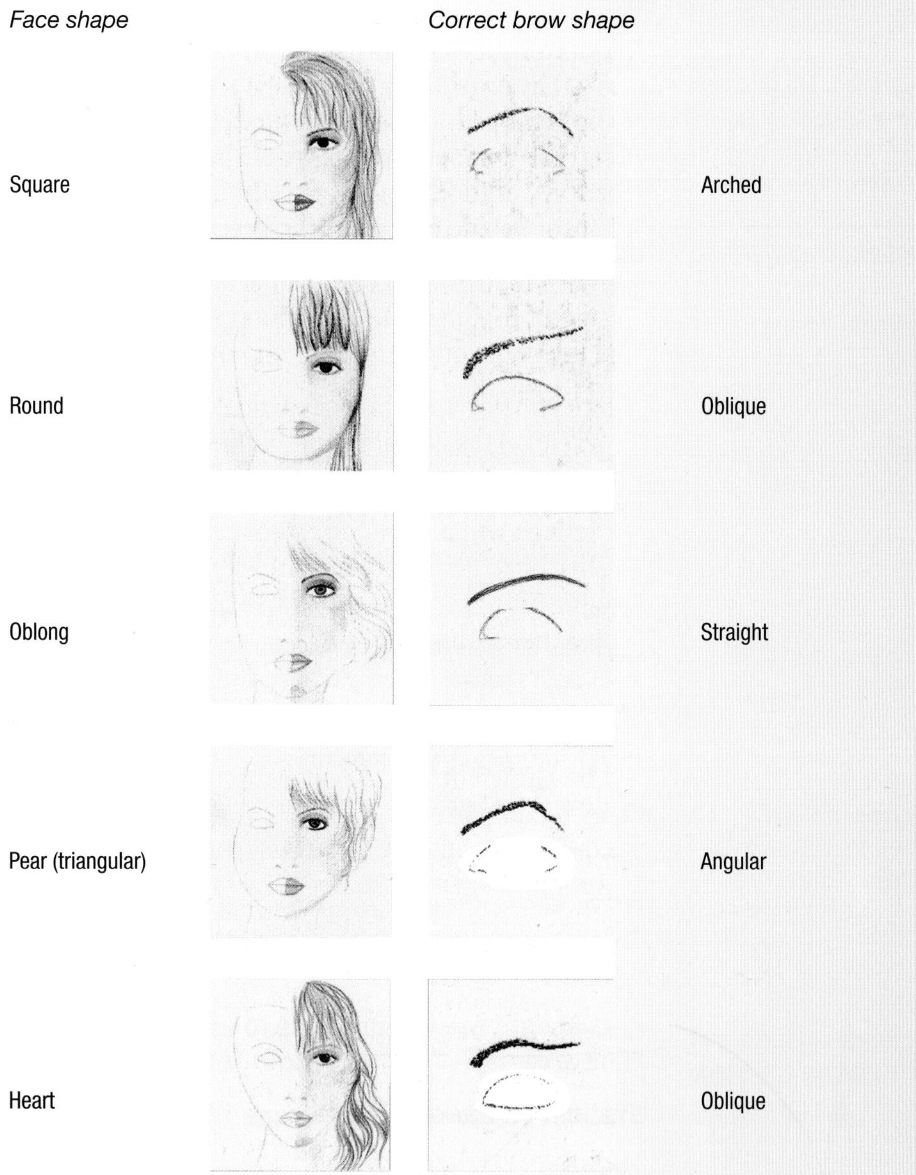

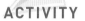

ACTIVITY

Correcting brow shapes through brow-shaping service

How would you correct the appearance of the following eye shapes:

- wide-set
- close-set?

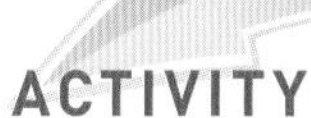

ACTIVITY

Correcting brow shapes

From magazines, collect pictures of faces showing different eyebrow shapes. Discuss which you think are correct and which incorrect for the person, explaining why.

ALWAYS REMEMBER

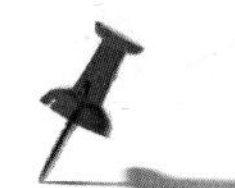

Accurately record your client's answers to necessary questions asked at the consultation.

Following the consultation, record all client details accurately on the client record card. A record card that can be used for the eye services follows.

The following record card is designed to record details of all **eyelash and brow treatments**.

A sample client record card

Date	Beauty therapist name	
Client name		Date of birth (identifying client age group)
Home address		Postcode
Landline phone number	Mobile phone number	Email address
Name of doctor	Doctor's address and phone number	
Related medical history (conditions that may restrict or prohibit service application)		
Are you taking any medication? (this may affect the condition of the skin or skin sensitivity)		

CONTRA-INDICATIONS REQUIRING MEDICAL REFERRAL
(preventing eye treatment application)

- ☐ severe skin conditions, (e.g. severe eczema in area)
- ☐ eye infections (e.g. conjunctivitis, styes)
- ☐ eye disease
- ☐ inflammation of the skin
- ☐ during chemotherapy and radiotherapy

EYE TREATMENT

- ☐ shaping eyebrows
- ☐ tinting eyebrows
- ☐ tinting eyelashes
- ☐ artificial eyelashes
- ☐ lash perming

BROW SHAPING TECHNIQUES

- ☐ brow shape selected following measurement of the client's natural brow and eye
- ☐ opening of the pores and hair follicle to facilitate removal
- ☐ keeping the skin taut
- ☐ removal of hairs in the direction of hair growth
- ☐ protection of the eye
- ☐ hair removed to complement the shape and proportions of client's natural brow, in relation to facial features and shape and to client's satisfaction

TREATMENT AREA

- ☐ eyebrows
- ☐ total reshape
- ☐ maintenance of original shape

CONTRA-INDICATIONS WHICH RESTRICT TREATMENT
(treatment may require adaptation)

- ☐ recent scar tissue
- ☐ eye disorders
- ☐ product allergies
- ☐ bruising
- ☐ undiagnosed lumps and swellings

EYELASH OR BROW TINTING

- ☐ skin sensitivity test carried out
- ☐ tint colour selection suited to client's colouring characteristics
- ☐ effectively protecting the surrounding skin
- ☐ timing, development and removal of tint adapted according to client's natural colouring characteristics
- ☐ manufacturer's instructions complied with

COLOURING CHARACTERISTIC

fair ☐ red ☐ dark ☐ white ☐

ARTIFICIAL EYELASHES

- ☐ skin sensitivity test carried out
- ☐ colour and length of lash type selected to meet agreed service requirement and effect to be achieved
- ☐ individual flare lash
- ☐ strip lash
- ☐ manufacturer's instructions complied with

EYELASH PERMING

- ☐ skin sensitivity test carried out
- ☐ rod size selected to suit client's lash length and effect to be achieved
- ☐ treatment application time in accordance with client's eyelash hair and manufacturer's instructions

Beauty therapist signature (for reference)

Client signature (confirmation of details)

A sample client record card (continued)

TREATMENT ADVICE

Eyebrow shape – *allow 15 minutes*
Eyebrow tint – *allow 10 minutes*
Eyelash tint* – *allow 20 minutes*
Eyebrow shape and eyelash tint* – *allow 30 minutes*
Perming* – *allow 45 minutes*
Eyebrow tint, shape and lash tint* – *allow 30 minutes*
Artificial eyelashes – *allow 20 minutes*
*Eyelash tint timing and perming may differ according to the system used. Always follow the manufacturer's instructions.

TREATMENT PLAN

Record relevant details of your treatment and advice provided for future reference.

Ensure the client's records are up to date, accurate and fully completed following treatment. Non-compliance may invalidate insurance.

DURING

Find out:

- what products the client is currently using to cleanse and care for the skin of the eye area
- satisfaction with these products

Explain:

- how the different eye products should be applied and removed

Note:

- any adverse reaction (contra-action), if any occur

AFTER

Record:

- results of service
- any modification to service application that has occurred
- what products have been used in the eyelash/eyebrow service
- the effectiveness of service
- any samples provided (review their success at the next appointment)

Advise on:

- product application and removal in order to gain maximum benefit from product use
- use of aftercare products following eye service
- use of skincare/make-up products following eye service
- maintenance procedures
- recommended time intervals between services

RETAIL OPPORTUNITIES

Advise on:

- progression of the service plan for future appointments
- products that would be suitable for the client to use at home to care for the eye area
- recommendations for further services
- further products or services that the client may or may not have received before

Note:

- any purchase made by the client

EVALUATION

Record:

- comments on the client's satisfaction with the service
- if poor results are achieved, the reasons why
- how you may alter the service plan to achieve the required service results in the future, if applicable

HEALTH AND SAFETY

Advise on:

- how to care for the area following service to avoid an unwanted reaction
- avoidance of any activities or product application that may cause a contra-action
- appropriate necessary action to be taken in the event of an unwanted skin or eye irritation

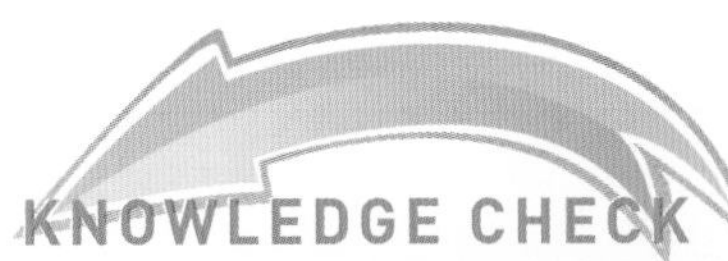

KNOWLEDGE CHECK

How can you determine the length of a client's eyebrows that will suit their facial features?

Need more time... refer to page 250 to help you.

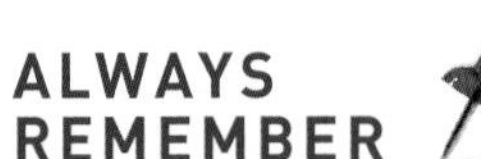
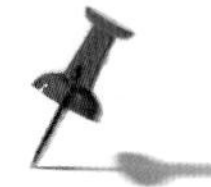

ALWAYS REMEMBER

Examples of eye service modification include:

Eyebrow shape

- Avoiding removing hair that is concealing a bald area, e.g. scar in the area.
- Hair removal when shaping a male client's eyebrows.

Eyelash tint

- Allowing further processing time to an area where the hair is more resistant to colour.

Artificial eyelashes

- Selecting an alternative lash length appropriate to the function of the lens, if the client wears glasses.
- If long-sighted, the lens will magnify the eye creating an unrealistic look if the artificial lash length is too long.

TOP TIP

Skin sensitivity test

It is acceptable for the salon receptionist – provided that they have been trained to do so – to carry out the skin sensitivity test.

ACTIVITY

Eyelash and eyebrow tinting
List reasons why clients would benefit from this service. Discuss the reasons with your tutor.

Tint eyebrow and lashes consultation

Reception

When making an appointment for this service, allow five minutes for a skin sensitivity test, ten minutes for an eyebrow tint, and 20 minutes for an eyelash tint. When the client is booking a service, ask them:

- to visit the salon 24 hours before the appointment for a skin sensitivity test
- if they wear contact lenses, to bring their lens container so that they can place the lenses in it during the tinting service

On average, a client will need their lashes tinted every six weeks, or sooner if for example they take a holiday in a climate where sun bleaches them. Eyebrow tinting, on the other hand, should be repeated when the client feels it to be necessary, perhaps every four weeks, as eyebrows seem to lose colour intensity more quickly than lash hair.

Skin sensitivity test

Some clients are sensitive to the tint, and produce an allergic reaction immediately on contact with it; others may become allergic later. For this you therefore need to carry out a **skin sensitivity test** before each lash- or brow-tinting service. (For the skin sensitivity test, a hypersensitivity test, or a predisposition test – see page 150.) This test should be given either on the inside of the elbow or behind the ear.

Two responses to the skin sensitivity test are possible – positive and negative:

- a **positive skin sensitivity test** result is recognized by irritation, swelling or inflammation of the skin – if this occurs, do not proceed with the service
- a **negative skin sensitivity test** result produces no skin reaction – in this case you may proceed with the service

The results should be recorded on the client's record card for insurance purposes.

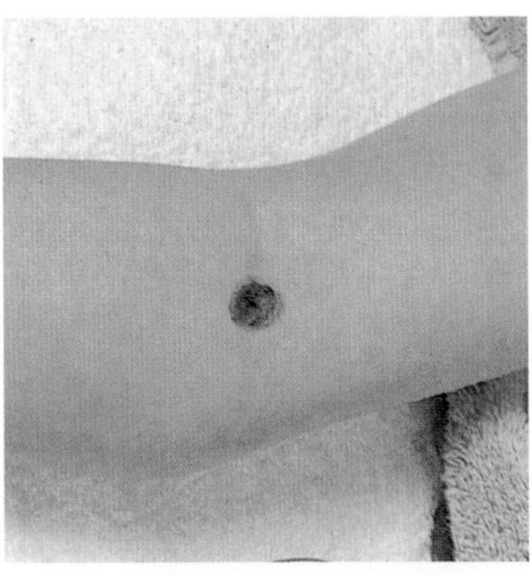

A skin sensitivity test for eyelash/brow tinting

Contra-indications

When a client attends for an eyelash or brow tinting service, the beauty therapist should always check that there are no contra-indications that might prevent service.

After completing the record card and inspecting the eye area, if you have found any of the following in the eye area, do not proceed with the tinting service:

- ***inflammation or swelling*** – the cause may be medical
- ***skin disease***
- ***skin disorder***, such as severe psoriasis or eczema
- ***cuts and abrasions*** – secondary infection and irritation of the skin could occur
- ***hypersensitive skin*** – the skin could become excessively red and swollen
- ***any eye disorders***, such as conjunctivitis, blepharitis, styes or hordeola, watery eye, or cysts
- ***a positive (allergic) reaction*** to the skin sensitivity test
- ***contact lenses*** (unless removed)

KNOWLEDGE CHECK

What details should be recorded on the client's record card?

Need more time... refer to pages 252–253 to help you.

Look back at the chart illustrating contra-indications to eye services on pages 246–247.

Remember you are not qualified to diagnose a contra-indication. Refer the client to their GP without causing unnecessary cause for concern.

A particularly nervous client would also be contra-indicated:

- it would be difficult for them to keep their eyes closed for ten minutes
- they might panic as the tint was applied, creating the possibility of tint entering the eye
- they might blink frequently, making preparation of the eye area and application of the tint both difficult and hazardous

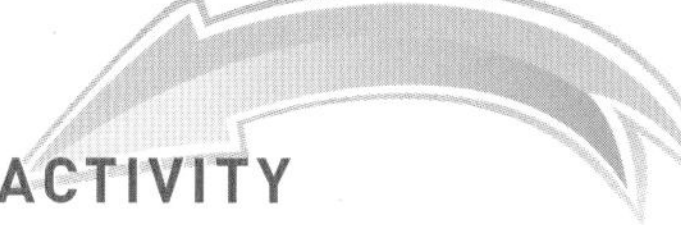

ACTIVITY

Allergic reactions
With colleagues, discuss the possible implications of ignoring a positive reaction to the skin test

Inform the client at consultation of any relevant contra-actions that may occur and the action to take.

Contra-actions

If the client complains of discomfort during the service, tint may have entered the eye. Take the following action:

1. Remove the tint immediately from the eye area, using clean, damp cotton wool pads in an outward sweep.
2. When you are satisfied that all excess tint has been removed (that is, when the cotton wool shows clean), carefully flush the eye with clean water. Repeat the rinsing process until discomfort has been relieved.
3. Apply a cool compress to cool and soothe the eye area.

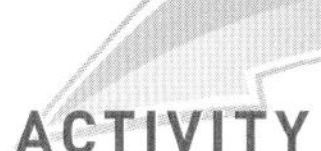

ACTIVITY

Explaining poor results
What reasons can you think of to explain why a permanent tint applied to the eyelashes or eyebrows has not coloured the hair successfully? Discuss your answers with your tutor.

If there is a noticeable sensitivity of the eye tissue after eyebrow or eyelash tinting it may be recommended that the client does not receive the service again. Alternatively, source an alternative tinting product to test compatibility. Record this on her record card so that the offending product may be avoided in the future.

In the event of an allergic contra-action the client should be advised to apply a cool compress and soothing agent to the skin to reduce redness and irritation. If symptoms persist they should seek medical advice.

HEALTH & SAFETY

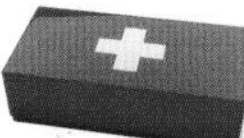

Contra-action: allergy to tinting product
Source an alternative manufacturer. The client may not be allergic to all products if the cause of the contra-action is allergy.

Planning the service

For the eyelashes and eyebrows, select a colour that complements the client's hair **colouring characteristics** (fair, red, dark and white), her skin colour, her age and her usual

KNOWLEDGE CHECK

When observing the area for eye services, what conditions would contra-indicate service?

Need more time... refer to pages 246–247 to help you.

eye cosmetics. Always discuss the choice of colour carefully with the client to discover her preference. You may ask certain questions in order to help you in your selection:

- 'What colour mascara do you normally wear?'
- 'How dark would you like your eyelashes/eyebrows?'
- 'Do you normally wear eyebrow pencil? What colour?'
- 'Have you had your eyebrows/lashes tinted before? Were you satisfied with the result?'

Artificial lashes consultation

Reception

When making an appointment for false eyelash application, find out why the client wants artificial lashes and determine which type would be most appropriate.

Allow 20 minutes for the application of individual eyelashes, and again allow a further 45 minutes if applying them in conjunction with a make-up.

Although individual flare lashes can be worn for up to six weeks, they look effective only for approximately three weeks. After this time, the appearance of the **artificial lashes** begins to deteriorate, the lash **adhesive** becomes brittle, and the eyelash area may become irritated.

Due to the cyclic nature of hair replacement, some individual flare lashes will be lost when the natural lash falls out. These lashes may be replaced each week, as necessary; the client is usually charged a price for each individual flare lash replaced. The client must be told of this service as part of the aftercare advice.

When a client makes an appointment for an artificial lash treatment, they should be asked the following questions:

- ***Have they had a similar treatment before in this salon?*** If they have not, they should visit the salon beforehand for a skin test to assess any sensitivity to the adhesive (see page 150). Commonly, a small amount of the eyelash adhesive is placed behind the ear. A positive skin reaction where the skin becomes reddened, irritated and swollen means that you cannot proceed with the service. A negative skin sensitivity test produces no skin reaction—in this case you may proceed with the treatment. Results should be recorded on the client record card for insurance purposes.
- ***Are they having the false eyelashes applied for any particular reason, such as a holiday or a special occasion?*** In deciding which type of false eyelash would be most appropriate, take into consideration the effect required and for how long the lashes are to be worn.

If the client wears glasses, the artificial lashes must not be so long as to touch the lenses. Also, if the lens magnifies the eye, this must be taken into account. Ask the client to bring their glasses with them to the salon.

Contra-indications

If following completion of the record card or inspection of the eye area you have found any of the following, do not apply false eyelashes:

- ***skin disease***
- ***skin disorder in the eye area***, such as severe psoriasis or eczema
- ***inflammation or swelling*** around the eye
- ***hypersensitive skin***
- ***any eye disorder***, such as styes or hordeola, conjunctivitis, blepharitis, watery eye, or cysts
- ***a positive (allergic) reaction*** to the adhesive skin test
- ***contact lenses*** (unless removed)

A chart is shown on pages 246–247 illustrating some contra-indications to eye treatment services.

Remember you are not qualified to diagnose a contra-indication. Refer the client to their GP without causing unnecessary cause for concern.

An unduly nervous client with a tendency to blink could also prove hard to treat in this way. Use your discretion in deciding on the suitability of a client for treatment.

Inform the client at consultation of any relevant contra-actions that may occur and the action to take.

Contra-actions

If, during application of artificial lashes, the eye starts to water, blot the tears with the corner of a clean tissue. The tears can cause the adhesive to take on an unsightly white crystallized appearance. Any possible irritation of the eyes should therefore be avoided, during both preparation of the eye area and application itself.

Never place eyelashes *underneath* the natural eyelashes – eye irritation would occur.

While practising individual eyelash application you may find at some point that you have accidentally glued a couple of the lower and upper natural lashes together. Apply adhesive **solvent** to a cotton wool-tipped orange stick, and gently roll this over the lash length to dissolve the adhesive.

If solvent or adhesive should accidentally enter the eye, remove excess product, rinse the eye thoroughly and immediately, using clean water. Repeat this until discomfort is no longer experienced.

The client should be shown through to the prepared work area after the record card has been completed.

Consult the record card and check the area for any contra-indications to service.

Remember always provide the opportunity for your client to ask any questions relating to the eye service.

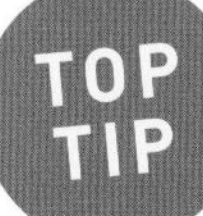

Fair lashes

If the client has fair lashes, you could promote an eyelash tint service before false eyelash application to achieve a more natural, realistic effect.

TOP TIP

Achieve a natural look

Individual flare lashes may be applied in a variety of lengths, short, medium and long, to create a natural look. The longest lashes are applied in the centre of the lashes.

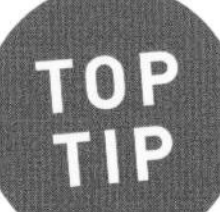

TOP TIP

Streaked lashes

Streaked lashes can be sourced, to give a more subtle effect for the mature client.

The record card should be signed and dated by the client and beauty therapist following the consultation to confirm the suitability and consent with the agreed service.

It is important that accurate records are kept and stored in compliance with the Data Protection Act for future reference.

Planning the service

A variety of artificial lashes are available, including lashes intended for corrective work as well as those simply intended to enhance the natural lashes. Lash length may be short, medium or long; their texture may be fine, medium or thick, with some having a feathered effect. Strips designed for use on the lower lashes are called **partial lashes**: here small groups of hairs are placed intermittently along the length of the false-lash base.

In a commercial salon, the most popular colours are usually black and brown. For special effects, however; strip lashes are available in fantasy colours, complete with glitter and jewels!

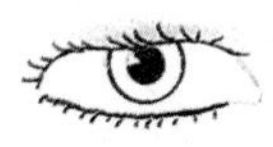

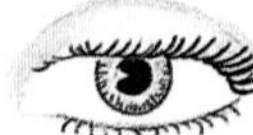

Short and stubby lashes

Factors when choosing false eyelashes

Before applying artificial lashes the beauty therapist should consider the following points, and advise the client accordingly.

The client's age Artificial lashes create a very bold, dramatic effect, which can make an older client look too hard. Remember that the skin colour and the natural hair colour change with age: the lash chosen must enhance the client's appearance.

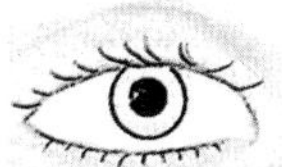

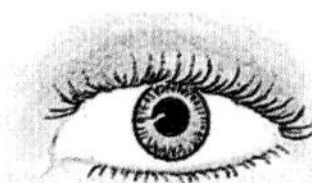

Sparse lashes

The client's natural lashes Does the client have short or long, sparse or thick, very curly or straight lashes? Choose an artificial lash to complement the natural lash. Here are some guidelines:

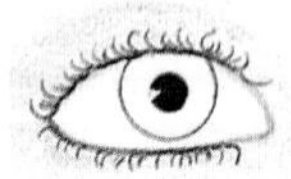

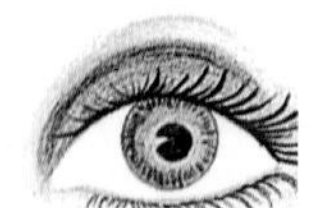

Curly eyelashes

- ***Short and stubby lashes*** These are commonly seen on older clients who have overhanging eyelids. Choose a medium lash length in a medium thickness at the outer corner of the eyelid; the lashes should become gradually shorter from the centre of the eyelid to the inner corner. Brush the artificial and natural lashes together after application to ensure that they blend.
- ***Sparse lashes*** Place individual short lashes along the natural lash line; or, to give a more natural appearance, you may wish to apply partial strip lashes to the upper eyelid.
- ***Curly eyelashes*** These are very common on African-Caribbean clients. Choose a longer, sweeping strip or individual artificial lashes, in black. The chosen lashes and colour should give emphasis and depth to the eye.

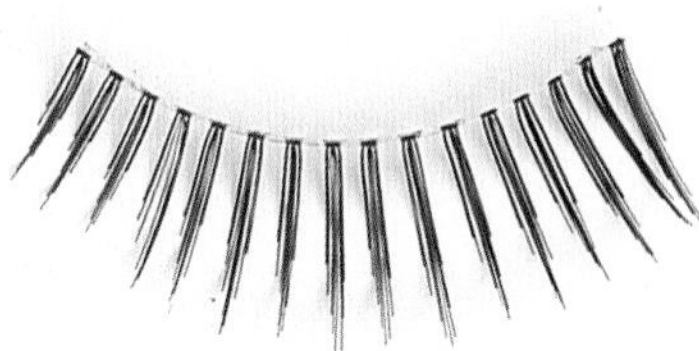

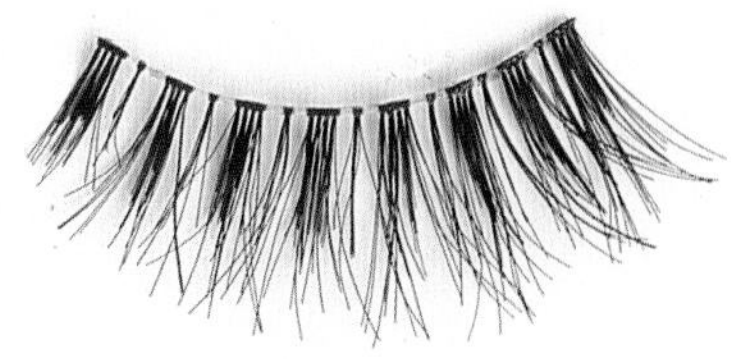

Artificial strip lashes

The natural eyelash colour Select artificial lashes that complement the hair and skin tone. Natural-hair false eyelashes offer the greatest choice of colour, but these are expensive and may be difficult to purchase.

Using false eyelashes for corrective purposes Here are some outlines of corrective techniques for various eye shapes.

Eye shape	Corrective steps
Small eyes 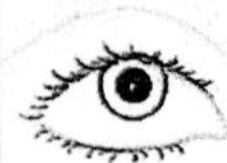 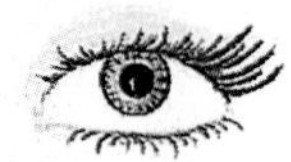	Place artificial lashes at the outer corners of the upper eyelid. These should be longer than the natural lashes.
Close-set eyes 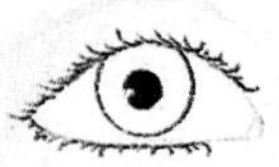 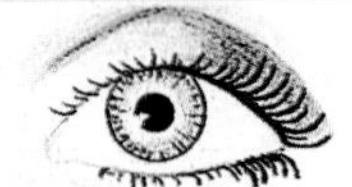	Place fine, long, individual or partial lashes at the outer third of the eye. They may be applied to the lower lashes as well as to the upper.
Wide-set eyes 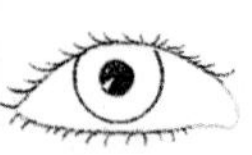 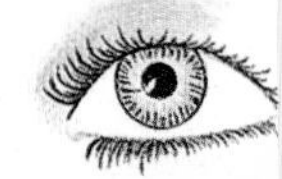	Apply medium-length lashes at the inner corner of the eye and to the centre, becoming slightly shorter towards the outer corner of the upper eyelid. This may be repeated on the lower lash also.
Downward-slanting eyes 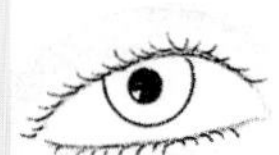 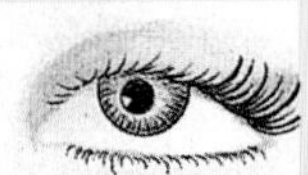	Apply longer lashes (individual or partial strip lashes) to the outer corners of the upper eyelid.
Round eyes 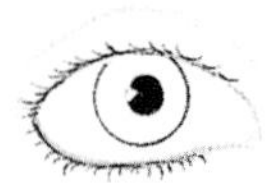 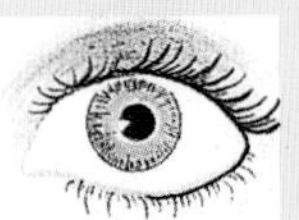	Individual or strip lashes should be used to lengthen the lash line. Apply the artificial lashes from the centre of the upper eyelid outwards.
Deep-set eyes 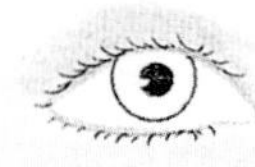 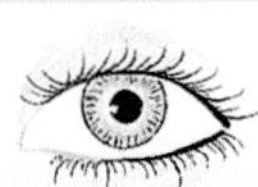	Apply fine lashes to the upper and lower lashes. The upper-lid artificial lashes should be longer, to draw attention to the eye.
Overhanging lids 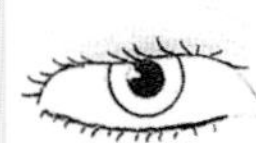 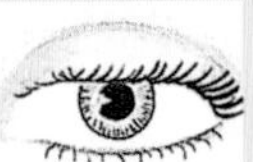	Apply longer lashes to the upper eyelid, from the outer corner and tapering to a shorter length at the centre of the lid and toward the inner corner.

ACTIVITY

Choosing eyelash colours

Suggest a choice of false eyelash colour for the clients below:

- a mature grey-haired client
- a young red-haired client
- a mature client with bleached hair
- a mature African-Caribbean client

KNOWLEDGE CHECK

Why is a skin sensitivity test needed before every tinting/perming and artificial individual flare lash service?

Need more time... refer to page 256 to help you.

On completion the artificial lashes should give a balanced and well-proportioned look complementing the client's eye shape, producing the agreed desired effect.

Eyelash perming consultation

Reception

When making the appointment for eyelash perming, recommend that the client has a skin sensitivity test. Ask them to visit the salon for this 24 hours before the appointment.

If they wear contact lenses, ask them to bring the lens container so that they can place the lenses in it during the eyelash perming treatment.

Advise the client that the treatment requires that they keep their eyes closed for a long time. Some clients may find this uncomfortable, and may choose not to have the treatment.

The client should not have an eyelash tint immediately before perming, as the colour for the lashes will be lightened by the treatment process. However, tinting is effective following eyelash perming and should be promoted. Allow a minimum of 24 hours following the eyelash perming treatment before tinting.

On average, a client will need their eyelashes permed every two to three months. A treatment takes approximately 45 minutes.

Contra-indications

When a client attends for an eyelash perming treatment, the therapist should always check that there are no contra-indications that might prevent the service.

If following completion of the record card or inspection of the eye area you have found any of the following, do not carry out eyelash perming:

- ***inflammation or swelling*** – the cause may be medical
- ***skin disease***
- ***skin disorder***, such as psoriasis or eczema
- ***cuts and abrasions*** – secondary infection and irritation of the skin could occur
- ***hypersensitive skin*** – the skin could become excessively red and swollen
- ***any eye disorders***, such as conjunctivitis, blepharitis, styes or hordeola, watery eye, or cysts
- ***a positive (allergic) reaction*** to the skin sensitivity test
- ***contact lenses*** (unless removed)
- ***considerable nervousness*** – a particularly nervous client may make application, fixing and removal hazardous.

Look back at the earlier chart illustrating contra-indications to eye services on pages 246–247.

Remember you are not qualified to diagnose a contra-indication. Refer the client to their GP without causing unnecessary cause for concern.

Inform the client at consultation of any relevant contra-actions that may occur and the action to take.

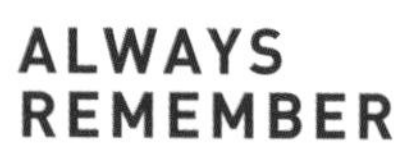

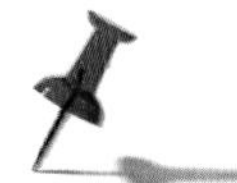

When not to perm

Permanent curling is not advisable if the lashes are:

- naturally curly (unnecessary treatment outcome)
- very short and sparse (the result will be ineffective)
- fragile (hair breakage may occur).

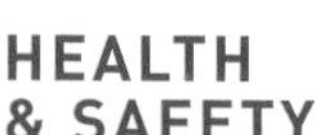

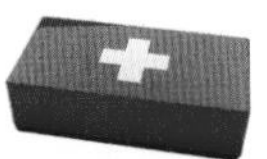

Lanolin

Some eyelash perming lotions contain lanolin. If using such lotions, ask the client before application of they are allergic to lanolin.

Skin sensitivity test

Some clients may be sensitive to the perm solution, and may produce an allergic reaction immediately on contact with it; others may become allergic later. For this reason, a skin sensitivity test must be carried out before each eyelash perming treatment. This is essential not just for new clients; but also if there has been a lengthy interval since the previous eyelash perming treatment.

1 Apply a small amount of the perm solution to the inside of the elbow or behind the ear; and a small amount of fixing lotion to the other.

2 Test the client tolerance to the adhesive by applying a small amount of the adhesive to the inside of the elbow or behind the ear.

Avoid immediate contact with clothing.

3 Advise the client how to recognise a positive skin reaction: skin reddening, itching and swelling. Advise them to apply a soothing agent if this occurs and to notify you. This reaction can then be recorded on the client's record card.

TOP TIP

Positive promotion

To maximize revenue and to enhance the client's treatment, offer the client another service whilst the eyelashes are being permed. Suitable treatments include manicure or hand treatment.

Contra-actions

If the client complains of discomfort during the treatment, perm lotion may have entered the eye. Take the following action:

1 Remove the perm lotion immediately from the eye area, using clean, damp cotton wool. Remove the perm rod, using the moisturising agent if necessary to facilitate.

2 Carefully flush the eye with clean water. Repeat the rinsing process until discomfort has been relieved.

3 Apply a cool compress to sooth the eye area

Record this information on their record card.

Discuss possible contra-actions that may occur during or after the eyelash perming service with your client at consultation.

Undesirable perm results	Possible cause	Preventative action
Hooked end	Incorrect positioning of the point of the eyelash hair around the curler	Ensure that the point of the eyelash is corrected if it appears crooked before application of the perm lotion. Use eyelash adhesive to secure hair into the desired position.
Poor curl result	Incorrect preparation of the lashes; oil present on the lashes Eyelashes too damp before perm lotion application. Uneven application of the perm/fixing/neutralizing lotion Incorrect curler size for the hair	Ensure that the lashes are clean and excess moisture removed before perm lotion application. Ensure that the lashes are brushed through to separate the ends before curler application. Be methodical in application of perm/fixing neutralizing lotions to ensure effective curl result. Select the correct curler size for the lash length and coarseness of the hair. Use a reliable timing device to ensure accuracy of the timing process.

Undesirable perm results	Possible cause	Preventative action
Hairs pointing in different directions	Incorrect placing of the eyelash hair along the eyelash curler	Ensure the hairs are evenly placed and secured along the eyelash curler.
Vertical not curled	This tends to occur on short lashes where small curlers have been selected and the perm lotion has been applied to the majority of the length of the hair: from the base of the lashes the hair stands vertically	Ensure correct application of the perm lotion.
Too curled	Curlers too small for the eyelash length	Ensure that the correct curler is chosen for the lash length and thickness.

Planning the service

The eyelash curler should be selected to suit the natural eyelash hair and length.

The eyelash curler should be measured against the client's eyelid and trimmed to the appropriate length.

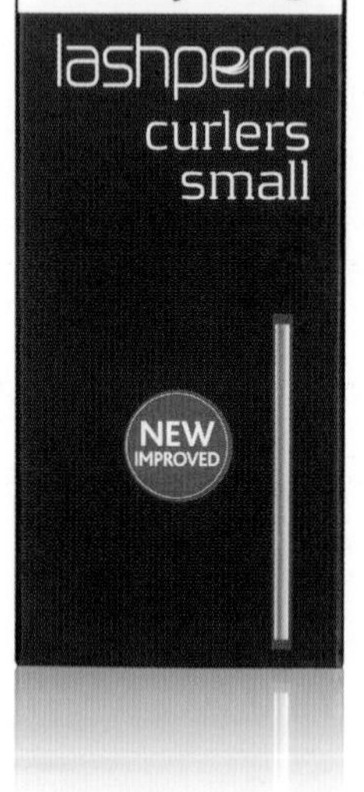

Small curlers are suitable for short eyelashes or if a tighter curl is required.

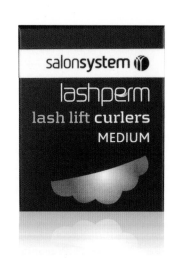

Medium curlers are suitable for average length lashes and will produce a defined curl.

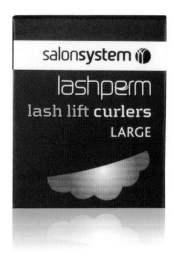

Large curlers are suitable for longer lashes and will produce a gently defined curl.

Eyebrow shaping

TOP TIP

It is often stated that before beginning shaping, the brows should be prepared with warm, damp cotton wool pads, to relax the hair follicles and soften the eyebrow tissue, thus making hair removal easier. During service, however, you will be wiping over the area with an antiseptic lotion, which has a cooling, soothing and tightening effect on the skin, so this preparation is often ineffectual but is relaxing for the client.

Outcome 2: Provide eyelash and brow treatments

Learn how to provide eyelash and eyebrow treatments

Practical skills

1. **Communicate and behave** in a professional manner.
2. Follow **health and safety working practices**.
3. Position yourself and the client correctly throughout the treatment.
4. Use **products, tools, equipment and techniques** to suit clients treatment needs.
5. Complete the treatment to the satisfaction of the client.
6. Record the results of the treatment.
7. Provide suitable **aftercare advice**.

Underpinning knowledge

1. State how to **communicate and behave** in a professional manner.
2. Describe **health and safety working practices**.
3. Explain the importance of positioning themselves and the client correctly throughout the treatment.
4. Explain the importance of using **products, tools, equipment and techniques** to suit clients treatment needs.
5. Describe how treatments can be adapted to suit client treatment needs and facial characteristics.
6. Describe the **normal reaction of the skin** to eyebrow shaping treatments.
7. State the **contra-actions** that may occur during and following treatments and how to respond.
8. Describe the chemical reaction which creates the tinting effect.
9. State the importance of completing the treatment to the satisfaction of the client.
10. State the importance of completing treatment records.
11. State the **aftercare advice** that should be provided.
12. Describe the structure and function of the skin and hair.
13. Describe diseases and disorders of the skin and hair.

HEALTH & SAFETY

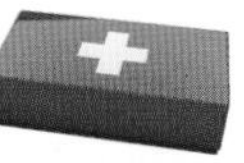

Cross-infection
Use a fresh cotton wool pad for each eyebrow to avoid cross-infection.

TOP TIP

Atchoo!
Occasionally clients start sneezing when you tweeze hairs at the bridge of the nose. If this happens, leave this area till last.

ALWAYS REMEMBER

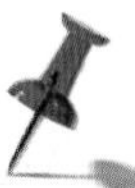

Twenty per cent of hairs are not visible above the skin's surface at any one time. Explain this to the client so that they understand why stray hairs may appear shortly after service.

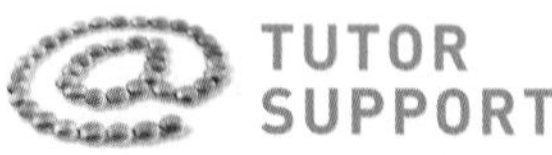

TUTOR SUPPORT

Activity 1: Methods of shaping project

Step-by-step: Eyebrow shaping

1 Position the cold-light magnifying lamp to give maximum visibility of the area.

2 Position the client on the couch or chair.

3 Clean your hands using an approved hand cleaning technique.

4 Secure a clean headband in place, to keep client's hair away from treatment area.

5 Working from behind the client, cleanse the eyebrow area, using a lightweight cleansing lotion or eye make-up remover. Apply a mild antiseptic lotion to two damp cotton wool pads, then gently wipe each eyebrow. (This removes all grease from the area, so that the tweezers will not slip.) The brow area should then be blotted dry, using a clean, folded facial tissue.

6 Brush the brow hair with the disposable brush, first ***against*** the natural hair growth, then with it. This enables you to define the brow shape and to observe the natural line.

7 Measure the brows (using the guidelines on page 250).

8 Place a clean piece of cotton wool in a convenient position for collecting the removed hairs, for instance at the top of the couch next to the client's head.

9 Best practice is to wear disposable gloves, as you may come into contact with body tissue fluid.

10 Begin tweezing, using a sterilized pair of automatic tweezers. These are designed to remove hairs quickly and efficiently, and are therefore used for the bulk of the hair identified for removal. It is usual to start at the bridge of the nose: the skin here is less sensitive than under the brow line.

11 Gently stretch the skin between the index and middle fingers, pressing lightly onto the skin. This will help you to avoid accidentally nipping the skin; it will also open the mouth of the **hair follicle** and minimize discomfort to the client.

12 Remove the hairs quickly, in the direction of growth. This prevents the hairs from breaking off at the skin's surface. Hair breakage can be seen to have occurred if a stubbly regrowth appears one or two days after shaping. Incorrect removal may also cause distortion of the hair follicle, or result in the hair becoming trapped under the skin as it starts to regrow (***ingrowing hair*** – see page 496).

Hairs should be removed individually, and the tweezers should be wiped regularly on the pad of clean cotton wool used to collect the removed hairs.

13 Remove the hairs from underneath the outer edge of the brow, working inwards towards the nose. It is advisable to work on each brow alternately. This ensures that the brows are evenly shaped; it also reduces prolonged discomfort in any one area during shaping. Hairs should ideally be removed only from ***below*** the brow, otherwise the natural line may be lost. It is sometimes necessary, however, to remove the odd stray hair growing ***above*** the natural line.

During shaping, show the client their brows and avoid removing too much hair.

14 At regular intervals during shaping, brush the brows to check their shape. Apply antiseptic lotion or gel to a clean, dampened cotton wool pad, and wipe this gently over the eyebrow tissue to reduce sensitivity and to sanitize the area.

15 When the bulk of excess hair has been removed, manual tweezers may be used to take away any stray hairs and to define the line. Long hairs may be trimmed with scissors if necessary. Any discoloured, coarse, long, curly or wavy hairs may be removed, as long as this does not alter the line or leave a bald patch.

Brush the brows into shape and show the client the finished effect. The client may wish further hairs to be removed. Ask them to identify these. If you think this would be unsuitable explain why.

16 On completion of brow shaping, wipe the eyebrows with the antiseptic soothing lotion or gel, applied with clean, damp cotton wool. Apply a mild antiseptic cream to the area, using clean, dry cotton wool, to reduce the possibility of infection.

17 The hairs that have been removed should be disposed of hygienically.

18 Record details of the service on the client's record card.

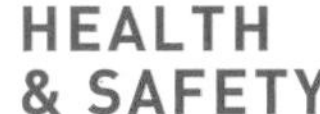
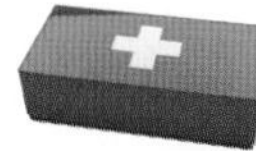

HEALTH & SAFETY

Soothing lotion

Care should be taken when applying soothing lotion. If too much is applied it may run and enter the eye, causing further discomfort.

It is often best to apply a small amount of soothing lotion to a clean cotton wool pad, using a separate one for each eye to avoid cross-infection.

4 Protecting client's hair with headband.

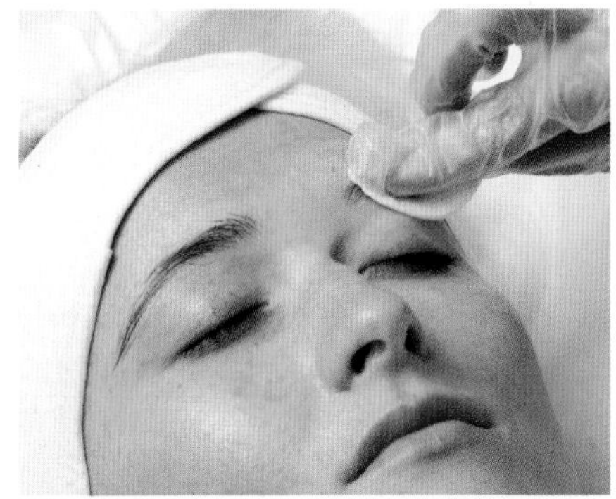

5 Cleansing the eyebrow.

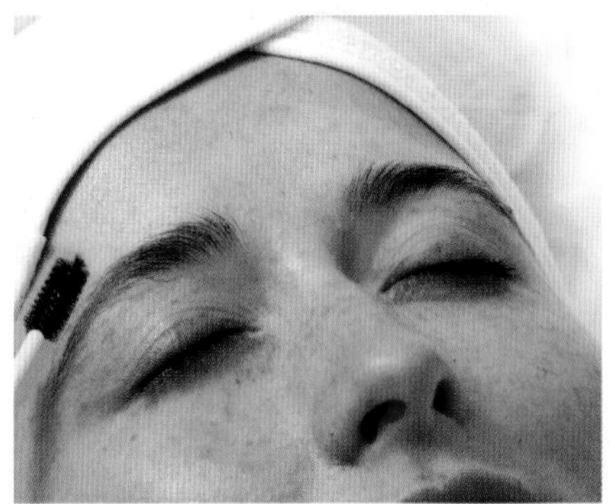

6 Brushing the eyebrow.

7 Measuring the eyebrow: the inner corner of the eye.

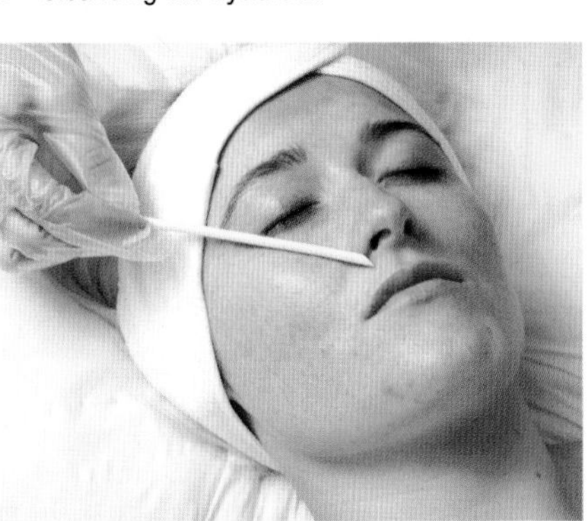

7 **continued** Measuring the eyebrow: the outer corner of the eye.

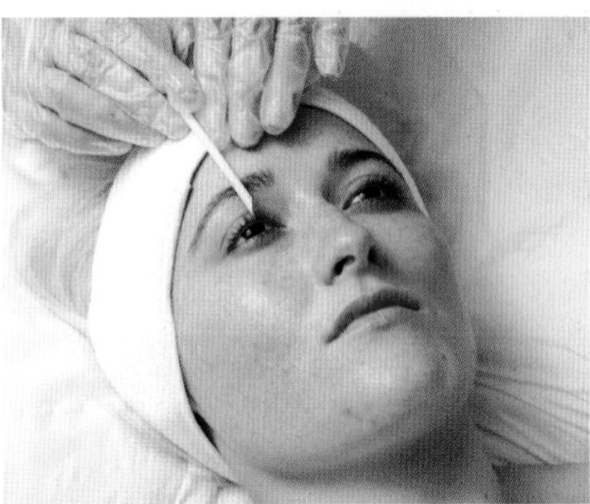

7 **continued** Measuring the eyebrow: the arch.

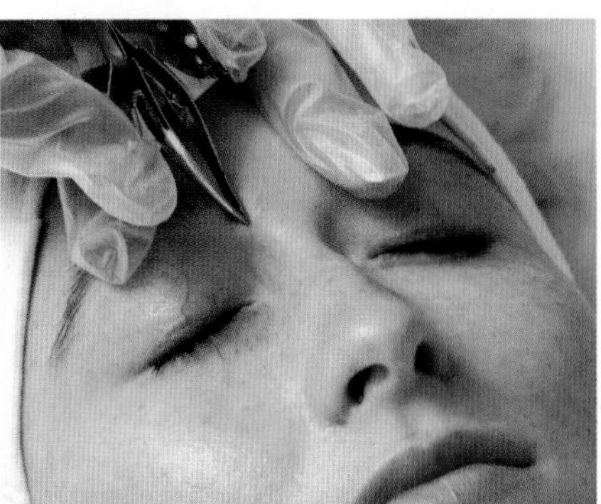

10 Tweezing at the bridge of the nose, using automatic tweezers.

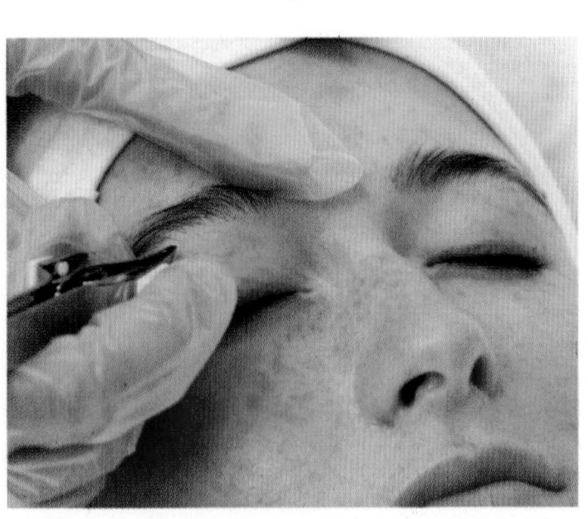

10 **continued** Tweezing at the outer corner of the eyebrow, using automatic tweezers.

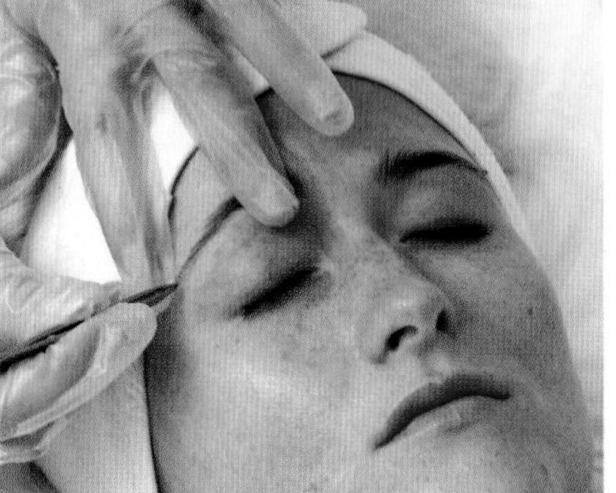

10 **continued** Tweezing using manual tweezers to define the finished eyebrow shape.

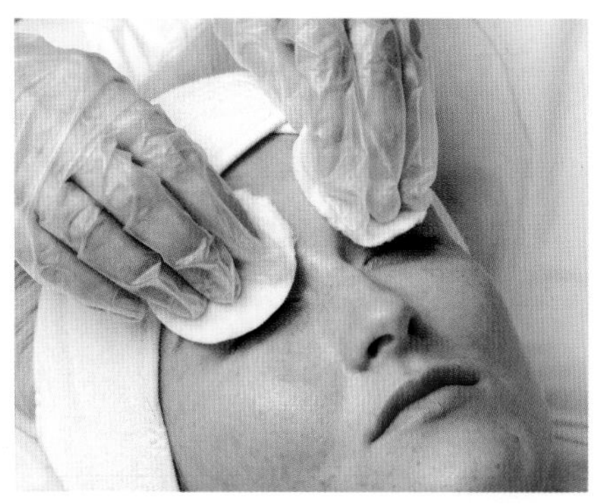
13 Applying antiseptic and soothing lotion.

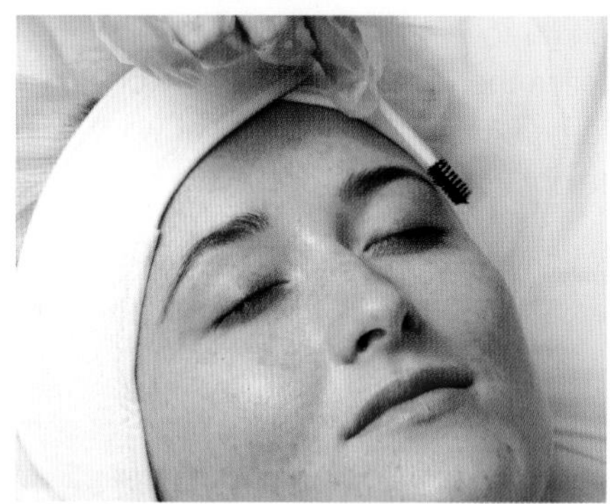
14 Brushing the eyebrow into shape.

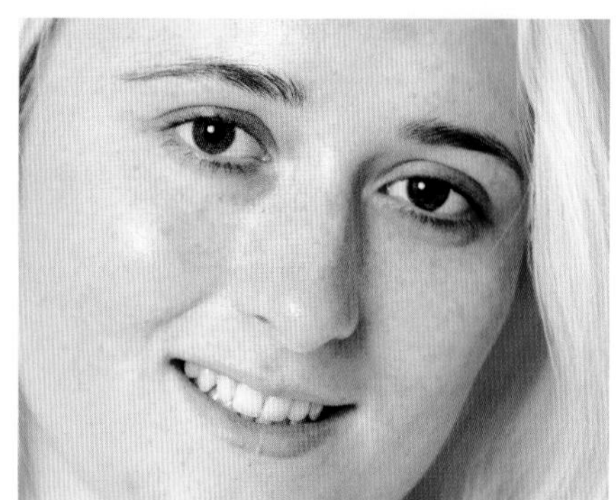
16 The completed eyebrows after shaping.

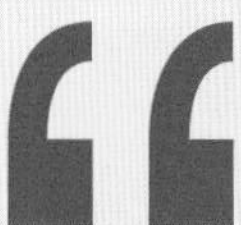

Think on your feet

For example, if a client is running late and there is a way to fit them in, then do it!

Be confident with who you are and your skill set. If you give confidence, you will create it around you.

Never agree to conduct a treatment that you do not feel is correct for the client. For example if the client wants to create something that you simply know will not suit her then be honest. She will appreciate it in the long run.

Shavata Singh

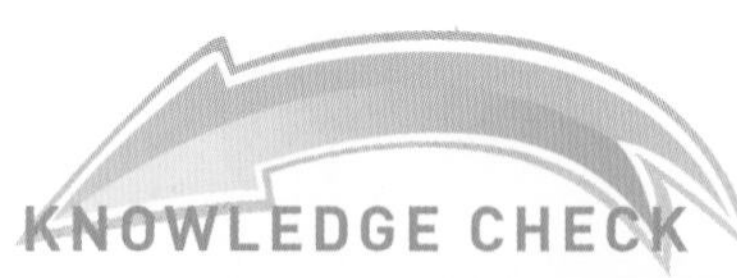

KNOWLEDGE CHECK

How can you ensure that the hairs are removed at their root ?

Need more time... refer to page 264 to help you.

ALWAYS REMEMBER

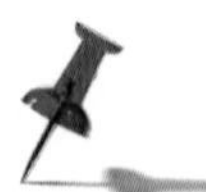

White hair

When selecting and using permanent tint for a white-haired client, note that the hair is very often resistant to colour. The processing time may need to be increased. Note any modification on the record card for future reference.

Tinting the eyebrows and lashes

How to prepare the client

The client should be shown through to the cubicle after the record card has been completed.

1. Position the client comfortably, in a flat or slightly elevated position. If they are wearing contact lenses, these must be removed.
2. Drape a towel across the client's chest and shoulders, and protect their hair with a clean headband.
3. Wash your hands, which assures the client that the service is beginning in a hygienic and professional manner.
4. Consult the client's record card, then check the area for any visible contra-indications or abnormalities before proceeding.
5. Cleanse the area to be treated with a cleansing milk to dissolve facial make-up (if worn). Then use a non-oily eye make-up remover to remove eye products: apply this with clean, damp cotton wool.
6. To ensure that the area is thoroughly clean and grease-free, apply a mild toning lotion, stroked over the lash or brow hair.
7. Blot the eyelashes or eyebrows dry with a clean facial tissue. This ensures that the tint is not diluted, and also prevents the tint from being carried into the eye.

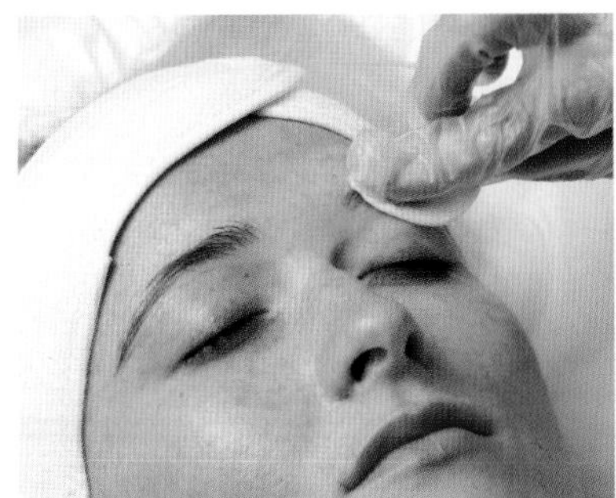
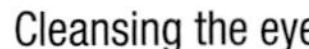
Cleansing the eye

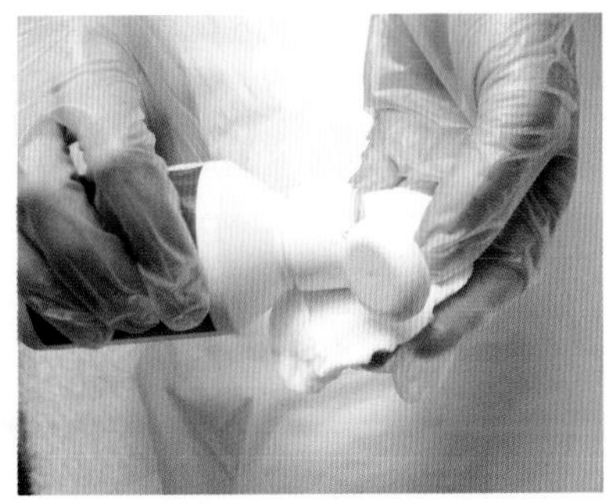
Apply a mild toning lotion

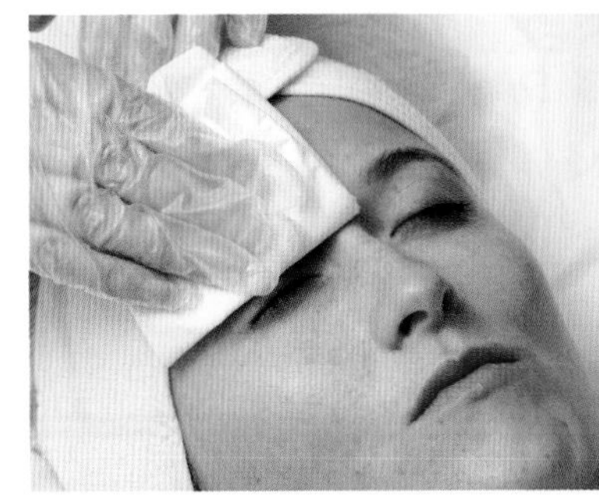
Blotting the brow hair to remove moisture

Brush through the brows to separate the hair using a disposable brush. Note the fair root at the lash base.

8 Prepare the pre-shaped eye shields by applying petroleum jelly to the inner surface of each eye shield (the surface that comes into contact with the skin).

9 Ensure that the light is not shining directly into the client's eyes. If it were, the eyes might water, carrying the tint into the eye or down the face (causing skin staining).

10 Finally, check that the client is comfortable before beginning tint application.

11 Best practice is to wear disposable gloves to avoid contact with the tint that could lead to skin staining and possibly **contact dermatitis**. If worn, put on at this stage.

A great manager will…

- have regular updates and meetings
- have newsletters that reward and make your team happy to be working with you
- be a team player too
- set high standards and lead by example
- be a good communicator

Shavata Singh

ALWAYS REMEMBER

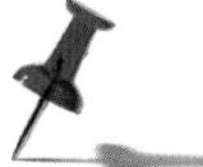

Tone and blot

The brows or lash hair to be tinted must be grease-free – the grease would be a barrier to the tint.

Step-by-step: Tinting the eyelashes

1 Remove some petroleum jelly from its container, using a new disposable spatula.

2 Working from behind the client, ask the client to open their eyes and to look upwards towards you. Using a disposable brush, apply petroleum jelly underneath the lower lashes of one eye, ensuring that it extends at the outer corner of the eye. (This is in case the client's eyes water slightly during service, which might otherwise lead to skin staining.) The petroleum jelly must not come into contact with the lash hair, where it would create a barrier to the tint.

3 Place the prepared eye shield on the skin under the lower lashes, ensuring that it adheres to the petroleum jelly and fits 'snugly' to the base of the lower lashes.

4 Repeat the above process for the other eye.

5 Ask the client to close their eyes gently. Instruct them not to open them again until you advise them to do so, in about ten minutes' time.

ALWAYS REMEMBER

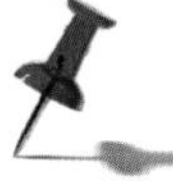

Cover surfaces

Make sure that work surfaces are protected with disposable coverings, to prevent permanent staining following spillages.

HEALTH & SAFETY

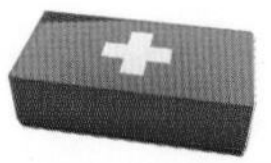

Maintaining hygiene
Do not use the same spatula in the container again, or you might contaminate the product.

6 Apply petroleum jelly to the upper eyelid, in a line on the skin at the base of the lashes.

7 Considering the length and density of the client's eyelashes, mix the required amount of tint with 10-volume (3%) hydrogen peroxide. As a guide, a 5mm length of tint from the tube, mixed with two or three drops of hydrogen peroxide, is usually sufficient. Mix the products to a smooth cream in the tinting bowl, using the disposable brush. Always recap bottles and tubes tightly after use, to avoid deterioration of materials.

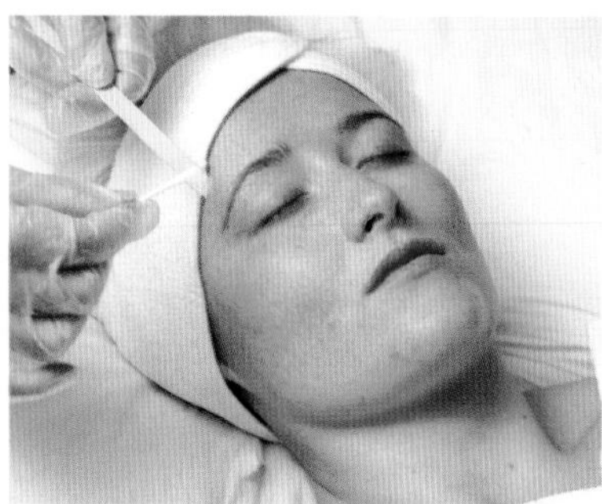

Use a disposable spatula for the petroleum jelly

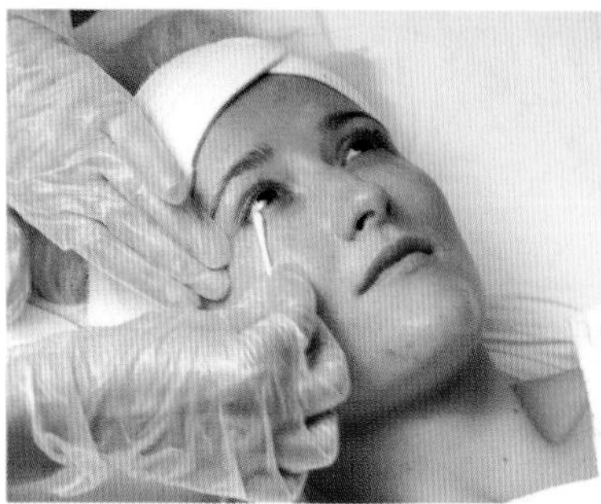

Apply petroleum jelly to prevent skin staining

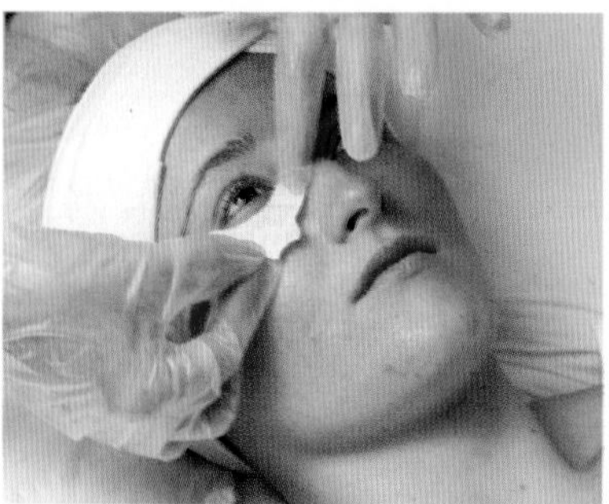

Placement of eye shield

BEST PRACTICE

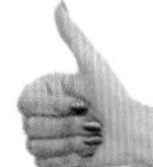

Client care
Speak to your client as you apply the eyelash tint. Check that they are comfortable and understand what you are doing. Remember: the eyes are very sensitive and will water readily.

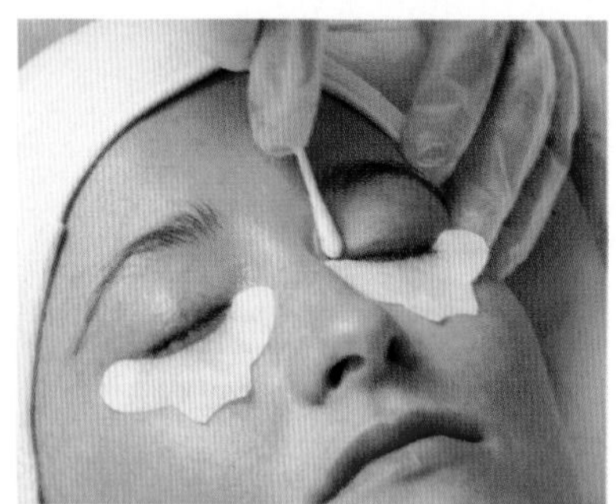

Application of petroleum jelly to upper eyelid

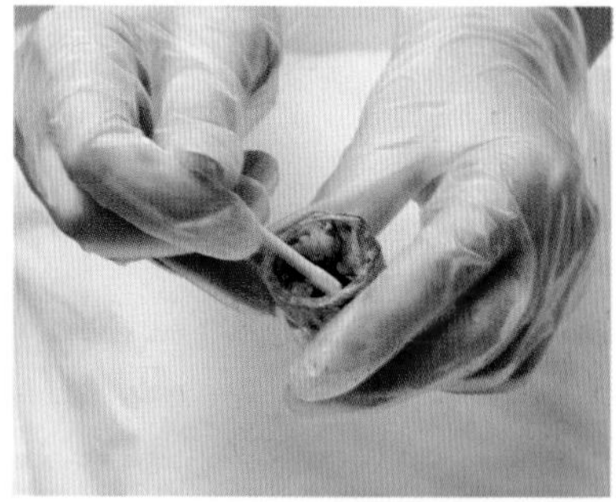

Mix the tint and hydrogen peroxide according to manufacturer's instructions

8 Wipe excess tint off the brush onto the inside of the bowl. Apply the tint thinly to each hair. Work from the base of the lash to the tip, ensuring that each hair is evenly covered. Press down gently with the applicator to ensure that the lower lashes also are covered. The few inner and outer lashes should also be covered, down to the base. Remove any excess tint from the skin with a clean cotton bud.

9 Allow the tint to process, for approximately five to ten minutes from the completion of application. Discard any unused mixture as soon as the tint has been applied.

10 On completion of processing, remove the eyelash tint by applying clean, damp cotton wool pads over each eye, wiping away most of the tint and removing the protective eye shield in one movement, an outward sweep. Using fresh dampened cotton wool pads, gently stroke down the lashes from roots to tips, until all excess tint has been removed. With a sweeping action on each eye and using one cotton wool pad, wipe from the side to the middle against the lash growth, while the other hand supports the eye tissue. ***All tint must be thoroughly removed before the client opens their eyes.***

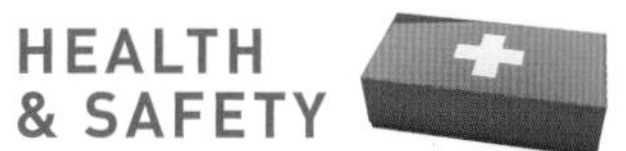

HEALTH & SAFETY

Client comfort

The client should not be left during the lash-tinting service. You must be available both to offer reassurance and to take the necessary action if the eyes water.

If the eyes do water while the eyes are closed, hold a tissue at the corner of the eye to soak up the moisture. Take further action if watering persists and the eyes begin to sting. See the contra-action description on pages 246–247.

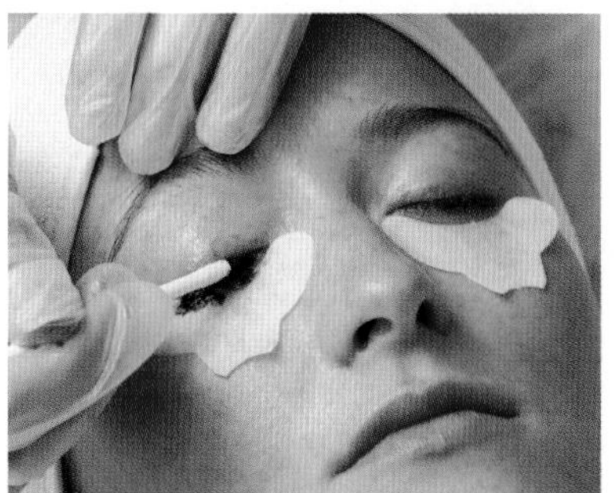

Applying the tint to the eyelashes

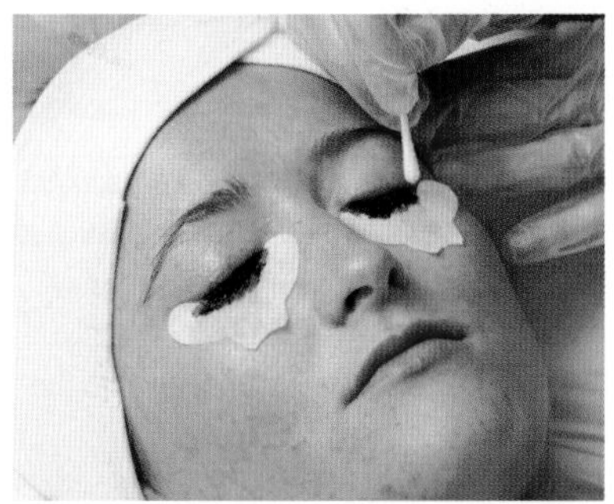

Removal of any excess tint with a cotton bud

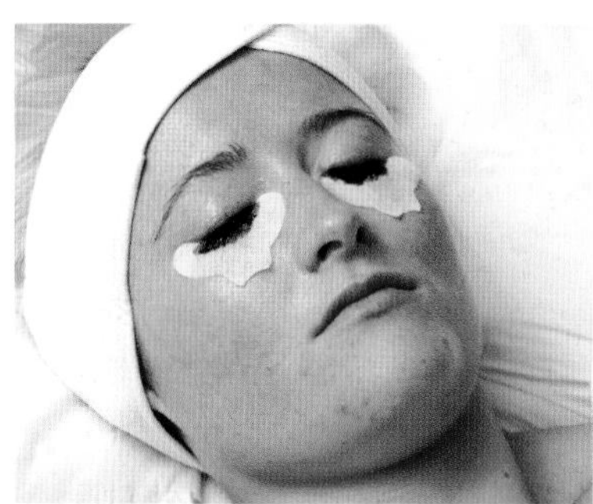

Processing the tint

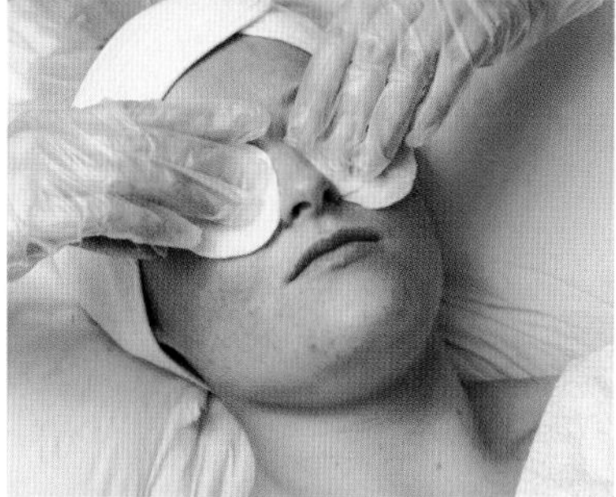

Removing the tint

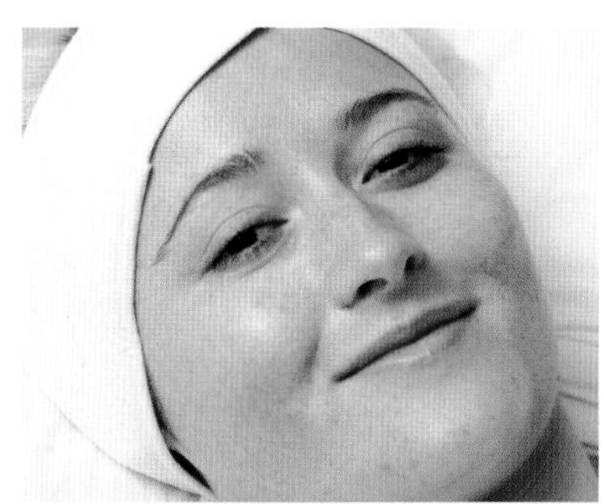

The completed eyelash tint

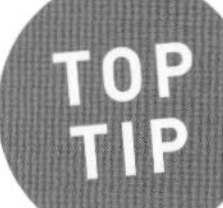

TOP TIP

Tint removal

Use a cotton bud to remove any excess tint from along the lash line on removal.

11 Ask the client to open their eyes. If removal has been correctly carried out, the lashes and their bases will be free from tint. (While training, if any tint remains at the base of the lashes after the eyes have been opened, ask the client to close her eyes again and finish the removal process using clean, damp cotton wool.) Check that every lash has been tinted, especially the base of each lash and the inner and outer corner lashes. Show the client the result, ensuring the colour is dark enough and that they are satisfied with the final effect.

12 Once you are satisfied that all tint has been removed, place a cool, damp cotton wool pad over each eye for two to three minutes to soothe the eye tissue.

13 Record details of the treatment on the client's record card.

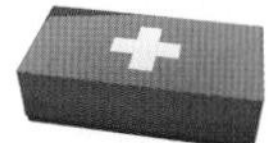

HEALTH & SAFETY

Using tints

Always read the manufacturer's instructions carefully before using a permanent tint.

Step-by-step: Tinting the eyebrows

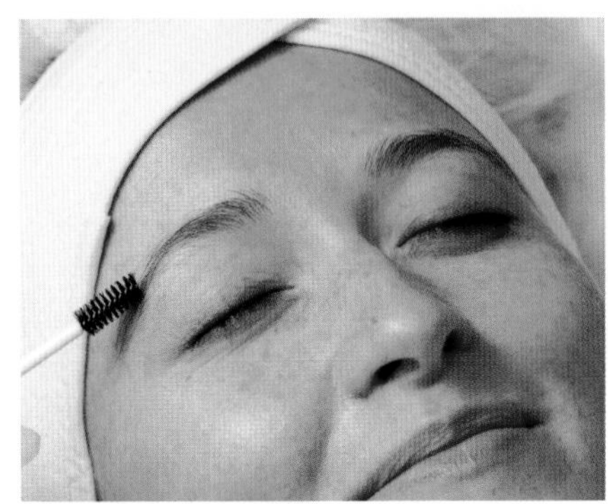

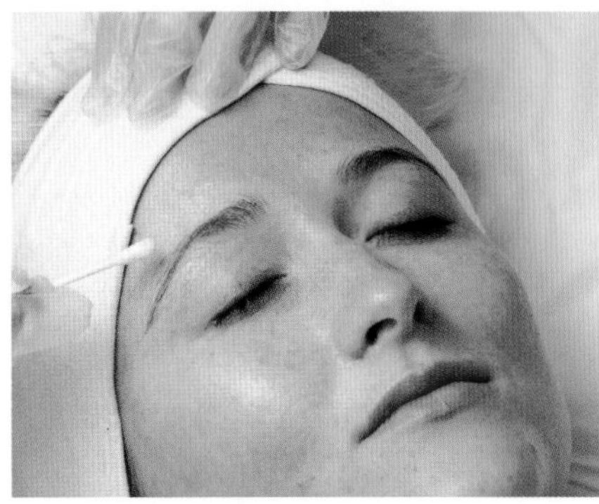

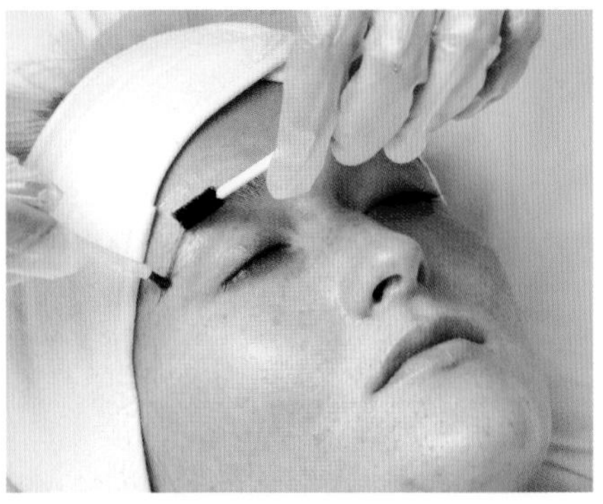

1 Remove some petroleum jelly from its container, using a new disposable spatula.

2 Brush the brow hair away from the skin, using a disposable brow brush (as shown in the picture).

3 Using a disposable brush, surround each eyebrow with petroleum jelly, as close as possible to the brow hair (to avoid skin staining).

4 Mix approximately 5mm of the chosen tint colour with two or three drops of 10-volume (3%) hydrogen peroxide in a tinting bowl. Ensure that the tint is mixed thoroughly to a creamy consistency, according to the manufacturer's instructions.

5 Wipe excess tint off the brush onto the inside of the tinting bowl. Apply the tint neatly and economically to the brow hair of the first eyebrow; ensuring that the brow hairs, from the base to the tips, are evenly covered (as shown in the picture).

TOP TIP

Application to brow hair

To ensure even coverage of brow hair, use a brush to lift the hair to enable application at the roots of the hair to mid-length of the hair shaft.

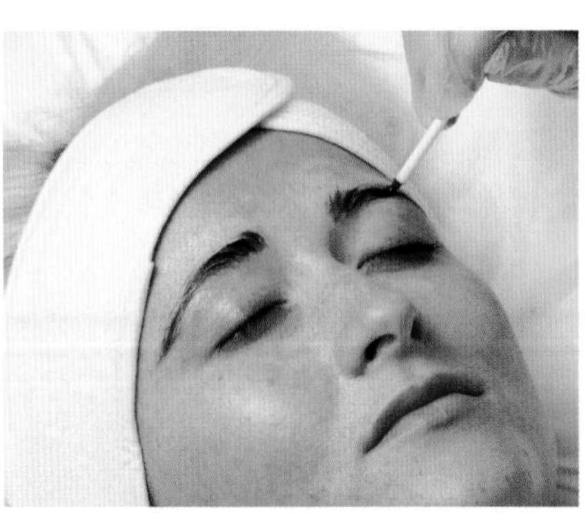

6 Apply the tint to the second eyebrow; following the same procedure.

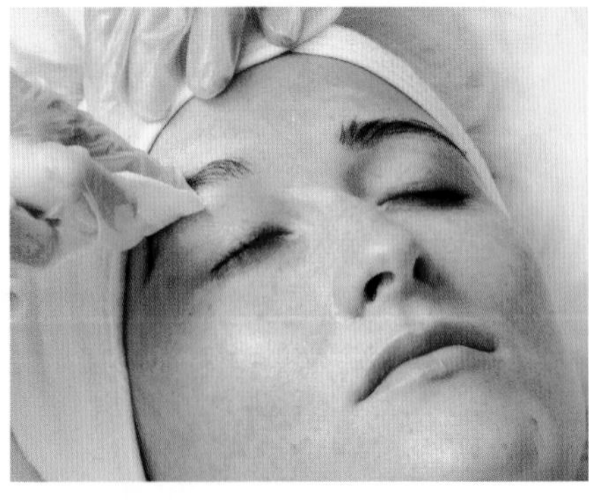

7 Immediately after application of the tint to the second eyebrow, remove the tint from the first eyebrow. Use a clean dampened cotton wool pad. Place it on the eyebrow, then wipe it across the eyebrow in an outward sweep, removing the excess tint. Ensure that all traces of excess tint have been removed, to prevent skin staining.

Never leave tint on the eyebrows for longer than two minutes. Eyebrow hair colour develops much more quickly than lash hair.

How should you select the tint colour when carrying out a permanent tinting service?

Need more time... refer to pages 255–256 to help you.

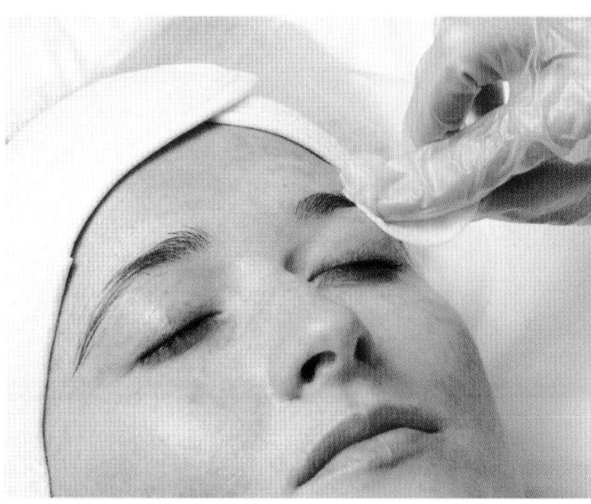

8 Remove the tint from the second eyebrow in the same way.

Show the client the effect of the tinted eyebrows. If the brow hair is not dark enough, reapply the tint to the eyebrow hair; following the same application and removal procedure. Note this on the client's record card.

When you are both satisfied with the colour of the tinted eyebrows, complete the client's record card by recording details of the service.

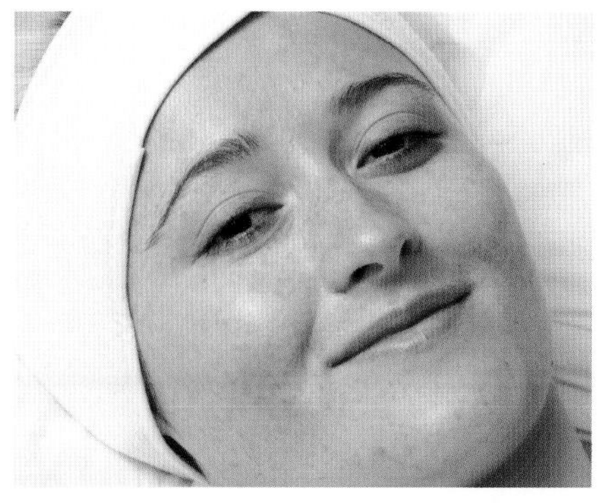

9 The completed effect, showing both eyelash and eyebrow tint.

HEALTH & SAFETY

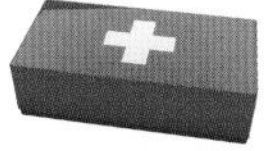

Skin stains

If skin staining accidentally occurs, use a professional skin stain remover designed for this purpose. Afterwards, use plenty of clean, dampened cotton wool pads to avoid skin irritation.

ALWAYS REMEMBER

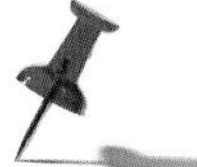

The effect of tinting depends on the natural colour:

- ***Blonde hair*** develops colour rapidly – if the tint is left on the eyebrow too long, a harsh, unnatural appearance will be created.
- ***Red/grey hair*** is more resistant to the tint, and developing will take a little longer – allow 15 minutes' processing time when tinting lash hair.
- ***Dark hair*** requires tinting to increase the intensity of the natural eyebrow colour, giving a glossy, conditioned appearance.

Step-by-step: Applying artificial lashes

How to prepare the client

Show the client through to the prepared work area after the record card has been completed. Consult the record card and check the area for any contra-indications to treatment.

1 Position the client comfortably on the treatment couch or beauty chair (which should be slightly elevated). If the client wears contact lenses, these must be removed before the treatment begins.

2 Drape a clean towel across the client's chest and shoulders. Protect their hair with a clean headband.

3 Wash your hands, which indicates to the client that treatment is beginning and in a hygienic and professional manner.

4 It is usual to carry out a full facial cleanse (rather than cleansing only the eye area), as make-up is usually applied to complement the false eyelashes. Use a cleansing milk to dissolve facial make-up, followed by a non-oily eye make-up remover to cleanse the eye area. Both products should be removed with clean, damp cotton wool.

5 To ensure that the eye tissue and eyelashes are thoroughly clean and grease-free, apply a mild oil-free toning lotion: stroke this over the skin using clean, damp cotton wool.

6 Blot the lashes dry, using a fresh facial tissue for each eye. (Any moisture left on the natural lashes will reduce the effectiveness of the eyelash adhesive.)

7 Apply make-up to complement the effect achieved. Brush the natural lashes to separate them before application.

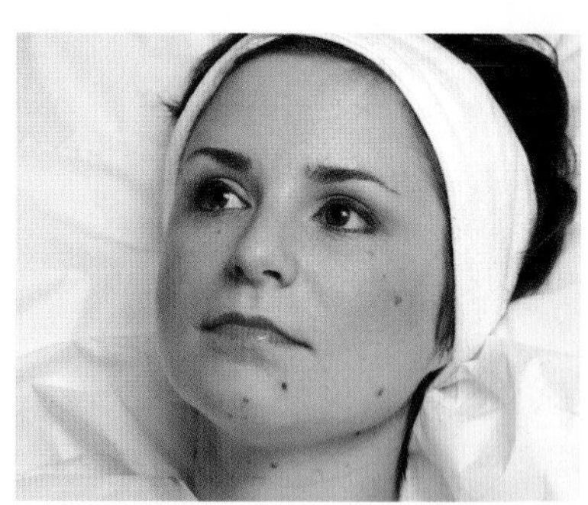

Special occasion make-up is applied before application of artificial eyelashes

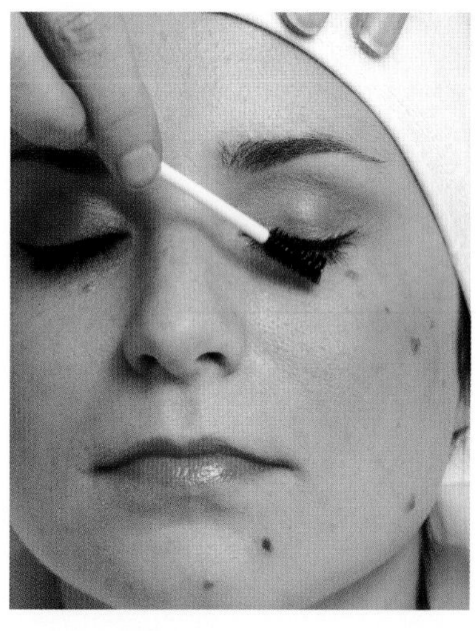

Brushing natural lashes before application

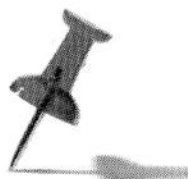

ALWAYS REMEMBER

Adhesive
Do not prepare the lash adhesive until you are ready to use it. It tends to dry on contact with air.

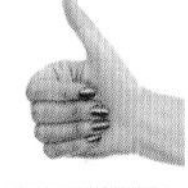

BEST PRACTICE

Clean tweezers
To ensure efficient application, don't get adhesive on the points of the tweezers.

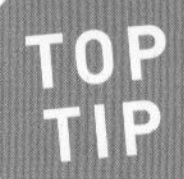

TOP TIP

Positioning
When applying the individual flare lashes to the inner portion of the eyelid, hold the skin taut, stretching the skin slightly. This will enable you to position the artificial lash more easily.

TOP TIP

Keep a grip
Use a clean pair of tweezers to remove the individual flare lashes from their container when required. Holding the tweezers firmly, grip each lash near its base (this avoids misshaping the outer lash hairs).

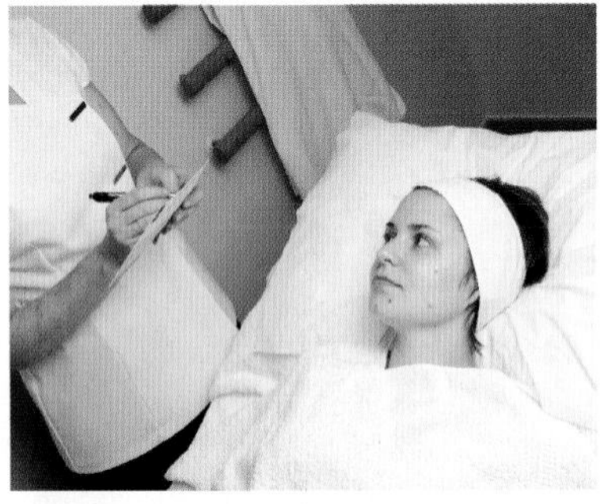

Explaining the service procedure

Adhesive application to individual flare artificial eyelashes

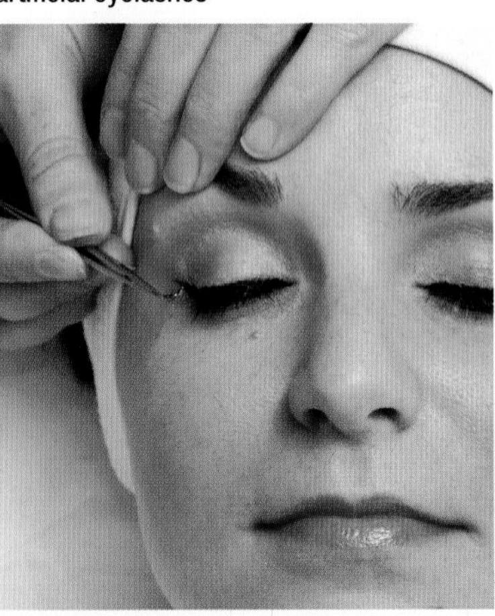

Application of individual flare artificial eyelash to outer eyelash hair

How to apply individual flare lashes

1 Check that everything you need is on the trolley.

2 Check that the back of the couch or beauty chair is slightly raised, at a height that is comfortable for you.

3 Discuss the service procedure with the client. Explain that they will be required to keep their eyes open during the service. Reassure them that they may blink during application. Very often clients feel that they shouldn't, and their eyes begin to water.

4 Ask them to tilt their head downwards very slightly. This tends to lower the upper eyelids, making application easier.

5 Depending on the effect required, you may start application of the individual flare lashes at different positions along the natural lash line. In general, apply shorter lashes to the inner corners of the eyelid, and longer lashes to the outer corners; this creates a realistic effect and ensures client comfort. If you are applying individual flare lashes to the entire upper lid, it is practical to start application at the inner corner of the eyelid and work outwards: this follows the natural contour of the eye.

6 With the sterile tweezers, select a lash from the package, holding it near its centre. Brush the underside of the individual flare lash, at the root, through the adhesive. The adhesive should extend slightly beyond the root. You need sufficient adhesive, but not too much – excess adhesive should be removed by wiping the lash against the inside of the adhesive container.

7 Working from behind the client, hold the tweezers at the angle at which the artificial lashes will be applied to the natural lash line. Hold the brow tissue with your other hand to steady the eyelid.

TOP TIP

Practice makes perfect
Positioning the individual flare lashes correctly requires experience. It is a good idea initially to practise application without adhesive.

Using a stroking movement, place the underside of the artificial lashes on top of the natural lash. Stroke the adhesive along the length of the natural eyelash. Guide the artificial lashes towards the base of the natural lash, so that the artificial lashes rests along the length of the natural lash. Wait a few seconds to allow the adhesive to dry (to prevent the lashes from sticking together). Continue placing further artificial lashes side by side until the desired effect is achieved.

During application, keep checking your work. If a lash is out of line, remove it while the adhesive is still soft. If the adhesive has set, the lash will need to be removed using adhesive solvent.

8 Apply the artificial lashes one at a time, to each eye alternately. This avoids sensitizing the eye, and makes it easier for you to create a balanced effect.

9 If the client requires artificial lashes to be applied to the *lower* lid, the application technique is slightly different.

Work facing the client, with the client looking upwards, their eyes slightly open. Follow the same general procedure for applying the false eyelashes; here, however, the lashes curve downwards and the adhesive is applied to the *upper* surface of the lash.

Lashes applied to the lower eyelid are usually shorter than those chosen for the upper lid, and more adhesive is required for the lashes to be secure and have maximum durability.

10 When you have completed the lash application, ask the client to sit up, and show them the completed effect.

11 If the client is satisfied with the result, you can apply a water- or powder-based eye make-up at this stage if desired. Do not apply mascara, as this will reduce the adhesion to the natural lash. Mascara also clogs the lashes together; and is difficult to remove without affecting the **eyelash adhesive**. There are specially formulated mascaras available to be used with artificial lashes. On completion, the lashes can be gently brushed – using a disposable brush – to remove particles of eye shadow.

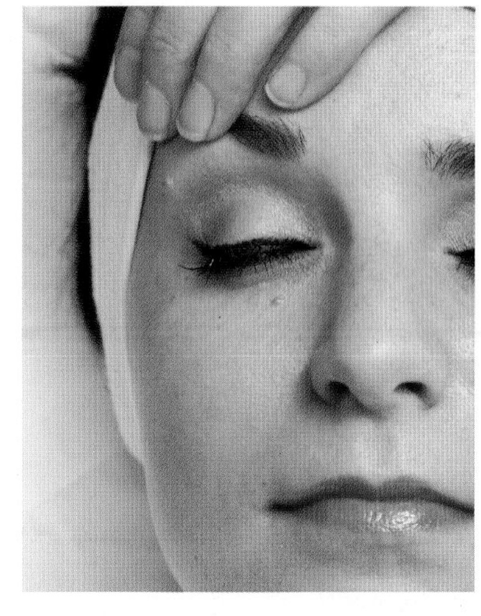

Artificial eyelash positioned

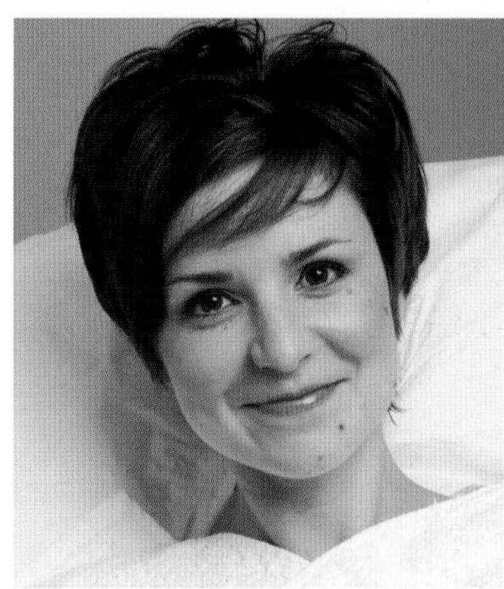

Short individual flare lashes applied to thicken the natural lashes

ALWAYS REMEMBER

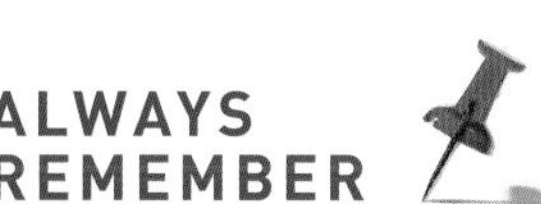

Bottom lashes don't last
Tell the client that artificial lashes applied to the lower lashes tend to fall off after one week. (This is probably due to the natural watering of the eye affecting the adhesive.)

How to apply strip lashes

Strip false eyelashes may be applied *before* carrying out the eye make-up – this avoids the eye make-up being spoilt if the eyes water slightly during application.

1 Check that everything required for the false eyelash application is available on your trolley.

2 Carefully apply moisturiser and foundation, taking care not to get any cosmetic products on the lashes. (If you do, gently wipe over the lashes with the non-oily eye make-up remover, and blot the eyelashes dry again with a clean facial tissue.)

3 Brush the lashes to separate them, using a clean disposable mascara brush. This makes artificial lashes application easier, and removes any fine particles of loose powder.

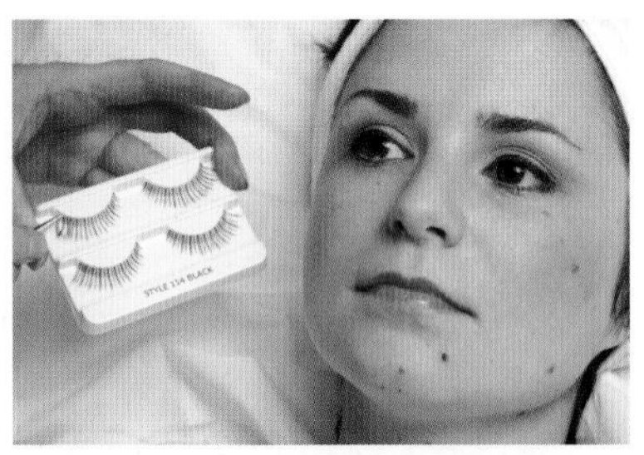

Removal of strip artificial lash from container

HEALTH & SAFETY

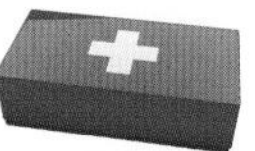

Lash length

If the lashes were not shorter at the inner corner of the eyelid, they would irritate the client's eye.

4 Remove the strip lashes from their container; and place them on a clean, disinfected palette. Each strip is designed to fit either the left or the right eye: remember which is which when placing them on the palette.

5 Check the length of the strip against the client's eyelid. The strip should never be applied directly from one corner of the eyelid to the other; but should start about 2mm from the inner corner of the eye, and end 2mm from the outer corner. This ensures a natural effect and maximizes the durability of the artificial lashes.

When you remove the strip lash from the package you will find that there is adhesive on the backing strip, which fixes the lash in the container: this adhesive is sufficient to hold the lash onto the client's natural lash while you measure the length.

TOP TIP

Dealing with downward growing lashes

If a client has straight eyelashes that grow downwards, curl them slightly using eyelash curlers. If you don't, a gap will be visible between the real lashes and the false strip lash.

BEST PRACTICE

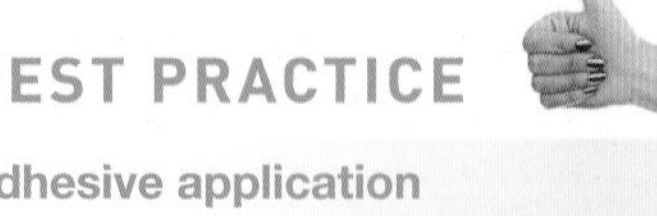

Adhesive application

With individual flare lashes, do not apply adhesive directly from the tube to the eyelash base – you would apply too much adhesive.

6 To trim the artificial strip lashes you require a sharp pair of scissors. First correct the length of the *strip* if necessary. Hold the lashes securely with one hand, and then trim the strip at the outer edge. Then trim the lashes themselves, if necessary. Never reduce the length of the lashes by cutting straight across them: the result would not look natural. Natural eyelashes are of varying lengths, due to the nature of the hair growth cycle; it is this effect that you must simulate. To shorten the lash, 'chip' into the lash. Use the *points* of the scissors to shorten the lash length. Cut the lashes so that the shorter lashes are at the inner corner of the eyelid, gradually increasing toward the outer corner.

7 The couch or beauty chair should be in a slightly raised position. During the treatment, you will be working from behind the client: the height must be comfortable for you.

8 Discuss the treatment procedure with the client. Explain to her that she will be required to keep her eyes open during the application. Ask her to tilt her head downwards very slightly – this lowers the upper eyelids, making application easier.

9 Using the sterile tweezers, remove one of the eyelash strips from the palette. Handle it very carefully, as it can easily become misshapen.

Remembering that the strip is designed to fit either the right or the left eye, place it against the appropriate eyelid and check the length (with the client's eyes closed).

10 Once satisfied that the length of the strip lash is correct (see step 5 for reducing the length), remove the adhesive tape used to hold it in the container.

11 Place a small quantity of strip lash adhesive on the disinfected palette.

12 Ask the client to look down slightly, with their eyes half open. With one hand lift their brow to steady the upper eyelid.

Holding the strip lash with the sterile tweezers at its centre, drag it at its base through the adhesive. (The adhesive must be moist.) It is usually white, but when it dries it becomes colourless.

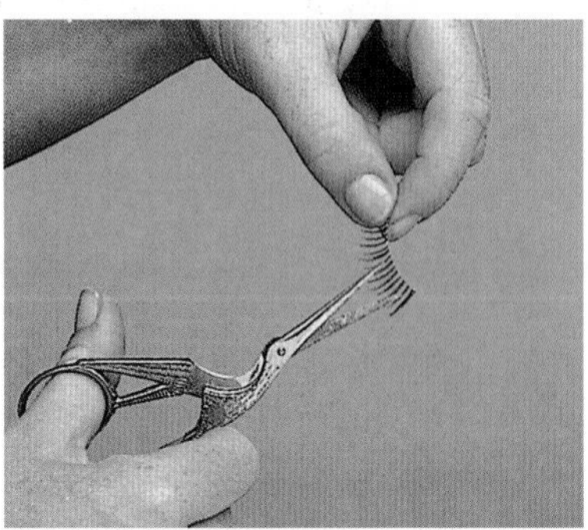

Trimming the strip lashes

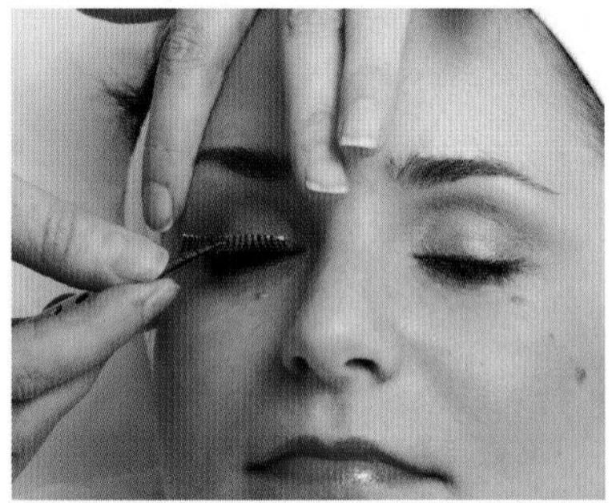

Applying to strip lash to the eye

Position the base of the strip lash as close as possible to the base of the natural eyelash, ensuring that it is about 2mm in from the inner and outer corners of the eye. *Gently* press the false and natural eyelashes together with your fingertips, along the length of the lash and at the outer corners.

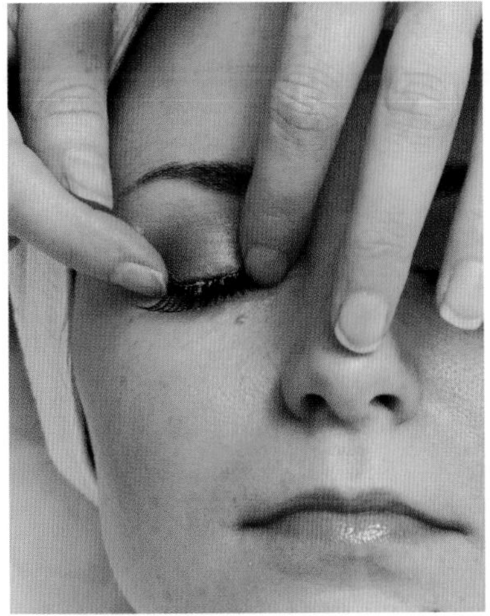

Positioning base of strip lash on the base of the natural lash line

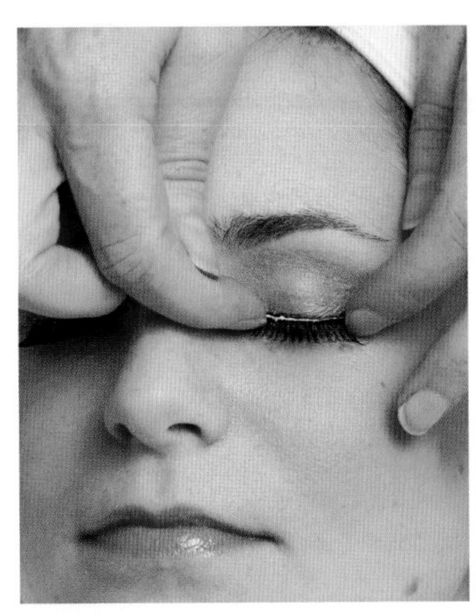

Making sure the strip lash is secure

TOP TIP

Prevent lifting

Extra glue (although not excessive) may be applied to the ends of the lashes to prevent lifting while wearing them.

TOP TIP

Continuing professional development

As part of your progression you may develop your skills further in the application of artificial lashes by learning the Level 3 Unit Single lash extensions.

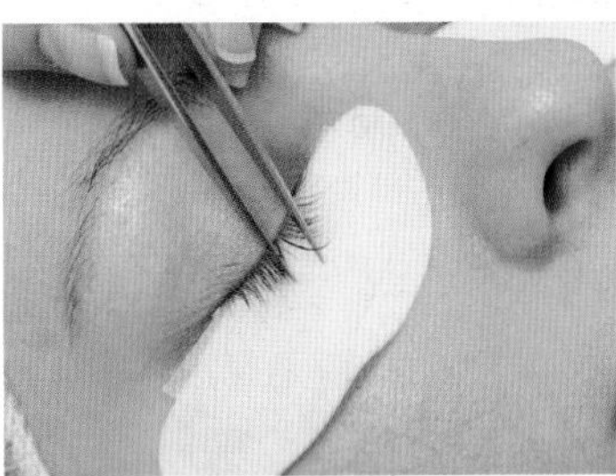

Single lash extensions

TOP TIP

Retail opportunity

Mascaras are available formulated to be worn with individual flare lashes. The product is more easily removed than regular non-waterproof mascaras.

13 When you are sure that the first strip lash is secure, apply the second in the same way.

14 If strip lashes are to be applied to the bottom lashes also, apply these now, in the same way as the upper lashes. (Strip lashes for the lower lids are fine, with an extremely thin base. These lashes should be trimmed as before to ensure comfort and durability in wear.)

15 Allow three to five minutes for the adhesive to dry.

16 Gently brush the lashes from underneath the natural lash line, using a clean disposable mascara brush. This will blend the natural and artificial lashes together Check that both sets of lashes are correctly positioned, and that a balanced look has been achieved.

17 Artificial lashes look more realistic if eyeliner is applied to the client's eyelid: this disguises the base of the strip lash.

18 Show the client the finished effect.

19 When you are satisfied, record the details on the client record card.

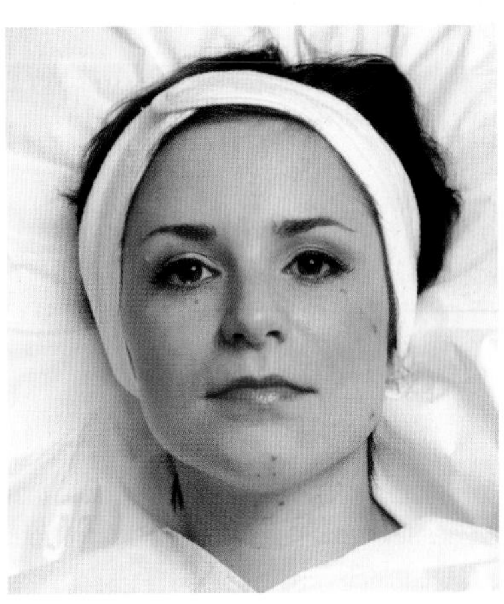

The completed effect

HEALTH & SAFETY

Client comfort

Check the eyelash application as you work. Ensure that the lower and upper lashes are not stuck together, and that the eyelashes are accurately and evenly applied.

Eyelash perming

How to prepare the client

The client should be shown through to the cubicle after the record card has been completed.

1 Position the client comfortably, in a flat or slightly elevated position. If they wear contact lenses, these must be removed.

2 Drape a towel across the client's chest and shoulders, and protect their hair with a clean headband.

3 Wash your hands. This assures the client that the treatment is beginning in a hygienic and professional manner.

4 Consult the client's record card, then check the area for any visible contra-indications or abnormalities before proceeding.

5 Cleanse the surrounding eye area with a suitable make-up cleanser (oil-free) to dissolve facial make-up. Then use a non-oily eye make-up remover to remove eye products: apply this with clean, damp cotton wool.

6 Blot the eyelashes dry with a clean facial tissue. This ensures that the perm lotion is not diluted, and also prevents the perm lotion being carried into the eye.

7 Explain the procedure to the client and tell them about the sensations they may experience during eyelash perming. Warn them that they will need to keep their eyes closed for a long period. Some clients may find this difficult, while others will enjoy this as a time of relaxation!

TOP TIP

Optimal results

If possible, after cleansing leave the eyelashes to dry for 10 minutes before perming, to ensure that the lashes are completely dry. Comb through the lashes to ensure they are evenly separated and dry. This will optimise the results.

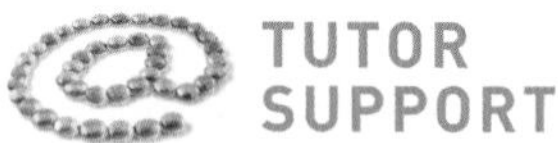

TUTOR SUPPORT

Activity 2: Eye treatments wordsearch

Step-by-step: Eyelash perming

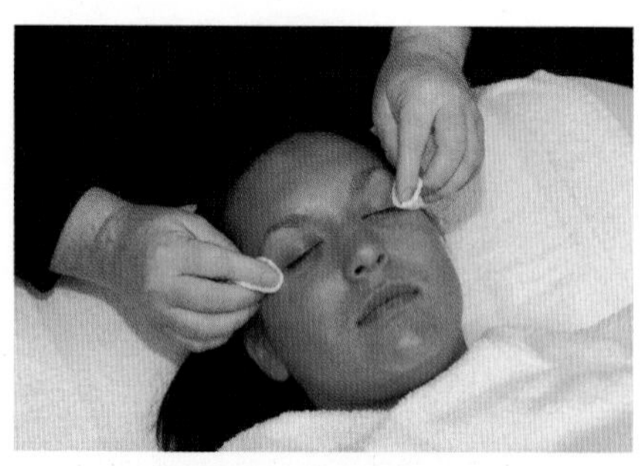

1 Comb through the lashes to ensure they are evenly separated and dry. This will optimize the results.

2 Cleanse the eye area.

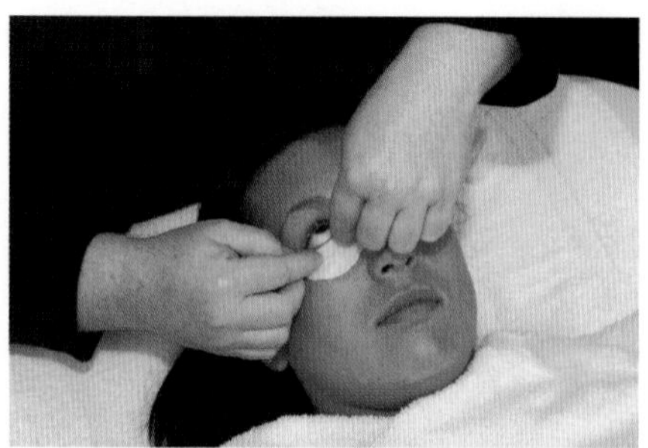

3 Ask the client to look upwards whilst you protect lower eyelashes with damp cotton wool or alternative suitable eye shield.

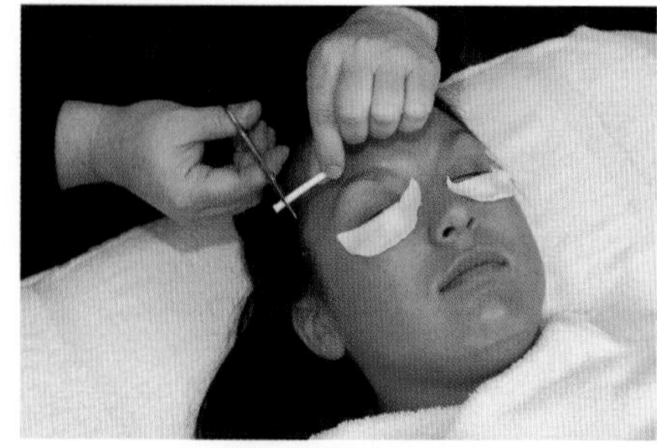

4 Select the correct size of curler for the client's lash length. Bend it so that it fits the contour of the eye. If the curler is too long it may be trimmed.

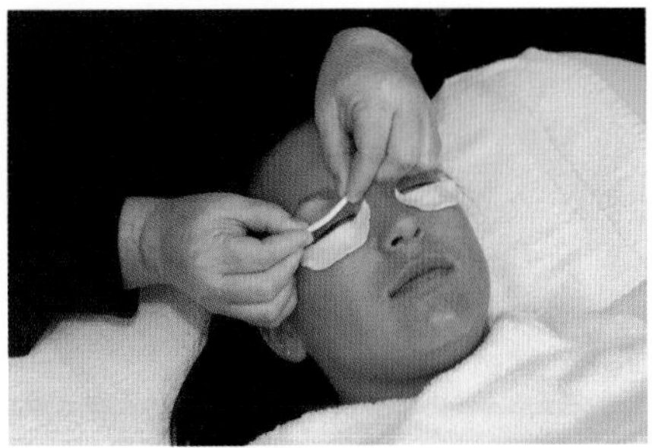

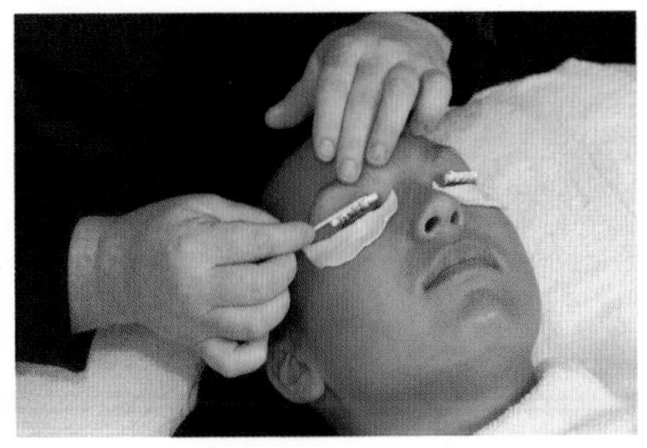

5 Place the curler at the base of the upper lashes, near the inner tear duct.

6 Gently curl the natural lashes around the curler, using the disposable stick. Ensure that the lashes do not overlap each other and are straight or the ends will be 'crooked', spoiling the overall effect and appearance. A specialized adhesive may be applied to secure the lashes to the curler and keep them even and straight so that the upper and lower lashes do not come into contact.

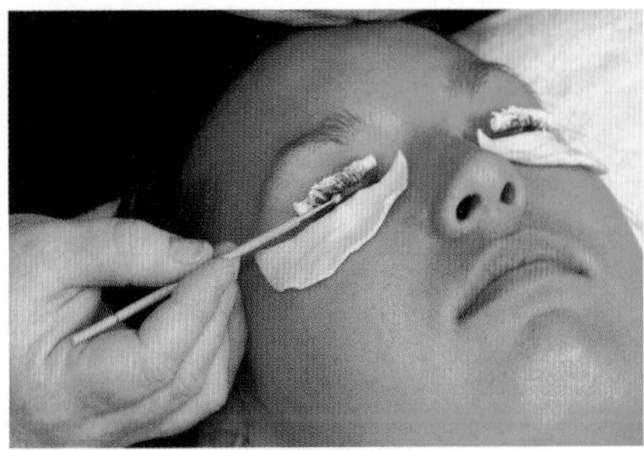

7 When you are satisfied that the lashes are straight and that the client is comfortable, apply the perm lotion evenly to the upper lashes, using a brush, avoiding contact with the skin.

The lashes may be covered with a plastic film (clear wrap) or dry lint pads. This creates warmth which aids the perming process. Allow:

- 7–10 minutes for fine or previously tinted hair;
- 10 minutes for coarse hair.
- Follow manufacturers guidance on timing as this may vary.

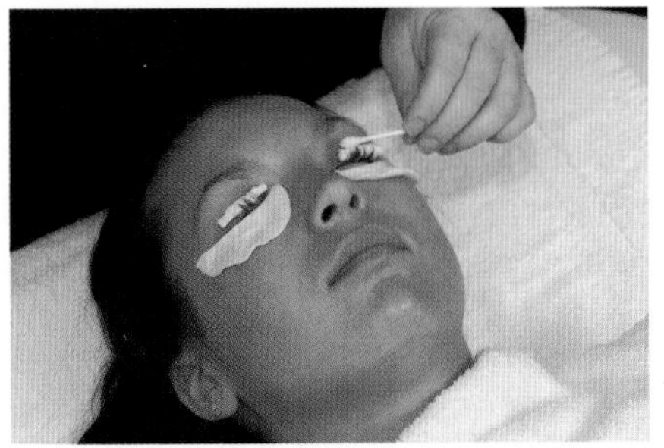

8 Check for the desired curl before removal. Separate a couple of eyelashes from the curler, leave for 2–3 minutes longer if the curl required has not been achieved.

9 Remove the perm lotion using dry lint free pads, gently blotting the lashes.

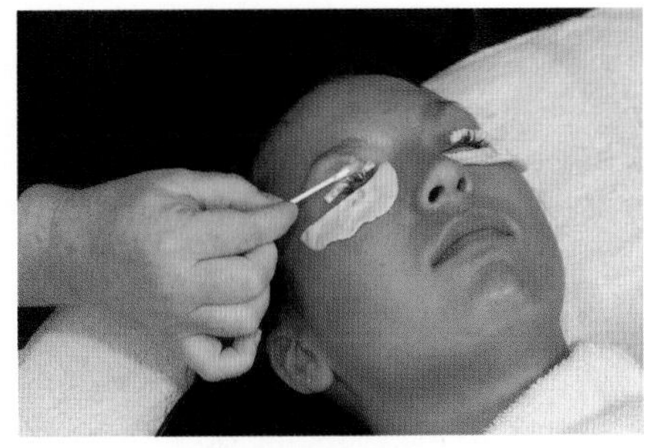

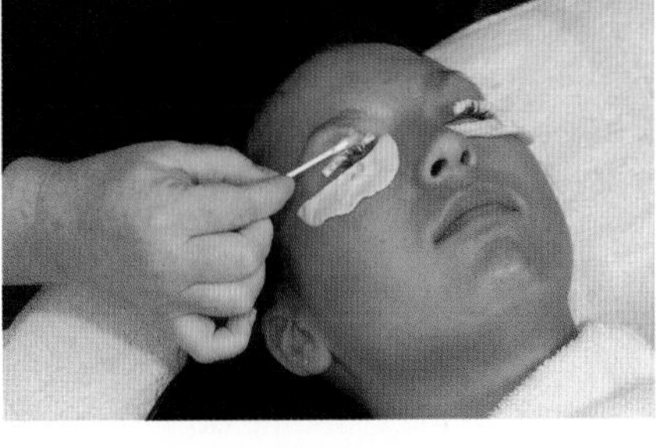

10 Apply the fixing/neutralizing lotion with a clean brush or applicator.

11 Cover the eyelashes with plastic film (clear wrap) or dry lint free pads for 10 minutes, following manufacturer's guidance.

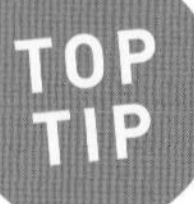

Protect lower lashes

A protective damp cotton wool pad may be placed over the lower lashes to form a barrier to the perm lotion when it is being applied to the upper lashes.

12 Gently remove the fixing/neutralizing lotion for the eyelashes, using dry lint-free pads.

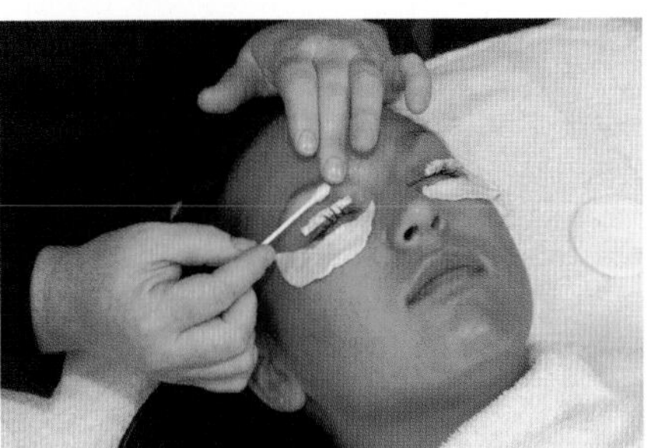

13 When all the fixing/neutralizing lotion has been removed, gently remove each curler, rolling downwards. A moisturising agent may be applied with a cotton bud to the eyelashes to aid the removal of the curlers. Wipe excess product from the lashes with damp, clean cotton wool. Brush gently though the eyelashes to define their shape and appearance.

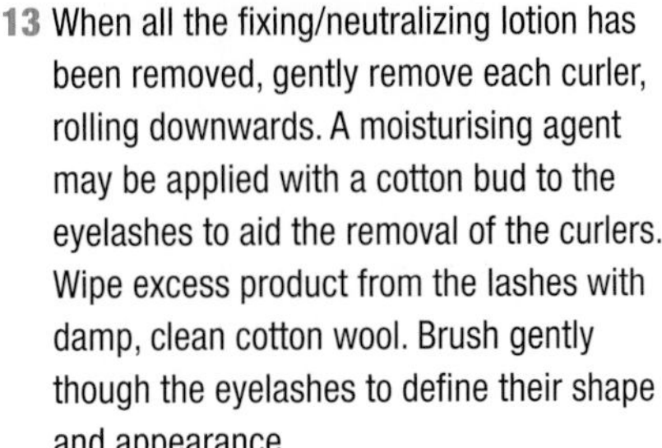

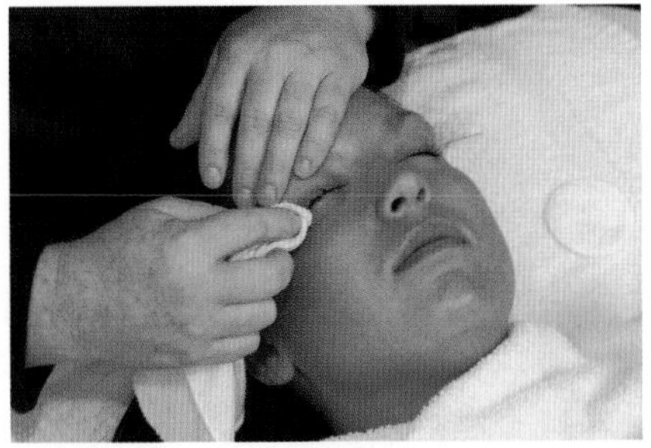

14 Show the client the effect of their permed eyelashes in a mirror. When you are both satisfied with the result, finalize details on the client's record card. Take the client to reception to book their next appointment.

What are the differences between the application of artificial strip lashes and the application of individual flare lashes?

Need more time... refer to pages 272–275 to help you.

HEALTH & SAFETY

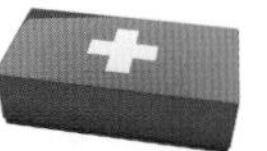

Cross-infection
Remind the client to avoid touching the area immediately following an eyebrow shaping treatment. This is because the area is susceptible to infection and the fingers may transfer dirt, causing secondary infection.

HEALTH & SAFETY

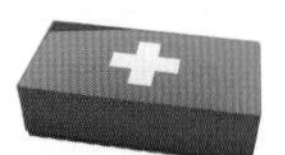

Avoiding infection
If excess antiseptic lotion or cream is left on the area, this may attract small particles of dust, which could cause infection.

Aftercare advice

Advise the client on skincare preparations to use at home to enhance the appearance of the eyebrows and lashes.

The following **aftercare advice**, specific to the eye service received, should be given to clients.

Eyebrow shape aftercare advice Advise the client to receive the treatment as follows:

- eyebrow maintenance every 1–2 weeks
- eyebrow re-shaping every 3–4 weeks

While a client receives an eyebrow shape it is an ideal opportunity to promote an eyebrow/eyelash tint.

An eyebrow pencil or powder cosmetic can be recommended to disguise bald patches, e,g. scars. Sparse eyebrows can be made to appear thicker. It can also be used to stimulate hairs, when the length needs to be increased.

Explain how to care for the area following the service to avoid an unwanted reaction – a contra-action. Advise the client not to wear eye make-up for at least six hours following the eyebrow-shaping service. The hair follicle has been damaged where the hair has been torn out: it will be susceptible to infection unless the area is cared for while it heals. It should not be necessary for the client to continue using antiseptic lotion at home, but they should be advised to carry out these instructions if discomfort or continued reddening occurs:

1. Explain to the client the action to take in the event of a contra-action.
2. Cleanse the eyebrow area using a mild antiseptic lotion or witch hazel, applied with a small piece of clean, dampened cotton wool.
3. Apply an antiseptic soothing lotion, cream or gel with clean, dry cotton wool.
4. Gently remove excess antiseptic lotion, cream or gel using a clean, soft facial tissue or clean damp cotton wool.
5. Repeat as necessary, approximately every four hours. ***If the reddening does not subside in the next 24 hours, contact the salon***.
6. Eye make-up may be worn as soon as the redness has gone – usually after eight hours.

Tint eyebrow and lash aftercare advice If an unwanted reaction occurs (a contra-action, e.g. irritation or redness), apply cool water or a damp cotton wool pad compress to the area.

If reddening continues after 24 hours contact the salon.

Advise the client to receive the service as follows:

- eyelash tinting every 4–6 weeks
- eyebrow tinting every 3–4 weeks

Artificial eyelash aftercare advice

- Provide advice on the action to take it an unwanted reaction, a contra-action, occurs.
- Avoid rubbing the eyes, or the lashes may become loosened.

- Do not use an oil-based eye make-up remover as its cosmetic constituents will dissolve the adhesive.
- Use only dry or water-based eye make-up (as these may readily be removed with a non-oily eye make-up remover).
- If the lashes are made of a synthetic material, heat will cause them to become frizzy. Advise the client to avoid extremes of temperature, such a hot sauna.
- Do not touch the eyes for 1½ hours after application, while the adhesive dries thoroughly.

If the client has had *individual* artificial flare lashes applied, the following homecare advice should be given on caring for the lashes:

- Use a non-oily eye make-up remover daily to cleanse the eyelids and eyelashes. Avoid contact with oil-based preparations in the eye area, such as moisturisers and cleansers – the oil content will dissolve the adhesive, and the lashes would become detached.
- Do not attempt to remove the artificial lashes – pulling at artificial lash will also pull out the natural eyelashes.
- After bathing or swimming, gently *pat* the eye area dry with a clean towel.
- A disposable spiral applicator brush may be used to comb through the lashes to separate.

Clients with individual false eyelashes should have the artificial lashes maintained by regular visits to the salon. Lost individual flare lashes can be replaced as necessary; this is often described as an eyelash *infill* service. Schedule this for every 10–14 days.

If the client wishes to have the individual artificial lashes removed, this should be done professionally.

How to remove individual eyelashes

1 Position the client lying on the couch.

2 Wash your hands.

3 Remove make-up from the eye area, cleansing the skin with a suitable eye make-up remover.

4 While the client's eyes are open, place a pre-shaped eye shield underneath the lower lashes of each eye. (This will protect the eye tissue from the solvent.) Position the eye shields so that they fit snugly to the base of the lower lashes.

5 Ask the client to close their eyes gently, and not to open them again until you tell them to do so.

6 Prepare a new disposable orange stick by covering it at the pointed end with clean, dry cotton wool (or alternatively a cotton bud may be used).

7 Moisten the cotton wool with the artificial eyelash adhesive solvent.

8 Treating one eye at a time, gently stroke down the false eyelashes with the adhesive solvent until the adhesive dissolves and the false eyelash begins to loosen.

9 When you are satisfied that the eyelash adhesive has dissolved, gently attempt to remove the false eyelash. Support the upper eyelid with the fingers of one hand,

HEALTH & SAFETY

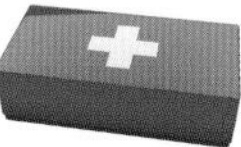

Solvents

Although solvents are formulated to remove artificial lashes from the natural lash, great care must be taken to avoid skin/eye irritation. Ideally this solution should be used to clean the artificial lashes after removal. Removal of artificial lashes should be with an oil-based eye make-up remover product.

TOP TIP

Solvent application

Disposable cotton buds may be used to apply eyelash adhesive solvent.

HEALTH & SAFETY

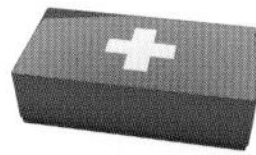

Eye care when using artificial lash glue solvent

Do not allow eyelash adhesive solvent to come into excessive contact with the eye tissue – it could cause irritation of the skin. Ensure that there is sufficient solvent only on the cotton wool: it should be moist but not dripping wet or the solvent might enter the eye.

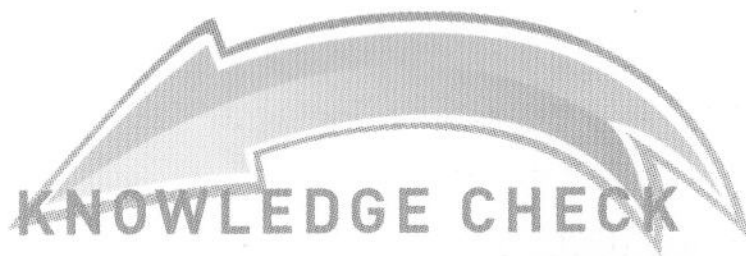

What aftercare advice should be given to a client following an eyebrow shaping treatment?

Need more time... refer to page 278 to help you.

using the other hand to remove the artificial lash with a sterile pair of manual tweezers. If the adhesive has been adequately dissolved, the eyelash will lift away easily from the natural eyelash. If there is any resistance, repeat the solvent application until the eyelash comes away readily.

10 As the artificial eyelashes are removed, collect them on a clean white facial tissue or a clean pad of cotton wool.

11 Having removed all of the artificial eyelashes from one eye, soothe the area by applying damp cotton wool pads soaked in cool water. (This will also remove any remaining solvent.) A damp cotton wool pad may be placed over the eye, while you remove the artificial lashes from the other eye.

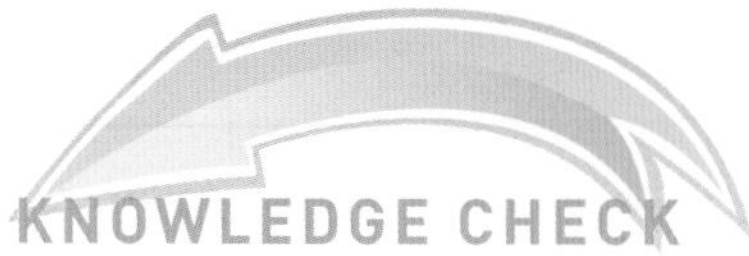

KNOWLEDGE CHECK

What aftercare advice should be given to a client following a permanent tinting service?

Need more time... refer to pages 278–279 to help you.

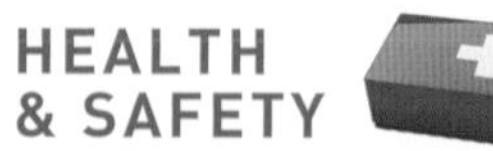

HEALTH & SAFETY

Client comfort

Never attempt to remove the artificial eyelashes until they have begun to loosen – if you do, the client's natural eyelashes will also be removed, causing them discomfort.

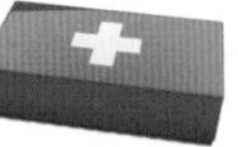

HEALTH & SAFETY

Client comfort

When removing the strip lash, avoid pulling the natural lashes with the artificial lashes.

How to remove strip lashes

If a client wears strip eyelashes, they will need instructions on how to remove and care for the artificial lashes themselves.

1 Use the fingertips of one hand to support the eyelid at the outer corner. With the other hand, lift the lash strip base at the outer corner of the eye. Gently peel the strip away from the natural lash, from the outer edge towards the centre of the eyelid.

2 Peel the adhesive from the backing strip, using a clean pair of manual tweezers. Take care to avoid stretching the strip lash.

3 Clean the strip lash in the appropriate way.

- ***Strips made from human hair*** Clean with a commercial lash cleaner or 70% alcohol. This removes the remaining adhesive and the eye make-up.
- ***Synthetic strips*** Place in warm, soapy water for a few minutes, to clean the lashes and remove the remaining adhesive. Rinse in tepid water.

4 After cleaning the strip lashes should be recurled.

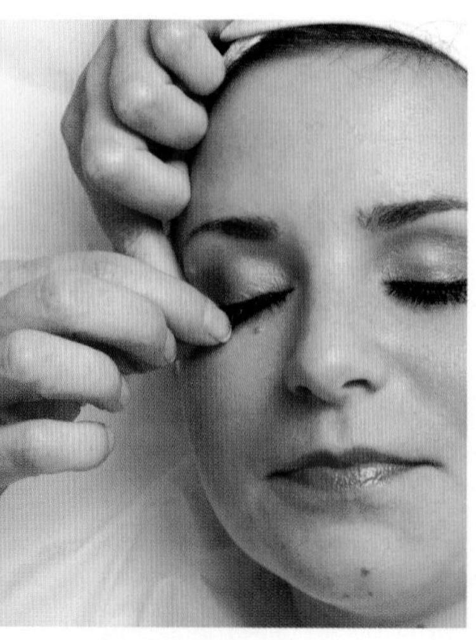

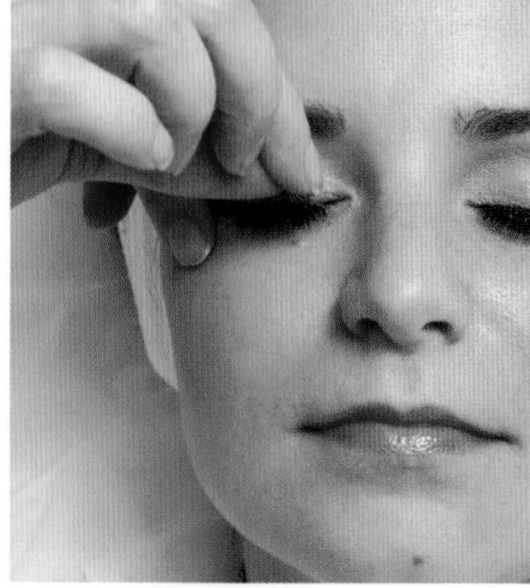

Removing strip lashes

How to recurl strip lashes

For reasons of hygiene and because of the time involved, this service will not be offered by the salon. The client, however; will need advice on how to recurl the lashes at home.

1. On removal from the water, place the lashes side by side, ensuring that the inner edges are together inside a clean facial tissue.
2. Wrap a tissue around an even, barrel-shaped object such as a felt-tip pen, and secure it with an elastic band.
3. The artificial lashes, inside the facial tissue, should then be rolled around this object. Keep the base of the lash straight, so that the whole lash length curls around the object.

Once recurled, the strip lashes can be returned to the contoured shelves in their original container and stored for further use.

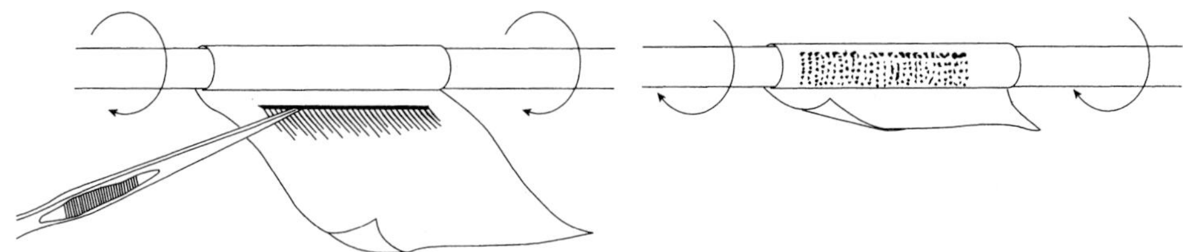

Recurling strip lashes

Eyelash perming aftercare

- Recommend that the client receives the service every 2-3 months.
- A skin sensitivity test is required before each perming service
- Advise your client not to apply make-up for at least 24 hours to the lash area.
- Similarly, they should not receive any other eye treatments for at least 24 hours.
- Subsequently however, eyelash tinting will enhance the effect of the newly permed lashes so you can promote this service to the client.

HEALTH & SAFETY

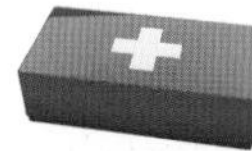

Semi-permanent lashes
The client should be advised to return to the salon for semi-permanent lashes to be removed professionally.

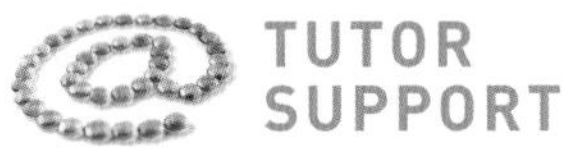

TUTOR SUPPORT

Activity 3: Re-cap and revision evaluation

KNOWLEDGE CHECK

What is the correct method for removing artificial strip lashes and individual flare lashes?

Need more time... refer to pages 279–280 to help you.

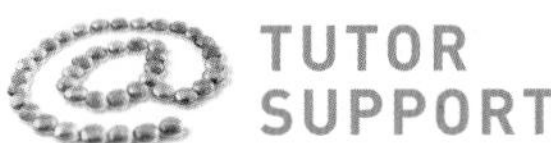

TUTOR SUPPORT

Activity 4: Multiple choice tests

GLOSSARY OF KEY WORDS

Adhesive specialized glue used to attach artificial lashes to the natural lashes. This glue differs in formulation according to the lash type strip or individual flare lashes.

Aftercare advice recommended advice given to the client following service to continue the benefits of the service.

Artificial lashes threads of nylon fibre which are attached to the natural hair. These are referred to as strip lashes, individual artificial lashes and single lash extensions.

Blepharitis inflammation of the eyelid caused by an infection or an allergic reaction.

Colouring characteristics the client's natural hair colouring, e.g. fair, red, dark or white.

Conjunctivitis a bacterial infection. Inflammation of the mucous membrane that covers the eye and lines the eyelid. The skin of the inner conjunctiva of the eye becomes inflamed, the eye becomes very red, itchy and sore, and pus may exude from the eye area.

Consultation assessment of a client's needs using different assessment techniques, including questioning and natural observation.

Contact dermatitis a skin disorder caused by intolerance of the skin to a particular substance, or a group of substances. On exposure to the substance the skin quickly becomes irritated and an allergic reaction occurs.

Contra-action an unwanted reaction occurring during or after service application.

Contra-indication a problematic symptom that indicates that the service may not proceed.

Cortex the thickest layer of the hair structure.

Cyst localized pocket of sebum that forms in the hair follicle or under the sebaceous glands in the skin. Semi-globular in shape, either raised or flat, and hard or soft. Cysts are the same colour as the skin, or red if bacterial infection occurs.

Disulphide bonds two chemical sulphur bonds joined together forming a chemical bond in the cortex of the hair.

Eyebrow shaping involves the removal of eyebrow hair to create a new shape (reshape) or to remove stray hairs to maintain the existing brow shape (maintenance). Small metal tools, called tweezers, are use to remove the hairs.

Eyelash adhesive used to apply strips and individual eyelashes.

Eyelash and eyebrow tinting definition of the brow and lash hair, achieved by the application of a permanent dye especially formulated for use around the delicate eye area.

Eyelash curlers small flexible rods around which the natural eyelashes are curled during eyelash perming treatment.

Eyelash perming a chemical treatment applied to the eyelashes to permanently curl the lashes, enhancing the appearance of the eyes.

Fixing/neutralizing lotion usually containing sodium bromate, which makes the curl produced during eyelash perming permanent.

Hair a long slender structure that grows out of, and is part of, the skin. Each hair is made up of dead skin cells, which contain the protein called keratin.

Hair follicle an appendage (structure) in the skin formed from epidermal tissue. Cells move up the hair follicle from the bottom (the hair bulb), changing in structure to form the hair.

Hydrogen peroxide (H_2O_2) an *oxidant*, a chemical that contains available oxygen atoms and encourages chemical reactions.

Negative skin sensitivity patch test a test where result produces no skin reaction. in this case you may proceed with the service.

Perm solution usually contains 6% thioglycollate, which when applied to eyelash hair softens and curls the hair into its new shape.

Positive skin sensitivity patch test an allergic reaction to the skin test. The skin appears red, swollen and feels itchy.

Service plan after the consultation, suitable service objectives are established to treat the client's conditions and needs.

Skin sensitivity test method used to assess skin tolerance/sensitivity to a substance or service.

Solvent a product designed to remove and clean artificial lashes without causing eye irritation.

Stye bacterial infection. Infection of the sebaceous glands of the eyelash hair follicles. Small lumps appear on the inner rim of the eyelid and contain pus.

Thioglycollate the active ingredient in perm solution.

Toluenediamine small molecules of permanent dye used in tinting service.

Tweezers small metal tools used to remove body hair by pulling it from the bottom of the hair follicle (small opening in the skin where the hair grows from). There are two types: *automatic* – designed to remove the bulk of the hair and *manual* – designed to remove the stray hairs.

Watery eye over-secretion of tears from the eyes, which would normally drain into the nasal cavity.

ASSESSMENT OF KNOWLEDGE AND UNDERSTANDING

You have now learnt how to provide eyelash and brow treatments in the beauty therapy workplace. To test your level of knowledge, answer the following short questions. These will prepare you for your summative (final) assessment.

1. An allergic reaction to a skin sensitivity test is known as a:
   a. positive skin sensitivity test
   b. negative skin sensitivity test

2. The following is a contra-indication that restricts an eyebrow shaping service:
   a. client is undergoing chemotherapy treatment
   b. diabetes
   c. conjunctivitis
   d. severe psoriasis

3. A skin sensitivity test is carried out:
   a. 48 hours before each treatment
   b. 24-48 hours before each treatment
   c. the first time the client ever has the treatment
   d. if the client has a sensitive skin

4. If the client has a round face, an unsuitable eyebrow shape would be?
   a. round
   b. straight
   c. oblique
   d. arched

5. The method of sterilization for tweezers is:
   a. an ultra-violet cabinet
   b. a chemical disinfectant
   c. a glass bead steriliser
   d. an autoclave

6. How often would you recommend that a client returns to the salon for an eyebrow trim?
   a. once a week
   b. every 2 weeks
   c. every 3 weeks
   d. every month

7. When applying artificial individual flare lashes, if the clients has close set eyes:
   a. place longer lashes at the outer third of the eyes
   b. apply medium length lashes at the inner corner of the eye and the centre of the lash line
   c. apply longer lashes along the length of the lash line
   d. apply shorter lashes at the outer corner of the lash line and medium from the centre to the inner third of the eye

8. The small dye molecules used in permanent tinting swell and join together, trapped permanently in the:
   a. cuticle of the hair
   b. the medulla of the hair
   c. the cortex of the hair
   d. the papilla

9. How often would you recommend that a client has their eye lashes permed?
   a. every month
   b. every 2–3 months
   c. every 2 weeks
   d. every 4–6 months

10. Hair maintains its shape and strength by chemical cross bonds in the cortex (the thickest layer of the hair) called what?

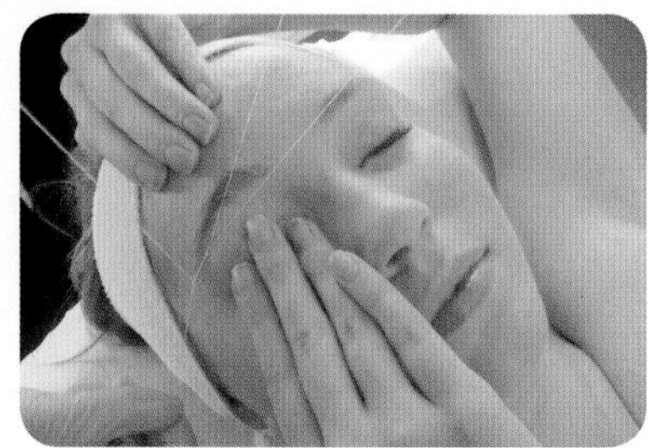

9 Threading

Learning Objectives

This chapter covers **VRQ Unit Provide threading treatments for hair removal.**

This unit is about removing hair from areas of the face using a variety of threading techniques. It will also include reference to shaping and maintenance of different eyebrow shapes. For brow shaping using the tweezer hair removal technique, see Chapter 8.

You will need to be able to consult with the client, prepare for the threading treatment and identify with the client the treatment objectives. You will also need to provide advice to the client including future treatment needs and aftercare advice.

There are **two** learning outcomes for this unit which you must achieve:

1 **Be able to prepare for threading**

2 **Be able to provide threading**

From the **range** statement, you must show you can:

- use **consultation techniques** to identify the treatment **objectives**
- use **products, tools and equipment** as appropriate
- ensure the **environmental conditions** are suitable
- identify **contra-indications**
- **communicate and behave** in an appropriate and professional manner
- use the threading **techniques** to remove hair
- follow all the **health and safety working practices**
- treat all **skin types and conditions**
- identify normal reactions of the skin and **contra-actions**
- provide relevant **aftercare advice**

You must be able to show you have the necessary practical skills and underpinning knowledge to provide threading services for hair removal.

This unit is linked to the Beauty Therapy NOS **Unit B34**.

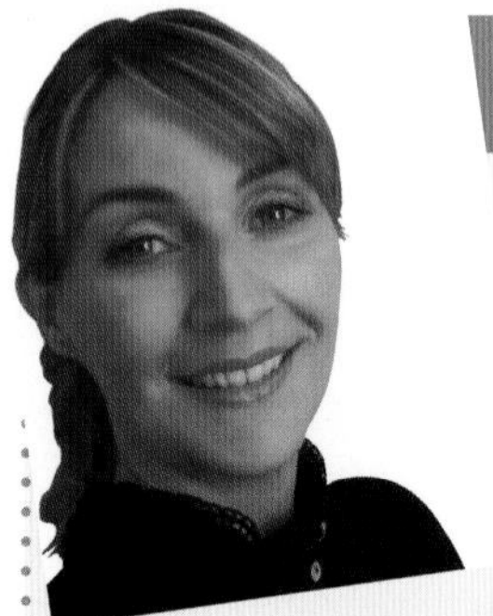

ROLE MODEL

Lorraine Onorato
Director
National School of Threading and Principal of The Surrey School of Beauty & Complementary Health

"Following a career in nursing I entered the beauty industry in 1995.

After many years as a therapist and salon owner I decided to follow my passion for education and began to lecture at a further education college in Surrey.

In the following six years I gained further professional skills and qualifications including writing examination questions for CIBTAC (Confederation of International Beauty Therapy and Cosmetology), achieving the Cert.Ed. teaching qualification and embarking on training to become a beauty therapy examiner.

I set up my first training company, The National School of Threading in 2006 in response to a growing demand for threading teachers and have since performed many demonstrations and exhibitions in London and participated in the World Skills Championships.

As a leading expert and role model in this field, I have been privileged enough to work alongside some high profile businesses to provide both training and consultative work. This has included working with Nails Inc – trade testing, training and launching their 'Get Lashed' brand, GMTTEC Training Education Consultancy and, more recently, Boots UK, where I was commissioned as a consultant to assist in the development of a new brand concept.

My plan for the future is to offer a wide range of short courses with my new training company – The Surrey School of Beauty and Complementary Health – to provide training for new and existing therapists across many therapies and to expand my threading expertise into Europe where the skill is still relatively unknown.

Essential anatomy and physiology knowledge requirements for this chapter are identified on the checklist chart on page 27.

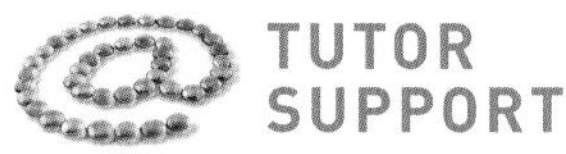

Activity 1: Promote threading treatments

Introduction

History

Threading has been used for many centuries. Its origin is a little uncertain but it is believed that it was originally used in Arabia, Turkey and India.

Threading is an ancient manual method of temporary hair removal, similar to tweezing. It involves the use of a loop of twisted cotton thread which is passed across the skin to trap the hairs and so 'pluck' them from their follicles. There are three main methods of threading: the mouth technique, neck technique and hand technique, which are discussed later in the chapter.

TOP TIP

Gentle on the skin

Threading has less effect on the skin than other hair removal treatments, e.g. waxing which can cause irritation from heat, allergic reactions and possible skin removal.

Benefits of threading

Threading is a simple, inexpensive and an efficient way of removing unwanted hair with minimal pain and skin irritation. Neat results are achieved, with hair regrowth in approximately two to four weeks. An advantage is that very short hair can be removed with little irritation to the area making it possible to go over the area more than once. Hair can be removed individually or in 'lines' to create a perfect shape and can be removed from both above and below the eyebrow giving the threaded eyebrow its characteristic groomed appearance. Threading is also good for individuals that have undergone strong acne treatments, e.g. roaccutane, retin A, where the skin becomes very delicate or those that have other contra-indications to waxing.

TOP TIP

Extra protection

Some specialist threading thread has an anti-bacterial coating added to it during the manufacture process to give protection to the skin while performing the treatment and so reduce the risk of infection.

Advantages	Disadvantages
● Only removes hair not skin. ● Good for short hairs. ● Can isolate one hair at a time. ● Can go over an area more than once without causing skin irritation. ● Sharp, defined shape can be achieved. ● Inexpensive to perform. ● Fast results. ● Ideal for eyebrows and facial hair. ● Minimal skin irritation – good for delicate, sensitive skin types.	● Some clients may experience side effects following the treatment. ● The area may be uncomfortable for a short while. ● Itching may occur following hair removal. ● Ingrowing hair may occur when the hair regrows or as a result of poor technique. ● Infections may occur (e.g. folliculitis), if homecare advice is not followed as the follicle will remain open for up to 24 hours following the treatment. ● Excessive skin reddening (erythema). ● Short-term puffiness of tissues treated can occur.

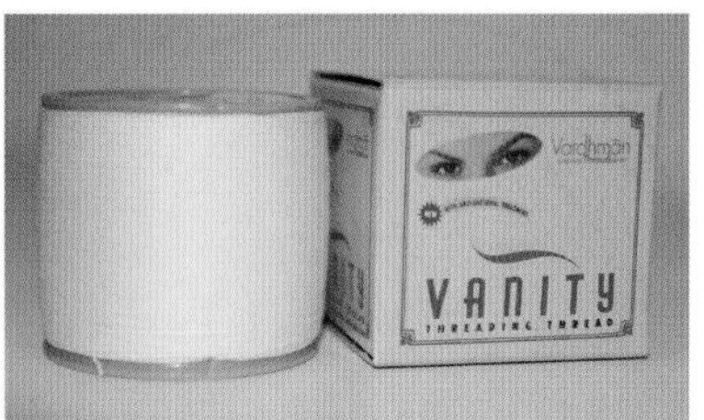

Specialist threading thread

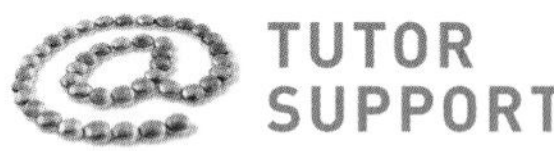
TUTOR SUPPORT

Activity 2: Research threading treatments

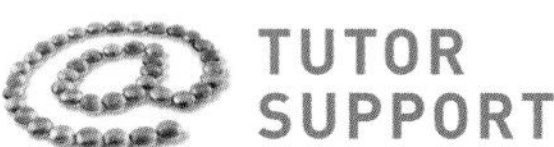
TUTOR SUPPORT

Activity 3: Comparing hair removal techniques

> It is good practice to use specialist threading thread to perform the treatment as this thread will be the correct strength and thickness to facilitate accurate technique and results. It should be placed back into its box or a sealed container when not in use to avoid contamination.
>
> **Lorraine Onorato**

What type of thread is used for threading?

A specialist 100 per cent cotton thread is used for threading. This thread allows strength but resilience during the treatment which is important in order to perform threading to a high standard.

What areas can be threaded?

Threading is mainly performed on the face (eyebrows, upper lip, chin, sides of face, nose, ears, neck and forehead) but can be used all over the body if desired.

Like tweezing, threading can be combined with other eye treatments to enhance the treatment. A good example would be to tint the eyebrows and lashes (ensure skin sensitivity test has been completed 48 hours in advance of the treatment with a negative result obtained) before performing the threading treatment.

To further enhance the eye area, artificial eyelashes may be applied.

For male grooming an eyebrow treatment can combine with a barbering treatment. Hair can also be removed from the tops of the cheeks, nose and ears.

What are the three layers of terminal hair called?

Need more time... refer to page 54 to help you.

Outcome 1: Be able to prepare for threading

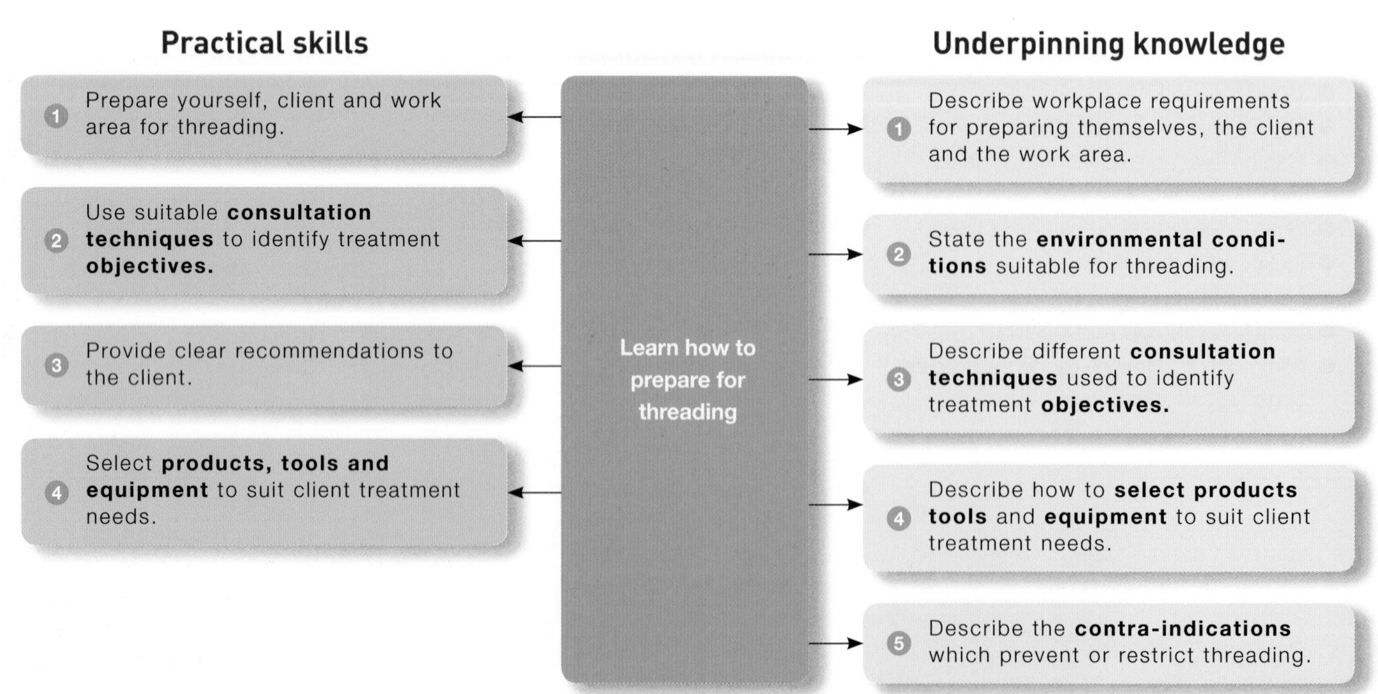

Practical skills
1 Prepare yourself, client and work area for threading.
2 Use suitable consultation techniques to identify treatment objectives.
3 Provide clear recommendations to the client.
4 Select products, tools and equipment to suit client treatment needs.
Learn how to prepare for threading
Underpinning knowledge
1 Describe workplace requirements for preparing themselves, the client and the work area.
2 State the environmental conditions suitable for threading.
3 Describe different consultation techniques used to identify treatment objectives.
4 Describe how to select products tools and equipment to suit client treatment needs.
5 Describe the contra-indications which prevent or restrict threading.

Preparing the work area

Before beginning threading, check that you have the necessary products, tools and equipment to hand and that they meet the legal hygiene and industry requirements for threading treatment.

PRODUCTS, TOOLS AND EQUIPMENT

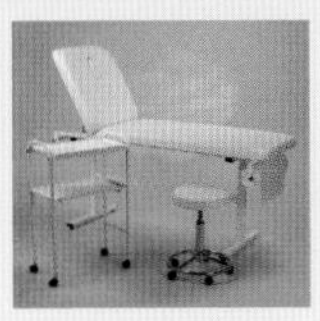

Couch or chair
With neck and foot support

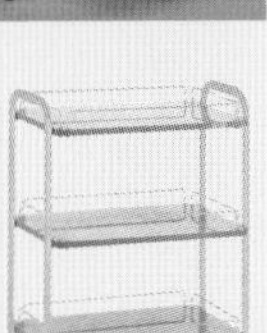

Trolley
On which to place everything

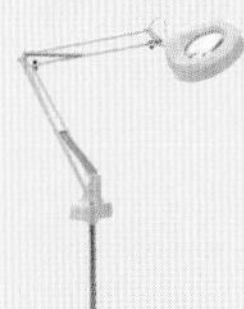

Bright lighting and magnifying lamp
To optimize visibility

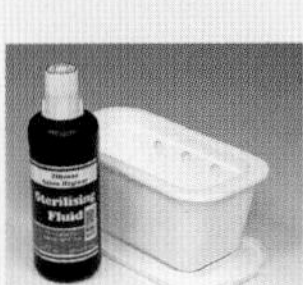

Disinfecting solution
For storing sterilized tweezers

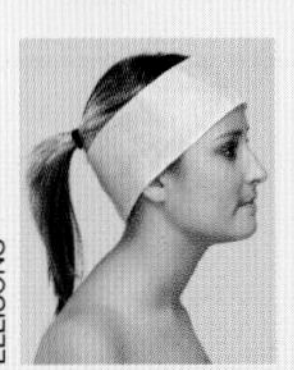

ELLISONS

Headband (or clips)
To hold the hair from the client's face

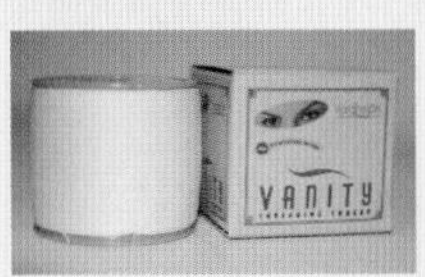

Specialist threading thread
To remove hair with threading techniques

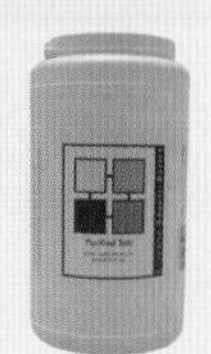

Powder
Purified talc or other specialist powder supplied by the manufacturer for threading

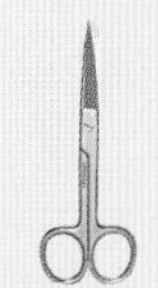

Scissors
Specialist stainless steel eyebrow trimming scissors for trimming long hairs

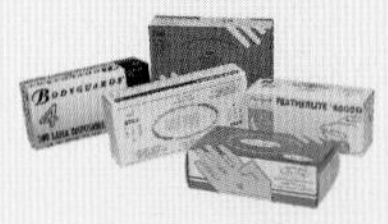

Disposable non-latex (synthetic) powder-free gloves
To be worn to prevent cross-contamination

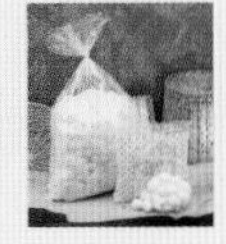

Cotton wool
To cleanse the treatment area

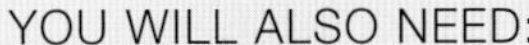

YOU WILL ALSO NEED:

Mirror To show the client the finished result

Skin disinfectant To cleanse and disinfect the client's skin

Antiseptic soothing lotion or gel With healing and anti-septic properties, suitable for facial skin

Medium sized towels (2) To protect the client's clothes

Client record card To record confidential details of each client registered to the salon including personal details, products used and details of the treatment

Eyebrow brush To brush the eyebrows into shape before and after treatment

Waste container This should be a lined metal bin with a lid

Disposable tissue (such as bedroll) To cover the work surface and couch or chair

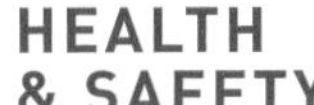
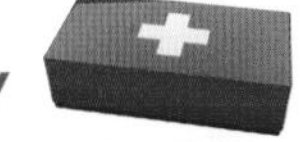

HEALTH & SAFETY

Waste
Contaminated waste must be disposed of in accordance with the environmental health department of the local council.

"Remember that you are an advert for your skill: maintain excellent eyebrow grooming and ensure that you are prepared for the treatment."

Lorraine Onorato

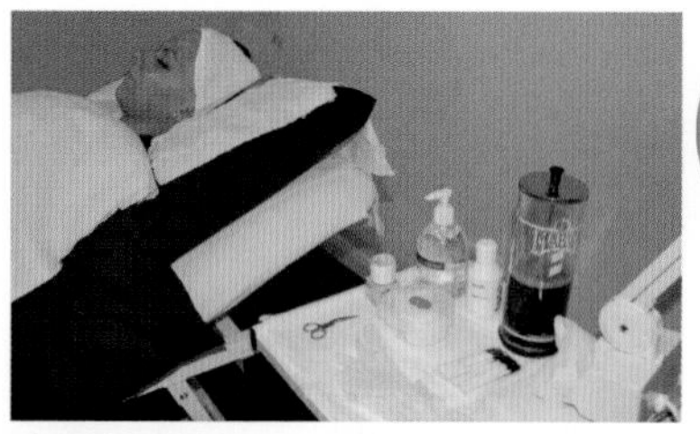

Prepared client and trolley

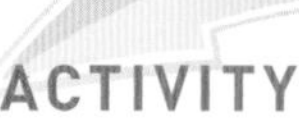

Hygiene

Disposable mascara wands can be used to brush the eyebrows as an alternative to a brow brush – which can then be hygienically disposed of immediately after use.

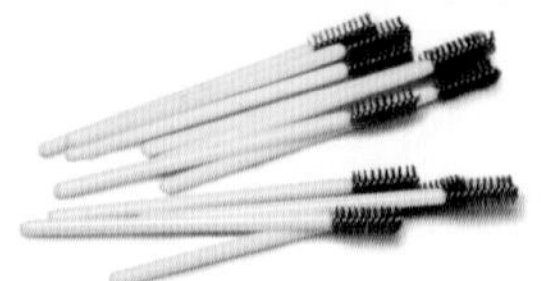

Disposable mascara wands

ACTIVITY

Collect magazines, look at images of eyebrows and see if you can identify which eyebrows have been threaded. You will need to look for a sharp and defined angular eyebrow.

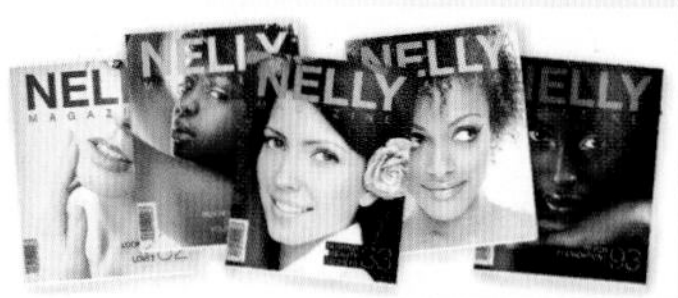

ISTOCK/© IZABELA HABUR

HEALTH & SAFETY

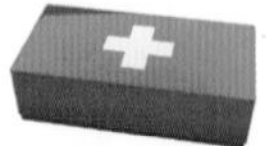

Contra-action

A contra-action is what may occur as a result of the treatment. This must be discussed at consultation and must be indicated on the client's record card where appropriate with action taken recorded.

TOP TIP

Powder

Cornflour is traditionally used as an alternative to talc, to dry the skin and lift the hair before the treatment. Some threading specialists use the powder to ensure the smooth gliding of the thread on the skin's surface.

Sterilization and disinfection

Hygiene must be maintained in a number of ways:

- Client hair and clothing is protected and any clothing and accessories are removed where necessary.
- Wearing disposable gloves to avoid cross-infection.
- Ensuring that the client's hands do not come into contact with the treatment area whilst stretching the skin.
- Selecting a new piece of thread for each treatment area.
- Maintaining accepted industry hygiene and safety practices throughout the treatment.

Reception

When a client makes an appointment for a threading treatment, the receptionist will need to check which area the client would like threading treatment to allow sufficient time.

As contact lenses should be removed when performing eyebrow threading, inform the client of this in order that they can store them safely on removal.

All staff, especially the staff communicating with clients at reception, should be familiar with the different pricing structures for the range of threading treatments and products available for retail.

Commercially, 10 minutes is allowed for threading to the upper lip or chin and 20 minutes for an eyebrow reshape.

Consultation

As with all treatments, consultation is essential and should be carried out in a comfortable and quiet area where the client is able to ask any questions and clarify points if necessary. All details should be recorded and signatures obtained.

Consult with the client ensuring there is a clear understanding of the area to be treated and what is realistically achievable both short- and long-term. Explain to the client that they will be required to support the skin to assist hair removal as instructed. You may wish to demonstrate this to confirm understanding at consultation. Encourage clients to ask questions to clarify any points.

Check client suitability, certain contra-indications will prevent or restrict threading.

If the client is a **minor** under the age of 16, it is necessary to obtain parent/guardian permission for the threading treatment. The parent/guardian will also have to be present when the treatment is received.

Contra-indications

Although threading is considered to be more suitable for individuals with skin sensitivities resulting from conditions like psoriasis, eczema, dermatitis and diabetes, as with all hair removal techniques **contra-indications** will apply and will be the same as other hair removal techniques (e.g. waxing and tweezing refer to Chapter 8 Eyelash and Brow Treatments and Chapter 14 Waxing Techniques).

There is also the possibility that **contra-actions** may arise. This can be avoided by ensuring a thorough consultation prior to the treatment to assess clients' suitability for the treatment and giving clear aftercare instructions on completion of the treatment.

Contra-actions

Examples of possible contra-actions:

- **folliculitis**
- **erythema**
- ingrowing hairs
- bruising
- blood spots
- broken hair
- histamine (allergic reaction)
- severe swelling
- severe erythema

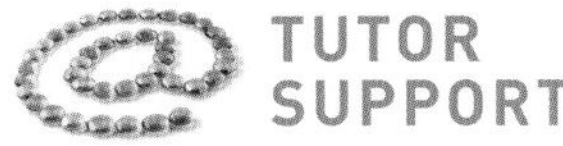

TUTOR SUPPORT

Activity 4: Threading wordsearch

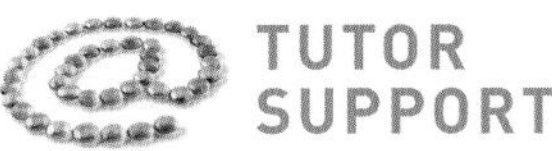

TUTOR SUPPORT

Activity 5: Threading wordsearch 2

The record card should be signed and dated following the **consultation** to confirm the suitability and consent with the agreed threading treatment. It is important that accurate records are kept and stored in compliance with the Data Protection Act for future reference. Any additional details are to be recorded on the reverse of the card. Existing clients will need to indicate whether there have been any changes since their last treatment, which must also be noted down on the record card.

Please refer to the sample client record card on pages 252–253.

Preparing the client

Preparation for the treatment is as important as the preparation of the beauty therapist (see page 288) and must be carried out thoroughly and professionally:

1 Escort the client to the treatment area and assist with removal of clothing/accessories in the area (e.g. jewellery, scarves, etc.) and help the client onto the couch where necessary. Ensure that they are comfortable and positioned at the correct height for you to work.

2 Confirm required hair removal discussed at consultation and advise where necessary.

3 Disinfect your hands and apply disposable gloves.

HEALTH & SAFETY

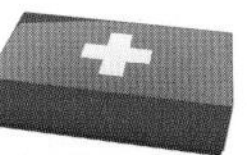

Contact lenses

Contact lenses must be removed as clients will be required to support the eye area during the threading treatment.

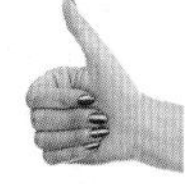

BEST PRACTICE

Cleanliness

Before beginning a new client wash your hands at the hand basin with antibacterial cleanser.

> Keep up to date with current developments in industry and be aware of changing fashion – we need to be ahead of our clients!
>
> **Lorraine Onorato**

> An eyebrow threading specialist must use their initiative to create the perfect eyebrow shape for each individual client. It may be necessary for the client to leave some areas of the eyebrow to grow in order to achieve a good result and this should be discussed and agreed during the consultation.
>
> **Lorraine Onorato**

HEALTH & SAFETY

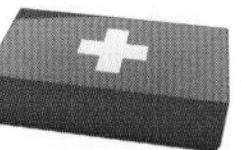

PPE

PPE should be worn to prevent cross and secondary infection.

Outcome 2: Be able to provide threading

Learn how provide threading

Practical skills

1. **Communicate and behave** in a professional manner.
2. Follow **health and safety working practices.**
3. Position themselves and client correctly throughout the treatment.
4. Use **products, tools and equipment** and **techniques** to suit clients treatment needs.
5. Complete the treatment to the satisfaction of the client.
6. Record the results of the treatment.
7. Provide suitable **aftercare advice.**

Underpinning knowledge

1. State how to **communicate and behave** in a professional manner.
2. Describe **health and safety working practices.**
3. State the importance of positioning themselves and the client correctly throughout the treatment.
4. State the importance of using **product, tools, equipment and techniques** to suit clients treatment needs, **skin types and conditions**.
5. Describe how treatments can be adapted to suit client treatment needs.
6. State the **contra-actions** that may occur during and following treatments and how to respond.
7. State the importance of completing the treatment to the satisfaction of the client.
8. State the importance of completing treatment records.
9. State the **aftercare advice** that should be provided.
10. Describe the structure and functions of the skin.
11. Describe the structure and function of the hair.

HEALTH & SAFETY

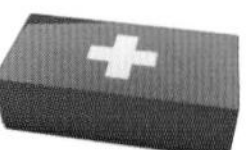

Disinfectant

Ensure chemical disinfectant is diluted as per the manufacturers' guidelines and wear disposable gloves when handling it as it is a skin irritant.

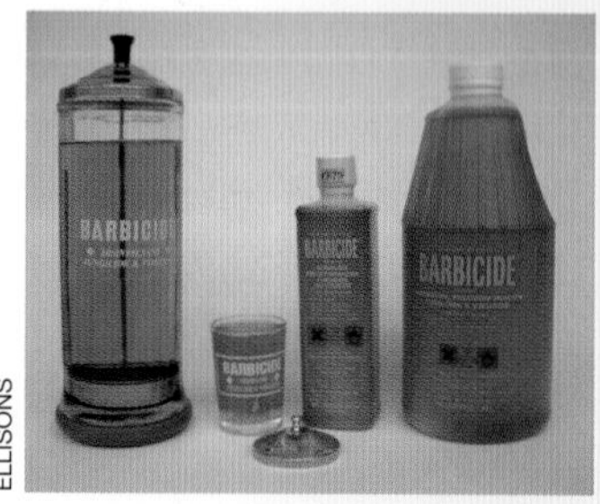

ELLISONS

Barbicide – chemical disinfectant

KNOWLEDGE CHECK

How should you prepare yourself hygienically for threading treatment?

Need more time... refer to page 288 to help you.

TOP TIP

Trimming hairs

Long eyebrow hairs are trimmed by first brushing the hair in an upwards direction. The point of the scissors should be angled towards the bridge of the nose with the shank laying flat to the skin's surface. The long hair is then trimmed to match to length of the other eyebrow hair. This process is then repeated underneath the eyebrow by brushing the hair in a downwards direction.

Step-by-step: Eyebrow threading

1 First remove any facial creams or cosmetic products from the area to be treated by using clean cotton wool and a disinfecting product, e.g. witch hazel, and then blot dry with a clean tissue, disposing of both in a lined metal waste bin. Moisture in the area will reduce the effectiveness of the thread gripping the hair.

2 For eyebrow shaping, brush the eyebrows in an upwards and then downwards direction to ensure the hairs are laying flat, and trim any long hairs that may spoil the finished result. Brush eyebrows back into place.

3 With a clean piece of cotton wool, apply a light dusting of powder (optional) to the area – this will enable the thread to glide over the skin and is particularly good when the skin is hot and moist.

4 Decide the method of threading to be used (examples are shown below) and prepare the cotton. Shorter lengths of thread are easier to handle whilst developing your skills or if you have smaller hands.

TOP TIP

Client assistance

If a client has arm mobility issues, then a pillow/support can be placed under the elbow to support the arm.

ALWAYS REMEMBER

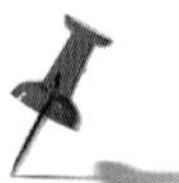

Personal space

Avoid invading your client's space during the treatment by working at approximately arm's length distance of the area.

HEALTH & SAFETY

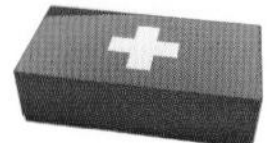

Repetitive stain injury

To avoid RSI (repetitive strain injury):

- Breaks should be taken every 30–45 minutes for at least five minutes.
- Stretch your arms, hands, neck, and back during breaks.
- Perform facial exercise when possible.
- Maintain posture alignment. Don't slouch.
- Adjust your chair or couch to avoid strain.

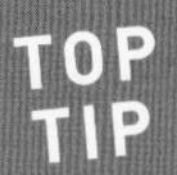

TOP TIP

Dealing with different hair

Different hair densities will require an adjustment of tension in the thread, e.g. male hair will need more tension to remove it from the root without snapping it.

Before threading, long hair will need to be trimmed first to approx ¼ cm to avoid discomfort to the client.

Hair removed from ears and noses will need to be trimmed first and the area supported.

5 The client must now support the area to be treated – for eyebrows one hand should be over the eye and one over the top of the eyebrow (see image below). The area should be supported firmly in order to avoid the skin being pinched or cut by the thread.

6 The hairs are removed against the direction of hair growth, with the thread firmly placed onto the skin ensuring even tension throughout the treatment. This will enable effective and accurate removal of the hair from the root, avoiding snapping while reducing any discomfort to the client.

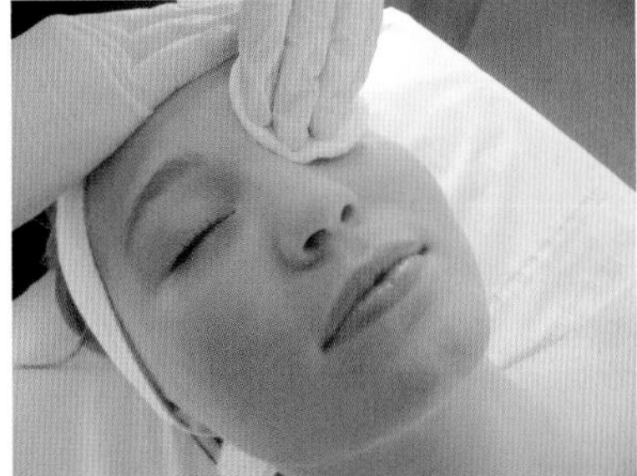

Cleanse the area to be treated

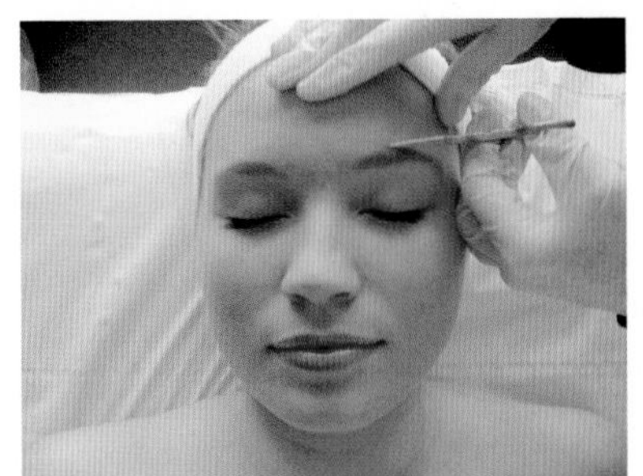

Trim long hairs if necessary

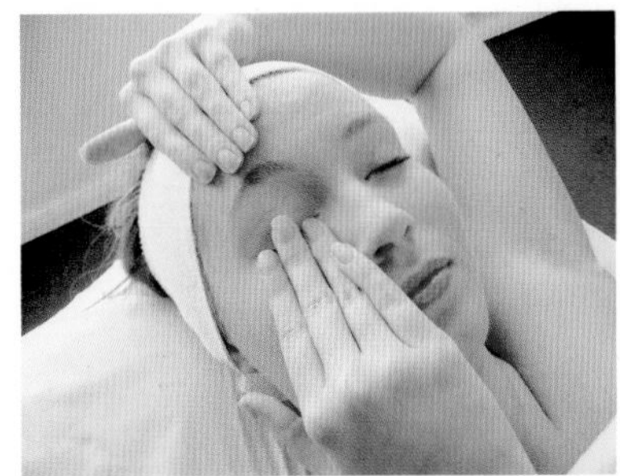

Get the client to support the area to be treated

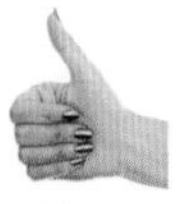

BEST PRACTICE

Client satisfaction
To ensure client satisfaction, especially when re-shaping a thick eyebrow shape, it is advisable to show the client the shape as it is developing.

7 Remove all hairs as necessary, using the thread to brush away any loose ones dropping onto the skin during the treatment. Keep checking the threaded area to ensure symmetry of both eyebrows. If completing a reshape show the client the eyebrow shape as the treatment progresses to ensure client satisfaction.

8 On completion of the treatment and when the treatment is to the satisfaction of the client, apply soothing aftercare lotion to the area using clean cotton wool to remove loose hairs and soothe the area and then dispose of in a lined bin.

9 Brush the eyebrows into shape and show client the finished result.

10 Assist client from couch and give appropriate homecare advice.

TOP TIP

Retail opportunities
On completion of the treatment you could recommend a retail product or further eye treatment e.g. a soothing massage to the eye area with a suitable aftercare cream to enhance the treatment.

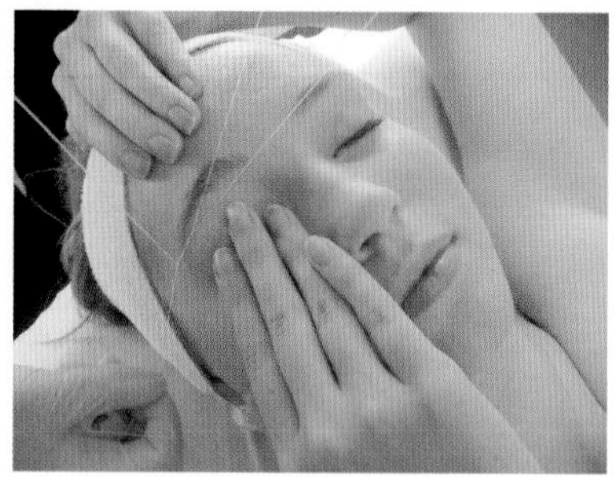

Thread against hair growth

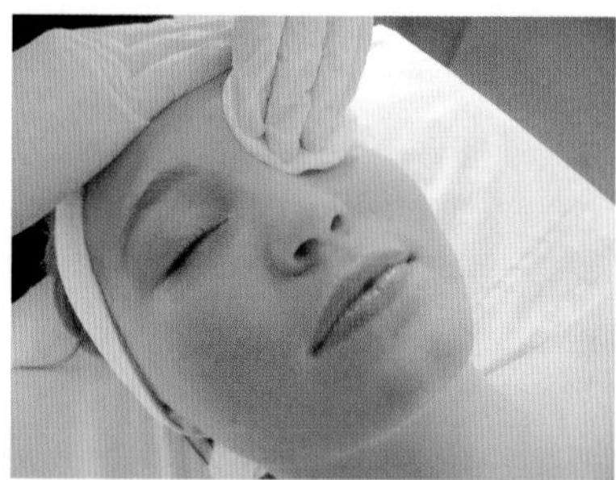

Wipe over area to remove loose hair and apply aftercare antiseptic, soothing product

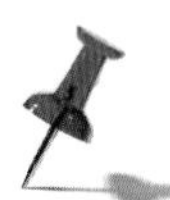

ALWAYS REMEMBER

Skin tags and hairy moles
Avoid skin tags and removal of hair from moles.

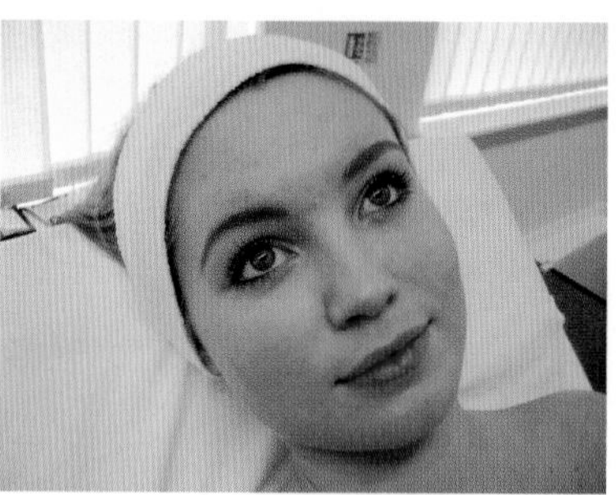

Brush eyebrow and show client finished result

ACTIVITY

For different areas, position the thread so that it will remove hair 'against' hair growth. Check your own working position and observe correct posture to avoid injury.

KNOWLEDGE CHECK

What is a contra-action? What is a contra-action to threading?

Need more time... refer to page 289 help you.

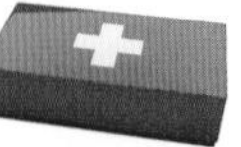

HEALTH & SAFETY

Cross-contamination
To avoid **cross-contamination**, ensure all disposables and waste are put immediately into the bin and not left on the trolley.

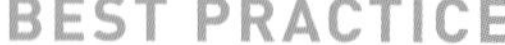

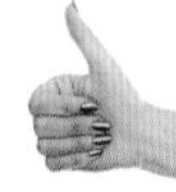

BEST PRACTICE

Ensure that you are removing hair against direction of hair growth.

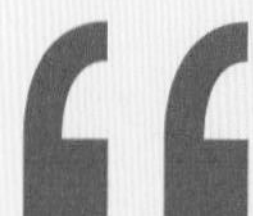

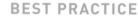

In order to enhance your chances of employment you should be able to perform an eyebrow thread to a high standard in 15 minutes. To achieve this you must be committed to practising your skill at every opportunity.

Lorraine Onorato

Threading techniques

There are three techniques that are commonly used:

1 ***Mouth technique*** – Hair removal using thread where one part of the thread is anchored in the mouth and the other part is looped in the hands. This is the most commonly used technique, originating from the Far East and is also know as the Asian or single looped method.

2 ***Neck technique*** – A substitute for the mouth technique where one part of the thread is anchored around the neck and the other part is looped in the hands. This technique originates from the Middle East and is also known as the Arabian or single looped method.

3 ***Hand technique*** – Hair removal using thread held and looped between both hands. Commonly used by practitioners on themselves. This technique is also known as cats cradle, doubled looped or self technique.

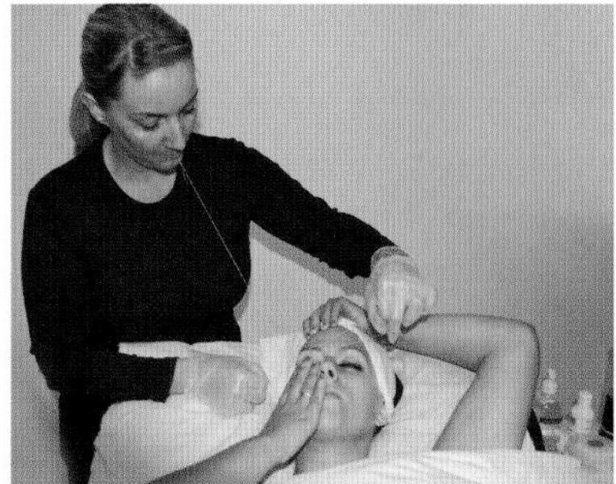
The mouth technique

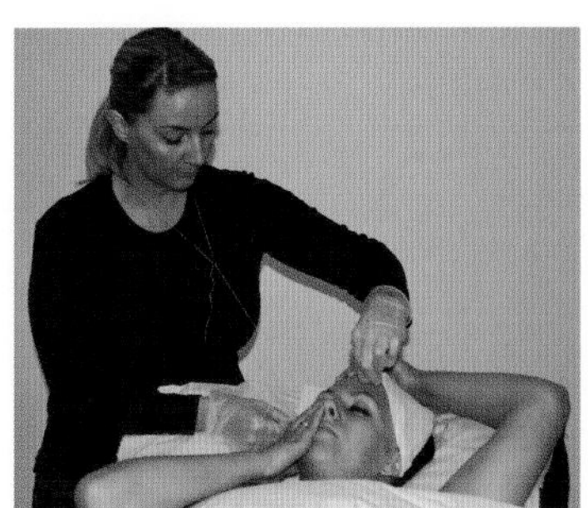
The neck technique

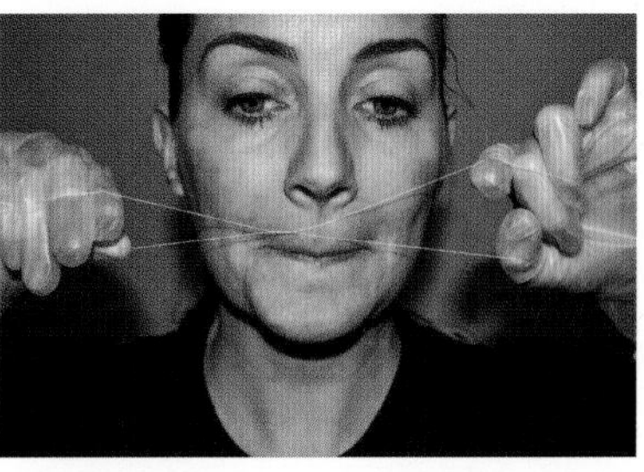
The hand technique (self-threading)

Aftercare advice

Aftercare advice and homecare advice are essential not only to avoid contra-actions but in order to maintain the treatment results. It is important to give general as well as specific advice.

For the next 12–24 hours it is important to avoid:

- swimming
- heat treatments, e.g. hot water, sauna, steam
- ultra-violet light exposure; natural or artificial
- perfumed products applied the area treated
- facial treatments/exfoliation
- touching the area
- excessive sweating
- applying make-up to the area

To avoid ingrowing hairs it is important to **gently exfoliate** the area after three days and twice weekly thereafter.

If needed the area can be soothed with either a recommended product or a soothing and calming product, e.g. aloe vera gel.

> Ensure you have related products to retail following the treatment for the client to maintain and enhance her eyebrows between appointments, e.g. brow make-up kits, brow setting mousse and tweezers.
>
> **Lorraine Onorato**

ALWAYS REMEMBER

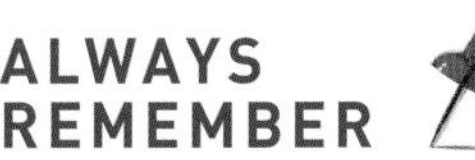

Appointments

To schedule the client's next appointment as part of the aftercare advice.

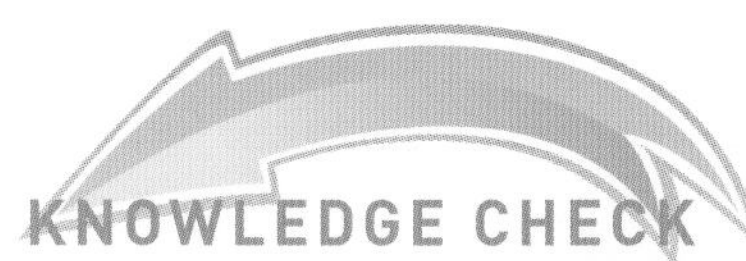

KNOWLEDGE CHECK

What are the three techniques of threading that you can use?

Need more time... refer to page 293 to help you.

If there is a contra-action following treatment, advise the client what appropriate action should be taken. Advise the client to receive the treatment in the specified time according to their hair growth cycle. Repeat bookings vary according to the natural hair regrowth and client requirements.

Ensure that the client's records are up to date, accurate and complete following the threading treatment. Provide written instructions in an aftercare leaflet.

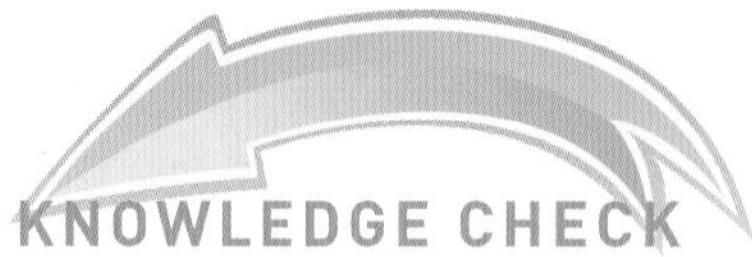

KNOWLEDGE CHECK

Why is exfoliation to the area following threading treatment important as part of the aftercare advice?

Need more time... refer to page 293 to help you.

GLOSSARY OF KEY WORDS

Contra-action an unwanted reaction occurring during or after treatment application.

Contra-indication a problematic symptom that indicates that the treatment may not proceed or may restrict treatment application. Further contra-indications identified for eye treatments are discussed in more detail in Chapter 8.

Cross contamination transfer of an infection directly or indirectly from one person to another.

Erythema reddening of the skin cause by increased blood circulation to the area.

Folliculitis a bacterial infection where pustules develop in the skin tissue around the hair follicle.

Hand technique threading hair removal using thread held and looped between both hands. This technique is also known as cat's cradle, double looped or self technique.

Mouth technique threading hair removal where one part of the thread is anchored in the mouth and the other part is looped in the hands.

Neck technique threading hair removal where one part of the thread is anchored around the neck and the other part is looped in the hands.

Threading hair removal using a length of thread, which is moved over the skin surface, gripping hairs and removing them from the skin against hair growth.

ASSESSMENT OF KNOWLEDGE AND UNDERSTANDING

You have now learnt how to provide threading treatments in the beauty therapy workplace. To test your level of knowledge, answer the following short questions. These will prepare you for your summative (final) assessment.

1. The part of the skin where the hair is removed from when performing threading is the
   a. papillary layer
   b. reticular layer
   c. subcutaneous layer
   d. cornified layer
2. The growing active stage of the hair growth cycle is known as:
   a. catagen
   b. telogen
   c. anagen
3. Hair that is coarse and usually pigmented is known as:
   a. terminal hair
   b. vellus hair
   c. lanugo hair
4. What are the three popular threading techniques for removal?
   a. mouth, neck and hand
   b. lip, chin and eyebrow
   c. mouth, neck and foot
   d. two-handed threading, hand and mouth threading

5. Good working practice will avoid RSI. What does this stand for?

6. What is a normal, expected skin reaction to hair removal threading?

7. To avoid hair breakage, coarse hair will require the thread tension to be:
   a. more
   b. less

8. Why is powder applied to the skin?

9. What is the best method of sterilization for threading scissors?
   a. a chemical disinfectant
   b. an autoclave
   c. an ultra-violet cabinet
   d. surgical spirit

10. As the thread moves along the skin it removes hair from the hair follicle:
    a. with hair growth
    b. against hair growth

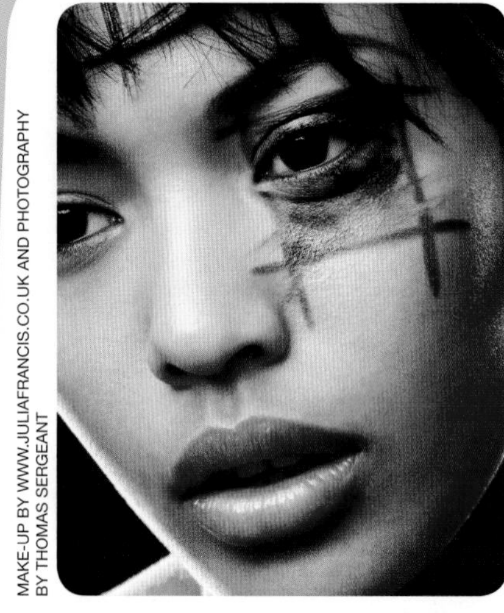

MAKE-UP BY WWW.JULIAFRANCIS.CO.UK AND PHOTOGRAPHY BY THOMAS SERGEANT

10 Make-up

Learning Objectives

This chapter covers **VRQ Unit Apply make-up**.

This unit is about how to apply make-up for a variety of occasions including day, evening and special occasions. The choice and application of make-up products and techniques to be applied will suit the client's skin type, condition and age.

At the of this chapter is case study for **VRQ Unit Create an image based on a theme within the hair and beauty sector** including a practical assignment for you to complete.

There are **two** learning outcomes for this unit which you must achieve:

1 Be able to prepare for make-up

2 Be able to apply make-up

From the range statement, you must show you can:

- use **consultation techniques** to identify treatment **objectives**
- use **products, tools and equipment** as appropriate
- treat all **skin types and conditions**
- apply make up to meet the **objectives** for different occasions
- ensure the **environmental conditions** are suitable
- identify **contra-indications**
- **communication and behave** in an appropriate and professional manner
- follow all **health and safety working practices**
- apply **corrective methods**, taking into account age, facial shape, eye and lip shape and if the client wears glasses or contact lenses
- provide relevant **aftercare** and **contra-action advice**

(continued on the next page)

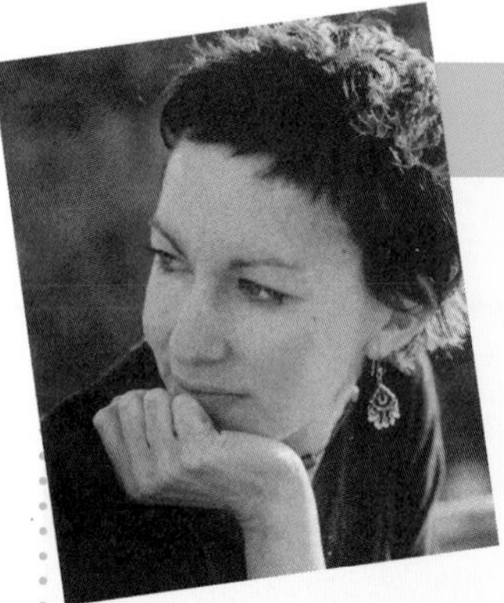

ROLE MODEL

Julia Francis

Make-up artist and body painter
www.juliafrancis.co.uk

"I have been a make-up artist for over ten years working with some of the industry's leading photographers, advertising agencies, directors, musicians and actors. For film and TV, my credits include *Star Wars*, *Hitchhiker's Guide to the Galaxy*, *Wimbledon* and *Eastenders*. My celebrity clients include Sir Tom Jones, Colin Firth and Jonathan Ross. Agencies and brands that I have worked with include Bacardi, Pantene, Olay, Gillette and Saatchi & Saatchi.

I am also an experienced teacher and make-up consultant and have been conducting workshops for many years. The monthly workshops offer students a unique opportunity to find out how to move forward in a career as a make-up artist.

Topics covered include:

- understanding the industry and the role of a freelance make-up artist
- areas of specialization – fashion, body painting, bridal, special effects, wigs, etc.
- advice on choosing make-up courses and qualifications required
- building up a make-up kit
- how to gain work experience, get work and make contacts
- how to create a portfolio, a show reel and a CV

To find out more about these workshops, please email me at workshops@juliafrancis.co.uk.

You must be able to show you have the necessary practical skills and underpinning knowledge to apply make-up.

This unit is linked to the Beauty Therapy NOS **Unit B8.**

Essential anatomy and physiology knowledge requirements for this chapter are identified on the checklist chart on page 27.

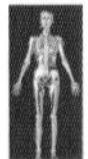

Make-up application

Make-up is used to enhance and accentuate the **facial features** to make us appear more attractive – which in turn makes us feel more confident. Make-up is used to create balance in the face, by skilful application of different cosmetic products to reduce or to emphasize facial features.

Each client is unique, so each requires an individual approach for their make-up. The overall effect should be attractive, complementing the client's personality, lifestyle and the context for which the make-up is to be worn.

Make-up products can also improve the appearance and condition of the skin. Products should be selected to suit the client's **skin type**, colouring condition and age.

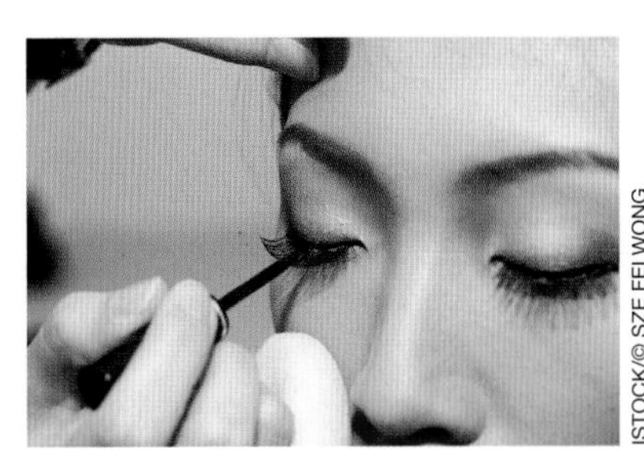

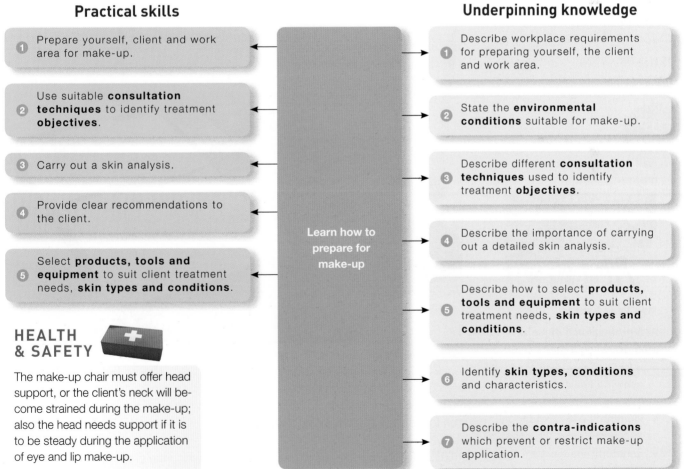

ISTOCK/© SZE FEI WONG

Outcome 1: Be able to prepare for make-up

Learn how to prepare for make-up

Practical skills

1. Prepare yourself, client and work area for make-up.
2. Use suitable **consultation techniques** to identify treatment **objectives**.
3. Carry out a skin analysis.
4. Provide clear recommendations to the client.
5. Select **products, tools and equipment** to suit client treatment needs, **skin types and conditions**.

Underpinning knowledge

1. Describe workplace requirements for preparing yourself, the client and work area.
2. State the **environmental conditions** suitable for make-up.
3. Describe different **consultation techniques** used to identify treatment **objectives**.
4. Describe the importance of carrying out a detailed skin analysis.
5. Describe how to select **products, tools and equipment** to suit client treatment needs, **skin types and conditions**.
6. Identify **skin types, conditions** and characteristics.
7. Describe the **contra-indications** which prevent or restrict make-up application.

HEALTH & SAFETY

The make-up chair must offer head support, or the client's neck will become strained during the make-up; also the head needs support if it is to be steady during the application of eye and lip make-up.

The height should be correct for you to avoid stretching and straining to avoid repetitive strain injury

Know your brands

You will always be asked advice on the best products for people. Although you can't know everything that is available, it is essential that you have a good knowledge of products and have enough variation of different brands to hand. Always check in advance if an actor/model is allergic to anything.

Julia Francis

Pack your kit well

The make-up artist's role is not only to apply make-up to actors, models, presenters, performers, etc. but also to look after people and have available anything from plasters to safety pins if you are asked for it. Your kit is very heavy and a suitable case on wheels is a good idea, especially if you don't drive to work.

Julia Francis

Preparing the work area

The make-up work area should be decorated in light, neutral colours to avoid creating unnecessary shadows. The area where the make-up is to be applied should be well lit, ideally with the same kind of light as that in which the make-up will be seen.

If provided, background music should be at a sound level that allows effective communication with your client.

Place all the products, tools and **equipment** required on the trolley or work surface, in front of a make-up mirror. If you are displaying the make-up on a trolley, place the cosmetic products on a lower shelf until required, when they can be moved to the top shelf. This avoids cluttering the working area.

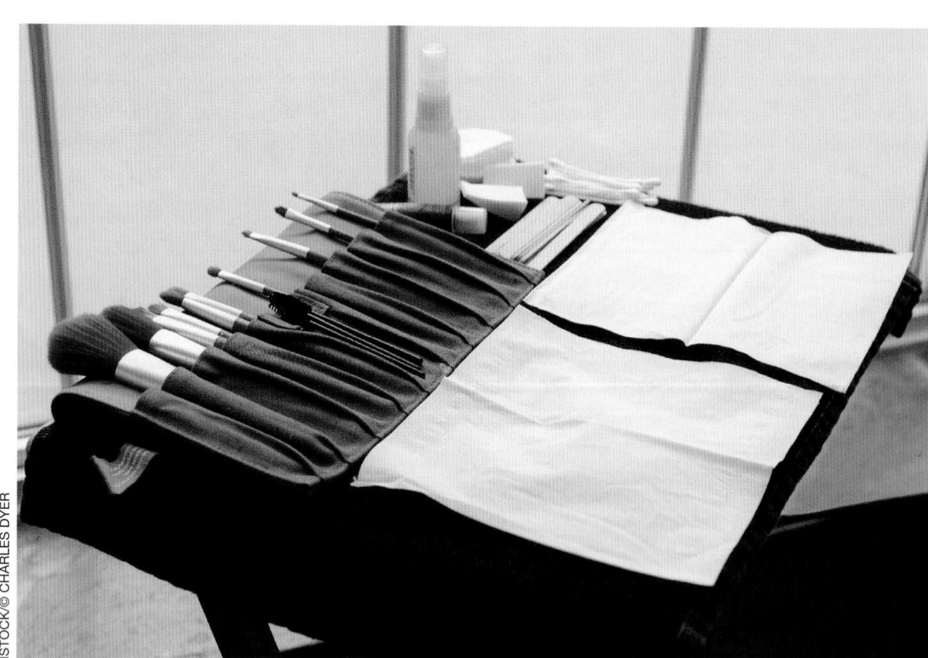

ISTOCK/© CHARLES DYER

Make-up work station

Keeping the work area tidy promotes an organized and professional image, and prevents time being wasted as you try to find resources. The work area should always be in a condition to provide further make-up treatments.

Lighting You need to know the *type* of light in which the proposed make-up will be seen: this is important when deciding upon the correct choice of make-up colours, because the appearance of colours may change according to the type of light. Is the make-up to be seen in daylight, in a fluorescent-lit office or a softly lit restaurant?

TOP TIP

A professional make-up station

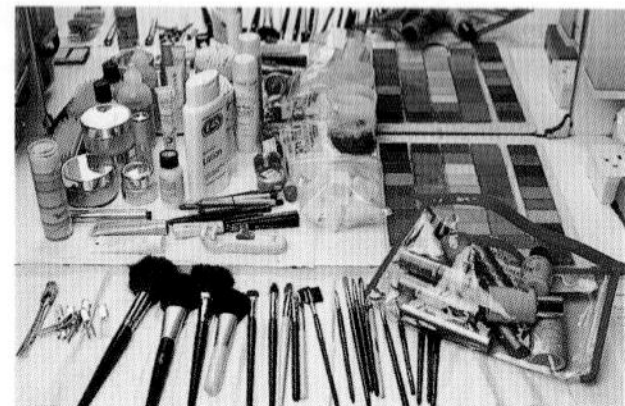

Make-up work station

At a professional make-up station:

- **a large mirror is provided, allowing full view of the head and shoulders**
- **illumination is provided by specialist make-up bulbs**
- **unnatural shadows are avoided by ensuring that light is reflected by the work shelf and overhead shelf**

White light (natural daylight) contains all the colours of the rainbow. When white light falls on an object, it absorbs some colours and *reflects* others: it is the reflected colour that we see. Thus, an object that we see as red is an object that absorbs the colours in white light except red. A *white* object reflects most of the light that falls on it; a *black* object absorbs most of the light that falls on it.

If the make-up is to be worn in natural light, choose subtle make-up products in neutral colours as daylight intensifies colours.

If the make-up is to be worn in the office, it will probably be seen under **fluorescent light**. This contains an excess of blue and green, which have a 'cool' effect on the make-up: the red in the face does not show up and the face can look drained of colour. Reds and yellows should be avoided, as these will not show up; blue-toned colours will. This light also sharpens colours. Don't apply dark colours, as fluorescent light intensifies these. Choose lighter textured products in natural and neutral colours.

Evening make-up is usually seen in **incandescent light** – light produced by a filament lamp. This produces an excess of red and yellow light, which creates a warm, flattering effect. Almost all colours can be used in this light, except that browns and purples will appear darker. Choose a lighter foundation than normal to reflect the light, and use frosted highlighting products where possible for the same reason.

Because it is necessary to choose brighter colours and to emphasize facial features using contouring cosmetics, evening make-up will appear very obvious and dramatic in daylight. Explain to the client the reasons for the effect created, so that when she leaves the salon in daylight she won't feel that the make-up is inappropriate.

Before beginning the make-up application, check that you have the necessary products, tools and equipment to hand and that they meet the legal hygiene and industry requirements for make-up application.

HEALTH & SAFETY

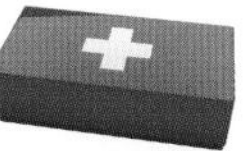

Ventilation
Good ventilation is important so that the client's skin does not become too warm. It is easier to apply make-up effectively to cool skin, and the make-up will be more durable.

Be calm under pressure

Always remain calm and professional even in situations where you are running out of time or are compromised in some way. There is often a tight schedule that you have to fit in to and you don't want the whole production to be waiting for you. An employable make-up artist is always a calm make-up artist.

Julia Francis

Understand the brief

It is essential that a make-up artist is able to create a look based on the context required and that the choice of products meets the client's requirements. For instance, it needs to be appropriate for the director's vision. You will need to know how long certain looks will take and what you need to have available in order to make them happen.

Julia Francis

PRODUCTS, TOOLS AND EQUIPMENT

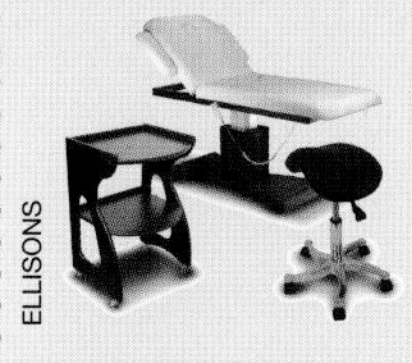
ELLISONS

Couch or make-up chair
With sit-up and lie-down positions and an easy-to-clean surface

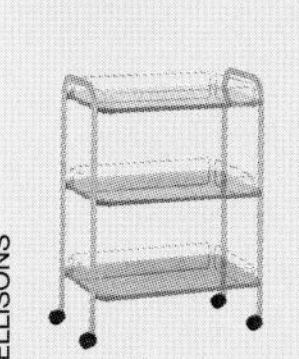
ELLISONS

Trolley
Or other surface on which to place everything

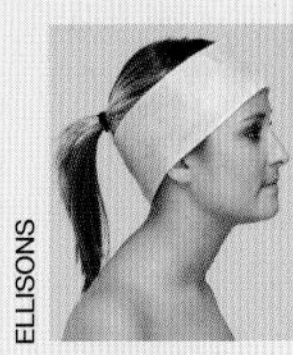
ELLISONS

Headband (clean) or hair clips
To protect the client's hair while cleansing the skin. Alternatively if the hair has been styled it will be necessary to secure the hair away from the face with hair clips

COURTESY OF DERMALOGICA

Cleansing lotion
To clean and prepare the skin for make-up application

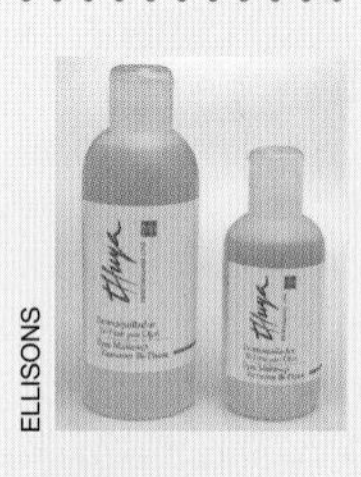
ELLISONS

Eye make-up remover
To remove eye make-up and prepare the skin for make-up application

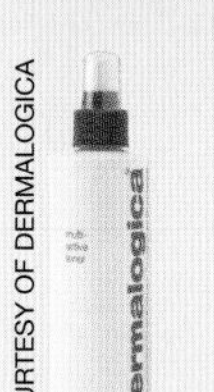
COURTESY OF DERMALOGICA

Toning lotion
To remove excess cleanser and restore the skin's pH balance

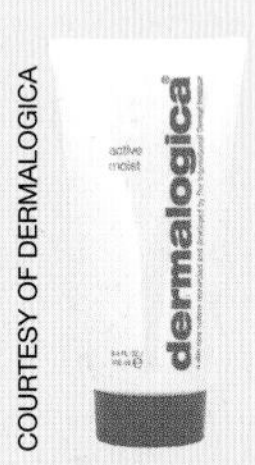
COURTESY OF DERMALOGICA

Lightweight moisturiser or primer
To facilitate make-up application and create a barrier between the skin and make-up

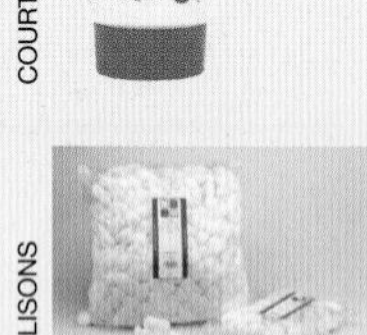
ELLISONS

Dry cotton wool
Stored in a covered jar, to apply loose face powder

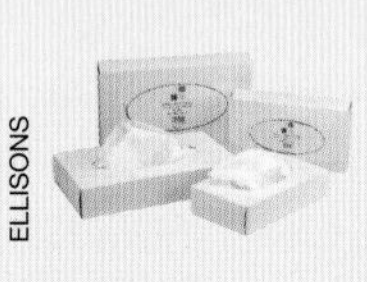
ELLISONS

Large white facial tissues
To blot the skin after facial toning, and to protect the skin during make-up application

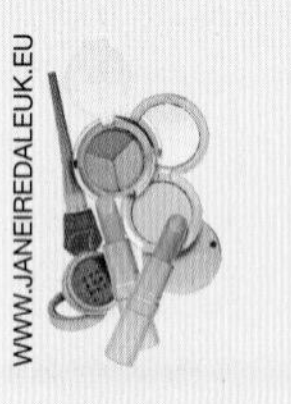
WWW.JANEIREDALEUK.EU

Make-up (a range)
To suit different skin types, tones and age groups

Bright lighting and magnifying lamp
To inspect the skin after cleansing and check for areas requiring special attention, e.g. broken capillaries that require concealer

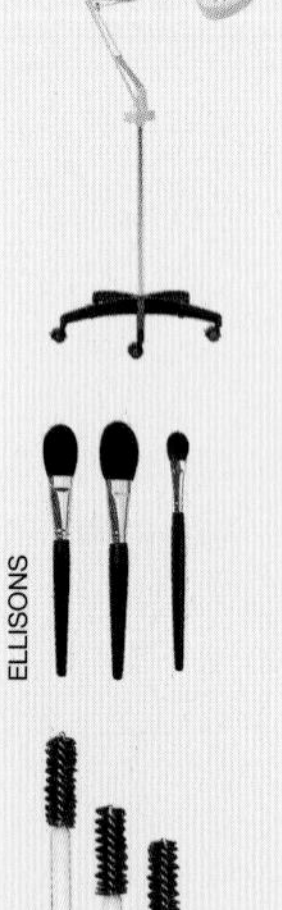
ELLISONS

Make-up brushes (assorted – at least three sets)
To allow for disinfection after use

ELLISONS

Applicators and brushes
Where possible use disposable, for example for mascara and the application of eye shadow and lipstick

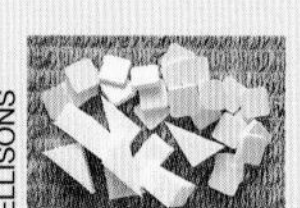
ELLISONS

Non-latex cosmetic sponges
For applying foundation and other facial cosmetic preparations

ELLISONS

Make-up palette
For preparing and dispensing cosmetic products prior to application

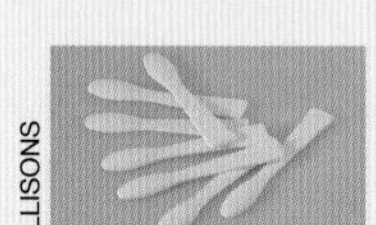
ELLISONS

Pencil sharpener
For cosmetic pencils

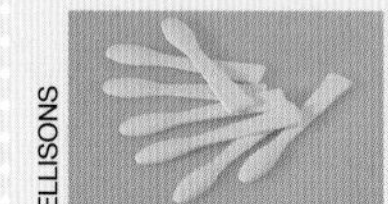
ELLISONS

Artificial eyelashes
To enhance the eyes as required

ELLISONS

Small spatulas (Several)
For removing make-up products from their containers

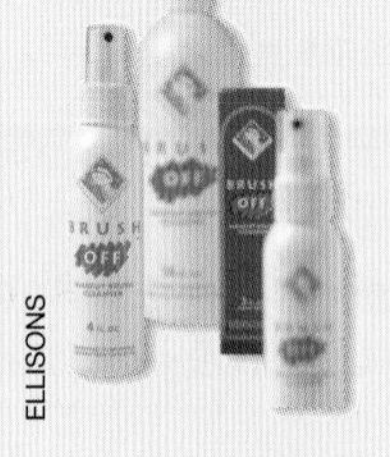
ELLISONS

Brush cleanser
A proprietary brand cleaner to care for and maintain brushes hygienically

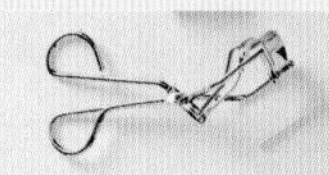

Eyelash curlers
Tool used to temporarily curl the eyelashes

YOU WILL ALSO NEED:

Disposable tissue (such as bedroll) To cover the work surface and the couch or beauty chair

Towels (2) Freshly laundered for each client – one to be placed over the head of the couch or chair, the other over the client's chest and shoulders to protect their clothing

Damp cotton wool Prepared for each client and used during skin cleansing

Bowls To hold the prepared cotton wool

Bowls and lined metal pedal bin For waste materials

Hand mirror (clean) To show client the make-up during and after application to ensure satisfaction

Client record card To record confidential details of each client registered at the salon, including the client's personal details, products used and details of the treatment.

You will need to have to hand a good range of make-up, suitable for clients with known skin allergies to cosmetics, for contact-lens wearers, for different skin types, conditions, ages and skin colours including:

- concealing and contouring cosmetics (shaders, highlighters and blushers)
- foundations
- translucent powders
- eye shadows
- eyeliners
- brow liners
- mascara
- lipsticks
- lip glosses
- lip liners

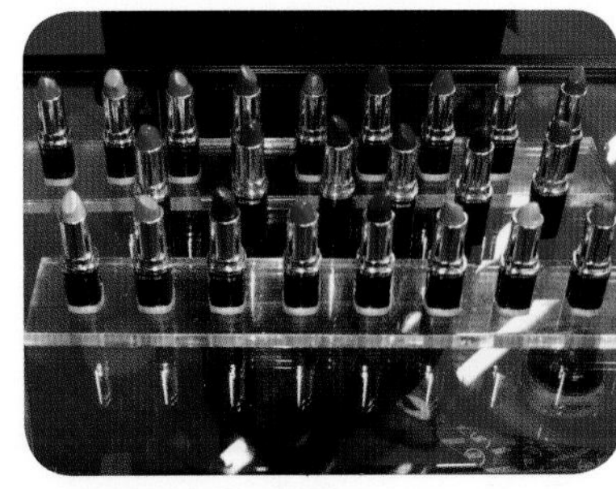

Lipstick retail products

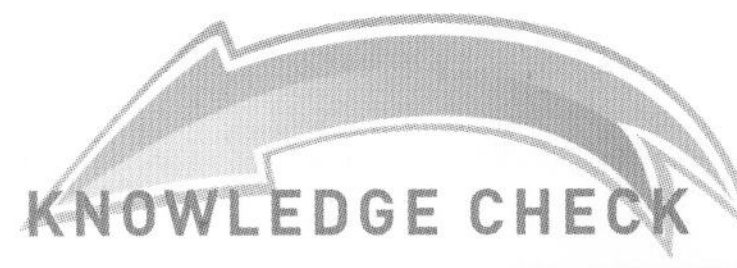

Why is it important to match lighting with the occasion for which the make-up is to be worn?

Need more time... refer to page 298 to help you.

BEST PRACTICE

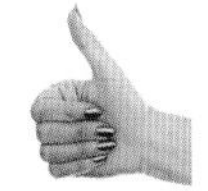

Positive promotion

Where possible, use make-up that you also sell in the salon, so that the client can buy the products for home use if they wish. Use attractive visual aids such as posters and displays to raise awareness and interest in the products.

Make-up brushes

Make-up brushes are made from different fibres, which may be synthetic or animal including camel, sable, squirrel, pony and goat. Synthetic brushes are better for the application of cream or gel textured products as they control the application of the product more. Powder and blusher brushes are usually made from soft animal hair but for the purposes of contouring and blending you will need firmer brushes.

When buying make-up brushes make sure the fibres are securely attached to the handle. Test the comfort of the fibres on the skin by stroking the brush on the back of your hand.

You will need to have more than one set of brushes so one set can be used whilst the other is being disinfected. To avoid cross-contamination all brushes must be cleaned after each use.

> **Clean your brushes**
>
> Always turn up to a job with clean brushes and a clean kit. Never use the same brushes on more than one person and always maintain high levels of health and hygiene standards.
>
> **Julia Francis**

Range of make-up brushes

Name	Description
Large face powder dusting brush	To remove excess face powder or to apply specialized powders such as bronzing and shimmer powders.
Foundation brush	To apply foundation to specific areas.

Range of make-up brushes (continued)

Name	Description
Contouring blush brush	To apply facial contouring products to highlight and shade areas of the face.
Blusher brush (large to medium)	To apply powder colour to the face and for blending.
Small flat angle-edged eye shadow brush	To apply and blend powder eye make-up products in the socket area of the eye.
Small rounded-edged eye shadow brush	To apply eye shadow, blend and shade.
Medium firm eye shadow blending brush	To blend powder eye colours and soften harsh lines and colour.
Small concealer brush	For exact placement of concealing product in areas such as around the nose and mouth.
Eyebrow brush	To remove excess make-up from the brow hair and to add colour, blend eyebrow pencil and groom the brow hair into shape.
Eyeliner brush	A fine brush used to apply make-up eye liner colour to contour the eyes, creating a precise line. A line and define brush is shown.
Mascara wand/comb	To apply mascara and remove excess mascara to separate the lashes.
Lip brush	To apply lip products and ensure a definite, balanced outline to the lips.

BEAUTY EXPRESS LTD

Sterilization and disinfection

Hygiene must be maintained in a number of ways:

- ensure that tools and equipment are sterile before use
- disinfect work surfaces after every client
- always follow hygienic work practices
- maintain a high standard of personal hygiene

TOP TIP

Make-up case

If you intend to apply make-up at different locations, buy a large make-up case so that you can transport the make-up easily and hygienically.

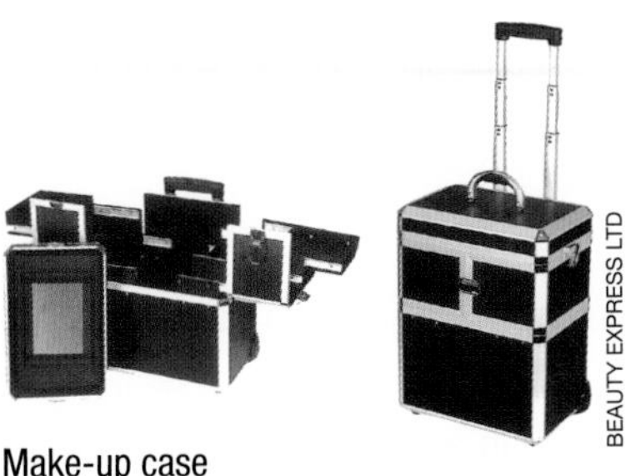

BEAUTY EXPRESS LTD

Make-up case

TOP TIP

Make-up instruction

If you provide make-up instruction to a client, do so in front of a large mirror so that the client can watch the various stages of make-up application.

Record the make-up used and the advice given on a separate record, for the client to take away with them.

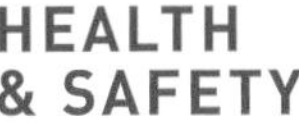

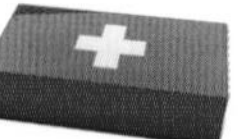

HEALTH & SAFETY

Maintaining hygiene

If you drop a make-up tool on the floor, discard it – don't use it again until it has been disinfected and sterilized.

Where possible, use disposable applicators during make-up application, costing these into the treatment price. Disinfect make-up brushes after each use: wash them in warm water and detergent, rinse them thoroughly in a disinfecting solution and then rinse in clean water, and allow them to dry naturally. Once dry, place the brushes in an ultra-violet light cabinet ready for use. An alcohol-based brush cleaner is recommended to clean and care for your brushes.

All cosmetic products should be removed from their containers using a clean spatula and placed on the clean plastic make-up palette before application. (This avoids contamination of the make-up with bacteria from unclean make-up applicators.)

The make-up palette should be cleaned with warm water and detergent, then wiped with a disinfectant solution applied using clean cotton wool. It should be stored in the ultra-violet cabinet.

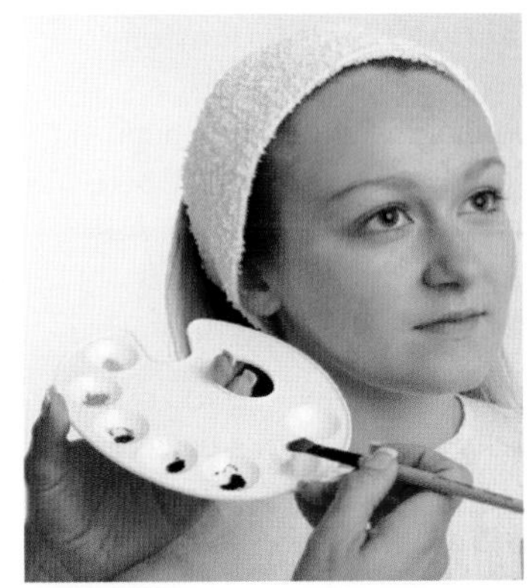

Make-up pallete and client prepared for make-up

Mascara should be applied using a disposable brush applicator, fresh for each client. Sharpen cosmetic pencils with a pencil sharpener before each use.

Make-up sponges should be disposed of after use, or washed in warm water and detergent, then placed in a disinfectant solution and rinsed. Allow them to dry, then place them in the ultra-violet cabinet, with each side being exposed for at least 20 minutes.

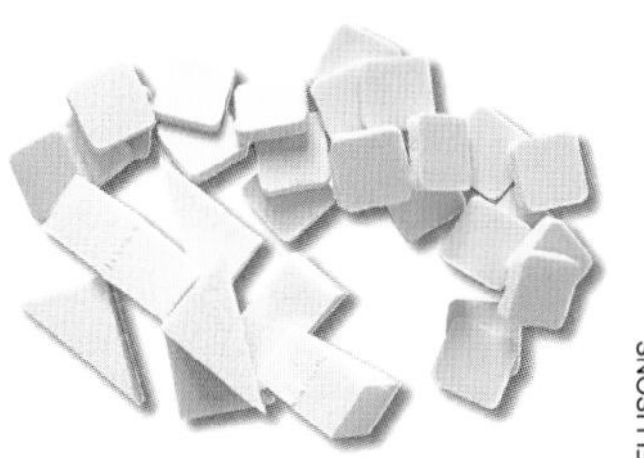

ELLISONS

Make-up sponges

Reception

When a client makes an appointment for make-up, the receptionist will need to check the purpose of the make-up application.

TOP TIP

Lighting

If working under artificial light, use warm white fluorescent light for day make-up, as this closely resembles natural light.

A diffuser may be used to cover the fluorescent tube. This softens the cool effect on the make-up and reduces the effects of shadows.

KNOWLEDGE CHECK

Give five examples of how the work area should be prepared for the next client following make-up application.

Need more time... refer to pages 298–303 to help you.

BEST PRACTICE

Effective communication
When applying make-up it is important that you fully understand the effect to be achieved. Good communication is essential. Ask the client what the final result should look like.

It is also important that you check that the client does not have allergies to any products to avoid a possible contra-action.

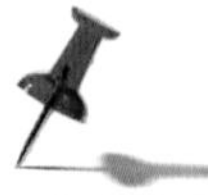

ALWAYS REMEMBER

Treatment timings

Make-up lesson: allow 1 hour.

Special occasion or evening make-up: allow 45 minutes to hour.

Day make-up: allow 45 minutes.

Make-up application is offered for different purposes, called make-up objectives.

- ***A make-up lesson*** A chance for the client to learn from a professional how to apply make-up that suits them.
- ***Special occasion make-up*** Applied to suit the occasion for which it is to be worn, such as a wedding. If the make-up is for a bride, advise the client to visit the salon for a consultation and a practice session so that you can decide together on appropriate make-up. Ask the client if possible to bring a swatch of the dress material with her, so that you can select colours to complement this and to co-ordinate with the accessories.
- ***Evening make-up*** Generally will be seen under artificial lighting. The effect this has on the appearance of the make-up will depend upon the light source, which must be considered when applying evening make-up. Generally evening make-up is heavier in application and stronger colours may be applied. Products to emphasize and highlight, such as frosted eye shadows and **lip glosses**, may be introduced.
- ***Remedial make-up*** May be applied for remedial purposes, to cover facial disfigurements or birthmarks, and the client can be taught how to do this themselves.
- ***Photographic make-up*** Applied for many reasons including magazine shoots, portrait work and fashion shows. Make-up application must be skilful to achieve the right end-result as the location may be a photographic studio or outdoors on location.
- ***A professional look*** Some clients simply wish to have their make-up professionally applied.

All staff, especially the staff communicating with clients at reception, should be familiar with the different pricing structures for the range of make-up treatments and products available for retail.

In the salon, advise the client that if they intend to have their hair washed and styled, this should be done before they have the make-up applied.

If a client requests a deep cleansing facial followed by make-up application, suggest that they have the facial at least five days prior to the make-up. The facial will stimulate the skin, increasing its normal physiological functioning. This will affect how long the make-up lasts; it may even cause the colour of the foundation to change.

Do not reshape the eyebrows at the same treatment as make-up application – secondary infection could occur; also the skin in the area will be come very red or darker, depending upon skin colour,, altering the colour and thus the effect of eye shadow. This is because of an increase in blood circulation in the local area.

The consultation Complete a record card noting the client's personal details. This will be used to record details of the make-up applied. A sample record card for make-up is found on pages 306–307.

If the client is a **minor** under the age of 16, it is necessary to obtain parent/guardian permission for the make-up treatment. The parent/guardian will also have to be present when the treatment is received.

Discuss your make-up plan with the client to ensure that the make-up will meet their requirements or treatment objectives. You may need to ask questions such as those that follow, but of course the questions depend on the purpose of the make-up application.

- 'Do you normally wear make-up?'
- 'For what occasion is the make-up to be worn?'
- 'What colour are the clothing and accessories to be worn on this occasion?'
- 'Are there any colours that you particularly like or dislike?'
- 'What effect would you like the make-up to create?' (This question may be asked in many contexts – the client may wish to achieve a natural or a glamorous effect, or to emphasize or diminish certain facial features.)
- Are there any products that you are allergic to?
- Do you wear contact lenses?

If the client wears glasses, check the function of the lens, as this can alter the effect of the make-up.

Provide the opportunity for your client to ask any questions relating to the make-up treatment.

The record card should be signed and dated following the **consultation** to confirm the suitability and consent with the agreed make-up treatment.

It is important that accurate records are kept and stored in compliance with the Data Protection Act for future reference.

Contra-indications

Certain **contra-indications** prevent make-up application. These include bacterial, fungal, parasitic and viral infections, which are described in more detail in Chapter 2, where contra-indications are illustrated and discussed. Check for these at the consultation, and if any of the following are present on inspection of the skin, do not proceed with make-up application.

Remember that not all contra-indications are visible – a current bone fracture, for example would not be. The following disorders may contra-indicate or restrict make-up applications. If you suspect the client has any disorder from the list below, do not attempt a diagnosis but refer the client tactfully to their GP without causing concern.

- ***pediculosis capitis (head lice)***
- ***pediculosis corporis (body lice)***
- ***acne vulgaris (active)***
- ***herpes simplex (cold sore)***
- ***impetigo***
- ***styes or hordeola***
- ***conjuncitivitis (pink eye)***
- ***watery eye or epiphora***
- ***blepharitis***

ALWAYS REMEMBER

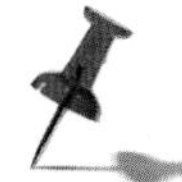

Accurately record your client's answers to necessary questions to be asked at consultation on the **record card**.

KNOWLEDGE CHECK

In order to select the correct skin care and make-up products to suit the clients skin, it is necessary to correctly identify the skin type. What are the facial skin characteristics conditions of the following skin types that you learnt about in Chapter 7 Facial Skincare:

- oily skin
- dry skin
- combination skin

Need more time... refer to pages 176–178 help you.

ACTIVITY

Recognizing contra-indications
What skin disorders can you think of that would contra-indicate make-up application?

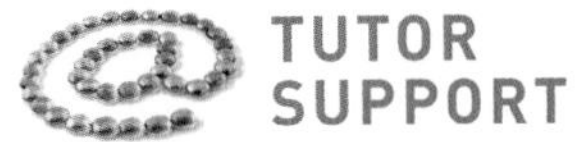

TUTOR SUPPORT

Activity 6: Client record card task

A sample client record card

Date | Beauty therapist name

Client name | Date of birth (identifying client age group)

Home address | Postcode

Email address | Landline phone number | Mobile phone number

Name of doctor | Doctor's address and phone number

Related medical history (conditions that may restrict or prohibit treatment application)

Are you taking any medication? (this may affect skin sensitivity)

CONTRA-INDICATIONS REQUIRING MEDICAL REFERRAL
(Preventing the application of make-up.)
- ☐ bacterial infections (e.g. impetigo, conjunctivitis)
- ☐ viral infections (e.g. herpes simplex)
- ☐ fungal infections (e.g. tinea corporis)
- ☐ parasitic infestations (e.g. pediculosis and scabies)
- ☐ severe skin conditions e.g. eczema and psoriasis

CONTRA-INDICATIONS WHICH RESTRICT TREATMENT
(treatment may require adaptation)
- ☐ cuts and abrasions ☐ bruising and swelling
- ☐ recent scar tissue ☐ eczema
- ☐ skin allergies ☐ vitiligo
- ☐ styes ☐ hyper keratosis
- ☐ watery eyes ☐ epilepsy

MAKE-UP CONTEXT
☐ day ☐ evening ☐ special occasion

SKIN TYPE
- ☐ normal ☐ dry
- ☐ oily ☐ combination

SKIN CONDITION
☐ sensitive ☐ mature ☐ dehydrated

CONCEALER
☐ cream ☐ stick ☐ liquid

FOUNDATION
- ☐ liquid ☐ compact
- ☐ stick ☐ cream
- ☐ mineral ☐ tinted moisturiser

POWDER
☐ loose ☐ compact ☐ mineral

BRONZING PRODUCTS
☐ powder ☐ gel ☐ liquid

EYE PRODUCTS FOR EYE AREA
- ☐ cream eye shadow ☐ powder eye shadow
- ☐ pencil eyeliner ☐ mineral and pigment eye shadows
- ☐ kohl eyeliner
- ☐ liquid eyeliner ☐ gel eye shadow
- ☐ cake eyeliner

EYE PRODUCTS FOR BROW AREA
- ☐ pencil ☐ liquid
- ☐ shadow ☐ eyebrow mascara

EYE PRODUCTS FOR EYELASHES
- ☐ waterproof mascara ☐ non-waterproof mascara
- ☐ false lashes ☐ lash curling

CHEEK PRODUCTS
☐ highlighter ☐ shader ☐ blusher

LIP PRODUCTS
- ☐ pencil lip liner ☐ lip gloss
- ☐ lipstick ☐ lip balm

Record of make-up products applied

Beauty therapist signature (for reference)

Client signature (confirmation of details)

A sample client record card (continued)

TREATMENT ADVICE
Make-up application – allow 45 minutes

TREATMENT PLAN
Record relevant details of your treatment and advice provided for future reference.
Ensure the client's records are up to date, accurate and fully completed following treatment. Non-compliance may invalidate insurance.

DURING
Find out:
- what products the client is currently using to cleanse and care for the skin of the face and neck

Discuss:
- the importance of a good skincare routine in relation to make-up application
- current satisfaction with the client's make-up technique
- tips and explain each stage of the make-up application to enhance the client's understanding

Note:
- any adverse reaction, if any occur

AFTER
Record:
- any modification to make-up application that has occurred
- what products have been used in the make-up application
- the effectiveness of the make-up result
- any samples provided (review their success at the next appointment)

Advise on:
- how to reapply products to achieve/maintain the result
- correct make-up removal technique

RETAIL OPPORTUNITIES
Advise on:
- products that would be suitable for the client to use at home to care for their skin
- the benefits of each make-up product clearly and logically during application
- recommendations for further make-up treatments
- further products or treatments that the client may or may not have received before

Note:
- any purchase made by the client

EVALUATION
Record:
- comments on the client's satisfaction with the treatment
- if poor results are achieved, the reasons why

HEALTH AND SAFETY
Advise on:
- avoidance of activities or product application that may cause a contra-action
- appropriate necessary action to be taken in the event of an unwanted skin reaction

ALWAYS REMEMBER 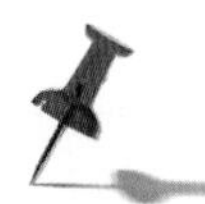

Examples of make-up application modification include:

- choice of make-up products and application techniques for corrective work
- choice of make-up to suit the client's skin type and condition
- disguising minor skin imperfections
- using hypo-allergenic products for a client with cosmetic sensitivity
- age of client, using light-reflecting make-up products for a mature skin or one showing signs of premature aging

HEALTH & SAFETY 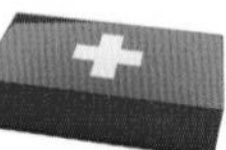

Hygiene at home

Advise clients to keep their own make-up clean. Dirty brushes spoil effective make-up application, and offer breeding grounds for bacteria.

Make-up generally has a shelf life of two years and is then past its best and becomes unhygienic. It is recommended that mascara be replaced every six months.

The following conditions also contra-indicate make-up application:

- ***skin disorders*** including those not listed in the above list, such as bacterial infections (e.g. boils), viral infections (herpes zoster), and fungal infections (e.g. tinea corporis)
- ***active psoriasis*** and ***eczema***
- ***bruising*** in the area
- ***recent haemorrhage***
- ***swelling and inflammation*** in the area
- ***recent scar tissue***
- ***sensory nerve disorders***
- ***cuts or abrasions*** in the area
- ***a recent operation*** in the area
- ***eye disorders*** including those not listed in the chart
- ***parasitic infestation*** such as pediculosis capitis and corporis and scabies

Ask the client whether they have any known allergies to cosmetic preparations. Note the answer on the record card. Care must be taken to avoid contact with an allergen.

Remember—never name a contra-indication, you may be wrong. Refer the client to their GP whose role it is to identify and advise.

In the case of the skin disorder herpes simplex, the make-up treatment may be received when the skin is healed and clear.

Contra-actions

Certain cosmetic ingredients are known to cause allergic reactions in some people. These ingredients are known as allergens. Allergens may cause irritation, severe erythema, inflammation and swelling, known as a **contra-action**. This may occur during or following treatment.

Known cosmetic allergens include the following:

- ***Lanolin*** This is similar to sebum, and is obtained from sheep's wool. It is added to many cosmetics as an emollient.
- ***Mineral oils*** Examples are oleic acid and butyl stearate.
- ***Eosin (bromo-acid dye)*** A staining **pigment**, used in some lip cosmetics and perfumes.
- ***Paraben*** An antiseptic ingredient, used as a preservative in facial cosmetics.
- ***Certain colourants*** One example is carmine.
- ***Perfume*** This is added to most cosmetics, and is a common sensitizer.

Products should be selected without the allergen where identified.

Other contra-actions include:

- ***Watery eyes*** The client's eyes water excessively. If the client has watery eyes a tissue may be placed at the corners until the irritation has ceased. If the client's eyes continue to water, remove eye make-up and discontinue treatment.
- ***Excessive perspiration*** Some clients may perspire, which will affect adherence of the make-up and its finished result. Blot the skin with soft facial tissue and apply more loose face powder to absorb perspiration. If the client continues to perspire, discontinue treatment.

External contact with an allergen may cause urticaria, also know as hives and eczema or dermatitis. If an allergy occurs, the product should be removed from the skin and a soothing substance applied. The client should be advised not to use the product again. Always record any allergies on the client's record card so that the offending product may be avoided in the future.

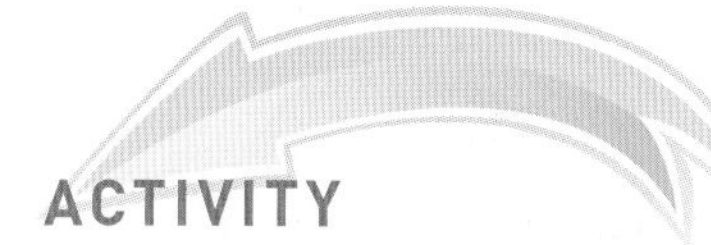

ACTIVITY

The record card
Why is it important to complete a record card? What information should be recorded on it?

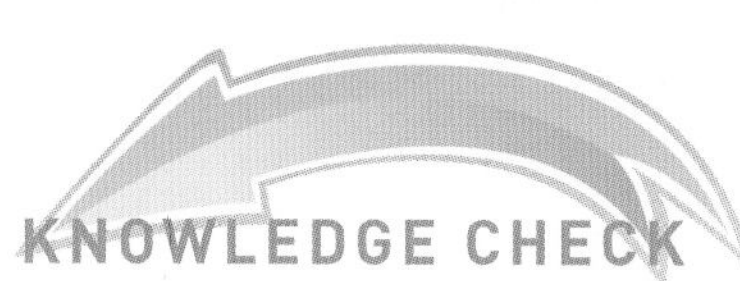

KNOWLEDGE CHECK

Name three skin disorders and three eye disorders that would contra-indicate make-up application.

Need more time... refer to page 308 to help you.

HEALTH & SAFETY

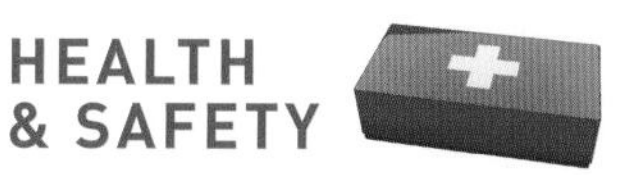

Allergies
Where possible, before using a new cosmetic, a client with known allergies should first receive a skin sensitivity test, or be given a small sample of a product to try on a less sensitive area of the skin, to assess the skin's tolerance. If an allergic reaction occurs, medical attention must be sought immediately.

It is possible that clients may grow out of an allergy to a given product. It is also possible, however, suddenly to become allergic to a product that has not given problems before.

Preparing the client

Take the client through to the make-up work area. Make-up application may take place either at the make-up chair, in front of a mirror, or at the treatment couch. Before you start the make-up, discuss and plan the make-up with the client, recording significant details on their record card.

Before preparing the client for the treatment, clean your hands using an approved hand cleansing technique in front of your client who will observe hygienic procedures being carried out. The client need remove only their upper outer clothing, to their underwear. Offer the client a gown, or drape a clean towel or make-up cape across their chest and shoulders. Place a headband or hairclips around the hairline, to protect the hair and keep it away from the face. Any jewellery in the treatment area should be removed. Refer to the record card to check for any known allergies to cosmetic products.

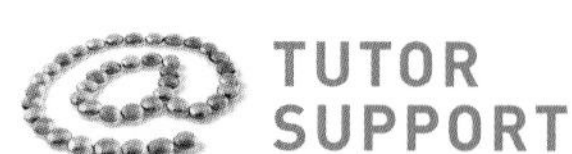

TUTOR SUPPORT

Activity 1: Skin tones task

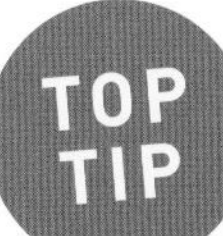

TOP TIP

Hair clips
If the client has had their hair styled it may be better to clip the hair out of the way rather than using a headband.

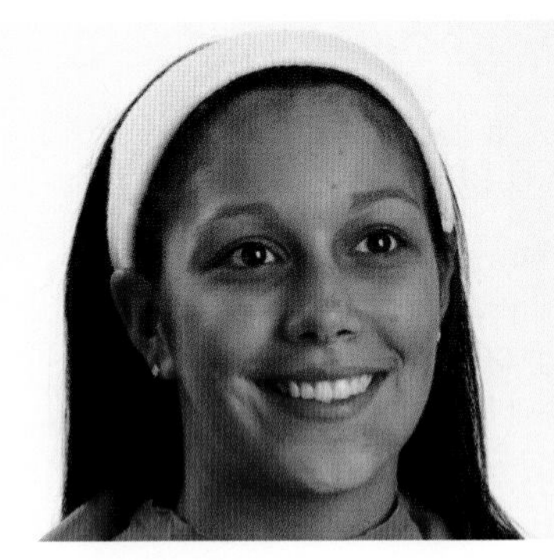

Client preparation

Ensure that the client is comfortable.

After preparing the client, and before touching the skin, clean your hands again. Now cleanse and tone the skin, using products appropriate to their skin type. Just as skincare products vary in their formulation to suit the various skin types, so make-up products are designed for different skins. Record all relevant details on the record card.

Perform a skin analysis by inspecting the skin using a magnifying lamp. Identify any areas that require specific attention, i.e. broken capillaries, pustules, papules, dark circles, hyper-pigmentation, hypo-pigmentation and scarring.

Apply a light-textured **moisturiser** before make-up application. This has the following benefits:

- it prevents the natural secretions of the skin changing the colour of the foundation
- it seals the surface of the skin, and prevents absorption of the foundation into the skin
- it facilitates make-up application by providing a smooth base

Remove excess moisturiser by blotting the skin with a facial tissue.

Special lotions may be applied to improve the skin texture and increase make-up durability. These include skin **primers** and oil control lotions.

Skin primers are silicone-based, creating a film on the skin's surface. They refine the skin's appearance, minimizing open pores and the appearance of fine lines. The formulations can vary to suit the client's skin type and may contain pigments to correct **skin tone**. The primer provides a base and acts as a barrier, preventing absorption of the make-up products into the skin. Primers are applied the same way as moisturiser, but less is required.

Oil control lotions contain powder ingredients which absorb the skin's natural oil, reducing shine and producing a matt finish. They are ideal to prepare an oily or combination skin before make-up application.

HEALTH & SAFETY

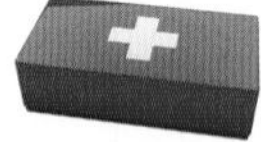

Contact lenses

If the client wears contact lenses, ask them whether they wish to remove them before the skin is cleansed. (The need for this will depend on the sensitivity of the eyes.)

TOP TIP

Removing eyeliner

Existing cosmetic eyeliner is sometimes difficult to remove. Use a cotton bud soaked in eye make-up remover: gently stroke this along the base of the lower eyelashes, in towards the nose.

TOP TIP

Headbands

If a headband is used, it is a good idea to remove it directly after the facial cleanse so that it doesn't flatten and spoil the hair.

ALWAYS REMEMBER

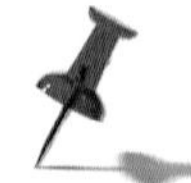

Erythema

Avoid excessive pressure and stimulation of the skin while cleansing and preparing the skin for make-up application.

The skin will become too warm, affecting durability and erythema of the skin will occur – skin reddening requires correction.

Outcome 2: Be able to apply make-up

Learn how to apply make-up

Practical skills

1. **Communicate and behave** in a professional manner.
2. Follow **health and safety working practices.**
3. Position yourself and client correctly throughout the treatment.
4. Use **products, tools, equipment** and techniques to suit clients treatment needs, **skin types and conditions.**
5. Complete the treatment to the satisfaction of the client to suit a range of occasions.
6. Record the results of the treatment.
7. Provide suitable **aftercare advice.**

Underpinning knowledge

1. State how to **communicate and behave** in a professional manner.
2. Describe **health and safety working practices.**
3. State the importance of positioning yourself and the client correctly throughout the treatment.
4. State the importance of using **products, tools, equipment** and techniques to suit clients treatment needs, **skin type and conditions.**
5. Describe how to use **corrective methods** to suit client treatment needs, **skin types and conditions.**
6. State the **contra-actions** that may occur during and following treatments and how to respond.
7. State the importance of completing the treatment to the satisfaction of the client.
8. State the importance of completing treatment records.
9. State the **aftercare advice** that should be provided.
10. Describe the structure and functions of the skin.
11. Describe diseases and disorders of the skin.
12. Explain how natural ageing, lifestyle and environmental factors affect the condition of the skin and muscle tone.
13. State the position and action of the muscles of the head, neck and shoulders.
14. State the names and position of the bones of the head, neck and shoulders.
15. Describe the structure and function of the blood and lymphatic system for the head, neck and shoulders.

ALWAYS REMEMBER

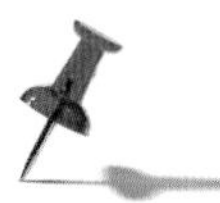

Order of application
Make-up is applied in a specific sequence to ensure:

- a balanced look is achieved
- products are applied effectively, i.e. cream on cream, powder on powder, which allows products to be blended and set appropriately
- the client's understanding, e.g. when carrying out a make-up lesson or demonstrating how to achieve a certain look
- durability and the optimum look of the make-up is maintained

Applying make-up products

The make-up sequence

The correct sequence for applying make-up is as follows.

1. Conceal any blemishes.
2. Apply foundation.
3. Contour the face (with cream liquid products).
4. Apply powder.
5. Contour the face (with powder products).
6. Apply blusher.
7. Apply eye shadow.
8. Make up the eyebrows.
9. Apply mascara.
10. Make up the lips.
11. Contour products, used to shade and highlight the face and features, can be applied in powder or cream formulation. Application sequence for contouring will depend upon product formulation chosen.

Age of the client

When applying make-up, consider how skin changes with age. This will influence the imperfections and skin conditions that may be present and require correction.

Appearance and age table

Age	Appearance
<15	Nearly perfect skin. Smooth texture, pores small.
15–24	Acne key factor in surface texture. Fine lines start to appear, pore size increasing.
25–45	More fine lines and appearance of first wrinkles (photodamage). Early signs of sagging near the eye. Some loss of elasticity. Adult acne.
46–55	More wrinkles, rough texture. Sallow yellow colour begins to appear. Pores and age spots enlarge and define. Sagging near eye and cheek.
56+	Wrinkles and fine lines in abundance. Uneven colour, pigmentation. Sagging worsens. Dark circles under eye.

DR. JOHN GRAY, THE WORLD OF SKIN CARE

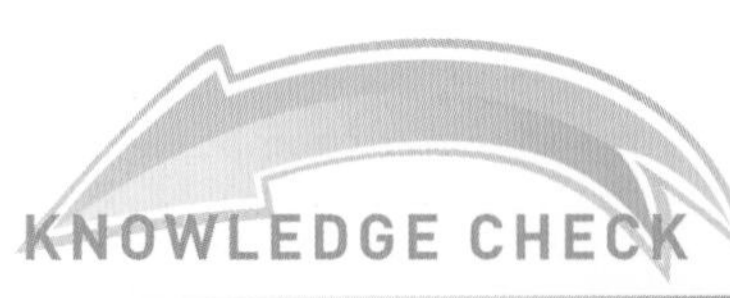

How should the skin be prepared before the make-up application?

Need more time... refer to page 310 help you.

ALWAYS REMEMBER

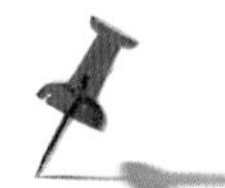

Manufacturers' instructions
Use all products following manufacturers' instructions to ensure the optimum make-up is achieved.

Concealer

Before you begin to apply make-up to the face, inspect the skin and identify any areas that require concealing, such as blemishes, uneven skin colour, dark circles under the eyes or shadows.

Foundation may be used to disguise minor skin imperfections, but where extra coverage is required it is necessary to apply a special concealer, a cosmetic designed to provide maximum skin coverage. The concealer may be applied directly to the skin after skin moisturising, or following application of the foundation.

Choose a concealer that is one to two shades lighter than the client's skin tone.

Concealers designed for use around the eye area are light in texture, lighter in colour than the foundation with a yellow tone to minimize the appearance of dark circles. Concealers designed for covering blemishes are unsuitable for application around the eyes.

Concealer can contain pigment to help correct skin tone.

- ***Green*** helps to counteract high colouring, and to conceal dilated capillaries.
- ***Lilac or pink*** counteract a sallow skin colour.
- ***Peach and pink*** counteract dark circles around the eyes and are suitable for darker skin tones.
- ***White or cream*** help to correct unevenness in the skin pigmentation.
- ***Yellow*** helps to counteract the appearance of dark circles around the eyes.

Concealers come in a range of colours and consistencies, to suit all skins and differences in skin texture. Mix different colours together to obtain the required colour.

Colour correctors target problem areas and contain pigments which balance skin tone. Select lighter shades, e.g. light pink for lighter skins, if the skin is darker select shades of peach. Peach is particularly effective to counteract bluish under-eye shadows. Green correctors counteract areas of redness. Yellow counteracts pink tones.

Correctors are applied like concealer and may be followed with concealer or foundation.

Applying concealer Remove a small quantity of the concealer from its container, using a clean disposable spatula. If it has a brush applicator attached to the product, for reasons of hygiene this cannot be used.

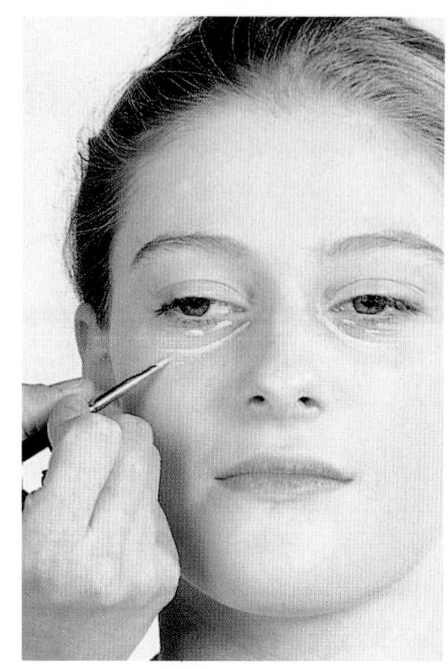

Applying concealer

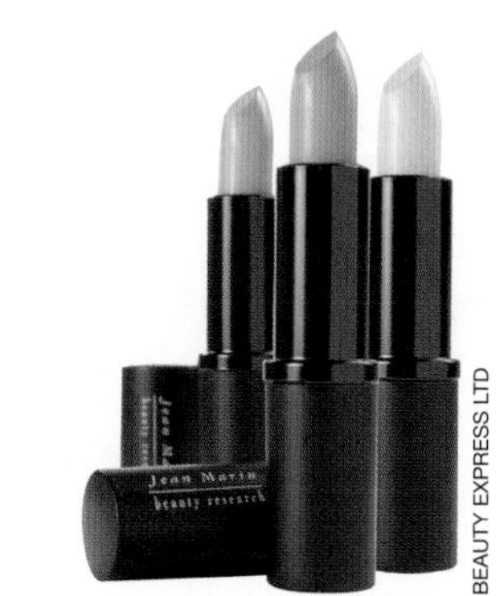

Concealing products

TOP TIP

Blending

Avoid rubbing the product while blending it, or it will wipe off.

ALWAYS REMEMBER

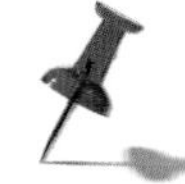

Common racial skin problems

- Caucasian – easily damaged by exposure to high temperatures and ultra-violet light, leading to broken veins and pigmentation disorders.
- Oriental – prone to uneven pigmentation on ultra-violet light exposure.
- Asian – often has uneven pigmentation skin tones; darker skin is often found around the eyes.
- African – melanin is present in all layers of the epidermis; this can cause scarring following skin damage, possibly leading to uneven pigmentation, vitiligo and keloids.

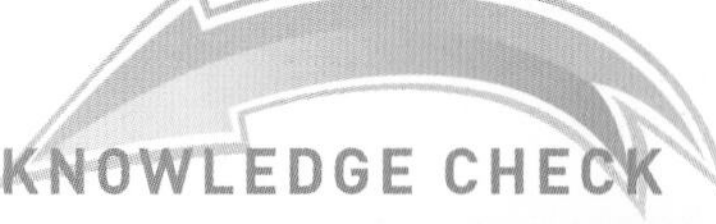

KNOWLEDGE CHECK

Why is it important that make-up is applied in a suitable sequence?

Need more time... refer to page 312 to help you.

Apply the concealer to the area to be disguised, using either a clean make-up sponge or a soft make-up brush. Blend the concealer to achieve a realistic effect. Reapply concealer as necessary until correction is achieved.

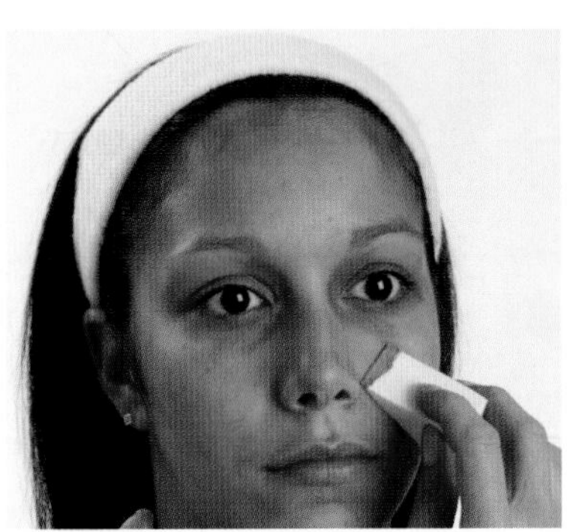

Foundation application

Foundation

Foundation is applied to produce an even skin tone, to disguise minor skin blemishes, and as a contour cosmetic. Black skin in particular often has an uneven skin tone, requiring certain parts of the face to be lightened and others darkened to produce an even skin tone.

Foundation is available as cream, liquid, compact stick, gel, cake, mousse, mineral-based and tinted moisturiser.

Foundations can contain **'anti-ageing' ingredients** such as vitamins A, C and E. These are to neutralize **free radicals**, natural chemicals thought to be responsible for damaging the skin and producing the signs of ageing – the lines and wrinkles! Sunscreens and moisturisers are commonly included in foundations to protect the skin from the environment.

Silica beads can be included in the formulations, especially for combination/oily skin, to absorb the skin's natural sweat and oil.

KNOWLEDGE CHECK

For what purpose would you apply a concealer?

Need more time... refer to page 313 to help you.

ACTIVITY

Comparing foundations

Compare the proportions of ingredients contained in foundations for each skin type. How, and why, are they different?

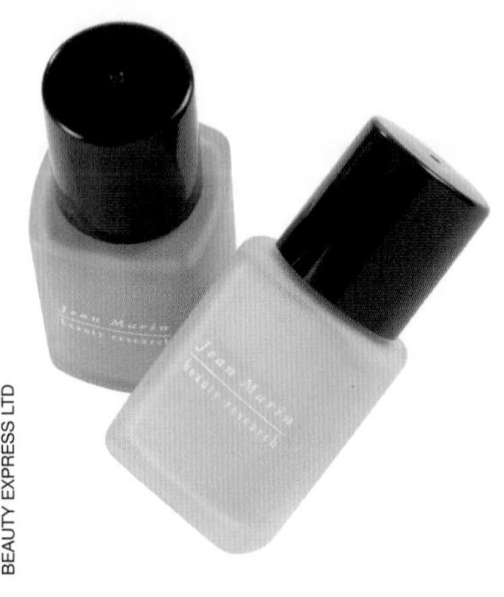

Foundation products

Kinds of foundations

Each foundation differs in its formulation to suit a particular skin type. The correct choice will guarantee that the foundation lasts throughout the day.

Cream foundation **Cream foundations** are oil-based and blend easily on application. They provide a heavy coverage, and have these specific treatment uses:

- dry skin
- normal skin
- mature skin

TOP TIP

Tinted moisturiser

To achieve a light, healthy, natural appearance, the client may apply a tinted moisturiser.

Liquid foundation **Liquid foundations** are oil- or water-based, providing light to medium coverage. Oil-based liquid foundations have these specific uses:

- dry skin
- normal skin
- mature skin
- combination skin (apply the foundation to the *dry* areas)

Water-based liquid foundations have the following uses:

- normal skin
- oily skin
- combination skin (apply the foundation to the *oily* areas)

Liquid foundations are composed of water, powder, oil, humectant (such as glycerol), pigments and additives.

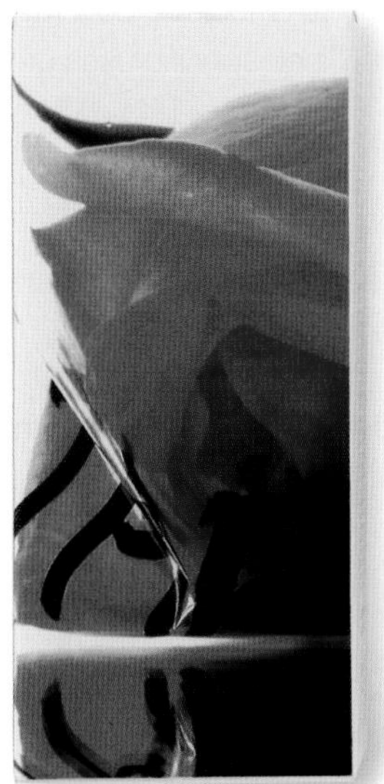

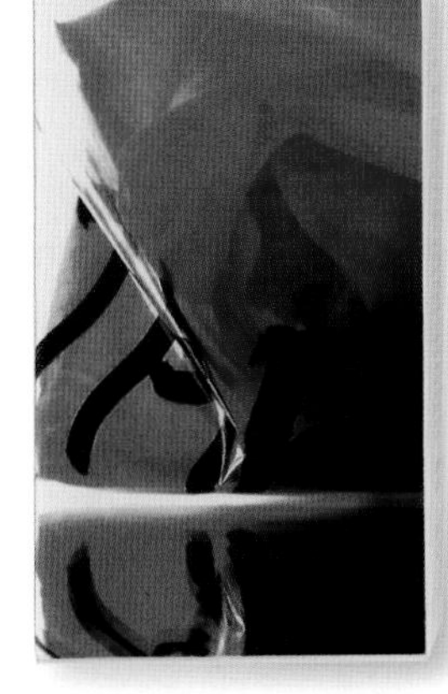

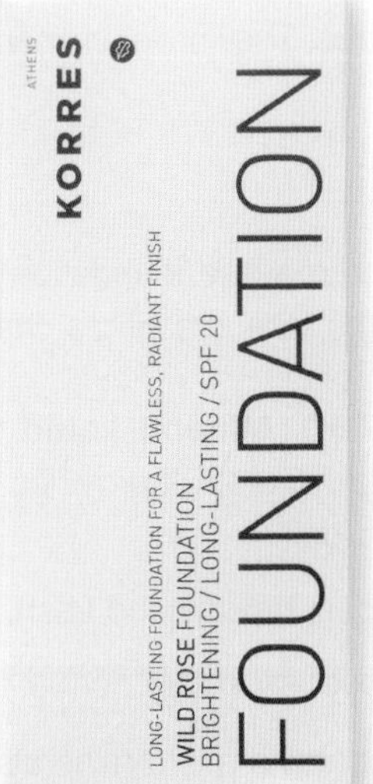

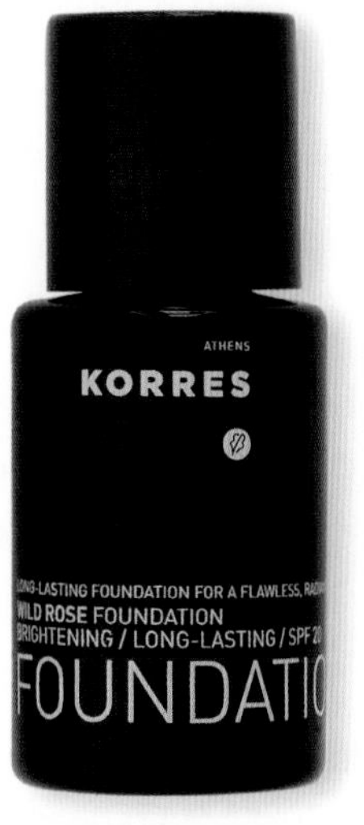

KORRES NATURAL PRODUCTS, WWW.KORRES.COM

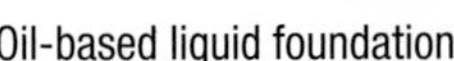

Oil-based liquid foundation

Water-based foundations do not spread very easily because the water content rapidly evaporates, so these foundations must be applied quickly.

Gel foundation **Gel foundations** provide sheer, oil-free non-greasy coverage and a matte finish. Light reflective properties are achieved through the addition of pigments. They have these specific uses:

- black, unblemished skin
- tanned skin
- skin on which a natural effect is required

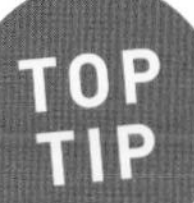

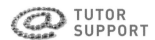

TUTOR SUPPORT

Activity 3: Foundation and concealer handout

TOP TIP

Dealing with wrinkles

Cream and cake foundation can settle in creases and accentuate wrinkles. Apply only a very fine film of such foundations over these areas.

TOP TIP

Specialist foundations

Special ingredients may be included in a foundation for oily skin, selected to avoid clogging the pores and thereby causing congestion.

On an ebony black skin, avoid powder-based foundations as these will make the skin look grey and dull. Use a transparent gel foundation instead.

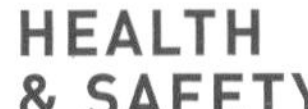

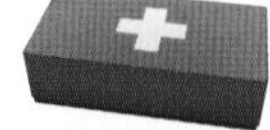

HEALTH & SAFETY

Choosing a foundation

- If the skin is oily and blemished, a *medicated* foundation may be used.
- If the client suffers from acne vulgaris, it is preferable not to apply foundation at all – bacterial infections might be aggravated.
- If the skin is sensitive, select a *hypoallergenic* foundation.

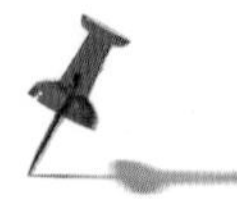

ALWAYS REMEMBER

Foundation colour

The skin's natural oils can change the colour of the foundation, making it appear darker.

A tester, if available, should be provided to ensure the correct colour is chosen.

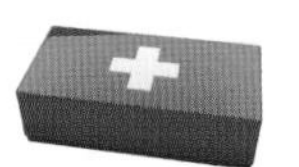

HEALTH & SAFETY

Product formulation MSDS sheets

Legally the manufacturer must produce a list of ingredients used in their product.

Request a Material Safety Data Sheet to refer to and ensure safe product selection.

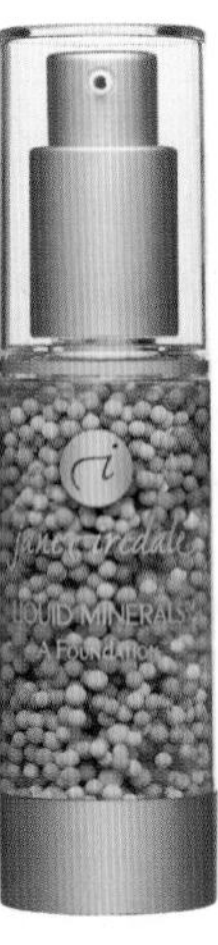

Liquid mineral

Compact skin or cake foundation

Compact skin or cake foundations may have an oil, wax or powder base. They give a heavy coverage, and have these specific uses:

- dry skin
- normal skin
- badly blemished or scarred skin

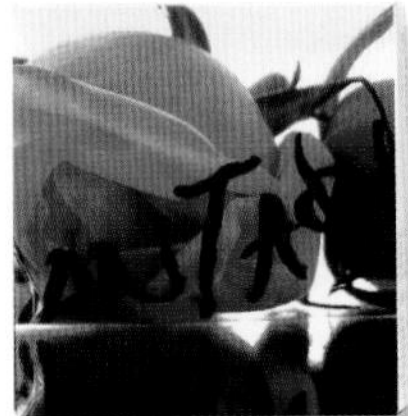

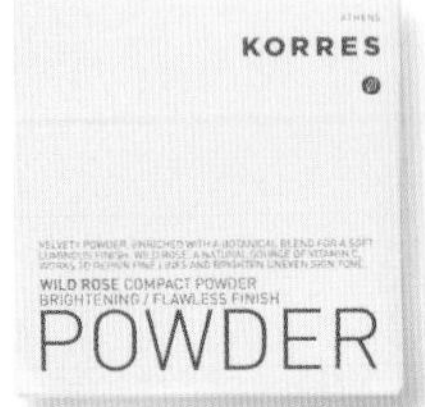

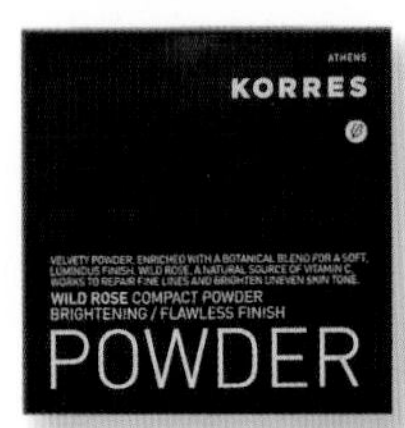

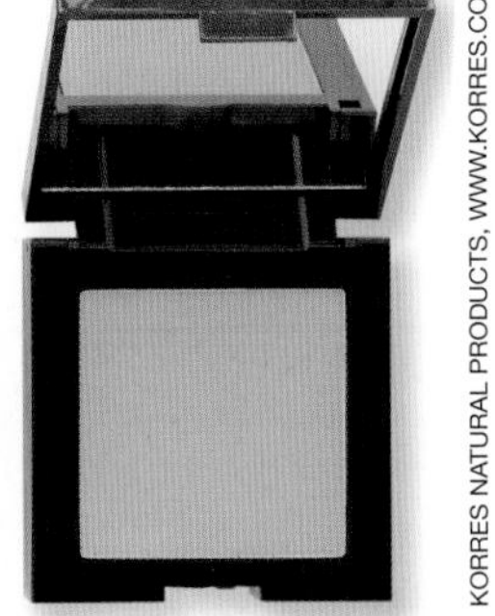

Compact foundation

KORRES NATURAL PRODUCTS, WWW.KORRES.COM

Mousse foundation

Mousse foundations provide light to medium coverage depending on application technique. They have a mineral oil base. Their specific uses are:

- normal skin
- combination skin

Care must be taken to apply the mousse foundation to an area of the skin and blend quickly or it may start to dry on the face, creating a chalky appearance.

Mineral-based foundation

Mineral liquid foundation contains the natural light-reflecting properties of micro-minerals. It provides a low to medium coverage, with a skin enhancing, slightly luminous look.

- It helps make the skin appear healthy and fresh.
- It is suitable for all skin types, especially normal to dry skin.

Mineral powder foundation contains micro-minerals in a solid powder with a binding ingredient such as algae. Again, suitable for all skin types providing a heavier coverage through layer application.

Mineral make-up is created from finely ground minerals, a process called micronization. Pure mineral make-up allows the skin to breathe as it does not contain synthetic powders and oils.

The make-up may contain a selection of the following minerals which all contribute an effect to the finished look of the make-up:

- Titanium oxide, a natural white mineral powder providing opacity – titanium is also an ingredient used in cosmetics for its sun protection factor (SPF) effect.
- Zinc oxide, a natural white mineral powder which enhances the appearance of the crystallized minerals; mica, a natural mineral which has light-reflecting properties showing a range of colours. (It also affects the finished formulation, providing slip to facilitate make-up application.)
- Bismuth oxychloride, a synthetic white mineral with a silvery metallic sheen providing coverage to the make-up; iron oxide, a synthetic mineral iron used to add colour.

Tinted foundation **Tinted foundation** provides a moist, light to medium coverage available in a range of shades. It offers protection from the environment with added sunscreen and skin moisturisers.

- It helps make the skin appear natural, healthy and fresh.
- It is suitable for all skin types in oil or oil free formulation.

ACTIVITY

Selecting a foundation

Name a suitable foundation for each of the following skin types:

- normal
- dry
- oily
- combination
- sensitive
- blemished

Foundation colour

The colour or shade of the foundation should match the client's natural skin colour. Test the foundation for compatibility on the client's jaw line or forehead. If an incorrect colour is selected, or if the foundation is insufficiently blended on application, there will be a noticeable **demarcation line**.

Skin tones may vary on the face with lighter and darker areas, especially on black skin. If the lighter tones are to be emphasized, a lighter coverage foundation product should be selected allowing the skin's natural tone to show. Multi-ethnic skin will require mixing products and shades to create a balanced look. Remember products can be layered to increase coverage.

Skin colour	Foundation colour
Fair	Ivory or light beige, with warm tones of pink or peach.
Olive	Dark beige or bronze.
Suntanned	Bronze.
Florid	Matt beige with a green tint.
Sallow	Beige with a pink tint.
Light brown	Light brown foundation with a warm tone.
Medium brown	Light brown with a yellow/orange tone.
Dark brown	Deep bronze foundation with a yellow/orange tone.
Black	Dark golden bronze (usually a gel).

TOP TIP

Mineral make-up

Mineral make-up can be applied following a facial as the blend of minerals and pigments form microscopic flat crystals due to its formulation which allows the skin to breathe and function.

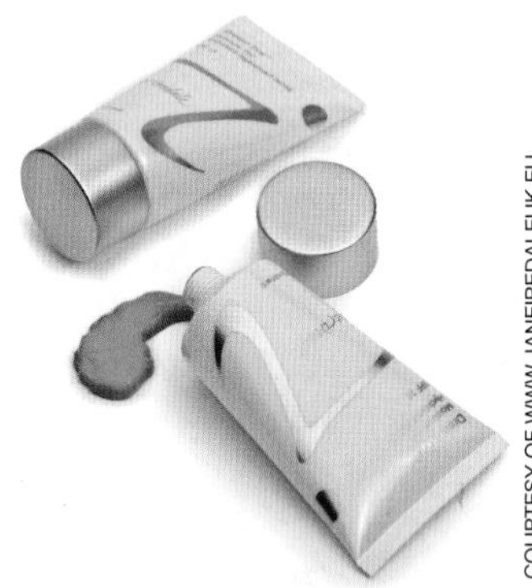

COURTESY OF WWW.JANEIREDALEUK.EU

Mineral make-up products

TOP TIP

Client application

A client may be advised to apply tinted foundation with the fingers which provides a sheer coverage. Instruct the client they must wash their hands before application.

TOP TIP

Using a palette

The make-up palette is useful when mixing foundations to match the colour of your client's skin.

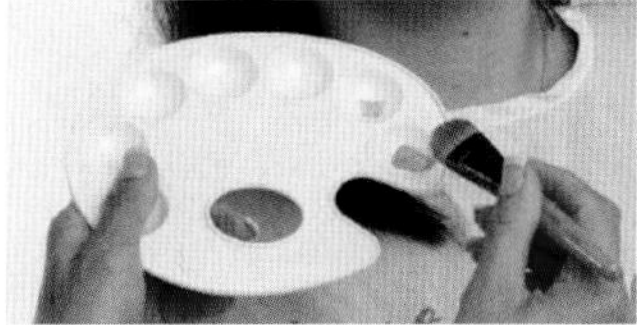

TOP TIP

Selection of foundation colour

If the foundation is too light it will appear ashen.

TOP TIP

Professional application

Professionally, avoid applying foundation with the fingers. Apart from being less hygienic, with this method the warmth of your hands may cause streaking.

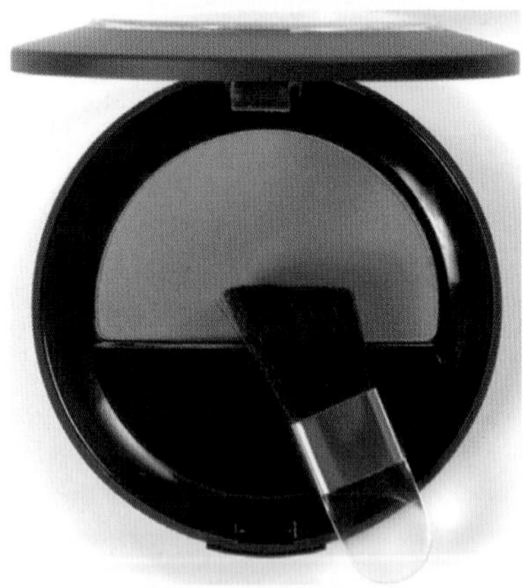

Blusher contour product

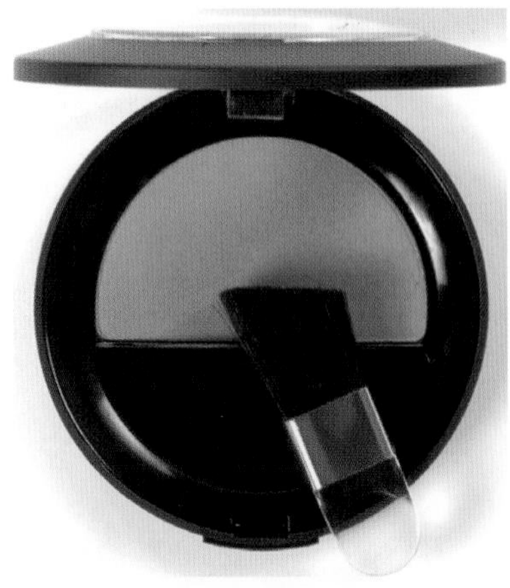

Shader/blusher contour product

Applying the foundation

If the foundation is in a jar, remove some from its container using a clean disposable spatula. Put it on a clean make-up palette.

Foundation may be applied using either a large soft foundation brush, which is stroked over the surface of the skin, or a cosmetic sponge. It should be applied to one area of the face at a time, with an outward stroking movement.

Also use a cosmetic sponge to blend the foundation. Take care that you blend it at the hairline and at the jaw line. Avoid clogging the eyebrows with foundation. The **cosmetic make-up wedge** is designed to apply varying amounts of pressure to the different areas of the face, and to ensure even coverage of the foundation.

When applying foundation around the eye area, use a small soft brush or the angular edge of a cosmetic sponge. This will help you achieve accuracy in application.

The extent of coverage can be controlled by the method of application. If the cosmetic sponge is damp, coverage is light and sheer. To achieve a heavier coverage, use a dry latex-free sponge.

Apply foundation to cover the entire face, including the lips and the eyelids. Do not extend the make-up past the jaw line unless the occasion requires this – for example, if a bride's dress exposes part of the upper chest – because the foundation will mark clothes at the neckline.

Trouble spots such as areas of pigmentation should be concealed with a concealing product.

Contouring

Contour cosmetics

Changing the shape of the face and the facial features can be achieved with the careful application of **contour cosmetics**. These products draw attention either towards or away from facial features, and can create the optical illusion of perfection.

Each face differs in shape and size, so each requires a different application technique.

Contour cosmetics include **highlighters**, **shaders** and **blushers**. They are available in powder, liquid and cream forms.

- ***Highlighters*** Draw attention towards – they emphasize.
- ***Shaders*** Draw attention away – they minimize.
- ***Blushers*** Add warmth to the face and emphasize the facial contours.

Some blushers appear very vibrant in the container, yet when they are applied to the skin they are subtle.

Before applying these products, decide on the effect you wish to achieve. Study the client's face from the front and side profiles, and determine what facial corrective work is necessary.

The colour should brighten the face. Hold different blusher shades next to the face to identify a suitable colour. Consider the age of the client: natural shades are preferable to bright fashion colours.

Blushers are available in powder, cream and liquid formulations.

Powder blushers Mineral powder blusher is formulated using pigments to add colour and warmth to the skin. Alternatively, synthetic or natural pigments are formulated with a face powder with a talc base to add bulk, and zinc stearate to bind the ingredients together with various skin conditioning agents. A softer look is achieved with powder blusher.

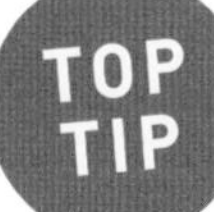

TOP TIP

Blusher

Blusher can be applied to the cheeks and temples to add warmth to the face.

Cream blushers A cream or wax base holds the pigment colour. Silicone is added to cream blushers to facilitate application.

Liquid blushers Pigment providing the tint shade is suspended in a liquid containing water, glycerine, silica and alcohol.

If liquid or cream cosmetics are used, these must be applied on top of a liquid or cream foundation before powder application. (If powder contour products are used, these should be applied after the application of the loose face powder. The rule of contour cosmetic application is: powder on powder; cream on cream.)

Mineral powder blushes Minerals are refined to a light-weight, sheer application where colour is achieved by layering. Ideal to use for a mature skin.

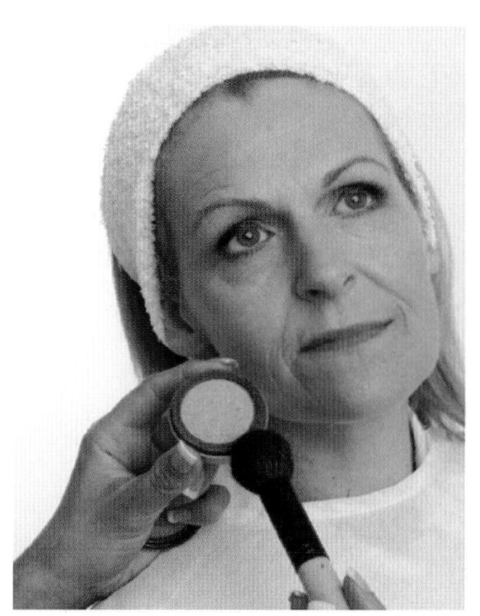

Applying mineral powder blush

How to apply powder blushers

Stroke the contour brush over the powder blusher. Tap the brush gently to dislodge excess blusher.

Apply the blusher to the cheek area, carefully placing the product according to the effect you wish to create. The direction of brush strokes should be upwards and outwards, towards the hairline. Keep the blusher away from the nose, and avoid applying blusher too near the outer eye. Ensure the edges of the blusher application are blended and softened.

Apply more blusher if necessary. The key to successful blusher application is to build up colour slowly until you have achieved the optimum effect.

If too much blusher is applied, tone down with the application of a loose face powder.

How to apply cream blushers

Remove the cream blusher hygienically from its container.

Apply the cream blusher after foundation application. Using the fingertips dot the cream blush colour sparingly onto the fullness of the cheek area and blend towards the hair line. Cream blusher is suited to all skin types except oily. Place a loose translucent powder over the cream blusher to set if required. Alternatively it can be left unpowdered for a 'dewy' effect.

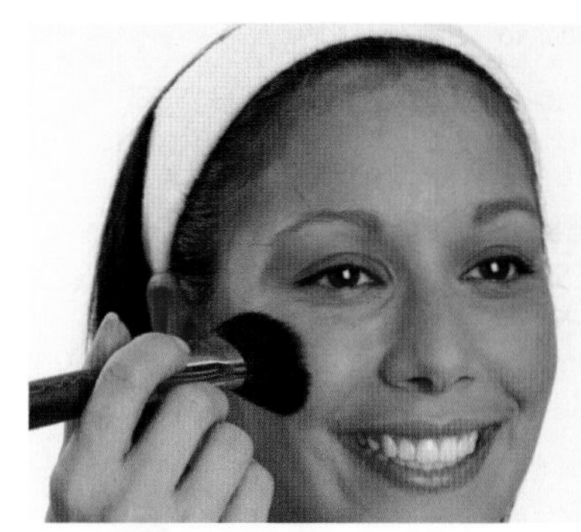

Applying blusher

How to apply liquid blushers

Liquid blusher provides a sheer to strong, stained look, dependent upon product usage. It is best to apply to a normal skin as it is difficult to blend and would be generally unsuitable on a dry skin type.

Dot the liquid blush on the cheek area and blend well. Remember it must be worked with quickly, if left in an area too long it will stain.

TOP TIP

Colour and balance
Check blusher result after each application. Look at the client from the front and from each side of the face to check depth of colour and balance in application.

ACTIVITY

Facial bone structure
Draw and label the main facial bones. It is the differing sizes and proportions of these bones that give us our individual features.

To discover the size of each facial feature, feel the bony prominences of your own face with your fingers.

ALWAYS REMEMBER

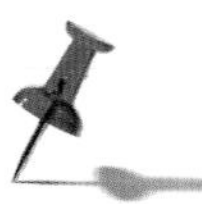

Less is more
Remember – it is easier to apply more blusher than to remove excess, which disturbs the foundation!

TOP TIP

Contouring with foundation
Foundation may be suitable as a contour cosmetic. Choose a foundation either two shades lighter (as a highlighter) or two shades darker (as a shader) than the base foundation.

Face shapes

To assess the client's **face shape**, take the hair away from the face – hairstyles often disguise the face shape. Study the size and shape of the facial bone structure. Consider the amount of excess fat and the muscle tone.

Oval ***Bone structure*** This is regarded as the perfect face shape.

Corrective make-up Corrective make-up application usually attempts to create the *appearance* of an oval face shape. Draw attention to the cheekbones by applying shader beneath the cheekbone, and highlighter above. Blusher should be drawn along the cheekbone and blended up towards the temples.

Round ***Bone structure*** Broad and short.

Corrective make-up Apply highlighter in a thin band down the central portion of the face to create the illusion of length. Shader may be applied over the angle of the jaw to the temples. Apply blusher in a triangular shape, with the base of the triangle running parallel to the ear.

Square ***Bone structure*** A broad forehead and a broad, angular jaw line.

Corrective make-up Shade the angles of the jawbone, up and towards the cheekbone. Apply blusher in a circular pattern on the cheekbones, taking it towards the temples.

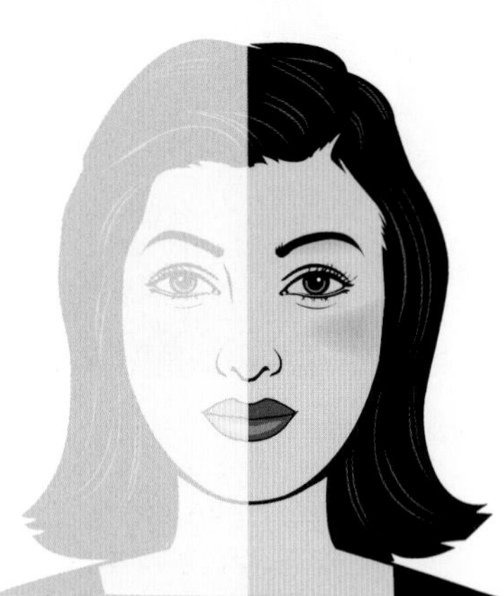

Oval face

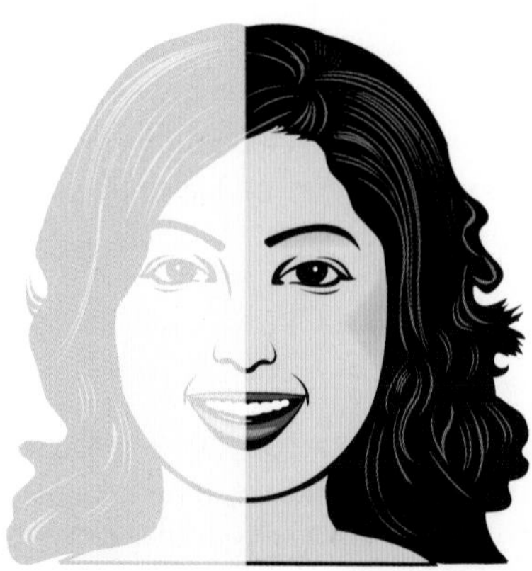

Round face

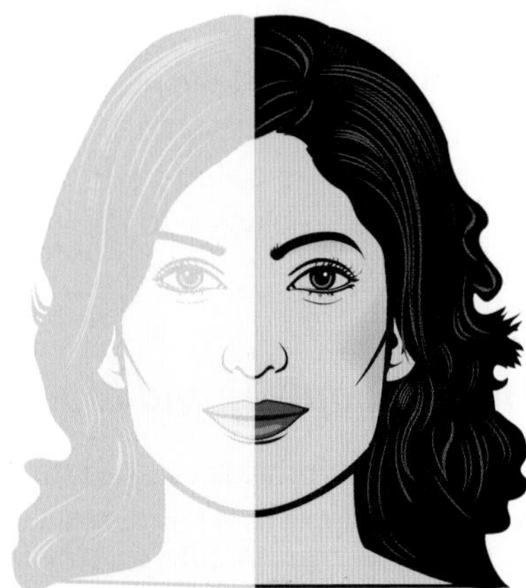

Square face

Heart ***Bone structure*** A wide forehead, with the face tapering to a narrow, pointed chin, like an inverted triangle (heart shape is also know as an inverted triangular – a triangle on its point).

Corrective make-up Highlight the angles of the jawbone and shade the point of the chin, the temples and the sides of the forehead. Apply blusher under the cheekbones, in an upward and outward direction towards the temples.

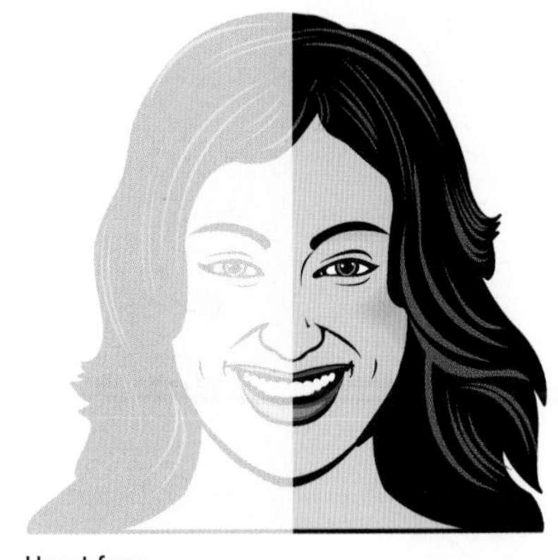

Heart face

Diamond ***Bone structure*** A narrow forehead, with wide cheekbones tapering to a narrow chin.

Corrective make-up Apply shader to the tip of the chin and the height of the forehead, to reduce length. Highlight the narrow sides of the temples and the lower jaw. Apply blusher to the fullness of the cheekbones to draw attention to the centre of the face.

Oblong ***Bone structure*** Long and narrow, tapering to a pointed chin.

Corrective make-up Apply shader to the hairline and the point of the chin to reduce the length of the face. Highlight the angle of the jawbone and the temples to create width. Blend blusher along the cheekbones, outwards towards the ears.

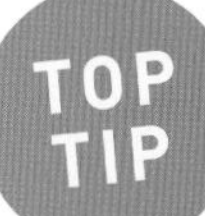

Blusher

Keep blusher away from the centre of the face to avoid accentuating the breadth of the face.

Pear ***Bone structure*** A wide jaw line, tapering to a narrow forehead. Also known as triangular face shape.

Corrective make-up Highlight the forehead and shade the sides of the chin and the angle of the jaw. Apply blusher to the fullness of the cheeks, or blend it along the cheek-bones, up towards the temples.

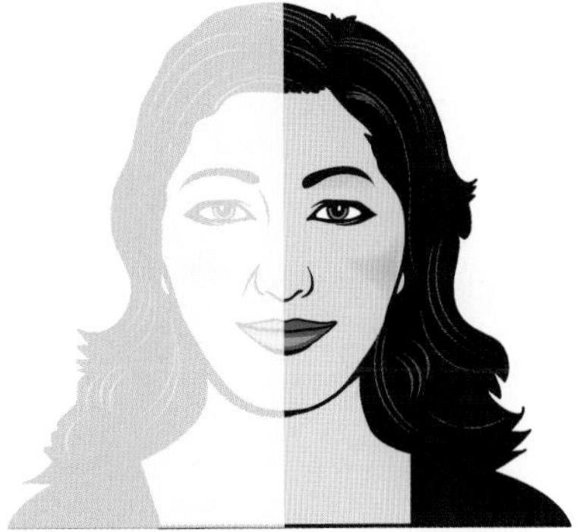

Diamond face

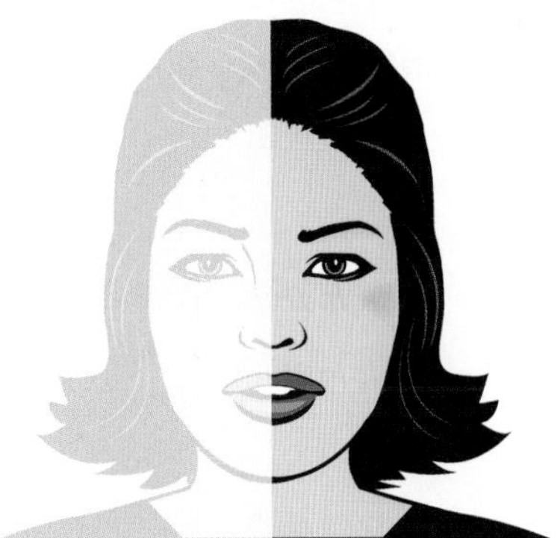

Oblong face

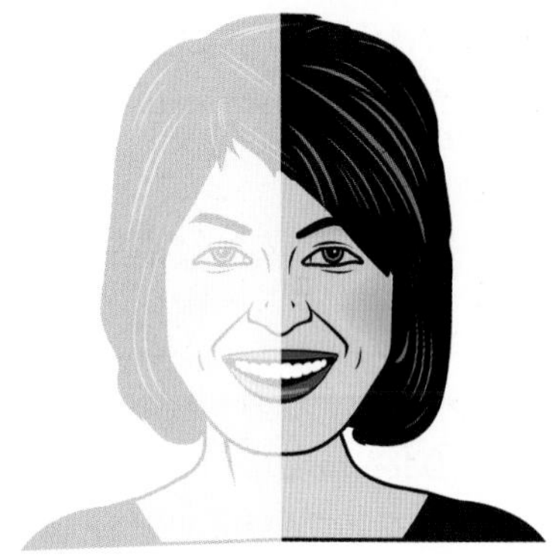

Pear face

Features

Noses

- **If the nose is too broad:** apply shader to the sides of the nose.
- **If the nose is too short:** apply highlighter down the length of the from the bridge to the tip.
- **If the nose is too long:** apply shader to the tip of the nose.
- **If there is a bump on the nose:** apply shader over the area.
- **If there is a hollow along the bridge of the nose:** apply highlighter the hollow area.
- **If the nose is crooked:** apply shader over the crooked side.

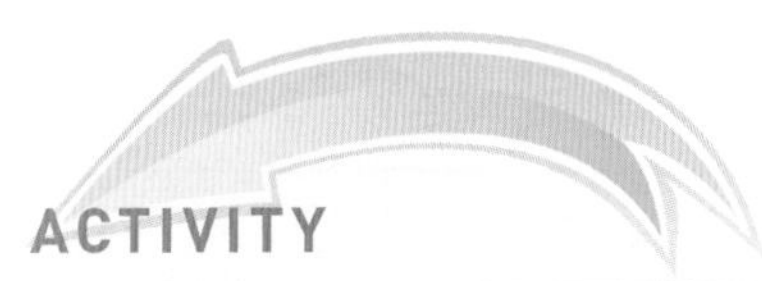

ACTIVITY

Contouring

Study three different clients or colleagues. Identify their face shapes. Where would you apply the contouring cosmetics for each face shape, and why?

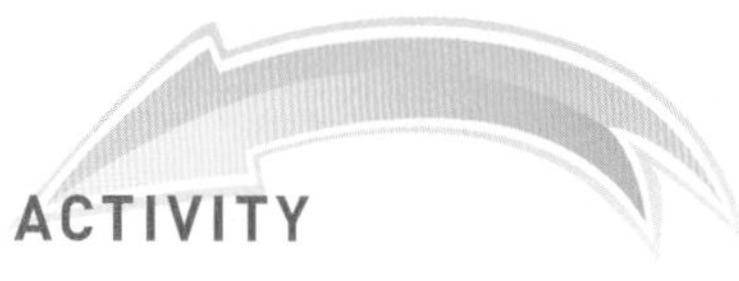

ACTIVITY

Correcting nose shapes
Think of the different nose shapes you may encounter, such as Roman, turned up, bulbous, or with a long tip. Which contour cosmetics would you select to correct each? Where would you apply them?

TOP TIP

Asian faces

An Asian face may appear as a flat plane: the skilful application of shading and highlighting products can create highs and lows.

Foreheads

- ***If the forehead is prominent:*** apply shader centrally over the prominent area, blending it outwards toward the temples.
- ***If the forehead is shallow:*** apply highlighter in a narrow band below the hairline.
- ***If the forehead is deep:*** apply shader in a narrow band below the hairline.

Chins

- ***If the jaw is too wide:*** apply shader from beneath the cheekbones and along the jaw line, blending it at the neck.
- ***If the chin is double:*** apply shader to the centre of the chin, blending it outwards along the jawbone and under the chin.
- ***If the chin is prominent:*** apply foundation to the tip of the chin.
- ***If the chin is long:*** apply shader over the prominent area.
- ***If the chin recedes:*** apply highlighter along the jaw line and at the centre of the chin.

TOP TIP

Foreheads

Foreheads can be improved by a flattering hairstyle:

- *Prominent forehead*: choose soft, flat, textured fringes.
- *Shallow forehead*: choose a shorter, soft fringe. Height will make the forehead appear longer.
- *Deep forehead*: choose a longer, soft fringe.

Necks

- ***If the neck is thin:*** apply highlighter down each side of the neck.
- ***If the neck is thick:*** apply shader to both sides of the neck.

Face powder

Face powder is applied to set the foundation, disguising minor blemishes and making the skin appear smooth and oil-free. It protects the skin from the environment by acting as a barrier. It also allows the application and smooth blending of other powder products such as blusher and eye shadow.

Most powders are based on **talc** as the main ingredient, but talc particles are of uneven size, and substitutes such as **mica** are now becoming popular. These give a more natural, flattering appearance to the skin.

Powder adheres to the foundation through the addition of **zinc, magnesium stearate** or **fatty esters**. These chemicals set the make-up and remove tackiness. Further powder products can then be applied to the skin.

Face powder contains absorbent materials such as **precipitated chalk, rice powder** or **nylon derivatives**. These absorb sweat and sebum throughout the day, reducing shine and giving the foundation greater durability.

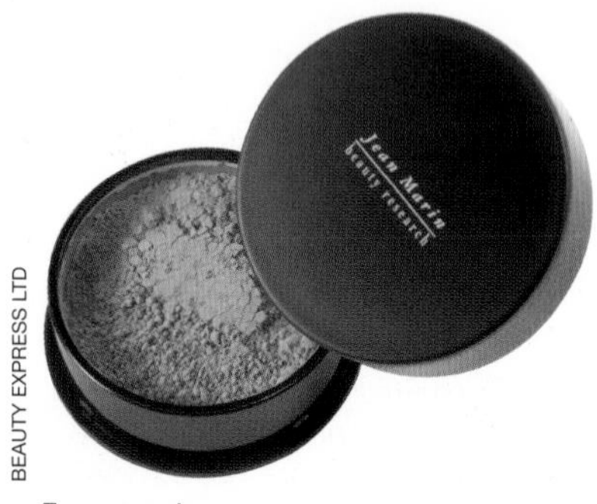

BEAUTY EXPRESS LTD

Face powder

Light-reflecting ingredients such as mica and moisturising ingredients are popular to reduce and soften the signs of ageing such as fine lines.

Shine control ingredients or 'blot powder' is created for use in professional situations and for touch-ups. Blot powder contains crystallized minerals and silica to absorb excess oils and reduce shine on the skin's surface.

HEALTH & SAFETY

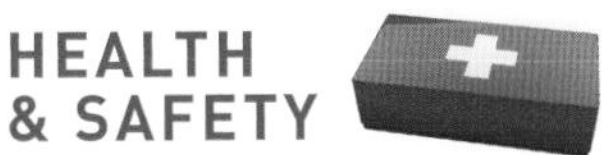

Avoiding contamination
Before application, always remove sufficient loose powder from the container. This minimizes the chances of bacteria entering the powder.

Kinds of face powders

There are two basic products: loose powders and compact powders.

Loose powders

Loose powders do not contain any oils or gums to bind the powder together. They are available in a range of shades, with different pastel pigments added to counteract skin imperfections. Colours include pink and lilac, which are flattering when viewed under artificial lights; yellow, which enhances a tanned skin; and green, which counteracts a red skin. Iridescent ingredients may be included to produce shimmering and highlighting effects.

Many cosmetic products contain **titanium dioxide**, an opaque white pigment, to provide coverage. When applied to black skin, this can give the skin a chalky appearance. When selecting products for black skin, bear in mind not just the shade but also the ingredients.

Compact powders

Compact powders contain a gum, mixed with the ingredients to bind them together. These powders provide a greater coverage, especially if they contain titanium dioxide. Pressed powders should be recommended mainly for a client's personal use, and then only to remove shine from the skin during the day, as required.

HEALTH & SAFETY

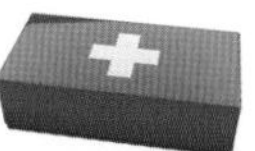

Home use
If the client uses a pressed powder, advise them to wash the powder applicator regularly to minimize the reproduction of bacteria.

How to apply powder

Face powder is applied ***after*** the foundation, unless a water-based foundation or a combination powder foundation has been selected. Select a matt powder for a daytime make-up, and an iridescent shimmer powder for an evening make-up.

Don't apply face powder to excessively dry skin, as it would aggravate and emphasize the dry skin condition. Beware of applying powder if a client has superfluous facial hair, as it may emphasize this. If the skin appears too pale apply a facial bronzer to correct. Oily skin can make the powder darker. If this occurs apply a lighter powder to correct.

Loose face powder

1 Remove the loose powder from its container, using a clean spatula or, if the powder is in a shaker, by sprinkling it out. Place the powder on a clean facial tissue.

2 Ask the client to keep their eyes closed. Using a clean piece of cotton wool or velour sponge, press into the powder and then press the powder all over the face.

TOP TIP

Mature skin

Some powders reflect light while appearing subtle and non-shiny. These are most flattering for mature skin, as wrinkles appear less obvious.

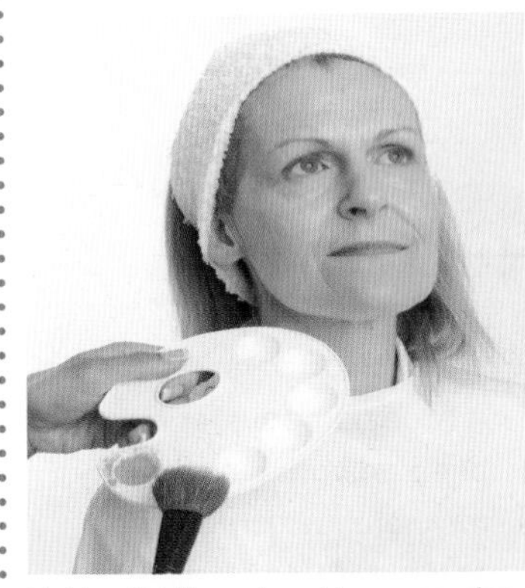

Light-reflecting mineral loose powder

3 Remove excess powder using a large, disinfected facial powder brush. Direct the brush strokes first up the face, which dislodges the powder, then down the face, which flattens the facial hair and removes the final residue of excess powder.

Compact powder Apply powder with a brush or velour powder puff.

Facial contouring using powder products may now be carried out.

Bronzing

Bronzing products are applied to create a healthy, natural or subtle tanned look. They are formulated to create a matt or shimmer effect and are also suitable as a highlighting contouring product.

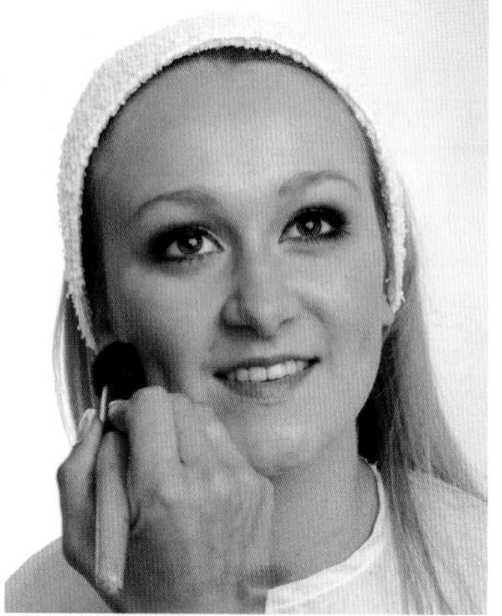

Applying bronzing product

Kinds of bronzing products

Bronzing products are available in powder, gel and liquid formulation. Powder bronzer, a tinted powder in different shades, gives skin natural colour effects and highlights. Ideal for enhancing a client's skin tone or tan and suitable for all skin types, although they can emphasize a dry or mature skin. Gel bronzer contains gel and glycerine in which the pigment is suspended. Gel bronzer is preferable for a dry, mature skin type and can be applied to the whole face or specific areas. Liquid bronzer is suitable for all skin types and contains a pearlized, light-reflective micro-fine powder with an oil-free formulation. Silicone enhances its application.

Apply bronzing products according to the effect you want to achieve after powder application or in the case of gel and liquid after foundation application. Remember you can use bronzers as a contour product also.

Powder Using a large powder brush apply the bronzer powder. Stroke the brush over the cheek area, followed by nose, chin and neck area.

Gel As for liquid blusher you need to blend the gel bronzer quickly over each area. Apply with the fingers or a damp sponge. Commence at the cheek area, forehead, nose and chin.

Liquid Apply as for gel bronzer.

Bronzers for males

A bronzing powder has been designed especially for males which is matt and natural.

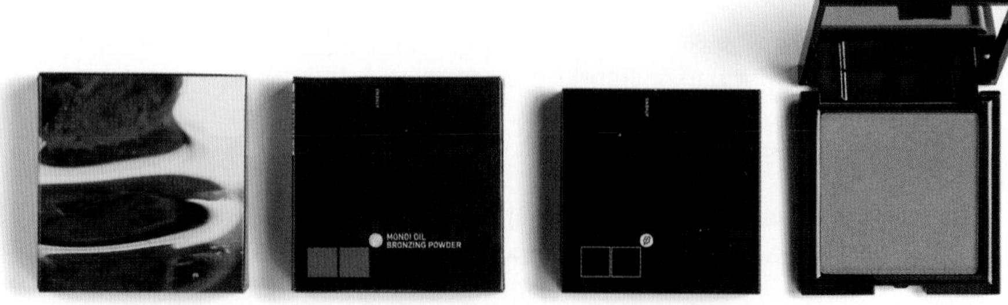

Bronzing products

KORRES NATURAL PRODUCTS, WWW.KORRES.COM

Eye make-up

Make-up is applied to the eye area to complement the natural eye colour, to give definition to the eye area, and to enhance the natural shape of the eye.

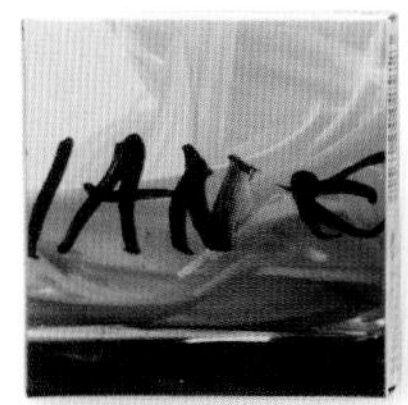

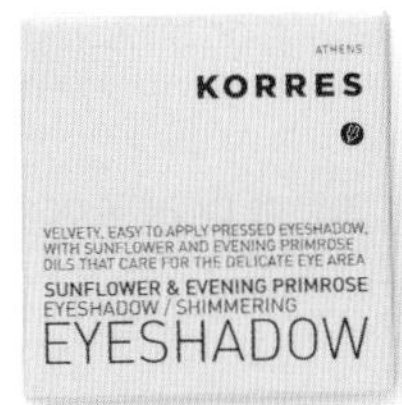

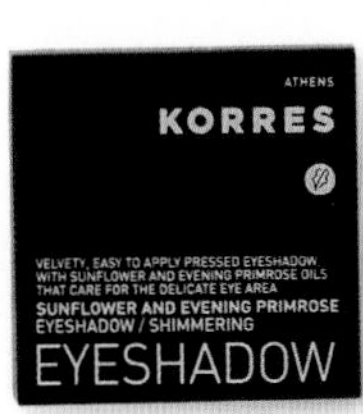

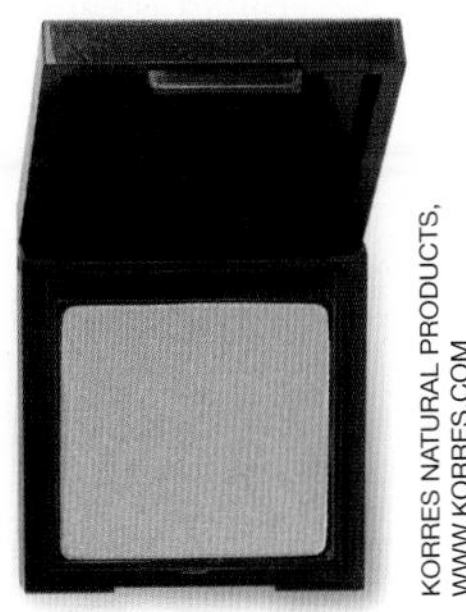

KORRES NATURAL PRODUCTS, WWW.KORRES.COM

Eye shadows

Eye shadow

Eye shadow adds colour and definition to the eye area. The different types include matt, pearlized, metallic and pastel. They are available in cream, crayon or powder form. Eye shadows are composed of either oil-and-water emulsions or waxes containing inorganic pigments to give colour.

- ***Powder eye shadows*** have a talc base, mixed with oils to facilitate application. Lighter shades are produced by the addition of **titanium dioxide** – avoid these on dark skin as they contrast too harshly with the natural skin colour.
- ***Cream eye shadows*** contain wax, oil and silica.
- ***Liquid eye shadows*** contain water, mica, glycerine and butylene glycol to achieve the correct viscosity.
- ***Crayon eye shadows*** are composed of wax and oil, and are similar in appearance and application to an eye pencil.

Pearlized mineral eye shadows are created by the addition of **bismuth oxychloride**, a fine crystalline powder or **mica,** a light-reflecting mineral powder; a *metallic* effect is created by the addition of fine particles of **gold leaf, aluminium** or **bronze**.

How to apply eye shadow

Eye shadow application will differ according to the eye shape of the client and the look to be achieved.

Powder eye shadow

1 Protect the skin beneath the eye with a clean tissue or loose powder to collect small particles of eye shadow that may fall during application.

2 Lift the skin at the brow slightly to keep the eye tissue taut, enabling you to reach the skin near to the base of the eyelashes.

3 Apply the selected eye shadow to the eyelid, using a sponge or a brush applicator.

HEALTH & SAFETY

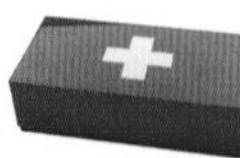

Eye cosmetics

The eye tissue is particularly sensitive. Eye cosmetic products should be of the highest quality, and be permitted for use according to the Cosmetics Products (Safety) Regulations (2008).

TOP TIP

Cream eye shadows

Cream eye shadows are less popular – they are difficult to blend and quickly settle into creases. They are usually used by clients who have dry, mature skin.

HEALTH & SAFETY

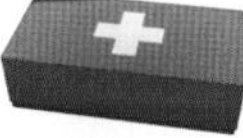

Contact lenses

It is preferable for the client not to be wearing contact lenses during eye shadow application.

ALWAYS REMEMBER

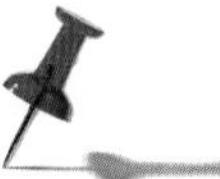

Too much powder

When applying powder colours, always tap the brush before application to remove excess eye shadow. If too much colour is deposited on the applicator, stroke it over a clean tissue to remove the excess.

Remember it is better to apply more product in stages until you create the look you want to achieve.

HEALTH & SAFETY

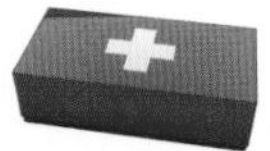

Eye pencil
A good-quality eye pencil will be quite soft when applied to the skin, to avoid dragging the delicate eye tissue.

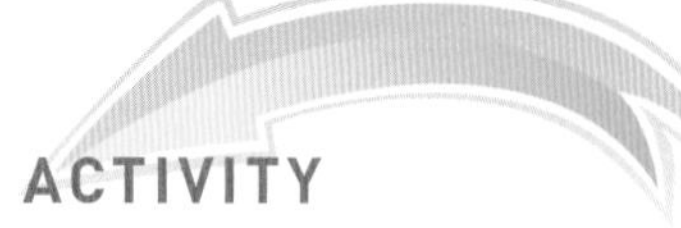

ACTIVITY

Eye shadow application techniques
There are many different looks that can be created by the placement of eye shadow. Consider 'smoky' and 'winged'. Collect different images of techniques and practise their application.

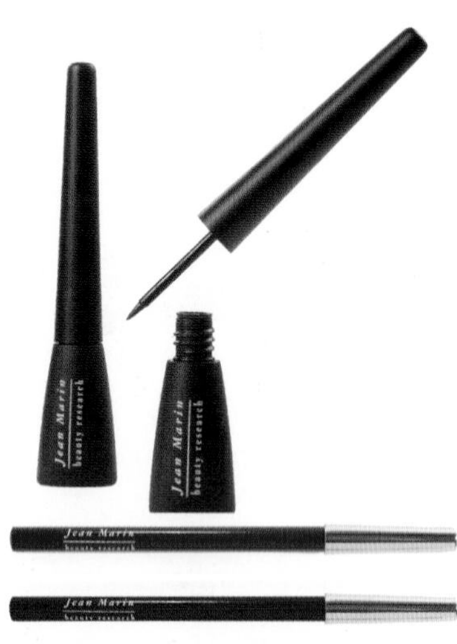

BEAUTY EXPRESS LTD

Eyeliners

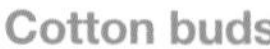

BEST PRACTICE

Cotton buds
Have a clean cotton bud available so that you can remove the powder from any minor mistakes during application.

4 Highlight beneath the brow bone.

5 Using a brush, apply a darker eye shadow to the socket area, beginning at the outer corner of the eye. Blend the colour evenly, to avoid harsh lines.

6 Ask your client to open her eyes during application so that you can look at the effect created.

Cream eye shadow Apply over a base to hold the cream shadow in place. It may be applied with a brush and blended with the finger or brush.

Liquid eye shadow Apply the liquid shadow pearly colour with a brush stroking and blending over the eyelid where required.

Eyeliner

Eyeliner defines and emphasizes the eye area. It is available in pencil, liquid or powder form.

- ***Eye pencil*** Made of wax and oil, and contains different pigments which give it its colour.
- ***Liquid and gel eyeliner*** A gum solution, in which the pigment is suspended.
- ***Powder eyeliner*** A powder base with the addition of mineral oil.

Powder eyeliner is the most suitable choice for a client who is exposed to a warm environment, as it will not smudge.

How to apply eyeliner If you are using a powder or liquid eyeliner, apply it with a clean eyeliner brush.

1 Lift the skin gently upwards at the eyebrows, to keep the eyelid firm and make application easier.

2 Draw a fine line along the base of the eyelashes (as close to the lashes as possible), as required.

3 If using an eye pencil or powder line, lightly smudge the eyeliner to soften the effect of the line. (This is not effective with liquid liner.) If required, a further application may be applied for a thicker line.

4 Eyeliner may be applied to the inner eye, usually accompanying a 'smoky' eye shadow look. This technique is unsuitable on small eyes as it would make them appear smaller.

TOP TIP

Kohl eyeliner

Kohl was used by the Ancient Egyptians, a black cosmetic containing stibium. This is now banned. Iron oxide is a mineral ion commonly used today.

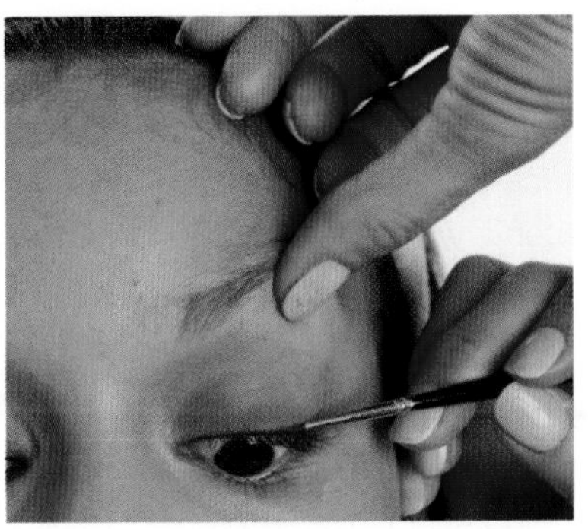
Applying eyeliner to the upper lashline

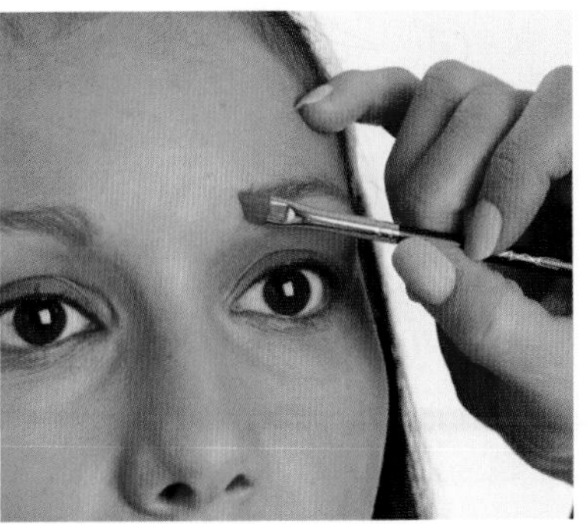
Applying eyebrow colour

TOP TIP

Lasting eyeliner
Powder eye shadow may be applied over the eye pencil application to increase its durability, as heat and moisture can disturb the wax/oil content of a pencil.

Eyebrow colour

Eyebrow colour emphasizes the eyebrow, darkens the hair, alters its shape, disguises bald patches and can make sparse eyebrows look thicker. It is available in pencil, liquid or powder form.

- ***Eyebrow pencil*** Firmer than an eye pencil, and is composed of waxes that hold the inorganic pigments.
- ***Powder brow colour*** Composed of a talc base, mixed with mineral oil and pigments.
- ***Liquid eyebrow*** A fluid, quick-drying eyebrow colour to define the brows.
- ***Eyebrow mascara*** Composed of mineral oil and waxes with pigment suspended in it. The mascara defines the brows and controls and shapes them.

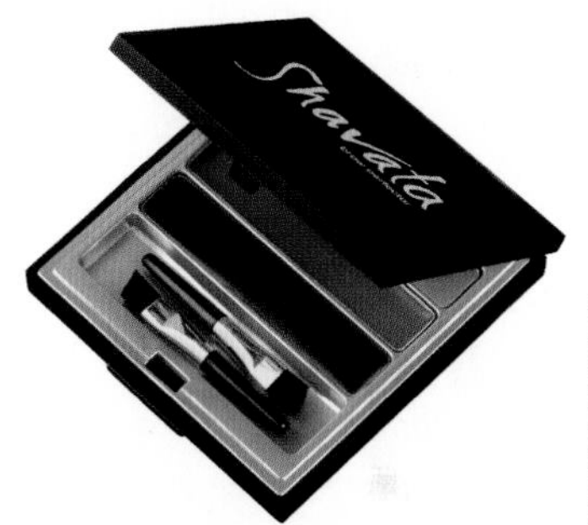

WWW.SHAVATA.CO.UK
Brow perfector

How to apply eyebrow colour

1 Select an appropriate colour of powder or eyebrow pencil. Brush the eyebrows with a clean brow brush to remove excess face powder and eye shadow. A specialized wax or gel can be applied which aids adherence of powder brow shadow and separates and defines the brow hair.

2 Simulate the appearance of brow hair by using fine strokes of colour, or disguise bald patches with a denser application. Use a pencil or liquid eyebrow to apply feathery strokes or alternatively using a brush apply powder to the prepared brow hair.

3 Brush the eyebrows into shape if necessary without disturbing product application.

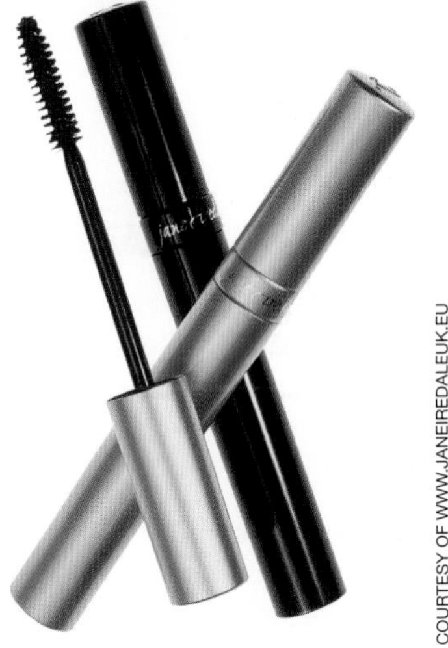
COURTESY OF WWW.JANEIREDALEUK.EU
Mascara

ACTIVITY

Brow colour
What brow colour product would you select for the following and how would you apply it:

- fair-haired client, day wear
- dark-haired client, evening make-up
- red-haired client, special occasion
- grey-haired client, sparse brow hair, day make-up?

TOP TIP

Eyelash curling
The eyelashes may be temporarily curled before mascara application to open up the eye area.

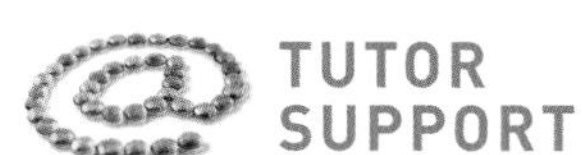

TUTOR SUPPORT

Activity 4: Make-up techniques wordsearch

HEALTH & SAFETY

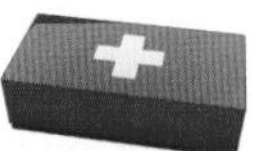

Mascara

Mascara when purchased is usually provided with a brush applicator. This applicator cannot be effectively cleaned and disinfected, however, so it should not be used. Instead use a disposable mascara brush for each client.

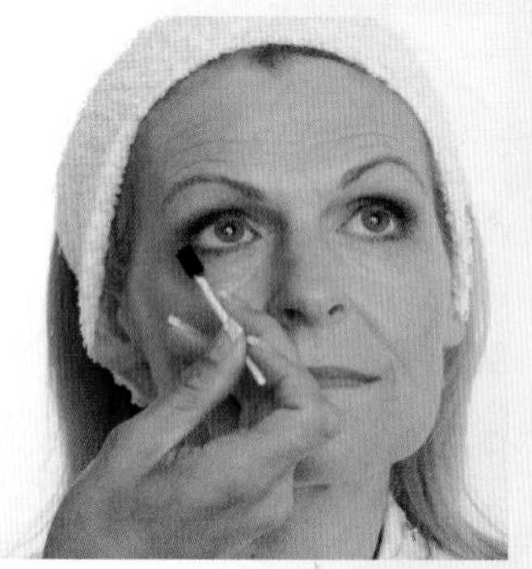

HEALTH & SAFETY

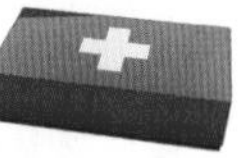

Allergies

If the client has hypersensitive eyes or skin, use hypoallergenic cosmetics that contain no known sensitizers.

Contact lenses

If the client wears contact lenses, don't use either lash-building filament mascaras or loose-particled eye shadows, which have a tendency to flake and may enter the eye.

TOP TIP

Clear mascara

Clear mascara makes the lashes appear thicker, while appearing very natural.

Mascara

Mascara enhances the natural eyelashes, making them appear longer, changed in colour and thicker. It is available in liquid, cream and block-cake forms. It is composed of waxes or an oil-and-water emulsion, and contains pigments which give it its colour. Other ingredients can be added to increase its durability, making it waterproof which will require a special eye make-up remover for waterproof mascara.

- **Liquid mascara** – a mixture of gum in water or alcohol; the pigment is suspended in this. It may also contain short textile filaments that adhere to the lashes and have a thickening, lengthening effect. Water-resistant mascara contains resin instead of gum, so that it will not run or smudge.
- **Cream mascara** – an emulsion of oil and water, with the pigment suspended in this.
- **Block mascara** – composed of mineral oil, lanolin and waxes, which are melted together to form a block on setting. It must be dampened with water before application.

How to apply mascara Using a disposable mascara brush, apply mascara to the eyelashes:

1. Hold the brush horizontally to apply colour to the length of the lashes. Where the lashes are short and curly, or difficult to reach, hold the brush vertically and use the point of the brush.
2. Place a clean tissue underneath the base of the lower eyelashes, and stroke the brush down the length of the lashes from the base to the tips.
3. Lift the eyelid at the brow bone. Ask the client to look down slightly while keeping their eyes open. From above, stroke down the length of the lashes from the base to the tips.
4. Using a zigzag motion, draw the brush upwards through the upper and lower surfaces of the lashes, from the base to the tips. Apply several coats to create a dramatic evening look.
5. Finally, separate the eyelashes with a clean brush or lash comb.

ALWAYS REMEMBER

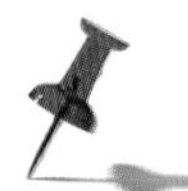

Curly lashes will require brushing, using a clean brush, both before mascara application and after each coat, to separate the lashes. A specialized gel may be applied before mascara application which, on drying, separates the lashes.

TOP TIP

Mascara accidents!

If you accidentally get mascara on the skin, remove with a cotton bud. If waterproof you may need a small amount of eye make-up remover on the bud. Apply any corrective make-up to follow and conceal.

Eye make-up for the client who wears glasses

If the client wears glasses, check the function of the lens, as this can alter the appearance and effect of the eye make-up.

- ***If the client is short-sighted, the lens makes the eye appear smaller.*** Draw attention to the eyes by selecting righter, lighter colours. When applying eye shadow and eyeliner, use the corrective techniques for small eyes. Apply mascara to emphasize the eyelashes.
- ***If the client is long-sighted, the lens will magnify the eye.*** Make-up should therefore be subtle, avoiding frosted colours and lash-building mascaras. Careful blending is important, as any mistakes will be magnified!

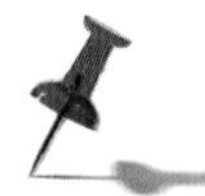

ALWAYS REMEMBER

Never pump the mascara wand when loading it with mascara. This encourages air to enter and makes the mascara dry out.

LEARNER SUPPORT

Corrective eye make-up diagram

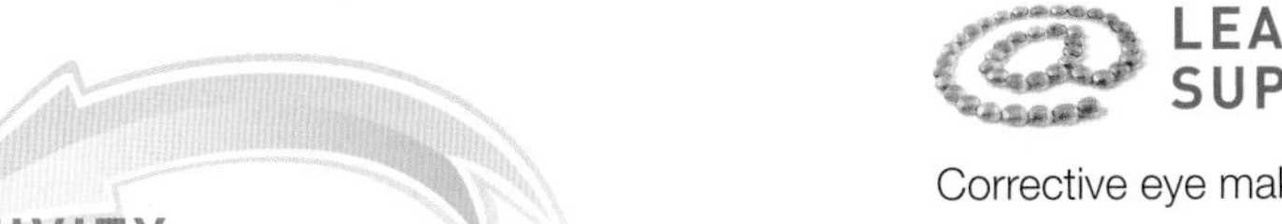

ACTIVITY

Choosing mascara
What colour mascara should be applied if the client has the following hair colouring: brown, red, black or grey?

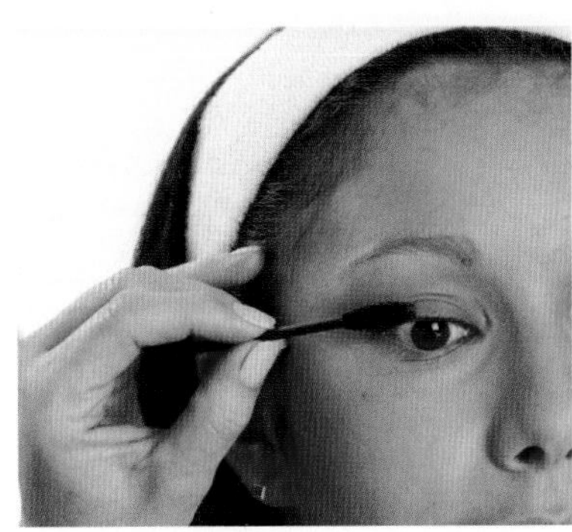

Applying mascara

How to apply corrective eye make-up

Dark circles

1 Minimize the circles by applying a concealing product.

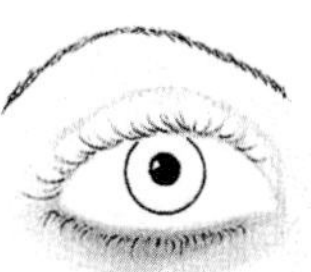
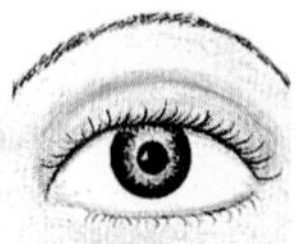

Dark circles

Wide-set eyes

1 Apply a darker eye colour to the inner portion of the upper eyelid.

2 Apply lighter eye shadow to the outer portion of the eyelid.

3 Apply eyeliner in a darker colour to the inner half of the upper eyelid.

4 Eyebrow pencil may be applied to extend the inner bowline.

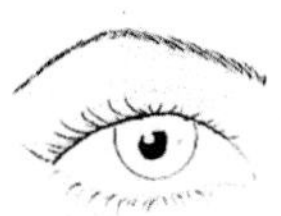
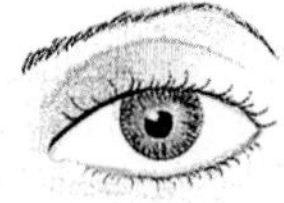

Wide-set eyes

Close-set eyes

1 Lighten the inner portion of the upper eyelid.

2 Use a darker colour at the outer eye.

3 Apply eyeliner to the outer corner of the upper eyelid.

4 Pluck brow hairs at the inner eyebrow – this helps to create the illusion of the eyes being further apart.

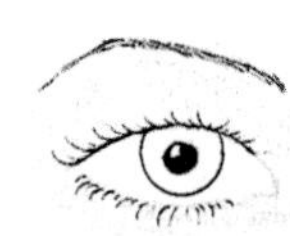
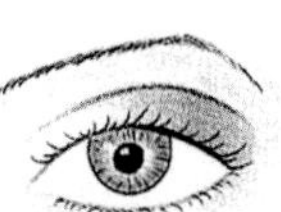

Close-set eyes

Round eyes

1 Apply a darker colour over the prominent central upper-lid area.

2 Elongate the eyes by applying eyeliner to the outer corners of the upper and lower eyelids.

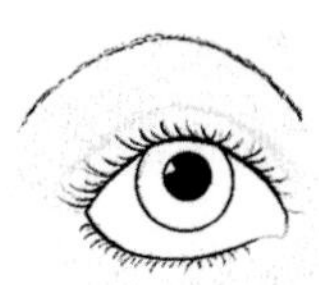
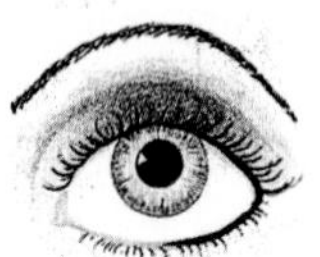

Round eyes

Prominent eyes

1 Apply dark matt eye shadow over the prominent upper eyelid.

2 Apply a darker shade to the outer portion of the eyelid, and blend it upwards and outwards.

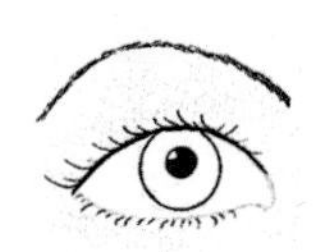
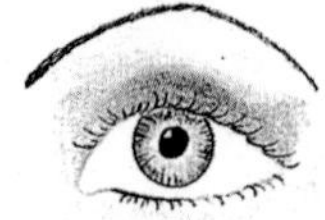

Prominent eyes

3 Highlight the brow bone, drawing attention to this area.

4 Eyeliner may be applied to the inner lower eyelid.

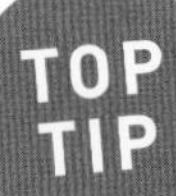

TOP TIP

Prominent eyes

To make the eyes appear less prominent, select matt eye shadows – pearlized and frosted eye shadows will highlight and emphasize the eye.

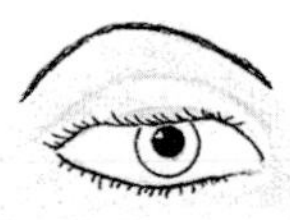

Overhanging lids

Overhanging lids

1 Apply a pale highlighter to the middle of the eyelid.

2 Apply a darker eye shadow to contour the socket area, creating a higher crease (which disguises the hooded appearance).

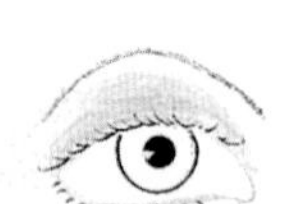
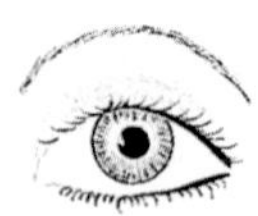

Deep-set eyes

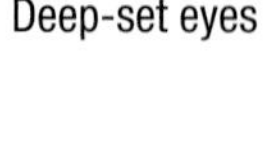

Deep-set eyes

1 Use light-coloured eye shadows.

2 Eye shadow may also be applied in a fine line to the inner half of the lower eyelid, beneath the lashes.

3 Apply eyeliner to the outer halves of the upper and lower eyelids, broadening the line as you extend outwards.

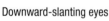

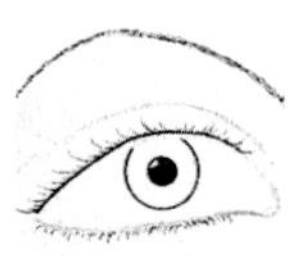
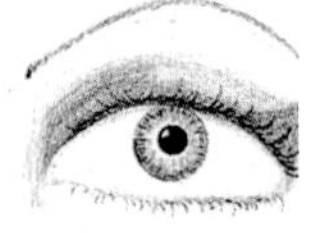

Downward-slanting eyes

Downward-slanting eyes

1 Create lift by applying the eye shadow upwards and outwards at the outer corners of the upper eyelid.

2 Apply eyeliner to the upper eyelid, applying it upwards at the outer corner.

3 Confine mascara to the outer lashes.

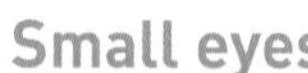

Small eyes

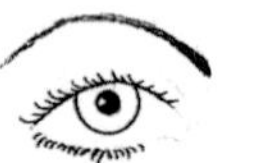
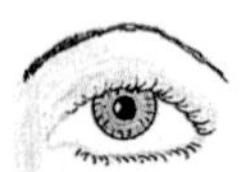

Small eyes

1 Choose a light colour for the upper eyelid.

2 Highlight under the brow, to open up the eye area.

3 Curl the lashes before applying mascara.

4 Apply a light-coloured eyeliner to the outer third of the lower eyelid.

5 A white eyeliner may be applied to the inner lid, to make the eye appear larger.

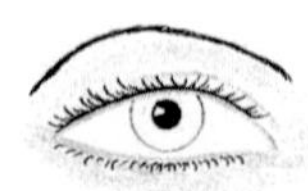
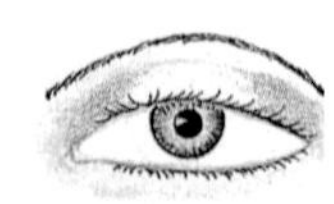

Narrow eyes

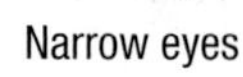

Narrow eyes

1 Apply a lighter colour in the centre of the eyelid, to open up the eye.

2 Apply a shader to the inner and outer portions of the eyelid.

Oriental eyes

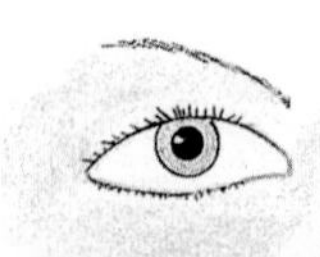
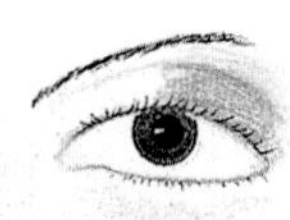

Oriental eyes

1 Divide the upper eyelid in two vertically. Place a lighter colour over the inner half of the eyelid and a darker colour at the outer half.

2 Apply a highlighter under the eyebrow.

3 White eyeliner may be applied at the base of the lash line, on the lower inner eyelid.

The eyelashes

To emphasize the eyelashes, making them appear longer temporarily, curl them using eyelash curlers. If performing after mascara application it must be dry.

How to curl the eyelashes

1. Rest the upper lashes between the upper and lower portions of the eyelash curlers.
2. Bring the two portions gently together with a squeezing action.
3. Hold the lashes in the curlers for approximately ten seconds, then release them.
4. If the lashes are not sufficiently curled, repeat the action.

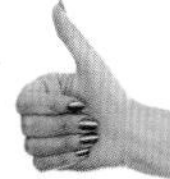

BEST PRACTICE

Artificial eyelashes
Artificial eyelashes should be available if you are applying an evening or special occasion make-up – you may wish to apply these to enhance the appearance of the eyes. Remember you will need to perform a skin sensitivity test in advance.

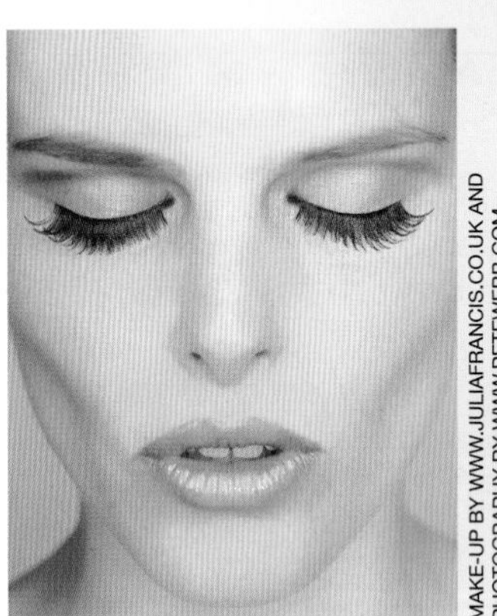

MAKE-UP BY WWW.JULIAFRANCIS.CO.UK AND PHOTOGRAPHY BY WWW.PETEWEBB.COM

Artificial eyelashes

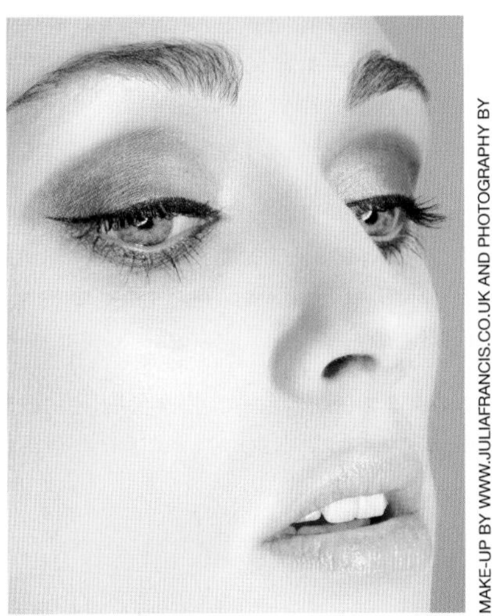

MAKE-UP BY WWW.JULIAFRANCIS.CO.UK AND PHOTOGRAPHY BY WWW.PETEWEBB.COM

Eye shadow on model

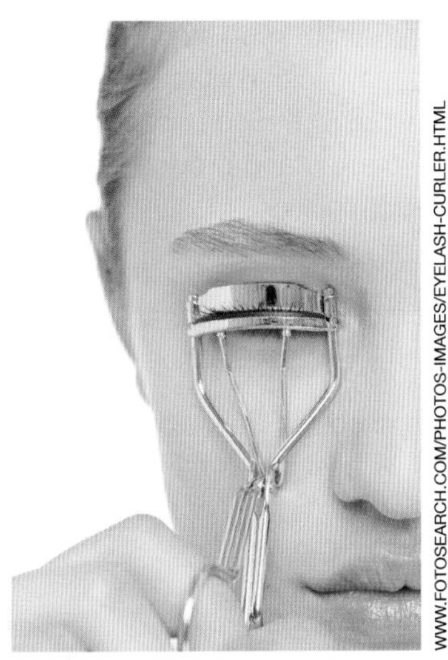

WWW.FOTOSEARCH.COM/PHOTOS-IMAGES/EYELASH-CURLER.HTML

Eyelash curler

TOP TIP

Oriental clients
Eyelash curling is beneficial for Oriental clients who have short lashes that grow downwards.

HEALTH & SAFETY

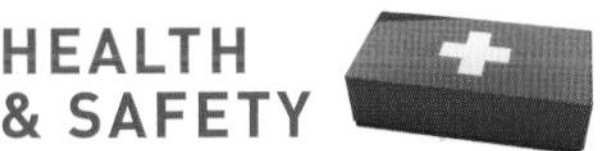

Eyelash curling
Repeated eyelash curling can lead to breakage. The technique should therefore be used only for special occasions.

The lips

Lip cosmetics add colour and draw attention to the lips. As the lips have no protective sebum, the use of lip cosmetics also helps to prevent them from drying and becoming chapped.

It is not uncommon for the lips to be out of proportion in some way. Using lip cosmetics and corrective techniques, symmetrical lips can be created. A careful choice of product and accurate application are required to achieve a professional effect.

The main lip cosmetics are lip liner, lipsticks, lip tints, lib balm and lip glosses. Sometimes the lips may be unevenly pigmented. The application of a lip toner or foundation over the lips corrects this.

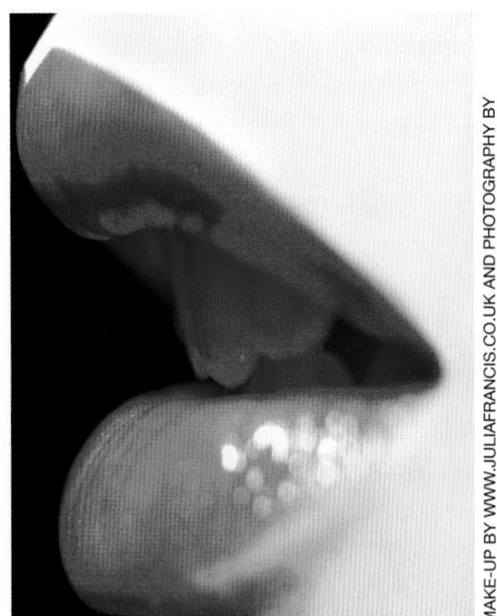

MAKE-UP BY WWW.JULIAFRANCIS.CO.UK AND PHOTOGRAPHY BY WWW.PETEWEBB.COM

Lip make-up

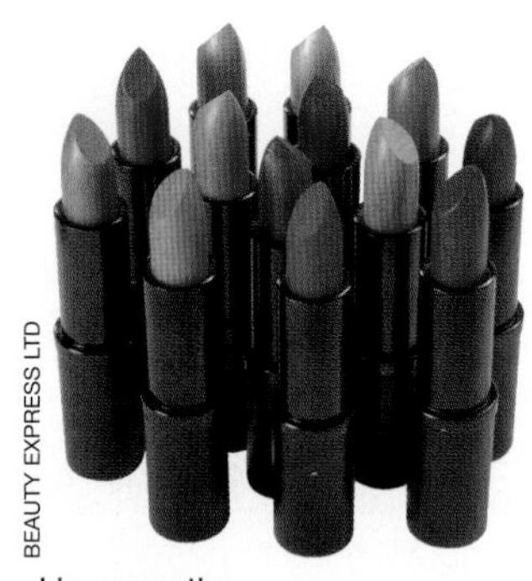
BEAUTY EXPRESS LTD
Lip cosmetics

HEALTH & SAFETY
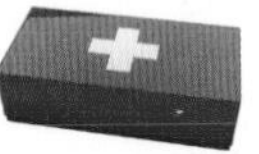

Lip pencils
Lip pencils are form of lip liner contained in wood. Always sharpen the lip pencil before use on each client, to provide a clean, uncontaminated cosmetic surface.

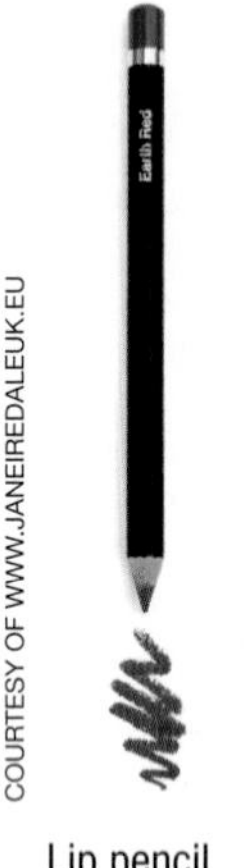
COURTESY OF WWW.JANEIREDALEUK.EU
Lip pencil

HEALTH & SAFETY
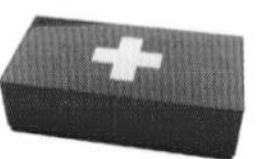

Lipstick
For reasons of hygiene, remove a small quantity of lipstick by scraping the stick with a clean spatula – don't apply the lipstick directly.

HEALTH & SAFETY
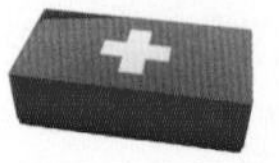

Allergies
Lipsticks often contain ingredients that can cause allergic reactions, such as lanolin and certain pigment dyes. If the client has known allergies, use a hypoallergenic product instead.

Lip liner

Lip liner is used to define the lips, creating a perfectly symmetrical outline. This is coloured in with another lip cosmetic, either a lipstick or a lip gloss. The lip liner also helps to prevent the lipstick from 'bleeding' into lines around the lips.

Lip liner has a wax base which does not melt and can be applied easily. It contains pigments which give the pencil its colour.

When choosing a lip liner, select one that is the same colour as, or slightly darker than, the lipstick to be used with it.

Lipstick

Lipstick contains a blend of oils and waxes, which give it its firmness, and silicone, essential for easy application. It also contains pigment, to add colour, an emollient moisturiser, to keep the lips soft and supple and perfume, to improve its appeal. In addition it may include vitamins, to condition the lips, or sunscreens, to protect the lips from ultra-violet rays. Some lipsticks contain a relatively large proportion of water – these moisturise the lips and provide a natural look. The coverage provided by a lipstick depends on its formulation.

Lipsticks are available in the following forms: cream, matt, frosted and translucent. Frosted lipstick has good durability, as it is very dry. Some other lipsticks also offer extended durability, and are suitable for clients who are unable to renew their lipstick regularly.

When choosing the colour of lipstick, take into account the natural colour of the client's lips (it is best if it is the same colour tone), the skin and hair colours, and the colours selected for the rest of the make-up.

Lip gloss

Lip gloss provides a moist, shiny look to the lips. It may be worn alone, or applied on top of a lipstick. Its effect is short-lived. Lip gloss is made of mineral oils, with pigment suspended in the oil.

Note that mature clients often have creases on the lips that extend to the surrounding skin. If lip gloss is used it will often bleed into these lines.

Lip stain

Lip stain adds intense colour to the lips and is made of water, glycerine, skin-conditioning ingredients and mineral pigments. Prepare the lip with lip liner. Apply to lips quickly, using the fingertips or a make-up sponge. Build up the colour to achieve the result required.

Lip balm

Lip balm is a lip moisturiser containing oil and beeswax, vitamins C and E to help prevent dryness and improve skin texture, and pigment to add colour and sheen. Following the lip liner, apply to the lips with a brush. A gloss may then be applied to enhance the lips.

Dry lips Sometimes the lips become dry and chapped. Recommend that the client keeps them moisturised at all times, especially in extremes of heat, cold or wind. Some facial exfoliants can be professionally applied over the lips to remove dead skin.

If the client does not like to wear make-up during the day, or if the client is male, recommend that the lips be protected with a lip-care product.

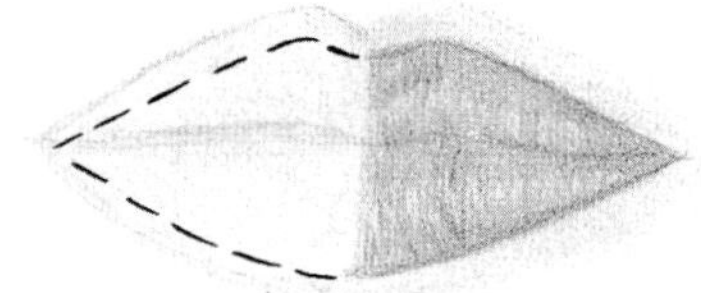
Thick lips

How to apply corrective lip make-up

Thick lips Select natural colours and darker shades, avoiding bright, glossy colours.

1 Blend foundation over the lips to disguise the natural lip line.

2 Apply a darker lip liner inside the natural lip line to create a new line.

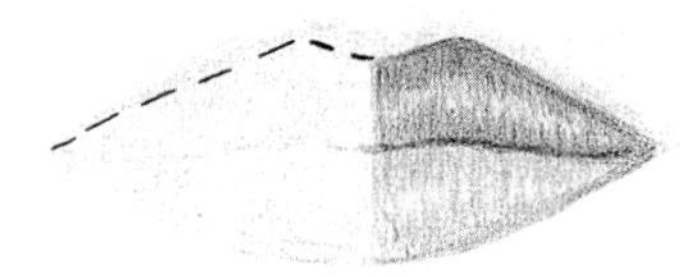
Thick upper lip

Thicker upper or lower lip

1 Use the technique described above to make the larger lip appear smaller.

2 Apply a slightly darker lipstick to the larger lip.

3 If the lips droop at the corners, raise the corners by applying lip liner to the corners of the upper lip, to turn them upwards.

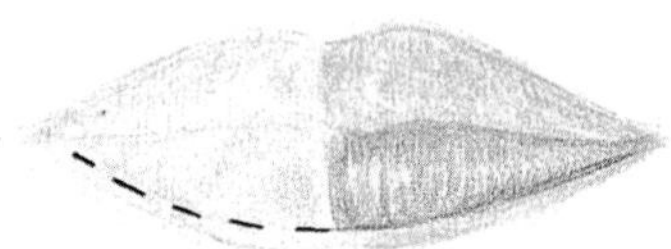
Thick lower lips

Thin lips Select brighter, pearlized colours. Avoid darker lipsticks, which will make the mouth appear smaller.

1 Apply a neutral lip liner just outside the natural lip line.

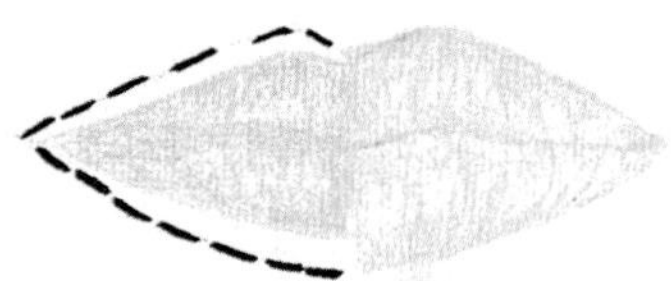
Thin lips

Small mouth

1 Extend the line slightly at the corners of the mouth, with both the upper and the lower lips.

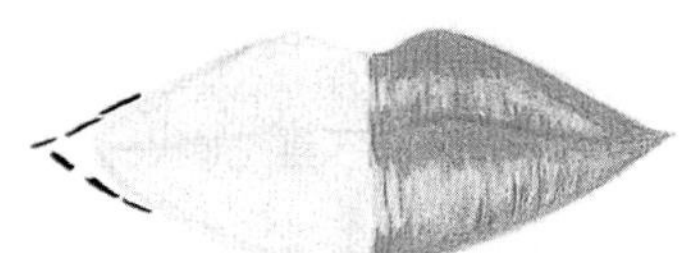
Small mouth

Uneven lips

1 Use a lip liner to draw in a new line.

2 Apply lipstick to the area.

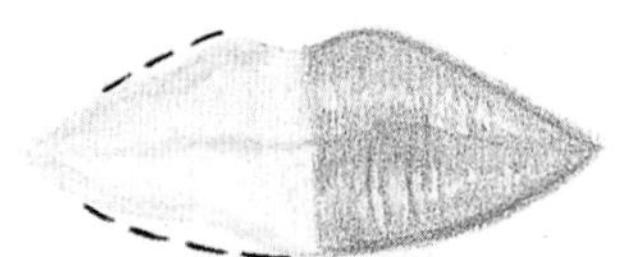
Uneven lips

Lines around the mouth

1 Apply lip liner around the natural lip line.

2 Apply a matt cream lipstick to the lips. (Don't use gloss, which might bleed into the lines around the mouth.)

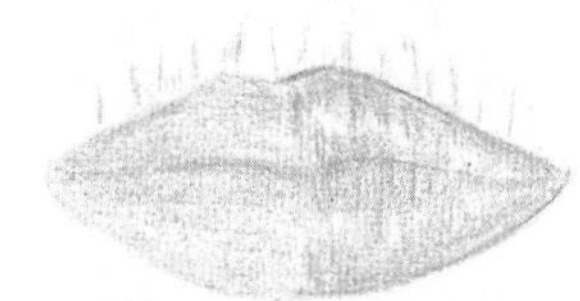
Lines around the mouth

How to apply lipstick

1 Select a lip pencil and lipstick to complement the client's colouring and the colour theme of the make-up.

2 Using a pencil sharpener, sharpen the lip pencil to expose a clean surface.

3 Ask the client to open her mouth slightly.

4 Outline the lips, carrying out lip correction as necessary. Begin the lip line at the outer corner of the mouth, and continue it to the centre of the lips. Repeat the process on the other side of the lip, commencing at the outer corner of the mouth.

5 Remove sufficient lipstick using a clean spatula.

HEALTH & SAFETY

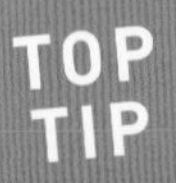

Lip brushes
Disposable lip brushes are available to enable lip cosmetics to be applied hygienically.

6 Using a disinfected lip brush, apply the lipstick to the lips.

7 Apply a clean facial tissue over the lip area, and gently press it onto the lips. This process, known as blotting, removes excess lipstick and fixes the colour on the lips.

8 The application of powder on the first application of lipstick will make the lipstick longer lasting.

9 A second light application of lipstick may then be applied.

10 If desired, lip-gloss may be applied over the lipstick to add sheen, again using a disinfected lip brush.

TOP TIP

Colour mixing
To obtain the correct colour of lipstick, you may need to mix different lipstick shades together.

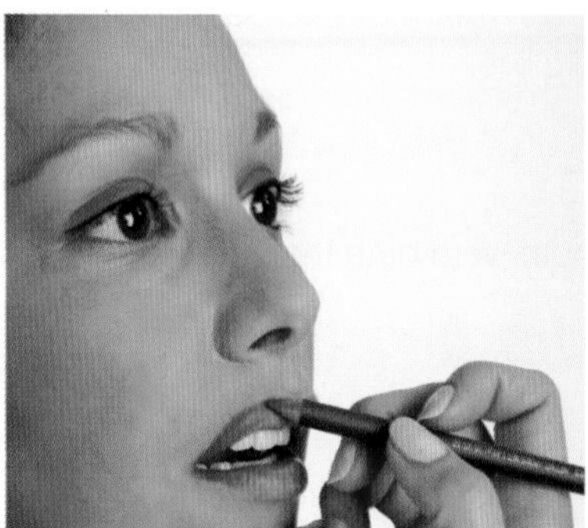

Applying lip liner

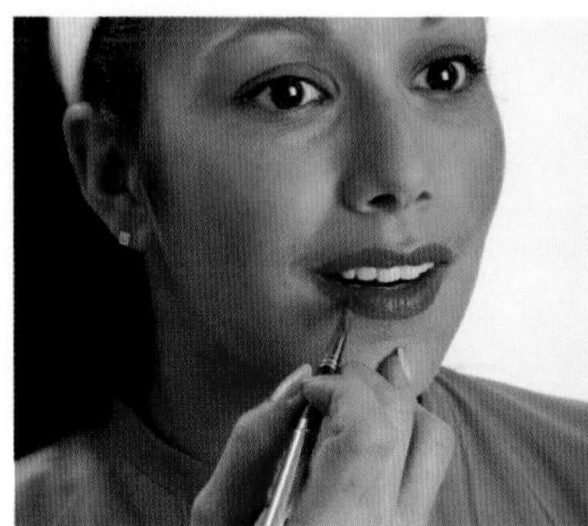

Applying lipstick

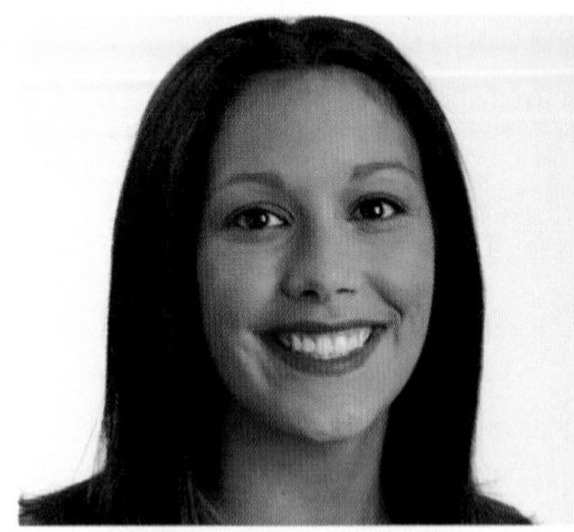

The finished day make-up

Finished make-up

After applying the make-up, fix the client's hair and then discuss the finished result in front of the make-up mirror.

Wash your hands. Record details of the treatment on the client's record card. Provide **aftercare advice**.

Aftercare advice

Following make-up application, recommend the correct skincare products to remove the products you have applied.

Eye cleansing advice

- Cleanse the eye area using a suitable eye make-up remover.
- Remove waterproof mascara, usually using an oily eye make-up remover.
- If false lashes have been applied, their removal must also be discussed (see pages 279–280).

Skincare advice

- Apply cleansing preparations to remove facial make-up with an appropriate cleanser in an upwards and outwards direction. Remove with damp cotton wool or clean facial sponges.
- Apply a suitable toner to suit skin type to remove excess cleanser.
- Apply day or night moisturiser, apply in small dots to the neck, chin, cheeks, nose and forehead. Quickly evenly spread a thin film over the face, using light upward, outward stroking movements.
- Blot the skin with a soft facial tissue to remove excess moisture.

Advise the client on application procedures to maintain the effect, e.g. removal of facial shine from the face with pressed powder, lip liner to stop 'bleeding', re-application of blusher to add warmth.

Explain to the client that you can offer a make-up lesson in which you would discuss the reason for the selection of make-up products and colours, and the techniques for applying them. Recommend the correct skincare products to remove the products you have applied.

Have retail products available for the client to purchase. These include the products that you have used during the make-up application and skincare products for preparation and removal of make-up.

Share tips that will ensure that the client gets the best out of any products purchased. Explain how to use the product hygienically and when it should be replaced.

Explain what action to take in the event of a contra-action.

Finally, at the end of the make-up treatment ensure that the client's records are updated, accurate and signed by the client and beauty therapist.

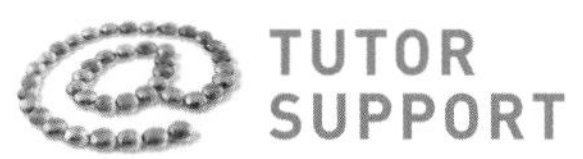

Activity 2: Case studies project

Make-up objectives

Day make-up

The effect should be natural. Any corrective work carried out should be very subtle and kept to the minimum, as natural light makes any imperfections appear obvious.

Select a foundation the same colour as the skin – aim to even out the skin tone. Set the foundation with a translucent face powder.

Apply a subtle, warm blusher or bronzing product to add colour to the face. Avoid strong colours of cosmetics, especially on the eyes. The mascara colour should be chosen to complement the client's natural lash and skin colours. Mascara should be used to emphasize, but not exaggerate, the length and thickness of the eyelashes. Eyeliner may be used, but it should be carefully placed and blended.

Line the lips in a colour that will co-ordinate with the lipstick to be applied, which again should be quite natural.

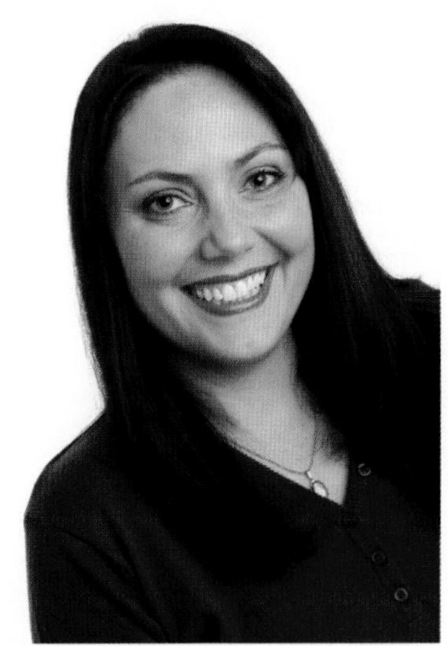

Day make-up

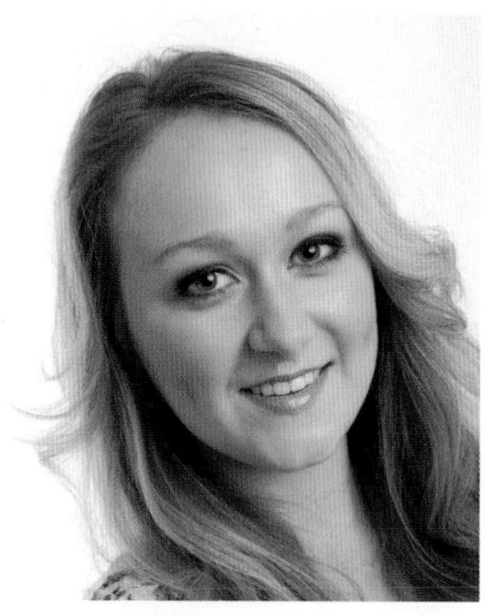

Evening make-up

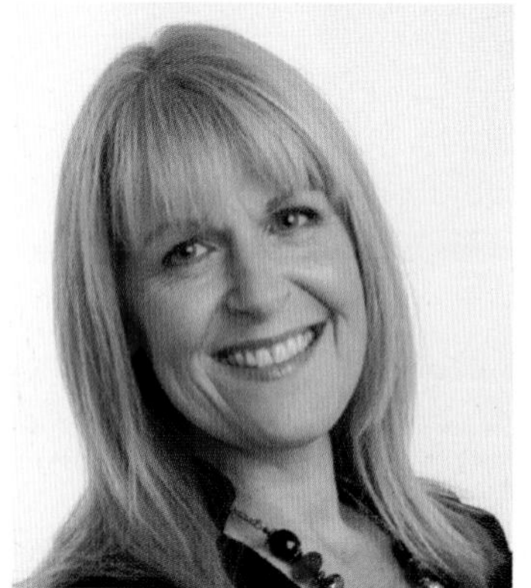

Special occasion make-up

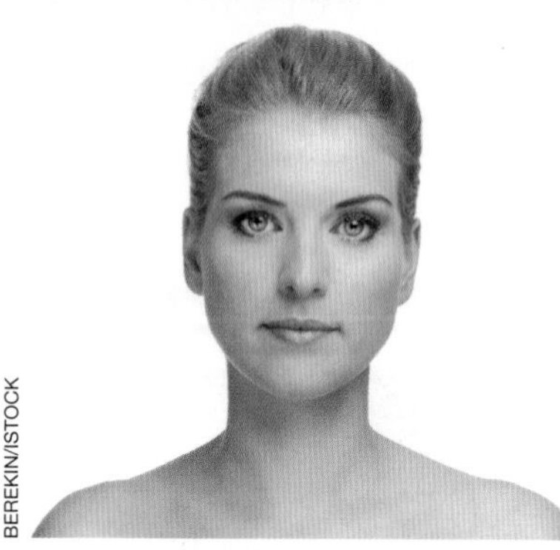

Fair skin

What aftercare advice should be given to a client following make-up application?

Need more time... refer to pages 334–335 to help you.

Evening make-up

This should be applied bearing in mind the type of lighting in which the client will be seen. Artificial light dulls the effect, and changes the colour of the make-up: dark shades lose their brilliance, appearing 'muddy', so you need to use brighter colours. Emphasize the facial features with the careful placement of contouring cosmetics.

Areas where shadows may be created, such as the eyes, should be emphasized using light, bright and highlighting cosmetic products. Add warmth to the face with an intense colour of blusher placed on the cheekbones. A highlighting or shimmer powder in a pearlized or metallic shade may be applied directly on top of or over the blusher. The client may like to try adventurous cosmetics such as metallics and frosted eye products.

Curl the eyelashes with eyelash curlers or apply false eyelashes to emphasize the eyes. Fashion shades of mascara may be selected, in purples, greens and blues, to complement the make-up and produce the effect required. Light shades of eyeliner may be used to frame the eyes and to 'open' them up.

Add a lip gloss to the lips, or apply a frosted lipstick to emphasize the mouth.

Colour the eyebrows, and carefully groom them to frame the eye area.

Special occasion make-up

A special occasion is usually an important event such as a wedding, day at the races, graduation ceremony or New Year's Eve party.

Whatever the occasion, whether daytime or evening, indoors or outdoors, you will need to consider the type of lighting the make-up will be viewed in – natural or artificial – and any other factors, such as how long it is to be worn for.

The selection of colours should co-ordinate with what the client will be wearing, and finally you need to know the effect they wish the make-up to create – should it be subtle or glamorous? Make-up products can then be selected and appropriately applied to suit the occasion.

Make-up to suit skin and hair colouring

Fair skin and blonde hair If the client has fair hair and fair skin, keep the skin colour natural. Apply a blusher in rose pink or beige.

Define the eyes with soft tones of browns and pinks. Apply a brown-black mascara.

Colour the lips with a rose-pink or peach lip-colour. Avoid lip colours lighter than the natural skin tone.

Oriental skin and black hair For creamy, sallow skin with dark hair, use blusher to add warmth and to brighten the skin, in either pink or brown.

The eyes are dark, with a prominent brow bone. Emphasize the socket of the eye with careful shading; extend this upwards and outwards. Place highlighter along the brow bone.

Pastel colours complement the eye colour. Select black mascara to emphasize the eyes. Deep pinks and orangey-reds suit the lips.

Fair skin and red hair Redheads usually have fair skin with freckles. The skin will flush and colour easily, probably requiring the application of a green-tinted moisturiser, concealer or face powder. Apply blusher in a warm rose or peach colour. Browns, rusts, greens and peach eye shadow colours suit this skin and complement the eyes. Brown mascara is preferable, to avoid making the eyes appear hard.

For the lips, select a lipstick in peach, golden rust or pink.

Black skin and black hair A yellow-toned foundation is required: it may be necessary to blend foundations to obtain the correct colour. Avoid pink-toned foundations, which make the skin appear chalky.

Women with dark skin tend to have dark brown to brown-black eyes, and can use a wide range of heavily pigmented colours, especially browns and bronzes. Dark shades of blusher in red and plum may be chosen; eyeliner and mascara can be black, or any other dark shade.

Avoid lip colours lighter than the skin tone. A lip liner darker than the lip colour may be used.

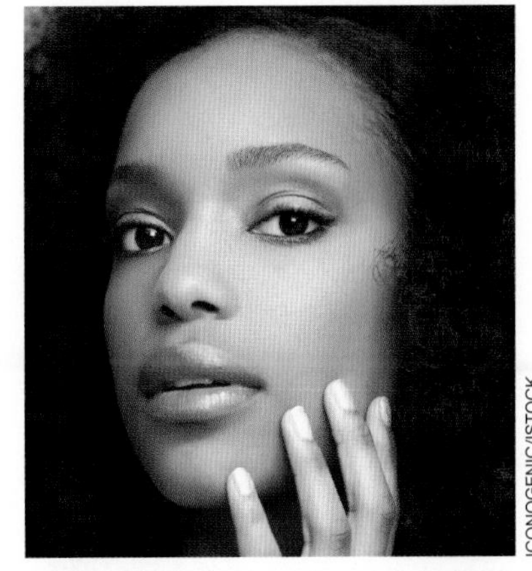

Black skin

Olive or fair skin and dark hair Select a foundation to suit the basic skin tone. If the skin is fair, choose an ivory base; if it is sallow, select a foundation with a rusty, yellow tone. (With a sallow skin, avoid the use of pinks on the eyes – they make the eyes look sore.)

A beige blusher suits this skin colour, and is complemented by the selection of brown or green shades for the eyes. Black mascara should be used for the eyelashes.

For the lips, choose warm reds or beige.

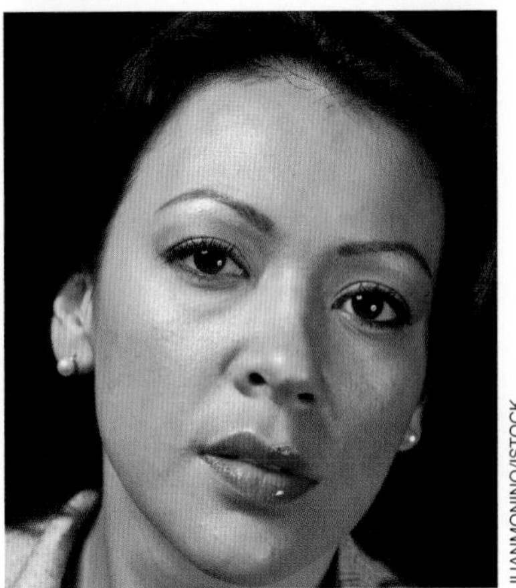

Olive skin

Make-up for mature skin

As the skin ages it becomes sallow in colour and appears thinner. Small capillaries can be seen, commonly on the cheek area, and small veins may appear around the eyes. Pigment changes in the skin become obvious, and remain permanently.

At the make-up consultation, discuss your ideas with your client. Very often a mature client will have been using the same colours and the same cosmetics for many years, and they may not even be complementary. You will need to advise them tactfully on a fresh approach.

Select a foundation that matches the skin colour yet enhances the skin's appearance. An oil-based foundation is appropriate for use on mature skin: it keeps the skin supple and prevents the foundation from settling into the creases and emphasizing the lines and wrinkles.

A concealer may be applied to cover obvious capillaries and small veins, or a foundation may be selected which provides adequate coverage.

A lighter foundation may be applied over wrinkled areas, to make them less obvious. These areas include:

- around the eyes (crow's feet)
- between the brows
- across the forehead
- between the nose and the mouth (nasolabial folds)
- around the mouth (the lip line)

With age, the contours of the face lose their firmness as the fat cells that plump the face reduce, and the facial muscles lose tone and sag. Poor muscle tone can be seen in the following areas:

- the cheek area
- loose skin along the jaw line
- loose skin under the brow and overhanging the lid
- loose skin on the neck

What are the differences in application between day, evening and special occasion make-up?

Need more time... refer to pages 335–336 help you.

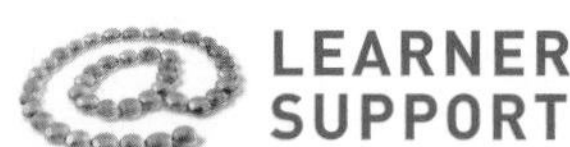

LEARNER SUPPORT

Make-up wordsearch

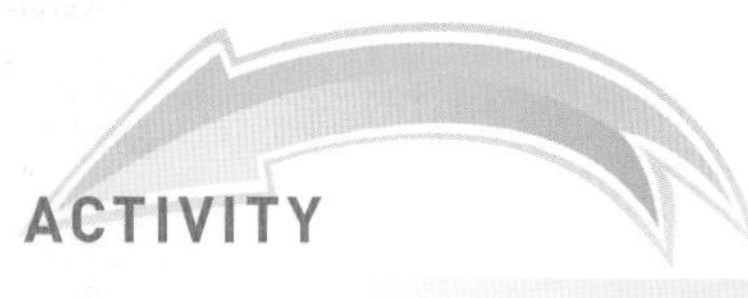

ACTIVITY

Shading

Where would you place the shading product in order to correct poor muscle tone in the areas discussed opposite?

ALWAYS REMEMBER

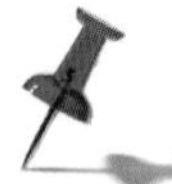

Cream eye shadow

Cream eye shadow settles into creases, which emphasize a crepey eyelid. Frosted or pearlized eye shadows also emphasize a crepey eyelid.

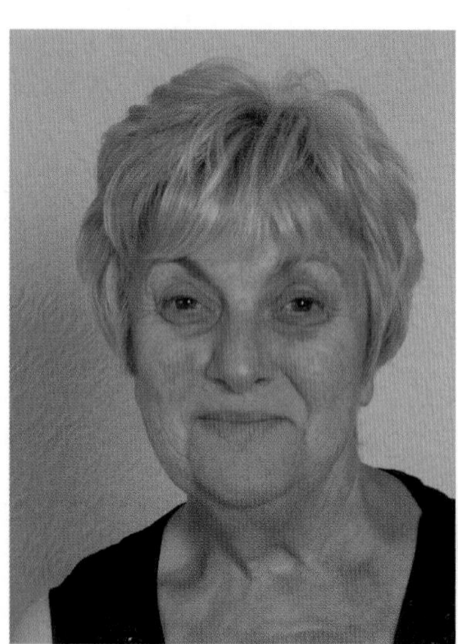

The client's skin has been cleansed, toned, moisturised and blotted to remove excess moisturiser.

ALWAYS REMEMBER

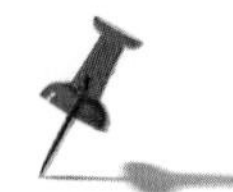

Dark circles under eyes

Dark circles under the eyes can be minimized with concealer. Select a concealer lighter than the foundation to be applied.

The application of a shader, subtly blended, can improve the appearance of such areas. Apply translucent powder. It may be preferable to avoid doing so in the eye area as it can emphasize lines around the eyes. To reduce the powdery effect, which may make the skin appear dry, you may direct a fine water spray from a suitable distance to set the make-up.

Apply a blusher with a warm tone – avoid harsh, bright shades. A cream blusher may be applied after the foundation. Place it high on the cheekbone and blend it upwards at the temples, drawing attention upwards rather than downwards.

The lip line becomes less obvious as one grows older, and lines often appear along it. Lip liner should be applied to redefine the lips and to prevent the lipstick from 'bleeding' into the lines. Select a lip liner that is the same colour as, or slightly lighter than, the lip colour. (A darker lip colour would create an unwanted shadow.) A special lip fixative may be recommended, and a durable cream lipstick applied. Avoid the use of a gloss lipstick, which emphasizes lines around the mouth.

The angle of the mouth may droop. Corrective techniques may be used to disguise this.

Powder matt eye shadows should be selected for use on the eyelid: these soften the appearance of any lines in the area. Choose natural, light shades. Dark colours can make the eyes appear small and tired.

Eyeliner should be used in neutral shades of brown and grey – avoid harsh, bright colours, which will give a hard appearance.

Eyebrows should be perfectly groomed, and arched to give lift to the eye. Bushy eyebrows give the eyes a hooded appearance. If eyebrow colour is required, select a colour that is slightly lighter than the brow colour, or a blend of two colours. If the client has grey hair, use grey and charcoal to provide a natural effect.

Eyelashes should be emphasized with a natural-looking shade of mascara, lightly applied. (If the eyelashes lose their colour, you can recommend that the client has their lashes professionally – and permanently – tinted. Individual false eyelashes may be recommended for corrective purposes.)

Step-by-step: Mature client special occasion make-up application

Make-up is to be applied to a Caucasian client to achieve a glamorous appearance for a social evening. We allowed 45 minutes to achieve this look.

TOP TIP

Positive promotion

If the client is visiting the salon for make-up, you could recommend that they have a professional make-up lesson – at which you could discuss ideas for a fresh approach to their make-up.

The client has dry skin as the sebaceous and sudoriferous glands have become less active as part of the ageing process. Noticeable facial **skin characteristics** include the following.

- Dark circles appear around the eyes area.
- Thin, delicate tissue is found around the eyes with small veins and capillaries showing through the skin.
- Habitual frown lines occur.
- Poor muscle tone has resulted in slack facial contours, e.g. double chin.
- Poor skin tone exists because the skin loses its elasticity, resulting in wrinkling and loss of firmness.
- Sallow skin colour is due to poor blood circulation.

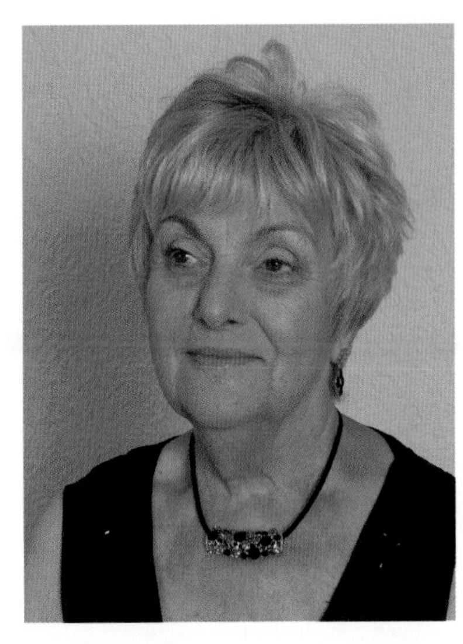

The finished special occasion make-up

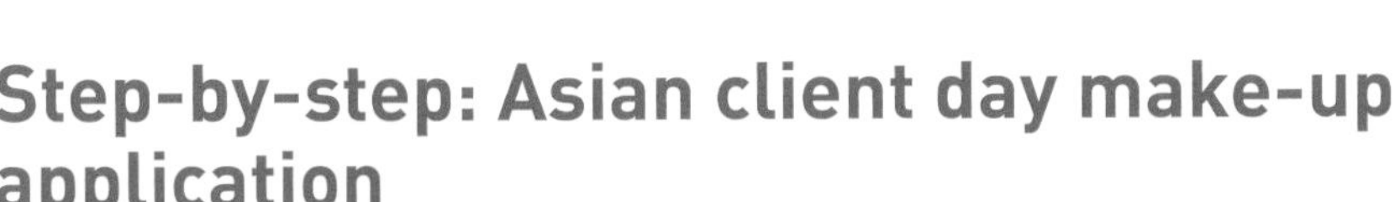

Step-by-step: Asian client day make-up application

Corrective work completed is subtle, as natural daylight makes any imperfections seem more obvious.

The client's skin has been cleansed, toned, moisturised and blotted to remove excess moisturiser. Thirty minutes were allowed to achieve the look.

This is an oily skin type, where over-activity of the sebaceous glands in the skin is creating a shiny, sallow appearance. Darker skin underneath the eye area requires concealer correction.

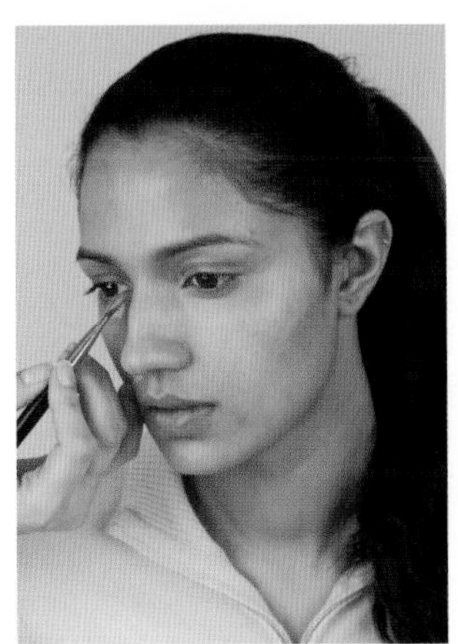

1 A concealer is applied with a brush underneath the eyes to disguise the darker skin tone.

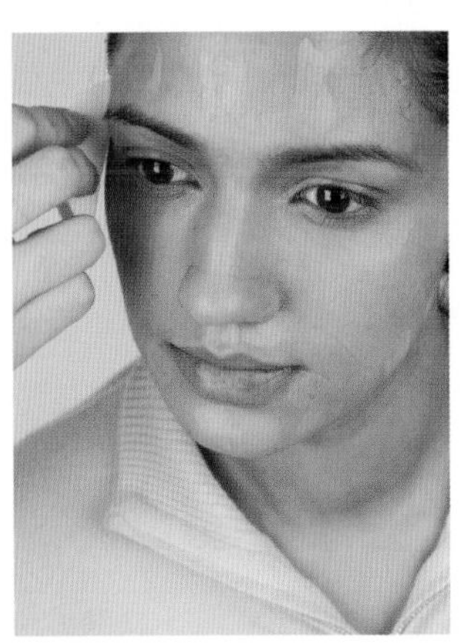

2 A liquid foundation matched to the client's skin tone is applied. Application is over the whole face, including the eyelids and lips, as this gives an even skin tone.

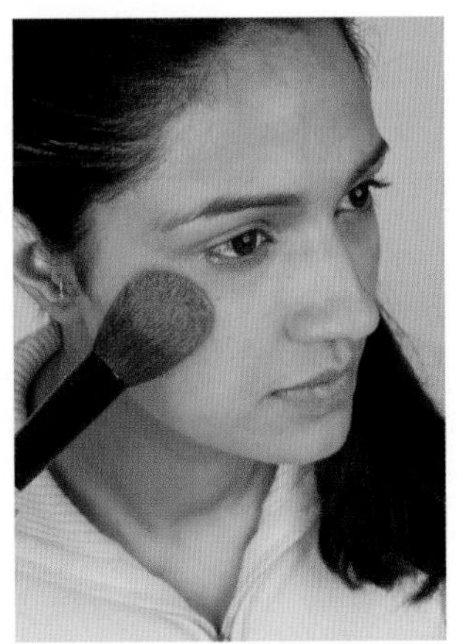

3 Following the application of loose powder, again matched to the client's skin tone, excess powder is removed using a large powder brush. Application is upwards and outwards.

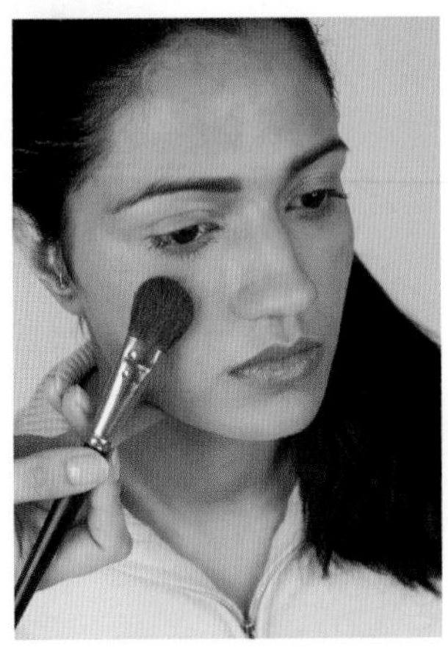

4 Blusher colour is applied to accentuate the cheek area and add colour to the face.

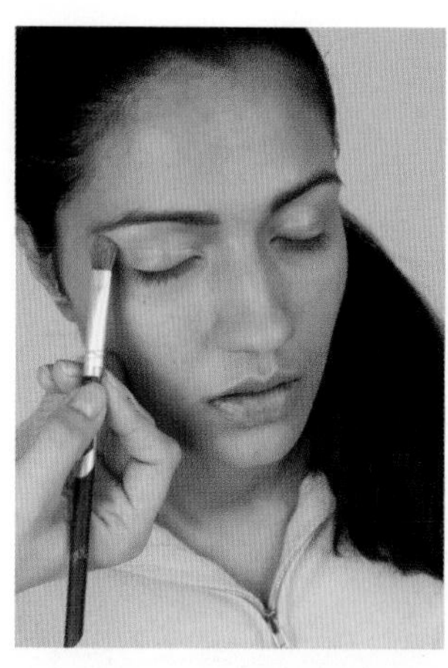

5 Colour applied to the eye emphasizes the eye area. We used complementary colours in a purple range. A highlighting colour accentuates the brow bone.

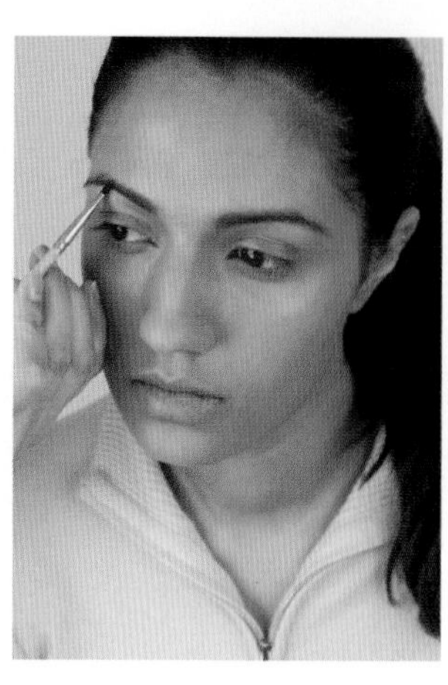

6 The eyebrows are accentuated using a dark matt brown colour applied with a stiff eyebrow brush. This gives definition to the eyebrow, disguising sparse hair and gaps.

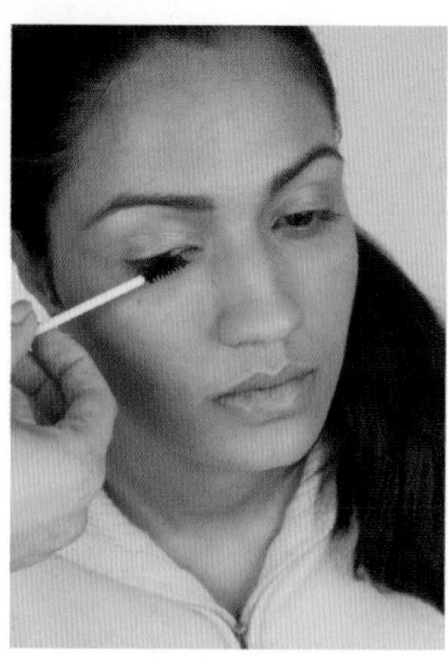

7 The lashes are lengthened using a lash-building mascara in black.

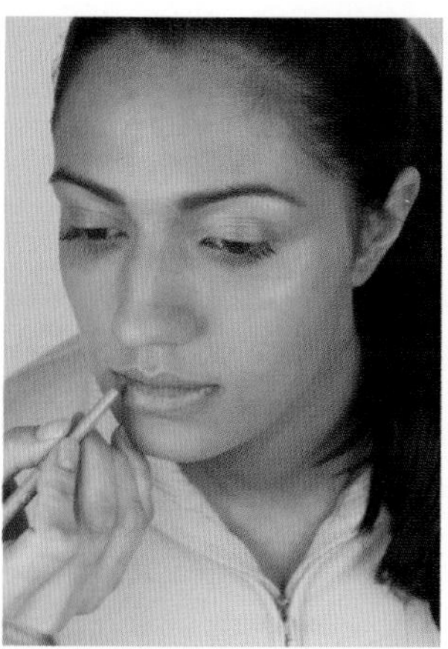

8 Lip liner colour is applied to define the desired lip contour. A co-ordinating lip colour is selected to match the lip liner and complement the eye make-up colour.

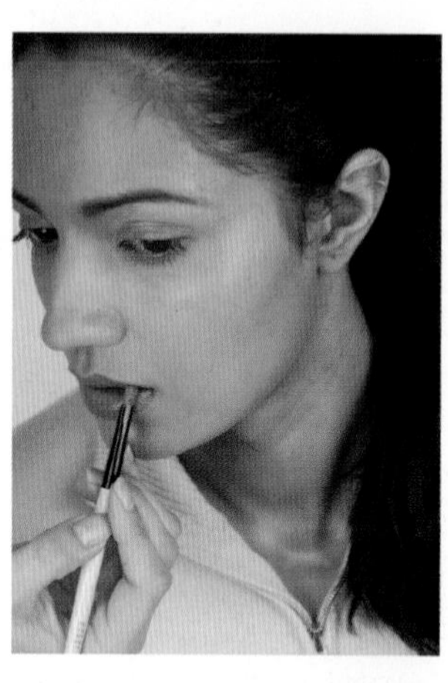

9 The lip colour is applied using a lip brush.

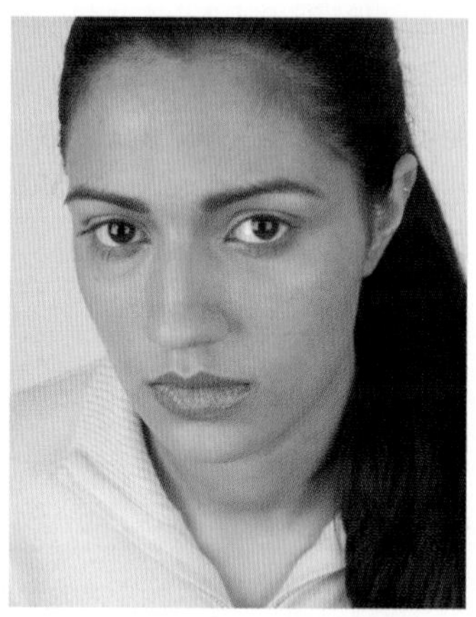

10 The final day make-up look.

Step-by-step: African client evening make-up application

Make-up which will be seen under artificial lighting is applied. Stronger pigmented make-up colours have been selected, and the make-up effect emphasizes facial features through the choice and application of make-up products. Forty-five minutes were allowed to achieve the look.

The client's skin has been cleansed, toned, moisturised and blotted to remove excess moisturiser.

This is a combination skin type and the sebaceous glands are overactive in the T zone – forehead, nose and chin – and the pores appear larger in this area. The sebaceous glands are less active in the cheek, which results in dry skin with tight pores.
Other noticeable facial characteristics include the following:

- the skin tone of the face has uneven pigmentation
- the face shape requires balance, which can be achieved using shaded contour colour

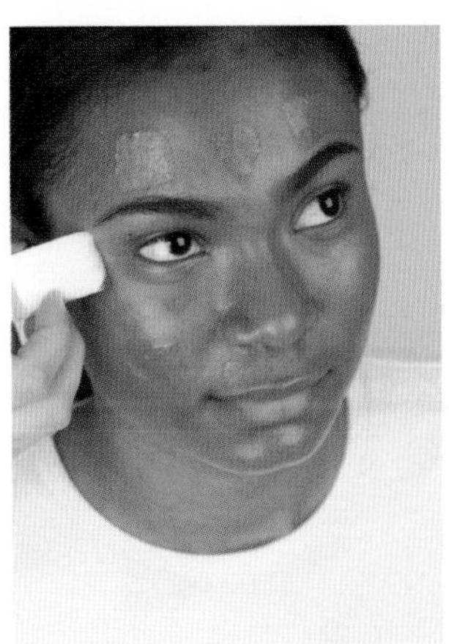

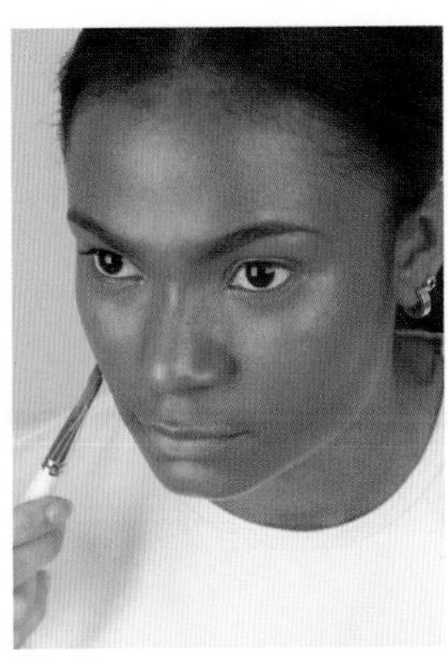

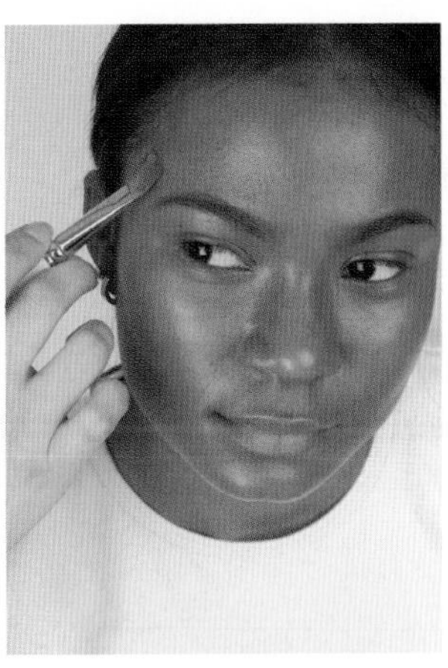

1 Foundation is selected to match the client's skin type and even the skin tone. A mousse foundation has been used to provide a medium coverage and has been blended quickly to avoid a chalky appearance.

2 A cream formulation shading product, in a darker shade than the foundation, is applied underneath the cheekbone and at the temples to accentuate the cheekbones and reduce the width of the face at the temples.

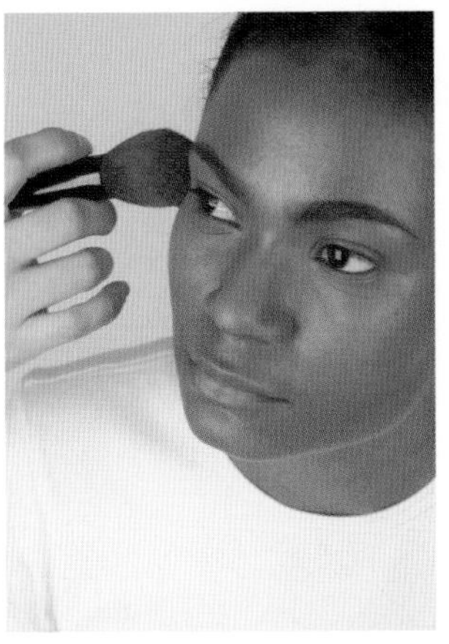

3 Loose powder matching the client's skin tone is applied to set the foundation and facilitate application of further powder products. Powder blusher is applied to the cheekbone.

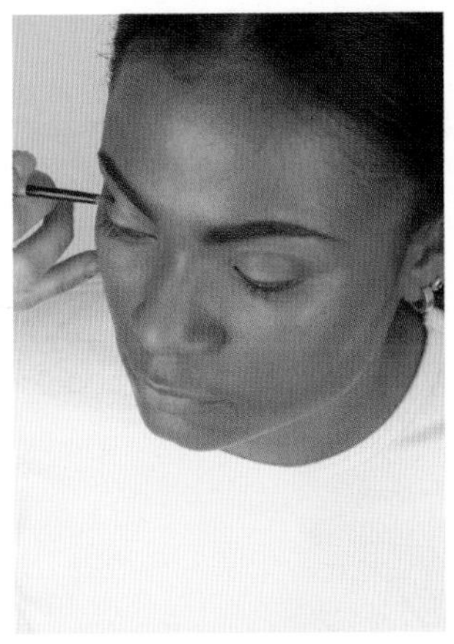

4 Following application of a neutral eye shadow matt colour, a darker shading product is used to emphasize the eye socket.

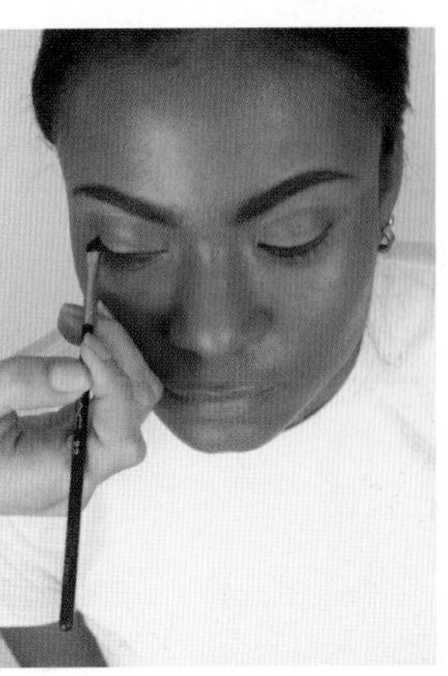

5 The natural lash line is accentuated by eyeliner application. A steady hand is required!

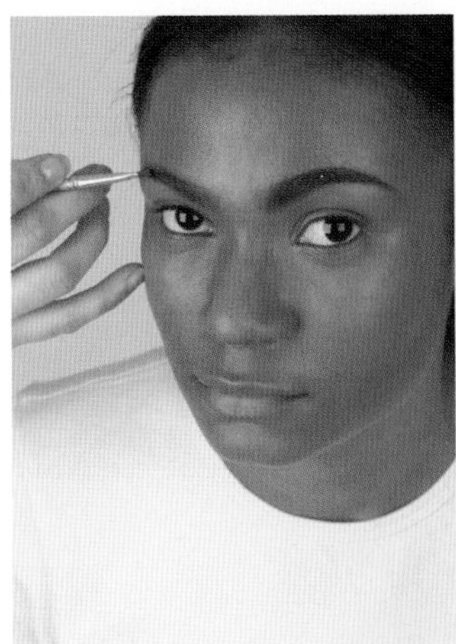

6 The brows are defined.

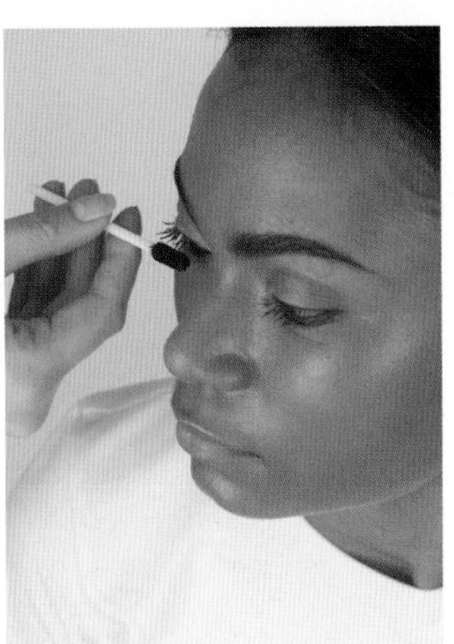

7 Mascara application draws attention to the eyes.

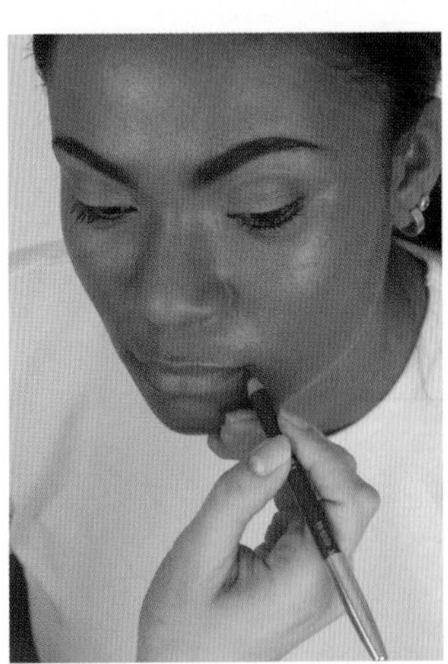

8 Lip liner is applied to define the perfect lip line.

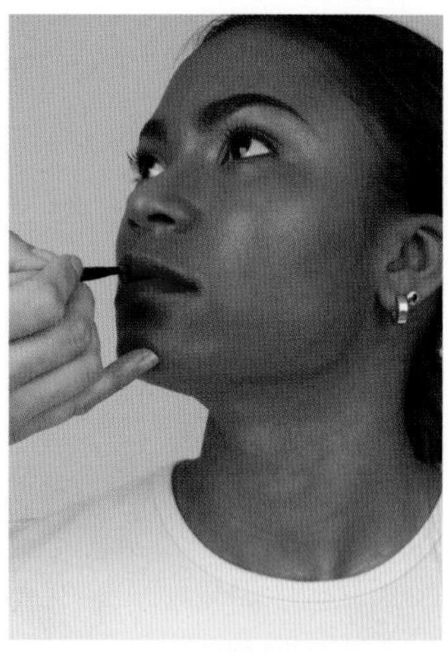

9 The lips are coloured in using a matt lipstick co-ordinated to suit the lip liner. Lip gloss achieves a final touch which will focus attention and add emphasis in darker lighting.

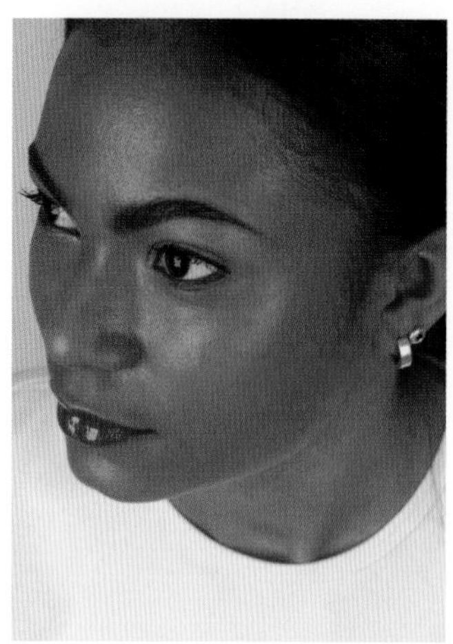

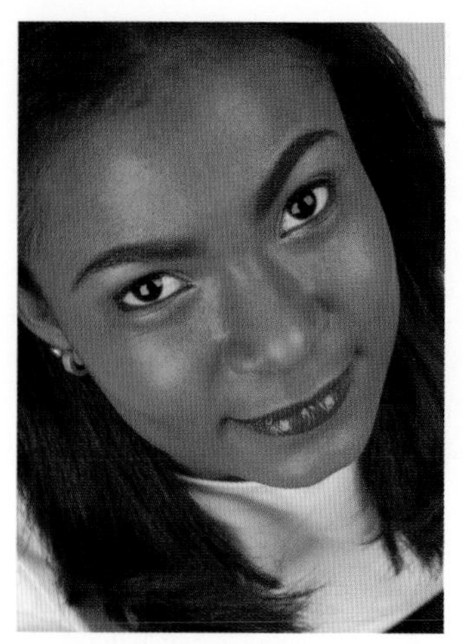

10 The final evening make-up look.

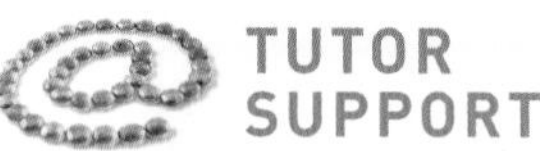

Activity 5: Re-cap, revision and evaluation

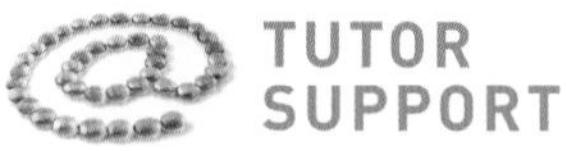

Activity 7: Multiple choice quiz

Developing your make-up ideas

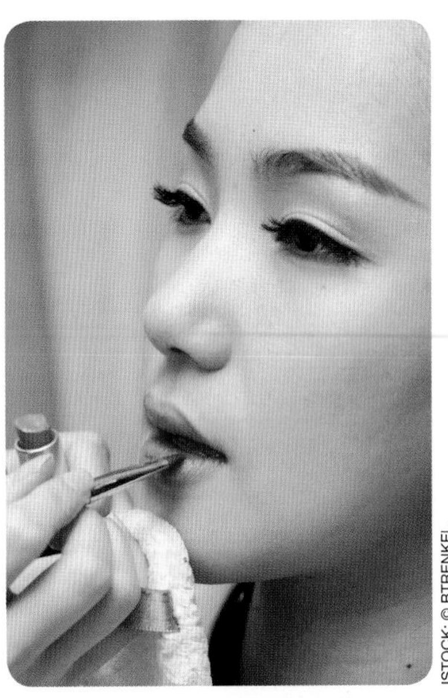

ISTOCK: © BTRENKEL

Learning Objectives

This case study covers **VRQ Unit 212 Create an image based on a theme within the hair and beauty sector**.

This unit is about developing your creative thoughts and ideas and consolidating these in order to present an image based on a theme. The image should be that which you feels best captures and represents the theme and your ideas. You may use this process for the purpose of advertising, and it is interesting to research the influences that led to the creation of different products in the beauty sector and how the final advertising image summarises the concept. The ability to research, plan and create a range of images to a given brief, in conjunction with others is required in this unit. The ability to evaluate the results against the design plan is also required.

To carry out this unit you will need to maintain effective health, safety and hygiene practice throughout your work. You will also need to communicate the design concepts or ideas effectively with others involved in the project.

There are **two** learning outcomes for this unit which you must achieve:

- **Be able to plan an image**
- **Be able to create an image**

From the range statement, you must show you can:

- **develop a mood board based on a theme** which clearly shows your ideas and influences and the research which guided you to create your final image to suit the requirements of the target audience

(continued on the next page)

ANDREA PERRY-BEVAN

ROLE MODEL

Andrea Perry-Bevan

Media and theatrical make-up artist and hair stylist (self-employed)

“I am a media and theatrical make-up artist and hair stylist, specializing in fashion and photographic make-up with 20 years of experience. I attended a three-year hair and beauty therapy course, then gained a theatrical and media qualification. I started out working as a hairdresser in salons part-time to fund my ever-growing kit and to help my career starting up as a media make-up artist. I joined a local model agency who helped me set up test shots to get my portfolio together and slowly gained paid work that way. I have done a lot of travelling, and have been lucky to work on amazing campaigns, editorials and have worked with celebrities. I work closely with photographers on shoot briefs to present to clients to give a better understanding of a final product. This can include gathering a mood board together of images and also a write-up of the connection between key points within the board. One of my career highlights was working with the designer Elizabeth Emanuel on her Archive Collection where I designed make-up and hair to fit in with the styles of the gowns, to add to this I also made headdresses to add to the drama of the look.

- explain the **purpose of a mood board**
- meet all **preparation requirements** for the implementation and presentation of the final theme based image
- **communicate and behave** in an appropriate and professional manner
- use **technical skills** to create a theme based image, for example hairstyling, make-up, nail art and nail enhancements
- follow all **safe and hygienic working practices**
- use different **methods of evaluating** feedback to assess the success of the treatment including observation, written, verbal, photographic and self evaluation

You must be able to show you have the necessary practical skills and underpinning knowledge to create an image based on a theme within the hair and beauty sector.

The unit will help you to plan and provide successful future promotional activities for the workplace. This will require the setting of clear objectives, realistic timescales to work to, attention to detail when planning and effective communication with all those involved with the activities implementation. Finally engaging successfully with your audience to ensure that the promotion is a success and achieves its objectives.

The hair and beauty sector

The world of hair and beauty is an exciting and ever-changing one. It is of the utmost importance to keep up to date with current fashion and trends. What may be fashionable one season can change the next, and quickly look outdated. This unit raises your awareness of how images used in advertising campaigns can raise client awareness of a particular product or treatment intending to increase interest. This unit will enable you to creatively develop images which can best be used to advertise or represent a particular theme. To demonstrate this activity we are going to look at the concepts behind creating and presenting make-up looks.

Outcome 1: Be able to plan an image

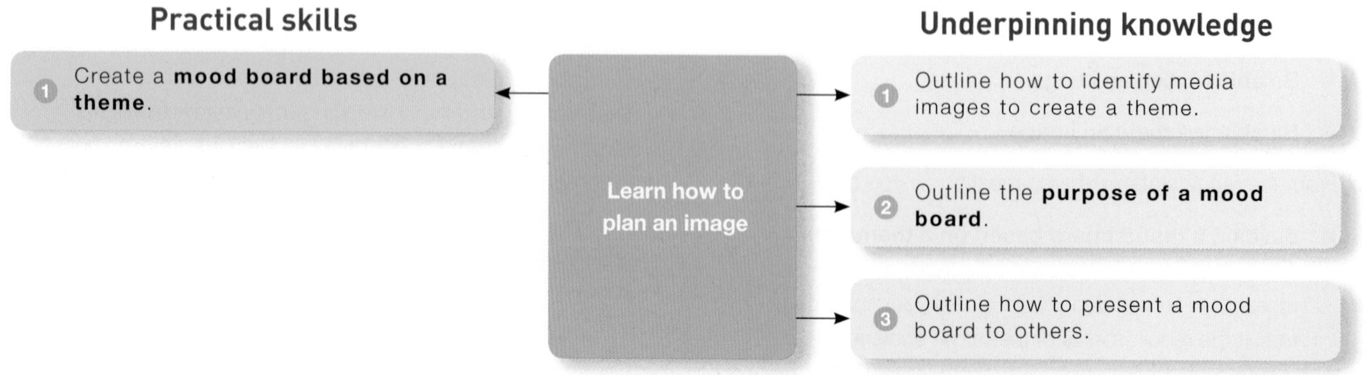
Practical skills
1 Create a **mood board based on a theme**.
Learn how to plan an image
Underpinning knowledge
1 Outline how to identify media images to create a theme.
2 Outline the **purpose of a mood board**.
3 Outline how to present a mood board to others.

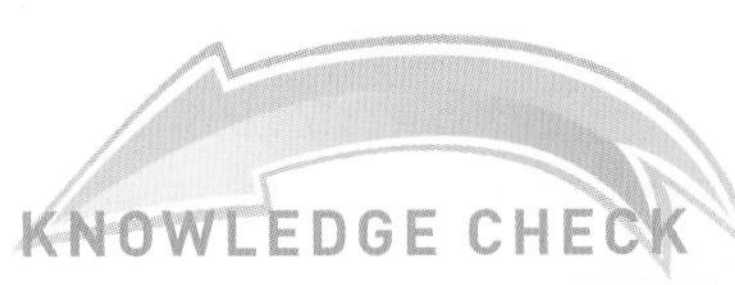

KNOWLEDGE CHECK

What are the health and safety requirements associated with make-up techniques?

Need more time... refer to pages 302–309 to help you.

Underpinning knowledge

(*Continued*) Learn how to plan an image

4 Describe the concepts of advertising to a target audience.

5 Describe the salon's requirements for **client preparation, preparing yourself and the work area**.

Planning an image

In the workplace it is usual for you to work on activities and events with other people. You must therefore develop skills to work closely with other people. It is important to all work towards, and aim for, the same agreed end result. Detailed and accurate planning is important so that no misunderstandings and subsequent waste of resources including time and money.

You may choose to create a period-inspired make-up look or to use your imagination and artistic skills to create a fantasy or high-fashion effect. Photographic commercial make-up is created for advertising purposes and must not detract from the subject/medium being advertised. If it is the make-up being advertised, do not distract from the make-up with too many other fussy accessories. Always consider the design, scale and proportion of the image as a whole. Bridal or special occasion make-up must suit and please the individual wearing it, as well as looking great for photographic purposes. The stages for fashion and special occasion make-up activities will always be similar, although the techniques and finished effects can be quite different. Your work in this area may include make-up looks for catwalk shows, music videos, commercials, bridal and special occasion make-ups.

Plan and design a make-up image based on a theme by:

1. agreeing your ideas and image to be created with the relevant person(s) prior to commencing your design plan
2. clearly identifying the intended themed activity for which the make-up is required
3. using suitable sources of information to research ideas on themes for the make-up design
4. accurately sourcing and using suitable information to create your design
5. creating a design plan which:
   - has clearly defined objectives which meet the requirements of the target audience
   - uses **mood boards** suitable for the look(s) required
   - identifies all resources required
   - states how any risks to health and safety can be reduced
   - takes into account any foreseeable problems and has noted ways of resolving them

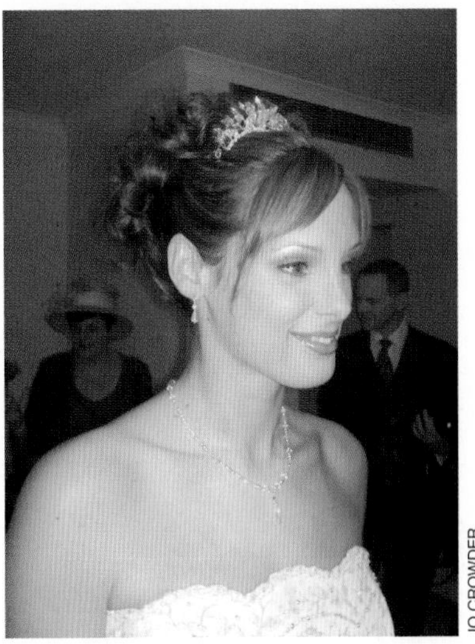

JO CROWDER

Bridal make-up

ACTIVITY

Target audience groups

From your current experience of working in the beauty sector, what target groups could be encouraged to engage with your salon treatments/products? How could you promote this using a theme based image?

HEALTH & SAFETY

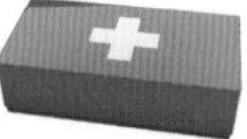

Hazards

- Recognize potential hazards in the workplace and warn other colleagues and clients of them.
- Recognize steps that can be taken to minimize the risk of injury and cross-contamination at any practical activity.

Preparation of products, tools and equipment

Make sure you are prepared, have everything you could possibly need, and that your tools, products and equipment are clean and well organized. Make sure the area is safe, comfortable and clean before you lay out your products, tools and equipment.

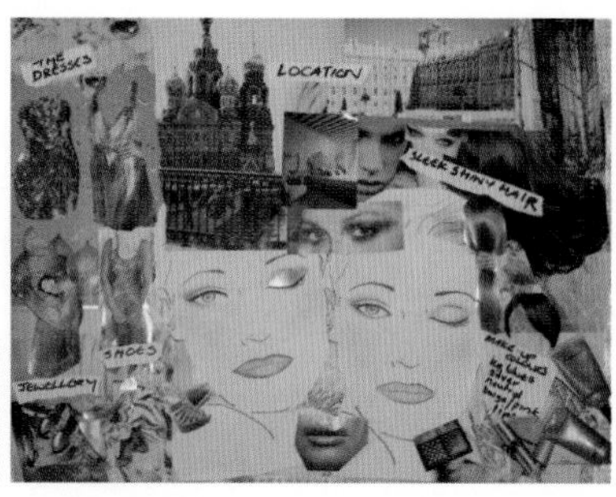

JO CROWDER

A metallic themed mood board

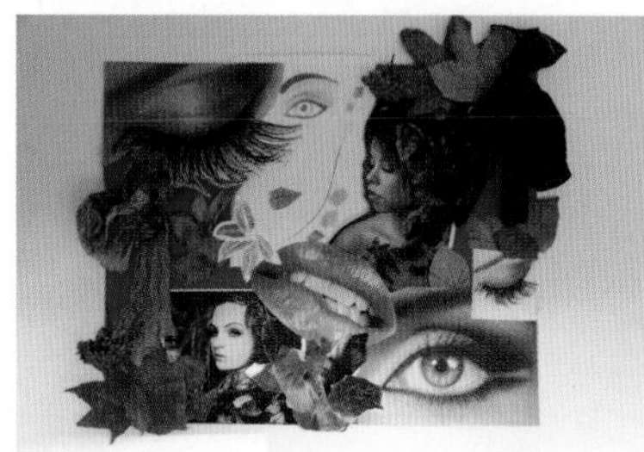

An autumn themed mood board

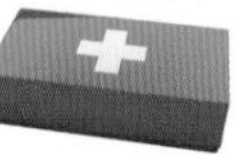

HEALTH & SAFETY

Cosmetics data

Be up to date with health and safety cosmetics data. Look out for certain synthetic colours like FD&C red no.6 and D&C green no.6 which should not be used too close to the eyes or on the lips.

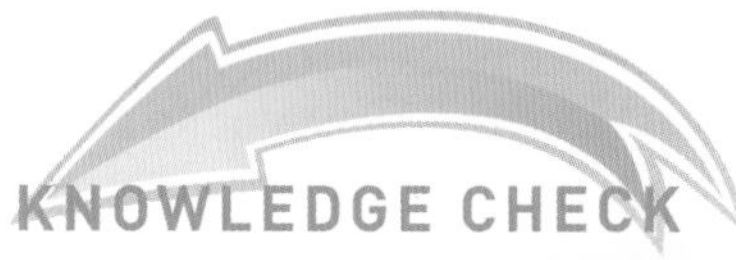

KNOWLEDGE CHECK

Why should you research and plan thoroughly prior to the job and explain how you have created your make-up design plan?

Need more time... refer to page 345 to help you.

When you have completed your make-up, you may need to keep a few products on hand, such as powder and a powder puff, cotton buds, tissues and lip colour required to maintain the make-up look dependant upon the intended purpose of the make-up activity.

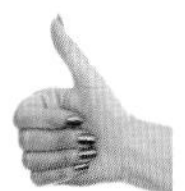

BEST PRACTICE

Keep your client safe

- When planning your make-up, always ask the client if they have any known allergies to cosmetic products.
- Perform a skin sensitivity **patch test** if you have any doubts if using special effects make-up, or are using non-cosmetic products such as gold leaf.
- Become familiar with ingredients in skincare preparations and make-up products and their purpose.
- Use products intended for their purpose, e.g. don't use chunky glitter intended for use on paper near someone's eyes as it will be very abrasive. Only use cosmetic grade glitters.

Mood boards

Having been told or decided upon the theme of the make-up you can then start to prepare and plan your ideas for the final look. This will require you to produce a **mood board,** which presents the ideas you have in mind and what you are trying to create/achieve for the overall image.

Mood boards may be also referred to as concept boards or theme boards. They will help you to express your overall ideas. The result will be a **collation**, or **collage**, of images which have inspired your innovation and creativity. Items may include objects and items such as photographs, fabric swatches and make-up colour samples – anything that has progressed your ideas. The mood board is used to communicate and share ideas with your target audience, who can view it and decide whether they like the concepts represented by the board for the design theme.

Use additional media wherever possible to enhance the final image and complement it, such as painting nails to colour coordinate, along with clothing, accessories (props, headdresses, jewellery) and hairstyling. Carefully chosen accessories can really improve the look of the overall look. Record these ideas on your mood board.

Be creative (as long as you comply with health and safety): products can be adapted to suit effects required, for example you may wish to dilute a creme foundation to make it into a tinted moisturiser, and lipstick could be used on eyelids, etc.

You may need to research extensively for your target audience, using references such as magazines, books and the internet. You must communicate your ideas effectively with the others before you agree to a final design plan and have your work checked over again at the end.

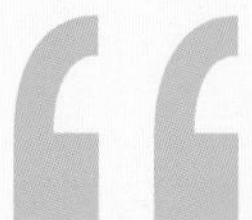

Be adaptable with the team or client you will be working with as many times you will be asked during the job for feedback on how you could improve on the initial brief.

Andrea Perry-Bevan

TOP TIP

Effective communication

- Always be respectful and aware of differences in culture, age, disability and gender. Always strive where practicable to meet the needs of your clients.
- Listen carefully to others, communicate your own ideas, take on board feedback and be prepared to make changes.

TOP TIP

Up your game!

If you are trained and proficient in hairstyling, fashion styling and/or nails, your chances of obtaining work will be increased, especially for smaller make-up assignments or where the budget is limited, as the client only has to pay one fee to one person. It pays to enhance your skills.

Developing images

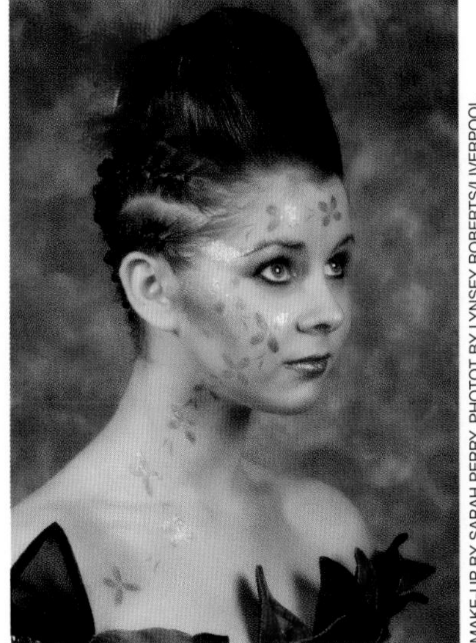

MAKE-UP BY SARAH PERRY, PHOTOT BY LYNSEY ROBERTS/LIVERPOOL

Spring fairy fantasy make-up

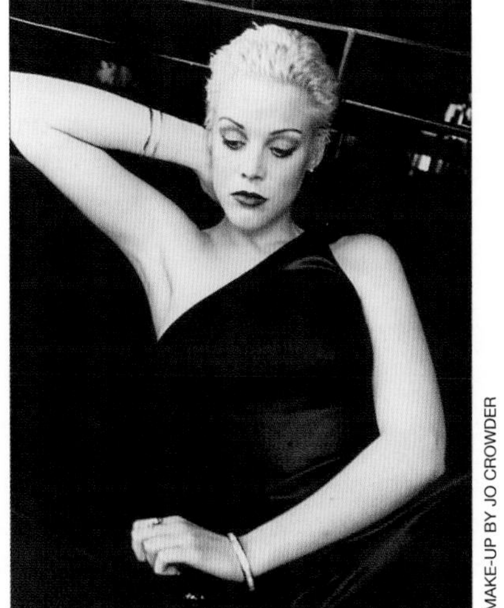

MAKE-UP BY JO CROWDER

Fashion shoot creating the required image/look

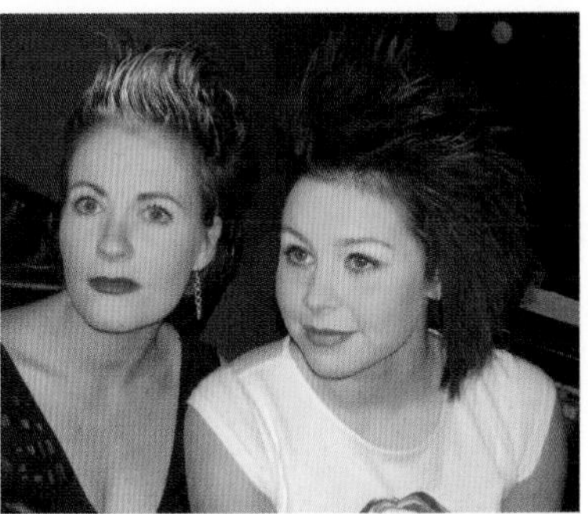

Catwalk make-up

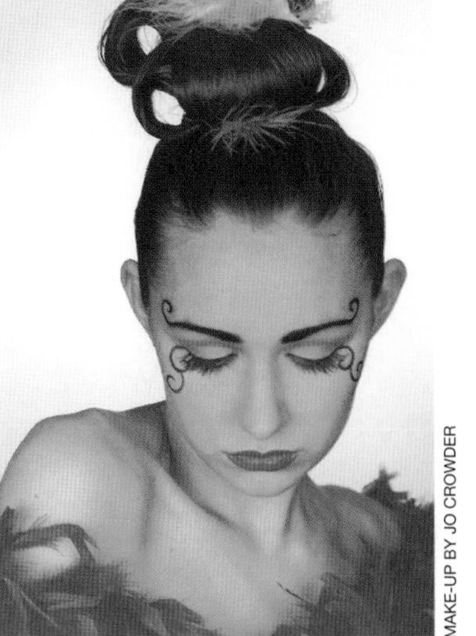

MAKE-UP BY JO CROWDER

Fantasy make-up for cosmetic promotion

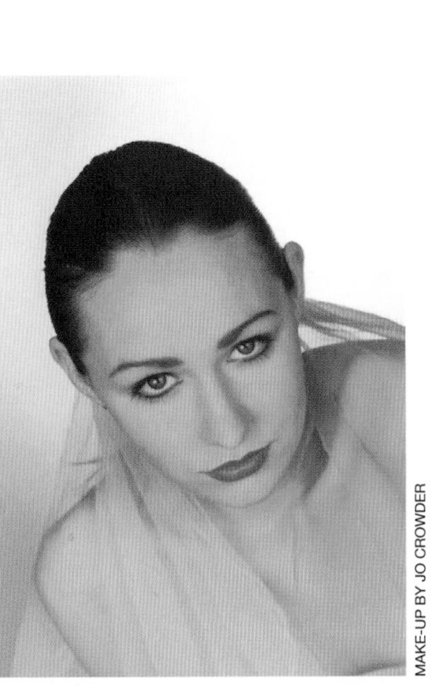

MAKE-UP BY JO CROWDER

Natural make-up for cosmetic promotion

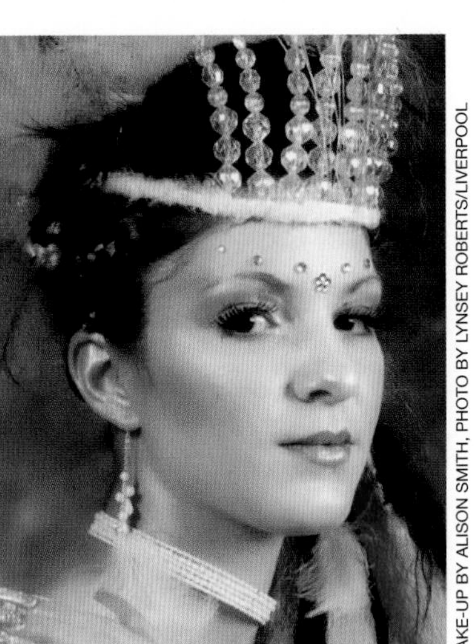

MAKE-UP BY ALISON SMITH, PHOTO BY LYNSEY ROBERTS/LIVERPOOL

Fantasy ice queen with use of additional media

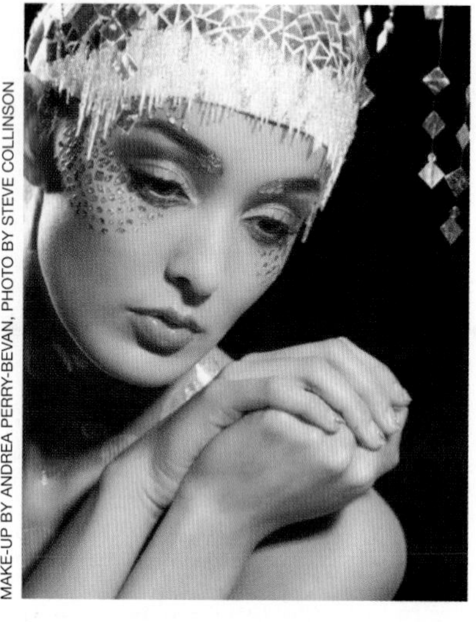

Fantasy with additional media

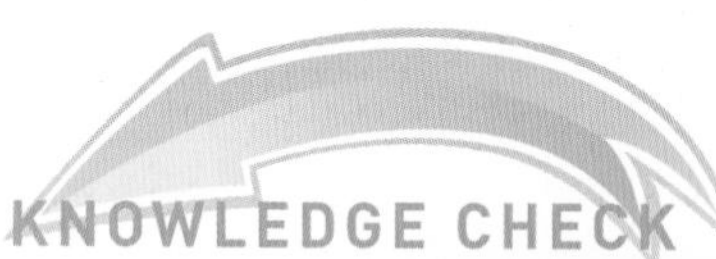

KNOWLEDGE CHECK

Name three contra-indications that could restrict make-up application.

Need more time... refer to page 308 to help you.

HEALTH & SAFETY

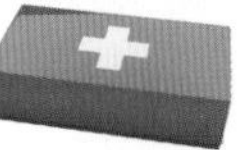

Contra-actions

If **contra-actions** occur, an unwanted reactions from the products, carefully remove make-up immediately and advise your client to seek medical advice if symptoms persist.

ACTIVITY

Research make-up trends from the Ancient Egyptians through to the present day. Include written information on how the make-up was applied, interesting ingredients used and colours worn in each era. Add as many images from each era as you can to build up your own photograph reference library.

Themes

You may need to interpret a theme, e.g. an icy winter scene could imply using colours such as silvers, blues, greys and white. Or you may want a make-up created in brighter colours to 'warm up' a winter's day.

Consider the use of other components apart from the make-up, which will be visible and enhance the overall image. These items are referred to as 'additional media' and include:

- clothing
- hair
- nails
- accessories and props

HEALTH & SAFETY

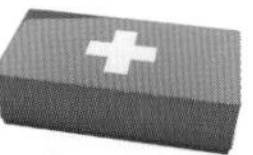

Contra-indications

Check your client for contra-indications. If they have the skin disorder herpes simplex for example, use disposables or their own brushes accompanied with hygienic practices, as you cannot cancel a shoot or wedding because of this!

HEALTH & SAFETY

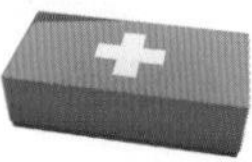

Hygiene

Use hygienic practices – wash hands regularly, and use antibacterial hand cleanser or disposable tissue cloths when on location, use clean gowns, disposable gloves if working on someone with contra-indications, keep tools and equipment clean and sterile, never dip tools straight into make-up – remove with a spatula, wipe down working areas with anti-bacterial cleaner. Try and keep an aseptic working environment. A work situation trying to eliminate bacteria.

Historical make-up looks

If creating an historical look, understanding the basic key make-up application points is important, such as:

- 1920s – pale skin, thin arched eyebrows, rounded eye shadow, blusher on the apples of the cheeks, red to dark red cupids bow style lips.
- 1940s – strong emphasis on the eyebrow shape and lips, typically lipstick was red.
- 1950s – strong angled eyebrows, thicker liner along the top eyelid, more eye shadow and lip colours available. Bright red glossy lips were popular.
- 1960s – pale skin, pale lipsticks, strong contouring in the eye socket in contrast with pale color on the eyelid with the addition of heavy artificial eyelashes.
- 1970s – from disco glam, glitter and gloss, through to early punk at the other end of the scale.
- 1980s – strong make-up applied to the cheekbones, eyes and lips using multiple vibrant colours on the eyes. Mineral pigments were popular and used to create metallic colors for the lips and eyes.

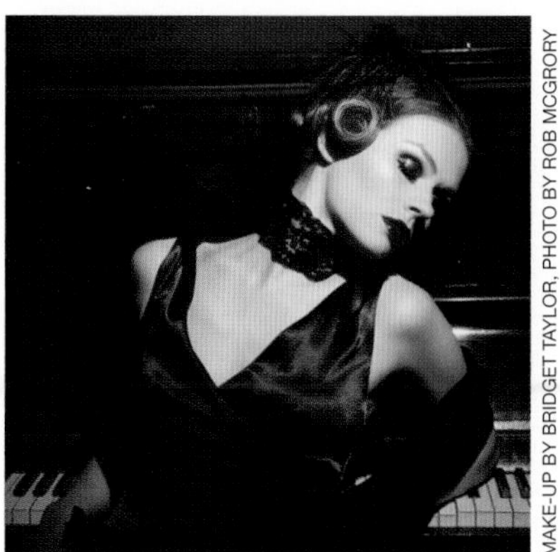
MAKE-UP BY BRIDGET TAYLOR, PHOTO BY ROB MCGRORY

1920s make-up

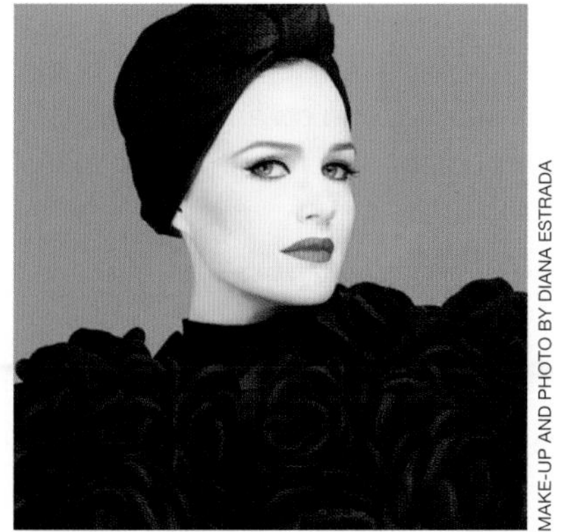
MAKE-UP AND PHOTO BY DIANA ESTRADA

1940s make-up

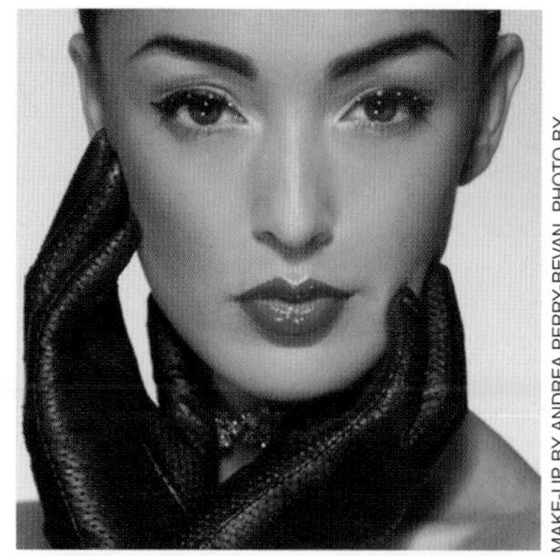
MAKE-UP BY ANDREA PERRY-BEVAN, PHOTO BY STEVE COLLINSON

1950s make-up

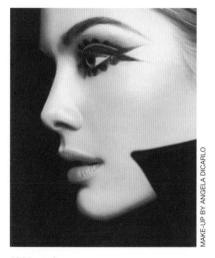
MAKE-UP BY ANGELA DICARLO

1960s make-up

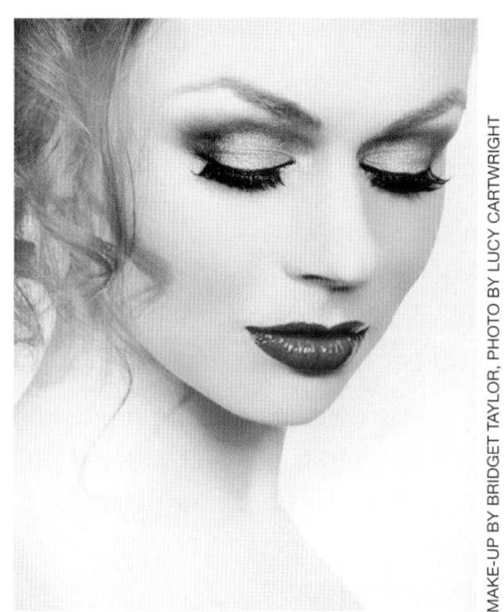
MAKE-UP BY BRIDGET TAYLOR, PHOTO BY LUCY CARTWRIGHT

1970s make-up

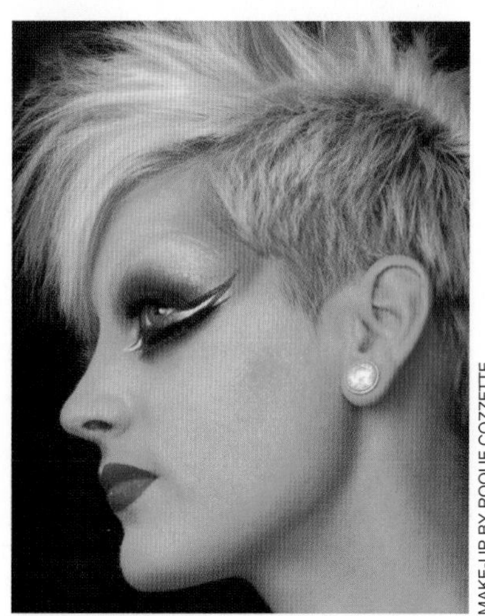
MAKE-UP BY ROQUE COZZETTE

1980s make-up

Creating the final look

Invariably, you will work with other colleagues (like hair stylists) to create your final look, therefore good communication is important to ensure the overall look/effect is achieved. Distance and lighting need to be taken into consideration to please the relevant people viewing your work, for example, consider the differences between make-up competition judges who will scrutinize your work in close up, or audiences at a catwalk show who will view work from a distance – usually under stronger and coloured lighting effects.

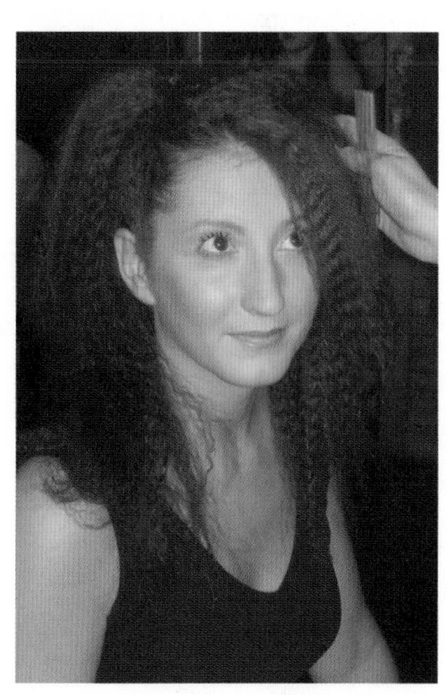

Make sure you have acquired any relevant props, make-up and hair equipment in preparation. If you need any other additions to your kit, allow plenty of time to source them, contacting relevant suppliers. Make-up products and equipment can be sourced from professional make-up suppliers and department stores. Additional items such as lace, feathers, gems, etc. can be sourced from art, haberdashery and fabric stores.

If the client has not had their make-up done by another person before, explain the procedure to reassure the client and make them feel comfortable.

You may wish to practice in advance and take your own photographs to check the make-up and, if styled, the hair. Digital cameras enable you to see results instantly. You can print these out and place them on your mood board. Evaluate the look and and its overall effectiveness, making any changes required. Make sure you have time and are able to adapt your design plan if any circumstances change.

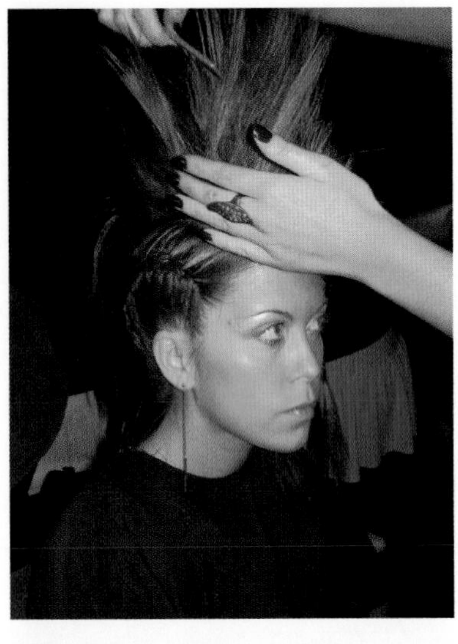

Adding finishing touches to the hair

As a result of evaluation through self evaluation, photographic evidence etc., you may see an opportunity to develop the initial image slightly. If you are working with a team, check with them before you go ahead and change anything as it is important that everybody is aware and in agreement with the change.

Retouching images

You should also be aware that today images are commonly 'retouched' or 'airbrushed', where the image taken is altered, often by the photographer or a graphic artist on a computer, generally using a 'Photoshop' programme, after the shots have been taken.

Retouching has been common practice for many years and you will find that most images in glossy magazines have undergone this process. This procedure explains images of people with completely flawless skin, lack of under eye shadows, wrinkles, slimline body, etc. Even the best make-up artist in the world cannot create that sort of magic!

You should, however, always aim for perfection using your make-up skills and never rely on your image being retouched afterwards.

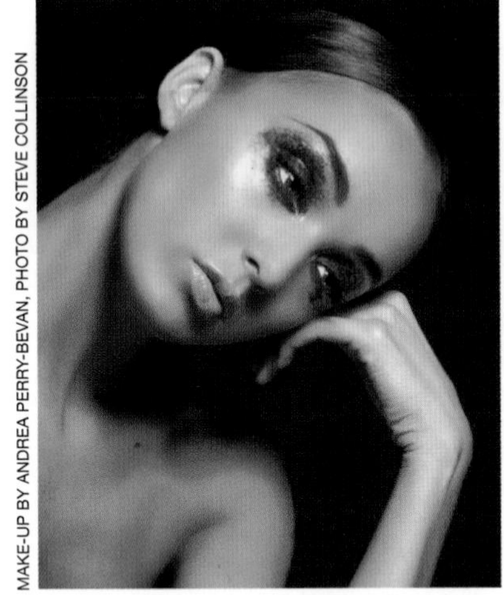

MAKE-UP BY ANDREA PERRY-BEVAN, PHOTO BY STEVE COLLINSON

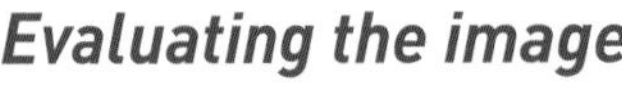

Evaluating the image

- Welcome feedback both positive and negative. Evaluate your make-up results. Ask for feedback from others as to the overall effectiveness and impact of your make-up, checking that it is conforming to the original design plan. If you are not 100 per cent sure of something, ask 'What do you think about this?'
- For your own self-development, check, evaluate and compare the development process and final result with the original themed image to identify opportunities for improvement in your design and application techniques. Is there anything you could have improved on? How? Have you used the products correctly to get the desired outcome?
- The final design should contribute to your professional profile.

Record the results of your evaluation for future reference. When you see the final image check everything carefully again.

Outcome 2: Be able to plan an image

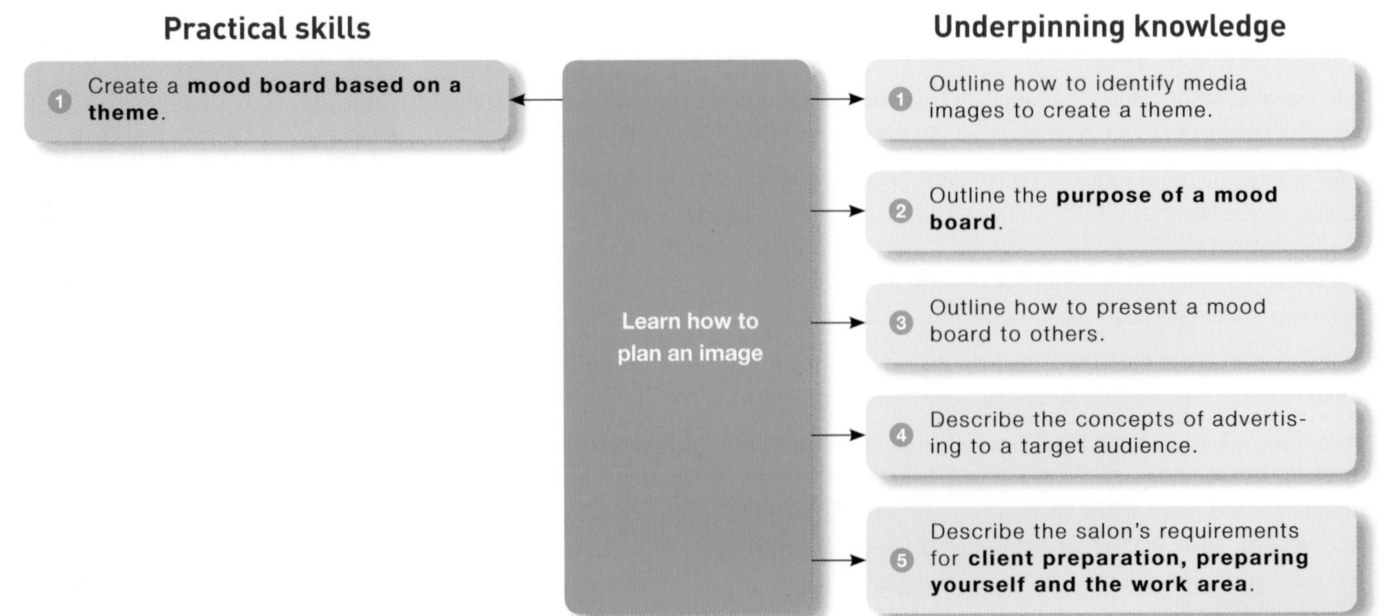

Practical skills
1 Create a mood board based on a theme.
Learn how to plan an image
Underpinning knowledge
1 Outline how to identify media images to create a theme.
2 Outline the purpose of a mood board.
3 Outline how to present a mood board to others.
4 Describe the concepts of advertising to a target audience.
5 Describe the salon's requirements for client preparation, preparing yourself and the work area.

Case study: Create an image based on a theme

Prepare and plan to create an image based on a theme. A make-up activity has been suggested but a choice could be made from any practical task within the hair and beauty sector.

- Develop a theme based make-up of your choice. Suggestions for consideration include future catwalk trends; period make-up; special occasion make-up; make-up for a product advertisement or make-up suitable for a competition brief (which you could enter!).
- Create a mood board to record your ideas and provide evidence of your research. Ensure this includes details of any additional media that you may be using.
- Do you have a budget to work to? If so, record what this is and itemise your expenditure.
- Provide a make-up work sheet that records the make-up products and application techniques you will use.
- Provide a brief description explaining and justifying how your make-up look promotes the chosen theme. Or, explain what the product stands for if it is to be used for an advertisement.
- Agree your final design plan with the relevant person/s and record their comments for evaluative purposes. It may be necessary to make amendments. Note any changes made and the reasons for these changes.

Complete the make-up

- Complete the make-up, meeting all safety and hygiene requirements.
- Take pictures of the final result and evaluate its effectiveness.
- If necessary make any changes and update your worksheet. Inform the relevant person/s of any changes made.
- Gather feedback from the relevant person/s; again you may want to make changes.

Summarise the success of the activity

- Where the objectives of the activity met?
- If working to a budget did you achieve this?
- Are you going to develop and use your image in the future?
- How could the idea be developed further?
- What have you learned or what experience have you gained?
- Did you encounter any issues and how were these were dealt with?

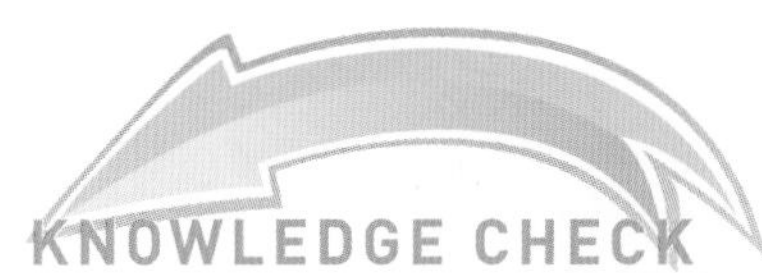

How would you identify the effectiveness of your theme based image and areas for improvement?

Need more time... refer to page 350 to help you.

GLOSSARY OF KEY WORDS

Aftercare advice recommendations given to the client following treatment to continue the benefits of the treatment.

Age groups the different classification of age groups: 16–30, 31–50 and over 50 years.

Artifical eyelashes threads of nylon fibre or real hair attached to the natural eyelash hair. There are two main types: individual or strip.

Blusher cosmetic applied to add warmth to the face and emphasize the facial contours.

Bronzing products make-up products applied to create a healthy, natural or subtle tanned look. They are formulated to create a matt or shimmer effect and are also suitable as a highlighting contouring product.

Cleanser a skincare preparation that removes dead skin cells, excess sweat and sebum, make-up and dirt from the skin's surface to maintain a healthy skin complexion. These are formulated to treat the different skin types, skin characteristics and facial areas.

Colour corrector make-up product applied to target problem areas. It contains pigments which balance skin tone.

Concealer cosmetic product used to disguise minor skin imperfections such as blemishes, uneven skin colour or shadows.

Consultation assessment of client's needs using different assessment techniques, including questioning and natural observation.

Contour cosmetics applied to cosmetically change and enhance the shape of the face and facial features.

Contra-action an unwanted reaction occurring during or after treatment application.

Contra-indication a problematic symptom that indicates that the treatment may not proceed or may restrict treatment application. Contra-indications identified for facial treatments are discussed in more detail in Chapter 3.

Equipment tools used within a make-up.

Eyebrow colour cosmetic applied to emphasize the eyebrows, alter their shape, and which can make sparse eyebrows look thicker.

Eyeliner cosmetic applied to define and emphasize the eye area.

Eye shadow cosmetic applied to the eye to complement the natural eye colour, to give definition to the eye area and enhance the natural shape of the eye.

Face shape the size and shape of the facial bone structure. Face shapes include oval, round, square, heart, diamond, oblong and pear.

Facial features the size of a person's nose, eyes, forehead, chin, neck, etc. When applying make-up products, make-up application can emphasize or minimize the appearance of facial features.

Foundation a make-up product applied to produce an even skin tone, to disguise minor skin blemishes and as a contour cosmetic.

Highlighter a make-up product that draws attention to and emphasizes features.

Hyperpigmentation increased pigment production.

Hypopigmentation loss of pigmentation.

Lip balm a lip moisturiser which may contain pigment.

Lip gloss cosmetic applied to the lips to provide a moist, shiny look.

Lip liner cosmetic used to define the lips, creating a perfectly symmetrical outline.

Lip stain make-up product which adds intense colour to the lips.

Lipstick cosmetic applied to the lips to add colour and keep the lips soft and supple.

Make-up cosmetics applied to the skin of the face to enhance and accentuate, or to minimize facial features. Make-up products create balance in the face.

Make-up products different cosmetics available to suit skin type, colour and condition, e.g. sensitive or mature. Make-up products include concealing and contour cosmetics, foundations, translucent powders, eye shadows, eyeliners, brow liners, mascaras, lipsticks, lip glosses, lip liners, etc.

Mascara cosmetic that enhances the natural eyelashes, making them appear longer, changed in colour and/or thicker.

Mineral make-up is created from finely ground minerals (a process called micronization). It is used in the formulation of different make-up products.

Minor a person classed as a child who requires by law to have a guardian or adult present.

Moisturiser a skincare preparation whose formulation of oil and water helps maintain the skin's natural moisture by locking in moisture, offering protection and hydration. The formulation is selected to suit the skin type, facial characteristics and facial area.

Mood board a collation or collage of images which have inspired or instigated innovation and creativity used to express your overall ideas. A mood board may include objects such as photographs, fabric swatches, make-up colour samples or anything else that has progressed your ideas.

Necessary action the action taken to deal safely with a contra-action or contra-indication.

Pigment the colour of skin and hair, called melanin. The amount of pigment varies for each client, resulting in different skin and hair colour.

Powder cosmetic applied to set the foundation, disguise minor skin blemishes and make the skin appear smoother and oil-free.

Primer provides a base for make-up and acts as a barrier preventing absorption of the make-up products into the skin.

Promotion ways of communicating products or treatments to clients to increase sales.

Record cards confidential records recording personal details of each client registered at the salon.

Shader a make-up product that draws attention away from and minimizes certain facial features.

Skin characteristics while looking at the skin type, additional characteristics may be seen. These include skin that may be sensitive, dehydrated, moist or oedematous (puffy), in addition to dry, oily or combination.

Skin tone the strength and elasticity of the skin.

Skin type the different physiological functioning of each person's skin dictates their skin type. There are four main skin types: normal (balanced), dry (lack of oil), oily (excessive oil) and combination (a mixture of two skin types, e.g. dry and oily).

Toning lotion a skincare preparation formulated to treat the different skin types: and facial characteristics. It is applied to remove all traces of cleanser from the skin. It produces cooling and skin-tightening effects.

Treatment objectives the context the make-up is to be applied for, i.e. day, evening and special occasion.

Treatment plan after the consultation, suitable treatment objectives are established to treat the client's conditions and needs.

ASSESSMENT OF KNOWLEDGE AND UNDERSTANDING

You have now learnt the knowledge and skills required for applying make-up in the beauty therapy workplace. To test your level of knowledge, answer the following short questions. These will prepare you for your summative (final) assessment.

1. A facial feature to be diminished (made to appear less noticeable) would require the application of:
   a. highlighter contour product
   b. powder product
   c. shader contour product
   d. blusher contour product
2. If the client has large, full lips, such as the ones below, how can these be made to appear smaller?

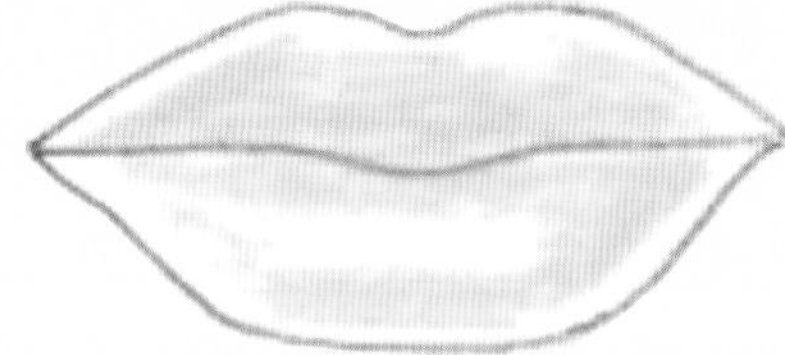

3. The most suitable brush to apply eyeshadow to cover the upper eyelid is:
   a. eyeliner brush
   b. medium firm eyeshadow blending brush
   c. small rounded-edged eyeshadow brush
   d. small flat-angle edged eyeshadow brush
4. To test the colour of the foundation you should test it:
   a. on the client's forehead
   b. on the back of the client's hand
   c. on the client's jawline
   d. on the client's cheekbone
5. If a cream blusher is to be applied, it should be applied:
   a. after the application of foundation
   b. after the application of powder
6. The following image shows dark circles under the eyes, these would be improved with the application of a __________ product.

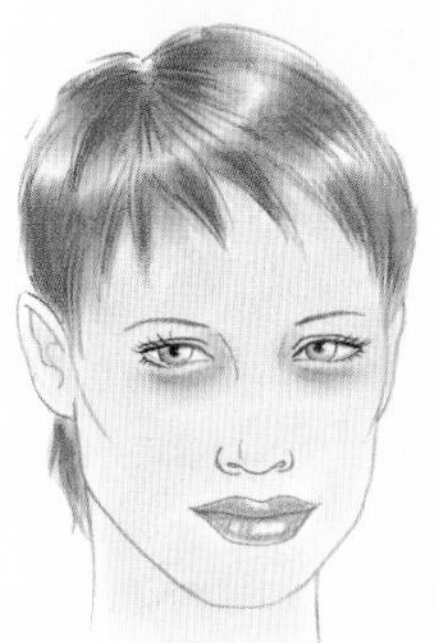

7. The client below has a narrow jaw line. How can this be improved to look fuller?

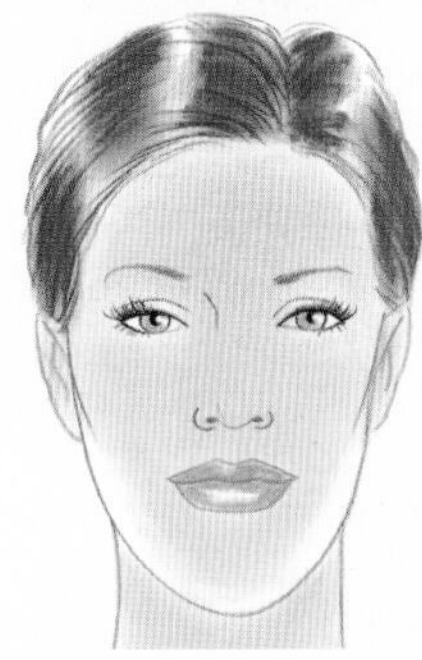

8. A contra-action to make-up application may result in:
   a. an allergic reaction
   b. severe eczema
   c. a dry skin type
   d. erythema
9. The contour product blusher is applied to emphasize the following bones:
   a. parietal
   b. zygomatic
   c. maxilla
   d. tibia
10. The muscle that raises the eyebrows is the:
    a. platysma
    b. orbicularis occuli
    c. corrugator
    d. frontalis

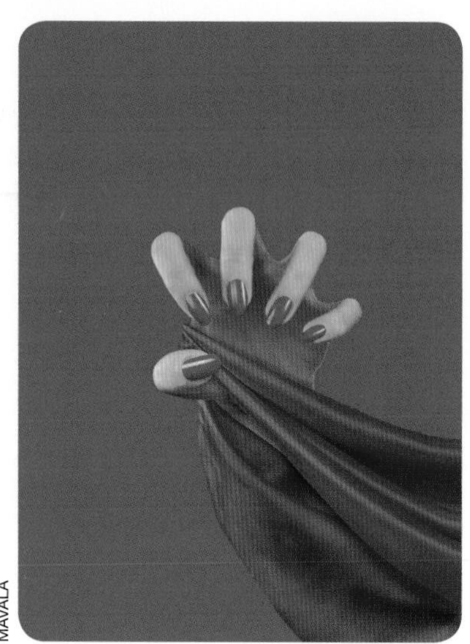
MAVALA

11 Manicure Treatments

Learning Objectives

This chapter covers **VRQ Unit Provide manicure treatments**.

This unit is all about improving and maintaining your client's hands, nails and surrounding skin. A manicure includes filing the nails to shape, buffing the nail plate surface, using specialized nail products, cuticle products and treatments, massaging the lower arm and hand and providing a complementary nail finish to suit the client.

There are **two** learning outcomes for this unit which you must achieve competently:

1 **Be able to prepare for manicure treatments**

2 **Be able to provide manicure treatments**

From the range statement, you must show you can:

- use **consultation techniques** to identify the treatment **objectives**
- use **products, tools and equipment** as appropriate
- treat all **skin types and nail conditions**
- ensure that the **environmental conditions** are suitable
- identify **contra-indications**
- **communicate and behave** in an appropriate and professional manner

(continued on the next page)

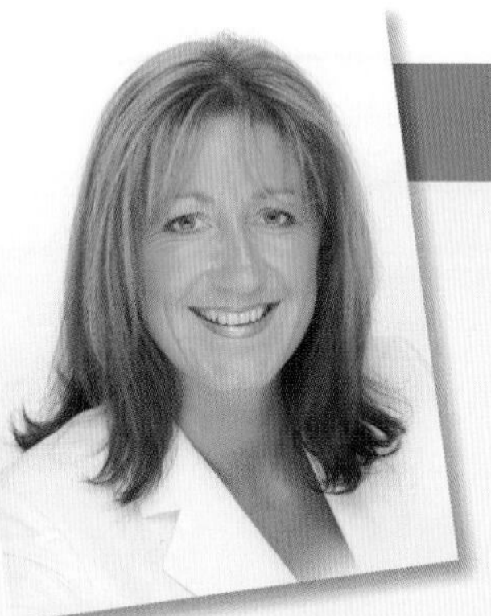

ROLE MODEL

Jacqui Jefford

Consultant and freelance session nail technician

"I have been in the nail and beauty industry for over 25 years, and am one of the leading figures in the industry in the UK and internationally. My work has taken me to many countries as a consultant in education, competitions (winning, designing and judging them), taking educational seminars and working in PR, TV and with the consumer press. I also have my salon, school and distribution company, and work with many FE colleges as a tutor, assessor and internal verifier. I have particularly enjoyed working at London and Paris Fashion Weeks as well as decorating the covers of top magazines such as Vogue. I have written four successful books and been involved in five DVDs. My passion has always been good education and I have worked alongside Habia on many projects over the last ten years.

- apply **massage techniques**
- follow all **health and safety working practices**
- provide relevant **aftercare** and **contra-action advice**

You must be able to show you have the necessary practical skills and underpinning knowledge to provide manicure treatments.

This unit is linked to the Beauty Therapy NOS **Unit N2.**

What are the functions of blood?

Need more time... refer to page 80 to help you.

Essential anatomy and physiology knowledge requirements for this unit are identified on the checklist chart in Chapter 2, page 27.

Manicure treatments

The word **manicure** is derived from the Latin words *manus*, meaning 'hand', and *cura*, meaning 'care'. A manicure therefore cares for the hands for the following reasons:

- to improve the hands' appearance
- to keep the nails smooth
- to keep the cuticles attractive and healthy
- to keep the skin soft

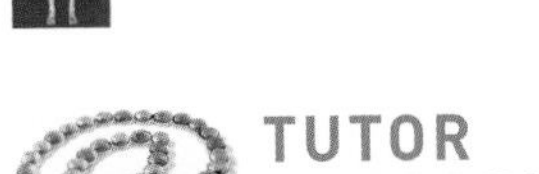

Activity 1: label the nail structure

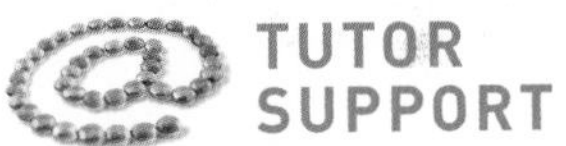

Activity 2: label the bones of the arm and hand

Preparing for the manicure

Outcome 1: Be able to prepare for manicure treatments

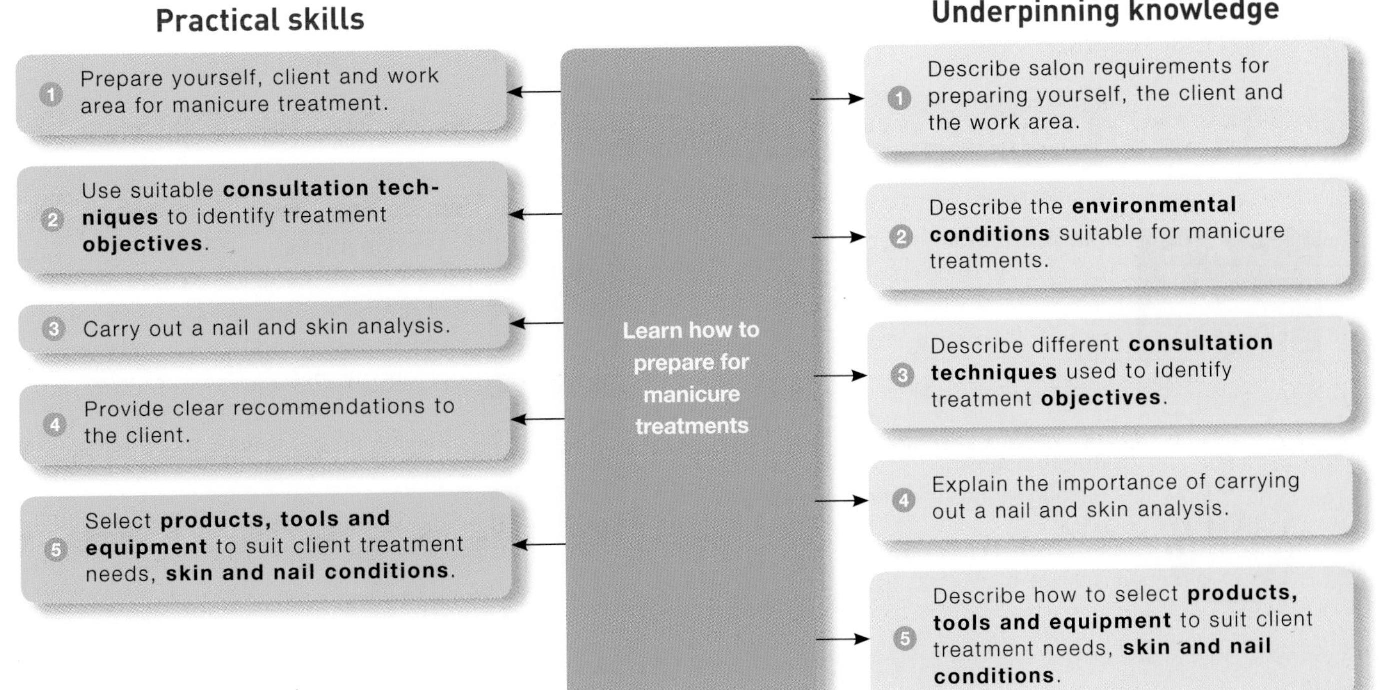

Practical skills
1 Prepare yourself, client and work area for manicure treatment.
2 Use suitable consultation techniques to identify treatment objectives.
3 Carry out a nail and skin analysis.
4 Provide clear recommendations to the client.
5 Select products, tools and equipment to suit client treatment needs, skin and nail conditions.
Learn how to prepare for manicure treatments
Underpinning knowledge
1 Describe salon requirements for preparing yourself, the client and the work area.
2 Describe the environmental conditions suitable for manicure treatments.
3 Describe different consultation techniques used to identify treatment objectives.
4 Explain the importance of carrying out a nail and skin analysis.
5 Describe how to select products, tools and equipment to suit client treatment needs, skin and nail conditions.

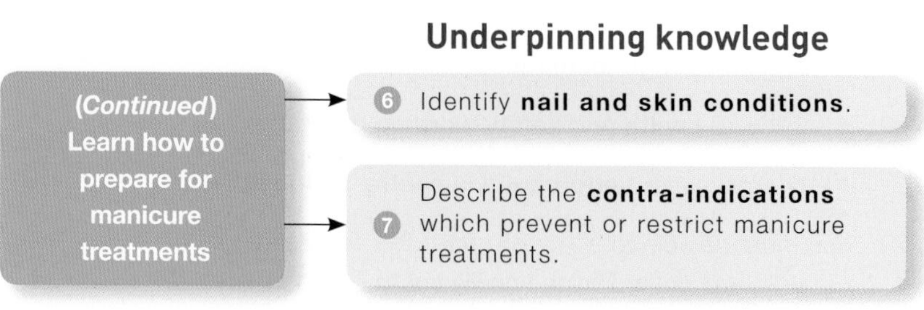

Underpinning knowledge
(Continued) Learn how to prepare for manicure treatments
6 Identify nail and skin conditions.
7 Describe the contra-indications which prevent or restrict manicure treatments.

Preparing the work area

Ensure that all manicure tools products and equipment are clean, sterilized and disinfected, as appropriate, and neatly organized on the work station which is suitably positioned.

Repetitive strain injury (RSI) is caused by repeated movements of a particular part of the body. This can result in injury to the skeleton and muscle of the upper body and limbs. A height adjustable chair with back support should be used ensuring that this is the correct height for the work station. Foot rests should be used for therapists who cannot place their feet flat on the floor. All equipment, products and tools should be easily accessible between knee and shoulder height. Regular breaks should be taken to avoid fatigue.

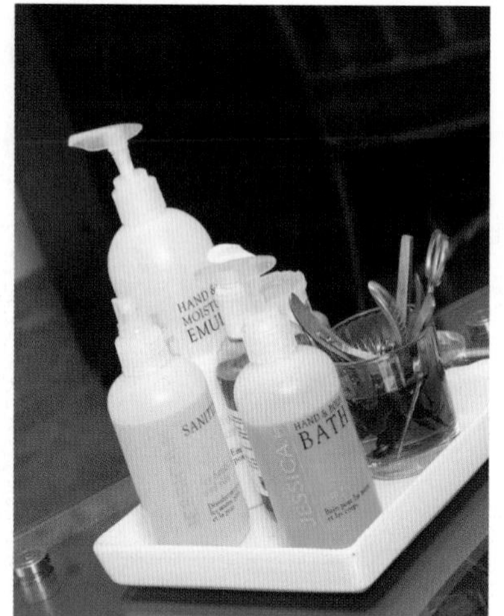
Manicure products, tools and equipment

Keeping the working area tidy promotes an organized and professional image, and prevents time being wasted as you try to find product, tools and equipment. It should always be left in a condition suitable for further nail treatments.

Place a towel over the work surface, then fold another towel into a pad and place it in the middle of the work surface. The pad helps to support the client's forearm during treatment. Place the third towel over the pad, with more of the towel on the manicurist's side – this is used to dry the client's hands during treatment.

A tissue or disposable manicure mat may then be placed on top of the towels, to catch any nail clippings or filings. This can be thrown away later, avoiding irritation to the client from filings. All towels should be replaced with freshly laundered ones following each treatment.

Before beginning the manicure, check that you have the necessary products, tools and equipment and that they meet legal hygiene and industry requirements for nail treatments.

PRODUCTS, TOOLS AND EQUIPMENT

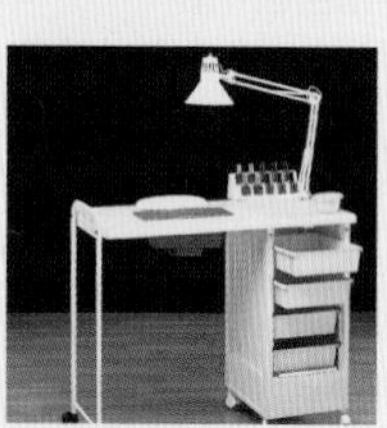

Manicure table or trolley
On which to place everything

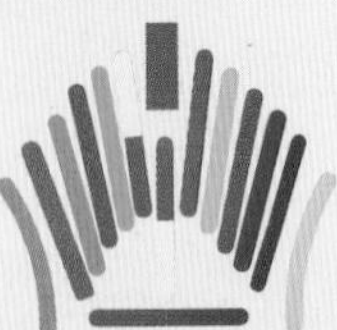

Emery boards
Used to shorten and shape the nail free edge

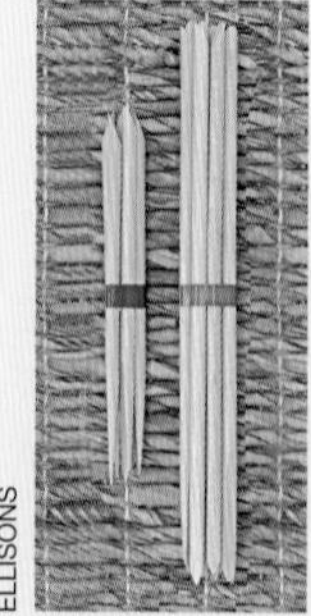

Orange sticks
(**Orange sticks** should be disposed of after each client, as they cannot be effectively sterilized.) Used to remove products from containers, and, when tipped at either end with cotton wool, to ease the cuticle back and clean under the free edge

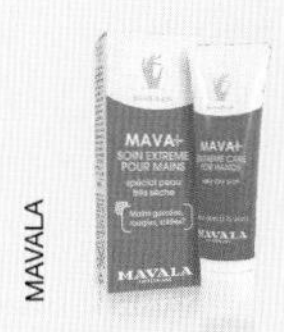
MAVALA

Hand cream or oil
Use hand cream or oil to massage the skin of the hand and arm

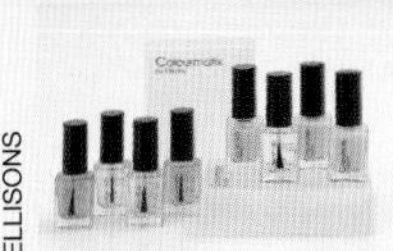
ELLISONS

Base coat
To prevent nail staining, improve appearance and health of the nail and provide an even surface to improve nail polish application and adherence

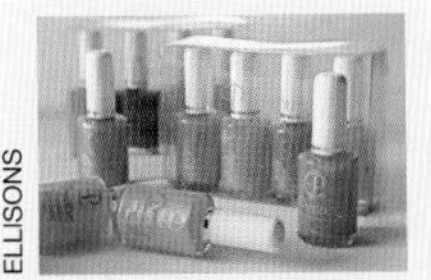
ELLISONS

Coloured nail polish (enamel)
A selection for the client to choose from in cream or pearlized (also termed crystalline) formulations

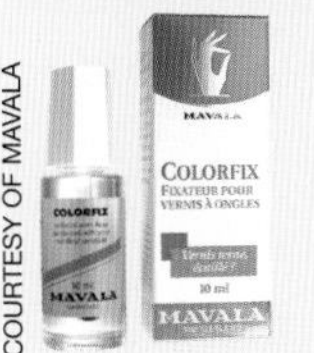
COURTESY OF MAVALA

Top coat
To provide shine and strength to protect the nail polish. Reduces peeling and chipping and increases durability of the nail polish

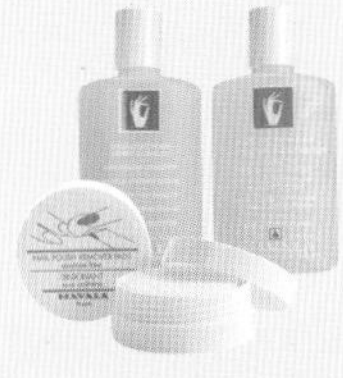

Nail polish remover
To remove nail polish and excess nail care and skincare preparations from the nail plate

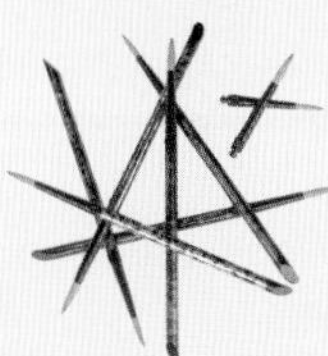

Hoof stick
To gently push back the softened cuticles

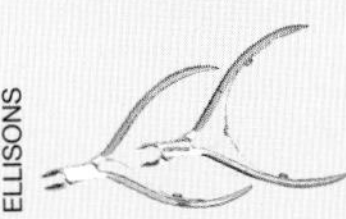
ELLISONS

Cuticle nippers
To remove excess cuticle and dead, torn skin surrounding the nail plate

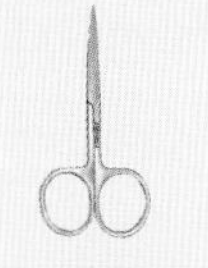

Nail scissors
To shorten nail length

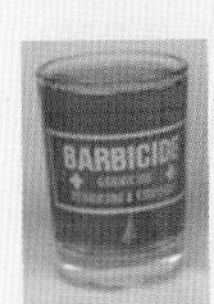

Disinfectant solution
To store small plastic and stainless steel sterilized tools

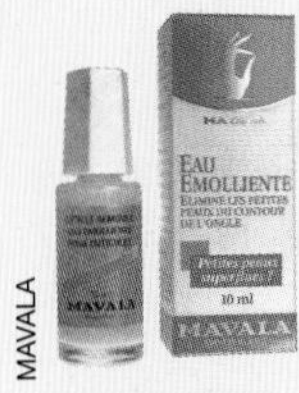
MAVALA

Cuticle remover
Used to soften the skin cells and cuticle so excess epidermal skin can be easily removed

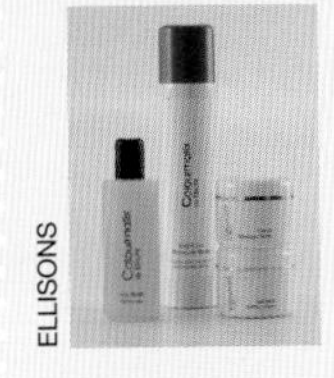
ELLISONS

Cuticle oil or cream
Used to condition and rehydrate the skin of the cuticle; especially beneficial for dry nails and cuticles

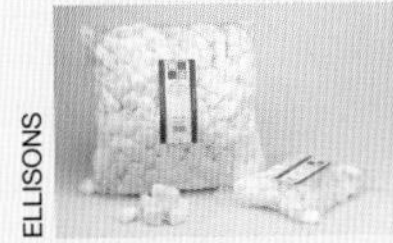
ELLISONS

Cotton wool
To remove nail polish and excess nail product preparations. Cotton wool may also be used to tip orange sticks for the purpose of nail product application and removal. Cotton wool filled gauze pads are also available which are more absorbent

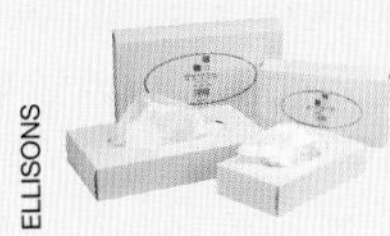
ELLISONS

Tissues
To protect client's clothing in the area, and for drying tools after immersion in disinfectant solution etc.

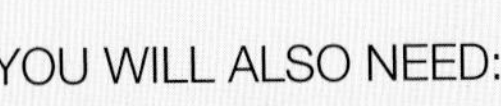

YOU WILL ALSO NEED:

Medium-sized towels (3) To dry the skin, nails, etc.

Small bowls (3) Lined with tissues for storage etc.

A finger bowl To place the fingers into a nail cleansing agent to soak, soften and cleanse the skin and nails

Cuticle knife To remove excess eponychium and perionychium from the surface of the nail plate

Buffers Buffers are used to improve nail shine, stimulate blood circulation and remove surface ridges when used with a buffing paste

Buffing paste Used to reduce the appearance of ridges on the nail plate surface in conjunction with a nail buffer tool

Disinfecting solution For all surfaces

Skin disinfectant To cleanse and disinfect the client's skin. Specialized sprays and gels are available for this purpose

Four-sided buffer To remove dead skin cells and impart shine improving the nail plate appearance

Products, Tools and Equipment (continued)

Client record card Used to record confidential details of each client registered at the salon to record the client's personal details, products used and details of the treatment provided.

Nail polish drier An aerosol or oil preparation applied to speed up the drying process of nail polish

Waste container This should be a lined metal bin with a lid to contain vapours from solvents

ADDITIONAL EQUIPMENT FOR FURTHER HAND AND NAIL TREATMENTS MAY INCLUDE:

Paraffin wax

Hand masks

Thermal mitts

Exfoliators and warm oil

TOP TIP

Hand/foot lotion/oil

Therapeutic ingredients may be added to the basic formulation, such as lavender essential oil which can soothe dry sensitive skin on the hands. Peppermint oil is a popular addition to foot lotion as it reduces redness and is refreshing, creating a cooling effect as it has vasoconstrictor properties.

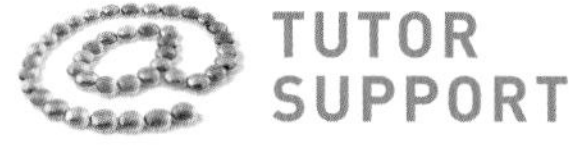

TUTOR SUPPORT

Activity 3: benefits of a manicure handout

ALWAYS REMEMBER

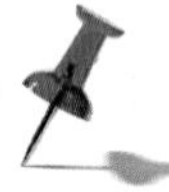

Pearlized polishes

Pearlized polishes are created by the addition of sparkling, reflective particles such as mica, a synthetic product.

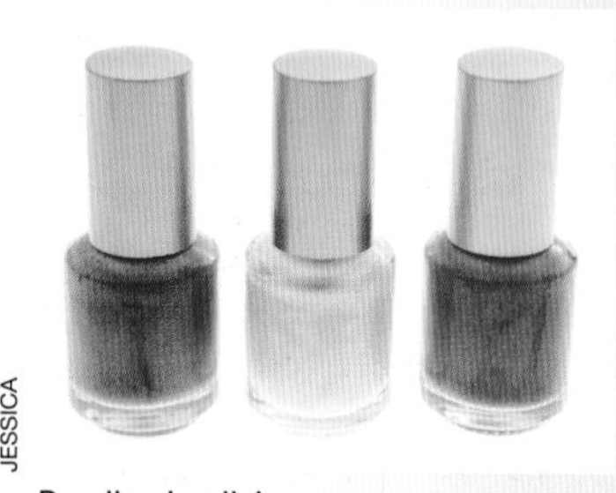

JESSICA

Pearlized polish

Products used in both manicure and pedicure treatments

The following is a list of products that are used in both manicure and pedicure treatments and should be referred to when studying pedicure in Chapter 12.

Product	Ingredients	Uses
Nail polish remover	Acetone or ethyl acetate – solvent Perfume Colour Oil – emollient to reduce drying effect of solvent	To remove nail polish To remove grease from the nail plate prior to applying polish
Hand/foot lotion/oil	Vegetable oils (e.g. almond oil) Perfume Emulsifying agents (e.g. beeswax or gum tragacanth) Emollients (e.g. glycerine or lanolin) Preservatives	To soften the skin and cuticles To provide slip during hand/foot massage
Nail bleach	Citric acid or hydrogen peroxide – bleaches the nail Glycerine – emollient Water	To whiten stained nails and the surrounding skin
Nail polish	Formaldehyde – film-forming plastic resin, improving adherence and flexibility Solvent – creates a suitable consistency when applying, and to help polish dry at a controlled rate Colour pigments – create nail polish colour Resin – improves adhesion of polish to nail plate and flexibility	To colour nail plates To provide some protection

Product	Ingredients	Uses
	Toluene – solvent which dissolves ingredients in nail polish Nitrocellulose – film-forming plastic which holds colour Plasticizers – to provide flexibility after the polish has dried, reducing chipping Pearlized particles – create a pearlized or crystalline effect	
Cuticle cream	Emollients (e.g. lanolin beeswax or glycerine) Perfume Colour	To soften the cuticles
Cuticle oil	Emollient oils such as lanolin and organic oils such as almond oil	To condition the nail and surrounding skin
Nail strengthener	Formaldehyde – film-forming plastic resin	To strengthen weak nails
Nail conditioners	Organic oils which are vitamin enriched and provide excellent emollient properties	Formulation designed to rehydrate improving the appearance and health of the nail, encouraging nail growth
Cuticle remover	Potassium hydroxide – a caustic alkali Glycerine – a humectant added to reduce the drying effect on the nail plate	To soften the skin of the cuticles
Buffing paste/ cream	Perfume Colour Abrasive particles (e.g. pumice, talc or silica) to remove surface cells	To provide a shine to the nail plate (used with a buffer)
Nail polish drier	Mineral oil – assists drying Oleric acid or silicone – lubricant	Increases the speed at which the polish hardens
Nail polish solvent	Ethyl acetate – thins nail polish consistency Toluene – solvent which dissolves nail polish ingredients	Thins nail polish that has thickened, restoring consistency

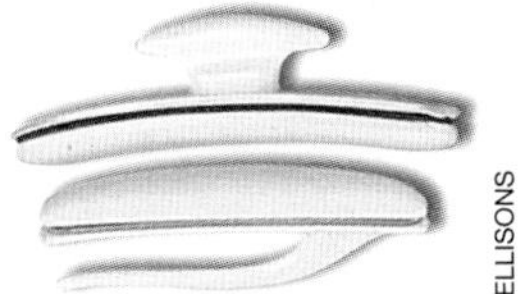

ELLISONS

Chamois nail buffers

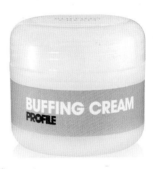

Buffing paste

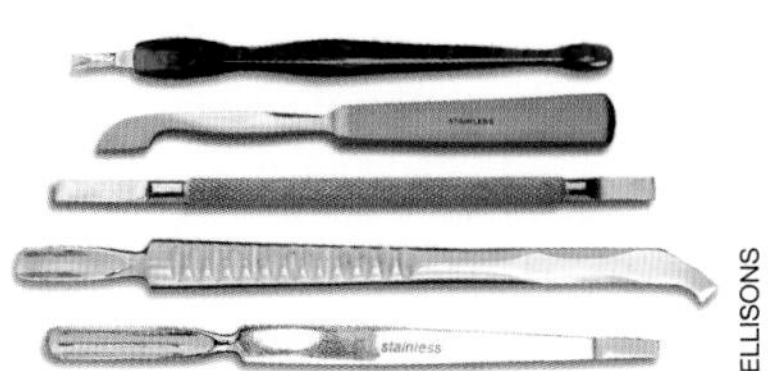

ELLISONS

Cuticle knives

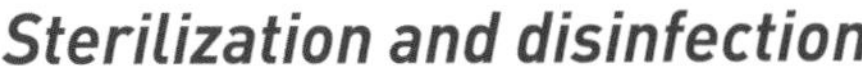

Sterilization and disinfection

Hygiene must be maintained in a number of ways:

- ensure that tools and equipment are clean and sterile before use
- having sterilized or disinfected tools and equipment store them in a chemical disinfectant or closed container until ready for use. Remember, they will remain clean but will not be sterile after 24 hours.

TOP TIP

Nail treatments legal requirements

Habia provide a Code of Practice for Nail Treatments. You should refer to this to ensure that you are complying with relevant health and safety legislation.

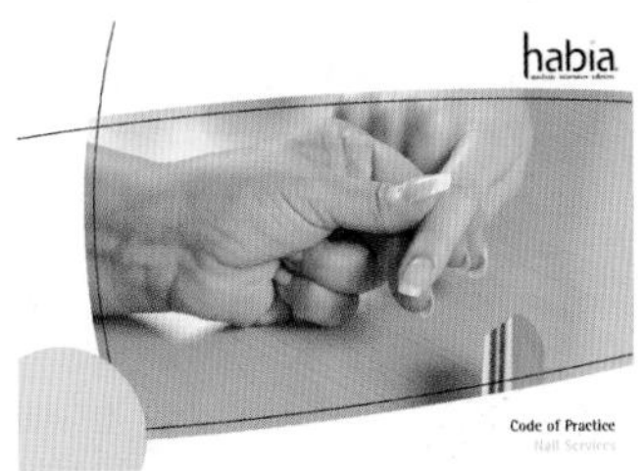

© HABIA

Habia Code of Practice guidance booklet

- dispense products, e.g. creams and lotions, from containers with a disposable spatula
- use disposable products wherever possible

Refer to Habia's Code of Practice for Nail Treatments for health and safety best practice guidance.

Manicure and pedicure tools and equipment can be disposable or can be sterilized or disinfected by the following methods:

Tool/Equipment	Method	Term used
Cuticle knife	Autoclave	Sterilization
Cuticle nippers	Autoclave	Sterilization
Orange stick	Throw away after use	Disposable
Callus file	Autoclave	Sterilization
	Chemical (e.g. disinfectant)	Disinfection
Bowl	Chemical (e.g. disinfectant)	Disinfection
Emery board	Throw away after use	Disposable
Buffer	Wipe handle with chemical disinfectant	Disinfection
	Wash buffing cloth in hot (60°C) soapy water	Cleaned
Towel	Wash in hot soapy water (60°C)	Cleaned
Spatula	Throw away after use	Disposable
Nail clippers	Autoclave	Sterilization
Scissors	Autoclave	Sterilization
Hoof stick	Immerse in chemical (e.g. disinfectant)	Disinfection
Trolley	Wipe with chemical (e.g. disinfectant)	Disinfection

Metal tools when ready for use should be placed in a disinfecting solution. After the manicure treatment they must be replaced and re-sterilized.

ALWAYS REMEMBER

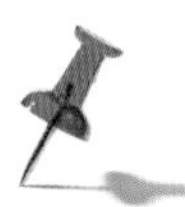

UV stabilizers
UV stabilizers are additives which prevent the polish changing colour on exposure to UV sunlight.

HEALTH & SAFETY

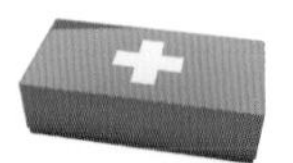

Disinfecting sprays
You can buy disinfecting sprays to disinfect the surface of the tools that the chemical agent comes into contact with. Any debris must first be removed using a detergent before the use of a disinfecting spray. Use in a well-ventilated area and avoid contact with flame and excessive heat.

HEALTH & SAFETY

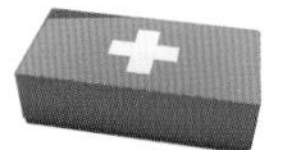

Metal in the autoclave
Any metal to be placed in the autoclave should be of a high-quality stainless steel, to prevent rusting. Always dry immediately to prevent damage.

> No one knows everything or can be everything, so teamwork is really important. We learn from those around us.
>
> **Jacqui Jefford**

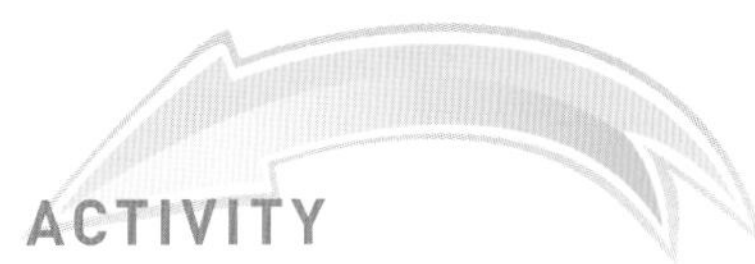

ACTIVITY

Stretching exercises to avoid RSI

Perform regular, daily stretching exercise to reduce tension and improve flexibility for the fingers, wrists, hands, arms, shoulder, neck and upper back.

Research simple stretching exercises for each of the above body areas.

Reception

When a client makes an appointment for a manicure treatment, the receptionist should ask a few simple questions that will help guide how long the treatment will take.

- Do they require nail polish? With drying time, this part of the treatment can last up to 20 minutes, so the client should be made aware of this.
- Are any nails damaged or in need of repair? Again extra time will need to be allowed for this work.
- Do they require any **hand and nail treatments** in addition to the manicure, such as exfoliation or paraffin wax? Allow extra time accordingly.
- Has the client had artificial nails applied previously which require removal? Allow approximately 20 minutes for this process.
- Commercial timing

Allow 45 minutes for a manicure treatment.

Allow up to one hour for a specialist hand-nail treatment.

All staff, especially the staff communicating with clients at reception should be familiar with the different pricing structures for the range of manicure treatments and products available for retail.

The receptionist should also check the age of the client. If the client is a minor under the age of 16, it is necessary to obtain parent/guardian permission for treatment. The parent/guardian will also have to be present when the treatment is received.

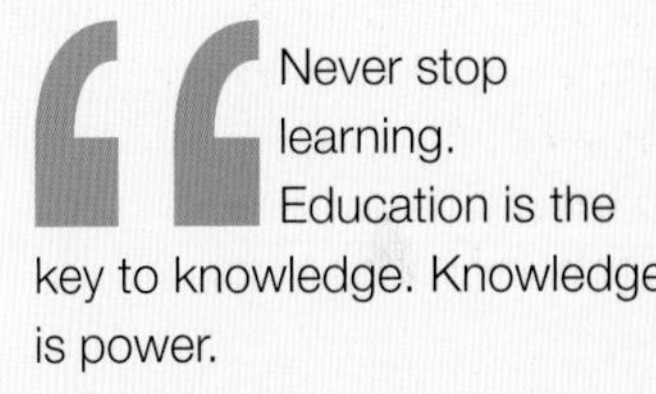

Never stop learning. Education is the key to knowledge. Knowledge is power.

Jacqui Jefford

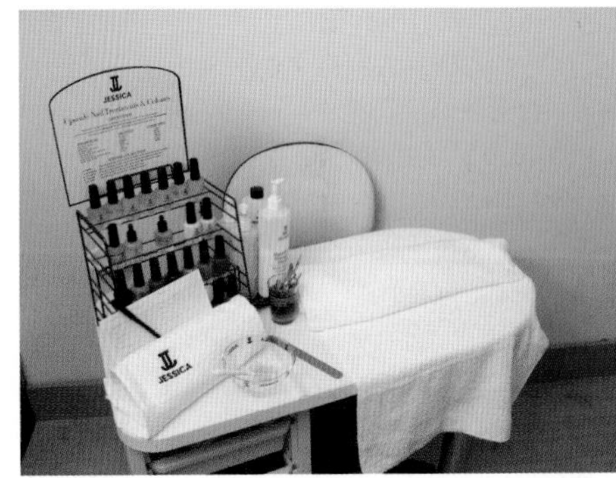

Work area

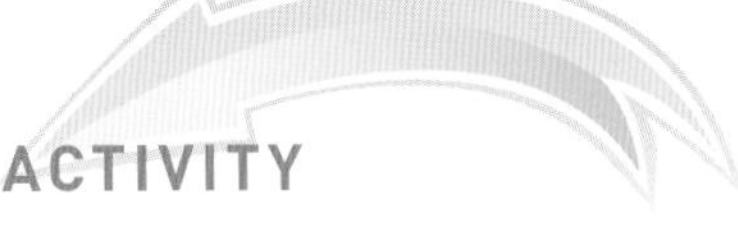

ACTIVITY

Making appointments

What questions could the receptionist ask when booking a client for manicure in order to make the appointments run more efficiently? Write down your answers.

An employer will always want someone who shows passion and initiative in all they do.

Jacqui Jefford

Consultation

Before carrying out a manicure treatment, it is necessary to assess the condition of the client's skin, nails and cuticles. This is done in order that the most appropriate hand and nail treatments and products may be chosen. Also, by correctly assessing and analyzing

ACTIVITY

Assessing the hands

Look closely at your own hands. Assess their condition and make notes about everything you see.

Then assess the hands of a colleague. How do they differ from your own?

Complete a record card and record the condition of the nails and surrounding skin. Design a suitable treatment plan for your client to meet their needs.

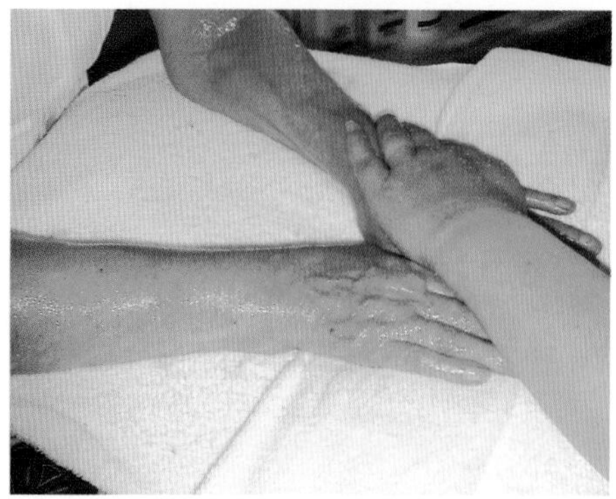

Specialist hand and nail treatment: warm oil application

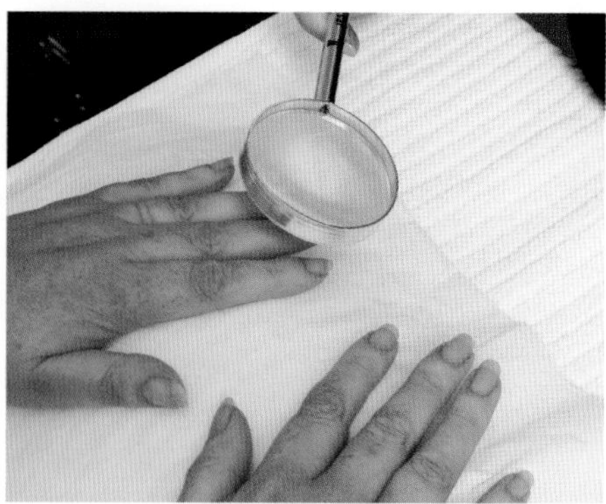

Assessing the nails and skin

the client's hand condition and writing this on their record card, you will be able to see over a period of time how the condition is improving and progressing.

Assess the condition of the following:

- ***The cuticles*** Are they dry, tight or cracked, or are they soft and pliable?
- ***The nails*** Are they strong or weak, brittle or flaking? Are they discoloured or stained? What shape are they – square, round, oval? Are they long or short? Are they bitten?
- ***The skin*** Is the skin dry, rough or chapped, or is it soft and smooth? Is the colour even?

While assessing the client's hands for treatment, you should also be looking for any *contra-indications* to manicure treatment.

ALWAYS REMEMBER

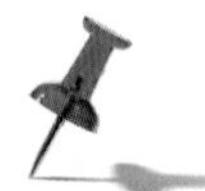

Artificial nails

If the client has had several new sets of artificial nails applied this will damage the natural nail.

The nail plate may be thin, ridges may appear upon the nail plate and the removal technique, using acetone, will cause dehydration. All of these effects will need to be discussed with your client at consultation and an appropriate treatment plan discussed.

Skin and nail disorders of the hands and nails

When a client attends for a manicure treatment, as part of the consultation and assessment of the client's needs, the therapist should always look at the client's skin and nails to check that no infection or disease is present which might contra-indicate treatment. These include bacterial, fungal, viral and parasitic infections. These are described in more detail in Chapter 2, where **contra-indications** are illustrated and discussed.

If the client is wearing nail polish, this must be removed before inspecting the nail plate.

Contra-indications The following disorders may contra-indicate or restrict manicure treatment. If you suspect the client has any disorder from the chart below, do not attempt a diagnosis, but refer the client tactfully to their GP without causing unnecessary concern.

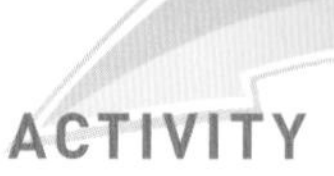

ACTIVITY

Communication skills

Communication is important. Give three examples of good communication techniques used when performing a manicure consultation.

Disorder	Description
Broken bones 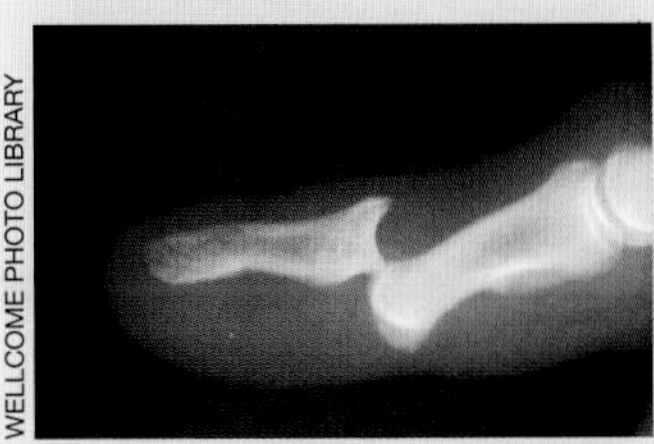 WELLCOME PHOTO LIBRARY	Injury resulting in a broken bone can often not be seen; confirm at consultation that there is no known injury in the treatment area.
Cuts or abrasions in the hands 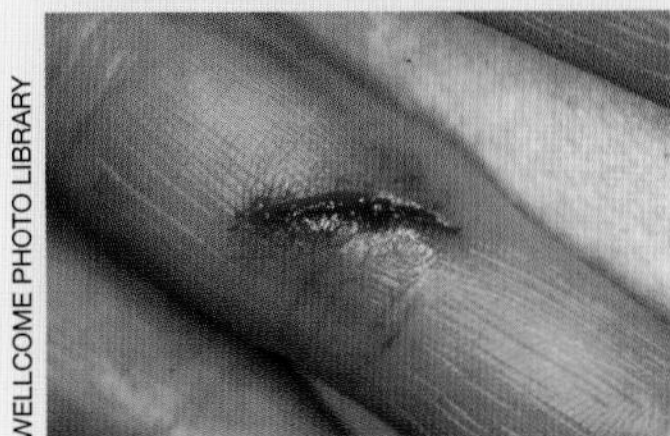 WELLCOME PHOTO LIBRARY	Broken skin. Any cut or abrasion could lead to secondary infection and the area should not be treated until healed.
Diabetes 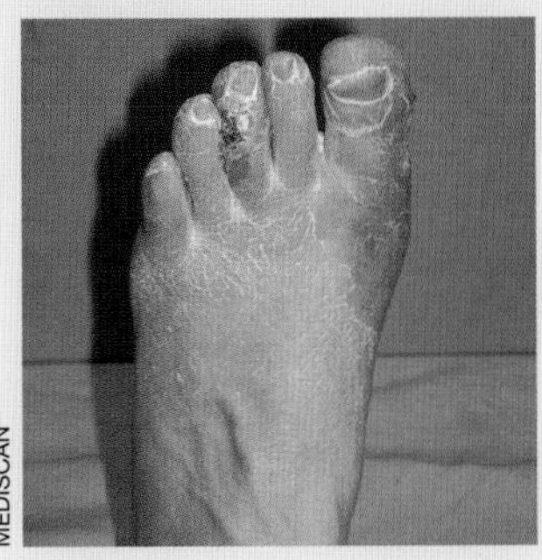 MEDISCAN	If a client has diabetic foot or hand condition, they are vulnerable to infection as they have slow skin healing. This could be problematic if the skin was accidentally broken during a pedicure treatment. Permission must be obtained from the client's GP before treatment can be received.
Paronychia 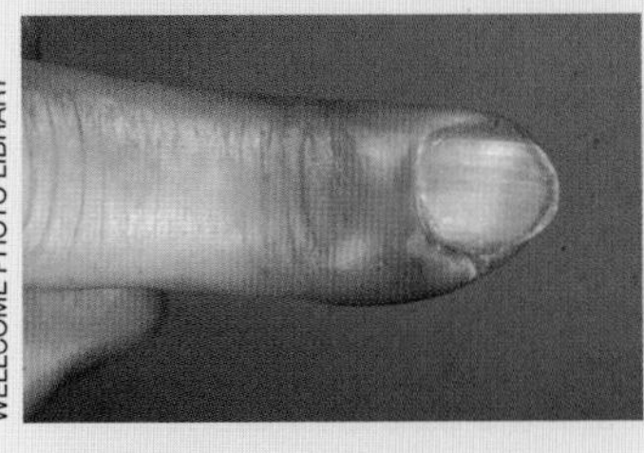 WELLCOME PHOTO LIBRARY	Infectious bacterial infection. Swelling, redness and pus appears in the cuticle area of the skin and surrounding the nail wall.
Scabies or itch mites 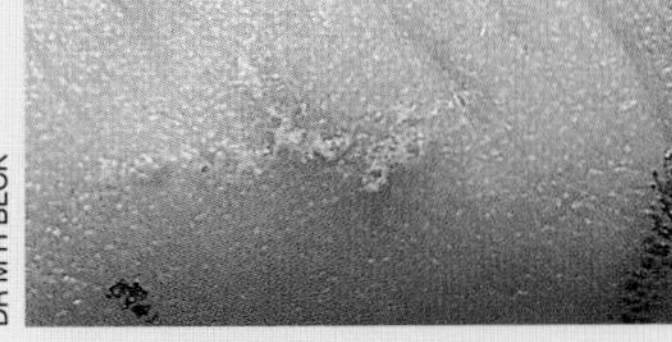 DR M H BECK	An infestation of the skin by an animal parasite. The animal parasite burrows beneath the skin and invades the hair follicles. Papules and wavy greyish lines appear, where dirt enters the burrows. Secondary bacterial infection may occur as a result of scratching the skin.

ALWAYS REMEMBER

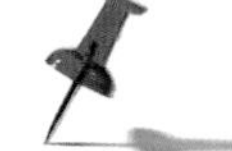

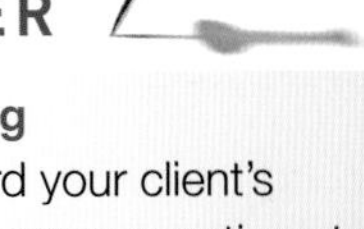

Record keeping

Accurately record your client's answers to necessary questions to be asked at consultations on the record card.

KNOWLEDGE CHECK

What is the cause of repetitive strain injury and how can this be avoided when performing manicure treatments?

Need more time... refer to pages 356 and 361 to help you.

Severe **eczema of the nail**

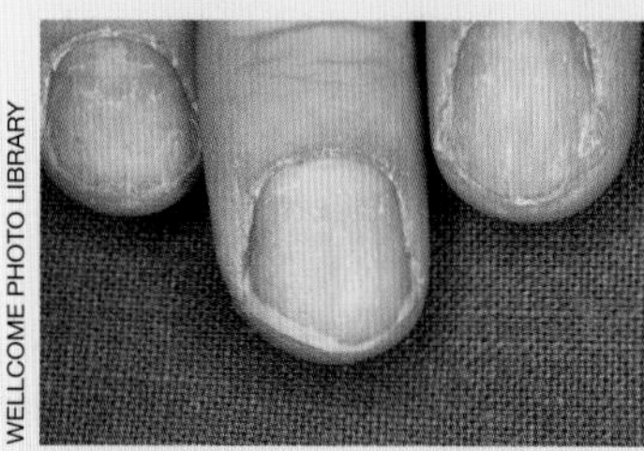
WELLCOME PHOTO LIBRARY

Inflammation of the skin occurs. Differing changes to the nail may occur, including the appearance of ridges, pitting, **onycholysis** or nail thickening (hypertrophy).

Severe eczema of the skin

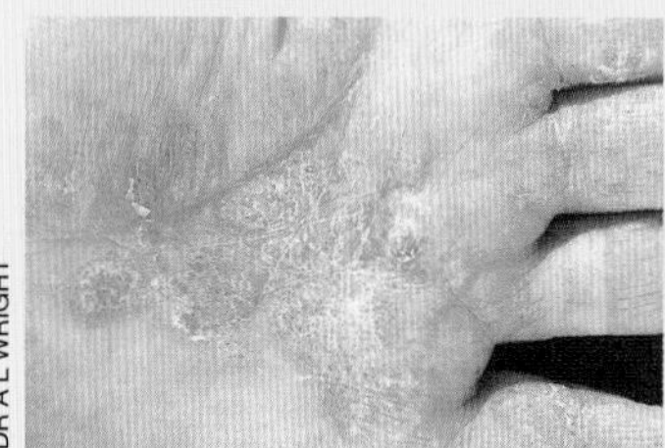
DR A L WRIGHT

Inflammation of the skin caused by contact internally or externally, with an irritant.
Reddening of the skin occurs with swelling and blistering; the blisters leak tissue fluid, which later hardens and forms scabs.

Severe nail separation (onycholysis)

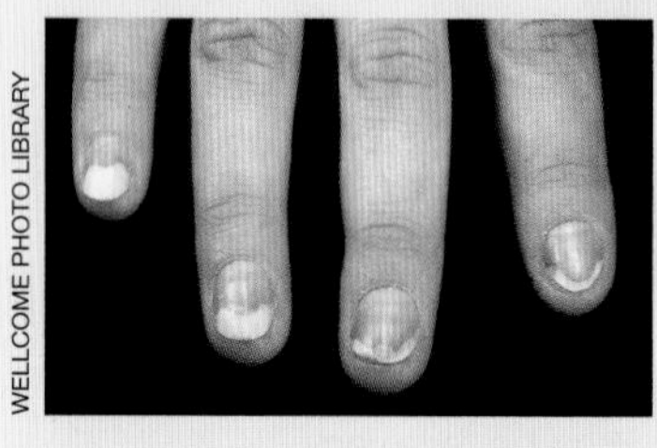
WELLCOME PHOTO LIBRARY

Lifting of the nail plate from the nail bed, may be caused by trauma or infection to the nail or surrounding area; where separation has occurred this appears as a greyish-white area on the nail as the pink undertone of the nail bed does not show.

Severe **psoriasis of the nail**

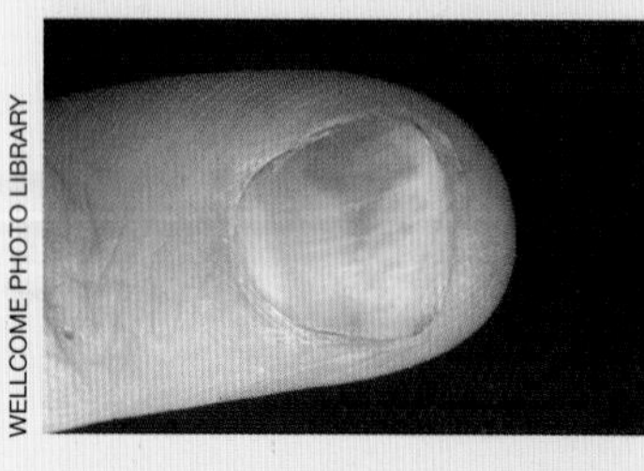
WELLCOME PHOTO LIBRARY

An inflammatory condition where there is an increased production of cells in the upper part of the skin.
Pitting occurs on the surface of the nail plate.
Nail plate separation from the nail bed (onycholysis) may also occur.

Severe psoriasis of the skin

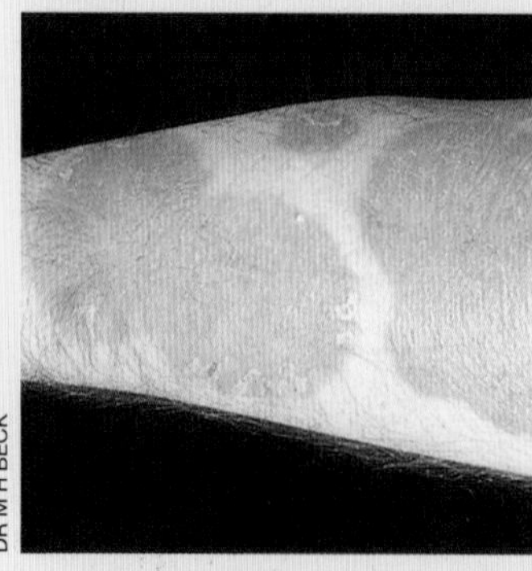
DR M H BECK

Red patches of skin appear covered in waxy, silvery scales.
Bleeding will occur if the area is scratched and the scales are removed.
The cause is unknown.

Disorder	Description
Tinea corporis (body ringworm) DR A L WRIGHT	Fungal infection of the skin, which may occur on the limbs. Small scaly red patches, which spread outwards and then heal from the centre, leaving a ring.
Tinea unguium WELLCOME PHOTO LIBRARY	Fungal infection of the fingernails. The nail plate is yellowish-grey. Eventually the nail plate becomes brittle, crumbles and separates from the nail bed.
Verrucae or warts 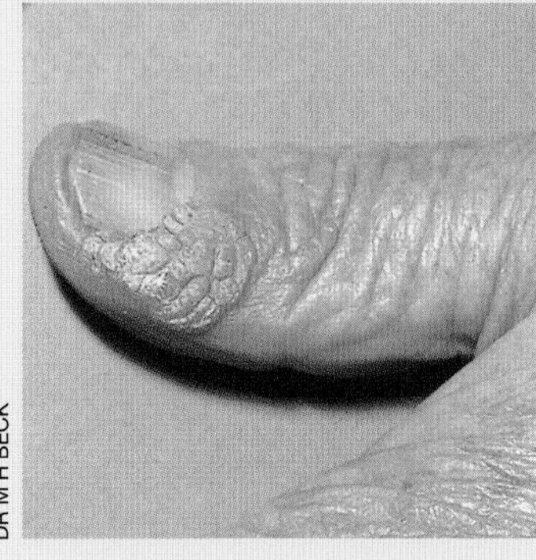 DR M H BECK	A viral infection. Small epidermal skin growths. Warts may be raised or flat depending upon their position. Warts vary in size, shape, texture and colour. Usually they have a rough surface and are raised. Plane wart – found on the surface of the hand.

Below is a list of common disorders that may be seen on the hands. Not all of these contra-indicate treatment but they may restrict treatment.

Disorder	Cause	Appearance	Salon treatment	Homecare advice
Blue nail WELLCOME PHOTO LIBRARY	Poor blood circulation in the area. Heart disease.	The nail bed does not appear a healthy pink colour but has a blue tinge.	Permission to treat to be received from the client's GP. Regular manicure, including hand treatment to improve circulation.	General manicure advice. Hand exercises and massage to improve circulation.
Bruised nails DR A L WRIGHT	Trauma to the nail (e.g. trapping it in a door); severe damage can result in loss of the nail.	Part of the nail plate may appear blue or black where bleeding has occurred on the new bed.	Although this disorder does not contra-indicate treatment, it is advisable to postpone manicuring the nails until the condition is no longer painful. Nail polish may be used to disguise the damaged nail.	Seek medical advice if swelling is present or if pain persists.

Disorder	Cause	Appearance	Salon treatment	Homecare advice
Eggshell nail WELLCOME PHOTO LIBRARY	Illness.	Thin, fragile, white nail plate, curving under at the free edge.	Permission for treatment to be received from the client's GP. Regular manicure.	General manicure advice. Strengthening base coats.
Hangnail DR A L WRIGHT	Biting the skin around the nails. Cracking of a dry skin or cuticle condition.	Epidermis around the nail plate cracks and a small piece of skin protrudes between the nail plate and the nail wall, sometimes accompanied by redness and swelling: this condition can become extremely painful.	**Warm-oil treatments** to soften the skin and cuticles. Remove the protrusion of dead skin with cuticle nippers: do not cut into live tissue.	Regular use of a rich hand cream. Wear rubber gloves when cleaning and washing up. Wear warm gloves in cold weather. Ensure a balanced diet.
Leuconychia DR A L WRIGHT	Trauma to the nail plate or matrix, due to pressure or hitting the nail with a hard object. Air pockets form between the nail plate and nail bed	White spots or marks on the nail plate: will grow out with the nail.	General manicure treatment. Coloured nail polish application will disguise their appearance until the damaged area disappears as it grows towards the free edge.	Be careful with the hands. Wear protective gloves when doing housework or gardening. Do not use the nails as tools!
Longitudinal ridges in the nail plate (corrugated nails) DR A L WRIGHT	Illness. Damage to the matrix. Age, associated with the ageing process.	Grooves in the nail plate running along the length of the nail from the cuticle to the free edge: may affect one or all nails.	Abrasive buffing paste applied to smooth out the ridges. Use of a **ridge-filling base coat** prior to nail polish application.	General manicure aftercare advice. Use of a ridge-filling base coat polish. Ensure a balanced diet.
Minor nail separation (onycholysis) WELLCOME PHOTO LIBRARY	Lifting of the nail plate from its bed. Can accompany a medical condition such as eczema or psoriasis or a fungal infection in the area.	Where separation has occurred this appears as a greyish-white area as the pink undertone of the nail bed does not show through the nail plate.	It is advisable to postpone manicuring for this nail until the condition is corrected. Refer the client to their GP to confirm cause.	Be careful to avoid infection of the nail bed. Protect the nail with a protective dressing.

Disorder	Cause	Appearance	Salon treatment	Homecare advice
Onychophagy DR A L WRIGHT	Excessive nail-biting.	Very little nail plate; bulbous skin at the fingertip; nail walls often red and swollen, due to biting of the skin surrounding the nails.	Regular weekly manicures. Cuticle treatment to maximize the visible nail-plate area. Nail conditioning treatments to prevent dry cuticles and hangnails.	Bitter-tasting preparations painted onto the nail plate. Wear gloves to avoid biting in bed.
Onychorrhexis DR A L WRIGHT	Using harsh detergents without wearing gloves. Poor diet. Not wearing gloves in cold weather.	Split, flaking nails.	Warm-oil manicures on a weekly basis.	Regular use of a rich hand cream. Always wear rubber gloves when cleaning or washing up. Always wear warm gloves in cold weather. Ensure a balanced diet. Prescribe nail base coat to protect split, flaking nails.
Pitting WELLCOME PHOTO LIBRARY	Eczema. Psoriasis.	Pitting resembling small irregular pin pricks appear on the nail plate.	Refer the client to their GP for permission to treat if required. Regular manicure with gentle buffing.	General manicure advice. Ridge-filling base coat polish.
Pterygium DR A L WRIGHT	Neglect of the nails.	Overgrown thickened cuticles, often tightly adhered to the nail plate: if left untreated, this may lead to splitting of the cuticle and subsequent infection.	Warm-oil or paraffin wax treatments weekly. Once softened, remove excess cuticle with cuticle nippers. If overgrown cuticle is excessive, refer client to their GP.	Regular use of a rich cuticle cream. Wear rubber gloves when cleaning and washing up. Gently push back the cuticles with a soft towel when softened, e.g. after bathing.
Transverse furrows in the nail plate (Beau's lines) DR A L WRIGHT	Temporary arrested development of the nail in the matrix, due to illness or trauma of the nail.	Groove in the nail plate, often on all nails simultaneously, running from side to side: this will grow out with the nail.	Regular manicure until normal cells replace the damaged cells.	General manicure advice. Ensure a balanced diet.

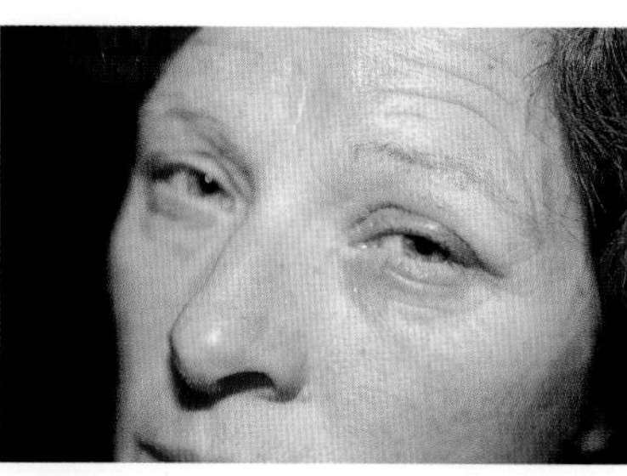
DR JOHN GRAY, THE WORLD OF SKIN CARE

Client with an allergic reaction that has affected the eyes, causing redness and swelling

HEALTH & SAFETY 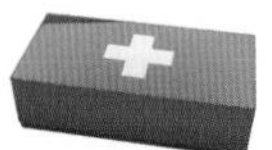

Diagnosis

You are not qualified to diagnose, this is the job of the GP.

Therefore if you are unsure about any nail or skin condition present refer the client to their GP.

HEALTH & SAFETY 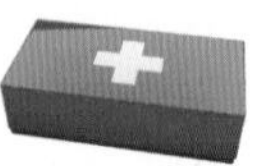

Contaminated waste

If there is any tissue damage during the manicure procedure resulting in bleeding, this is *contaminated waste* and must be disposed off in accordance with disposal of contaminated waste regulations.

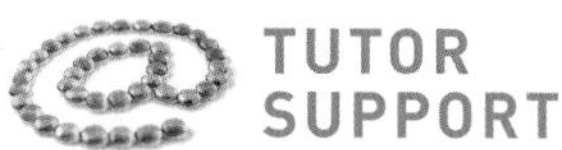
TUTOR SUPPORT

Activity 4: Promoting luxury treatments

KNOWLEDGE CHECK

What is the name of the infectious bacterial infection that may occur if the skin is broken as a result of the manicure treatment?

Need more time... refer to page 363 to help you.

Contra-actions

Certain cosmetic ingredients are known to cause allergic reactions in some people. This is known as a **contra-action**, this may occur during or following treatment.

The client – or the manicurist – may at some time develop an allergy to a manicure product that has been successfully used previously. This could be for a number of reasons, including new medication being taken or illness.

The symptoms of an allergic reaction could be:

- excessive redness of the skin (erythema)
- skin irritation i.e. itching
- swelling
- raised blisters

The symptoms do not necessarily appear on the hands. In the case of nail polish allergy, the symptoms often show up on the face, which the hands are continually touching.

In the case of an allergic reaction:

- Remove the offending product immediately, using water or, in the case of polish, nail polish solvent.
- Apply a cool compress and soothing agent to the skin to reduce redness and irritation.
- If symptoms persist, seek medical advice. If the client receives medical advice, ask them to inform you of the advice and/or treatment received so you can include this in your records.

Always record any allergies on the client's record card, so that the offending product may be avoided in future.

Further contra-actions may occur as a result of poor manicure techniques, e.g. failing to check the temperature of **paraffin wax** before application, which if too hot could cause skin sensitivity, even burning! Tissue damage could result in blood loss e.g. incorrect nipping removal technique when using cuticle nippers may result in pulling and tearing the skin. Incorrect positioning and use of the cuticle knife may lead to piercing the cuticle with the knife blade.

Avoid cutting the nails too short as again this can result in possible damage to the hyponychium the part of the epidermis under the free edge of the nail. This may affect its protective function leading to possible infection.

Treatment plan

After analyzing the client's nails and adjacent skin, a **treatment plan** should be considered and agreed with the client. In order to correct skin and nail problems, the client should attend the salon weekly. They should also be advised of the appropriate treatment preparations to use at home, so as to support the salon treatment. Specialist nail treatments to use will depend upon the nail and skin condition; they include:

- ***Nail strengthener*** This is used on brittle, damaged nails, to strengthen, condition and protect them against breaking, splitting or peeling.
- ***Ridge filler*** This is used on nails with ridges to provide a more even surface, creating a bond between the **base coat** and polish, allowing a smoother application of polish.
- ***Nail oil*** This contains ingredients to rehydrate the nail and soften the cuticle.
- ***Cuticle creams*** These nourish the skin and restore the condition of the cuticle.

A sample client record card

Date	Beauty therapist name	
Client name	Date of birth (identifying client age group)	
Home address	Postcode	
Email address	Landline phone number	Mobile phone number
Name of doctor	Doctor's address and phone number	
Related medical history (conditions that may restrict or prohibit treatment application)		
Are you taking any medication? (this may affect the sensitivity of the skin to the treatment)		

CONTRA-INDICATIONS REQUIRING MEDICAL REFERRAL
(preventing manicure treatment application)

- ☐ bacterial infections (e.g. paronychia)
- ☐ viral infections (e.g. plane warts)
- ☐ fungal infections (e.g. tinea unguium)
- ☐ parasitic infections, (e.g. scabies)
- ☐ severe nail separation
- ☐ severe eczema and psoriasis
- ☐ severe bruising
- ☐ severe skin conditions

CONTRA-INDICATIONS WHICH RESTRICT TREATMENT
(treatment may require adaptation)

- ☐ minor nail separation
- ☐ product allergies
- ☐ recent scar tissue
- ☐ severely damaged nails
- ☐ broken bones
- ☐ recent fractures and sprains
- ☐ undiagnosed lumps or swellings
- ☐ minor eczema and psoriasis
- ☐ severely bitten nails
- ☐ minor bruising or swelling
- ☐ minor cuts or abrasions

PRODUCTS, TOOLS AND EQUIPMENT

- ☐ nail and skin treatment tools
- ☐ abrasives (e.g. buffing cream)
- ☐ cuticle softeners
- ☐ nail and skin products
- ☐ nail conditioners (e.g. cuticle cream/oils)
- ☐ skin conditioners (e.g. hand cream)
- ☐ nail, skin and cuticle corrective treatments (e.g. paraffin wax)
- ☐ consumables

HAND AND NAIL TREATMENTS

- ☐ warm oil hand mask
- ☐ paraffin wax
- ☐ thermal mitts
- ☐ exfoliators

NAIL FINISH

- ☐ light colour
- ☐ dark colour
- ☐ French manicure
- ☐ buffing

COURSE OF TREATMENT

	Date	Date	Date
☐ improvement of skin condition products used	____	____	____
☐ improvement of nail condition products used	____	____	____

NAIL, CUTICLE AND SKIN CONDITION

Nails

- ☐ healthy
- ☐ dry
- ☐ ridged (horizontal or longitudinal)
- ☐ brittle
- ☐ weak
- ☐ split
- ☐ bitten (onychopagy)

Nail shape

- ☐ oval
- ☐ tapered
- ☐ square
- ☐ squoval
- ☐ claw
- ☐ fan
- ☐ pointed

Cuticle

- ☐ healthy
- ☐ dry
- ☐ split
- ☐ hangnails
- ☐ overgrown (pterygium)

Skin

- ☐ healthy
- ☐ dry
- ☐ hard

MASSAGE MEDIUMS

- ☐ creams
- ☐ oils
- ☐ lotions

Beauty therapist signature (for reference)
Client signature (confirmation of details)

A sample client record card (continued)

TREATMENT ADVICE

Manicure – *allow 45 minutes*

Specialized hand/nail treatment – *allow up to 60 minutes*

TREATMENT PLAN

Record relevant details of your treatment and advice provided for future reference.

Ensure the client's records are up to date, accurate and fully completed following treatment. Non-compliance may invalidate insurance.

DURING

Discuss:

- details that may influence the client's nail condition, such as their occupation
- the products the client is currently using to care for the skin of the hands and nails, and the regularity of their use
- the client's satisfaction with these products
- relevant manicure procedures (e.g. how to file the nails correctly)

Note:

- any adverse (unwanted) reaction, if any occur during or after the manicure treatment

AFTER

Record:

- results of treatment
- any modification to treatment application that has occurred
- what products have been used in the manicure treatment
- what hand and nail treatments have been used
- the effectiveness of treatment
- any samples provided (review their success at the next appointment)

Advise on:

- product application in order to gain maximum benefit from product use
- specialized products following manicure treatment for homecare use
- general hand/nail care and maintenance
- the recommended time intervals between treatments
- the importance of a course of treatment to improve nail/skin conditions

RETAIL OPPORTUNITIES

Advise on:

- progression of the treatment plan for future appointments
- products that would be suitable for the client to use at home to care for the skin of the hands and nails
- recommendations for further treatments
- further products or treatments that the client may or may not have received before

Note:

- any purchase made by the client

EVALUATION

Record:

- comments on the client's satisfaction with the treatment
- if poor results are achieved, the reasons why
- how you may alter the treatment plan to achieve the required treatment results in the future, if applicable

HEALTH AND SAFETY

Advise on:

- appropriate necessary action to be taken in the event of an unwanted skin or nail reaction

- ***Creams and lotions*** These nourish the skin preventing the skin becoming dry.
- ***Specialist hand and nail treatments*** These may also be recommended within the manicure treatment to improve the appearance of the skin texture, nail and cuticle condition and provide a number of physiological benefits. These may be offered each time the client has a manicure treatment to maintain the condition of the nails and hands.

Provide the opportunity for your client to ask any questions relating to the manicure treatment plan.

The record card should be signed and dated by the manicurist following the consultation to confirm the suitability and consent with the agreed manicure treatment.

It is important that accurate records are kept and stored in compliance with the Data Protection Act for future reference.

Preparing the client

Ensure that the client is warm and comfortable when preparing them for a manicure.

Lighting must be good to avoid eyestrain and to allow the treatment to be performed competently. Avoid positioning the work station in direct sunlight however to prevent discomfort to client and manicurist. Heat can also spoil many manicure preparations. Always store and handle products in the recommended way.

Background music, if provided, should be at a sound level that allows effective communication with your client.

Consider the clients comfort with the location of the manicure treatment area. Some clients may require a more private area than a busy area with lots of traffic (people walking past). Check suitability with your client.

A lightweight gown may be offered to the client to cover their clothing. This will prevent damage to their clothes from accidental spillage of products during treatment. Ask them to remove any jewellery from the area to be treated, to prevent the jewellery being damaged by manicure products and to avoid obstructing massage movements. Place the jewellery where the client can see it. Alternatively, ask the client to take possession of it for safe-keeping – follow your salon security policy. Ensure that the client is seated at the correct height, and close enough to avoid having to lean forward.

When the client is comfortably seated, clean your hands using an approved hand cleaning technique – preferably in view of the client, who will then observe hygienic procedures

TOP TIP

Examples of manicure treatment adjustments

Following your consultation, you may need to adjust your manicure to meet your client's need by modifying:

- **the depth of massage pressure when applying hand and arm massage and choice of massage movements applied, e.g. an elderly client's skin is thinner and has less elasticity and they may have reduced joint mobility**
- **the choice of massage medium, e.g. when client has excessively hairy arms**
- **the choice of nail polish product including base, colour and top coat to improve the nail condition and appearance**

HEALTH & SAFETY

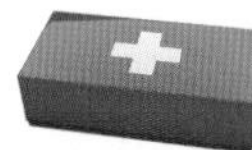

Contact dermatitis

Contact dermatitis is a skin problem caused by intolerance of the skin to a particular substance or a group of substances. On exposure to the substance the skin quickly becomes irritated and an allergic reaction occurs. This may occur when a manicurist's skin is exposed to dust and chemicals on a regular basis. Follow all HSE guidelines to reduce the risk of developing this skin disorder which could result in the need for a career change!

Always follow manufacturers' guidelines on the use of products.

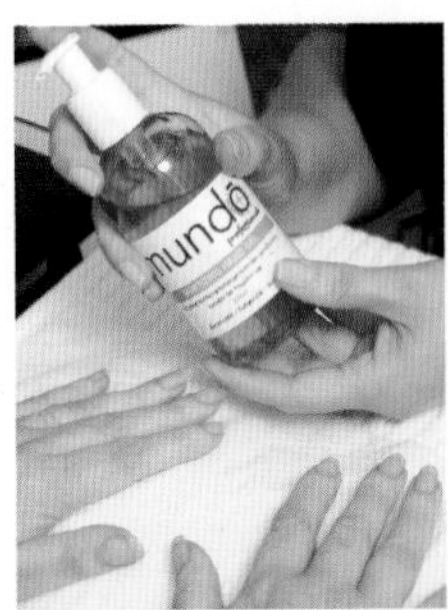

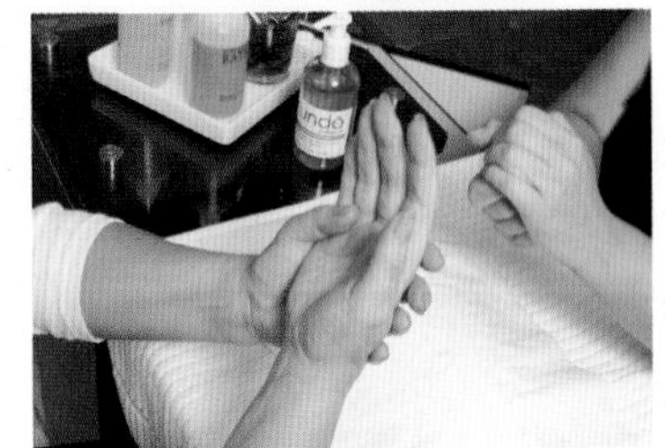

Cleaning the hands

Client consultation

being carried out. This will assure them that they are receiving a professional service. The client should also wash their hands before the treatment commences. The client's skin can also be cleaned with a disinfectant gel or spray.

Consult the client's record card, and begin the treatment.

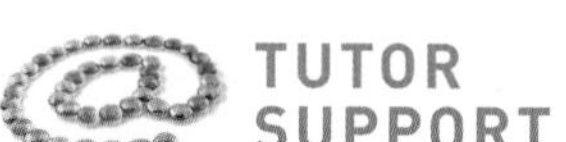

TUTOR SUPPORT

Activity 5: Hand and nail treatments handout

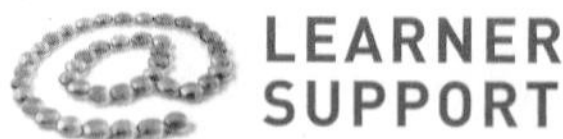

LEARNER SUPPORT

Nails true or false

BEST PRACTICE

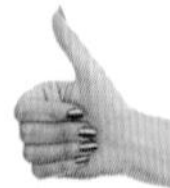

Removal of artificial nails or UV cured gel polish

These are removed using a solvent containing acetone that softens the product, allowing removal from the natural nail. However, it is particularly drying to the natural nail which will later require rehydrating.

Procedure

- Remove any nail polish from artificial nails, and trim any excess length using clippers.
- Soak the nails in the recommended removal product. For artificial nails this is usually acetone for approximately 20 minutes, until the product has thoroughly softened.
- Remove the softened product with an orange stick.
- Wash the hands and nails thoroughly to remove acetone.
- The surface of the nail may require to be buffed lightly with a gentle abrasive file to remove excess product and provide a smooth nail surface.
- Continue with manicure treatment selecting products and treatments to restore nail condition.

Carrying out manicure treatments

Outcome 2: Be able to provide manicure treatments

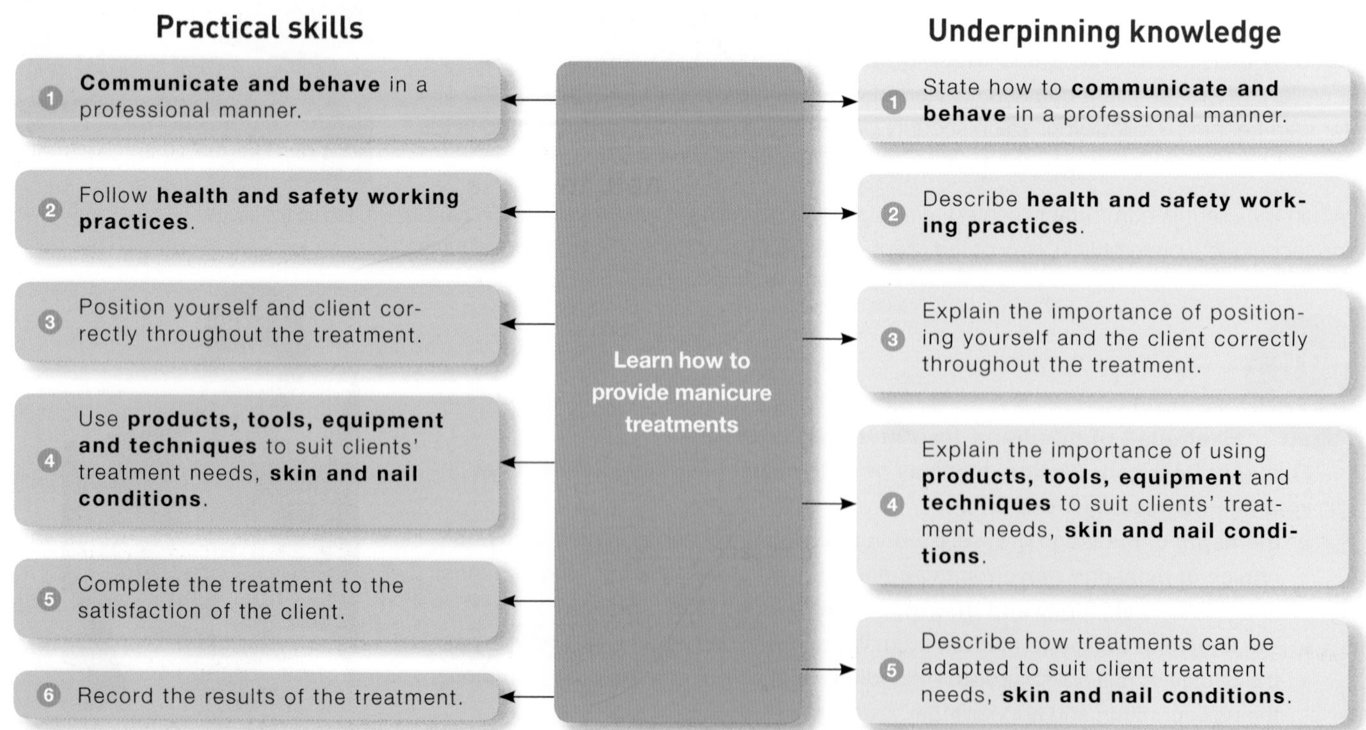
Practical skills
1 Communicate and behave in a professional manner.
2 Follow health and safety working practices.
3 Position yourself and client correctly throughout the treatment.
4 Use products, tools, equipment and techniques to suit clients' treatment needs, skin and nail conditions.
5 Complete the treatment to the satisfaction of the client.
6 Record the results of the treatment.
Learn how to provide manicure treatments
Underpinning knowledge
1 State how to communicate and behave in a professional manner.
2 Describe health and safety working practices.
3 Explain the importance of positioning yourself and the client correctly throughout the treatment.
4 Explain the importance of using products, tools, equipment and techniques to suit clients' treatment needs, skin and nail conditions.
5 Describe how treatments can be adapted to suit client treatment needs, skin and nail conditions.

(*Continued*)
Learn how to provide manicure treatments

Practical skills

7 Provide suitable **aftercare advice**.

Underpinning knowledge

6 Describe the different **massage techniques** and their benefits.

7 State the **contra-actions** that may occur during and following treatments and how to respond.

8 State the importance of completing the treatment to the satisfaction of the client.

9 State the importance of completing treatment records.

10 State the **aftercare advice** that should be provided.

11 Describe diseases and disorders of the nail and skin.

12 Describe the structure and functions of the nail and skin.

13 Describe the structure and function of the muscles of the lower arm and hand.

14 Describe the structure and function of the bones of the lower arm and hand.

15 Describe the structure and function of the arteries and veins of the arm and hand.

16 Describe the structure and function of the lymphatic vessels of the arm and hand.

ALWAYS REMEMBER

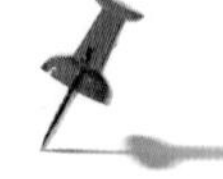

GP referral

A client referred from their GP will usually have a letter. This would be in the case when confirmation of suitability for treatment has been requested. This should be retained with the client's record card.

> Treat nails as jewels whether it be a manicure or nail enhancements. They are fashion accessories.
>
> **Jacqui Jefford**

Step-by-step: Manicure procedure

This procedure briefly shows the stages in the manicure. Each step is discussed in detail later in the chapter. The procedure may start with the right or left hand.

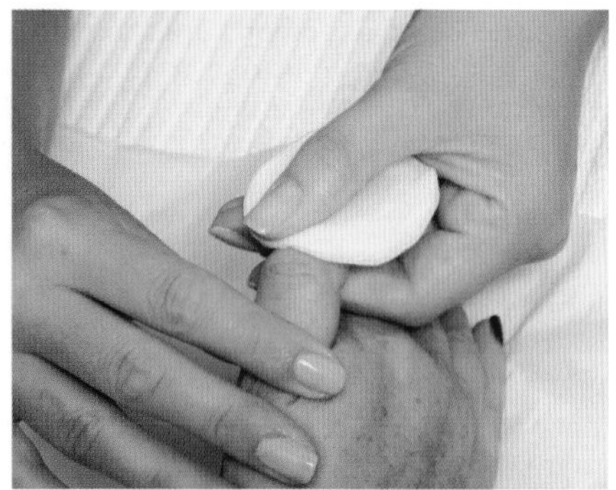

1 Remove any existing nail polish with nail polish remover, using fresh cotton wool for each hand. Replace cotton wool as required to maintain its effectiveness.

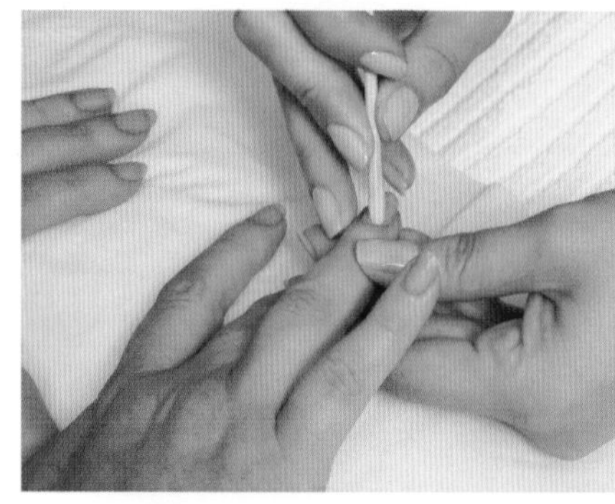

2 Use a cotton wool tipped orange stick to apply nail polish remover around the cuticle area if necessary to remove any excess nail polish. Avoid unnecessary contact with the skin to avoid drying out.

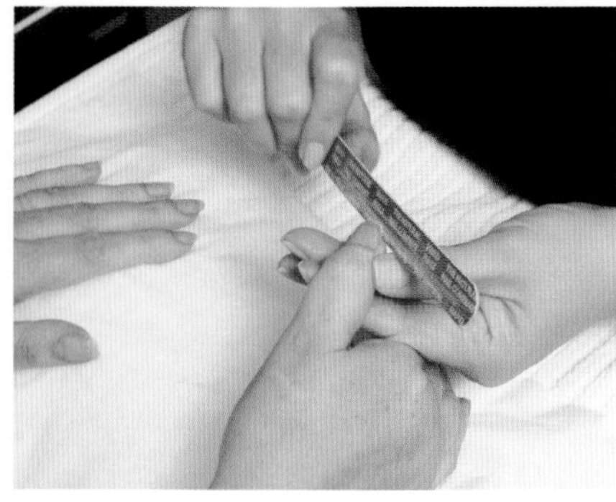

3 File the nails of the right hand to the desired length and shape.

Ensure the free edge is smooth by performing upward strokes with the file often referred to as **bevelling**.

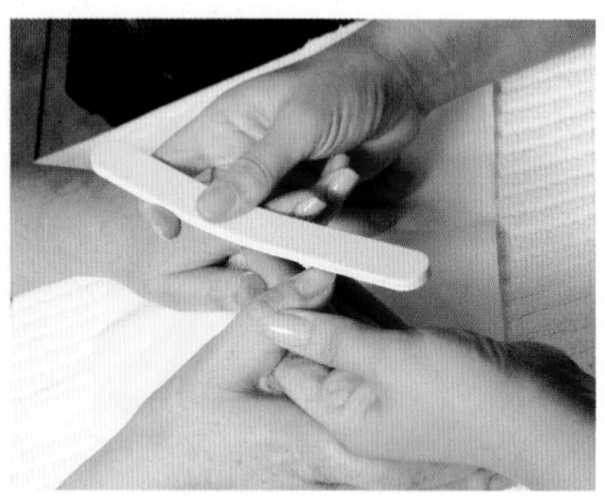

4 Buff the nail plate of the right hand.

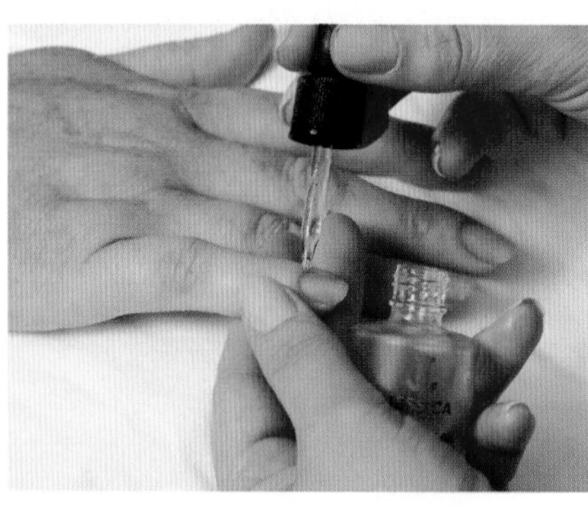

5 Apply cuticle cream or oil to the cuticle area.

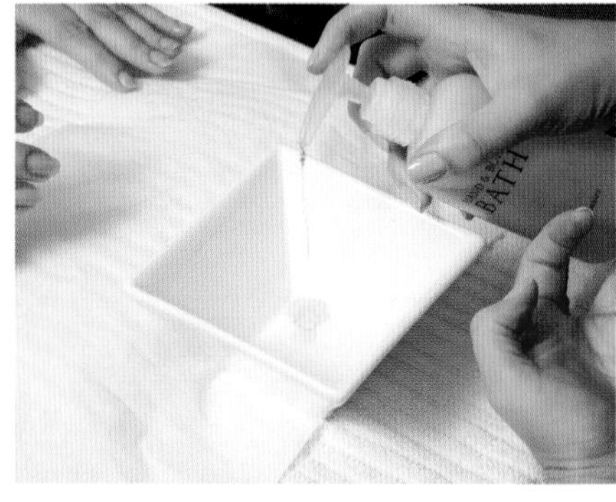

6 Place a small amount of liquid soap formulated for use in manicures and add warm water when ready to use.

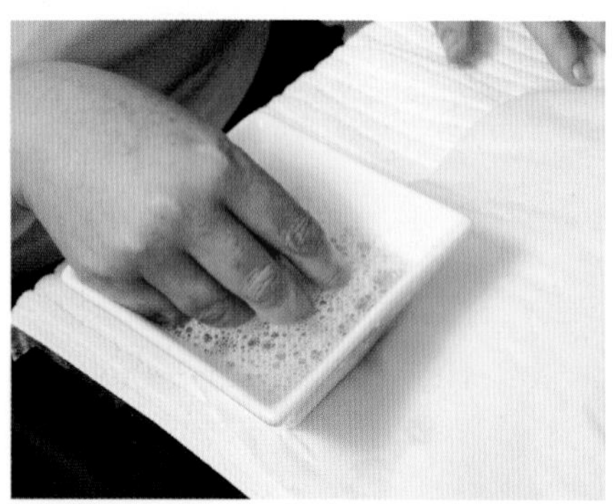

7 Place the right hand in the manicure bowl containing warm water and liquid soap. Repeat steps 3, 4, 5 and 7 for the left hand.

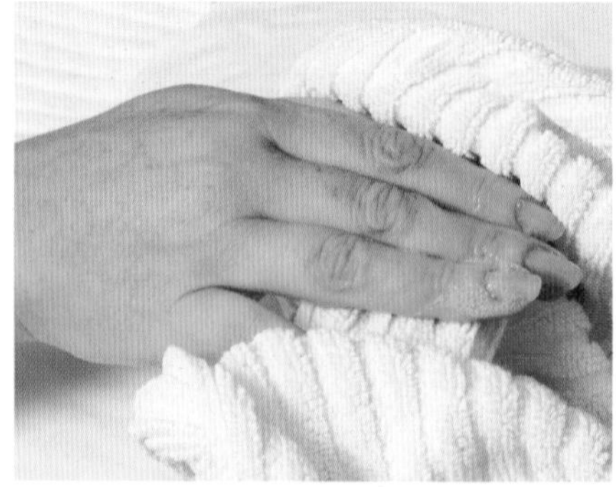

8 Remove the right hand from the manicure bowl and dry with a towel. Place the left hand into the manicure bowl.

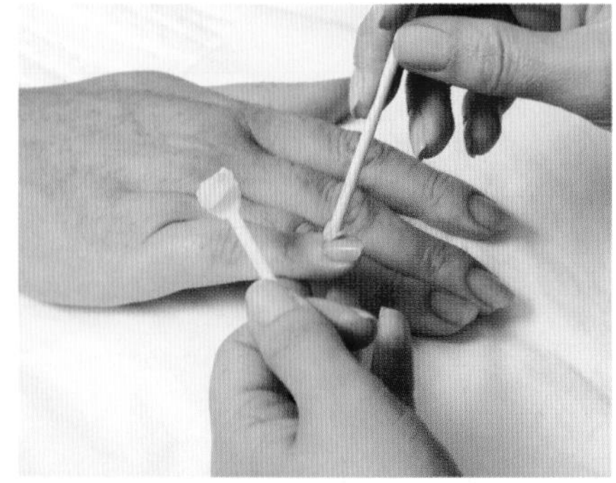

9 Apply cuticle remover to the right hand.

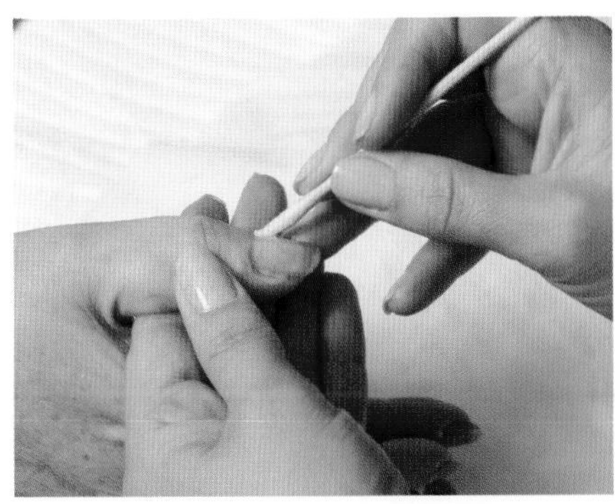

10 Push back the cuticle with a cotton wool-tipped orange stick or hoof stick.

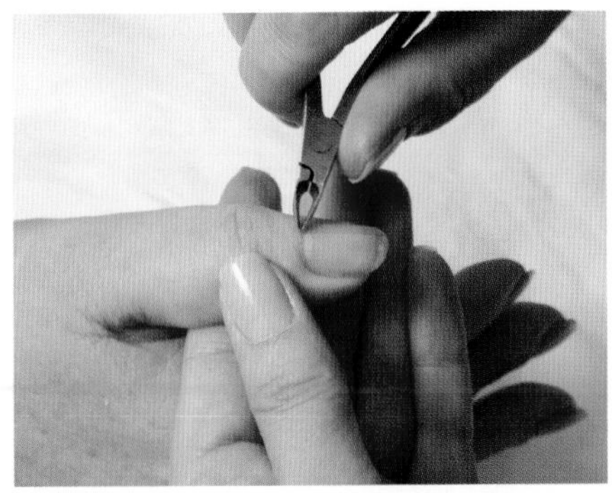

11 Remove excess cuticle with nippers.

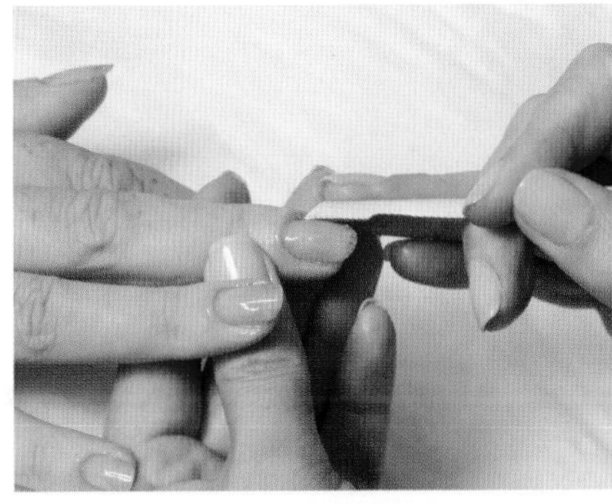

12 Remove excess eponychium with a cuticle knife.

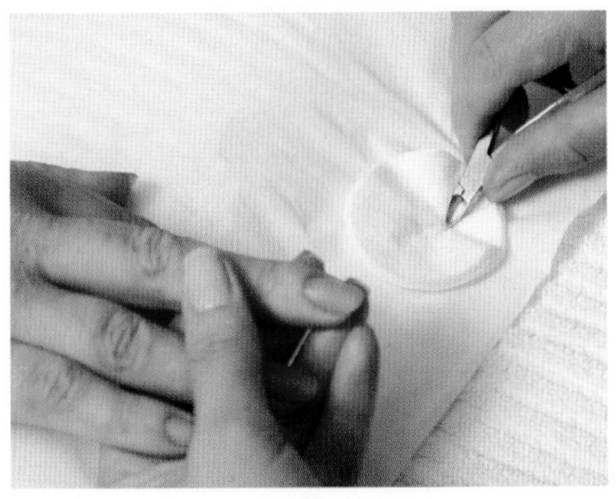

13 Collect excess skin tissue on a clean piece of cotton wool and dispose of it immediately following completion of this stage of the treatment.

Wipe the nails with damp cotton wool to remove excess cuticle remover.

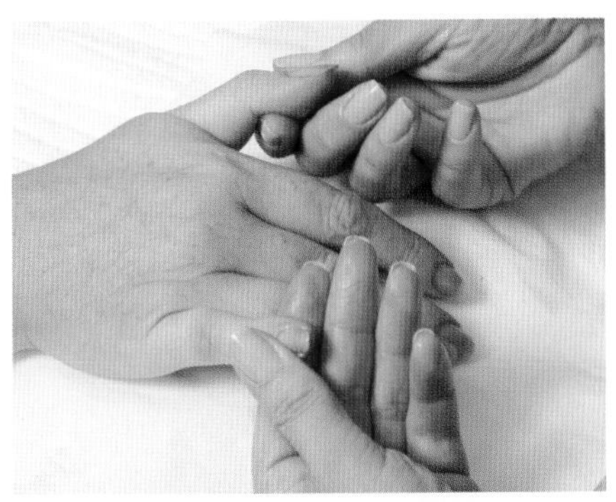

14 Apply cuticle oil and massage it in with your thumbs. Repeat steps 9–13 for the left hand. Apply massage routine to both hands and forearms.

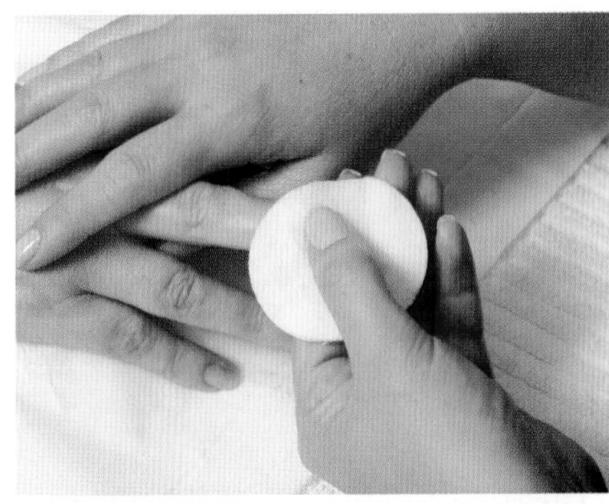

15 Remove grease and excess nail products from the nail plate with a cotton wool pad soaked in nail polish remover.

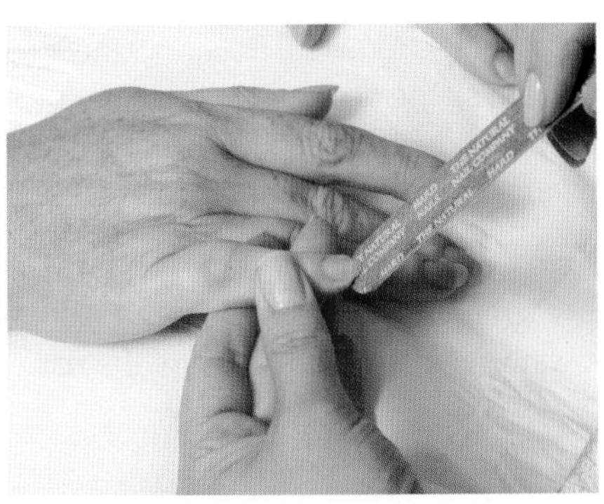

16 Refile the nails as necessary to ensure they are smooth and even.

17 The client may find it convenient to pay for her treatment at this stage, to avoid smudging her polish later. Also, if jewellery has been removed ask her to replace it to avoid damage to the polish after application.

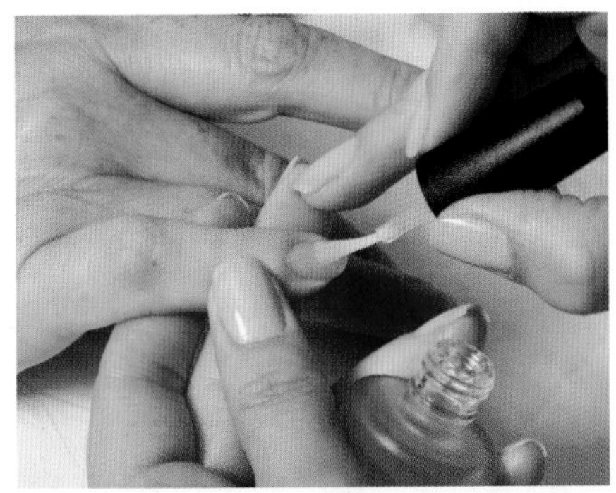

18 Confirm and apply the nail finish. If applying polish, apply: base coat (once); polish (twice); and top coat (once). If a pearlized polish is used, a top coat is *not* required and a third coat of polish may be applied. If the client doesn't want polish, buff to a shine with buffing paste or use a four-sided buffer.

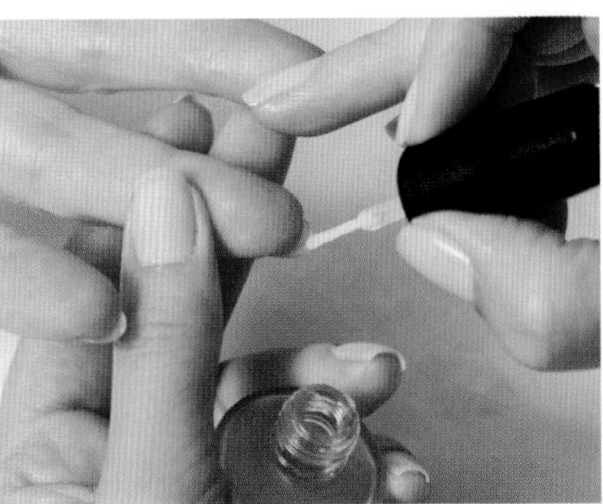

19 Base coat may be applied under the edge of the nail to create a protective seal.

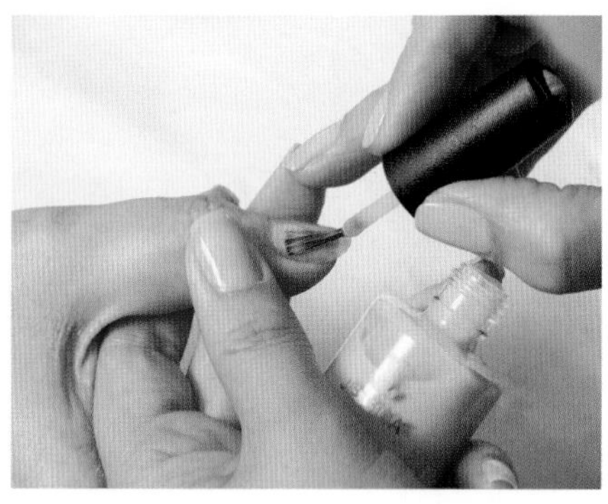

20a French manicure polish application shown: neutral nail polish applied in soft beige to evenly cover the surface. Apply one or two coats.

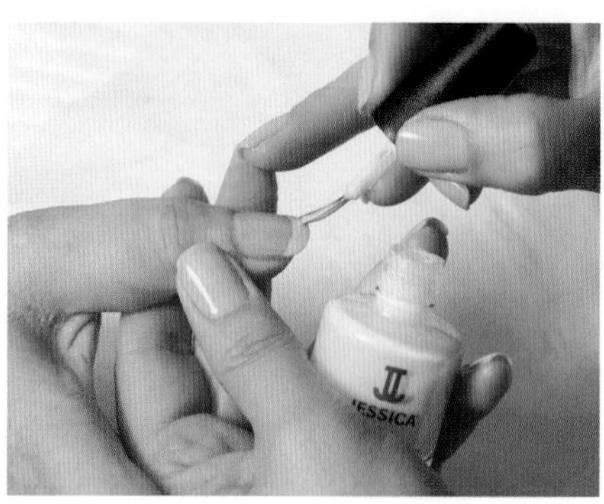

20b The free edge is painted white ensuring that the line is even. Apply one coat. If the nails are particularly stained the reverse of the free edge may be painted also.

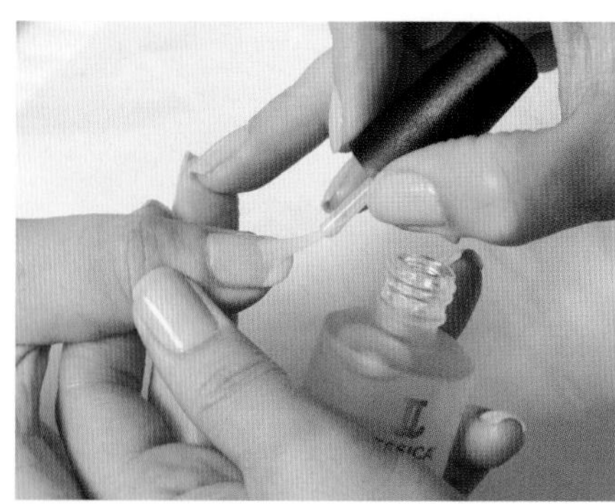

20c Apply a top coat to seal and protect the nail polish.

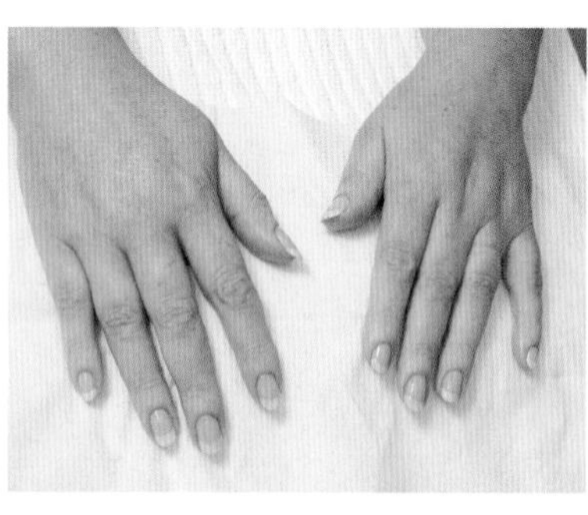

21 The completed French manicure.

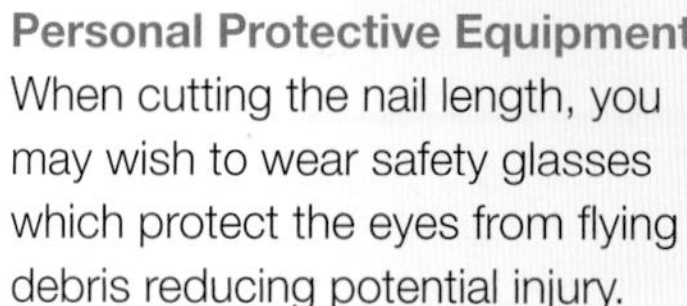

HEALTH & SAFETY

Personal Protective Equipment
When cutting the nail length, you may wish to wear safety glasses which protect the eyes from flying debris reducing potential injury.

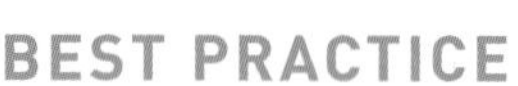

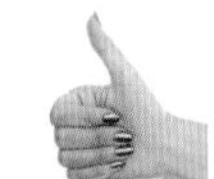

BEST PRACTICE

Client's jewellery
Keep the client's jewellery in full view throughout the treatment so they don't forget it when they leave.

Filing

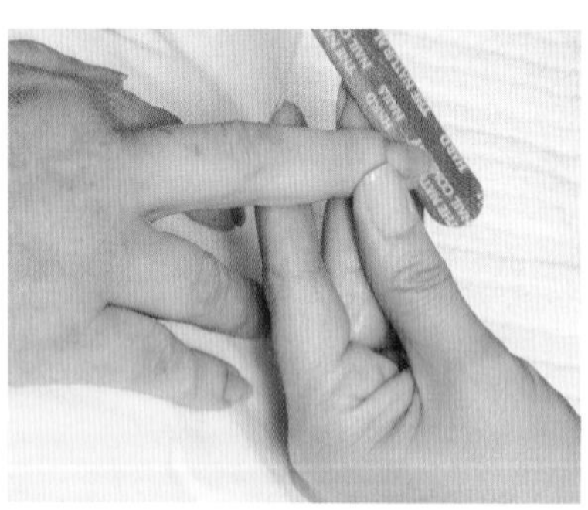

Filing the nails

The part of the nail that is filed is called the the free edge. This should be filed to complement the nail and hand shape and the nail condition. When filing the natural nail, use a fine **emery board**. Very often emery boards have different degrees of coarseness on either side, indicated by different colours. Use the darker, rougher side to remove excess length, and the lighter, smoother side for shaping and removing rough edges. A flexible emery board is preferable to a stiff one as it generates less friction.

When shaping the nail always file the nails from the side to the centre, with the emery board sloping slightly under the free edge. If a square shape is required, file straight across the free edge in one direction to create a uniform square shape and then smooth the outside edges to remove roughness which may lead to accidental damage and breakage. Use swift, rhythmical strokes. Avoid a sawing action – this would generate friction and might cause the free edge to split.

Never file completely down the sides of the nail, as strength is required here to balance the free edge. Always allow about 4mm of nail growth to remain at the sides of the nail.

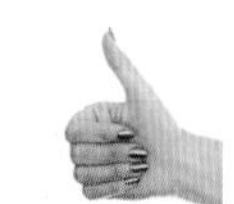

BEST PRACTICE

Emery boards
Cost the emery board into the manicure treatment it is a consumable, and cannot be used again. The client can keep the emery board for personal use. Instruct the client on how the nails should be filed to avoid nail damage.

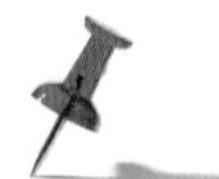

ALWAYS REMEMBER

Nail shapes
When filing the nails ensure that the finished appearance complements the client's nail/hand.

If the fingers are long and thin, select a rounded/square shape and keep the nail length short.

If the fingers are short and fat, the nails should be filed into an oval shape and the nail length should be longer to elongate the fingers.

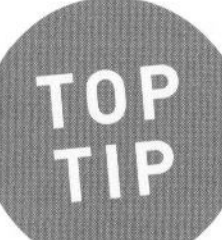

Nail filing

Some nail product suppliers consider the nails best filed after specialized oil application. It is considered less damaging than when filing the natural nail when dry.

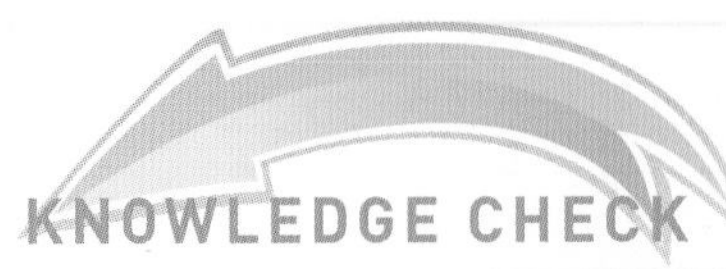

KNOWLEDGE CHECK

What shape are the nails shown in Step 21?

Need more time... refer to page 376 to help you.

Cutting the nails Where it is necessary to reduce nail length, it is more efficient to do so by cutting the nail free edge. This is performed using nail **scissors** or sometimes nail clippers, which have been sterilized before use on each client. Support the nail wall with one hand on the free edge being cut. This minimizes client discomfort. Dispose of the trimmed nail plate hygienically in the metal lined waste bin.

Nail shape

The nail shape should complement the client's fingers and hand length and size. The shape of the free edge that will most compliment a client's nails is one that is similar to the shape of the nail at the base of the nail plate.

Oval The ideal nail shape is oval. This is the shape that offers the most strength to the free edge.

Square A fashionable shape chosen by many clients. The client should be informed, however, that if they have severe corners on the nails they will be more likely to catch and break them.

Pointed One nail shape that should never be recommended is the pointed nail. This leaves the nail tip very weak and likely to break.

Squoval A combination of oval and square nail shape. The nail is filed to a square finish at the free edge and is then gently curved or rounded at the corners.

Round The free edge is rounded and is an ideal shape for short nails. This style is popular with male clients.

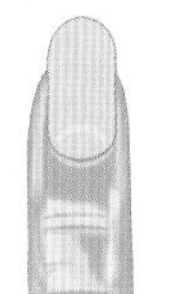

Oval shape

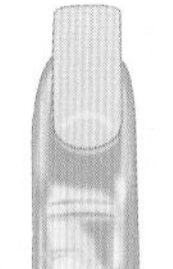

Square shape

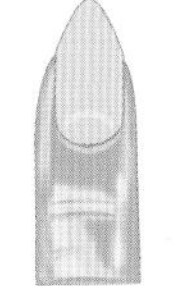

Pointed shape

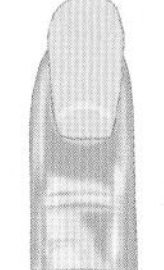

Squoval shape

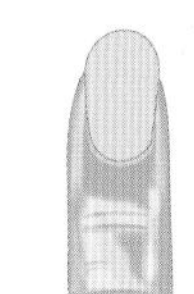

Round shape

Correcting natural nail shapes

Sometimes the natural nail shape will require filing into a suitable shape to maintain nail strength, improve the look of the nail and create overall balance.

Fan The nail becomes broader as it grows towards the free edge, appearing as a fan shape. The wider sides of the nail at the free edge should be shaped to achieve an oval shape.

Tapered nail The free edge part of the nail plate is slimmer than that at the cuticle area which makes it weaker in strength. The free edge should be filed to a squoval shape to maintain strength.

Claw nail Also referred to as hook or convex nail. The nail is excessively curved at the free edge. The nail should be kept short and filed to a round shape. Often this nails shape can occur as a result of nail injury.

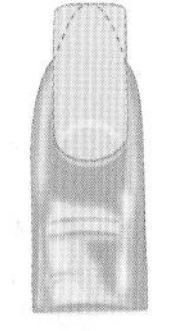

Fan shape

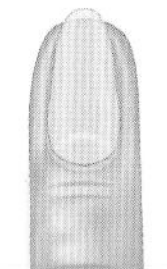

Tapered shape

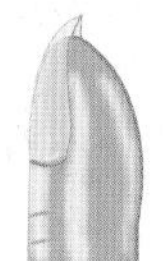

Claw shape

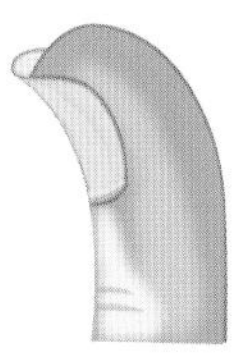

Spoon shape

Spoon shape Also referred to as ski jump or concave. The nail plate curves upwards as it grows from the free edge. File into an oval or squoval nail shape.

Buffing

In manicure, **buffing** is used for these reasons:

- to give the nail plate a sheen
- to stimulate the blood supply in the nail bed, increasing nourishment and encouraging strong, healthy nail growth
- to smooth any surface irregularities

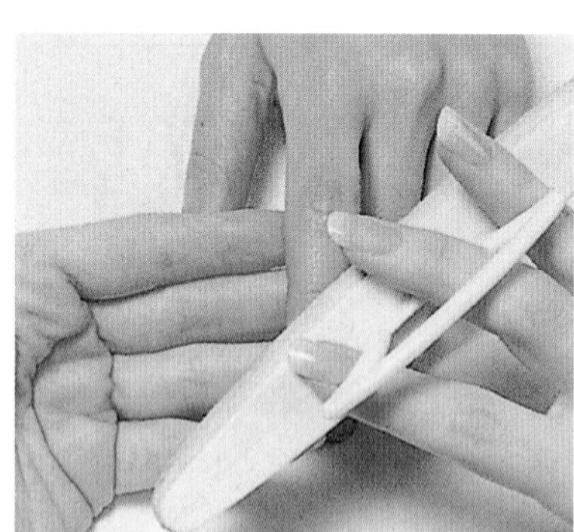

Buffing using a traditional chamois leather covered buffer

A buffer should have a handle made of plastic and a replaceable convex pad covered with chamois or soft leather. **Buffing paste** is the cream used to help smooth out surface irregularities, and thereby give the nail a shine. It contains abrasive particles such as pumice, talc or kaolin.

The **four-sided buffer:** this is shaped like a thick emery board and has four types of surface, ranging from slightly abrasive to very smooth. It can be used to bring the nail to a shine without the need for buffing paste. It cannot be effectively sterilized, however, and must therefore be discarded after use on one client.

Buffing is carried out after filing to stimulate healthy nail growth and before the nails are soaked in the finger bowl. It could also be used instead of polish at the end of the manicure, or as a nail finish. It is popular when performing a male manicure treatment as an alternative finish to nail polish application.

If it is being used, **buffing paste** is applied by taking a small amount out of the pot with a clean orange stick and applying this to each nail plate. With the fingertip, use downward strokes from the cuticle to the free edge to spread the paste without getting it under the cuticle (which would cause irritation). With the buffer held loosely in the hand, buff in one direction only from the base of the nail to the free edge, using smooth, firm, regular strokes. Use approximately six strokes per nail. Avoid excessive strokes which would cause friction and heat to the nail plate causing drying.

Cuticle work

Cuticle work is carried out to keep the cuticle area attractive, healthy and also to prevent cuticles becoming overgrown and adhering to the nail plate, which could lead to splitting of the cuticle as the nail grows forward, and subsequently to infection of the area.

KNOWLEDGE CHECK

What is the nail condition where the cuticle becomes overgrown and thickened on the nail plate?

Need more time... refer to page 367 to help you.

HEALTH & SAFETY

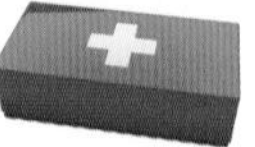

Clinical waste

If you accidentally cut the skin causing bleeding at the cuticle area, protect you hands with disposable gloves and wipe the skin with an antiseptic wipe. Any waste is classed as clinical contaminated waste and should be disposed of in a yellow medical sealed bag in accordance with the **Environment Act 1990**.

See the *Habia Hygiene in Beauty Therapy* booklet for further guidance.

The work is carried out after soaking the nails in warm soapy water. This step loosens dirty particles from the free edge and softens the skin in the cuticle area.

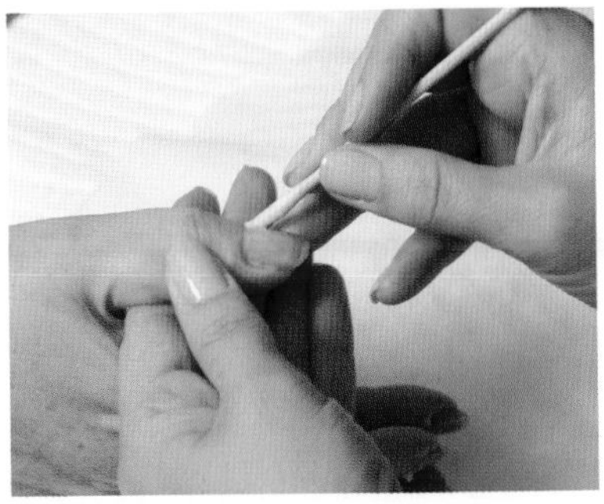

Pushing back cuticles using a cotton wool tipped orange stick

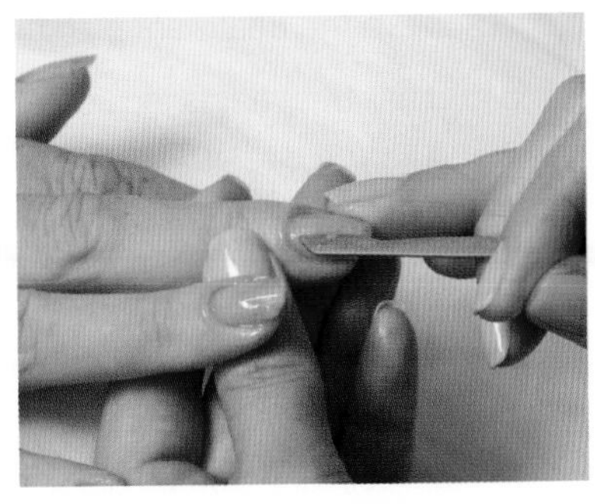

Using a cuticle knife

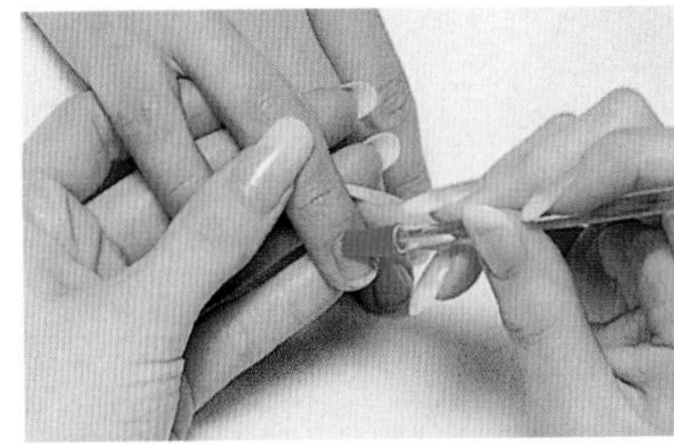

Pushing back cuticles using a hoof stick

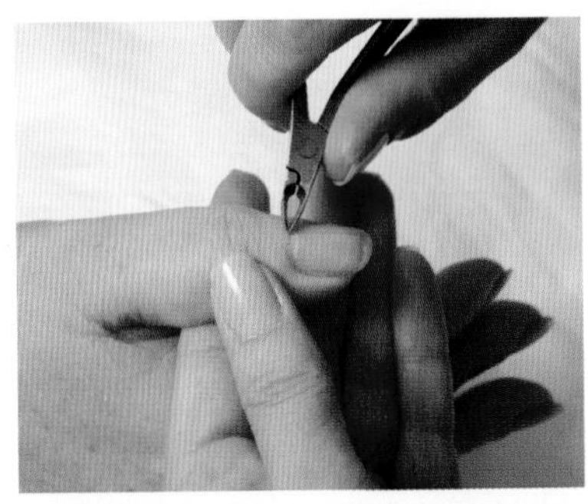

Using cuticle nippers

HEALTH & SAFETY

Hygiene

Use a fresh orange stick for each part of the manicure treatment, and when working on different hands, to prevent cross-infection. The orange stick is disposed of after use.

How to provide cuticle work

1 Take the fingers from the soapy water and pat them dry with a soft towel.

2 Apply cuticle remover to the cuticle and nail walls, using the applicator brush. (Cuticle remover is a slightly caustic solution that helps soften and loosen the cuticles and the eponychium from the nail plate.)

3 Gently push back the cuticle with a cotton wool-tipped orange stick or **hoof stick**. (The cotton wool is to avoid splinters from the wood, and also may be easily replaced if necessary.) Use a gentle, circular motion to push back the cuticle, holding the orange stick like a pen.

4 Hold the cuticle knife at 45° to the nail plate and stroke it in one direction only, gently loosening any eponychium and perionychium that has adhered to the nail plate: do not scratch it backwards and forwards. The **cuticle knife** should have a fine-ground flat blade which can be re-sharpened when necessary. Dampen it regularly in the manicure bowl to prevent scratches occurring on the nail plate.

5 Hold the nippers comfortably in the palm of the hand, with the thumb resting just above the blades – this gives firm control over what can be a dangerous instrument. Use the cuticle nippers to remove any loose or torn pieces of cuticle, and to trim excess dead cuticle. ***Do not cut into live cuticle:*** if you do, it will bleed profusely and will be very uncomfortable for the client. Not every client will require the use of **cuticle nippers** – use them only when needed. Avoid over trimming the cuticle, which can lead to overgrown, thickened cuticle.

TOP TIP

Choosing cuticle nippers

Cuticle nippers should have finely ground cutting blades to give a clean cut and to avoid tearing the cuticle. Check the quality of your nippers before you purchase, they should be of good quality and durable.

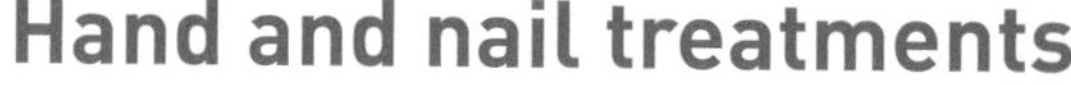

Hand and nail treatments

In addition to a manicure, further hand and nail treatments may be included as appropriate to achieve the treatment plan aims.

Hand and nail treatments include:

Warm-oil treatment

- Warm-oil treatment involves gently heating a small amount of organic oil (such as almond oil) and soaking the cuticles in it for ten minutes. This nourishes the nail plate, softens the cuticles and the surrounding skin, and is an excellent treatment for clients with dry, cracked cuticles.
- Warm oil may also be applied to the skin of the hand and forearm to improve skin texture, colour and blood circulation in the area.

KNOWLEDGE CHECK

Which manicure tools are used to improve the condition and appearance of the cuticles?

Need more time... refer to page 379 to help you.

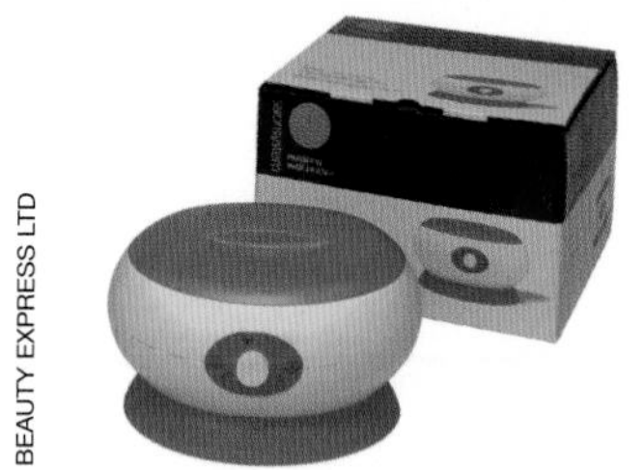

BEAUTY EXPRESS LTD

An oil/wax heater

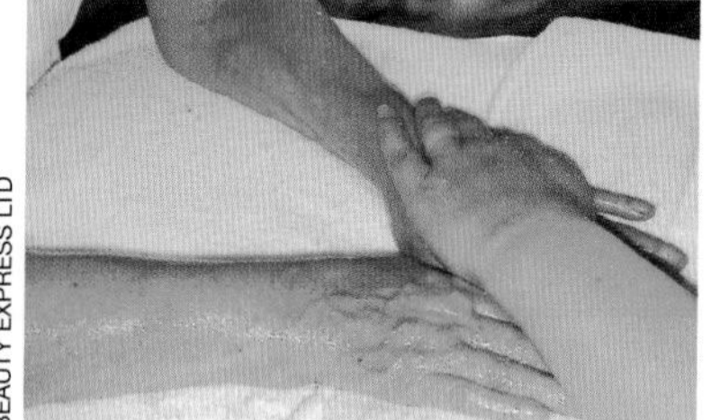

BEAUTY EXPRESS LTD

Warm oil application

Exfoliating treatment

Exfoliating treatment is carried out as part of the massage routine. The massage is performed as usual, using an **exfoliant** a mildly abrasive cosmetic product. It may be applied prior to hand and arm massage also to expose new cells and aid the absorption of the massage oil/cream. This treatment offers the following benefits:

- the removal of dead skin cells
- improvement of the skin texture
- improvement of the skin colour
- increased blood circulation
- increased lymph circulation

The abrasive particles must be thoroughly removed with hot, damp towels before continuing with the rest of the manicure.

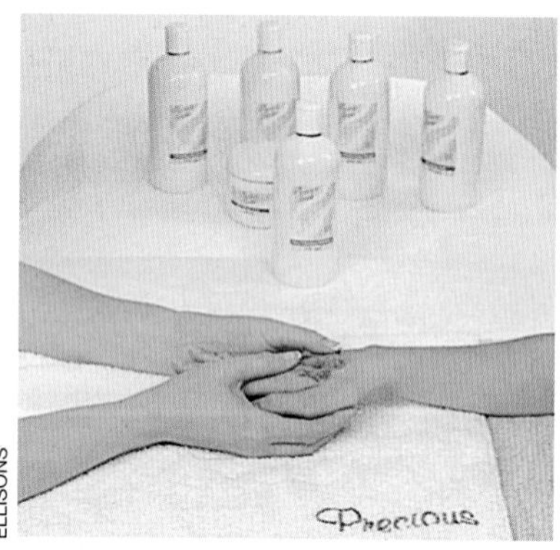

ELLISONS

An exfoliating treatment

Hand treatment mask

An appropriate treatment **mask** may be applied, according to the client's treatment requirements. This may be either stimulating and rejuvenating, or moisturising. The hands may be placed inside thermal mitts or hand gloves for ten minutes to enable the mask to penetrate the epidermis. Several layers are applied. The mask is then removed, and followed with treatment massage cream. Some products may also be used as the massage medium.

ELLISONS

A hand treatment mask

Paraffin wax treatment

The paraffin wax is heated in a special bath to a temperature of 50–55°C. It is then applied to the hands and usually over the wrists too with a brush. It is then, covered with a plastic protective covering and left to set for 10–15 minutes before removal. Several layers are applied. This offers the following benefits:

- the heating effect stimulates the blood and lymph circulation
- eases discomfort of arthritic and rheumatic conditions
- softens the skin; improving the appearance and condition of the nails and dry skin
- soothes sensory nerve endings

After use the wax is disposed of.

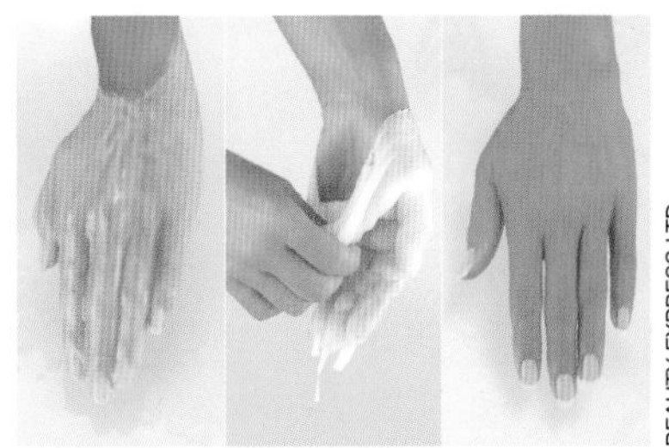

BEAUTY EXPRESS LTD

Paraffin wax application and removal

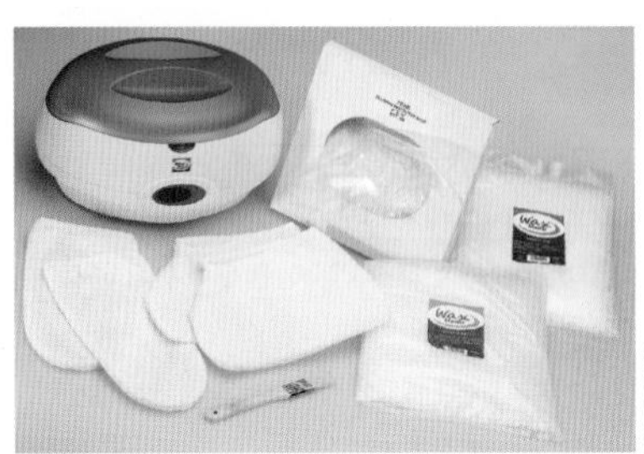

ELLISONS

Paraffin wax resources

Thermal mitts

These are electrically heated gloves in which the hands are placed for approximately 10–15 minutes.

They are usually used following the application of a treatment within the manicure routine e.g. a hand treatment mask. The hands are prepared by wrapping them in a plastic protective covering before placement in the mitts.

The treatment has the following benefits:

- decreases joint stiffness in the case of a client suffering from arthritis
- improves the condition of dry skin of the cuticles and hands by increasing the absorption of moisturising products
- improves skin colour and blood and lymph circulation

Always follow manufacturers' guidelines in the application procedure for hand and nail treatments.

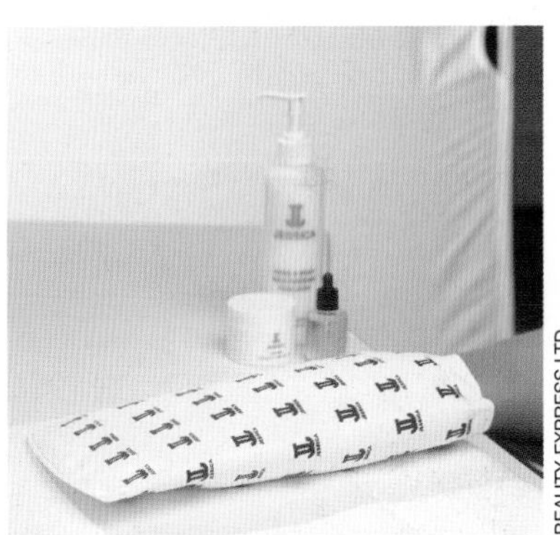

BEAUTY EXPRESS LTD

Thermal mitts

Step-by-step: Specialist hand and arm treatment

Specialist treatments should be offered to your client when there is a specific treatment need or if they feel they would like to benefit from such a treatment.

Specialist training in these advanced techniques is usually offered by major product companies.

The model for this specialist hand and arm treatment is a mature client who suffers from the medical condition rheumatoid arthritis where the joints become inflamed and painful.

The following hand and arm treatment will:

- stimulate the blood and lymph circulation
- have a skin cleansing action
- remove dead skin cells (desquamation)
- improve the moisture content of the skin
- minimize discomfort caused by an arthritic, rheumatic condition

Your treatments should be adapted the meet the treatment objectives for the client.

Allow 30 minutes for this specialist hand and arm treatment.

KNOWLEDGE CHECK

Why would you choose to include exfoliation in your manicure treatment?

Need more time... refer to page 380 to help you.

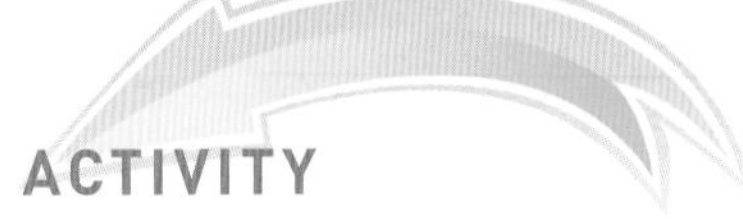

ACTIVITY

Researching treatments

Research other types of hand and nail treatments. Write down the details of your research, and try out the treatments on clients.

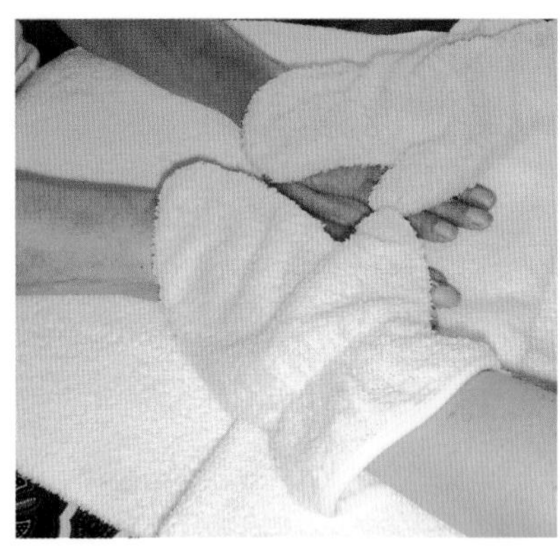

1 The hands and arms are cleansed using warm towelling mitts infused with lime oil for its therapeutic, refreshing and energizing properties.

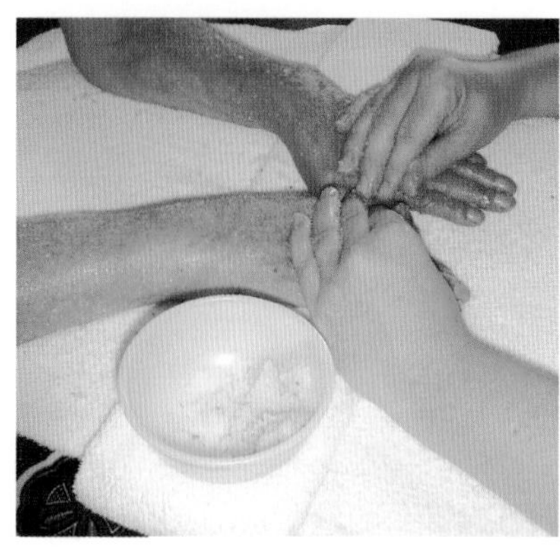

2 The hands are exfoliated to remove all dead skin cells and brighten the skin. A salt-based preparation with emollient, skin-softening ingredients is applied to the skin of each hand and is rubbed gently over the skin's surface.

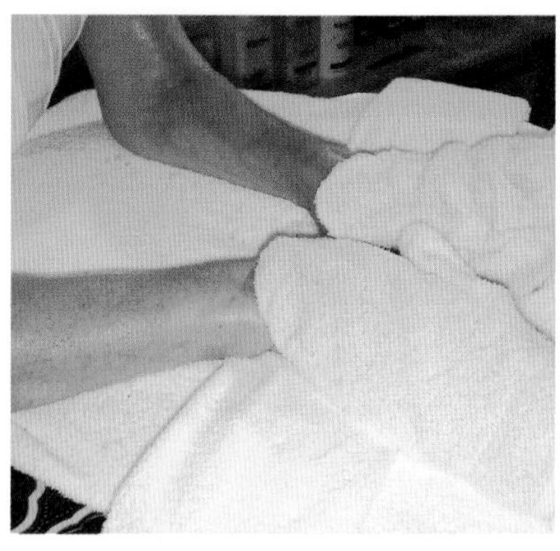

3 Towelling mitts are used to remove the exfoliating treatment. These have been steamed and are warm when used.

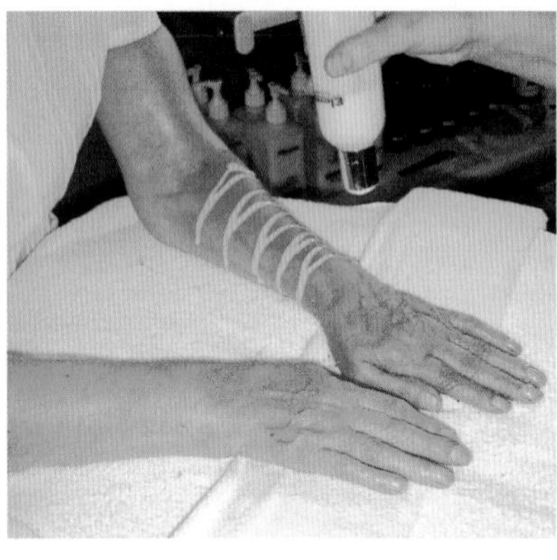

4 A skin-nourishing milk lotion is applied to each arm using a 'drizzling' technique. The milk is particularly beneficial for dry, sensitive skin.

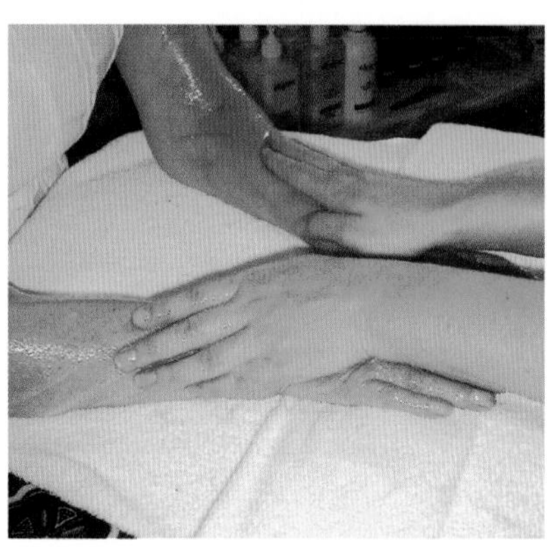

5 Massage movements are applied using effleurage and petrissage massage manipulations.

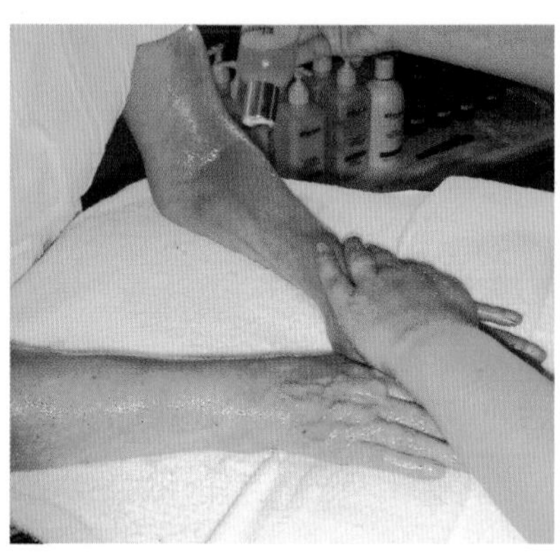

6 A further skin treatment product, warm oil, is applied and massaged into the skin. This will act as a treatment mask for the skin.

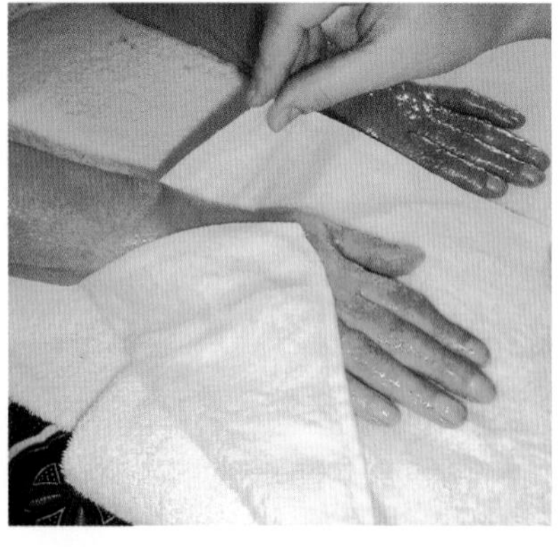

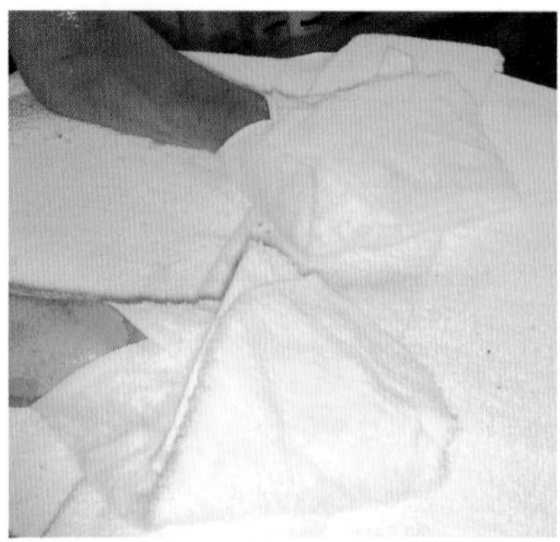

7 The hands are then placed in steamed towels and encased in a plastic bag and dry towelling mitten for 10–15 minutes. Remove mittens and continue with nail polish application if desired.

> You can only sell if you believe in what you are selling.
>
> **Jacqui Jefford**

Hand and forearm massage

Hand massage is generally carried out near the end of the manicure treatment, just prior to nail polish application. It can also be carried out on its own if the client wants the effects of the massage but does not need or want treatment to their nails.

The massage incorporates classic massage movements, each with different effects:

- **Effleurage** – a stroking movement, used to begin the massage as a link manipulation, and to complete the massage sequence.
- **Petrissage** – movements including **kneading** where the tissues are lifted away from the underlying structures and compressed. Pressure is intermittent, and should be light yet firm.
- **Tapotement** – also referred to as percussion. Performed in a brisk, light and stimulating manner. Rhythm is important as the hands break contact with the skin. Movements include tapping used to increase blood supply and muscle/skin in the area.
- **Joint manipulations** – the joints of the wrists and hands are manipulated through their range of movement dependant upon the type of joint. This helps to maintain good mobility within the range of movement but must be avoided if the client has any joint disorders.
- **Frictions** – small circular movements using the pads of the fingers or thumbs. The skin and muscle below is massage against the underlying bone. This can be used to loosen any adhesions in the tissues.

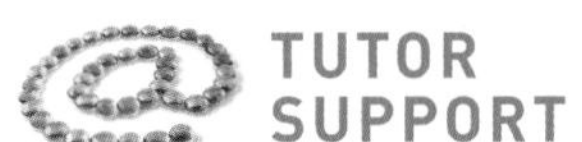

Activity 6 & 7: Manicure word searches

The beauty therapist can adapt the massage application according to the needs of the client. Either the **speed of application** or **depth of pressure** can be altered.

The reasons for offering massage during a manicure are as follows:

- to moisturise the skin with massage medium, improving skin hydration
- to increase blood circulation, transporting oxygen and nutrients to the lower arm and hand
- to increase lymph circulation, transporting waste products in the lymph from the lower arm and hand
- to help maintain joint mobility
- to ease discomfort from arthritis or rheumatism
- to relax the client
- to help remove dead skin cells (desquamation), exposing new cells

BEST PRACTICE

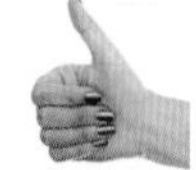

Positive promotion

Hand massage can be included during a facial while the mask is applied, maximizing treatment benefits and client relaxation. It also gives you the opportunity to promote another product or service to the client.

Step-by-step: Hand and forearm massage

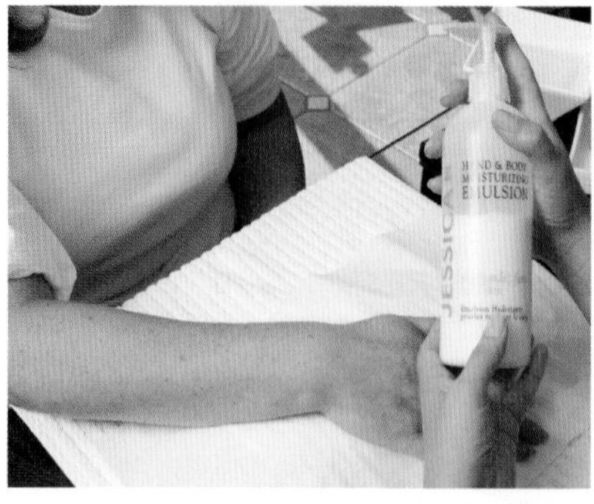

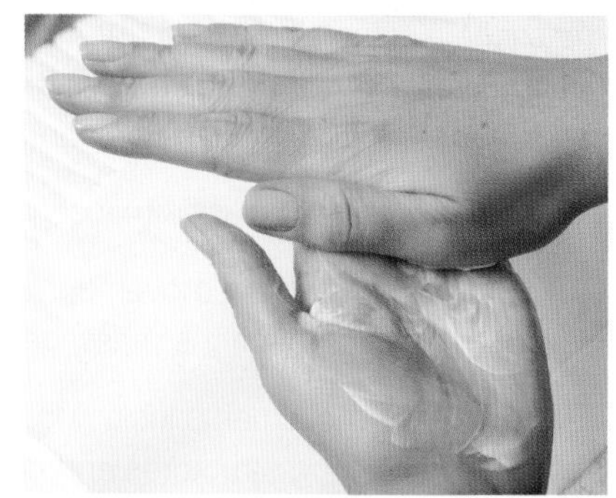

1 Dispense the chosen massage medium into the hands, warm the product over the palms and apply to the client's skin using effleurage technique.

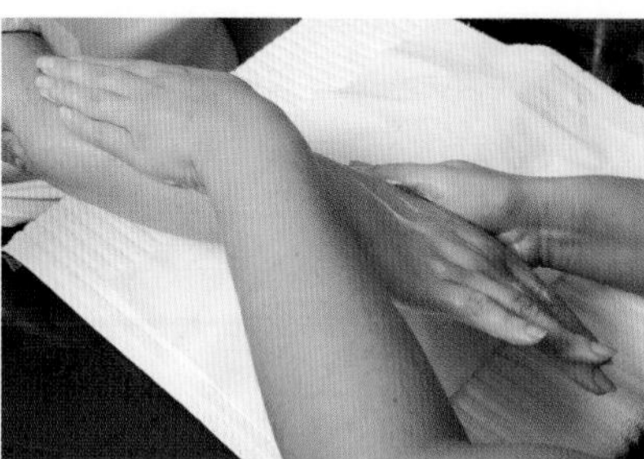

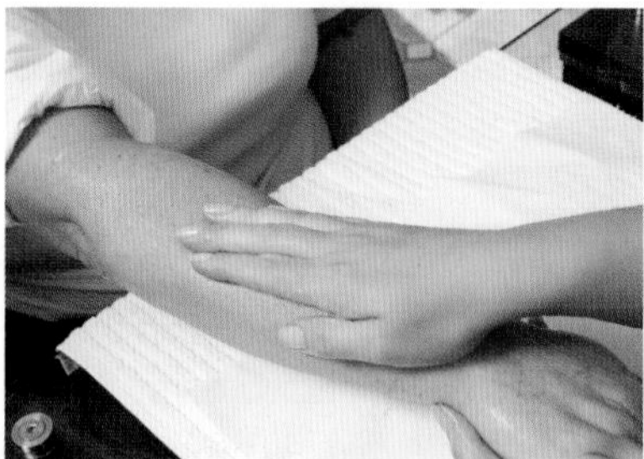

2 **Effleurage to the whole hand and forearm** Use long sweeping strokes from the hand to the elbow, moving on both the outer and the inner sides of the forearm.

Repeat step 2 a further 5 times.

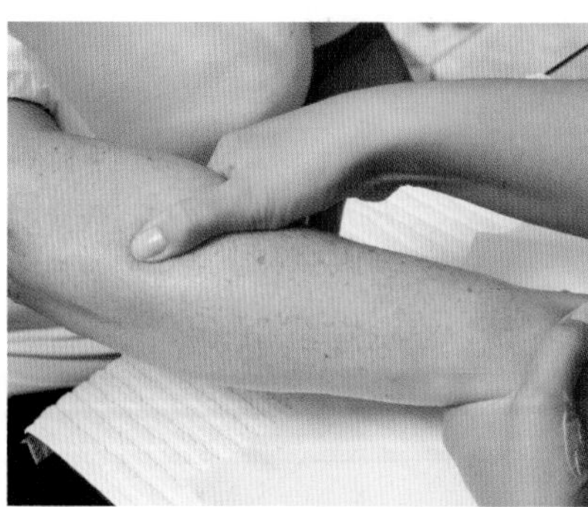

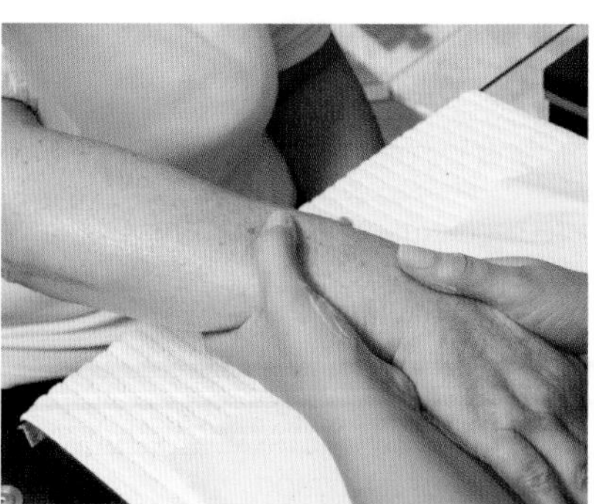

3 Using a **petrissage movement** pick up the flexor and extensor muscles of the lower arm.

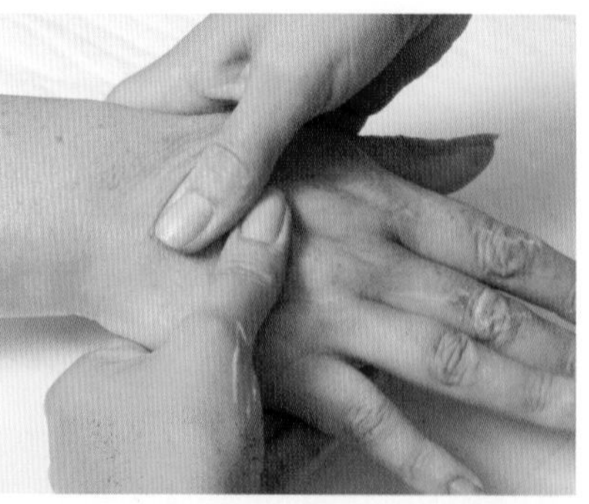

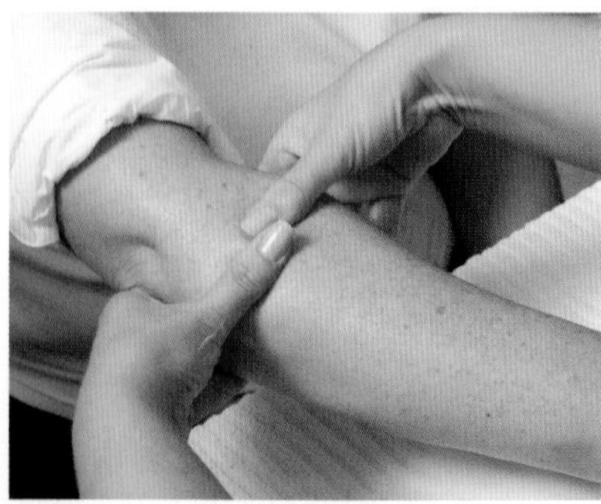

4 **Thumb kneading to the back of the hand and the forearm** Use the thumbs, one in front of the other, and rotate each thumb one in a clockwise direction, the other anti-clockwise. In a gently kneading action between each metacarpal bone. Move from the hand towards the elbow massaging over the interosseus membrane located between the radius and ulna bone, then slide the thumbs back down to the hands.

Repeat step 4 a further 2 times.

KNOWLEDGE CHECK

What is the name of the lymph node the therapist is massaging located in the elbow area?

Need more time... refer to page 85 help you.

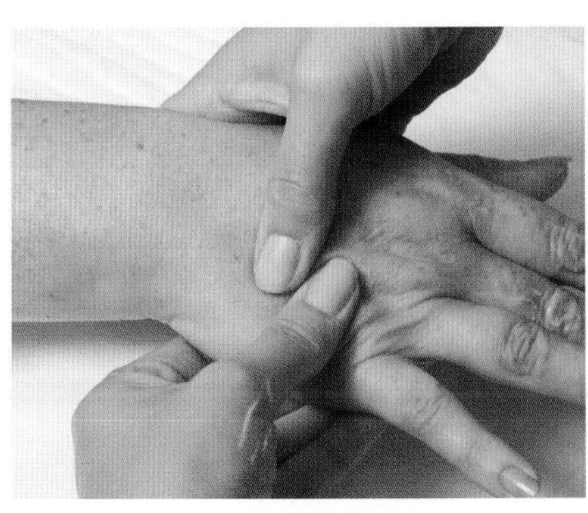

5 **Perform a scissoring, friction movement** using both thumbs between each metacarpal bone in the hands.

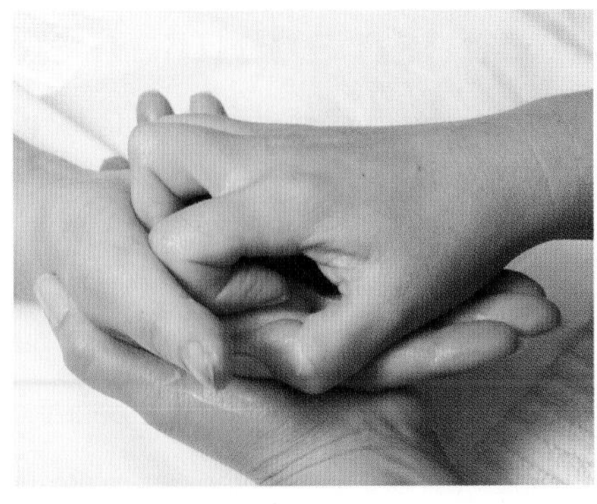

6 **Perform a 'knuckling' petrissage movement** rotating the fingers in a small fist shape against the muscles in the palms of the hand.

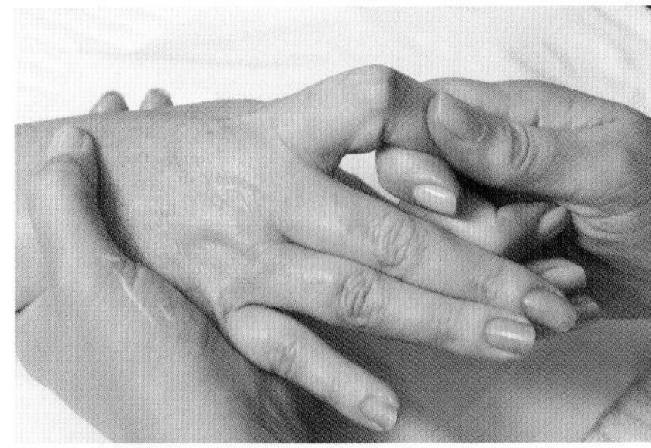

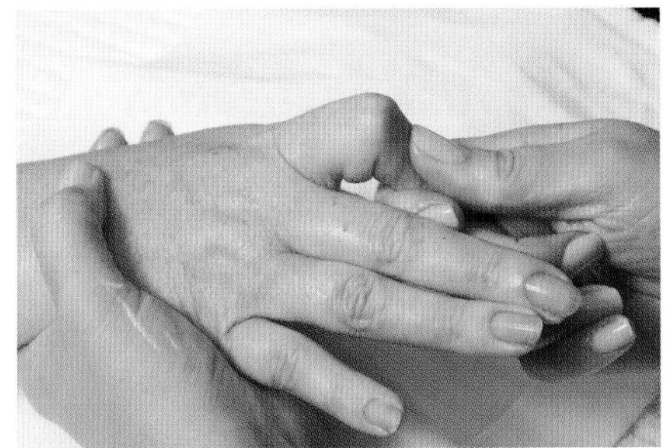

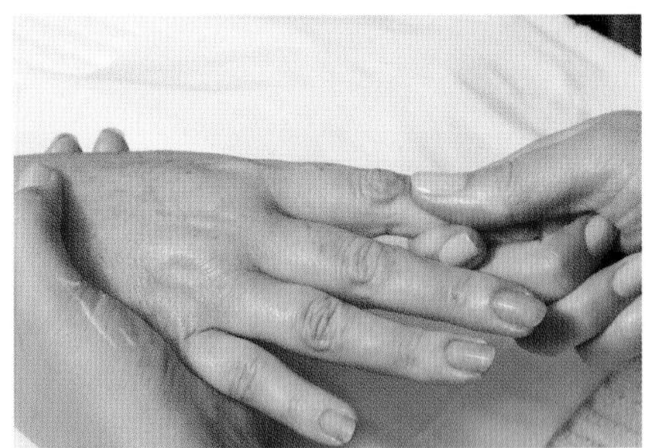

7 **Perform joint manipulations (Steps 7–9). Move the phalange bones of each finger**, bending the finger at each joint and then straightening in a resistance movement.

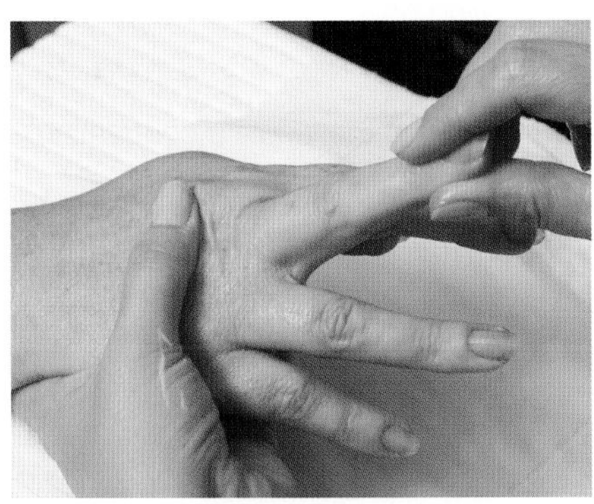

8 **Finger circulations, supporting the joints** Supporting the knuckles with one hand, hold the fingers individually and gently take each through its full range of movements, first clockwise and then anticlockwise. Move from the little finger to the thumb.

Repeat step 8 a further 2 times.

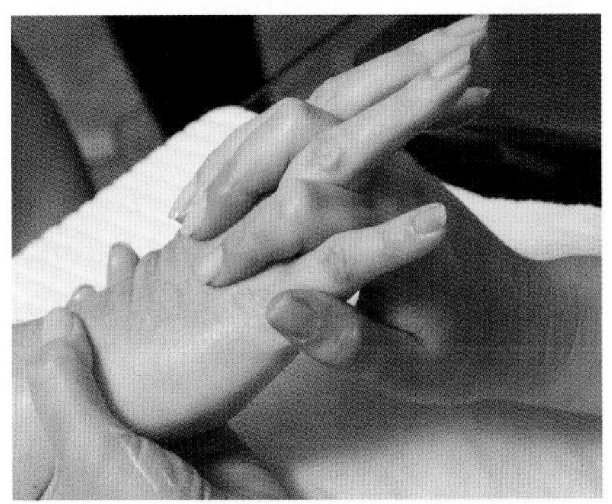

9 **Wrist circulations, supporting the joints** Support the wrist with one hand and put your fingers between the client's, gently grasping his/her hand. Move the wrist through its full range of movement, first clockwise and then anticlockwise.

Repeat step 9 a further 2 times.

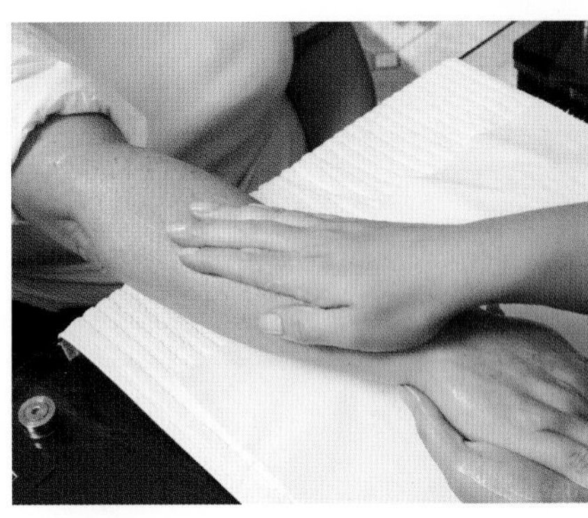

10 **Effleurage to the whole hand and forearm** Use the same movement as in step 2.

Repeat step 10 a further 5 times.

HEALTH & SAFETY

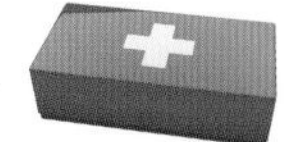

Joint mobility

If the client has any joint mobility restrictions, e.g. arthritis, you will need to modify your massage technique avoiding joint manipulation movements.

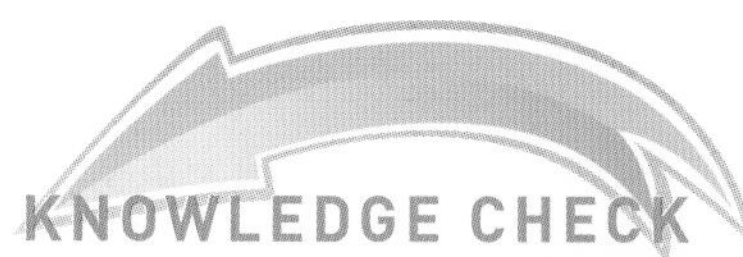

What are the terms used for the different types of massage used in manicure?

Need more time... refer to page 383 to help you.

Nail polish application

Nail polish is used to coat the nail plate for a number of reasons:

- to adorn the nail
- to disguise stained nails
- to add temporary strength to weak nails
- to improve the condition or appearance of the natural nail
- to co-ordinate with clothes or make-up
- to create designs and effects, called 'nail art'

Before nail polish is applied, the client's hand jewellery may be replaced, to avoid smudging afterwards.

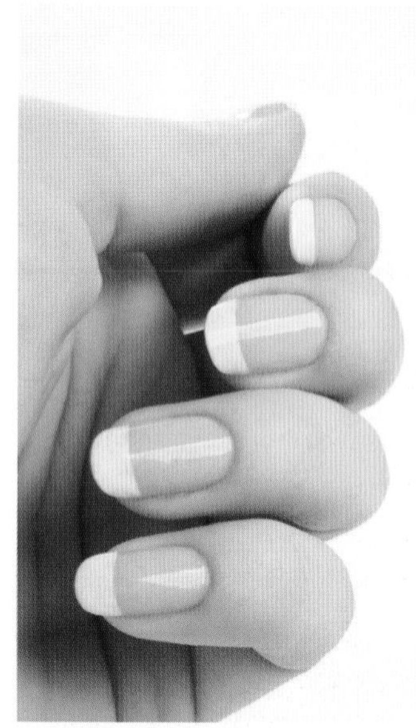

Manicured nails with french application

Styles of polish application

- ***Traditional application*** This style is the one most commonly requested by clients: the entire nail plate is covered with polish in a block colour.
- ***French manicure application*** This style involves painting the nail plate of the nail bed pink or pale beige, and the free edge white. This can be adapted by painting a narrow block of colour along the free edge which is more complimentary for a shorter nail. This technique can also provide product strength to a weaker nail.
- ***Free lunula application*** This style involves applying polish over the whole nail plate except the area of the lunula.
- ***Painted lunula application*** This style involves painting the lunula a contrasting colour.
- ***Application to give the appearance of longer nails*** This style creates an optical illusion that the nails are longer than they really are. The whole nail plate is painted, leaving a slightly larger gap than usual (usually 1.5mm) along the nail walls.

Tips for nail painting

- Ensure the surface of the nail is grease-free. If grease is present this will result in nail polish peeling or chipping.
- Select colours that suit the client's nail length, condition and skin colour.
- Dark colours will draw attention to the nails, and will make small/short nails appear smaller/shorter.
- If the nails are very broad leave a margin at the sides of the nail's wall free of polish, this will help them to appear slimmer.
- Avoid pearlized polish if the client's nail surface is uneven or ridged. The polish will emphasize the imperfection.
- Always apply a good quality base coat suited to the client's nail condition. This helps to prevent staining from pigment in the polish, and may strengthen the nail or smooth ridges depending on its formulation.

TOP TIP

Fast-drying products

A nail 'fast-drying' product may be applied to reduce the time taken for the polish to dry.

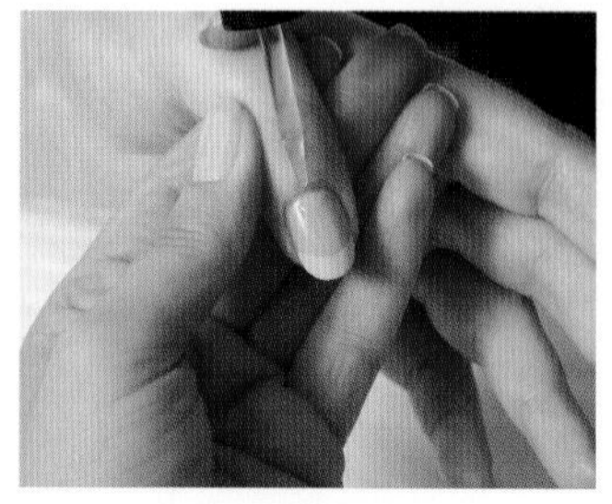

- When applying nail polish colour, apply two coats, allowing the nails to dry between each coat to prevent the appearance of brush marks.
- Ensure good colour coverage.
- Ensure your polish is a good quality. If it has become thickened use a specialised solvent to restore to the correct consistency. This should be done 20 minutes prior to use to ensure an even consistency.
- Allow nail polish to dry before **top coat** application.
- Always follow manufacturer recommendations for their nail polish application.

ALWAYS REMEMBER

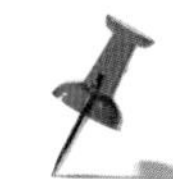

Maintaining the quality of your nail polish

Always clean the neck of the nail polish bottle after used with nail polish remover to ensure that it can be closed tightly. If the lid is not tightened the solvents that maintain its consistency can evaporate and it will become thickened.

Reasons for peeling and chipping nail polish

Chipping may be explained by any of the following:

- The nail polish was not thick enough because of over-thinning with solvent.
- No base coat was used.
- Grease was left on the nail plate prior to painting.
- The nail plate is flaking.
- The polish was dried too quickly by artificial means.

Peeling polish may have the following explanations:

- No top coat was used.
- Successive coats were not allowed to dry between applications.
- The nail polish was too thick, due to evaporation of the solvent.
- Grease was left on the nail plate prior to painting.

Nail polish storage Nail polish should be stored in a cool, dark place, to avoid thickening, separation and fading. The caps and the rims of bottles **must** be kept clean, not only for appearance but also to ensure that the bottle is airtight. Always use stock rotation to ensure that the oldest product is used first, remember FILO – first in, last out.

If polish does thicken, **solvent** may be added to restore the correct consistency.

HEALTH & SAFETY

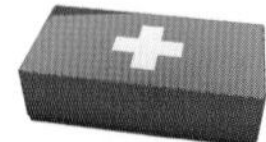

Stock storage

Always check MSDS recommendations to ensure that stock is stored safely and to maintain its quality.

BEST PRACTICE

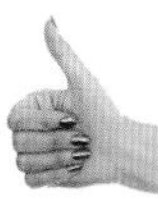

Choosing nail polish colours

For short nails, select a pale, neutral colour. Darker, more dramatic colours suit healthy, long nails, especially on clients with darker skin tones. Remember it is always the client's choice, but you will often be asked to recommend.

ALWAYS REMEMBER

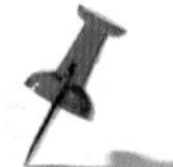

Essential nail polish qualities

Nail polish should:

- adhere to the nail plate and be flexible to resist peeling and chipping
- have good durability on exposure to water, detergents and other chemicals it may come into contact with
- not stain the nail plate
- flow freely onto the nail plate and be easy to apply

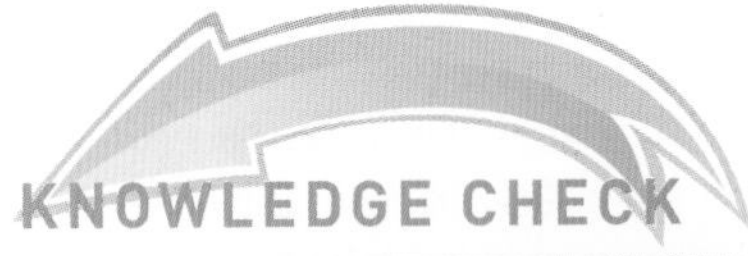

KNOWLEDGE CHECK

Identify the nail painting techniques shown:

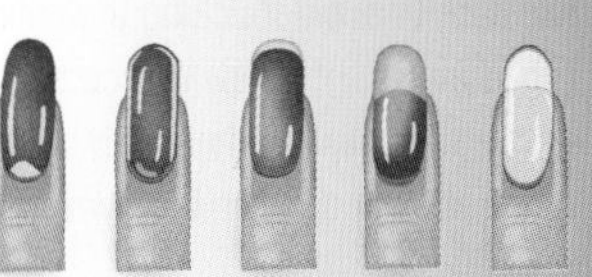

Need more time... refer to page 386 to help you.

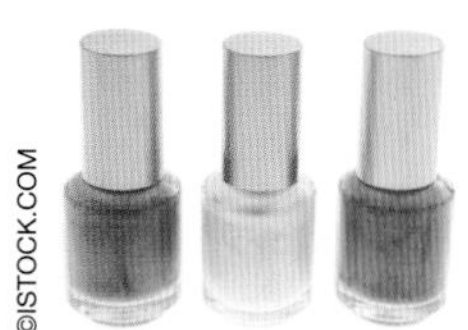

©ISTOCK.COM

Cream and pearlized nail polish

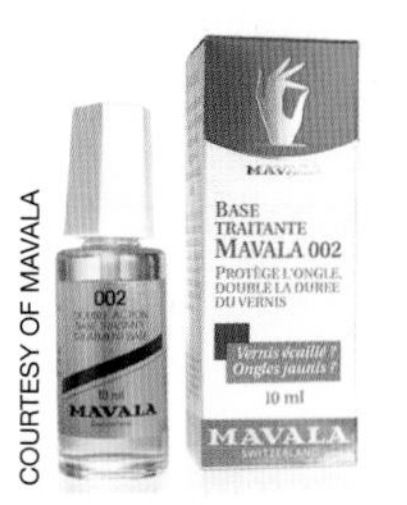

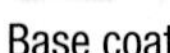

COURTESY OF MAVALA

Base coat

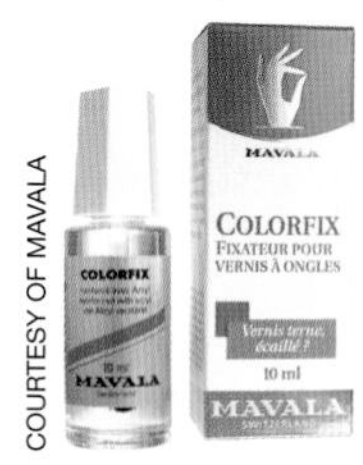

COURTESY OF MAVALA

Top coat

TOP TIP

Cleaning the nail plate before polish application

Use a lint-free pad as cotton wool may leave fibres, which may spoil the application of nail polish.

Types of polish The following types of polish may be used:

- ***Cream*** This has a matt finish, and requires a top coat application to give a sheen.
- ***Pearlized, also known as crystalline*** This has a frosted, shimmery appearance due to the addition of natural fish scales or synthetic ingredients such as bismuth oxychloride.
- ***Base coat*** This protects the nail from staining by a strong-coloured nail polish; it also gives a good grip to polish, and smooths out minor surface irregularities. Many base coats are formulated using ingredients to treat different nail problems such as weak, brittle, peeling or ridged nails.
- ***Top coat*** This gives a sheen to cream polish, and adds longer wear as it helps to prevent chipping.

Contra-indications to nail polish Do not apply polish in these circumstances:

- if there are diseases and disorders of the nail plate and surrounding skin
- if the client is allergic to nail polish

In addition, pearlized nail polish should not be applied to excessively ridged nails as it may appear to exaggerate the problem. Short or bitten nails should be painted only with pale polishes, to avoid attracting attention.

Step-by-step: Dark polish application

Confirm the client's choice of nail colour. A cream formulation has been demonstrated.

Ensure the free edge is smooth and the cuticles are neat and smooth.

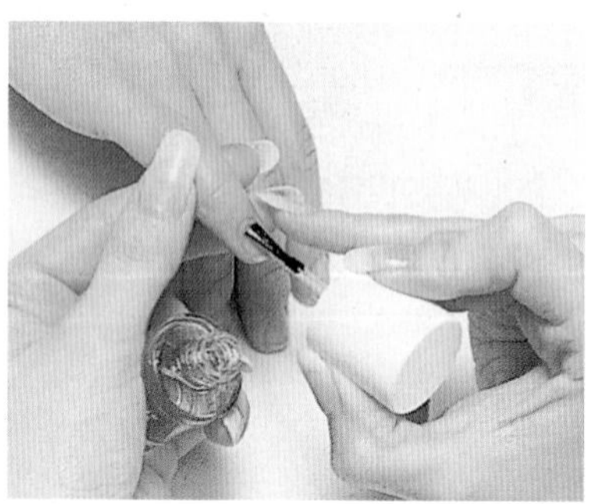

1 Ensure that the nail plate is free from grease. Starting with the thumb, apply three brush strokes down the length of the nail from the cuticle to the free edge, beginning in the centre, then down either side close to the nail wall.

Take care to avoid touching the cuticle or the nail wall. If flooding occurs, remove the polish immediately with an orange stick and polish remover.

Apply one coat of base coat.

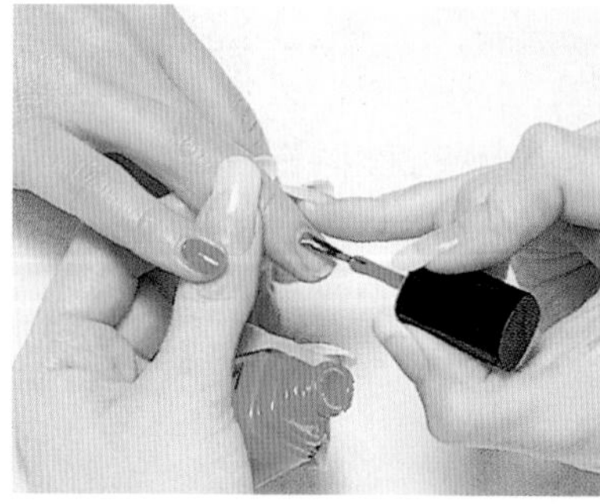

2 Apply the coloured polish, two coats are applied, followed by one coat of top coat.

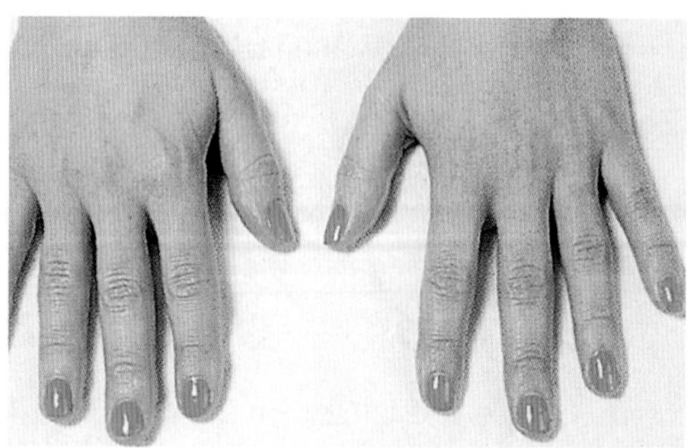

3 The complete dark polish application.

Confirm with the client that the finished result is to their satisfaction.

Complete details on the client's record card.

HEALTH & SAFETY

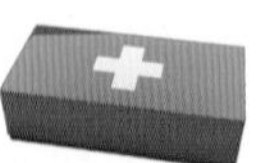

Environment

Ensure the area is well ventilated to avoid inhalation of excessive fumes. Lighting should be good to enable you to avoid eyestrain. It is a good idea to use a table lamp when painting the nails.

Manicure for a male client

A man's hands differ slightly from a woman's usually in size, being larger, and there may be coarse terminal hair on the fingers. Males tend to wear their nails shorter too. Consider the following in your treatment plan:

- File the nails to a shorter length.
- Usually coloured nail polish is omitted. A nail treatment base coat may be included if advised or requested.
- Shape the nails square rather than oval.
- Buff the nails with paste, if a shine is required.
- Use unperfumed lotion for massage.
- Use a lotion or an oil rather than cream for massage, to avoid dragging body hair.
- Use deeper movements during hand and arm massage as the arms are more muscular.

ACTIVITY

Comparing hands

Write down as many differences as you can between the appearance of a male and female client nails, hands and lower arms.

From your observations, can you think of any further adaptations or recommendations that may be necessary when manicuring a man's hands?

Step-by-step: Male manicure

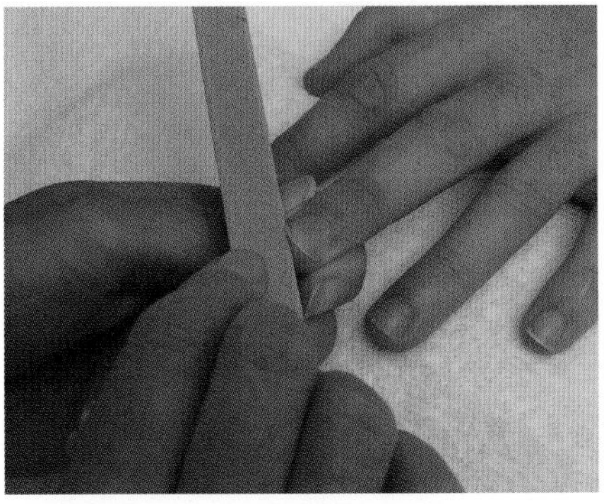

1 File the nails to a shorter length. The nails are usually filed to a square shape rather than oval.

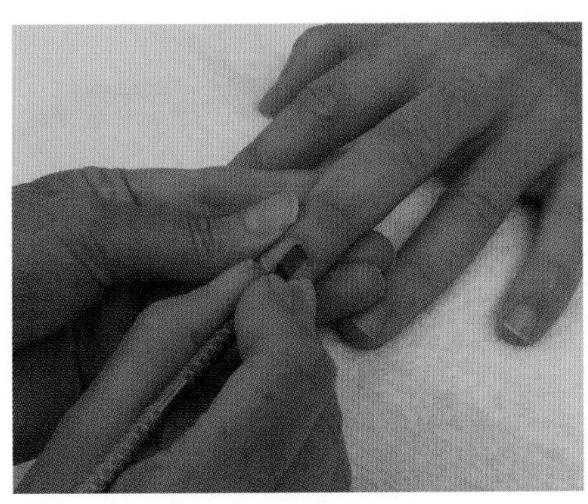

2 Improve the appearance of the cuticles. Push back the cuticles gently.

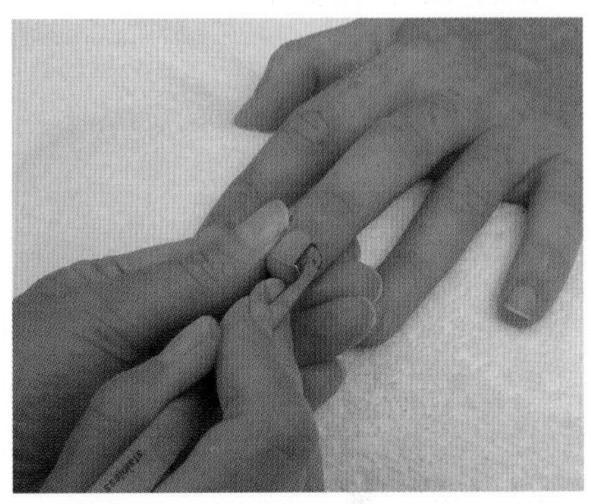

3 A cuticle knife is used to remove the excess eponychium from the cuticle area. Remember to keep the blade dampened to avoid scratches to the nail plate.

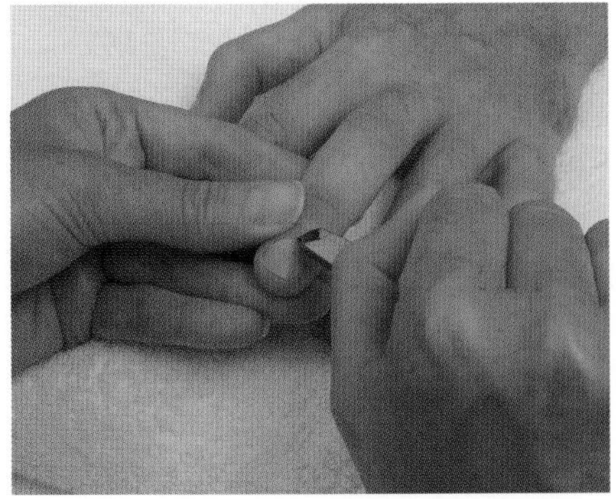

4 Remove excess cuticle using cuticle nippers.

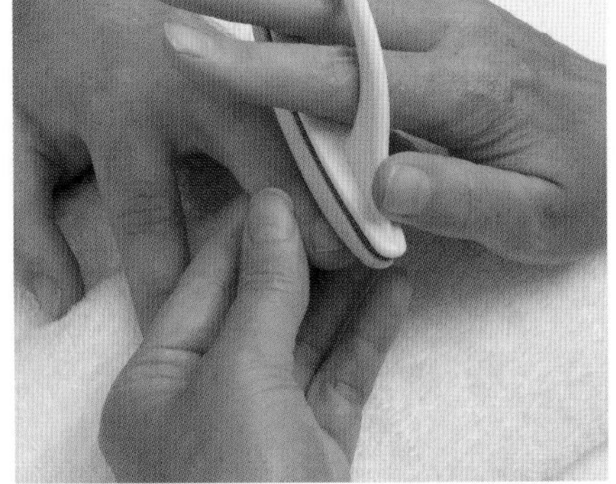

5 Buff the nails to improve blood circulation to the nail bed, giving a healthy appearance to the nail. Buff the nails with a buffing paste if a shine is required. This may be included at this stage or at the end of the manicure as a nail plate finish.

6 Specialist hand and arm treatments may be included if required. A hand massage is shown overleaf but you may wish to include massage to the lower arm also.

After massage, the nail plate is cleaned with acetone if buffing is required as a finish, or a specialist nail polish finish is applied.

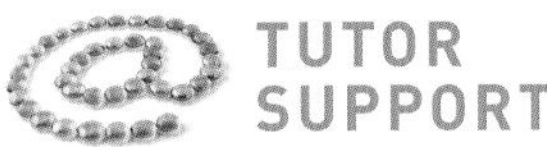

TUTOR SUPPORT

Activity 9: Manicure evaluation task

Step-by-step: Hand massage

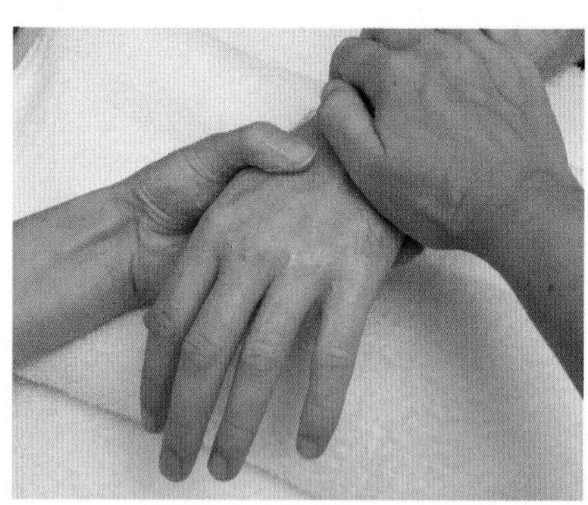

1 Effleurage to the hand and forearm. This movement starts and concludes the hand and arm massage. Use long, sweeping strokes from the hand to the elbow, moving on both the outer and inner sides of the forearm.

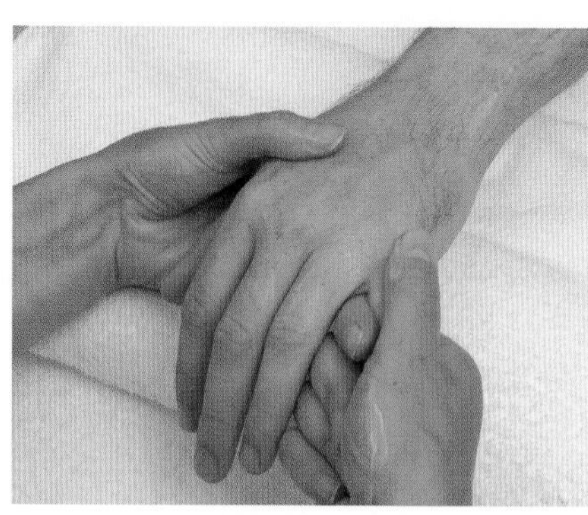

2 Finger twists movement. Gently apply a rotary petrissage movement to each finger.

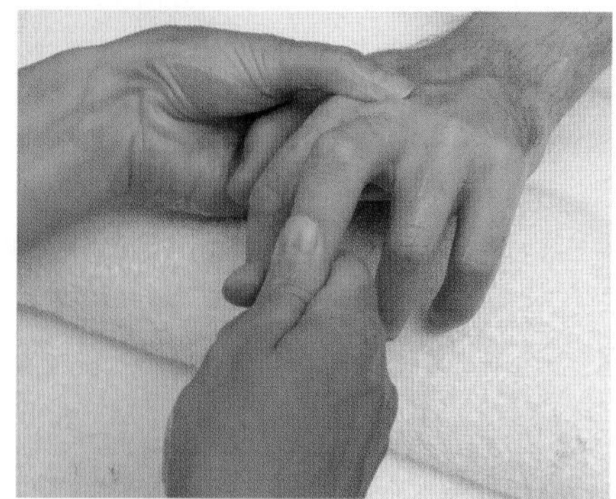

3 Finger resistance movement. Move each finger backwards through its range of movement to exercise the joints.

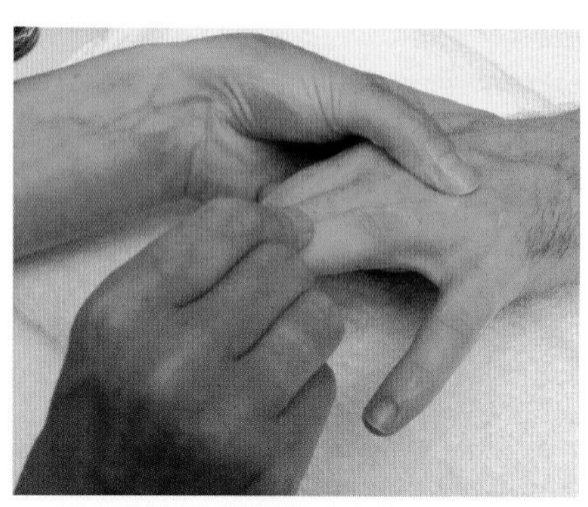

4 Finger rotary movement. Circle each finger in a rotary movement clockwise and then anticlockwise. Move the little finger to the thumb.

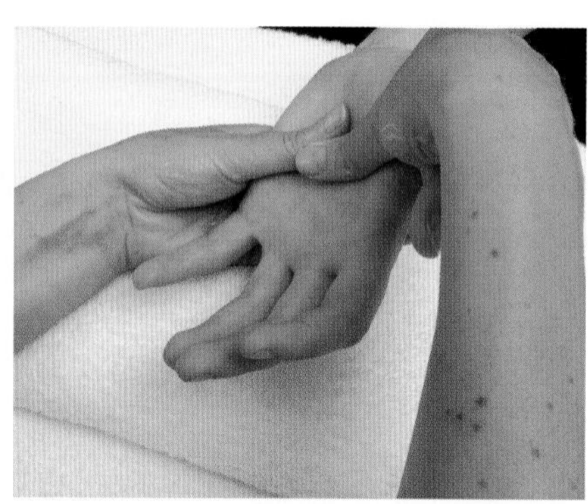

5 Thumbs kneading movement to the palm of the hand.

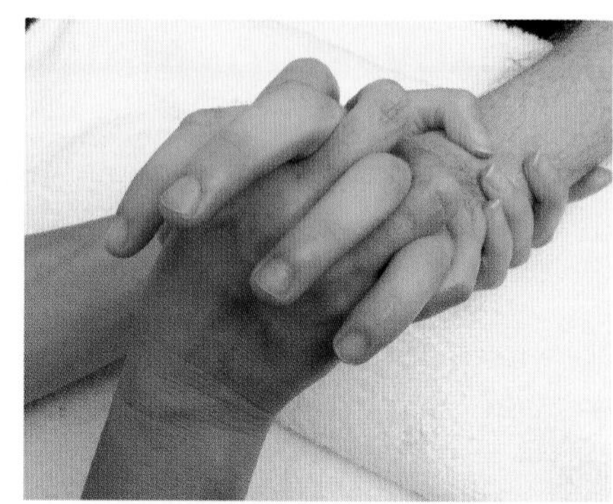

6 Wrist circulations movement, supporting the joints. Support the wrist with one hand and put your fingers between the client's, gently grasping their hand. Move the wrist through its full range of movement, first clockwise and then anti-clockwise. Repeat Step 1 effleurage to conclude the massage.

> Always know the features and benefits of what you are trying to sell whether it be a product or a treatment.
>
> **Jacqui Jefford**

Aftercare advice

It is important when carrying out a manicure that the client knows how to care for their nails and hands at home. It is your duty as a therapist to ensure that the correct **aftercare advice** is given. If it isn't, the client may unwittingly undo all the good work you have done during the treatment.

When giving aftercare advice you have a good opportunity to recommend retail products, such as nail treatment, polish or hand cream, thereby enhancing retail sales and the salon's profit.

Aftercare advice will differ slightly for each client, according to individual needs, but generally it will be as follows:

- Wear rubber gloves when washing up to avoid contact with harsh detergents, which may dehydrate the nails and skin.
- Wear protective gloves when gardening or doing domestic chores to avoid accidental damage.
- Always wear gloves in cold weather: this will help maintain healthy blood circulation in the area.
- Dry the hands thoroughly after washing, and apply hand cream. Some hand creams contain UV filters which reduce hyperpigmentation (seen as darker areas of skin) to the backs of the hands occurring.
- Avoid harsh soaps when washing hands.
- Advising the client on how to file their nails.
- Do not use the fingernails as tools (for instance, to prise lids off tins).
- Advising on appropriate nail/skincare products to remedy the problems present, e.g. dry skin, weak nails.
- Advising the client on what other professional treatments you could recommend.
- Advising the client on a treatment plan to improve the nail/skin condition and the time intervals recommended between each treatment.

It is also necessary to tell the client what to do in the event of a contra-action (see page 388).

Have retail products available for the client to purchase. These include emery boards, coloured nail polishes, **nail polish remover** and nail/skin treatment products.

It is a good idea to have available the nail polish colours that you have used. The client can then touch up any accidental chips themselves.

Recommend the use of top coat applied every three to four days to protect the nail polish, increase its durability and impart shine.

Finally, at the end of the manicure treatment ensure the client's records are updated, accurate and signed by the client and manicurist. Ensure that the finished result is to the client's satisfaction and meets the agreed treatment plan.

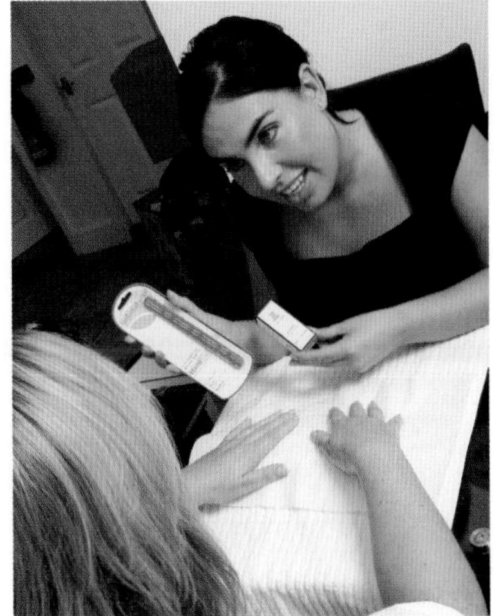

Recommending aftercare products to meet the client's needs

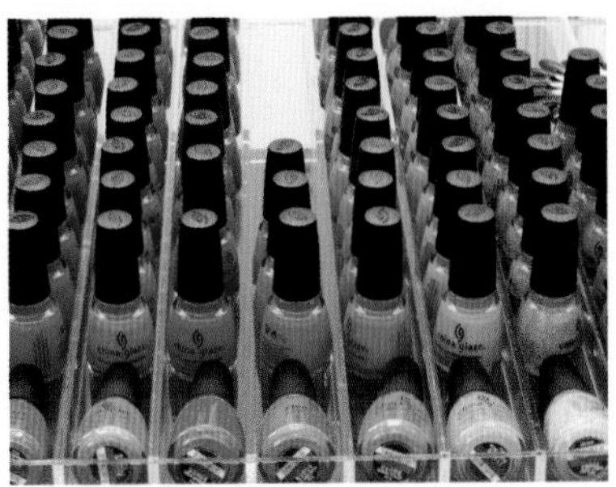

A range of nail polishes for retail

ACTIVITY

Designing an aftercare leaflet

Devise an aftercare leaflet for clients, advising a suitable homecare routine. It is good practice to provide the client with an aftercare leaflet outlining all recommendations following treatment.

ACTIVITY

For each of the clients below, suggest a treatment routine. Detail the treatment plan to include: cause of the condition, aims of the treatment, products used, treatments recommended, relevant retail sales and aftercare advice.

- A hairdresser with very soft, weak, stained nails.
- An engineer with a bruised nail, overgrown cuticles and cracked skin on the fingers.
- A teenager with badly bitten nails.
- An elderly client with strong, ridged nails and dry skin on the hands.

Exercises for the hands

Hand exercises play an important role in the homecare advice given to clients, for the following reasons:

- They keep the joints supple, allowing greater movement.
- Blood circulation is increased, encouraging healthy nail and skin growth.

TOP TIP

Hand exercises

Remember, hand exercises should be performed by the manicurist also to keep the hands supple, reducing the possibility of the effects of RSI in the hands.

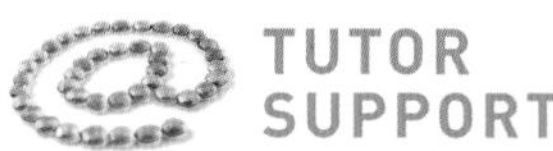

Activity 8: Re-cap, revision and feedback

- Good blood circulation helps to prevent cold hands.
- Exercises keep the client interested in their hands, and so more likely to keep regular salon appointments.

Exercise routine

1. Rub the palms together, back and forth, until warm.
2. Make a tight fist with each hand, then slowly stretch out all the fingers as far as possible.

   Repeat step 2 a further 3 times.
3. With the fingers extended, rotate the wrists slowly in large clockwise circles.

   Repeat step 3 a further 3 times.
4. With the fingers extended, rotate the wrists slowly in large anticlockwise circles.

   Repeat step 4 a further 3 times.
5. Play an imaginary piano vigorously with the fingers for ten seconds.
6. With the hands together as if praying, gently widen the fingers as far as possible, then relax.

   Repeat step 6 a further 3 times.

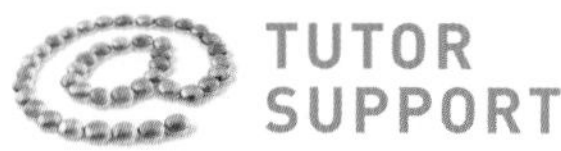

Activity 10: Multiple choice quiz

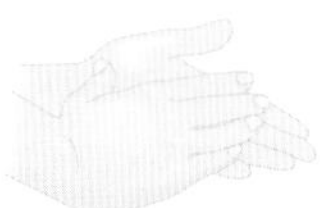
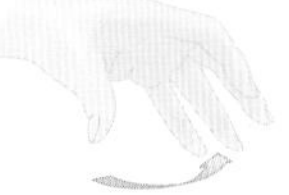
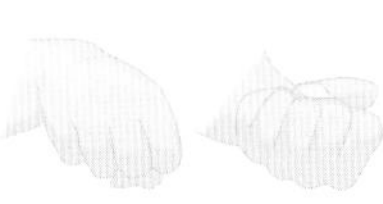
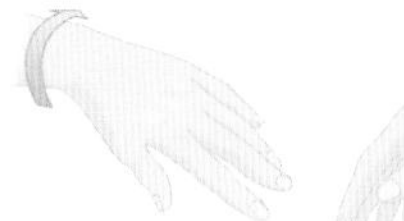

Hand exercises

GLOSSARY OF KEY WORDS

Aftercare advice recommendations given to the client following treatment to continue the benefits of the treatment.

Base coat a nail polish product applied to protect the natural nail and prevent staining from coloured nail polish.

Bevelling a nail filing technique used at the free edge of the nail to ensure it is smooth.

Blue nail nail condition where the nail bed has a blue tinge rather than a healthy pink colour due to poor blood circulation in the area.

Bruised nail nail condition where the nail appears blue/black in colour where bleeding has occurred on the nail bed following injury.

Buffer a manicure tool with a handle made of plastic and a pad with a replaceable cover, used on the nail to give a sheen, increase blood supply to the area and, if used with the gritty cream buffing paste, to help smooth out nail surface irregularities.

Consultation techniques assessment of client's needs using different assessment techniques, including questioning and natural observation.

Contact dermatitis a skin disorder caused by intolerance of the skin to a particular substance, or a group of substances. On exposure to the substance the skin quickly becomes irritated and an allergic reaction occurs.

Contra-action an unwanted reaction occurring during or after treatment application.

Contra-indication a problematic symptom that indicates that the treatment may not proceed.

Cuticle cream or oil a cosmetic preparation used to condition the skin of the cuticle.

Cuticle knife a metal tool used on the nail to remove excess eponychium and perionychium (the extension of the skin of the cuticle at the base of the nail).

Cuticle nippers a metal tool used to remove excess cuticle and neaten the skin around the cuticle area.

Cuticle remover a cosmetic preparation used to soften and loosen the skin cells and cuticle from the nail.

Eczema of the nail inflammation of the skin, causing changes to the nail including ridges, pitting, nail separation and nail thickening.

Effleurage a stroking massage movement, used to begin the massage, as a link manipulation and to complete the massage sequence.

Eggshell nail nail condition where thin, fragile white nails curve under at the free edge.

Emery board a nail file used to shape the free edge of the nail.

Exfoliant a mild abrasive cream applied and massaged over the skin's surface to remove dead skin cells and improve the appearance and texture of the skin.

Frictions massage technique using small circular massage movements using the pads of the fingers or thumbs. The skin and muscle below is massaged against the underlying bone. This can be used to loosen any adhesions in the tissues.

Hand and nail treatments specialized products and equipment designed to improve the condition and appearance of different nail and skin conditions.

Hand cream/oil a cosmetic mixture of waxes and oils applied to soften the skin of the hands and cuticles.

Hangnail nail condition where small pieces of epidermal skin protrude between the nail plate and nail wall, accompanying a dry cuticle condition.

Hoof stick a nail tool used to gently push back the softened cuticles.

Joint manipulations massage technique where the joints of the hand are manipulated through their range of movement dependant upon the type of joint.

Leuconychia nail condition where white spots or marks appear on the nail plate.

Longitudinal ridges nail condition where grooves appear in the nail plate, running along the length of the nail from the cuticle to the free edge.

Manicure a treatment to care for and improve the condition and appearance of the hands and nails.

Mask a treatment mask applied to the skin of the hands to treat and improve the condition of the skin. This may include properties to stimulate, rejuvenate and moisturise.

Nail finish the product finally applied to the natural nail to enhance its appearance, i.e. buffed nail or nail polish application.

Nail polish a clear or coloured nail product that adds colour/protection to the nail. Cream polish has a matt finish and requires a top coat application. Pearlized polish produces a frosted, shimmery appearance and top coat is not required.

Nail polish drier an aerosol or oil preparation applied following nail polish application to increase the speed at which the polish hardens.

Nail polish remover a solvent used to remove nail polish and grease from the nails prior to applying polish.

Nail polish solvent used to thin nail polish and restore its consistency.

Nail strengthener a nail polish product that strengthens the nail plate, which has a tendency to split.

Necessary action the appropriate action to take in the case of a contra-action or contra-indication to ensure the welfare of the client.

Onycholysis nail condition where the nail plate separates from the nail bed.

Onychophagy nail condition where a person bites their nails excessively.

Onychorrhexis nail condition where the person has split, flaking nails.

Orange stick a disposable wooden tool used around the cuticle and free edge of the nail and to apply products to the nail.

Paraffin wax this is heated and applied to the skin of the hands to provide a warming effect. It improves skin functioning, aids the absorption of products and is beneficial to ease the discomfort of arthritic and rheumatic conditions.

Paronychia bacterial infection where swelling, redness and pus appear in the cuticle area of the nail wall.

Petrissage massage movements, including kneading, where the tissues are lifted away from the underlying structures and compressed. Pressure is intermittent, and should be light yet firm.

Psoriasis of the nail an inflammatory condition where there is an increased production of cells in the upper part of the skin. Pitting occurs on the surface of the nail plate.

Pterygium nail condition where the cuticle is thickened and overgrown.

Ridge-filler a nail product used on ridged nails that improves the nail's appearance and provides a more even surface.

Scissors nail tools used to shorten the length of the nail before filing.

Tapotement also known as percussion, massage movements performed in a brisk, stimulating manner to increase blood supply and improve tone of the skin and muscles.

Thermal mitts electrically heated gloves in which the hands are placed following the application of a skin treatment product such as a mask. The heat aids the absorption of the product and improves skin functioning.

Tinea unguium fungal infection of the nails. The nail is yellowish-grey in colour.

Top coat a nail polish product applied over another nail polish to provide additional strength and durability to the finish.

Transverse furrows nail condition where grooves appear on the nail, running from side to side.

Treatment plan after the consultation, suitable treatment objectives are established to treat the client's conditions and needs.

Verruca or wart a viral infection where small epidermal skin growths appear, either raised or flat depending upon their location, and have a rough surface.

Warm-oil treatment involves gently heating a small amount of oil and soaking the nails and cuticles in it to nourish the nails and soften the cuticles and surrounding skin.

ASSESSMENT OF KNOWLEDGE AND UNDERSTANDING

You have now learnt about the knowledge and skills for providing manicure treatment for the beauty therapy workplace. To test your level of knowledge, answer the following short questions. These will prepare you for your summative (final) assessment.

1. The nail condition shown below is called

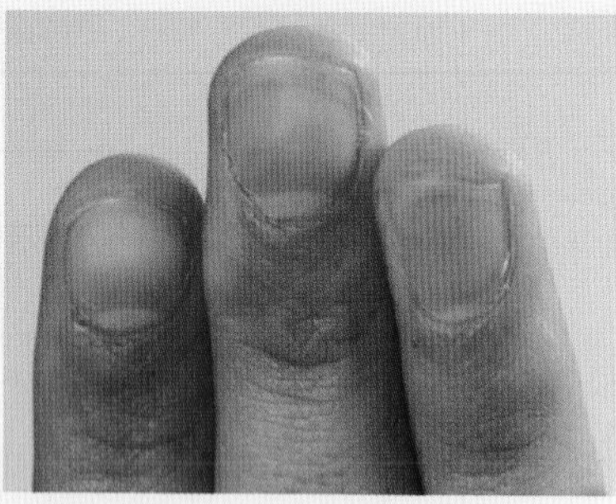

   a. onychia
   b. onycholysis
   c. onychopagy
   d. onychorrhexis

2. A hangnail is best removed with:
   a. cuticle nippers
   b. nail scissors
   c. cuticle knife
   d. an exfoliation product

3. Name the arteries shown on the diagram below.

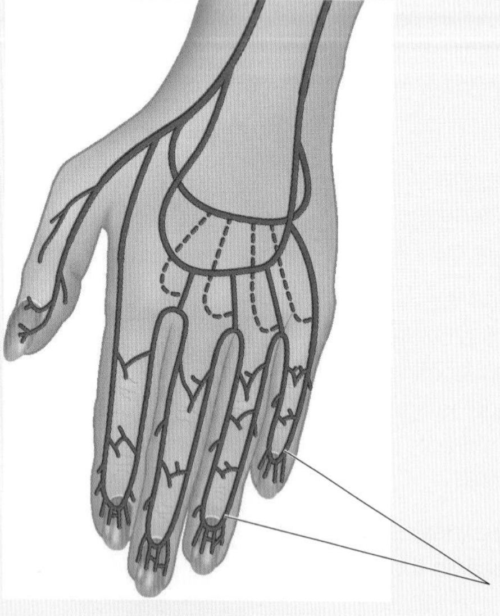

4. The part of the epidermis found under the free edge of the nails is called:

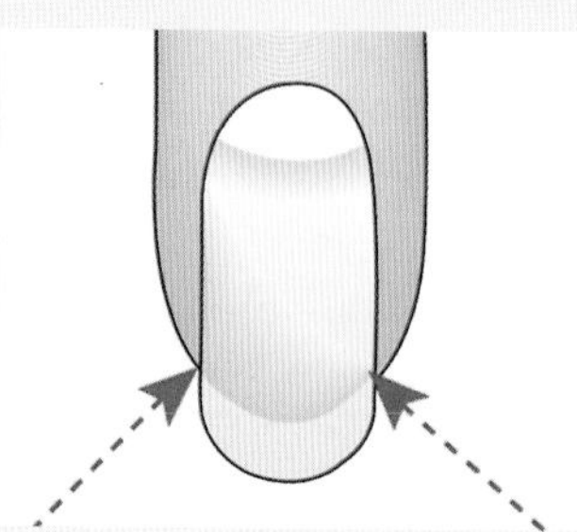

   a. perionychium
   b. cuticle
   c. hyponychium
   d. eponychium

5. The image below shows a nail polish finish using:

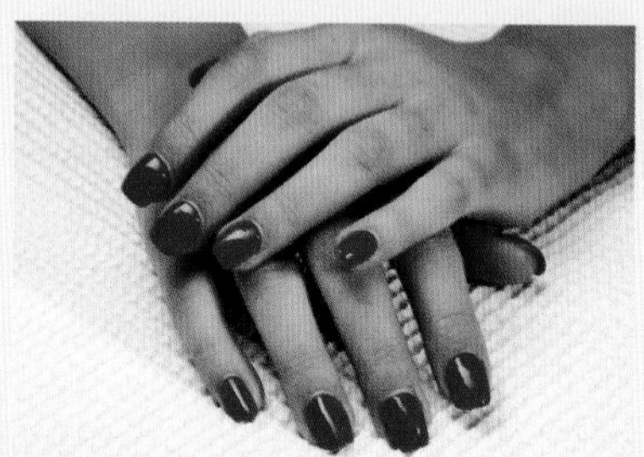

   a. cream polish
   b. pearlised (crystalline) polish

6. Match the following tools with their use in manicure:

1) orange stick	a) used to trim away dead skin tissue
2) hoof stick	b) used to gently push back softened cuticle
3) cuticle nipper	c) used to add shine to the nail plate and smooth out ridges
4) chamois buffer	d) used to apply product, treating cuticle tissue or to clean under the free edge
5) scissors	e) used to shorten the free edge
6) cuticle knife	f) used to remove excess eponychium and perionychium from the nail plate

7. The nail product designed to loosen dead tissue from the nail plate so that it can be more easily removed from the nail plate is:
   a. acetone
   b. cuticle oil
   c. cuticle remover
   d. cuticle cream

8. The massage manipulation that is used when starting and ending the hand and arm massage is called:
   a. vibrations
   b. frictions
   c. petrissage
   d. effleurage

9. The nail is made of a hard protein called what?

10. To ease the discomfort of joint stiffness, which specialist hand and arm services would be best to use?
    a. paraffin wax
    b. exfoliating treatment
    c. thermal mitts
    d. hand mask

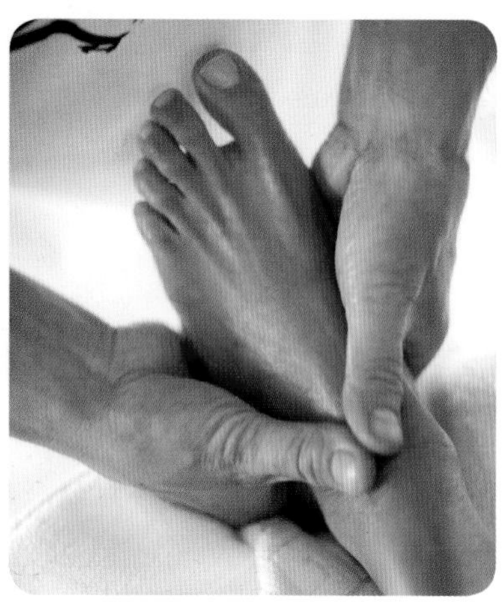

12 Pedicure Treatments

Learning Objectives

This chapter covers **VRQ Unit Provide pedicure treatments**.

This unit is all about improving and maintaining your client's feet, nails and surrounding skin condition. A pedicure includes filing the nails to shape, using specialized nail, cuticle products and foot treatments, massaging the lower leg and foot and providing a complementary nail finish to suit the client's treatment objectives.

There are **two** learning outcomes for this unit which you must achieve competently:

1 **Be able to prepare for pedicure treatments**

2 **Be able to provide pedicure treatments**

From the range statement, you must show that you can:

- use all **consultation techniques** to identify the treatment **objectives**
- use all listed **products, tools and equipment** as appropriate
- ensure that the **environmental conditions** are suitable
- identify and treat **skin and nail conditions**
- complete a consultation and skin inspection to identify any **contra-indications**
- **communicate and behave** in a professional manner
- use a variety of **massage techniques**
- follow all **health and safety practices**
- provide relevant **aftercare** and **contra-action advice**

You must be able to show you have the necessary practical skills and underpinning knowledge to provide pedicure treatments.

This unit is linked to the Beauty Therapy NOS **Unit N3**.

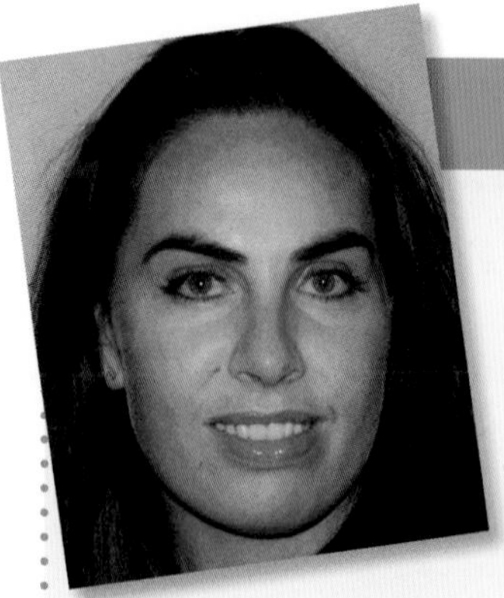

ROLE MODEL

Vicky Ann Kennedy

Paramedical skin practitioner and beauty therapist

"I have been the principal owner of a very successful beauty clinic since 1991. I knew the career path I wanted to take by the age of 12, but had to wait until the age of 19 before it became a reality. I trained at Bolton College under Lorraine Nordmann, and became Student of the Year when I left. I have carried on striving to achieve every day since.

Before starting my own business, I had not worked in many other places, but I already knew how I wanted things to be done and how standards should be followed.

I think that if your heart is in it, working in the beauty industry is very rewarding and a beauty salon is a lovely, happy place to work. I have no regrets and after nearly 20 years, still enjoy every day.

Essential anatomy and physiology knowledge requirements for this unit are identified on the checklist chart on page 27.

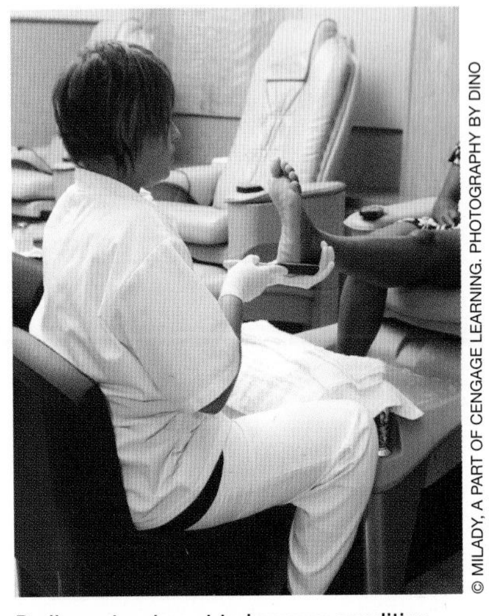

Pedicure treatment to improve condition of the feet

The purpose of a pedicure

The word **pedicure** is derived from the Latin word *pedis*, meaning 'foot' and *cura*, meaning 'care'. The treatment is very similar to manicure except that it is carried out on the feet instead of the hands. A pedicure is carried out for many reasons:

- to improve the appearance of the foot
- to reduce the amount of hard skin
- to relax tired, aching feet
- to keep the nails smooth and healthy

Keep your standards up

Always make sure that you keep your standards high, especially when dealing with hygiene and avoiding cross-infection. Remember the good practices that you learnt at college and always use them.

Vicky Ann Kennedy

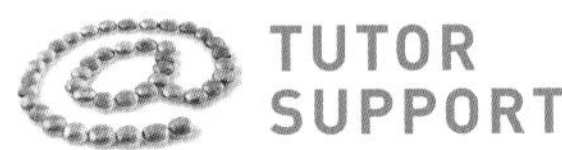

TUTOR SUPPORT

Activity 6: Benefits of foot and nail treatments

Preparing for a pedicure

Outcome 1: Be able to prepare for pedicure treatments

Learn how to prepare for pedicure treatments

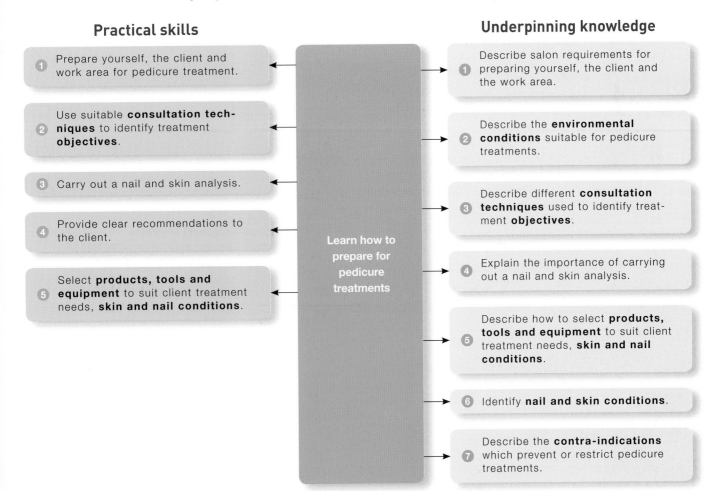

Practical skills

1. Prepare yourself, the client and work area for pedicure treatment.
2. Use suitable **consultation techniques** to identify treatment **objectives**.
3. Carry out a nail and skin analysis.
4. Provide clear recommendations to the client.
5. Select **products, tools and equipment** to suit client treatment needs, **skin and nail conditions**.

Underpinning knowledge

1. Describe salon requirements for preparing yourself, the client and the work area.
2. Describe the **environmental conditions** suitable for pedicure treatments.
3. Describe different **consultation techniques** used to identify treatment **objectives**.
4. Explain the importance of carrying out a nail and skin analysis.
5. Describe how to select **products, tools and equipment** to suit client treatment needs, **skin and nail conditions**.
6. Identify **nail and skin conditions**.
7. Describe the **contra-indications** which prevent or restrict pedicure treatments.

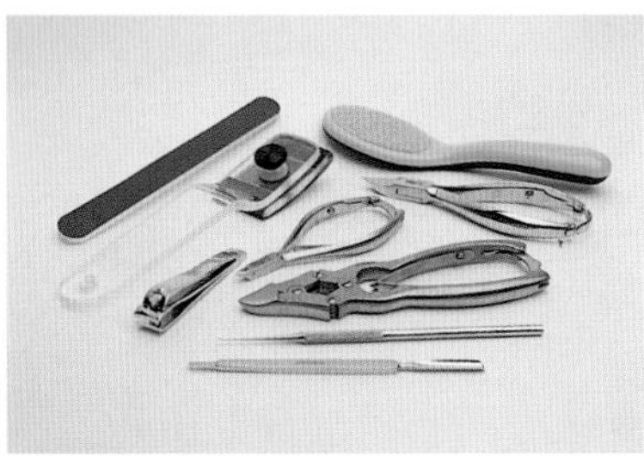
ELLISONS

Pedicure tools and equipment

Preparing the working area

All metal tools should be sterilized in the autoclave prior to use. Non-metal instruments should be disinfected by immersing them in a suitable disinfecting fluid. Prepare the products, tools and equipment neatly on the work station so that everything you need is to hand and the client need not be disturbed during treatment.

The work area should remain in a condition suitable for further nail treatments during the working day.

Place a towel on the floor between you and the client. The foot bowl or foot spa containing warm, soapy water should be placed on this towel. Exactly how you arrange the work area will depend upon how your work area is equipped to deliver the treatment resources.

Towels should be placed on your lap: one is for protection, the other is for drying the client's feet. Keep the other towels close by for wrapping the client's feet. Alternatively, the pedicure may be performed on a beauty couch or at a pedicure station. In this case towels are only required for drying and wrapping up feet.

When cutting the client's nails and removing hard skin, disposable tissue should be placed on your lap and then removed before continuing treatment.

Personal protective equipment, e.g. safety glasses and synthetic powder-free gloves may be worn for protection from skin and nail debris at this stage.

When the client is comfortably seated, clean your hands using an approved hand cleaning technique, preferably in view of the client, who will observe hygienic procedures being carried out. This will assure them that they are receiving a professional treatment.

Before beginning the pedicure, check that you have the necessary tools, products and equipment to hand and that they meet the legal hygiene and industry requirements for nail treatments.

TOP TIP

Foot spa

Foot spas help to relax the feet by a combination of massage provided by an integral vibration feature, aeration of the water, creating a bubbling effect, and heating of the water.

PRODUCTS, TOOLS AND EQUIPMENT

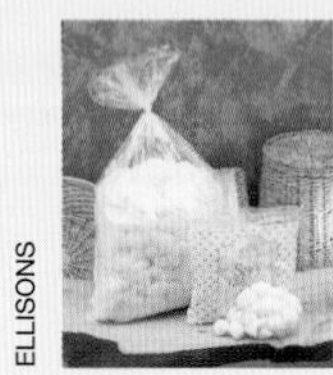
ELLISONS

Cotton wool
To remove nail polish and excess nail product preparations. Cotton wool may also be used to tip orange sticks for the purpose of nail product application and removal. Cotton wool filled gauze pads are also available and are more absorbent

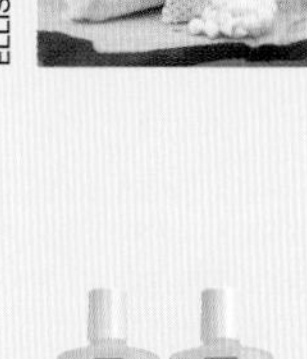

Nail polish remover
To remove nail polish and excess nail care and skincare preparations from the nail plate

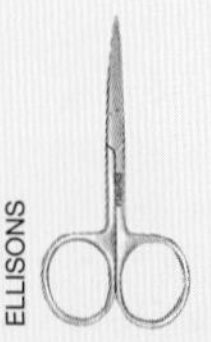
ELLISONS

Scissors or toenail clippers
To shorten nail length

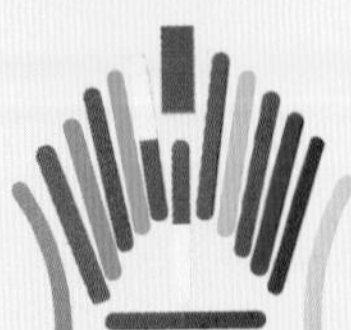

Emery boards
To shorten and shape the nail free edge

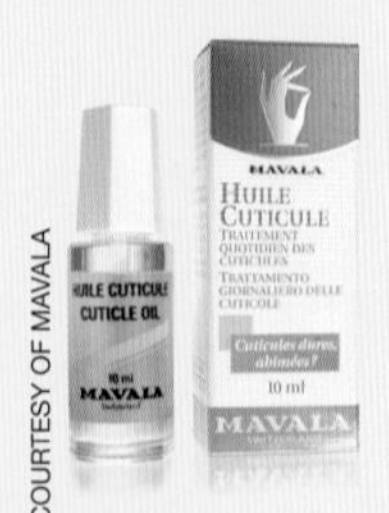

COURTESY OF MAVALA

Cuticle oil or cream
Used to condition and rehydrate the skin of the cuticle; especially beneficial for dry nails and cuticles

Cuticle remover
Used to soften the skin cells and the cuticle so excess epidermal skin can be easily removed

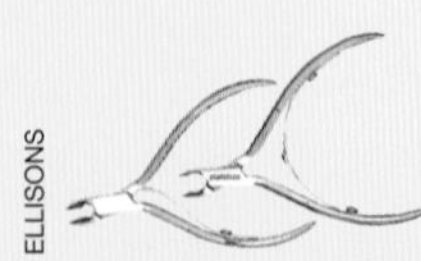
ELLISONS

Cuticle nippers
To remove excess cuticle and dead, torn skin surrounding the nail plate

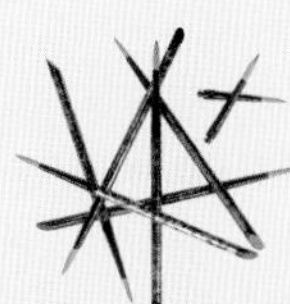

Hoof stick or cuticle pusher
To gently push back the softened cuticles

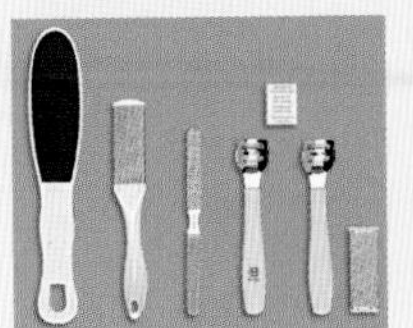

Foot rasp or callous file
To remove excess dead skin from the foot

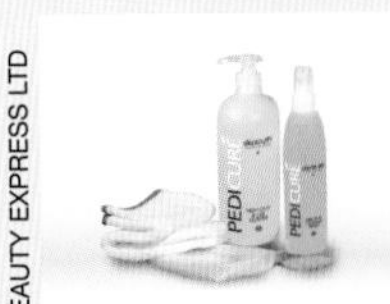
BEAUTY EXPRESS LTD

Foot massage lotion or oil
To massage the skin of the foot and lower leg

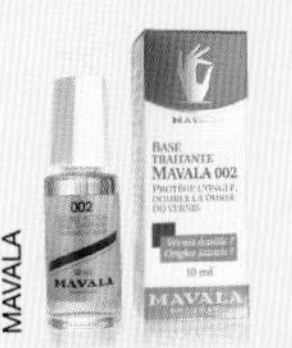
MAVALA

Base coat
Provides an even surface to improve nail polish application and adherence and prevent nail staining. Depending upon its formulation, it can also improve the appearance and health of the nail

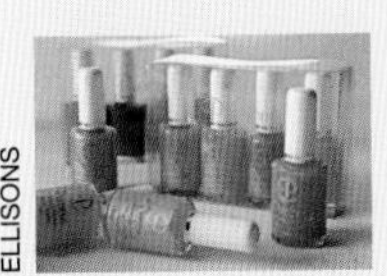
ELLISONS

Coloured nail polish (enamel)
A selection for the client to choose from in cream or pearlized (also termed crystalline) formulations

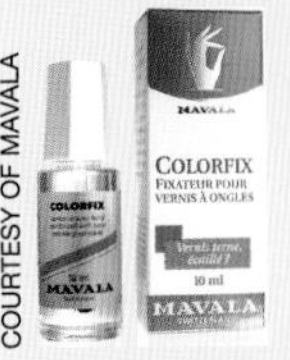
COURTESY OF MAVALA

Top coat
To provide shine and strength to protect the nail polish, reduces peeling and chipping and increases durability of the polish

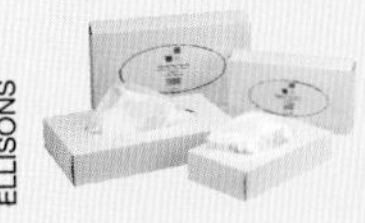
ELLISONS

Tissues
To protect client's clothing in the treatment area and for drying tools after immersion in disinfectant solution

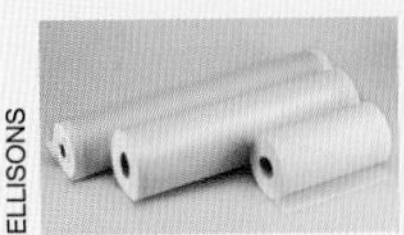
ELLISONS

Disposable bedroll tissue
To collect waste and be replaced as necessary during the treatment

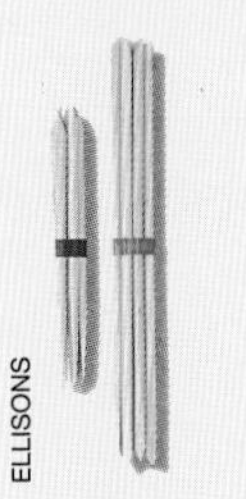
ELLISONS

Orange sticks
Used to remove products from containers and, when tipped at either end with cotton wool, to ease the cuticle back and to clean under the free edge. Orange sticks should be disposed of after each client as they cannot be effectively sterilized

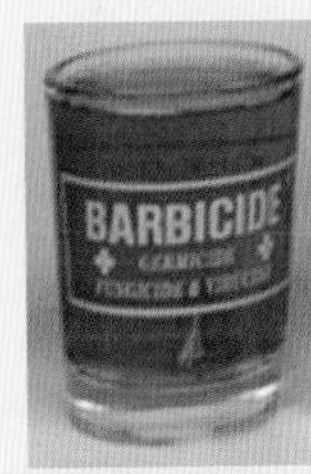

Disinfectant solution
To store small plastic and stainless steel sterilized tools

YOU WILL ALSO NEED:

Pedicure bowl or foot spa To soak and cleanse the foot. The foot spa also revitalizes and refreshes the skin by stimulating of the sensory nerve endings, and encouraging blood and lymph circulation

Small towels (5) Used for protection and to dry the client's skin

Small bowls (3) For storage, etc.

Liquid soap Specialized foot cleaning products to cleanse, soften and deodorize the feet

Skin disinfectant To cleanse and disinfect the client's skin. Specialized sprays and gels are available for this purpose

Cuticle knife To remove excess eponychium and perionychium from the nail plate

Client's record card Used to record confidential details of each client registered at the salon to record the client's personal details, products used and details of the treatment provided

Nail polish drier An aerosol or oil preparation applied to speed the drying process of nail polish

Disposable toe separators Used to keep the toes separated during nail polish application. Alternatively, disposable items such as cotton wool or tissues may be used for this purpose

Disposable footwear (optional) Enabling the client to move without smudging the nail polish application

Disinfecting solution For all surfaces

Foot and nail treatment equipment Including paraffin wax, foot masks, thermal boots and exfoliators

Waste container This should be a lined metal bin with a lid to contain vapours from solvents

Products used in pedicure treatments

For full details of products used for both manicures and pedicures, their ingredients and uses, see the table on pages 358–359. In addition to these, an exfoliating pedicure scrub may also be used for the feet (see below).

Product	Ingredients	Use
Exfoliating pedicure scrub	Abrasive ingredients such as pumice, sea salt, detergent, water and water-soluble ingredients, added moisturisers, refreshing agents, e.g. peppermint oil.	To remove dead skin cells, cleanse the skin, condition, soften and refresh the skin, improving blood circulation in the area.

COURTESY OF BEAUTY EXPRESS LTD

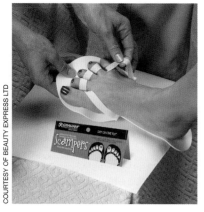

Disposable toe separator footwear

Sterilization and disinfection

Hygiene must be maintained in a number of ways:

- ensure that tools and equipment are clean and sterile before use
- having sterilized or disinfected tools and equipment stored in a chemical disinfectant or closed container until ready for use. Remember, they will remain clean but will not be sterile after 24 hours.
- dispense products from containers, e.g. creams and lotions, with a disposable spatula

ACTIVITY

Why is personal presentation and hygiene important to create a good impression?

Refer to the Habia *Code of Practice for Nail Services* to research recognized examples of good personal presentation and hygiene at www.habia.org.

Pedicure tools and equipment can be disposable or can be sterilized and disinfected by the methods shown on page 359–360.

Refer to the Habia Code of Practice for Nail Services for health and safety best practice guidance.

Reception

When a client makes an appointment for a pedicure treatment, the receptionist should advise the client how long the treatment will take. This will include sufficient time for the nail polish to dry before replacing footwear.

To allocate the appropriate length of time ask if they require a specialist foot treatment with their pedicure.

Ask the client whether they are currently receiving treatment from a chiropodist for conditions such as verrucas or athlete's foot. These would contra-indicate treatment: the receptionist should advise the client to wait until the condition has cleared.

If the client is a minor under 16 years of age, it is necessary to obtain parent/guardian permission for treatment. The parent/guardian will also have to be present when the treatment is received.

Commercial timing:

- *Allow 45 minutes for a pedicure treatment.*
- *Allow up to 1hour for a specialist foot treatment.*

All staff, especially the staff communicating with clients at reception should be familiar with the different pricing structures for the range of pedicure treatments and products available for retail.

It is important that accurate records are kept and stored in compliance with the Data Protection Act for future reference.

Keeping your appointments on time

Clients like to be seen promptly so try not to run behind with your appointments. To keep the treatment area ready for the next client, always ask your clients to bring flip flops with them, then they can leave the treatment area as soon as you have finished, without having to wait until toenails are dry.

Vicky Ann Kennedy

ALWAYS REMEMBER

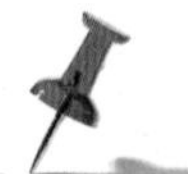

GP referral

A client referred from their GP will usually have a letter. This would be in the case when confirmation regarding suitability for treatment has been requested. This should be retained with the client's record card.

HEALTH & SAFETY

Avoiding RSI

Remember to consider your posture and prevent any awkward movements during delivery of the pedicure treatment. Ensure the work station is at the correct height to avoid stretching and straining your upper body and limbs.

Preparing the client

Ensure that the client is seated at the correct height, so that you can work comfortably and healthily and the client can enjoy the treatment without strain to the muscles and joints of the leg.

Ensure that the client is warm and comfortable when preparing for the pedicure. Client privacy and modesty should also be considered. Not all clients would be happy to be on view while receiving the treatment. Ensure that lighting is good to avoid eye strain and to enable the treatment to be performed competently. Avoid positioning the work station in direct sunlight however, to prevent discomfort to the client and pedicurist.

A sample client record card

Date | Beauty therapist name

Client name | Date of birth (identifying client age group)

Home address | Postcode

Email address | Landline phone number | Mobile phone number

Name of doctor | Doctor's address and phone number

Related medical history (conditions that may restrict or prohibit treatment application)

Are you taking any medication? (this may affect the sensitivity of the skin to the treatment)

CONTRA-INDICATIONS REQUIRING MEDICAL REFERRAL
(preventing pedicure treatment application)

- ☐ bacterial infections (e.g. paronychia)
- ☐ viral infections (e.g. plantar warts)
- ☐ fungal infections (e.g. tinea unguium, tinea pedis)
- ☐ parasitic infestations (e.g. scabies)
- ☐ severe skin conditions
- ☐ severe toenail separation
- ☐ severe skin disorders such as severe eczema or hyperkeratosis conditions such as psoriasis
- ☐ severe bruising
- ☐ diabetes

CONTRA-INDICATIONS WHICH RESTRICT TREATMENT
(treatment may require adaptation)

- ☐ minor toenail separation
- ☐ minor eczema and psoriasis
- ☐ recent scar tissue
- ☐ broken bones
- ☐ recent fractures and sprains
- ☐ minor cuts or abrasions
- ☐ minor bruising or swelling
- ☐ undiagnosed lumps and swellings
- ☐ broken capillaries
- ☐ moles
- ☐ product allergies
- ☐ varicose veins
- ☐ cuts and abrasions
- ☐ circulatory conditions such as phlebitis or thrombophlebitis

PRODUCTS, TOOLS AND EQUIPMENT

- ☐ toenail and skin treatment tools (scissors/clippers, foot file/rasps, cuticle knife, cuticle nippers and hoof sticks)
- ☐ abrasives (e.g. buffing paste)
- ☐ cuticle softeners
- ☐ toenail conditioners (e.g. cuticle cream/oils)
- ☐ skin conditioners (e.g. foot cream)
- ☐ toenail, skin and cuticle corrective treatments (e.g. paraffin wax)
- ☐ consumables

FEET AND TOENAIL TREATMENTS

☐ paraffin wax ☐ foot masks
☐ thermal booties ☐ exfoliators

TOENAIL FINISH

☐ light colour ☐ dark colour ☐ French manicure

COURSE OF TREATMENT

	Date	Date	Date
☐ improvement of skin condition products used	____	____	____
☐ improvement of toenail condition products used	____	____	____

TOENAIL, CUTICLE AND SKIN CONDITION

Toenails

☐ normal ☐ brittle ☐ dry ☐ weak ☐ ridged

Cuticle

☐ normal ☐ dry ☐ split ☐ overgrown ☐ hangnails

Skin

☐ normal ☐ dry ☐ hard

MASSAGE MEDIUMS

☐ creams ☐ oils ☐ lotions

Beauty therapist signature (for reference)

Client signature (confirmation of details)

A sample client record card (continued)

TREATMENT ADVICE
Pedicure – *allow 45 minutes*
Specialized foot/nail treatment – *allow up to 60 minutes*

TREATMENT PLAN
Record relevant details of your treatment and advice provided for future reference.
Ensure the client's records are up to date, accurate and fully completed following treatment. Non-compliance may invalidate insurance.

DURING
Discuss:

- details that may influence the client's toenail condition, such as the client's occupation
- the products the client is currently using to care for the skin of the feet and toenails
- the client's satisfaction with these products
- relevant pedicure procedures (e.g., how to file the toenails correctly)

Note:

- any adverse (unwanted) reaction, if any occur during or after the pedicure treatment

AFTER
Record:

- results of treatment
- any modification to treatment application that has occurred
- what products have been used in the pedicure treatment
- what foot treatments have been used
- the effectiveness of treatment
- any samples provided (review their success at the next appointment)

Advise on:

- product application in order to gain maximum benefit from product use
- specialized products following pedicure treatment for homecare use
- general foot/toenail care and maintenance
- the recommended time intervals between treatments
- the importance of a course of treatments to improve toenail/skin conditions

RETAIL OPPORTUNITIES
Advise on:

- progression of the **treatment plan** for future appointments
- products that would be suitable for the client to use at home to care for the skin of the feet and toenails
- recommendations for further treatments
- further products or treatments that the client may or may not have received before

Note:

- any purchase made by the client

EVALUATION
Record:

- comments on the client's satisfaction with the treatment
- if poor results are achieved, the reasons why
- how you may alter the treatment plan to achieve the required treatment results in the future, if applicable

HEALTH AND SAFETY
Advise on:

- appropriate necessary action to be taken in the event of an unwanted skin or nail reaction

TOP TIP

Pedicure spa chair

Pedicure spa chairs provide comfort and luxury for the client. The client immerses their feet in a tray equipped with hydrotherapy jets to massage the feet, while the chair also features a vibrating massage system.

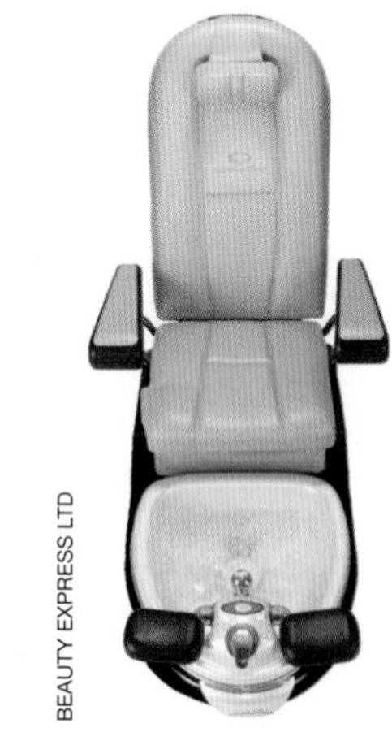

BEAUTY EXPRESS LTD

Before treatment begins, ask the client to remove their tights or socks, and any clothing that might restrict their lower leg movement, such as jeans or trousers. Cover their upper legs with a clean towel or provide a gown. This will help them to be more comfortable and allow you to work without restriction.

Ask them to remove any jewellery from the area to be treated, to prevent the jewellery being damaged by creams and to avoid obstructing massage movements. Place the jewellery where the client can see it. Alternatively ask the client to take possession of it for safe keeping – following your salon security policy.

When the client is comfortably seated, clean your hands using an approved hand cleaning technique – preferably in view of the client, who will observe hygienic procedures being carried out. This will assure them that they are receiving a professional treatment.

Keep aware when working

Always check during treatment that your client is comfortable and not feeling any discomfort. Don't soak feet for too long as they may become too soft making it more likely that you will accidentally remove too much callous.

Vicky Ann Kennedy

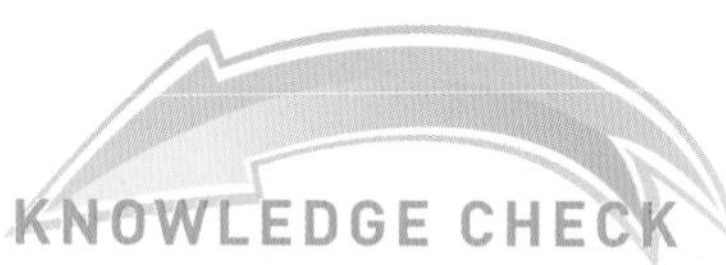

KNOWLEDGE CHECK

How many bones are there in the foot? How many can you name?

Need more time... refer to page 78 to help you.

Consultation

Before carrying out a pedicure treatment, it is necessary to assess the condition of the client's skin, nails and cuticles. This is done in order that the most appropriate **foot and nail treatments** and products may be chosen. Also, by correctly assessing and analyzing the client's foot condition and writing this on their record card, you will be able to see over a period of time how the condition is progressing.

Assess the condition of the following:

- ***The cuticles*** Are they dry, tight, cracked or overgrown, or are they soft and pliable?
- ***The nail*** Are they strong or weak, thickened, discoloured or stained? Sometimes this may indicate a nail disorder. The nails of the foot should be filed straight across into a square shape. Shaping the nails at the corners can cause **ingrowing toenails.**
- ***The skin*** Is the skin dry, rough or cracked, or is it soft and smooth? Is the colour even? Also check the skin between the toes.

TOP TIP

Footwear

Advise the client to wear open-toed shoes or sandals on the day of the pedicure to allow time for polish to dry completely before putting on shoes.

While assessing the client's feet, you should also be looking for any contra-indications to the treatment.

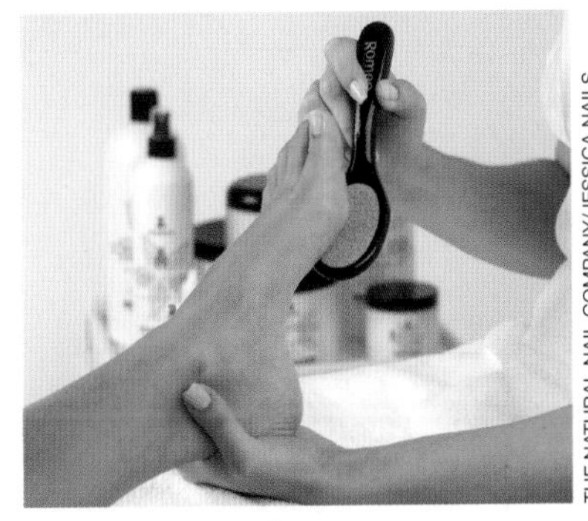

Ensure client is sat at the correct height so they can enjoy the treatment without strain to the leg

Skin and nail disorders of the feet

When a client attends for a pedicure treatment, as part of the consultation and assessment of the clients needs, the therapist should always look at the client's skin and nails to check that no infection or disease is present which might contra-indicate treatment.

These include bacterial, fungal, parasitic and viral infections, which are described in more detail in Chapter 2, where **contra-indications** are illustrated and discussed.

If the client is wearing nail polish, this must be removed before checking.

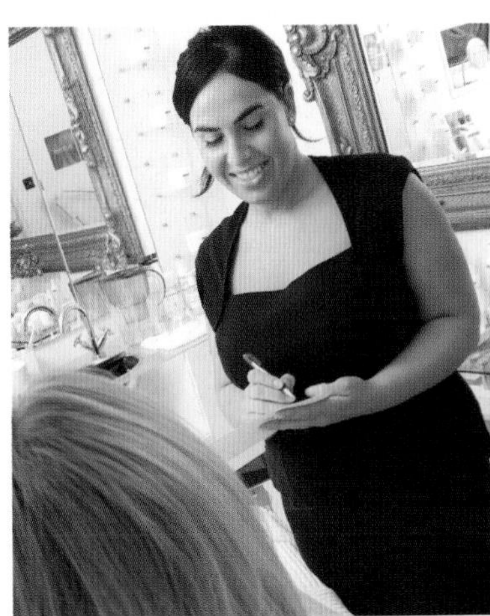

Consultation

Contra-indications

The following disorders contra-indicate pedicure treatments. If you suspect the client has any disorder from the chart below, do not attempt a diagnosis, but refer the client tactfully to their GP or a **chiropodist** without causing unnecessary concern.

Disorder	Description
Broken bones Cuts or abrasions on the feet Diabetes Paronychia Scabies or itch mites Severe eczema of the nail Severe eczema of the skin	*For full details, see page 363.*
Severe nail separation (onycholysis) Severe psoriasis of the nail Severe psoriasis of the skin Tinea corporis (body ringworm) Tinea unguium	*For full details, see page 364.*
	Phlebitis Recognized by swelling and pain in the leg caused by inflammation of the vein wall (veins transport blood from the tissues back towards the heart). If a vein becomes inflamed a blood clot commonly forms inside the inflamed area (termed **thrombophlebitis**) Venous problems can also lead to skin ulceration. Massage to the lower leg may cause a blood clot to move through the bloodstream, causing a blockage elsewhere which could prove fatal!

> **Keep a check on your client's health**
>
> Always check for contra-indications before commencing with any part of the pedicure treatment. Do your consultation thoroughly and especially find out whether your client is diabetic or on any medication.
>
> **Vicky Ann Kennedy**

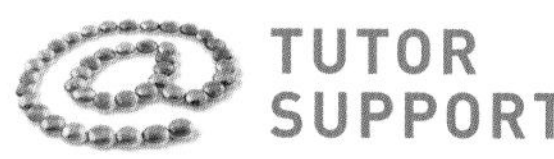

TUTOR SUPPORT

Activity 1: Label the bones of the leg and foot

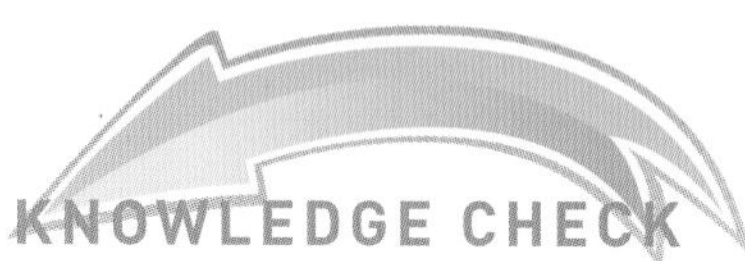

KNOWLEDGE CHECK

What information should be recorded following a pedicure treatment on the record card?

Need more time... refer to pages 402–403 to help you.

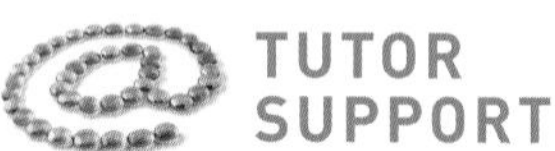

TUTOR SUPPORT

Activity 2: Label the nail structure

Disorder	Description
Ingrowing toenail 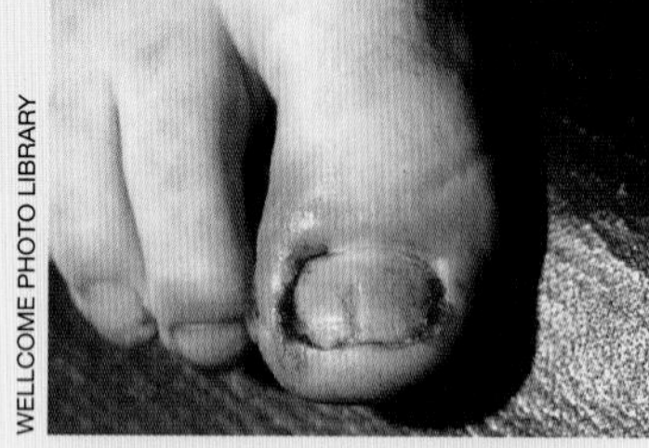 WELLCOME PHOTO LIBRARY	The sides of the nail penetrates the nail wall: redness, inflammation and pus may be present, depending on the severity of the condition. The client should be referred to chiropodist for appropriate treatment. To prevent ingrowing toenails clients should be advised to cut the toenails straight across, and not too short.
Tinea pedis (athletes' foot) 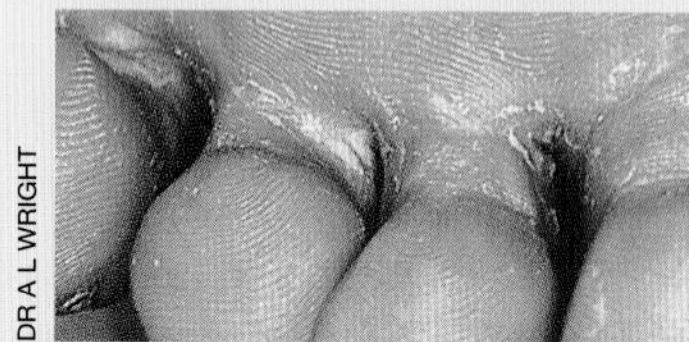 DR A L WRIGHT	Fungal infection of the foot occurring in the webs of the skin between the toes Small blisters form, which later burst. The skin in the area can become dry, with a scaly appearance.
Verrucae or plantar warts on the feet 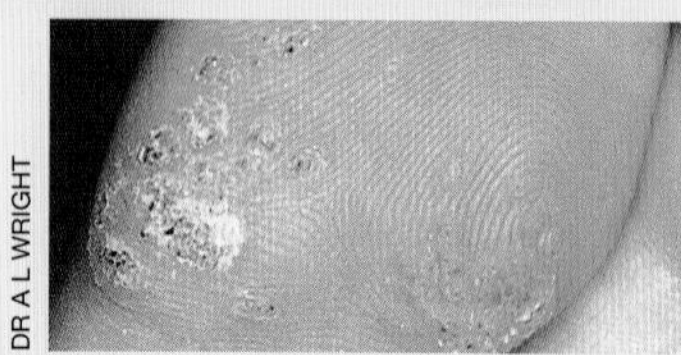 DR A L WRIGHT	A viral infection Small epidermal skin growths. Warts occurring on the sole of the foot grow inwards,due to the pressure of body weight. Warts vary in size, shape, texture and colour. Usually they have a rough surface and are raised. Plantar wart – found on the sole of the foot.

TOP TIP

The role of the chiropodist

A chiropodist is a person who is trained and qualified to treat minor foot complaints. Refer the treatment of non-cosmetic foot conditions to a chiropodist, e.g. conditions such as excessive hard skin.

KNOWLEDGE CHECK

Why is diabetes considered a contra-indication to pedicure treatments?

Need more time... refer to page 373 to help you.

Charge the correct fee

When you become self-employed, always remember that 'business is business' and start as you mean to carry on. A lot of clients do become your friends, but this should not interfere when charging. You may be happy to set a family discount at the beginning, but don't forget that your time (and your wages) are just as important to you as they are to everyone else.

Vicky Ann Kennedy

Below is a list of common disorders that may be seen on the feet. Not all of these contra-indicate treatment. See also **bruised nails**, on page 365.

Disorder	Cause	Appearance	Salon treatment	Homecare advice
Blue nail (shown on the fingernail) 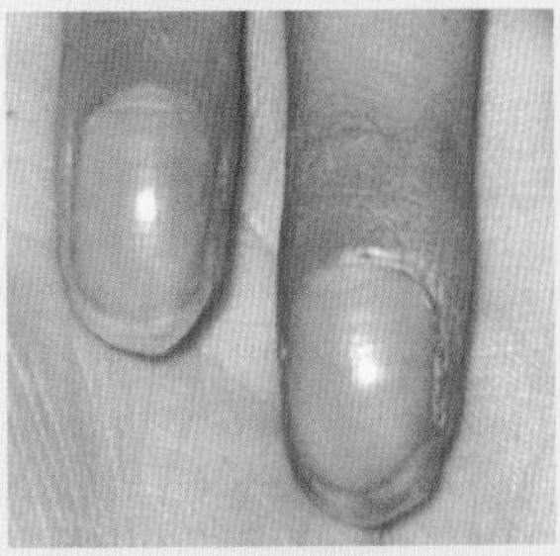 WELLCOME	Poor blood circulation in the area. Heart disease.	The nail bed does not appear a healthy pink colour but has a blue tinge.	Permission to treat to be received from the client's GP. Regular pedicure including foot treatment to improve circulation.	General pedicure advice. Foot exercises and massage to improve circulation.
Bunions 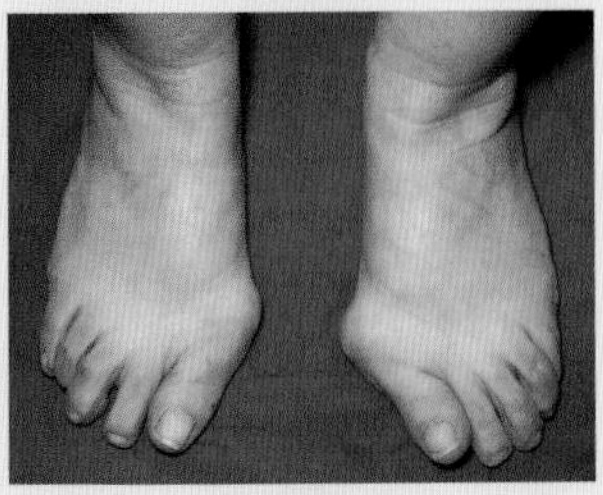 MEDISCAN	Long-term wear of ill-fitting shoes, especially those with high heels or pointed toe areas. A weakness in the arches of the feet.	The large joint at the base of the big toe protrudes, forcing the big toe inwards towards the other toes.	None – refer the client to a chiropodist if the bunion is painful; gentle massage may help to ease any pain or discomfort.	Try to keep pressure off the affected area.
Calluses 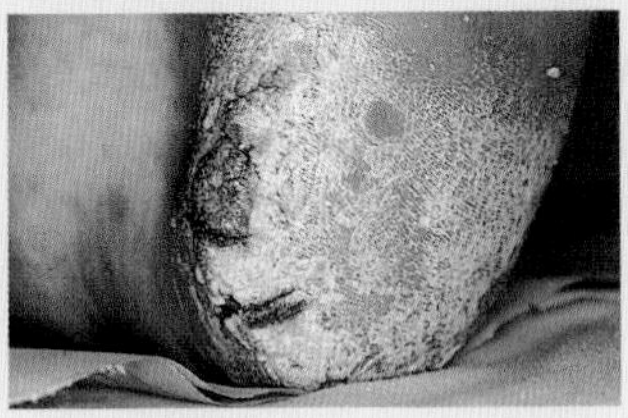 DR A L WRIGHT	Incorrect footwear.	Thick, yellowish, hardened patches of skin, usually found on prominent areas of the foot such as the heel and the ball of toe: may be painful.	Use a rasp or pumice stone gently to remove any build-up of hard skin: painful calluses should be treated by a chiropodist.	Ensure that shoes fit correctly. Avoid standing for long periods. Alternate style of footwear regularly Keep the skin of the foot moisturised with a specialized skin conditioner for the feet. Use a pumice stone regularly to remove excess skin.
Chilblains 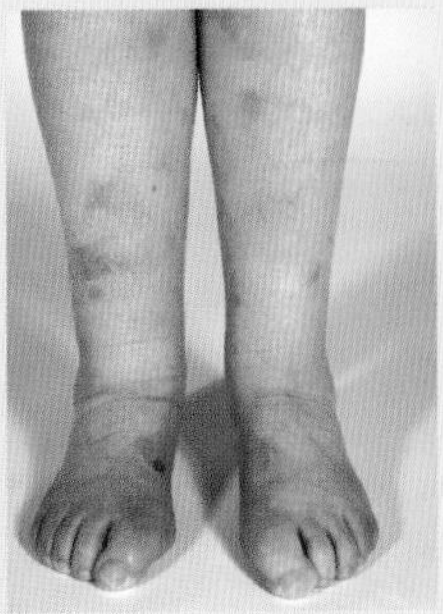 MEDISCAN	Poor blood supply to the hands and feet, aggravated in cold weather.	Fingers and toes may be red, blue or purple in colour; the client may complain of painful or itchy area.	Regular pedicures, with special attention paid to massage which will help to improve the circulation.	Keep affected areas warm and dry. Avoid tight footwear, which might restrict the circulation. If the condition is severe, seek medical advice.

Disorder	Cause	Appearance	Salon treatment	Homecare advice
Corns DR A L WRIGHT	Incorrect footwear (corns are often found on toes which have been squeezed together by tight shoes).	Similar to calluses except that the affected area is smaller and more compact; corns often look white, and may be extremely painful.	Small corns may be treated in the same way as a callus, but if the client has large or painful corns they should be treated by a chiropodist.	Ensure that shoes fit correctly. Avoid standing for long periods. Alternate style of footwear regularly.
Pitting (shown on the fingernail) WELLCOME	Eczema and/or psoriasis.	Pitting, resembling small, irregular pin pricks, appear on the nail plate.	Refer the client to their GP for permission to treat if required. Regular pedicure with gentle buffing.	General pedicure advice. Ridge-filling base coat polish.

HEALTH & SAFETY

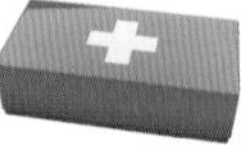

Contact dermatitis

Contact dermatitis is a skin problem caused by intolerance of the skin to a particular substance or a group of substances. On exposure to the substance the skin quickly becomes irritated and an allergic reaction occurs. This may occur when a manicurist's skin is exposed to dust and chemicals on a regular basis. Follow all HSE guidelines to reduce the risk of developing this skin disorder which could result in the need for a career change!

Always follow manufacturers' guidelines on the use of products.

ALWAYS REMEMBER

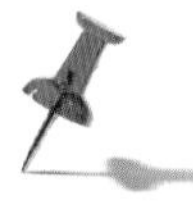

Consultation

Accurately record your client's answers to necessary questions to be asked at consultation on the record card.

Contra-actions

Certain cosmetic ingredients are known to cause allergic reactions in some people.

The client – or the pedicurist – may at some time develop an allergy to a pedicure product that has been successfully used previously. This could be for a number of reasons, including new medication being taken or illness. This is known as a **contra-action**. This may occur during or following a pedicure treatment.

The symptoms of an allergic reaction could be:

- excessive redness of the skin (erythema)
- skin irritation, e.g. itching
- swelling
- raised blisters

The symptoms do not necessarily appear on the feet. In the case of nail polish allergy, the symptoms often show up on the face.

In the case of an allergic reaction:

- Remove the offending product immediately, using water or, in the case of polish, nail polish solvent.
- Apply a cool compress and soothing agent to the skin to reduce redness and irritation.
- If symptoms persist, seek medical advice. If the client receives medical advice, ask them to inform you of the advice and/or treatment received so you can include this in your records.

Always record any allergies on the client's record card, so that the offending product may be avoided in future.

Further contra-actions could occur as a result of incorrect use of pedicure tools, e.g. sore, sensitized skin following hard skin removal or sore, reddened skin in the cuticle area due to excessive trimming of the cuticle. Tissue damage could result in blood loss, e.g. incorrect nipping removal technique when using cuticle nippers may result in pulling and tearing the skin. Incorrect positioning and use of the cuticle knife may lead to piercing the cuticle with the knife blade.

Avoid cutting the nails too short as again this can result in possible damage to the hyponychium the part of the epidermis under the free edge of the nail. This may affect its protective function, leading to possible infection.

Carrying out pedicure treatments

Outcome 2: Be able to provide pedicure treatments

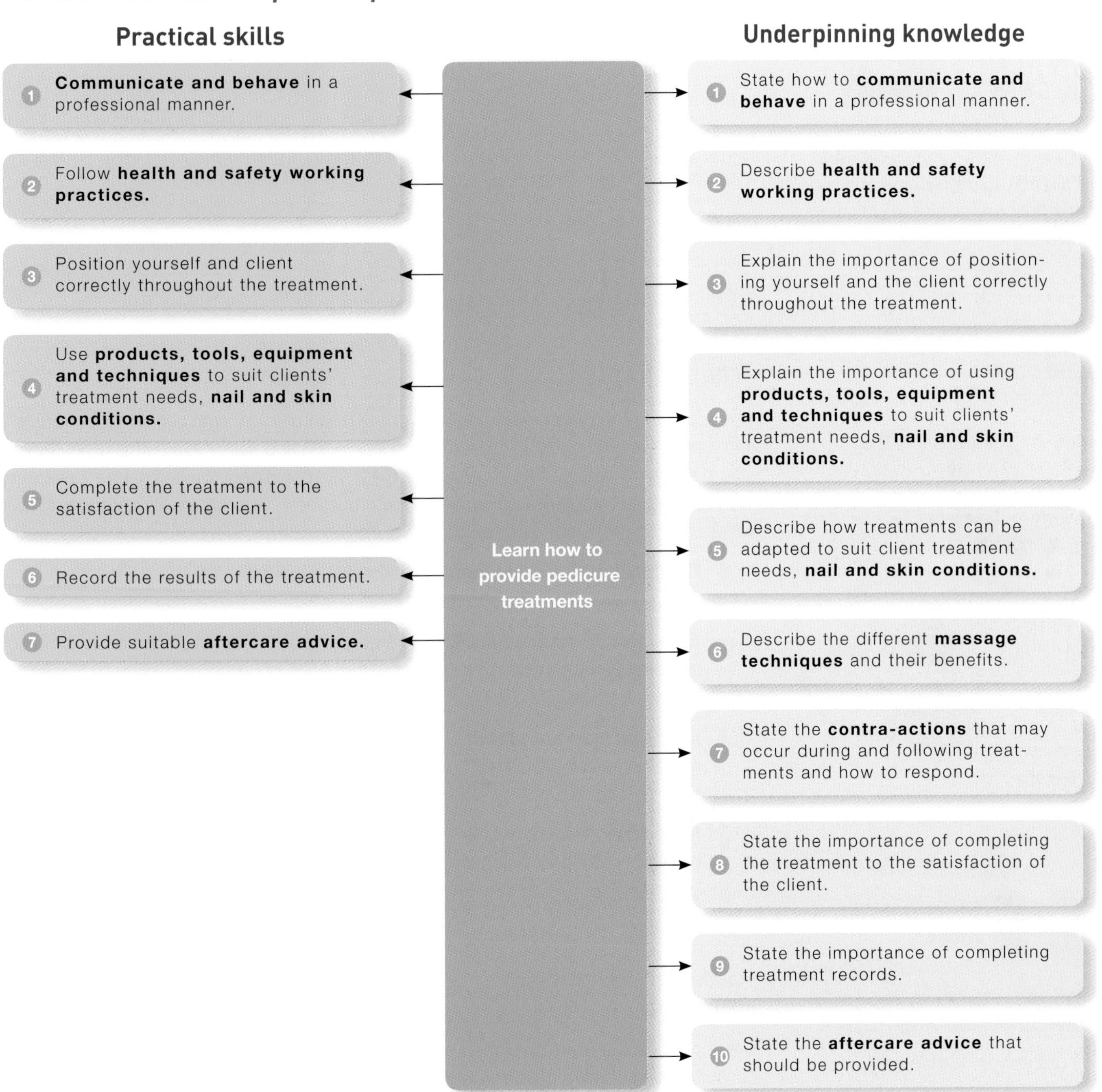

Practical skills
1 Communicate and behave in a professional manner.
2 Follow health and safety working practices.
3 Position yourself and client correctly throughout the treatment.
4 Use products, tools, equipment and techniques to suit clients' treatment needs, nail and skin conditions.
5 Complete the treatment to the satisfaction of the client.
6 Record the results of the treatment.
7 Provide suitable aftercare advice.
Learn how to provide pedicure treatments
Underpinning knowledge
1 State how to communicate and behave in a professional manner.
2 Describe health and safety working practices.
3 Explain the importance of positioning yourself and the client correctly throughout the treatment.
4 Explain the importance of using products, tools, equipment and techniques to suit clients' treatment needs, nail and skin conditions.
5 Describe how treatments can be adapted to suit client treatment needs, nail and skin conditions.
6 Describe the different massage techniques and their benefits.
7 State the contra-actions that may occur during and following treatments and how to respond.
8 State the importance of completing the treatment to the satisfaction of the client.
9 State the importance of completing treatment records.
10 State the aftercare advice that should be provided.

What advice would you give to a client who developed an allergic reaction to a product following a pedicure treatment?

Need more time... refer to page 408 to help you.

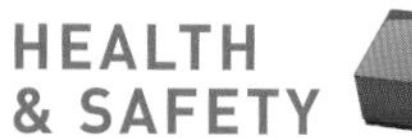

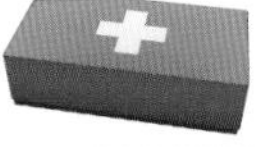

Contamination
Always remove products hygienically from containers to avoid contamination and cross-infection.

Underpinning knowledge

(Continued) Learn how to provide pedicure treatments

- ⑪ Describe diseases and disorders of the nail and skin.
- ⑫ Describe the structure and functions of the nail and skin.
- ⑬ Describe the structure and function of the muscles of the lower leg and foot.
- ⑭ Describe the structure and function of the bones of the lower leg and foot.
- ⑮ Describe the structure and function of the arteries and veins of the lower leg and foot.
- ⑯ Describe the structure and function of the lymphatic vessels of the lower leg and foot.

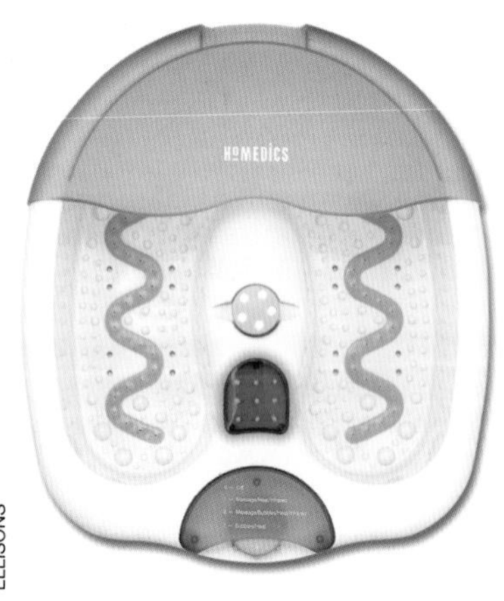

ELLISONS

Foot spa

> **Sterilize your tools**
> Never use tools that are not completely sterile. Use disposable products where possible.
> **Vicky Ann Kennedy**

Treatment plan

After analyzing the client's nails and adjacent skin, a treatment plan should be considered and agreed with the client. In order to correct any skin and nail problems the client should attend the salon weekly. They should also be advised of the appropriate treatment preparations to use at home, so as to support the salon treatment. Specialist foot treatments to use will depend upon the skin and nail condition; they include:

- ***Revitalizing foot spa agents*** These may be in tablet form or as a foaming soak. They are dissolved in warm water, in which the feet are then immersed.
- ***Exfoliator*** This is used following immersion of the feet in the foot spa. It removes surface dead skin cells, preventing the formation of callus (excess dead tissue) tissue.
- ***Massage lotion or cream*** This is a massage preparation which includes refreshing essential oils such as peppermint. It is recommended for the relief of tired, aching feet.
- ***Foot mask*** A mask may be applied to cool and to refresh the feet. Booties may be worn while the mask penetrates the epidermis.
- ***Foot gel or spray*** This may be applied to create an immediate cooling, refreshing effect.

Provide the opportunity for your client to ask any questions relating to the pedicure treatment plan.

The record card should be signed and dated by the client and pedicurist following the consultation to confirm the suitability and consent with the agreed pedicure treatment.

Step-by-step: Pedicure procedure

This process briefly shows the stages in the pedicure. Each step is discussed in detail later in the chapter. The procedure may start with either the right or left foot.

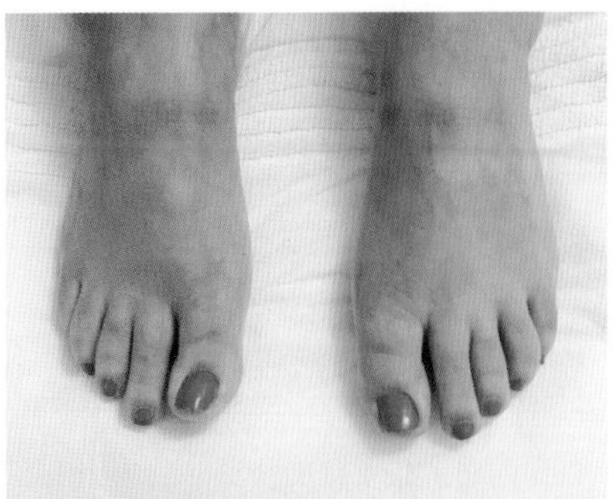

1 Nails before pedicure procedure.

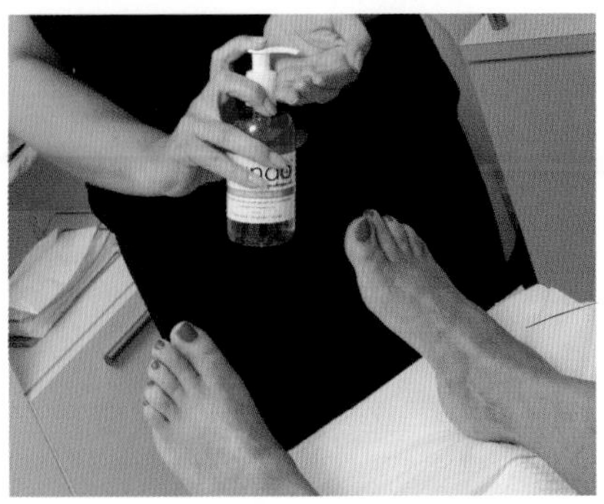

2 Clean your hands using an approved hand cleaning technique.

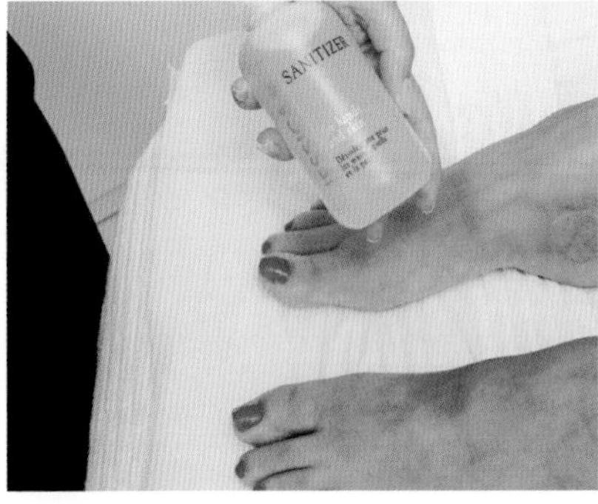

3 Wipe both feet (including between the toes) with cotton wool soaked in skin disinfectant (product example shown here) or a specialized hygiene spray for the feet. Use separate pieces of cotton wool for each foot.

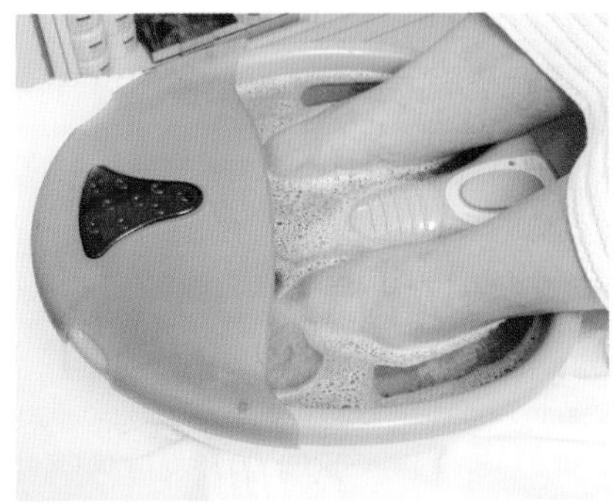

4 Soak both feet in warm water to which a liquid soap or a similar appropriate product has been added. Take out left foot and towel dry it.

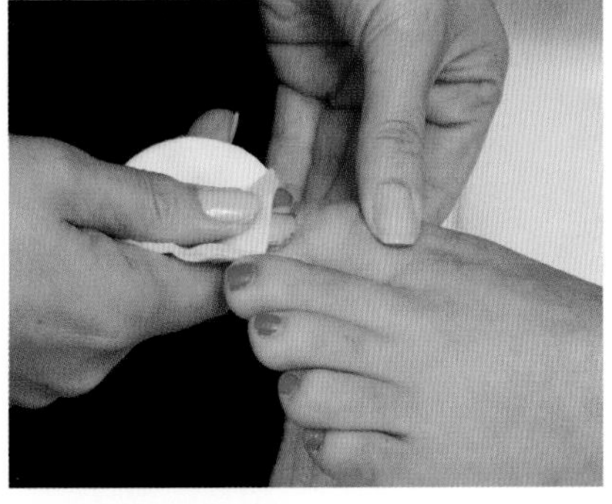

5 Remove any existing nail polish, and check again for contraindications below the nail plate. (If a nail contra-indication is present treatment must not continue. Tactfully explain why and give appropriate referral advice.)

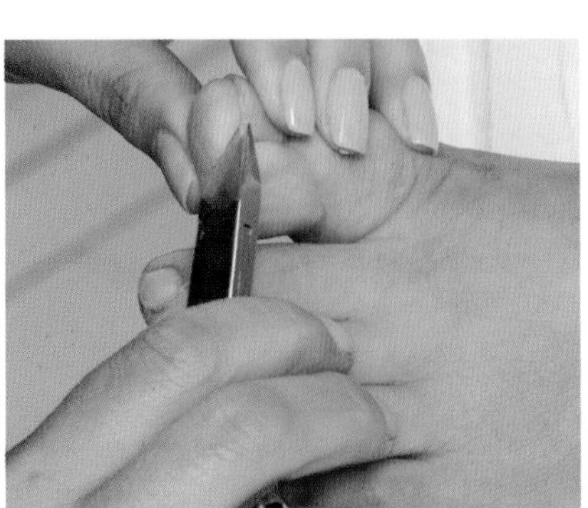

6 Cut the toenails straight across, using toenail clippers or scissors.

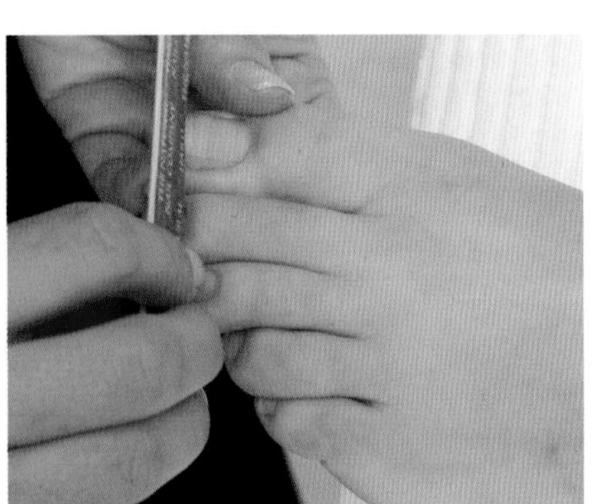

7 File the nails smooth with the coarse side of the emery board. Again do not shape the nails at the sides to avoid ingrowing nails.

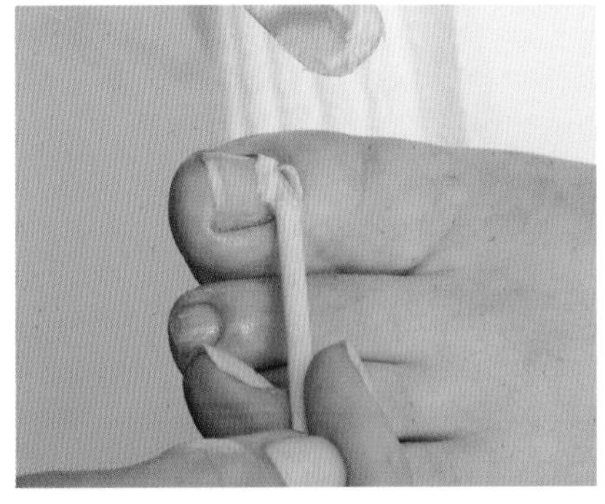

8 Apply cuticle massage cream or oil.

9 Place the foot back in the water.

10 Remove the right foot and repeat steps 5–10.

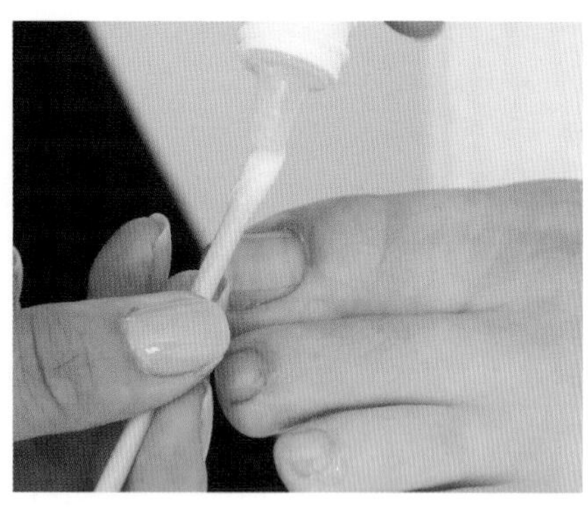

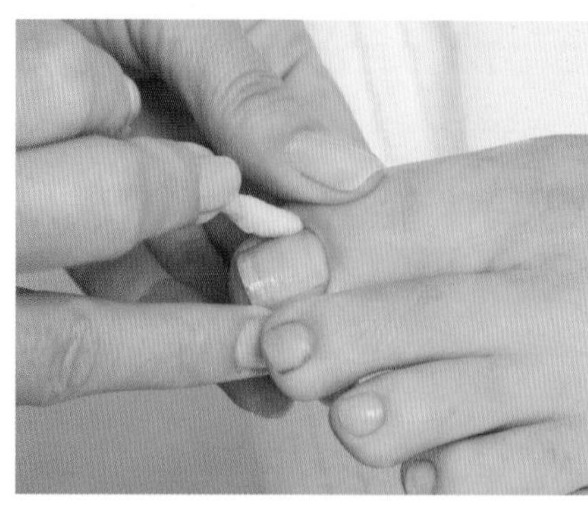

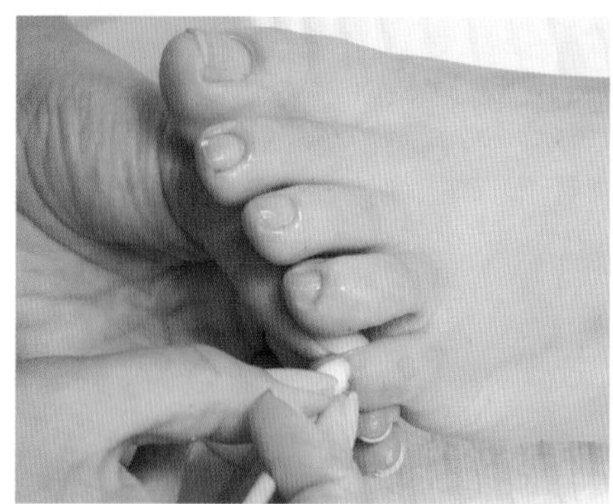

11 Dry the left foot and apply **cuticle remover**.

To avoid excessive application and contaminating the applicator apply to a cotton wool-tipped **orange stick**.

12 Push back the cuticles with a cotton wool-tipped orange stick, hoof stick or cuticle pusher.

13 Clean under the free edge with a separate cotton wool-tipped orange stick.

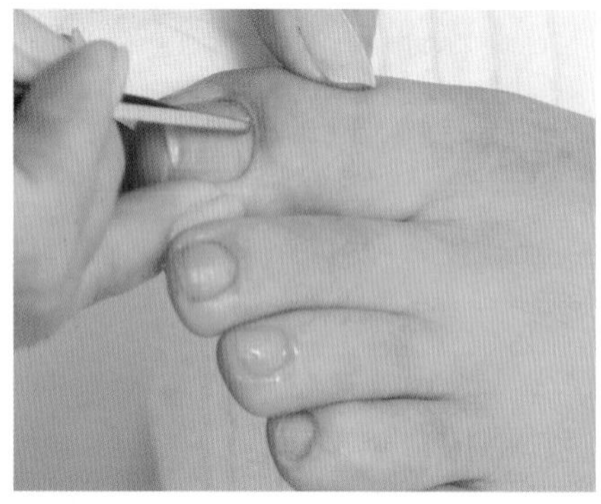

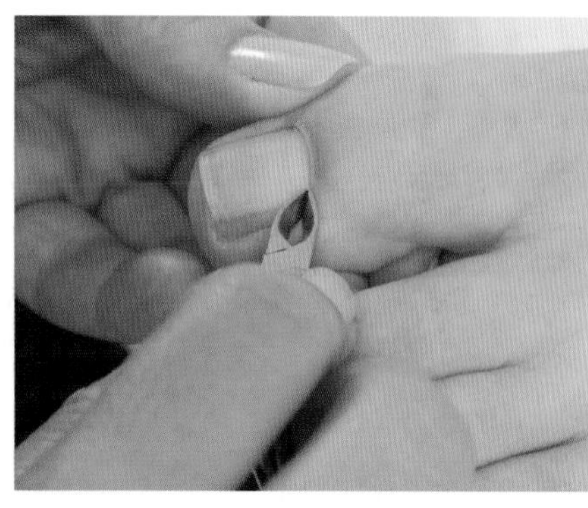

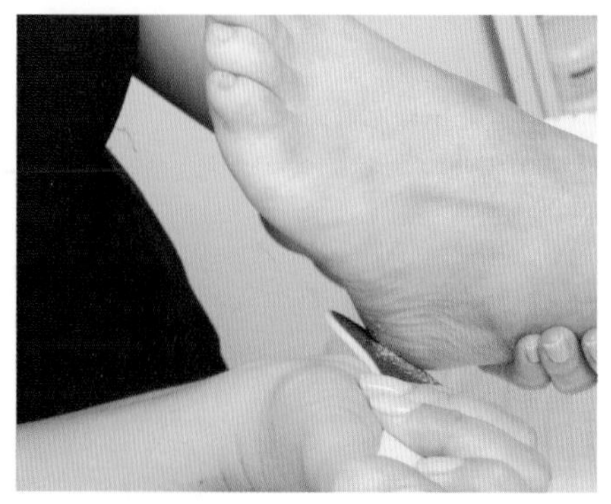

14 Use the **cuticle knife** where indicated to remove excess eponychium and peri-onychium. Collect excess skin in a tissue or a clean piece of cotton wool and dispose of immediately.

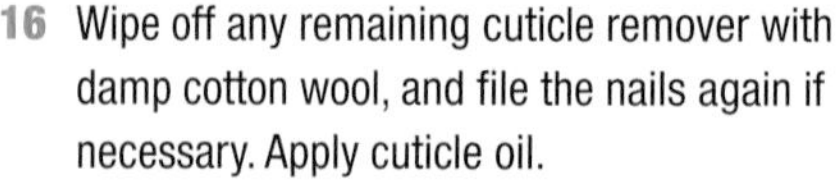

15 Use cuticle nippers where necessary to remove excess cuticle.

16 Wipe off any remaining cuticle remover with damp cotton wool, and file the nails again if necessary. Apply cuticle oil.

17 Remove any hard skin. This may be done with exfoliating cream, pedicure callous file or a rasp, depending on the severity of the excess dry skin condition.

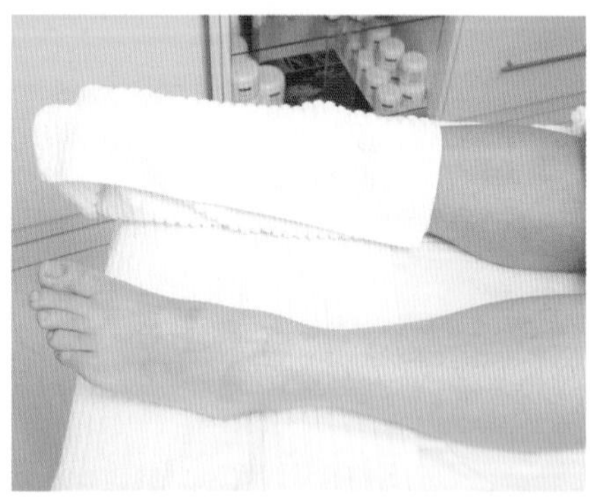

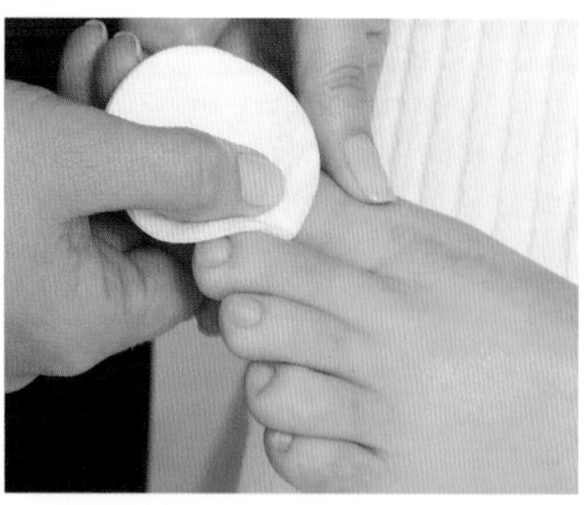

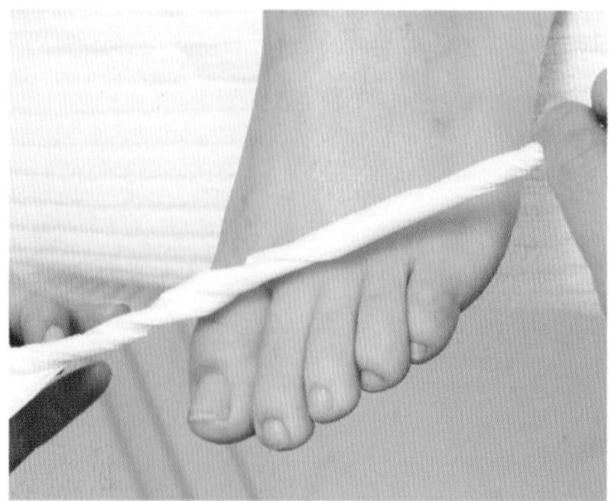

18 Wrap the foot in a dry towel and to keep it warm.

19 Repeat steps 12–19 for the other foot.

20 Remove the foot bowl from the working area.

21 Perform a foot and lower leg massage. (See pages 418–419.)

22 Remove any grease from the nail plates with a cotton wool pad soaked in nail polish remover. Refile the nails as necessary to ensure they are smooth and even.

23 Place disposable toe separators or other hygienic equivalent to separate them and facilitate polish application.

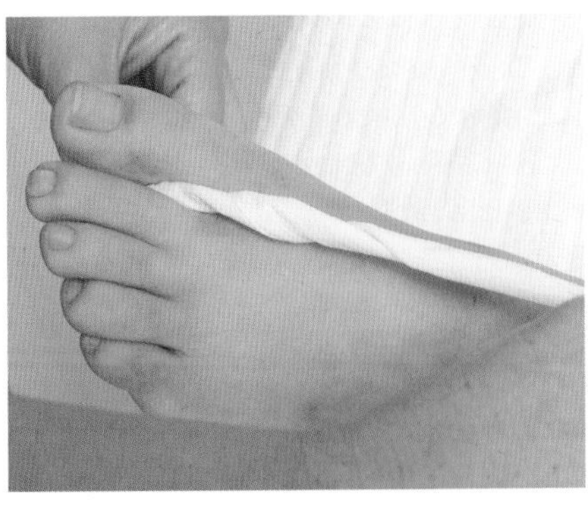

23 Continued.

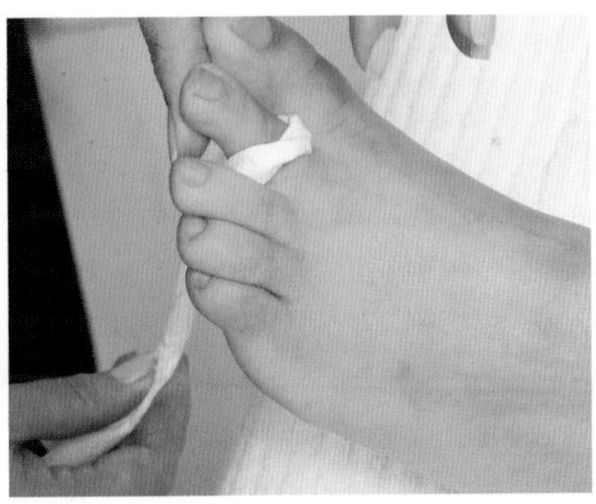

23 Continued.

24 Apply the polish: base coat (once), cream polish (twice) and top coat (once) where indicated. If a pearlized polish is used a top coat is not required and a third coat of polish may be applied.

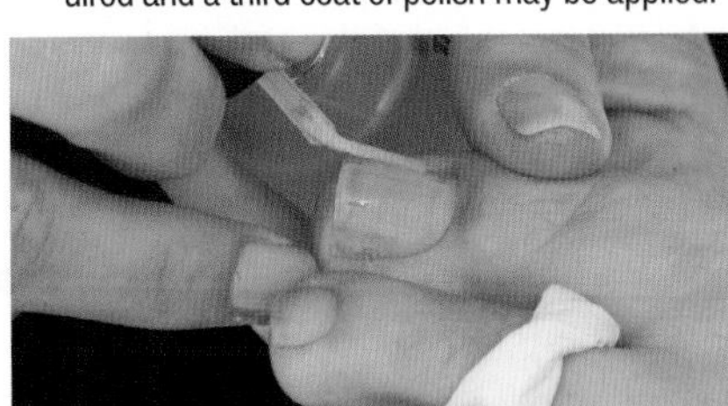

24a Application of base coat.

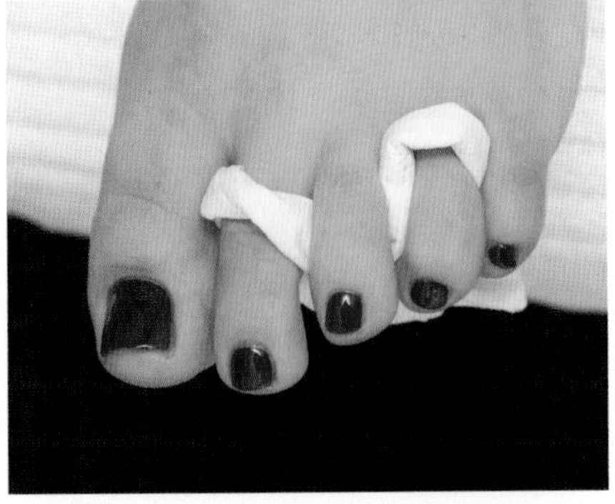

24b Application of first coat of coloured cream polish

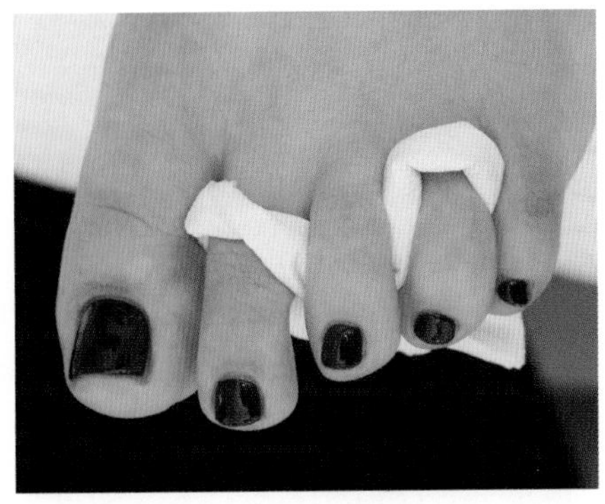

24c Application of second coat of coloured cream polish.

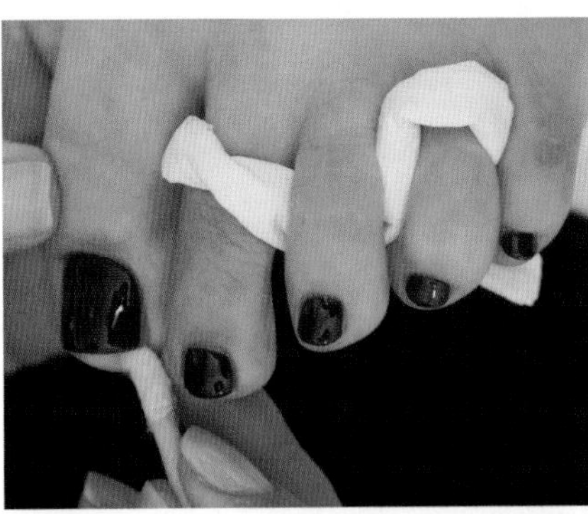

A cotton wool-tipped orange stick may be used to apply nail polish remover to remove any excess polish from the surrounding skin.

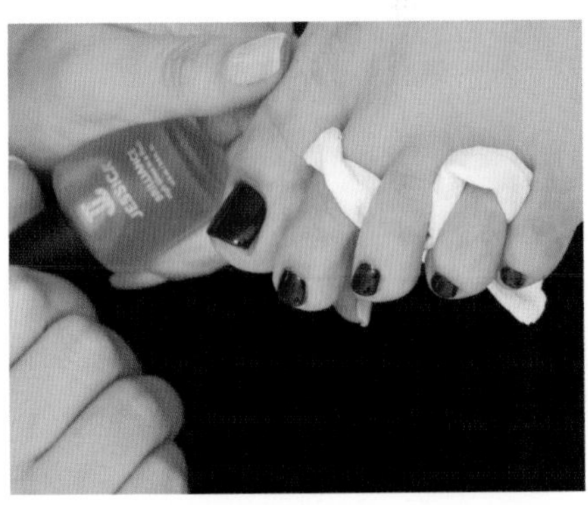

24d Application of top coat as the product is a cream polish, requiring a top coat.

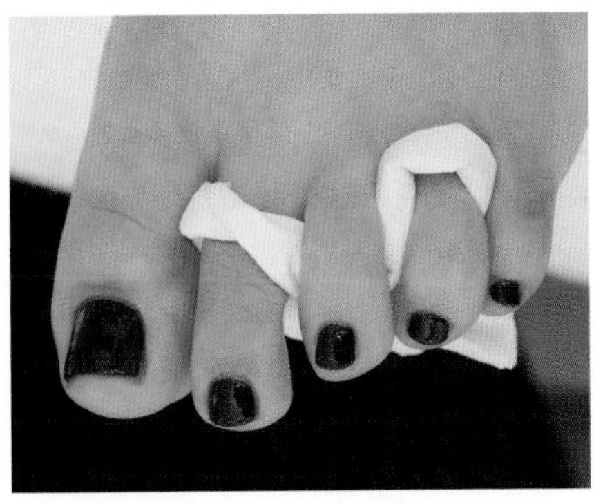

25 The complete dark polish pedicure

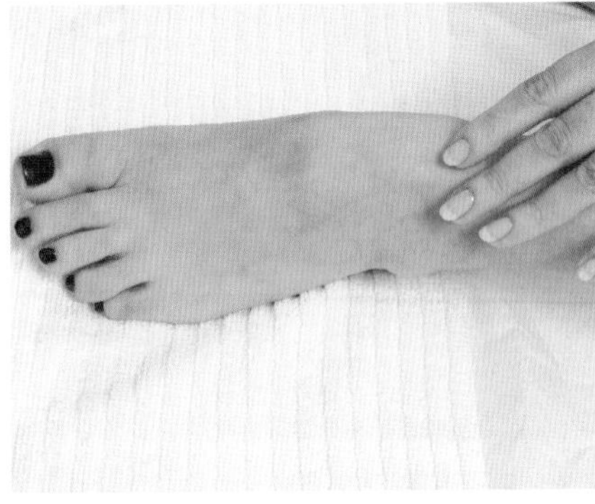

Complete nail treatment. (French polish application shown is illustrated on page 386.)

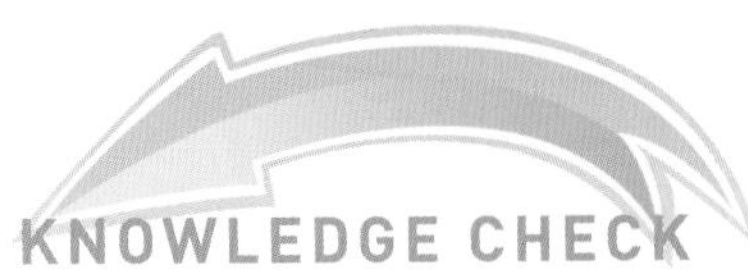

KNOWLEDGE CHECK

If you accidentally caused tissue damage resulting in bleeding which legislation must you comply with in the disposable of any contaminated waste?

Need more time... refer to page 110 to help you.

HEALTH & SAFETY

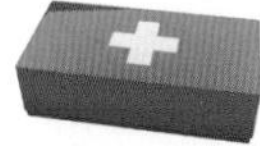

Disposing of waste

All waste should be disposed of as instructed by your local authority environmental agency requirements and the Industry Code of Practice for Nail Services.

HEALTH & SAFETY

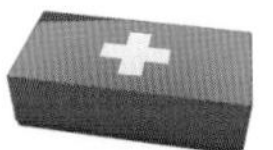

Cutting toenails
Never cut toenails down at the sides. This increases the chance of ingrowing toenails, and may lead to infection.

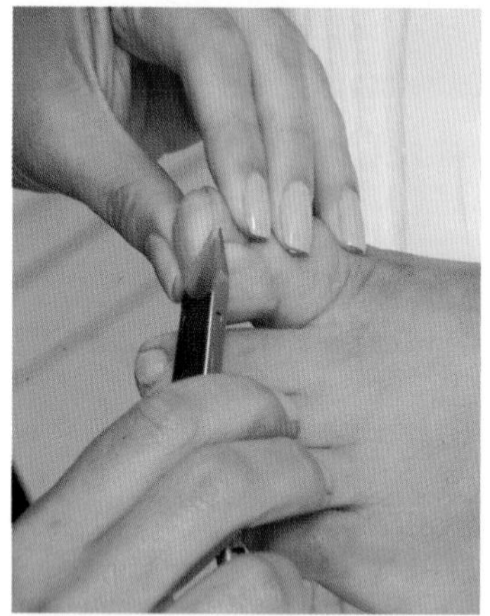

Cutting toenails

Cutting and filing toenails

Toenails should be cut straight across, using nail clippers or strong sharp scissors, then filed smooth using the coarse side of the emery board. This helps to avoid ingrowing toenails. Do not cut too short to ensure there is adequate protection at the free edge to avoid discomfort and infection.

Cuticle work Cuticle work is carried out to keep the cuticle area attractive, healthy and also to prevent cuticles from becoming overgrown and adhering to the nail plate, which could lead to splitting of the cuticle as the nail grows forward, and subsequently to infection of the area.

The work is carried out after soaking the feet in warm soapy water. This step loosens dirty particles from the free edge and softens the skin in the cuticle area.

HEALTH & SAFETY

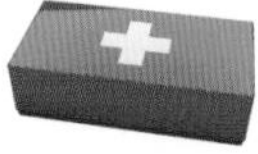

If you accidentally cut the skin, causing bleeding at the cuticle area, protect you hands with disposable gloves and wipe the skin with an antiseptic wipe. Any waste is classed as clinical waste or contaminated waste and should be disposed of in a yellow medical bin liner in accordance with the **Environmental Act (1990)** and **Controlled Waste Regulations (1992).**

See Habia *Hygiene in the Beauty Therapy* booklet for further guidance.

Pushing back the cuticles

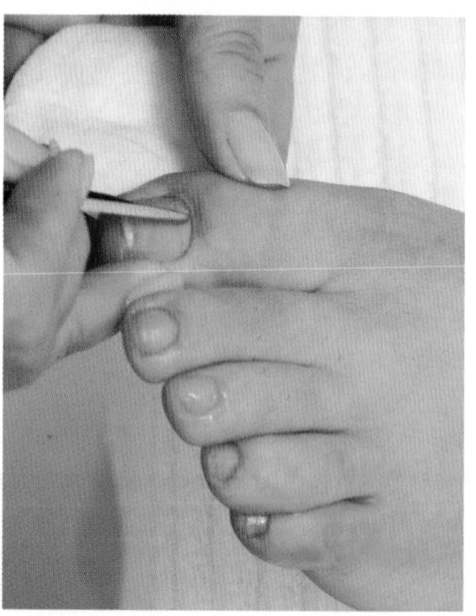

Using a cuticle knife

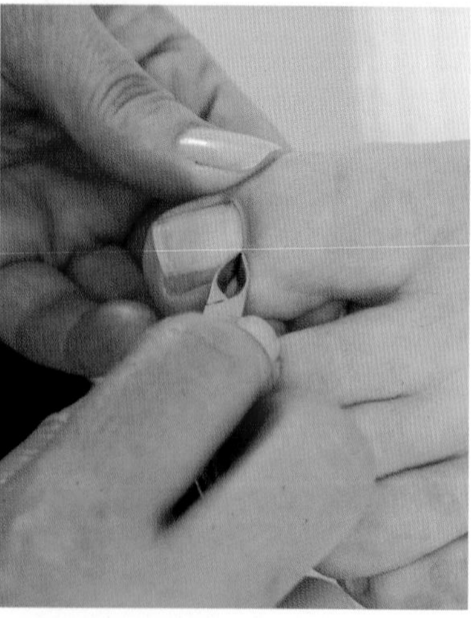

Using cuticle nippers

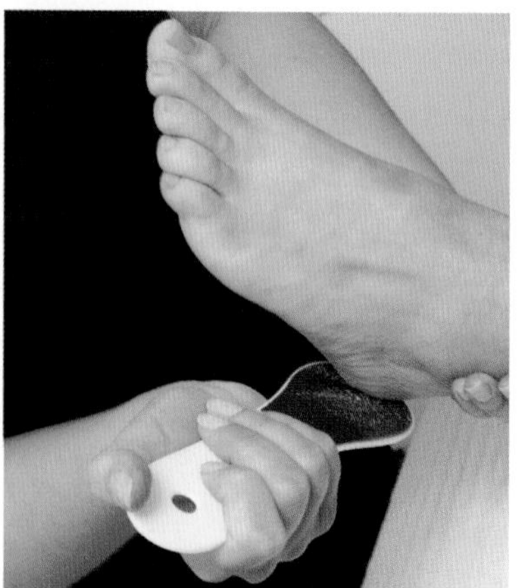

Removing hard skin with a pumice file

How to provide cuticle work Cuticle work on the feet follows the same principles and cuticle work on the hands. For a detailed description, see pages 378–379.

Removing hard skin

Hard skin, develops on the feet as a form of protection, either from friction from footwear or from standing for long periods of time.

It is therefore not advisable to remove *all* the hard skin from an area, as this would remove the protective pad. Hard skin should be removed only to improve the appearance of the feet. Hard skin build-up that causes pain or discomfort should be referred to a chiropodist for treatment.

Excess hard skin may be removed from the feet in a number of ways, including exfoliators, pumice stones, callus files, chiropody sponges, and corn planes. Exfoliators should be used with a deep circular massage movement: they are ideal when only a very small build-up of hard skin is present. Files, pumice stones and the rest should be used with a swift stroking movement in one direction only (similar to buffing). Sawing back and forth would lead to friction, and discomfort for the client.

Always finish off a hard skin removal procedure with the application of a specialized foot moisturiser or lotion, to soften the newly exposed skin.

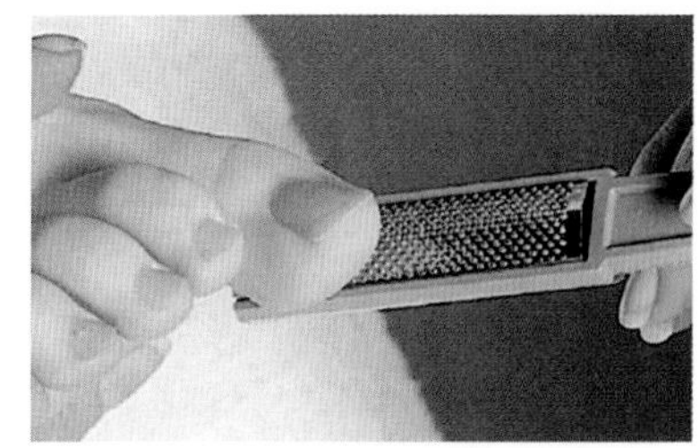

Removing hard skin with a rasp

Foot and nail treatments

In addition to the pedicure, further treatments may be added as appropriate. Here are some examples:

- ***Exfoliating treatment*** is carried out prior to massage or as part of the massage routine. An abrasive massage product is massaged over the skin of the foot in circular movements, concentrating over the ball and heel of the foot. Exfoliation removes dead skin, increases blood and lymph circulation and improves the condition and appearance of the skin and the absorption of further treatment products.
- ***Foot treatment mask*** is applied according to the client's treatment requirements. The mask is applied to the skin, then covered with a plastic protective cover and the feet can then be wrapped in warm **thermal booties** to aid the absorption of the mask. The mask removes dead skin cells, improves blood circulation and improves the condition of the skin of the feet.
- ***Paraffin wax treatment*** – this wax is heated in a special bath to a temperature of 50–55°C. The heating effect stimulates the blood and lymph circulation, eases the discomfort of arthritic and rheumatic conditions, soothes sensory nerve endings and softens the skin, improving the appearance and condition of dry skin.

  After checking the client's tolerance to the wax temperature, the client's whole foot and ankle is covered with paraffin wax. The liquid wax is usually applied with a brush. The initial wax application quickly sets, becoming solid and then further layers of paraffin wax are applied to provide a waterproof covering. Once applied the feet should then be placed in a plastic protective covering and covered with towelling booties. The wax may be removed after 10–15 minutes. It is a good idea to remove the wax with the plastic covering, which is usually in one action. After use the wax is disposed of.
- ***Thermal booties*** are electrically heated booties. They are used to stimulate, rejuvenate and moisturise the skin of the feet. The feet are prepared with the application of a foot treatment mask, protected in a plastic covering and placed inside warm booties for ten to fifteen minutes to enable the mask to penetrate the skin of the epidermis.

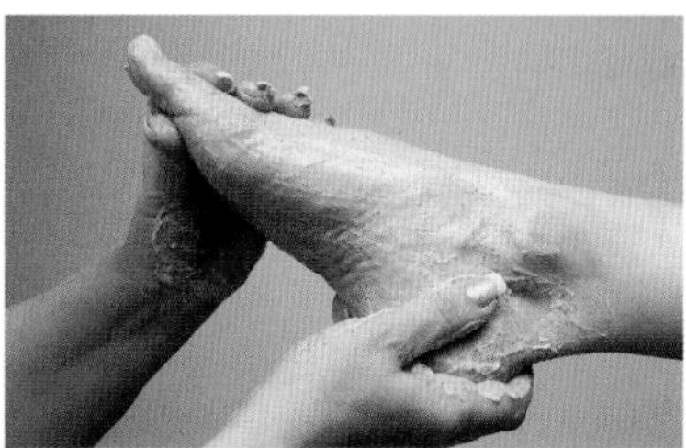

Exfoliating treatment

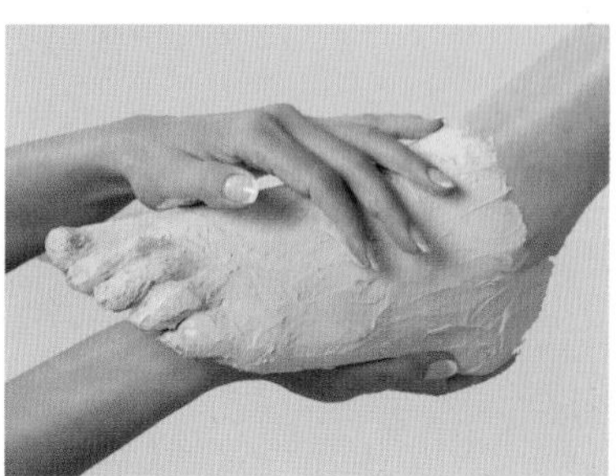

Foot treatment mask

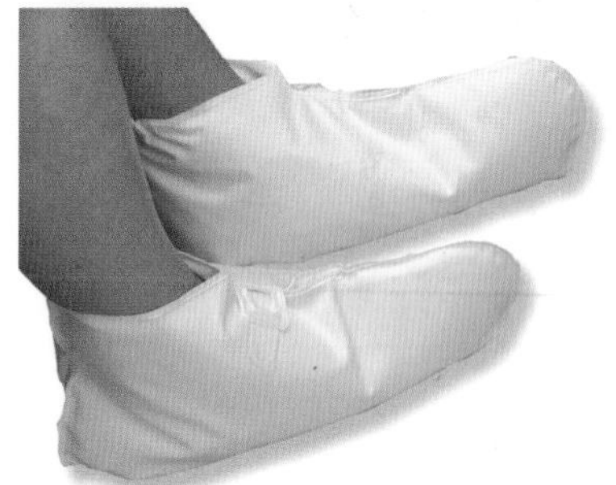

ELLISONS

Thermal booties

Always follow manufacturers' guidelines in the application procedure for feet and nail treatments.

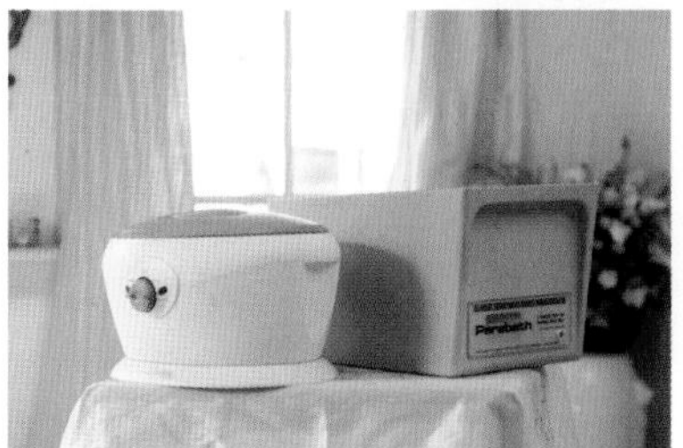

Paraffin wax tools and equipment

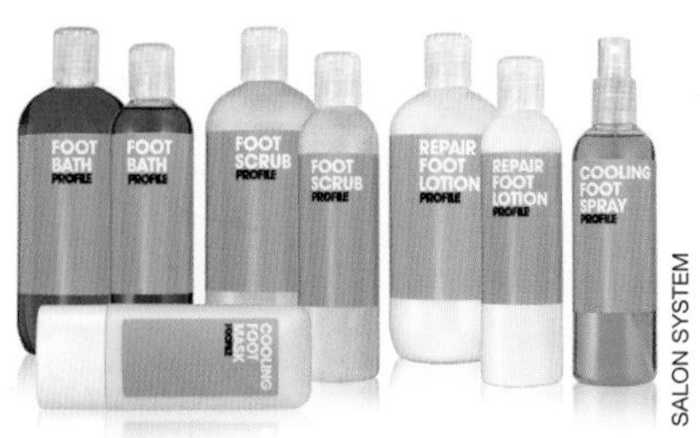

SALON SYSTEM

Pedicure products

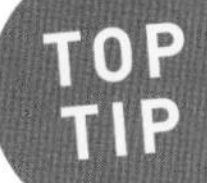

TOP TIP

Paraffin wax

Heat the wax at least half an hour before the client arrives to ensure it has melted properly. Paraffin wax may have essential oils added to enhance the therapeutic effects.

Step-by-step: Specialist foot and leg treatment

Specialist treatments should be offered to your client when there is a specific need or if they feel they would like to benefit from such a treatment. Specialist treatment training in these advanced techniques is usually offered by major product companies.

The model for this specialist foot and leg treatment is a client who regularly visits the gym and wished to benefit from a spa therapy revitalizing treatment following a workout.

The following foot and leg treatment will:

- stimulate the blood circulation
- aid with the removal of toxins and waste products
- have a skin-cleansing action
- remove dead skin cells (desquamation)
- improve the moisture content of the skin
- relax tense/stiff muscles in the foot and leg

Your treatments should be adapted the meet the treatment objectives for the client. Allow 30 minutes for the specialist foot and leg treatment below.

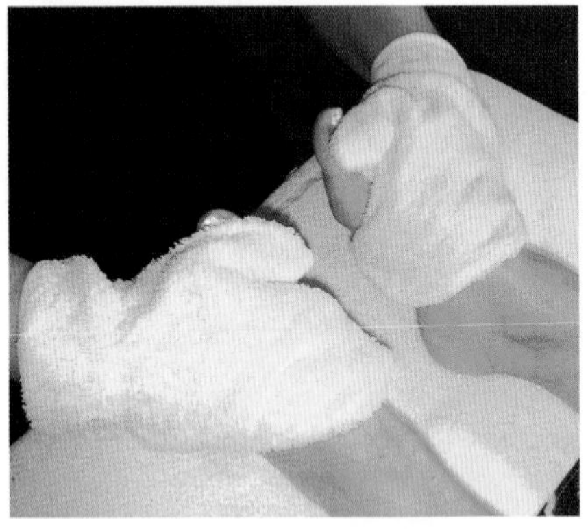

1 The skin of the feet and legs is cleansed using warm towelling mitts infused with lime oil for its therapeutic refreshing and energizing properties.

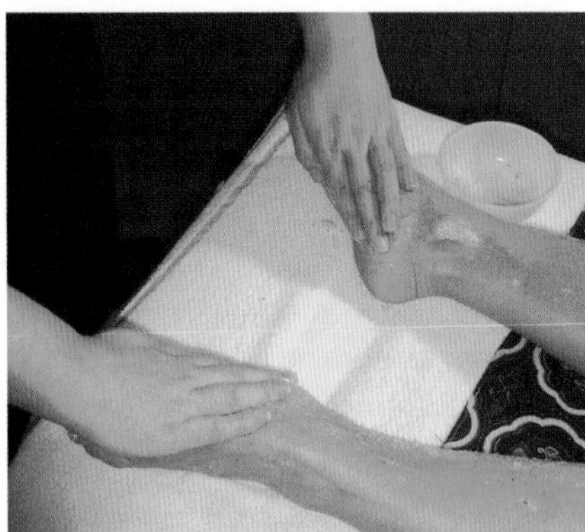

2 The feet and legs are exfoliated to remove all dead skin cells and brighten the skin. A sea salt-based preparation with emollient, skin softening ingredients is applied to each foot and leg.

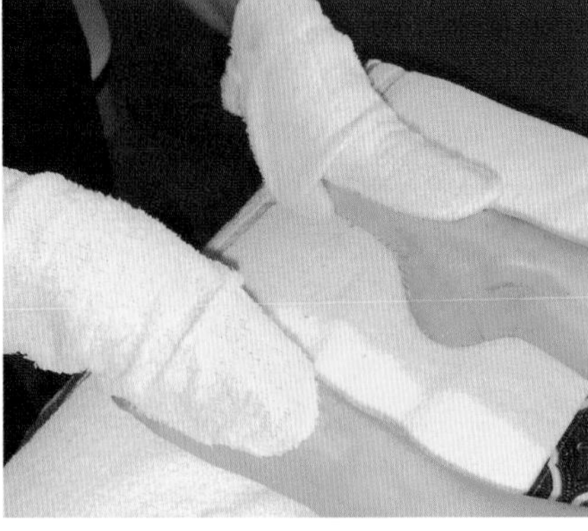

3 Towelling mitts are used to remove the exfoliating treatment. These have been steamed and are warm when used.

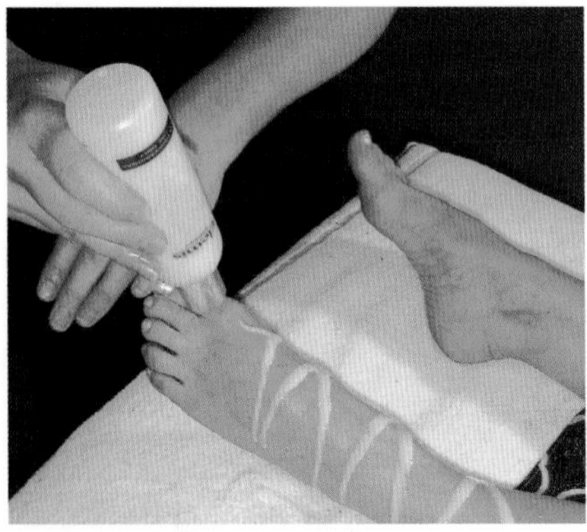

4 A skin-nourishing milk lotion is applied to each foot and leg using a 'drizzling' technique. The milk is particularly beneficial for dry skin.

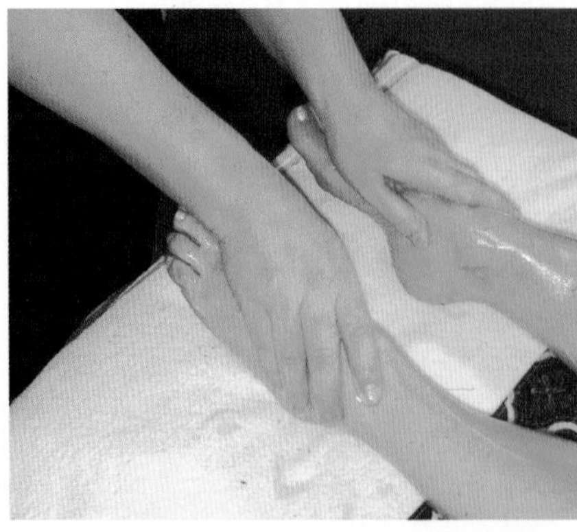

5 Massage movements are applied using **effleurage** and **petrissage** manipulations to introduce the massage medium into the skin.

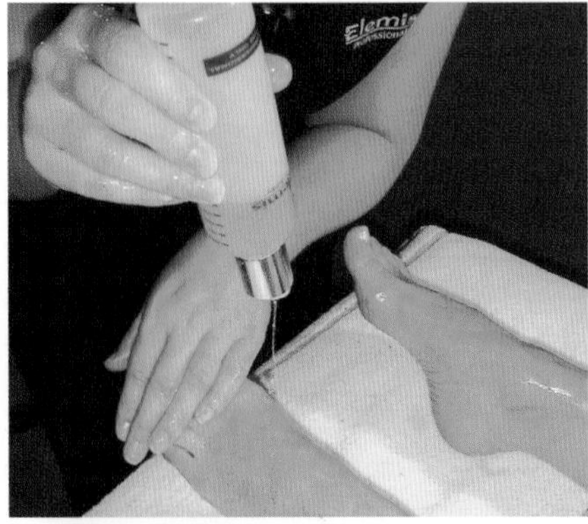

6 A further skin treatment product oil is applied and massaged into the skin. This will act as a treatment mask for the skin to soften and condition.

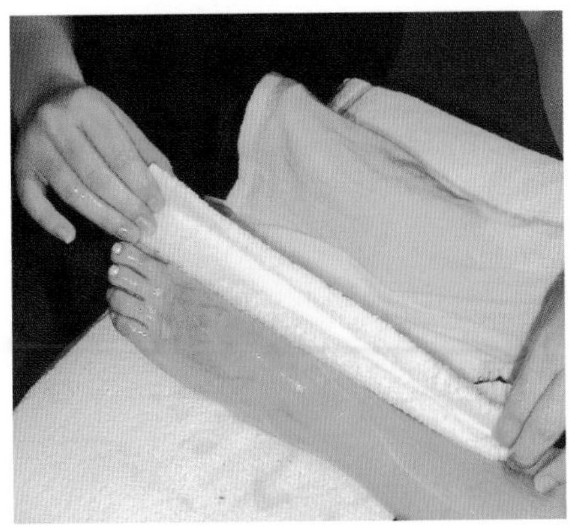
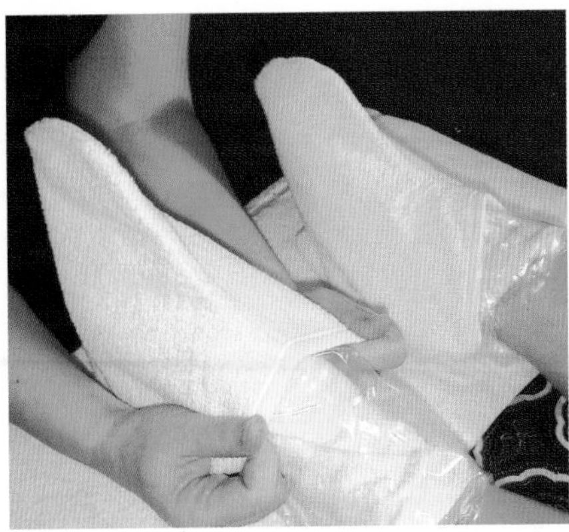

7 The feet are then placed in steamed towels, encased in a plastic bag and dry towelling foot bootie for 10–15 minutes.

Foot and lower leg massage

As with a manicure massage, the pedicure massage is carried out near the end of the treatment, prior to nail polishing. The pedicure massage includes the foot and the lower leg, and offers the following benefits to the client as follows:

- moisturises the skin with the massage medium, cream, lotion or oil, improving skin hydration
- increases blood circulation transporting oxygen and nutrients to the lower leg and foot
- increases lymph circulation, transporting waste products in the lymph away from the lower leg and foot
- helps maintain joint mobility
- eases discomfort from arthritis or rheumatism
- relaxes the client
- muscle tone is improved as the muscles receive an improved supply of oxygenated blood, essential for cell growth
- helps remove any dead skin cells (desquamation) exposing new cells

The massage incorporates classic massage movements, each with different effects:

- **Effleurage** – a stroking movement, used to begin the massage as a link manipulation, and to complete the massage sequence.
- **Petrissage** – movements, including **kneading**, where the tissues are lifted away from the underlying structures and compressed. Pressure is intermittent, and should be light yet firm.
- **Tapotement**, also known as **percussion**, may be included – **tapotement** movements are performed in a brisk, stimulating manner to increase blood supply and improve tone of the skin and muscles. Movements include clapping and tapping.
- **Joint manipulations** – ankle joints and toes are manipulated through their range of movement, dependant upon the type of joint. This helps to maintain

good mobility within the range of movement but must be avoided if the client has any joint disorders.

- **Frictions** – small circular movements using the pads of the fingers or thumbs. The skin and muscle below is massage against the underlying bone. This can be used to loosen any adhesions in the tissues.

The beauty therapist can adapt the massage application according to the needs of the client. Either the *speed of application* or *depth of pressure* can be altered.

Step-by-step: Foot and lower leg massage

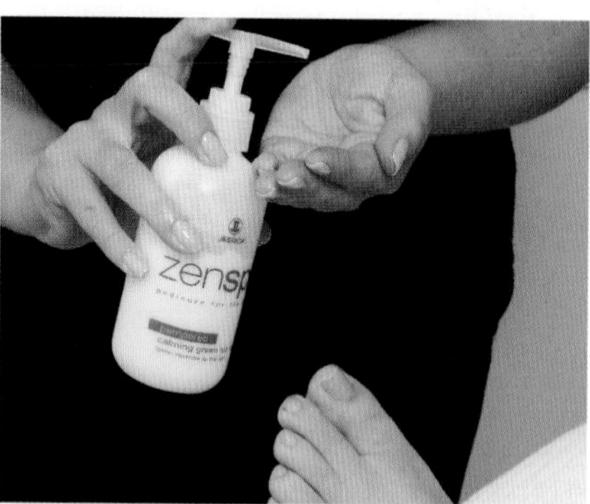

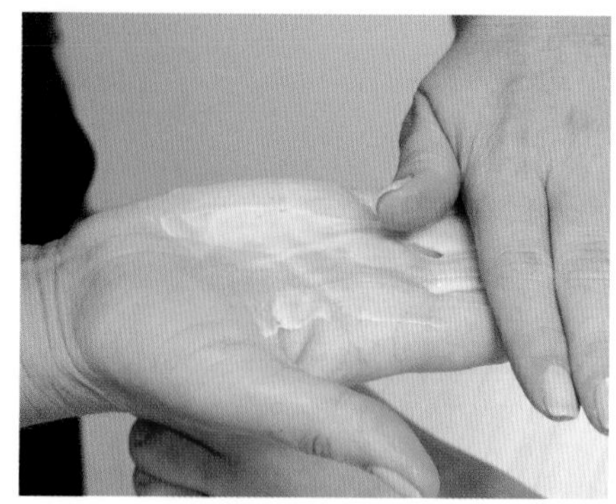

1 Dispense the massage medium into the hands, warm the product over the palms and apply to the client's skin using effleurage technique.

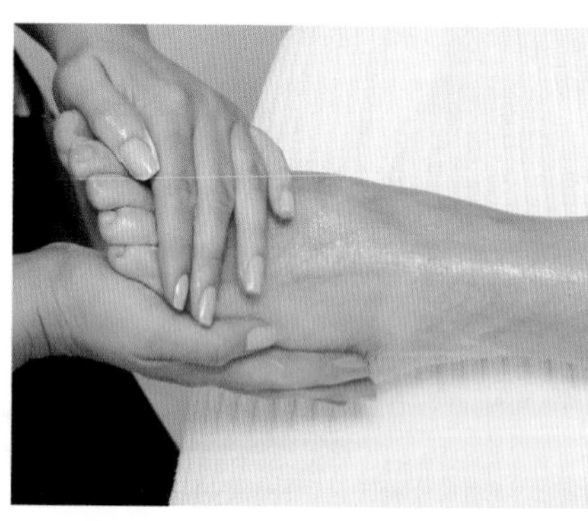

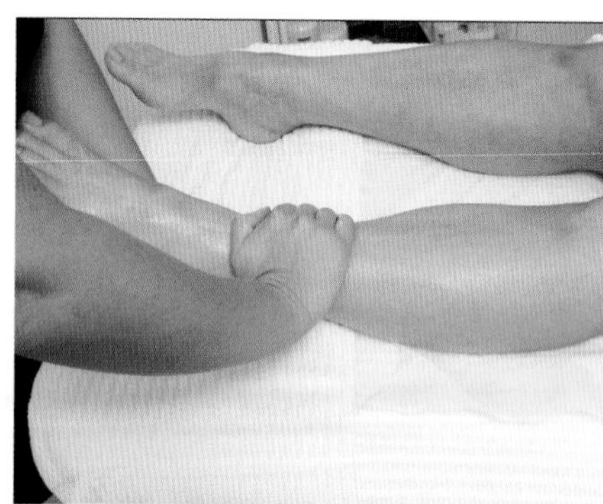

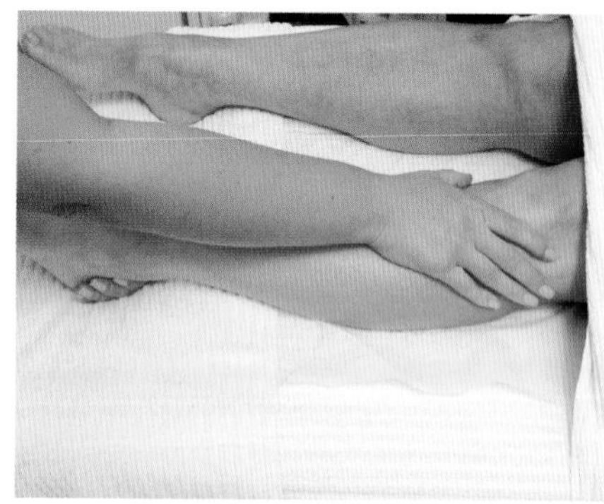

2 **Effleurage from the foot to the knee** Use long sweeping strokes from the toes to the knee, moving on both the back and the front of the leg.

Repeat step 2 a further 5 times.

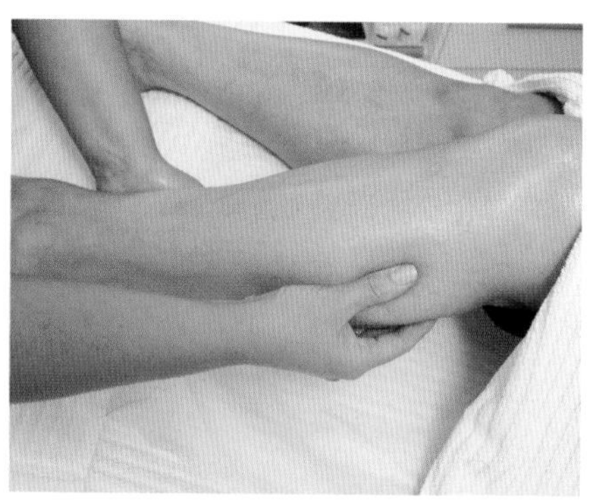

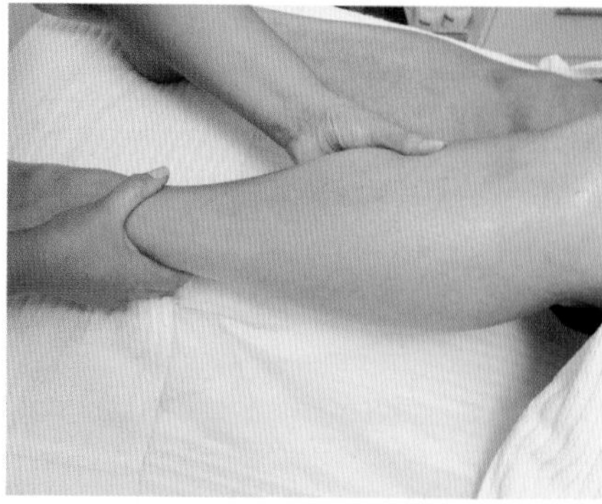

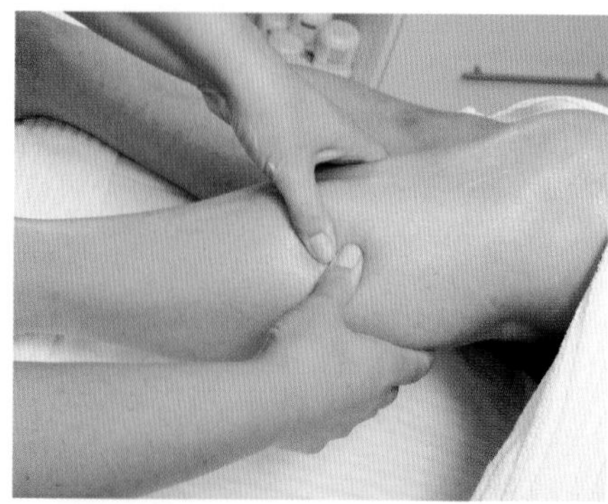

3 Flex the client's knee and using a petrissage movement in an upwards direction pick-up, and gently squeeze the gastrocnemius muscle.

4 Slide the palm down to the ankle and using the thumbs knead gently upwards along the tibialis anterior muscles on the outer shin.

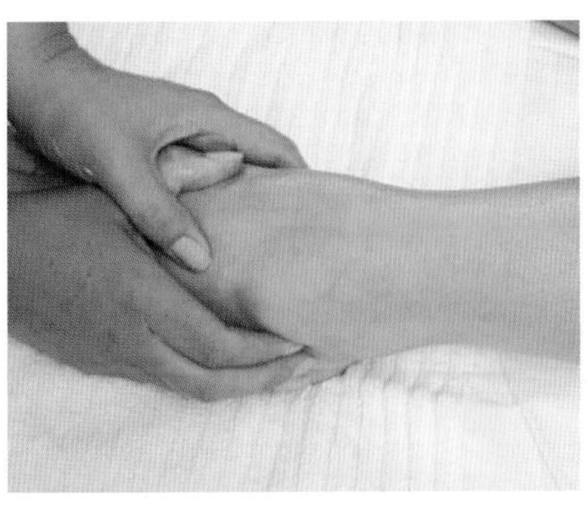

5 Using the pads of the fingers perform small circular kneading movements around the malleolus (ankle) bone. Massage both sides of the ankle bone at the same time.

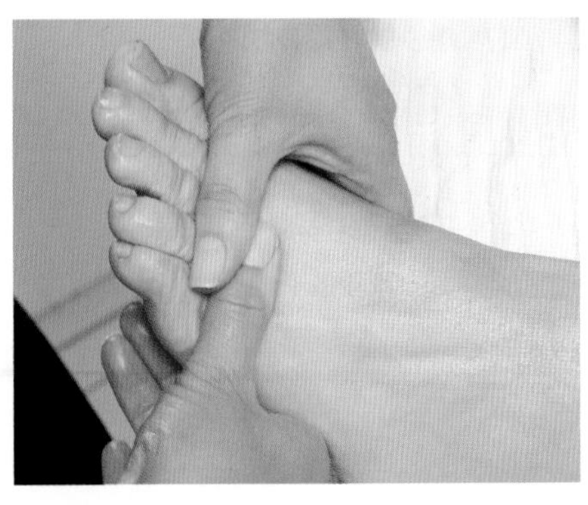

6 **Thumb frictions to the dorsal aspect of the foot** Use the thumbs, one in front of the other, and move backwards and forwards in a gentle sawing action between each metatarsal bone. Move from the toes to the ankle, then slide back down to the toes.

Repeat step 6 a further 2 times.

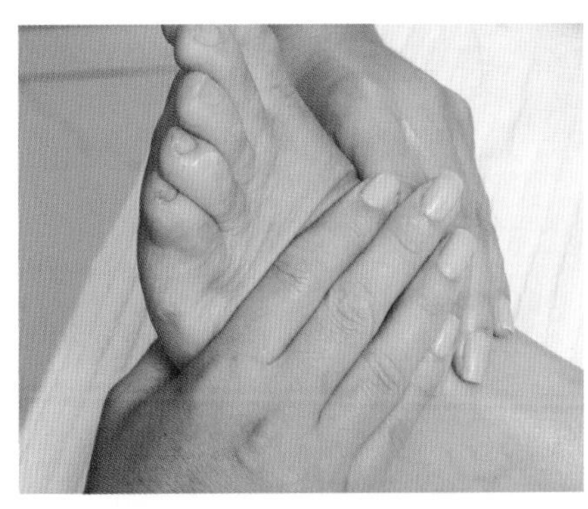

7 **Thumb frictions to the plantar aspect of the foot** Use the same movement as in step 6, but on the sole of the foot, moving from the toes to the heel.

Repeat step 7 a further 2 times.

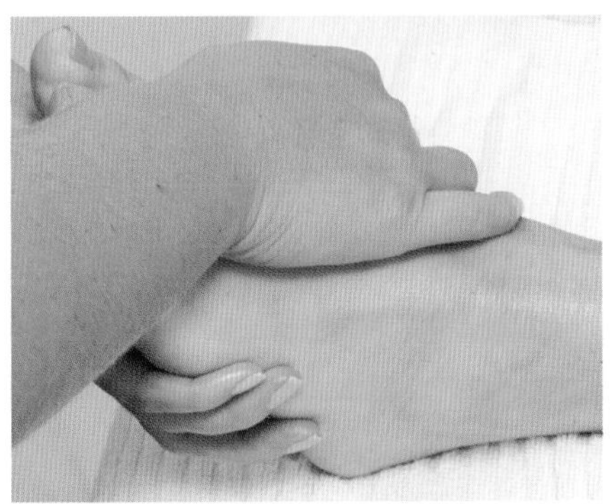

8 **Palm kneading to the plantar surface of the foot** Place the heel of the hand into the arch of the foot and massage with deep circular movements.

Repeat step 8 a further 5 times.

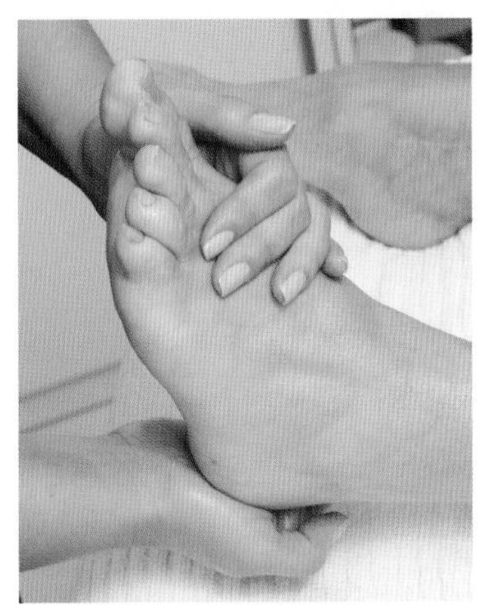

9 Support the foot with one hand perform joint manipulations, using the palm cup the heel and perform a circular kneading movement.

KNOWLEDGE CHECK

Which specialized foot treatment/s would be best for an elderly male client who has little movement in his ankle joints and slightly distorted joints in his toes?

Need more time... refer to pages 417–418 to help you.

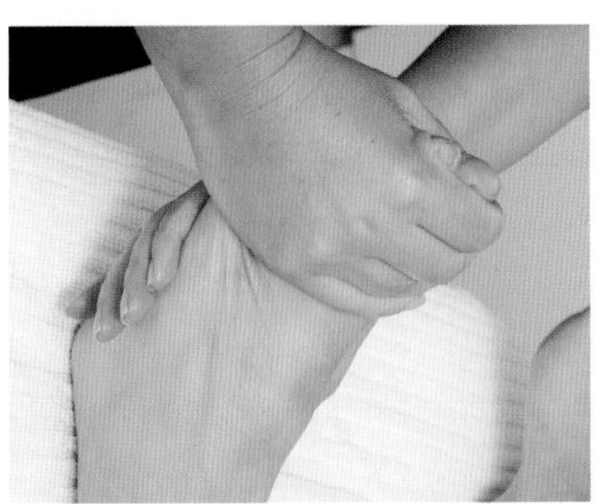

10 Perform joint manipulations to the toes. Place the hand either side of the toes; gently press together and rotate all the toes three times clockwise and three times anticlockwise.

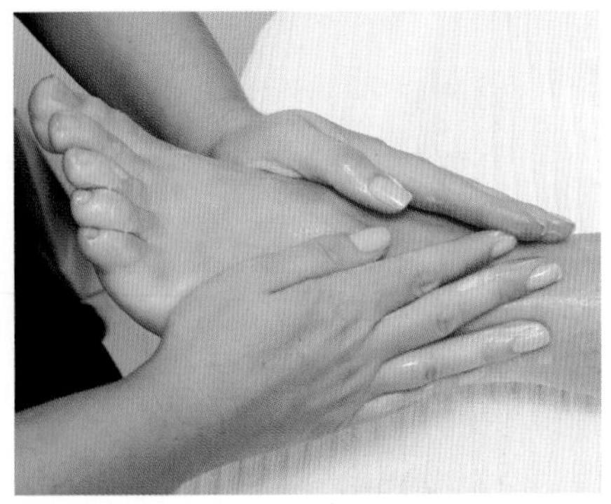

11 Effleurage from the foot to the knee. Use the same movements as in step 2.

Repeat step 11 a further 5 times.

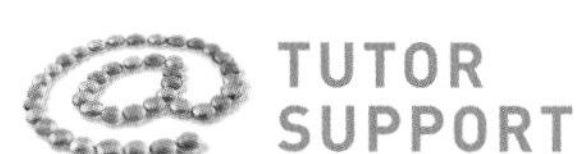

TUTOR SUPPORT

Activity 3: Home care advice handout

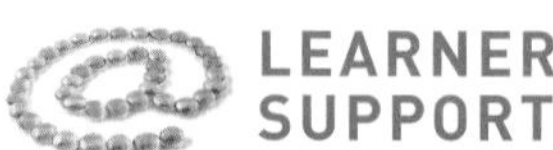

LEARNER SUPPORT

Pedicure true or false

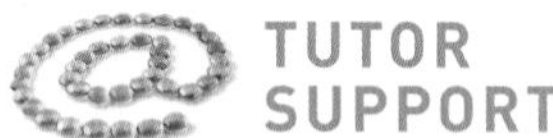

TUTOR SUPPORT

Activity 4: Pedicure word search

BEST PRACTICE

Advise on further professional treatments

If a client has dry skin on their heels, take the opportunity to recommend an **exfoliant** treatment for their next appointment.

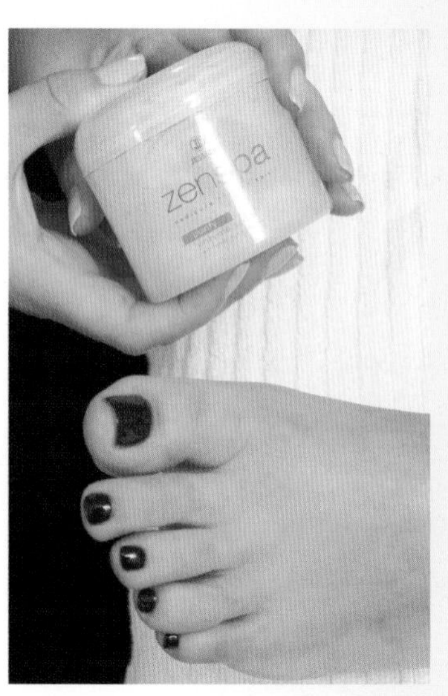

Nail polish application

Different types of nail polish are discussed on page 388. Nail polish is applied to coat the nail plate for a numbers of reasons:

- to adorn the nail
- to disguise stained toenails
- to improve the condition and appearance of the nail
- to co-ordinate with clothes
- to create designs and effects called 'nail art'

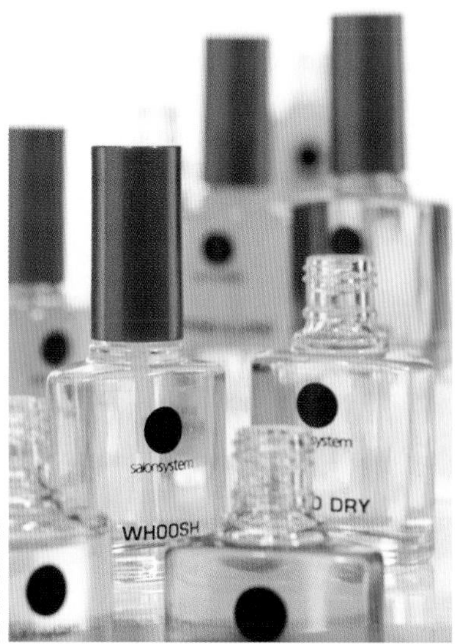

SALON SYSTEM

Nail polishes

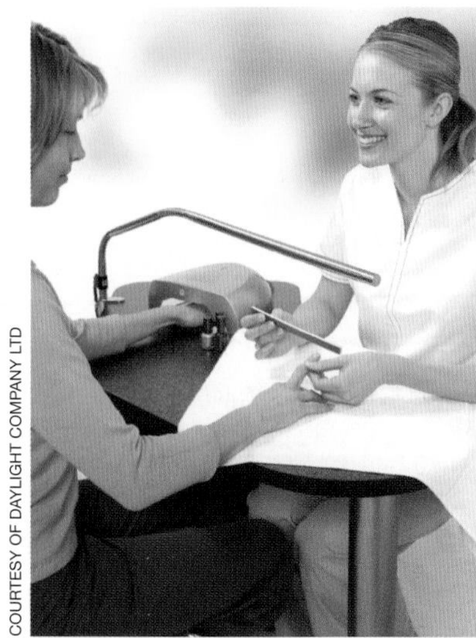

COURTESY OF DAYLIGHT COMPANY LTD

A nail work station with lamp

HEALTH & SAFETY

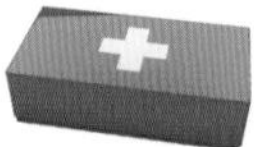

Lighting and ventilation

Ensure the area is well ventilated to avoid inhalation of excessive fumes. Lighting should be good to enable you to avoid eyestrain. It is a good idea to use a table lamp when painting the nails.

Styles of polish application

- ***Traditional application*** – This style is one of the most commonly requested by clients: the entire plate is covered with polish.
- ***French application*** – This style involves painting the nail plate of the nail pink or pale beige, and the free edge white.

See pages 386–388 for further information about nail polish application, including tips why it may chip or peel, and how to store.

Contra-indication to nail polish Do not apply polish in these circumstances:

- if there are diseases and disorders of the nail plate and surrounding skin
- if the client is allergic to nail polish

Step-by-step: Nail polish application

Confirm the client's choice of nail polish colour. A dark cream formulation has been demonstrated. Ensure the free edge is smooth and the cuticles are neat and smooth. Before nail polish is applied, any jewellery worn in the area should be replaced to avoid smudging the polish afterwards.

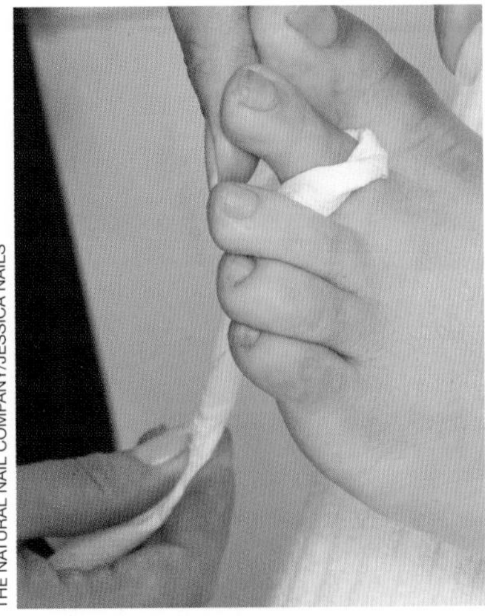

1 Place disposable toe separators or other hygienic equivalent to separate them and facilitate polish application.

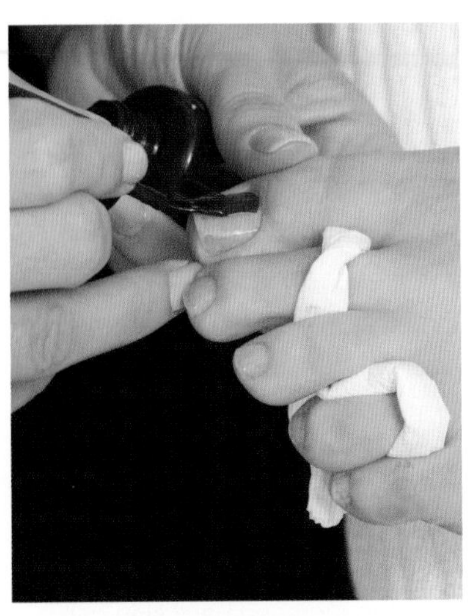

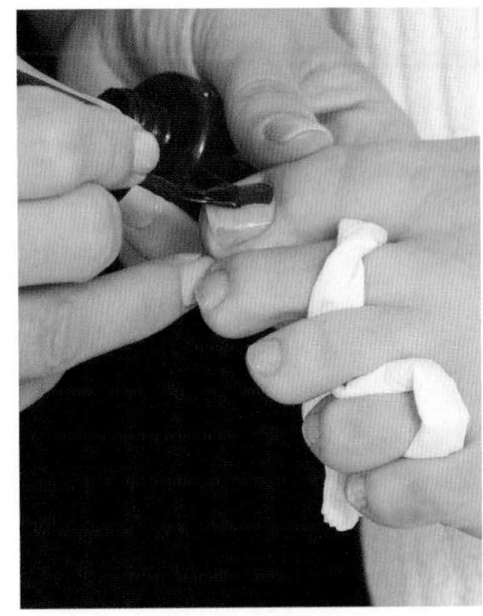

2 After ensuring that the nail plate is free from oil, start with the big toe. Apply three to four brush strokes down the length of the nail from the cuticle to the free edge, beginning in the centre, then down either side close to the nail wall.

Take care to avoid touching the cuticle or nail wall. If flooding occurs, remove the polish immediately with an orange stick and nail polish remover.

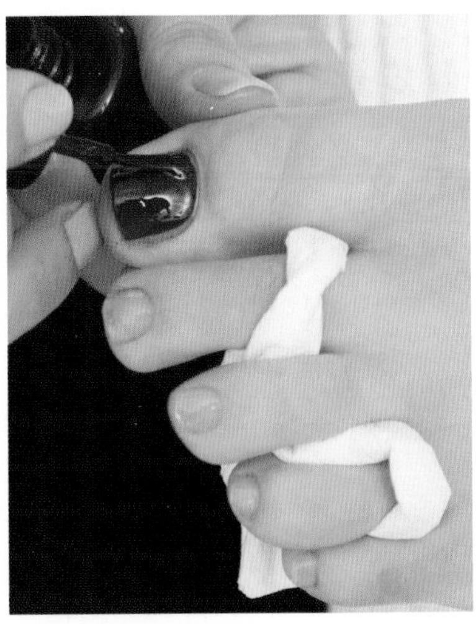

2 Continued.

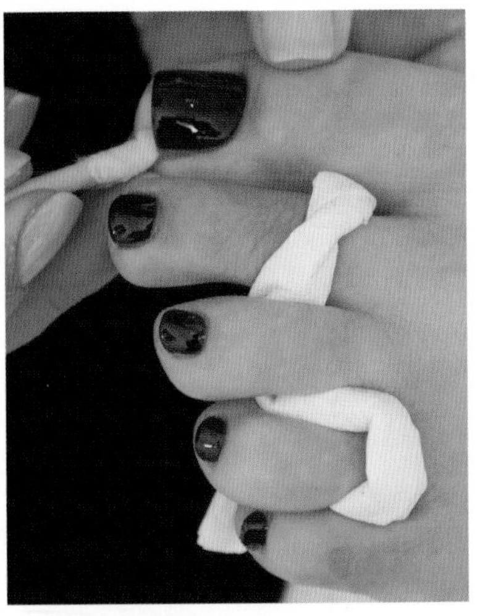

3 Apply one base coat, two coats of coloured polish and one top coat. Top coat is required only after using cream polish; pearl polish does not need a top coat but a third coat of polish may be applied.

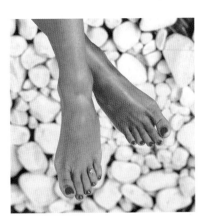

Ready for the holidays

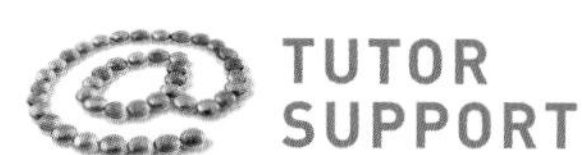

Activity 5: Promote luxury pedicure task

KNOWLEDGE CHECK

Can you list three retail products that you could recommend that a client uses at home?

Need more time... refer to page 422 to help you.

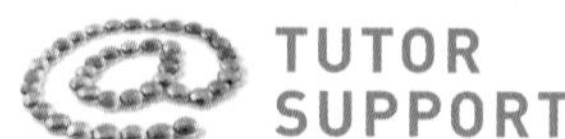

Activity 7: Re-cap, revision and evaluation

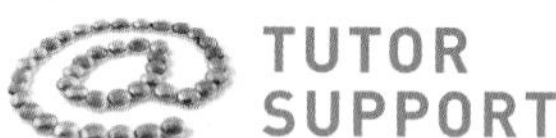

Activity 8: Multiple choice quiz

Aftercare advice

Offering **aftercare advice** at the end of a pedicure treatment will help the client to look after their feet between salon visits, and is also an ideal opportunity to recommend retail products.

Aftercare advice will differ slightly for each client according to individual needs, but generally it will be as follows:

- Change socks or tights daily.
- Apply moisturising lotion daily to the feet, preferably after bathing when the skin is softened.
- Ensure that the feet are thoroughly dry after washing, especially between the toes.
- Apply talcum powder or a special foot powder between the toes to help absorb moisture.
- Foot sprays containing peppermint or citrus oil to cleanse and refresh are useful to refresh the feet during the day.
- Go barefoot wherever it is safe and practical to do so.
- Ensure that footwear fits properly. Foot problems such as bunions can be aggravated by incorrect footwear.
- Avoid wearing high heels for long periods of time. They can cause postural problems and increase hard skin callus formation.
- Advise on appropriate nail/skincare products to remedy the problems present, e.g. dry skin, nails, stained nails.
- Advise the client of any other professional treatments you could recommend.
- Advise the client on a treatment plan to improve the nail/skin condition and the time intervals recommended between each treatment.
- When filing the nails, always file straight across in one direction.
- If any pain is felt in the feet visit a chiropodist.
- It is also necessary to advise the client what to do in the event of a contra-action (see page 408–409).

Have retail products available for the client to purchase. These include emery boards, coloured nail polishes, nail polish remover and nail/skin treatment products.

It is a good idea to have the nail polish colours that you have used available for purchase. The client can then buy the matching colour to touch up any accidental chips themselves.

Recommend the use of top coat applied every three to four days to protect the nail polish, increase its durability and impart shine.

Finally, at the end of the pedicure treatment ensure the clients records are updated, accurate and signed by the client and pedicurist. Ensure the finished result is to the client's satisfaction and meets the agreed treatment plan.

Exercises for the feet and ankles As part of the homecare advice given to a pedicure client **foot exercises** should be mentioned – these can play a very important role in keeping the client's feet healthy. They help:

- to stimulate blood and lymph circulation
- to keep joints mobilized, allowing a greater range of movement in the toes and ankles
- to keep muscles strong, reducing the chance of fallen arches (flat feet)

Here are some examples of exercises:

1 Sitting on a chair with the feet flat on the floor raise the toes upwards and then relax
2 Stand on tiptoes, and relax down again
3 Sitting on a chair with the feet flat on the floor, lift one leg slightly and draw a circle with the toes so that the ankle moves through its full range of movement
4 **Dorsiflexion:** bending the foot backwards towards the body
5 **Plantar flexion:** pointing the foot down towards the ground
6 **Inversion:** moving the foot inwards towards the middle of the body
7 **Eversion:** moving the foot out towards the side of the body

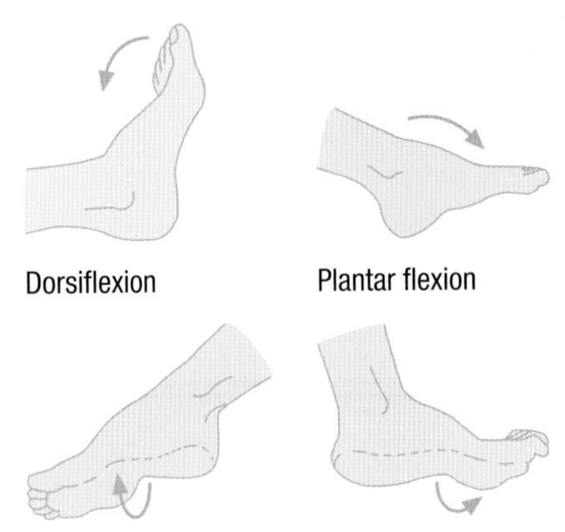

GLOSSARY OF KEY WORDS

Aftercare advice recommendations given to the client following treatment to continue the benefits of the treatment.

Base coat a nail polish product applied to protect the natural nail and prevent staining from coloured nail polish.

Blue nail nail condition where the nail bed has a blue tinge rather than a healthy pink colour due to poor blood circulation in the area.

Bruised nail nail condition where the nail appears blue/black in colour where bleeding has occurred on the nail bed following injury.

Bunion a foot condition. The large joint at the base of the big toe protrudes, forcing the big toe inwards towards the other toes.

Callus foot condition, displaying thick, yellowish hardened skin, usually found on prominent areas of the foot such as the heel.

Chilblains poor blood supply where the toes become red, blue or purple in colour and the area may become painful and itchy; aggravated in cold weather.

Chiropodist a person who is trained and qualified to treat minor foot complaints.

Consultation assessment of client's needs using different assessment techniques, including questioning and natural observation.

Contact dermatitis a skin disorder caused by intolerance of the skin to a particular substance, or a group of substances. On exposure to the substance, the skin quickly becomes irritated and an allergic reaction occurs.

Contra-action an unwanted reaction occurring during or after treatment application.

Contra-indication a problematic symptom that indicates that the treatment may not proceed.

Corn small areas of thickened skin on the foot. Often white in appearance.

Cuticle cream or oil a cosmetic preparation used to condition the skin of the cuticle.

Cuticle knife a metal tool used on the nail to remove excess eponychium and perionychium (the extension of the skin of the cuticle at the base of the nail).

Cuticle nippers a metal tool used to remove excess cuticle and neaten the skin around the cuticle area.

Cuticle remover a cosmetic preparation used to soften and loosen the skin cells and cuticle from the nail.

Diabetes a disease that prevents sufferers breaking down glucose in their cells.

Eczema of the nail inflammation of the skin; different changes to the nail may occur including ridges, pitting, nail separation and nail thickening.

Effleurage a stroking massage movement, used to begin the massage, as a link manipulation and to complete the massage sequence.

Emery board a nail file used to shape the free edge of the nail.

Exfoliant a mild abrasive cream applied and massaged over the skin's surface to remove dead skin cells and improve the appearance and texture of the skin.

Foot and nail treatments specialized products and equipment designed to improve the condition and appearance of different nail and skin conditions.

Foot cream lotion/oil a cosmetic mixture of waxes and oils applied to soften the skin of the feet and cuticles.

Foot rasp a pedicure tool used to remove excess dead skin from the foot.

Foot spa a foot bath incorporating massage and water aeration, creating a bubbling effect to cleanse and relax the feet.

Frictions massage technique using small circular massage movements using the pads of the fingers or thumbs. The skin and muscle below is massage against the underlying bone. This can be used to loosen any adhesions in the tissues.

Hoof stick a nail tool used to gently push back the cuticles when softened.

Ingrowing toenails nail condition where the side of the nail penetrates the nail wall; redness, inflammation and pus may be present.

Joint manipulations massage technique where the joints of the foot are manipulated through their range of movement dependant upon the type of joint.

Mask a treatment mask applied to the skin of the feet to treat and improve the condition of the skin; this may include stimulating, rejuvenating or moisturising properties.

Nail finish the product finally applied to the natural nail to enhance its appearance, e.g. choice of polish application.

Nail polish a clear or coloured nail product that adds colour/protection to the nail. Cream polish has a matt finish and requires a top coat application. Pearlized polish produces a frosted, shimmery appearance and top coat is not required.

Nail polish drier an aerosol or oil preparation applied following nail polish application to increase the speed at which the polish hardens.

Nail polish remover a solvent used to remove nail polish and grease from the nails prior to applying polish. Nail polish solvent used to thin nail polish and restore its consistency.

Necessary action the appropriate action to take in the case of a contra-action or contra-indication to ensure the welfare of the client.

Onycholysis nail condition where the nail plate separates from the nail bed.

Orange stick a disposable wooden tool used around the cuticle and free edge of the nail and to apply products to the nail.

Paraffin wax this is heated and applied to the skin of the feet to provide a heating effect. This improves skin functioning, aids the absorption of treatment products and is beneficial to ease the discomfort of arthritic and rheumatic conditions.

Paronychia bacterial infection where swelling, redness and pus appears in the cuticle area of the nail wall.

Pedicure a treatment to care for and improve the condition and appearance of the skin and nails of the feet.

Petrissage massage movements, including kneading, where the tissues are lifted away from the underlying structures and compressed. Pressure is intermittent, and should be light yet firm.

Phlebitis recognised by swelling and pain in the leg caused by inflammation of the vein wall (veins transport blood from the tissues back towards the heart).

Psoriasis of the nail an inflammatory condition where there is an increased production of cells in the upper part of the skin. Pitting occurs on the surface of the nail plate.

Scissors nail tools used to shorten the length of the nail before filing.

Tapotement, also known as percussion, massage movements performed in a brisk, stimulating manner to increase blood supply and improve tone of the skin and muscles. Movements include clapping and tapping.

Thermal booties electrically heated boots in which the feet are placed following the application of a skin treatment product such as a mask. The heat aids the absorption of the product and improves skin functioning.

Thrombophlebitis inflammation of a vein related to a blood clot (see **phlebitis**).

Tinea corporis or body ringworm fungal infection of the skin where small scaly red patches, which spread outwards and then heal from the centre, leave a ring.

Tinea pedis or athlete's foot fungal infection of the foot occurring in the webs of the skin between the toes. Small blisters form, which later burst. The skin in the area can become dry with a scaly appearance.

Tinea unguium fungal infection of the nails. The nail is yellowish-grey in colour.

Top coat nail polish product applied over another nail polish to provide additional strength and durability to the finish.

Treatment plan after the consultation, suitable treatment objectives are established to treat the client's conditions and needs.

Verruca or plantar wart a viral infection where small epidermal skin growths appear, either raised or flat depending upon their location, and have a rough surface.

ASSESSMENT OF KNOWLEDGE AND UNDERSTANDING

You have now learnt the knowledge and skills for providing pedicure treatments in the beauty therapy workplace. To test your level of knowledge, answer the following short questions. These will prepare you for your summative (final) assessment.

1. The image below shows the nail being shortened with nail clippers. Nails are cut straight across to avoid causing _________ nails.

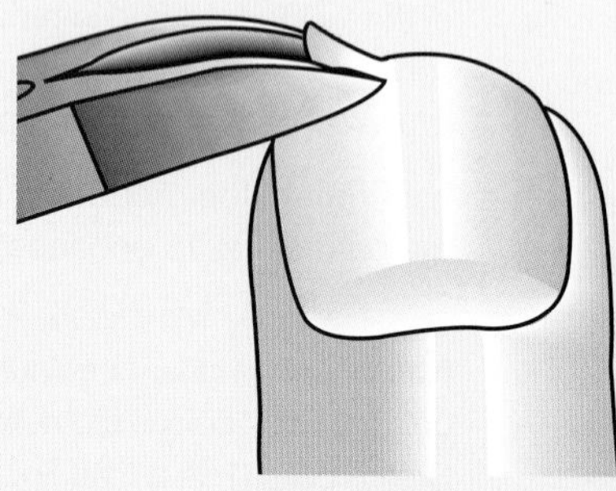

2. A cuticle pusher is shown performing cuticle work. The image shows the removal of cuticle at the sides of the nails, this is known as:

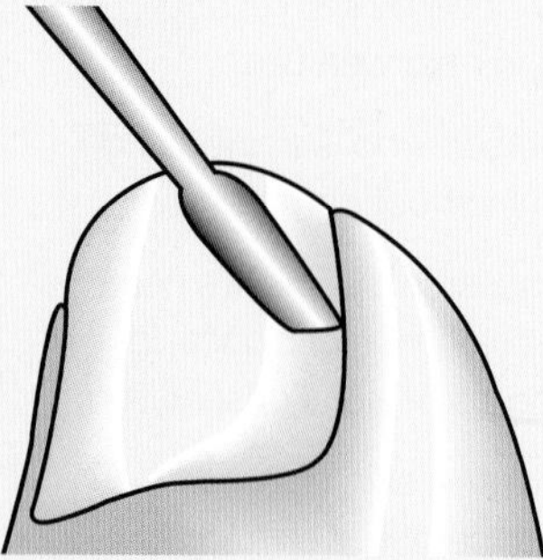

   a. cuticle
   b. hyponychium
   c. perionychium
   d. eponychium

3. One of the functions of a top coat is to make the nail polish:
   a. dry more quickly
   b. adhere to nail plate
   c. resistant to chipping
   d. appear smooth if uneven

4. A condition in which a blood clot forms under the nail plate, forming a dark purplish mark, usually due to injury, is called:
   a. eggshell nail
   b. bruised nail
   c. onycholysis
   d. pterygium

5. Thickened skin between the fingertip and free edge of the nail plate is the
   a. hyponychium
   b. eponyichium
   c. nail mantle
   d. nail grooves

6. Thick-walled, large elastic tubes that carry oxygenated blood away from the heart are called the:
   a. capillaries
   b. arteries
   c. veins
   d. vessels

7. The image shown is called tinea unguium, this is a:

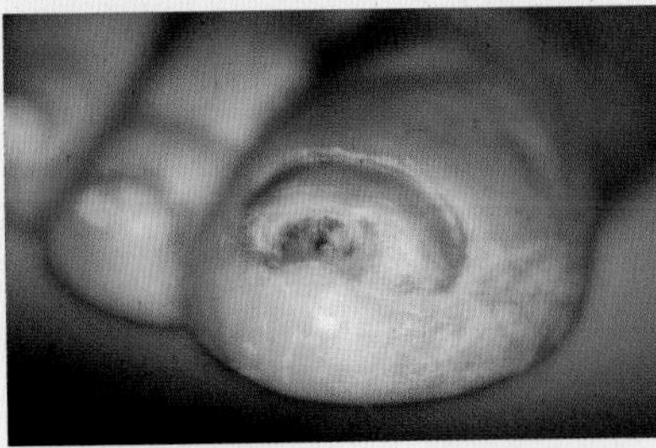

   a. bacterial nail condition
   b. viral nail condition
   c. fungal nail condition
   d. sebaceous gland disorder

8. The massage manipulation also known as percussion, performed in a brisk, stimulating manner to increase blood supply and improve tone of the skin and muscles is called:
   a. effleurage
   b. vibrations
   c. frictions
   d. tapotement

9. What are the names of the two bones of the lower leg labelled below?

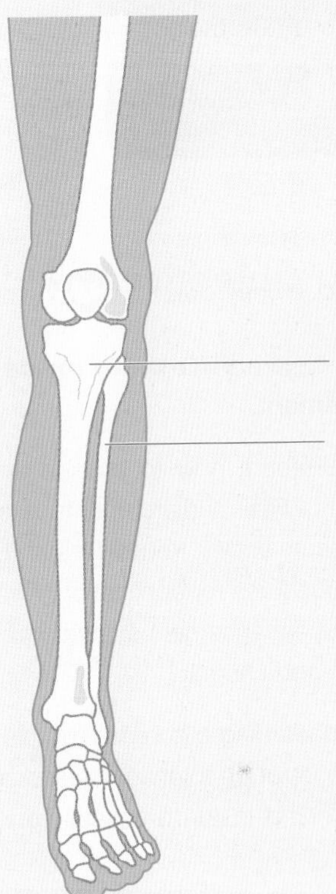

10. Rearrange the following steps to place them in the correct order of sequence that they would be performed in the pedicure treatment:
    - cut the toenails
    - massage the foot
    - remove excess cuticle with cuticle nippers
    - exfoliate the skin of the foot

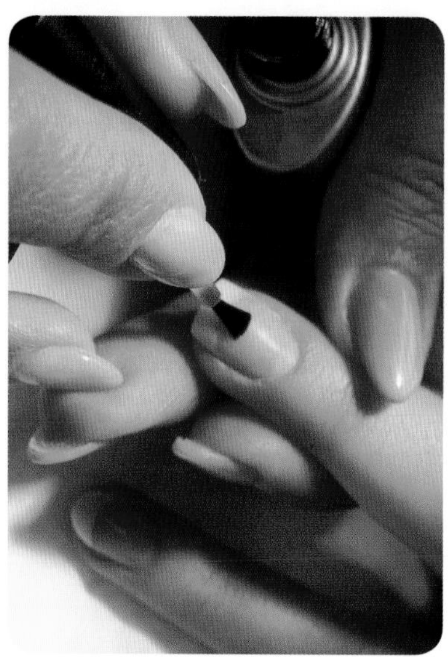

13 Provide and Maintain Nail Enhancement

Learning Objectives

This chapter covers **VRQ Unit Provide and maintain nail enhancement.**

This unit is all about now to provide and maintain nail enhancements. Nail enhancements are an important part of the beauty sector. You will learn about a variety of technique procedures for application, removal and maintenance of nail enhancement systems including nail tips, wraps, acrylic and UV gel.

There are **two** learning outcomes for this unit which you must achieve through practical tasks and knowledge and understanding tasks to assess your capability and knowledge:

- **Be able to prepare for nail enhancement services**
- **Be able to provide nail enhancement services**

From the range statement, you must show that you have:

- ensured that the **environmental conditions** are suitable
- used all **consultation techniques** to identify the treatment **objectives**
- met all requirements in client preparation for treatment
- completed a consultation and skin inspection to identify any contra-indications
- shown how to communicate and behave in a professional manner
- followed all **health and safety working practices**

(continued on the next page)

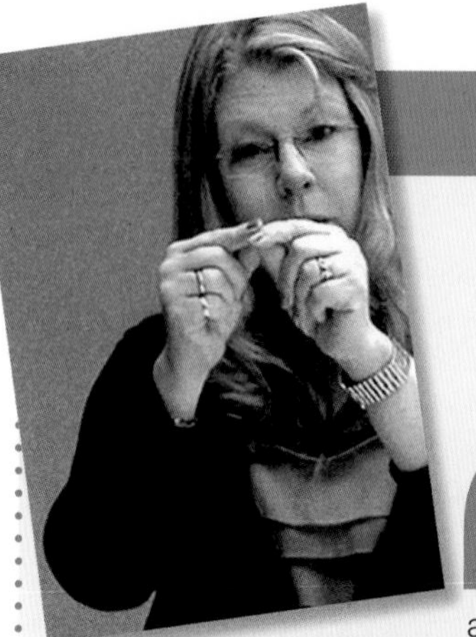

ROLE MODEL

Marian Newman

Professional nail technician

"I started my career in the nail industry in 1987 by opening a salon and since then have worked alongside some of the biggest names in fashion and beauty.

After three successful editions of my book *The Complete Nail Technician*, I still feel very strongly about the standards of education and skills of nail technicians working in the professional industry. I have over 20 years experience in training and education and now have my own consultancy company offering bespoke training services and courses. Nail enhancement is a highly technical subject which also requires a large dose of creativity, so these chapters are only the start!

- used all listed **products, tools and equipment**
- adapted treatments to suit different objectives and **nail conditions** and nail shapes
- provided all types of relevant **aftercare and contra-action advice**

You must be able to show that you have the necessary practical skills and underpinning knowledge to provide and maintain nail enhancement.

This unit is linked to the Nail Services NOS **Units N5**, **N6**, **N7** and **N8.**

Essential anatomy and physiology knowledge requirements for this unit are identified on the checklist chart in on page 27.

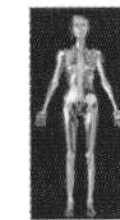

The purpose of nail enhancement

Nail enhancement treatments can provide the following benefits to the client:

- improve the appearance of the natural nail shape
- strengthen the natural nail
- improve the appearance of the fingers (e.g. short stubby fingers, by lengthening the free edge)
- motivate a nail-biter to break the habit – an acrylic/gel overlay or nail wrap will strengthen the nail and improve its appearance
- provide temporary length to the nails for a special occasion
- repair, in the case of flaking nails, free edge or flesh line break or severed free edge – the client can have the nail appearance balanced using the most appropriate nail **system**
- disguises a disfigured nail (that is not contra-indicated to treat) – a nail system can be applied for camouflage purposes
- an overlay placed over nail polish extends its durability.

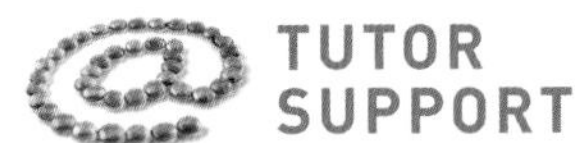

Activity 2: Design a promotional poster

Outcome 1: Prepare for nail enhancement services

Practical skills

1. Prepare yourself, client and work area for nail enhancement services.
2. Use suitable **consultation techniques** to identify service **objectives**.

Learn how to prepare for nail enhancement services

Underpinning knowledge

1. Describe salon requirements for preparing yourself, the client and the work area.
2. Describe the **environmental conditions** suitable for nail enhancement services.

Practical skills

3 Carry out a nail and skin analysis.

4 Provide clear recommendations to the client.

5 Select **products, tools and equipment** to suit client treatment needs and **nail conditions**.

(Continued) Learn how to prepare for nail enhancement services

Underpinning knowledge

3 Describe different **consultation techniques** used to identify service **objectives**.

4 Explain the importance of carrying out a detailed nail and skin analysis.

5 Describe how to **select products, tools and equipment** to suit client treatment needs and **nail conditions**.

6 Identify **nail conditions**.

7 Describe the **contra-indications** which prevent or restrict nail enhancement services.

BEST PRACTICE

Minimum dimensions for the work area

The minimum worktop space needed is approximately 75cm wide and 35cm deep. The width should be not so wide that you need to stretch to reach the client's hands if the client is sitting back in their chair, nor should it be so narrow that it causes you to bend your neck down too far.

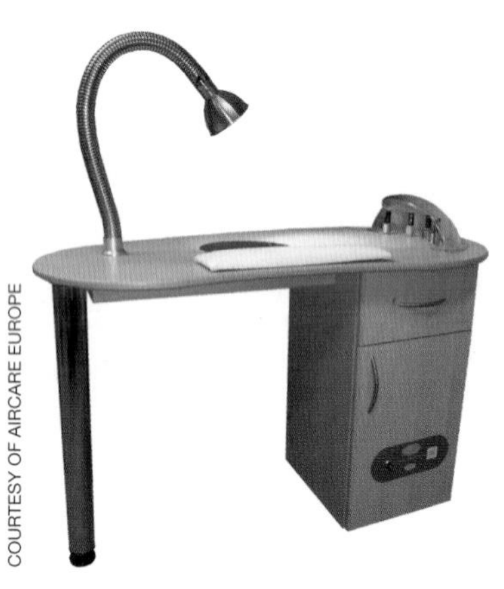

COURTESY OF AIRCARE EUROPE

A nail work station

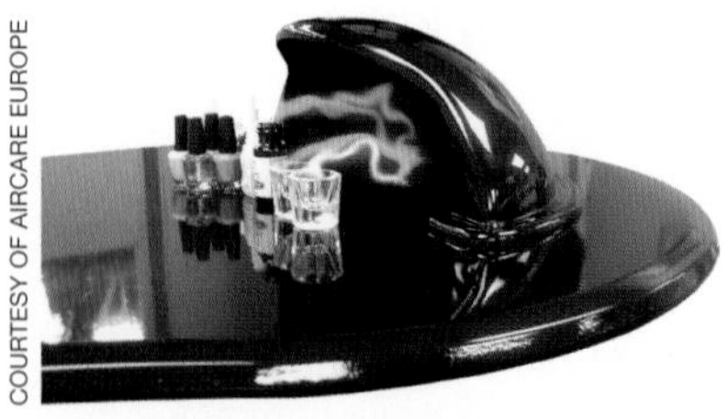

COURTESY OF AIRCARE EUROPE

Work station with built-in dust and vapour extractor

Preparing for nail enhancement treatments

Whether the technician is working in a nail salon, a client's home, a beauty salon or a hair salon, a minimum amount of space is needed. Assess the space available before purchasing equipment. All equipment must be durable and easy to clean.

Ensure that all tools and equipment are clean, disinfected and hygienic using the methods described on page 360, and that that all necessary products, tools and equipment are neatly organized and easily accessible.

The nail work station

When thinking about the space required for a nail technician in a salon, the work station is the first consideration. Ideally, the work station should have a couple of drawers for storage, and be very stable in construction.

Dust is one of the most important issues in health and safety for nail technicians. It is potentially more hazardous than any of the volatile products that are used. Dealing with the control of dust at the source, i.e. extraction of the dust at the work station, is the best method. Many nail work stations are available with built-in dust extraction systems. Whether built-in or independent to the work station, the dust extraction system should be on during treatment while any dust is being created so a good flow of air is generated.

HEALTH & SAFETY

Cleaning the dust extractor

Ensure that the filter is cleaned (according to manufacturer's instructions) very frequently. If it is an efficient extractor the filter will be full at the end of each day. The best system is made up of a fan that removes the dust that drops down into it combined a fan that takes the finer airborne dust (that is the most hazardous) from above the working area.

Good working practices will minimize vapours generated from working with nail products. However, it is always worth the investment in a system that helps remove these vapours from the atmosphere, again, at the source.

Seating

A comfortable seat is very important for both technician and client as you will be sitting for long periods of time. There are several exercises that a technician can do at various times throughout the day to help prevent strain, but, more than anything, sitting in the correct position and staying relaxed at all times is essential.

The chair for the client is as important as the one for the technician. The client must feel comfortable, as the could spend up to two hours in the same chair, but must also be in the right position for the technician. The height of the seat should be such that the client can rest their arms on the desk easily while keeping them and their shoulders in a relaxed position. They should also be able to get close enough to the desk so that their arm is still supported if they lean back into the chair. Make sure the client is sitting straight in front of the desk. This is important for the treatment because if the client is sitting at an angle, their hand will not be held straight in front of the technician. This could result in nail enhancements being applied unevenly.

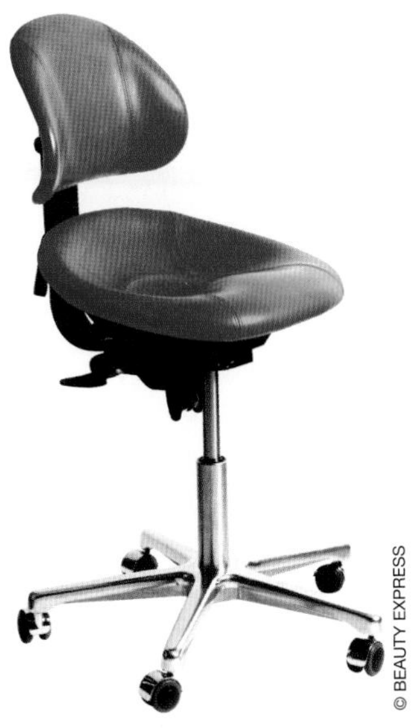

Nail technician's chair

BEST PRACTICE

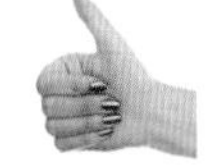

Choice of chair
A chair must have the correct support for the user. The seat should be padded and of a depth that supports the legs. The tilt of the seat also affects how we sit. The backrest should give support to the back and the combination of the back and seat should encourage the user to sit upright with a slight hollow in the lower back. There are also 'posture' chairs available, on wheels and incorporating a rocking motion, that are designed to help those working at a desk.

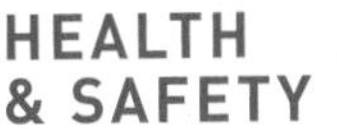

HEALTH & SAFETY

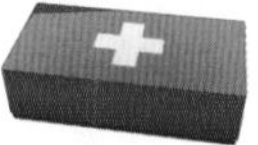

Always sit square to the desk without crossing your legs or leaning on one arm.

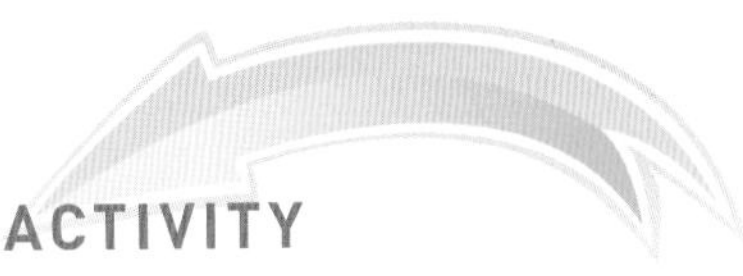

ACTIVITY

There are several exercises that a technician can do at various times throughout the day, examples shown below.

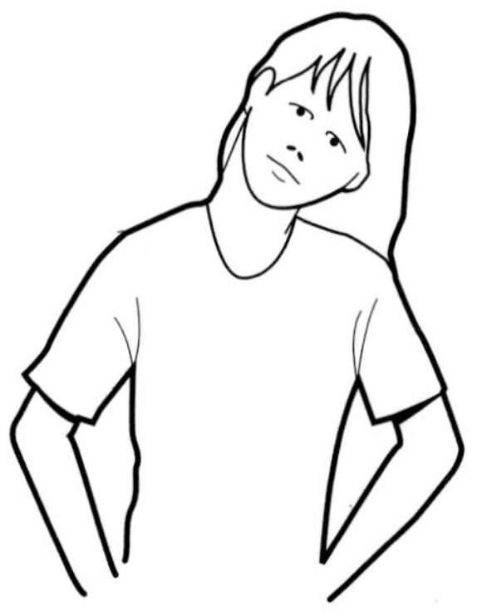

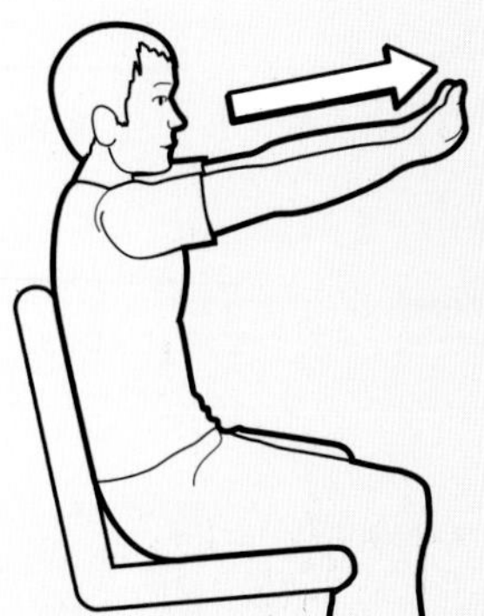

Research some further simple postural exercises that you could learn.

HEALTH & SAFETY

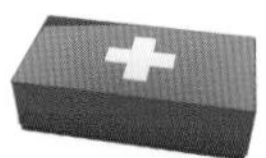

Electrical equipment
Make sure all electrical equipment is subject to regular certified checks.

TOP TIP

Retail opportunity
Make sure there is plenty for the client to look at while they are sitting at your desk, especially retail lines. It will be something interesting for them and should encourage questions that could lead to sales.

Lighting

It is essential to have excellent light, without glare, when providing any nail treatment to avoid eye strain and to be able to examine artificial nails for imperfections. This should be provided by a desk lamp, preferably one specifically designed for nail work. It is best to use halogen or low energy bulbs which do not get too hot when working with volatile products.

HEALTH & SAFETY

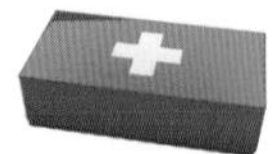

Trip hazards
Trailing wires in a workplace are a safety hazard, leading to trips and falls and should be avoided. Many work stations have a plug socket attached to them for electrical equipment. Always cover floor wires with a rubber conduit.

Before beginning the nail enhancement treatment make sure you have the necessary products, tools and equipment to hand and that they meet the legal, hygiene and industry requirements. Refer to the list on page 360 for details on the appropriate methods of sterilization and disinfection for this equipment.

PRODUCTS, TOOLS AND EQUIPMENT

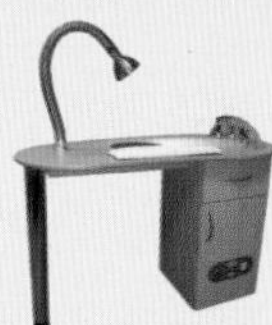

Nail work station
On which to place everything

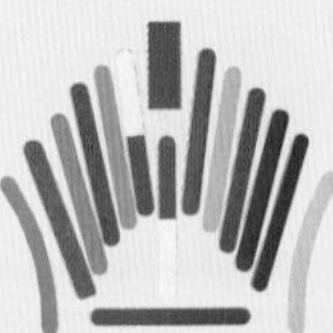

Files and buffers
Medium file (180 grit) used for shaping or removing overlays and shortening artificial nails. Fine file (240–360 grit) used for shaping natural nails. Buffers (400+ grit) used to refine the shape and smooth the surface of the artificial nail

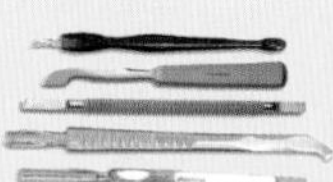

Cuticle knife
To remove excess eponychium and perionychium from the nail plate

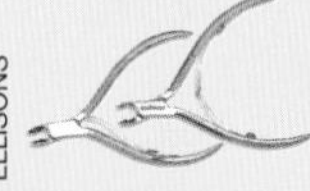

ELLISONS

Cuticle nippers
To remove excess cuticle and dead, torn skin surrounding the nail

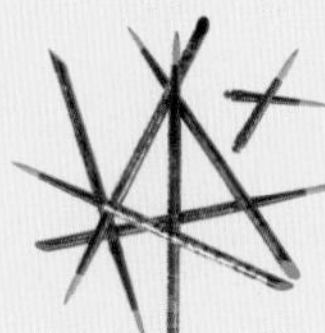

Hoof stick
Used to gently push back the softened cuticle

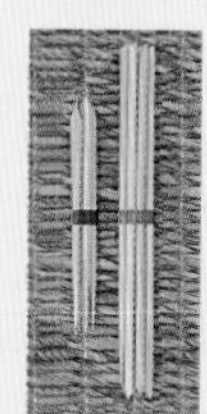

Orange sticks
Used to remove products from containers and, when tipped at either end with cotton wool, to ease the cuticle back and clean under the free edge

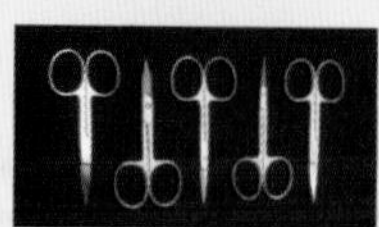

Scissors
A variety of scissors are used for cutting nails, artificial tips and fibre mesh for fibre overlays

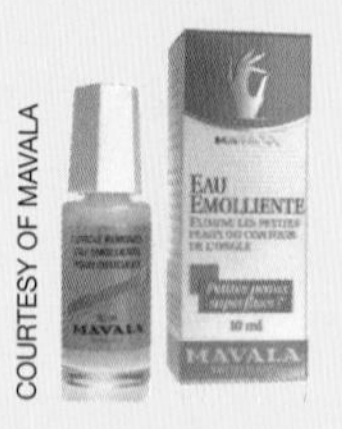

COURTESY OF MAVALA

Cuticle remover
Used to soften the skin of the cuticle so excess skin can be easily removed

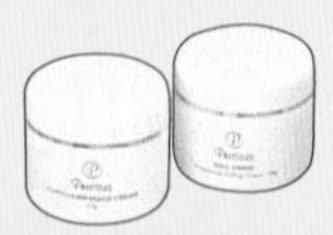

Cuticle oil or cream
Used to condition the skin of the cuticle

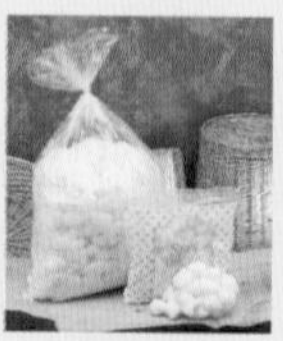

Cotton wool
To remove nail polish and excess nail preparations

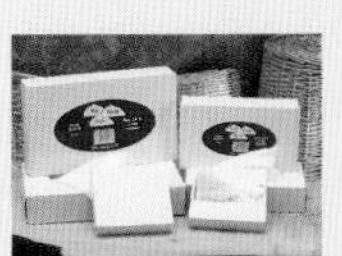

Tissues or disposal towels
To protect client's clothing in the area etc.

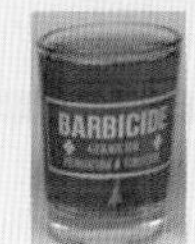

Disinfectant solution
To store small stainless steel sterilized tools

YOU WILL ALSO NEED:

Medium sized towels (3) To dry the skin, nails etc.

Skin disinfectant To cleanse and sanitize the client's skin and nails

Waste container This should be a lined metal bin with a lid to contain vapours from solvents

Small bowls (3) Lined with tissues for storage etc.

Client record card To record the client's personal details, products used and details of the treatment

Product safety

Irritants and corrosive materials

The majority of nail products come under the category of **hazardous** chemicals and many of them are classed as **irritants**. Care must be taken when using these types of products. There are some irritants that are also classified as **corrosive** and these will cause a bad reaction with everyone.

- A common example of this type of chemical in the nail industry is an acid-based primer. This is a product, as the name suggests, is an acid that will sting and itch on contact with skin. Washing in running water will remove the chemical, but it is likely that the skin will be temporarily damaged. However, most modern products do not require the use of a primer.
- Many other commonly used products are irritants – for example, nail adhesive is an irritant, and every bottle and tube should carry a warning. The adhesive will bond to skin very easily and can cause injury to the skin if it is not removed carefully – acetone will debond the skin safely. If adhesive is spilt onto clothing and penetrates through to the skin, very severe burns can be caused. The chemicals in the adhesive react with fibres in clothing and burns requiring cosmetic surgery have been known as a result of this accident.
- It is a legal requirement for there to be warnings on many labels, but the absence of a warning does not necessarily mean a product is safe. All products should be treated with respect and all potentially hazardous products should have a Material Safety Data Sheet (MSDS) available from the supplier (see Chapter 3 Health and Safety).
- As many nail products are classed as irritants, it is possible for individuals to develop a sensitivity (also known as a contra-action) to them at some time. As no one can tell how long this will take or how much of a specific product needs to come into contact with a person, it is important to take measures to avoid the possibility of a sensitivity occuring. It is also just as important to be able to recognize the signs – itchy skin, rash, headaches, etc. This happens when an individual has been exposed to too much of the product. Nail technicians can avoid developing a sensitivity by following good working practices. However,

HEALTH & SAFETY

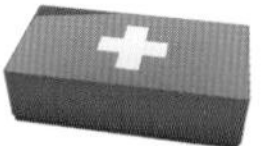

Secure lids
Make sure nail adhesive container lids are on securely and that there are no air pockets in the application nozzle that could cause the adhesive to spurt out. Clean the nozzle with remover before replacing the lid.

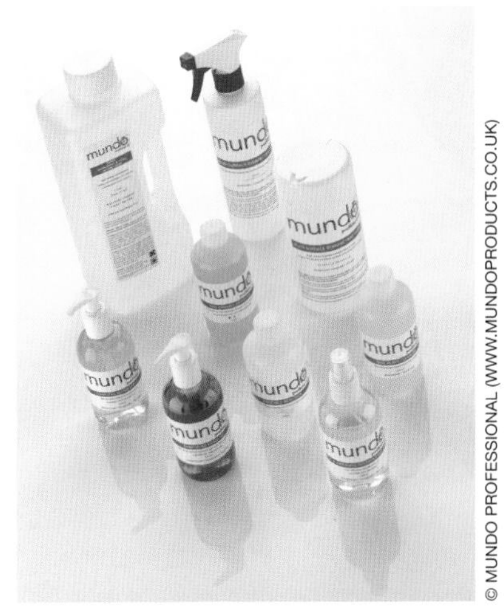

Ensure that you have a MSDS for all chemicals in the salon

HEALTH & SAFETY

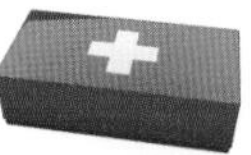

PPE

PPE should always be the last resort. COSHH assessments must be carried out, precautions taken, all information recorded and the situation reviewed on a regular basis.

once a sensitivity has started, gloves must be worn when handling the relevant products. If a client develops a sensitivity, all the products must be removed immediately. Once the product has been removed, the condition may disappear. If the condition does not disappear within a few days or if it seems to get worse after the removal of all products, the technician or client affected should seek medical advice. Always note down the details of the allergic reaction and the action taken on the client's record card. If the client is willing, a different system could be tried which may be successful. If the initial reaction is severe, however, it would be a good idea to do a skin sensitivity patch test to test skin tolerance first. Record the results of the skin sensitivity patch test on the client's record card.

There are three ways that potentially harmful chemicals can enter the body and if each of these **'routes of entry'** is prevented as far as possible, all hazards are avoided. The 'routes' are:

1. **Inhalation**: that is, *breathing in* vapours or dust.
2. **Ingestion**: that is, *through the mouth*.
3. **Absorption**: that is, chemicals can enter *through the skin*.

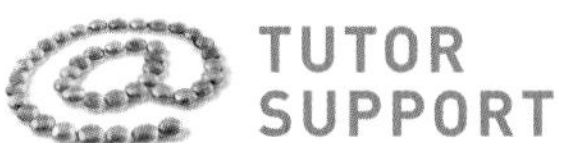

TUTOR SUPPORT

Activity 3: Nail enhancement wordsearch 1

HEALTH & SAFETY

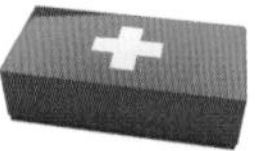

Dust masks

Wearing a disposable dust mask will not protect anyone from vapours. Chemical molecules that are present in the air are much smaller than dust particles and the mask is not a barrier to them. There are vapour masks available, but these are much larger pieces of equipment and are costly to buy. They are also very off-putting to clients!

ALWAYS REMEMBER

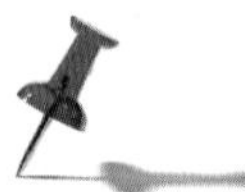

Low odour products

'Low odour' products are products that do not smell as much as others. This does not mean they do not produce vapours!

Inhalation

Vapours

- Many nail products involve *volatile chemicals* and even the tidiest technician cannot totally prevent some of the **vapours** escaping into the air. Vapours are molecules of chemicals in the air and, although most nail products have strong odours, if there is no obvious smell it does not mean the vapour is not there. Adequate ventilation is therefore essential using efficient filtration of the air through several specific filters, usually activated carbon or charcoal.
- *Contact lenses*: Never wear contact lenses when working with nail products. It is possible that vapours can be absorbed by soft lenses and seriously affect the eye.
- *Safety glasses*: Wearing plain safety glasses is highly recommended to protect eyes from harmful vapours and dust.

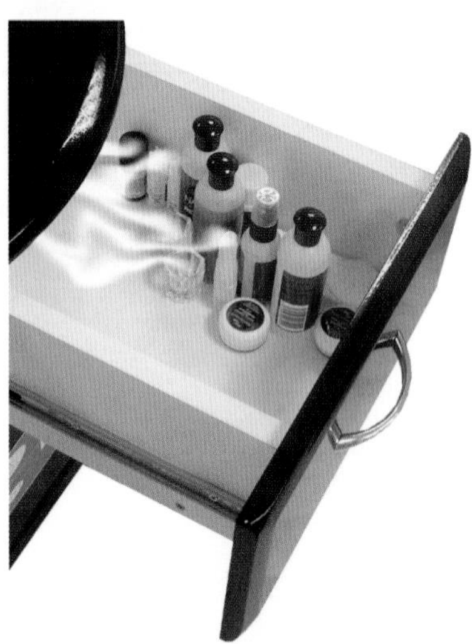

Vapours might be present even if there is no obvious odour; adequate ventilation is essential

Keep vapours to a minimum There are a few simple rules that can be followed to keep vapours to a minimum:

- Keep all bottles and jars closed.
- Keep any dishes covered at all times other than for the few seconds you are using them.

- Do not wipe your liquid and powder brush on a tissue. If you need to wipe your brush have a small wipe dampened with an alcohol-based liquid on the desk for this purpose.
- Clean your brush in monomer after every use, wipe it dry with a pad and discard this pad in a metal bin with a lid.
- Store your brushes flat in a closed container in a drawer, not open on the desk.
- Have a metal waste bin with a lid at every nail desk.
- Put all nail wipes/cotton wool straight into the bin after use.
- Change the paper towel under client's hands after each stage and put into the bin.
- Wipe up spills immediately with absorbent paper and put paper in an outside waste bin.
- When using a solvent to remove artificial nails, keep the bowl covered with a towel and remove directly after use.
- Keep the use of sprays to a minimum.
- Discard all unwanted solvents and nail monomers immediately by soaking in absorbent paper and placing in a covered waste bin; larger quantities should be placed in a safe place in the open and allowed to evaporate – do not pour down sinks or lavatories.
- Maintain adequate ventilation at all times, and make sure the salon is not too hot.
- Follow all these rules if working in a client's home and have several windows open.

ACTIVITY

Make a chart listing all the products you are using. Create a column for:

- safe storage
- safe and correct usage (e.g. methods of decanting, personal protective equipment (PPE) if required, etc.)
- spillage removal from hard surfaces
- any specific health hazard
- comments.

ALWAYS REMEMBER

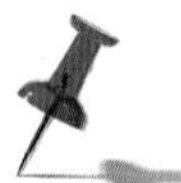

Reduce the risk
Reducing the risk of evaporation while working is the best method to avoid vapours. There is no system that can completely purify the air that will suit a salon's commercial budget.

HEALTH & SAFETY

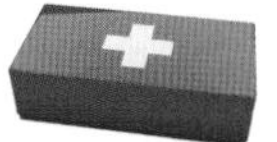

Eye bath
Always have an eye bath with several small bottles of distilled water available in case of accidents involving eyes.

KNOWLEDGE CHECK

What are the three ways that potentially harmful chemicals can enter the body?

Need more time... refer to page 432 to help you.

Dust

Dust is a major problem in the salon. Although the amount of dust can be minimized by correct working procedures, it is impossible to avoid the production of quantities of dust.

- Dust falls into two categories: the dust you can see and the dust you cannot see. All dust is potentially harmful, but the dust you can see is slightly less harmful than the dust you cannot see. Larger dust particles will settle on surfaces and not float around in the air to be breathed in.
- Particles that cannot be seen can be so small that they can be inhaled right into the lungs. Inhaled dust is an irritant and excess dust can cause respiratory problems.

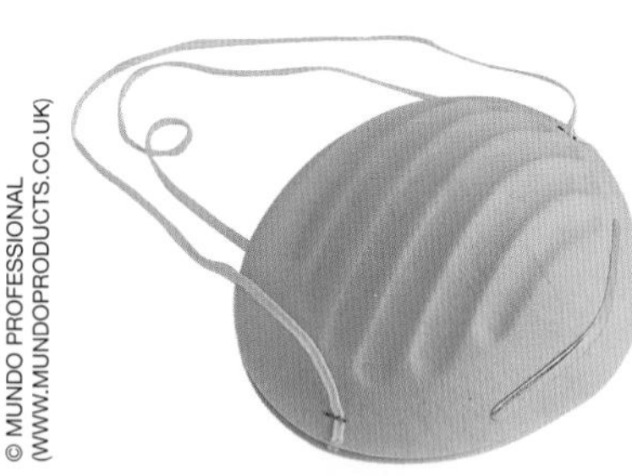
© MUNDO PROFESSIONAL (WWW.MUNDOPRODUCTS.CO.UK)

Disposable dust mask

Avoiding excess dust There are a number of ways that excess dust can be avoided using appropriate extraction units. Collected dust should be disposed of correctly according to the manufacturers' guidelines. For those technicians who feel particularly susceptible to dust, a disposable mask can be worn. Dust masks are only effective if they are worn correctly.

Ingestion

To avoid ingestion of dust and vapours:

- Do not drink hot liquids at the work station; it is possible for them to absorb vapours from the air.
- Avoid placing any drinks on the work station, as the container could collect dust.
- Wash your hands before eating anything.

TOP TIP

Hot drinks

It is safe for a client to drink a hot drink at the work station as they are in the salon so infrequently.

Absorption

Every time a chemical touches the skin or nails, some of it will be absorbed into the skin. Some chemicals are recognized by the skins cells as harmful and a skin reaction will occur as it defends itself.

- The most obvious reaction is irritated skin in the area of absorption.
- Local irritation is not always the first sign of an allergic reaction. Puffy or itchy eyes could be a reaction to a product on the nails. Headaches, tiredness, mood swings, nosebleeds, dizziness, coughs, or a sore throat can also be signs of a reaction to chemicals via any of the routes of entry.

Ways to avoid **sensitization:**

- Nail products are designed for the nail therefore keep them off the skin.
- Do not touch the skin with your brush. If you find this difficult when applying a liquid and powder overlay, use a smaller brush.
- Do not wipe your brush on the towel your hand is resting on.
- When removing the sticky inhibition layer (which is uncured monomer, one of the most active allergens in nail products) on a **UV light cured** material start with the smallest nail up to the largest nail to avoid putting the residue on the skin.

HEALTH & SAFETY

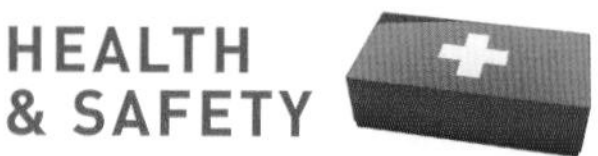

Contact with a skin irritant

If the irritating chemical is removed, the symptoms should also disappear. They will, however, reappear if the chemical is reintroduced, as once the body is sensitized it will always be sensitized to that substance. From the point of view of a technician, if this sort of sensitivity is created to a commonly used product it may be difficult to find an alternative. This could mean you can no longer work in the industry without appropriate PPE. If a client develops a sensitivity it could mean they can no longer receive nail enhancements.

- Wipe the nail away from the cuticle area towards the free edge.
- Make sure all the inhibition layer is removed as this will fall into your hand as you are shaping the overlay.
- Wear protective gloves if you are susceptible to allergic reactions and always wear gloves if you notice any redness or itching of your skin.

Allergic reactions

Although allergies can be caused by just about any product, they are more common when providing nail enhancement treatments because of the products involved. Following simple working procedures will help minimize the possibility for both the technician and their clients.

- Keep the nail desk clean and free from dust.
- Change the disposable towel between clients and several times during the treatment when dust is created.
- Avoid any skin contact with the liquid monomer:
  - Avoid the skin surrounding the nail during application.
  - Do not touch the brush with your fingers.
  - Do not have a patch wet with monomer where you have wiped your brush and then lean in it.
- If using 'low odour' or UV-cured liquid and powder systems, be aware of the dust on the client's fingers, your fingers and in the palm of your hand that is holding the client's finger. This usually has some unreacted monomer in it and can cause problems.
- Wipe away the inhibition layer on light-cured gels starting with the smallest finger first and wipe from cuticle to the free edge and avoid smearing uncured monomer onto the skin.

ACTIVITY

Would you like to see how much dust is generated during an artificial nail treatment?

Start with a clean nail desk and equipment. Provide an artificial nail treatment, such as applying tips and overlays or a maintenance treatment without using any local dust extraction and just a towel on the desk.

When you have finished, get a vacuum cleaner and 1–3 sheets of kitchen roll. Layer the sheets and push the centre down inside the hose, then attach the small flat attachment of the vacuum (the number of sheets will depend on their thickness and the size of the hose and its attachment). Make sure the corners of the sheet are outside the hose and held firmly in place. Vacuum your desk and towel. Then remove the vacuum attachment very carefully and tip out the contents of the sheets!

HEALTH & SAFETY

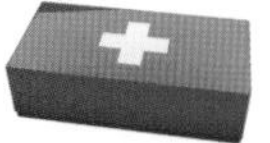

Follow manufacturers' instructions

Always read the manufacturer's instructions carefully and follow them exactly. For tools, it is usual that a fresh disinfectant solution must be made every day. When dealing with any disinfectant solution you should wear protective equipment as they are always irritants.

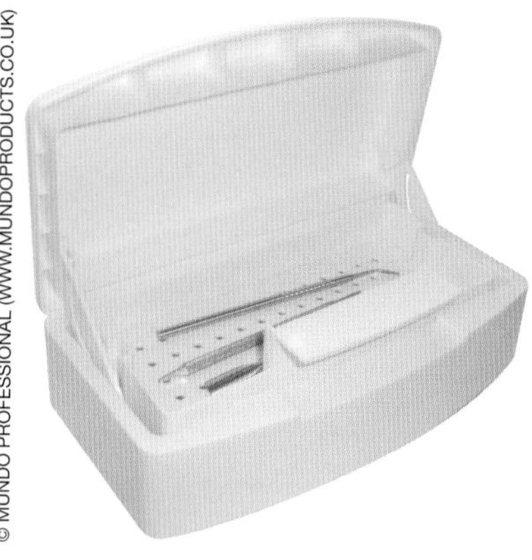

Store sterilized tools in a clean, covered container before use

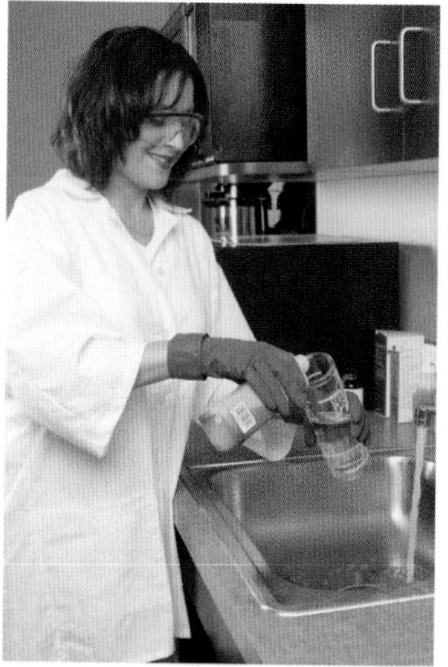

Wear gloves and saflety goggles while handling disinfectant

Sterilization and disinfection

Hygiene must be maintained in a number of ways:

- Ensure all tools and equipment are cleaned and disinfected or sterilized before use (see pages 359–360 for detailed information on the appropriate methods of disinfecting specific tools and equipment).
- Disinfect work surfaces after every client.
- Use disposable products and tools wherever possible.
- Always follow hygienic working practices.
- Maintain a high standard of personal hygiene.

Technicians' hands should be washed before and after every treatment for the safety of themselves and their clients. It not only limits the spread of bacteria but also removed traces of artificial nail products and dust.

Clients should also have clean hands and nails. A huge amount of debris can collect under the free edge and on the surface of the nail. Ask the client to wash their hands with soap and water before treatment. To ensure that under the nails are clean, ask the client to use a nail brush that is provided at the sink. Have a dish with clean nail brushes for this purpose plus a dish for used brushes. Disinfect these brushes at the end of the day.

As an extra precaution, both the technician and the client should use a hand sanitizer at the work station.

BEST PRACTICE

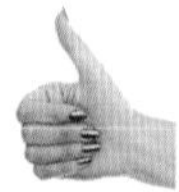

Disinfection

Have a clean, covered container for clean tools and another for used tools. Then the disinfecting process can be carried out at the end of the day.

When tools are removed from the disinfectant follow the manufacturer's instructions then pat dry and store in the 'clean container' ready for use.

Remember UV cabinets do NOT disinfect tools. They maintain a clean environment for the storage of disinfected tools.

Nail technician personal presentation

There is a large aspect of 'nails' that is connected with image and a professional working within that type of industry should promote a good image. It is not always necessary for a technician to wear a clinical white uniform, unless the workplace has such a dress code, but a technician should be suitably dressed in clean and pressed clothes. A technician's nails should be well cared for and immaculate. Jewellery on the hands should be kept to a minimum for the safety of the technician (products could get trapped under jewellery and cause a skin reaction) and hair should be worn in a way that does not impede working.

TOP TIP

Hair in your face

Hair that is continually being tucked behind the ears could create an allergic reaction on the face. Tie or clip it back.

Consultation

Reception

When a new client makes an appointment for nail enhancement treatment, the receptionist should ask the client:

- If they have had nail enhancements before.
- What type of extension do they have (acrylic, gel, etc.)?
- Do they require application or maintenance?

This will guide you on the time required to complete the treatment.

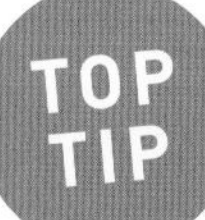

Client communication

When dealing with the public, especially in the service industries, you must have good communication skills. Your approach, while professional, should also be friendly and interested. You should make the client feel at ease and comfortable, and genuinely important. Use the time during a treatment usefully and educate your client in understanding what they need to do with their nails, hands and feet.

Client consultation and assessment

A thorough client consultation will help you to provide the best possible service for your client. Assessing the client for treatment is a very important part of every client's appointment and the keeping of records is a requirement for insurance purposes. A full client consultation should provide a great deal of important information, including:

- **Occupation**: to give an idea of the type of nails a client could cope with. It could also offer clues to any nail and skin problems.
- **Medical history**: with nail treatments, it is unnecessary to go into any medical history in any depth. There are some that are relevant in a general way and the main questions that should be asked are:
  - **Allergies**: If a client is prone to allergies, there is a good chance that they may be allergic to some of the products that will be used. If this is the case, it would be a good idea to carry out a skin test on a test nail.
  - **Diabetes**: if a client suffers from this condition great care must be taken with all treatments. Circulation is often poor and consequently diabetics are slow to heal approval from their doctor before embarking on any course of treatment.
  - **Other**: a general enquiry of the client should be made to ascertain whether there is any other condition that may be relevant to nail treatment.
- **Previous nail treatments**: ask if the client has received nail treatments in the past. Results from these treatments would be useful to know, as a sensitivity to products may have occurred or the client may be unable to keep on artificial nails owing to lifestyle or habits (like nail biting or picking).
- **The condition of the skin and nails**: this should be noted on the client's record card at this early stage. If everything looks healthy and in good condition, it should be noted in case something changes at a later stage. If there is any indication of a skin or nail condition, whether it restricts treatment or not, *it must be noted*.

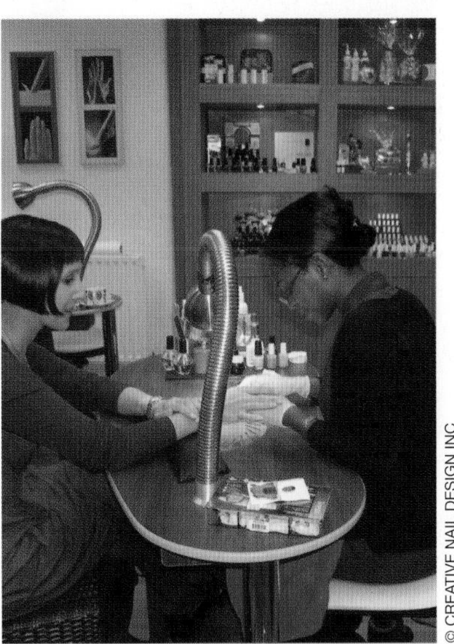

Examine the client's nails carefully before every nail enhancement treatment

Skin and nail disorders

It is important to be able to recognize various nail and skin conditions. There are many common conditions that do not prevent the application of nail enhancements, others which restrict and, less commonly, some which prevent treatment.

It is worth pointing out that if a client has an obvious medical condition of the skin or nails and is treated by a technician without an agreement from their GP or specialist, the technician's insurance can be void and he or she would be directly responsible for any claim against them should problems arise.

For detailed information on specific nail disorders refer to pages 363–367 and 405–409.

ALWAYS REMEMBER

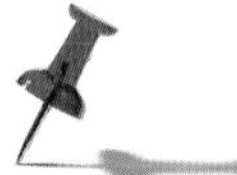

Do not diagnose
Always remember the two key rules:

1. Professional technicians are not doctors or dermatologists and therefore should not diagnose a medical condition.
2. If there is any doubt about a condition, do not continue, but suggest the client sees a specialist.

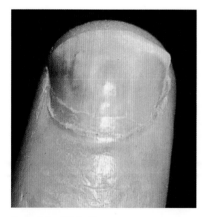

Bacterial nail infection

Contra-indications

Contra-indications that prevent treatment include fungal infection, bacterial infection, viral infection, infestations, severe nail separation, severe eczema, severe psoriasis and severe skin conditions.

Contra-indications that restrict treatment include broken bones, recent scar tissue, skin allergies, cuts and abrasions, diabetes, skin disorders, recent fractures and sprains, undiagnosed lumps and swellings, product allergies.

Treatable nail conditions

These are conditions of the hands, feet and nails that do not prevent treatment, but an understanding of each condition is important as suitable care and the appropriate action needs to be taken. These include pterygium, onychopaghy, weak, dry, brittle, split nails, hang nails, longitudinal or horizontal ridges and allergies to products.

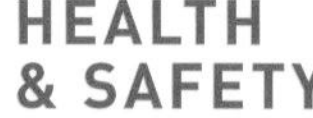

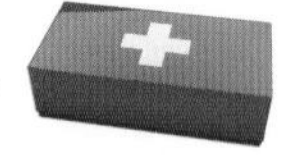

Client aftercare advice
The client should be advised to return if they notice any lifting of the artificial nail structures. It is possible to have a bacterial infection after just a few days of lifting!

Common and avoidable nail conditions

1 **Bacterial infection** This is, unfortunately, a common condition seen during nail treatments. This is caused by an overlay lifting from the nail plate and bacteria entering. The warm, moist environment is a perfect condition for the bacteria to grow. It is seen as an area that is discoloured. This starts as a faint yellow and can progress, if left untreated, to a very dark green. This colour is a by-product of the bacteria and not the bacteria itself. It will remain as a stain on the nail plate even after the bacteria has gone. If this is treated early it will not cause any long-lasting problem. But, if left, can, eventually destroy the nail plate!

This is virtually always associated with an area of lifted overlay and can be treated by a technician if caught early. To do this, remove all the existing overlay by gently buffing or soaking in **acetone** depending on the type of overlay. Throw away the buffer used and the disposable towel that has caught the dust. Then dehydrate the nail. Now the environment does not support the bacterial life. The stain will remain until it grows out but should not change in colour or size. It is safe to reapply the overlay.

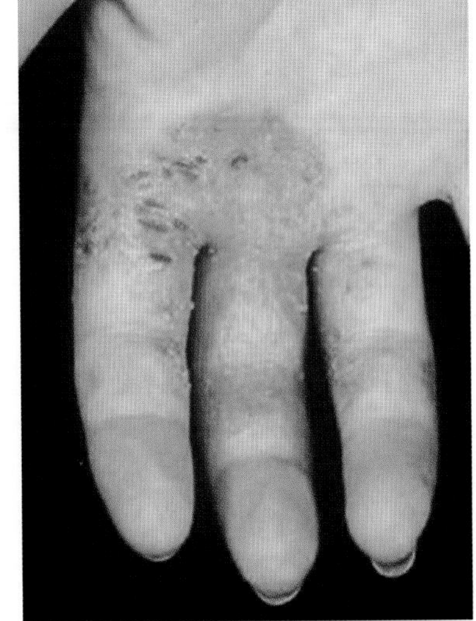

HSE

Contact dermatitis

Other common skin conditions

1 **Dermatitis:** this is a general term that describes a non-specific inflammation of the skin. This is common with nail technicians and often due to overexposure. This type is called allergic contact dermatitis. This is not necessarily localized and can be anywhere on the skin. There is another type commonly seen in salons. That is irritant contact dermatitis. This is caused where the skin has been irritated by contact with some substances.

BEST PRACTICE

Treating clients with dermatitis

If a client already has dermatitis then any nail treatments will need some restrictions. The client will probably be aware of what products affect their skin so these should be avoided. If they do not know what causes their condition all skin products should be avoided. If the skin around the nail is unaffected, treatments that treat just the nail can be provided but extra care must be taken to avoid touching the skin.

Treatment plan

The information obtained from the consultation should enable the technician to provide clear treatment recommendations to the client. An important piece of information to find out is exactly what the client expects from the treatment. Include discussion of the possible contra-actions and the appropriate action to be taken by the client.

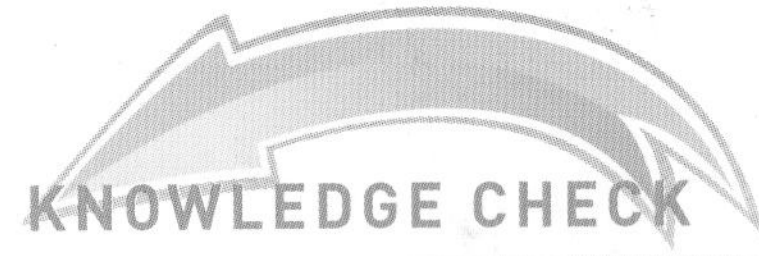

KNOWLEDGE CHECK

Name five functions of the skin.

Need more time... refer to Chapter 2 Anatomy and Physiology pages 30–31 to help you.

Contra-actions

A contra-action to nail enhancement is an adverse or unwanted condition. Examples include:

- allergies
- infection
- lifting of the nail enhancement product.

It is best practice to provide the client with a written aftercare instructions.

Once this discussion has taken place it is worth reminding the client of all the options available in order that both parties are sure the correct choice is being made. The technician should note down on the record card what the treatment is and what the client's expectations are. This can be referred to later to see if the expectations were fulfilled and it is also useful if another technician treats the client. The client should then sign this and a note made of which technician carried out the treatment.

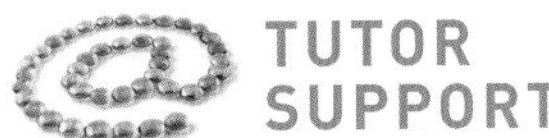

TUTOR SUPPORT

Activity 1: Contra-actions for nail enhancement

A sample client record card

Date | Nail technician name

Client name | Date of birth (identifying client age group)

Home address | Postcode

Email address | Landline phone number | Mobile phone number

Name of doctor | Doctor's address and phone number

Related medical history (Conditions that may restrict or prohibit treatment application.)

Are you taking any medication? (This may affect the sensitivity of the skin to the treatment.)

CONTRA-INDICATIONS REQUIRING MEDICAL REFERRAL
(Preventing nail enhancement application.)

- ☐ bacterial infections (e.g. **paronychia**)
- ☐ viral infections (e.g. plane warts)
- ☐ fungal infections (e.g. **tinea unguium**)
- ☐ parasitic infections, (e.g. scabies)
- ☐ severe nail separation
- ☐ severe eczema and psoriasis
- ☐ severe bruising
- ☐ severe skin conditions

CONTRA-INDICATIONS WHICH RESTRICT TREATMENT
(Treatment may require adaptation.)

- ☐ minor nail separation
- ☐ minor eczema and psoriasis
- ☐ recent scar tissue
- ☐ severely bitten nails
- ☐ severely damaged nails
- ☐ broken bones
- ☐ recent fractures and sprains
- ☐ minor cuts or abrasions
- ☐ minor bruising or swelling
- ☐ undiagnosed lumps or swellings
- ☐ product allergies
- ☐ diabetes

NAIL ENHANCEMENT SYSTEM

- ☐ liquid and powder
- ☐ fibre
- ☐ UV gel

NAIL ENHANCEMENT TREATMENT

- ☐ full set
- ☐ infill
- ☐ re-balance
- ☐ natural nail overlays
- ☐ removal

EQUIPMENT AND MATERIALS

- ☐ nail enhancement application tools
- ☐ nail cleanser
- ☐ cuticle softener
- ☐ nail dehydrator
- ☐ plastic nail tips
- ☐ adhesives
- ☐ liquid monomer and powders
- ☐ primers

NAIL, CUTICLE AND SKIN CONDITION

Nails

- ☐ healthy
- ☐ brittle
- ☐ split
- ☐ dry
- ☐ weak
- ☐ bitten (onychopagy)
- ☐ ridged (horizontal or longitudinal)

Cuticle

- ☐ healthy
- ☐ split
- ☐ overgrown (pterygium)
- ☐ dry
- ☐ hangnails

Skin

- ☐ healthy
- ☐ dry
- ☐ hard

CONTRA-ACTIONS FROM PREVIOUS TREATMENT

- ☐ artificial nail fitted incorrectly
- ☐ tip fitted incorrectly
- ☐ overexposure
- ☐ natural nail infected
- ☐ accidental damage
- ☐ mechanical damage
- ☐ lifting
- ☐ structural damage
- ☐ chemical damage
- ☐ contamination
- ☐ missing nail(s)
- ☐ chipping
- ☐ discolouration

NAIL SHAPE

- ☐ oval
- ☐ tapered
- ☐ square
- ☐ squoval
- ☐ claw
- ☐ fan
- ☐ pointed

Nail technician signature (for reference)

Client signature (confirmation of details)

A sample client record card (continued)

TREATMENT ADVICE
Full set – *allow 120 minutes*
Maintenance (infill or re-balance) – *allow 90 minutes*
Removal – *allow 60 minutes*
Natural nail overlays – *allow 75 minutes*

TREATMENT PLAN
Record relevant details of your treatment and advice provided for future reference.
Ensure the client's records are up to date, accurate and fully completed following treatment. Non-compliance may invalidate insurance.

DURING
Discuss:

- details that may influence the client's nail condition, such as their occupation
- previous nail treatments and current condition of any existing nail enhancements
- the client's satisfaction with previous treatments
- relevant nail care procedures (e.g. oiling cuticles daily)

Note:

- any adverse (unwanted) reaction, if any occur during or after treatment

AFTER
Record:

- results of treatment
- any modification to treatment application that has occurred
- what products have been used
- the effectiveness of treatment
- any samples provided (review their success at the next appointment)

Advise on:

- product application in order to gain maximum benefit from product use
- specialized nail products following nail enhancement for homecare use
- general nail care and maintenance
- the recommended time intervals between treatments

RETAIL OPPORTUNITIES
Advise on:

- products that would be suitable for the client to use at home to care for the nails
- recommendations for further treatments
- further products or treatments that the client may or may not have received before

Note:

- any purchase made by the client

EVALUATION
Record:

- comments on the client's satisfaction with the treatments
- if poor results are achieved, the reasons why
- how you may alter the treatment plan to achieve the required treatment results in the future, if applicable

HEALTH AND SAFETY
Advise on:

- appropriate necessary action to be taken in the event of an unwanted skin or nail reaction

Client preparation

After the client consultation has finished, prepare the client for the chosen nail enhancement treatment. The hands and nails of the technician and client should be clean as discussed.

Outcome 2: Be able to provide nail enhancement services

Practical skills
1 **Communicate and behave** in a professional manner.
2 Follow **health and safety working practices** and industry Code of Practice for Nail Services.
3 Position yourself and client correctly throughout the service.
4 Use **products, tools, equipment** and techniques to suit clients' service needs and **nail conditions**.
5 Complete the service to the satisfaction of the client.
6 Record the results of the service.
7 Provide suitable **aftercare advice**.
Learn how to provide nail enhancement services
Underpinning knowledge
1 State how to **communicate and behave** in a professional manner.
2 Describe **health and safety working practices** and industry Code of Practice for Nail Services.
3 Explain the importance of positioning yourself and the client correctly throughout the service.
4 Explain the importance of using **products, tools, equipment** and techniques to suit clients service needs, **nail and skin conditions**.
5 Describe how services can be adapted to suit client service needs and **nail conditions**.
6 Describe how to maintain and remove nail enhancements.
7 State the **contra-actions** that may occur during and following service and how to respond.
8 State the importance of completing the service to the satisfaction of the client.
9 State the **aftercare advice** that should be provided.
10 Describe the chemical process involved in the nail enhancement system.
11 Describe the structure and functions of the nail and skin.
12 Describe the different natural nail shapes.

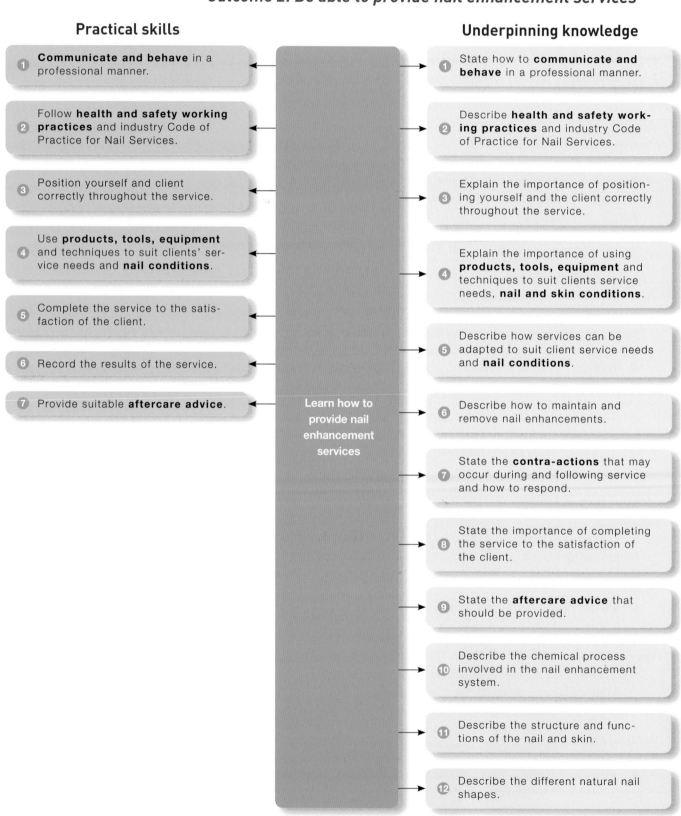

Applying tips to the nails

The application of plastic tips is relevant to all the different nail systems, as it forms the basis of this method of applying artificial nails.

Plastic tips come in many shapes and sizes, colours and lengths.

Good quality tips are made from 'virgin' ABS plastic; a plastic within the acrylic family. Some tips are made from another type of plastic called acetate, which is often cheaper but these are unsuitable for artificial nail systems as they are difficult to blend into the natural nail and have a higher oil content that ABS tips that may affect the overlay.

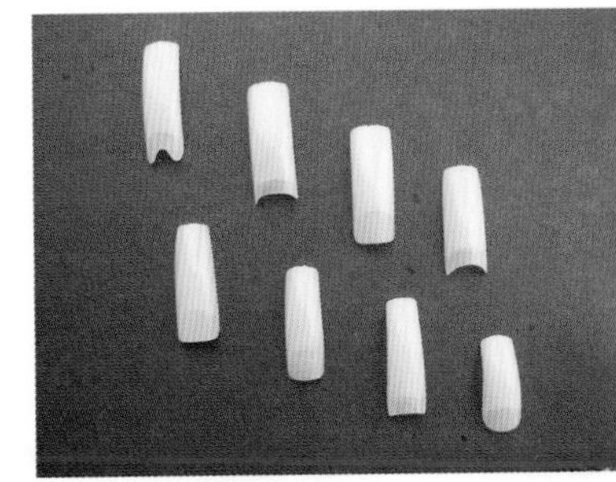

Various tip shapes

Every tip, whatever its shape or size, has a number of features that are relevant to the technician:

1. **Contact area or well**. This is a thinner area and the part that is in contact with the natural nail.
2. **Stop point**. This is the demarcation point of the contact area and the actual tip. When the tip is properly blended, this line will produce a natural-looking smile line.
3. **Side walls**. Tips either have parallel or tapered side walls to suit the natural shape.
4. **Upper arch**. Tips have differently curved upper arches from flat to very curved. Choose the one that fits the natural nail shape or, if the natural upper arch is flat, it will need some correcting and a tip with a curved upper arch will help. If the nail has a high arch, a curved tip will exaggerate this even more so a flatter tip will help compensate.
5. **Lower arch**. A tip needs to have a lower arch so that it looks as if it has grown from the finger and not been stuck on top.
6. **'C' curve**. As with the upper arch, this can vary between types of tip, and the shape of the natural nail should dictate which is most suitable. Unlike the upper arch, it is not advisable to choose a shape that is different from the natural 'C curve. The tip needs to sit on the nail comfortably without distorting the shape of the tip.

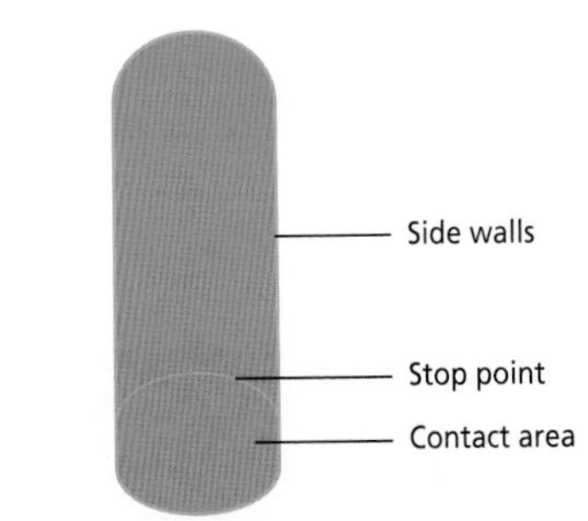

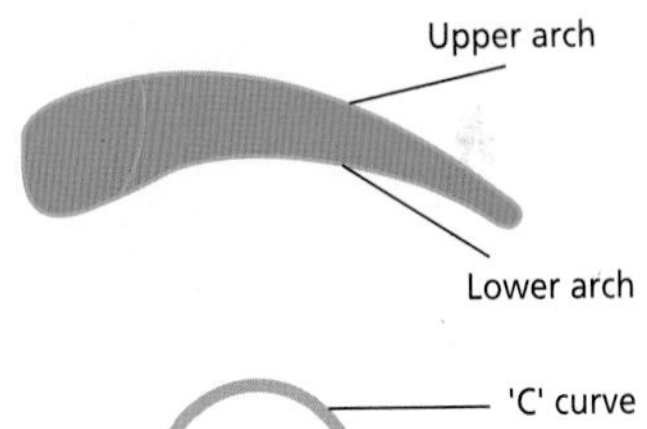

Features of tip (a) the front (b) the side (c) the end

Choosing the correct tip

Some guidelines

- The first thing to look for when choosing the correct tip is the 'C curve of the natural nail. Match the shape of the natural nail.
- The next area to take into account is the natural upper arch. Again, match the natural shape, or choose a tip to correct an over- or under-exaggerated arch.

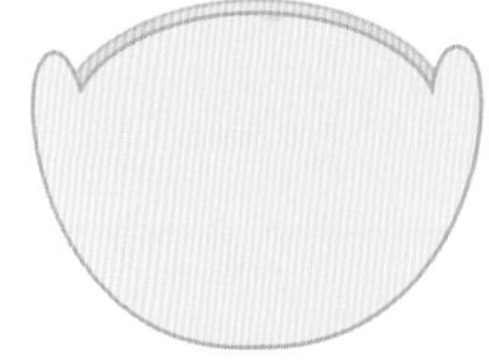

'C' curve of a nail looking from the nail down the length of the finger

Size and width Choose the right size or width must. Most tips come in 10 or 11 different sizes with 0 being the biggest and 10 the smallest. Sizes 4–6 are the most commonly used.

When choosing the correct size, the width of the contact area must be ignored as it is the width at the stop point that is important. This must be exactly the same width as the nail at the smile line (also referred to as the onychodermal band) without any gaps when the skin is pulled back from the sides.

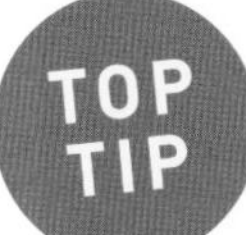

TOP TIP

Shape to fit

Always pre-tailor or shape a tip to fit before application as it cannot be changed when it is on the finger.

ACTIVITY

Problem nail shapes

Research techniques for customizing tips and methods for applying tips to problem nail shapes, including:

- ski-jump or spoon shaped nail
- fan shaped nail
- hooked or claw nail
- bitten nails.

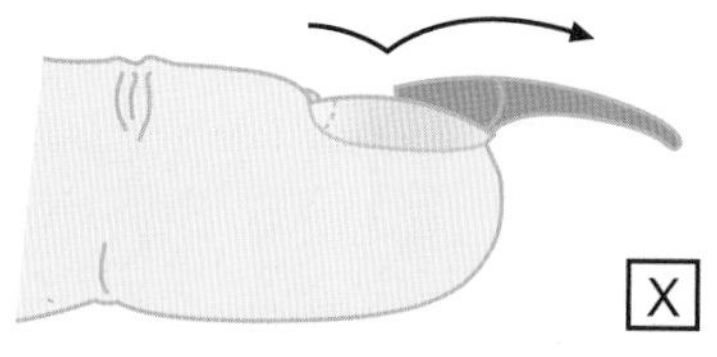

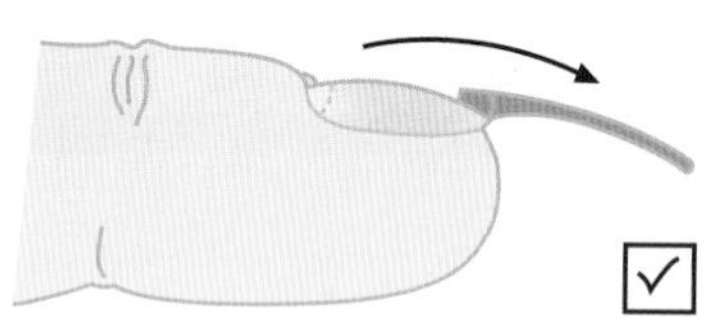

Tip and upper arch (a) tip with complete contact area producing wrong upper arch curve (b) tip with reduced contact area producing correct upper arch

If one size is too wide and the next is too narrow, choose the wider one and file away a very small amount from either side until it fits perfectly.

Full contact area versus reduced contact area Many tips have a full contact area. These can be applied directly to the nail plate with adhesive or they can be tailored beforehand.

There are two methods of removing the contact area:

1 *Using a file*. By holding the tip and the file at the appropriate angle (see picture), the contact area can be removed very quickly leaving a curved edge. By leaving this shape as opposed to a straight edge, the side walls of the free edge of the natural nail are provided with extra protection and support.

2 *Using scissors or clippers*. Scissors with a curved blade are ideal for snipping around the contact area, following the shape of the stop point. Nail clippers can also be used to cut out a 'V shape.

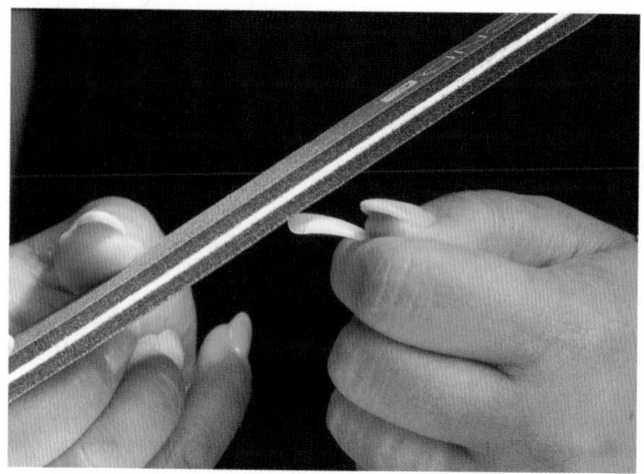

Removal of contact area using a file

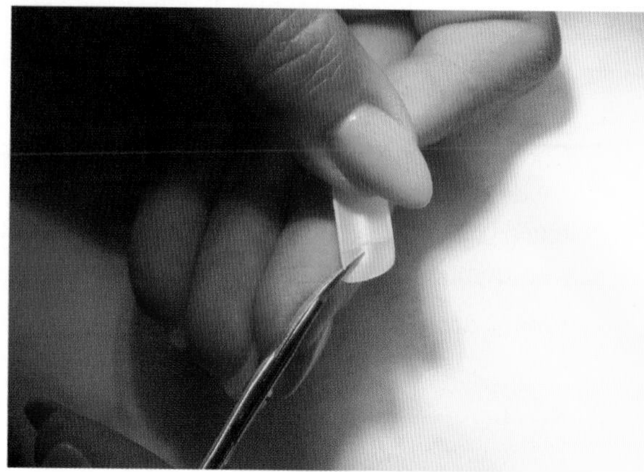

Removal of contact area using scissors

ALWAYS REMEMBER

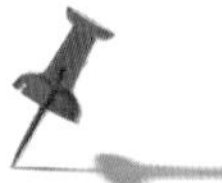

Bonded skin

If any skin is accidently bonded together with adhesive cotton wool soaked in acetone on an orange stick will quickly solve the problem.

Step-by-step: Preparing the natural nail

Before any artificial product is applied to natural nails, they must be carefully prepared.

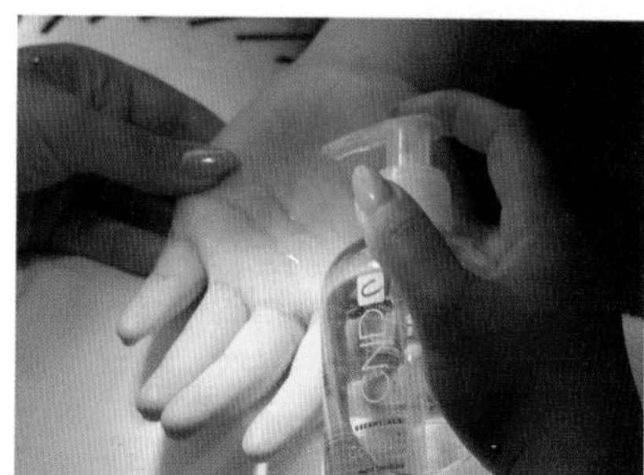

1 Sanitize the hands and the nail plate. Clean the nail plate of surface debris and oils using a solvent applied from free edge to cuticle.

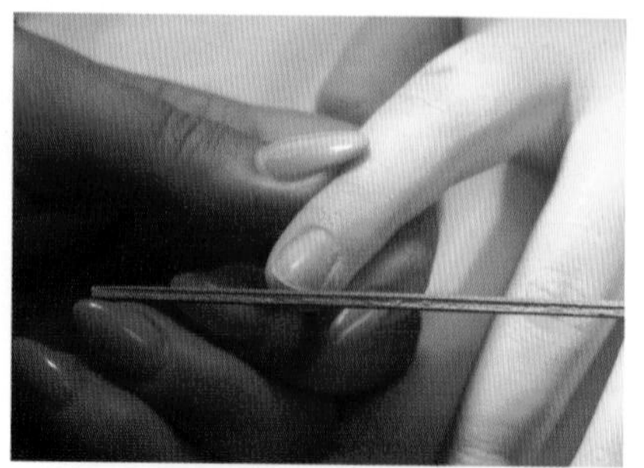

2 Shape the nail to fit the 'stop point' of the tip, which is the demarcation point between the contact area and the rest of the tip.

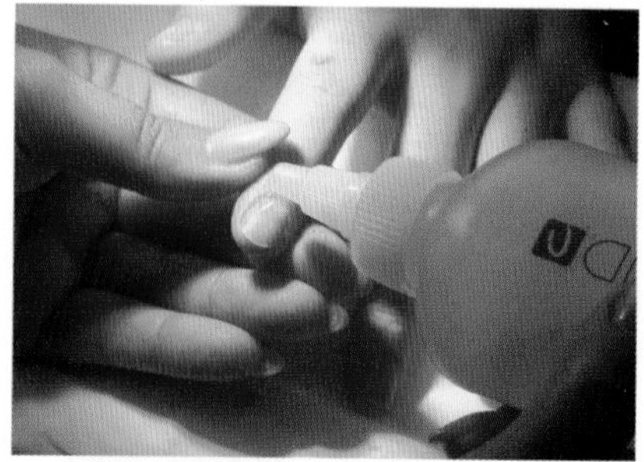

3 Apply cuticle remover to soften the cuticle.

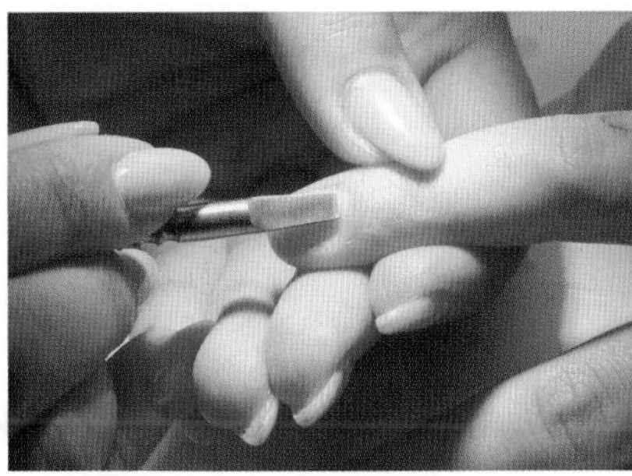

4 Remove all traces of cuticle from the nail plate with a clean cuticle knife. Carefully check the whole nail for cuticle, paying special attention to the sides of the nails.

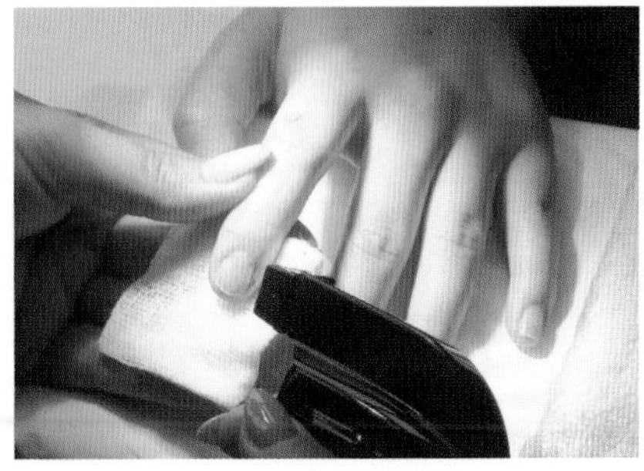

5 Wash the nail to remove cuticle remover. Dry the nail thoroughly. Careful preparation is essential to avoid potential problems later.

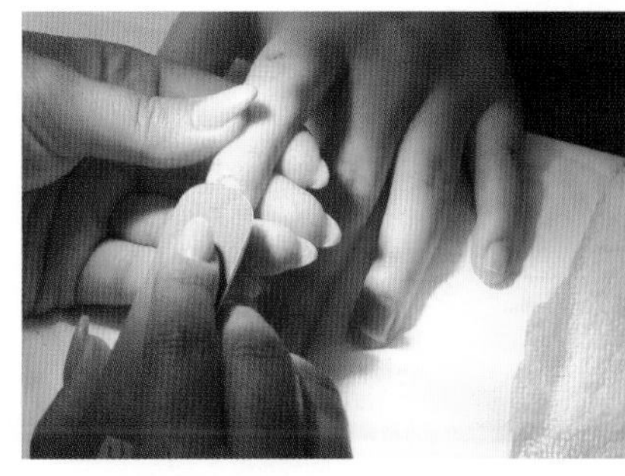

6 Two shiny surfaces do not bond together well as there is not enough 'grip', so the shine on the surface of the natural nail must be carefully removed (but only the shine). Use the end of a 240 grit file (the lowest grit that should be used on the natural nail) with gentle strokes from cuticle to free edge. Make sure the file is angled down towards the side walls. There should not be any scratches on the nail.

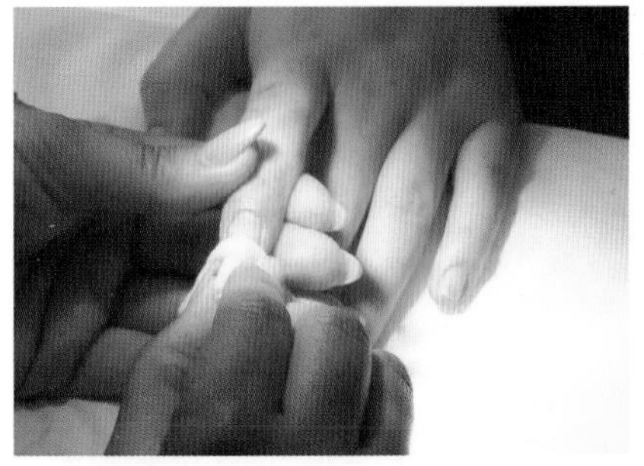

7 **Dehydrate** the nail plate with a specialist dehydrator to remove all traces of oil or moisture.

TOP TIP

Nail preparation

If the nail system to used does not involve a UV lamp for curing, it is best for each hand to be prepared and all artificial nails applied before the next hand is started. In this way, the client has one hand free and there is no chance of contaminating the prepared nails. If a UV system is being used, both hands must be prepared, as one hand is worked on while the other is under the lamp. The technician must ensure that the nails are kept away from any contamination.

Exactly the same process applies when enhancing toenails but remember that the feet are often the perfect environment for infections and toenails are often 'wetter' than fingernails.

Where will you find the Industry Code of Practice for Nail Services and what is it?

Need more time... refer to page 359 to help you.

Adhesives

Tips are attached to the nails with an adhesive. The adhesives used in the nail industry are cyanoacrylates, specifically ethyl cyanoacrylates. It is widely used in artificial nails, as it is used for applying tips and is also the basis of the **resin** in the fibre system. Nail adhesive is available in different viscosities (thicknesses) and curing speeds. You should always use a high grade adhesive but the viscosity and speed is up to personal preference. Nail adhesives are broken down by solvents, the most efficient being acetone.

Cutting the tip

Use clippers or scissors to cut each side separately, never straight across. If the clipper is angled under the client's hand it will cut a slightly curved shape at the tip. The more upright the clipper is held, the straighter the edge.

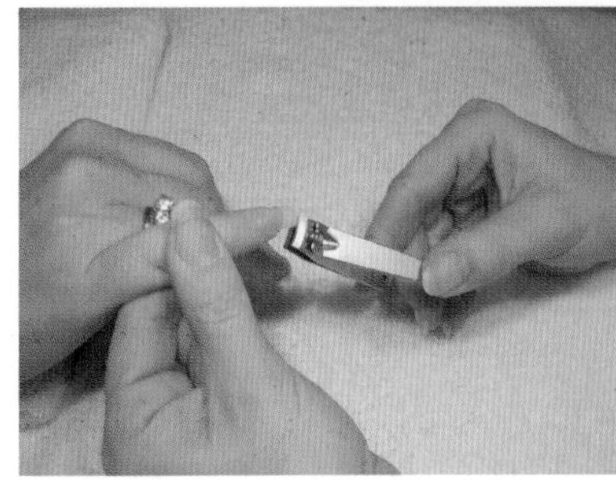

Cutting tips with clippers

Blending the tip

Once all the tips have been applied to the nails with adhesive and cut to the required length the tips must be blended to the natural nails. The result should be perfectly natural in appearance and look as if the nail grew there. More importantly, there must be no damage to the nail plate.

There are two methods of blending the tip: manually with a file (shown in step-by-step below) or chemically with acetone or a branded tip blender which melts the plastic when applied to the contact area. A fine file is then used to file away the melted plastic when it appears shiny.

In addition to the resources listed on page 430–431, you will require the following products, tools and equipment for applying tips to the nails.

PRODUCTS, TOOLS AND EQUIPMENT

ADDITIONAL EQUIPMENT FOR APPLYING TIPS

Tissues or disposable towels To cover the work area and protect the client's clothing

Nail tips A selection of tips in assorted sizes, styles and colours

Adhesive To attach the tip to the natural nail

Tip cutters To cut the tip to the desired length

Files (240 and 180 grit) To file the tip to the desired length and shape and blend the tip with the natural nail

Step-by-step: Applying tips to the nails

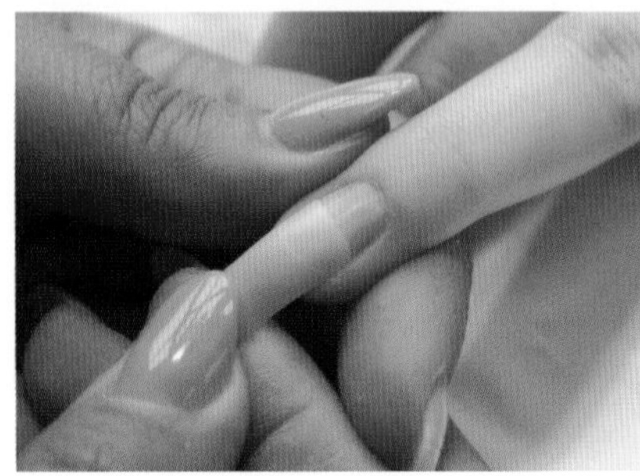

1 Choose the correct tip for the nail and pre-tailor by removing the contact area. Shape the sides if necessary.

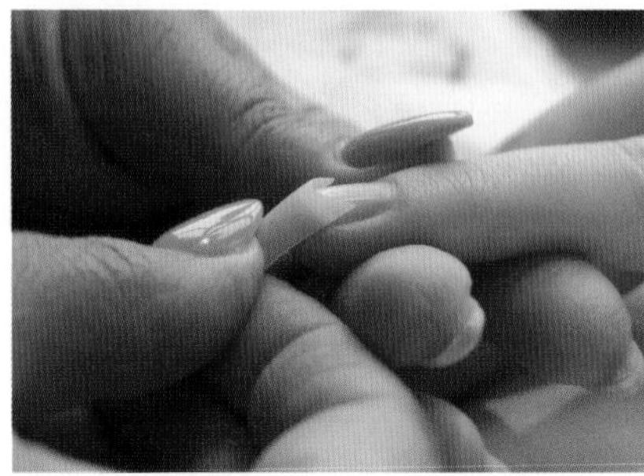

2 Place a small amount of adhesive in the contact area of the tip. Fit the free edge into the stop point at a 45 degree angle, as shown (this will avoid air bubbles under the tip).

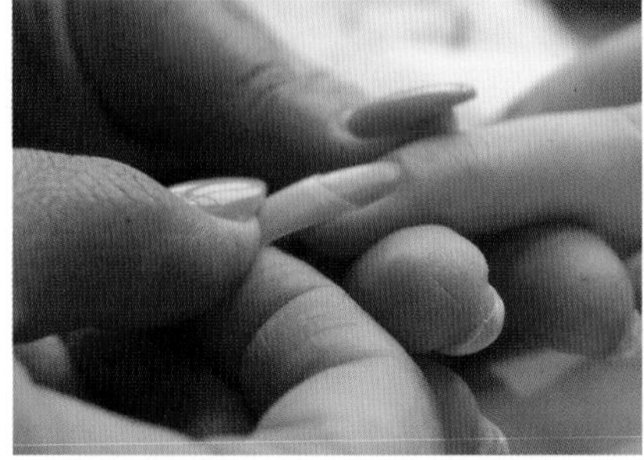

3 Lift the end of the tip so the contact area closes down onto the nail plate pushing out any bubbles that may be under the tip. Make sure the angle of the tip on the nail is correct by looking at the side view. Hold in place for a few seconds pushing the finger up from underneath by the hand that is holding it.

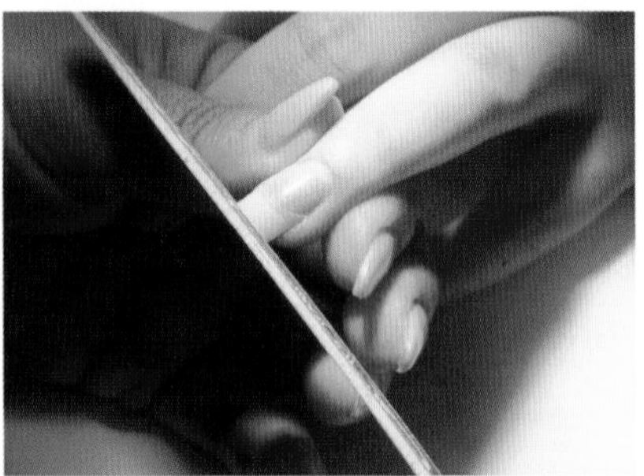

4 Cut the tip to the chosen length and roughly shape the free edge.

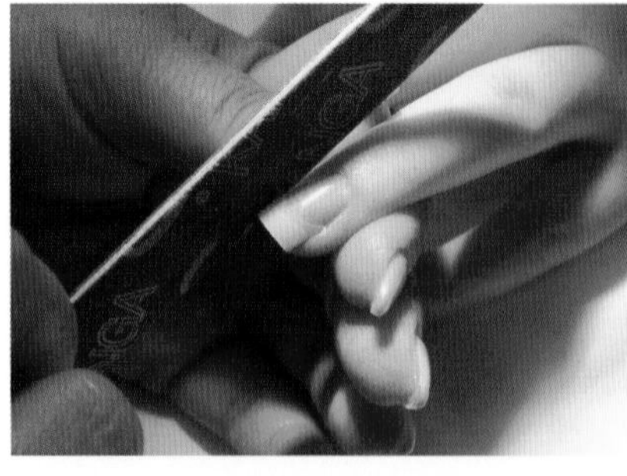

5 Using a thin file and holding the file parallel to the side walls, blend the side walls first so that the tip is the same width as the nail plate.

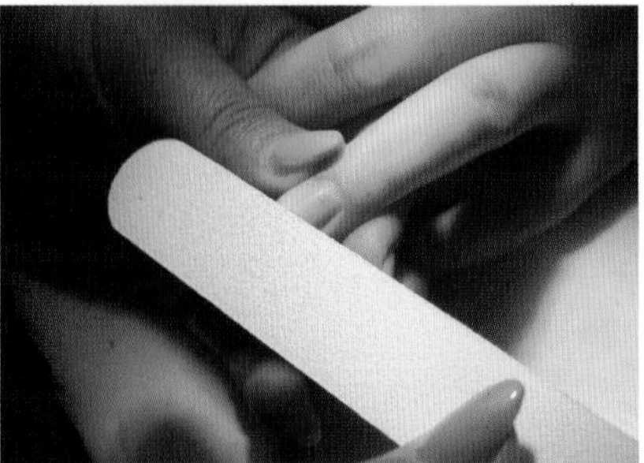

6 Using two-thirds of a 240 grit file blend the tip contact area taking great care to avoid the nail plate. Gently blend until there is no sign or shadow of the tip contact area. Refine the shape. Check the upper arch and lower arch is correct and even. Refine the 'smile line' to produce a neat, natural looking effect. The dust created from filing must be removed from the nails.

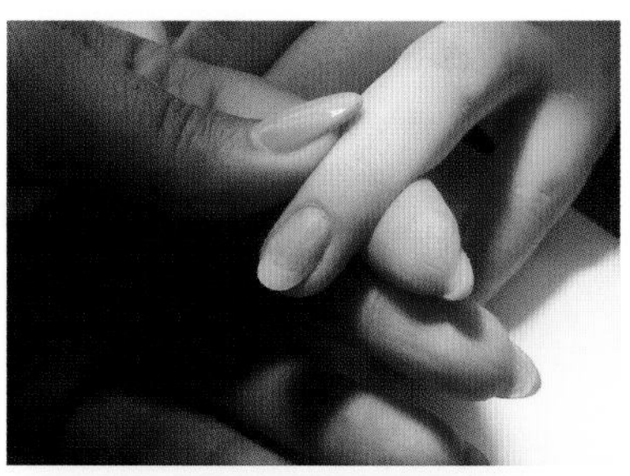

7 The finished nail. The tip should look like it 'grew there'! Perfect fit. Note the side walls are perfectly in line.

HEALTH & SAFETY

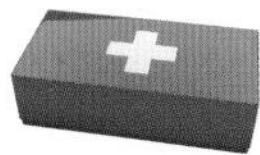

Only a fine grit of 240 or more should be used on the natural nail. Great care must be taken to avoid buffing the nail plate. This is the stage that causes many problems for beginners and removing the contact area of the tip may help.

TOP TIP

Nail wraps

An overlay can be applied to a natural nail (without an artificial tip) to strengthen and protect the nail. Some clients like to wear a natural nail overlay just to keep their nail varnish in perfect condition as it does not chip. Fibre mesh may sometimes be used under the free edge to seal the nail and strengthen it. This treatment is often called a nail wrap and the process is exactly the same as applying an overlay to a nail with a blended tip.

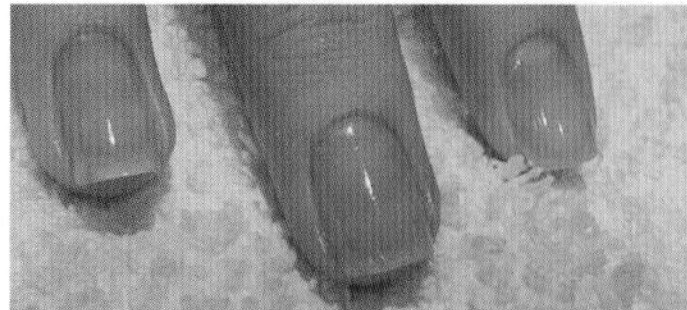

Nails protected by overlay

Applying overlays

The perfect foundation has been created with the application of tips. Now is the time to create the perfect artificial nail that looks good and is very durable and strong. The tip has provided the required length, now the overlay on that tip will provide the required strength.

All products in artificial nails belong to the acrylic family of chemicals. Acrylics are a vast family of various types of plastic. The word 'system', when it is related to artificial nails, describes the specific method and type of acrylic that produces the overlay.

We will look at the following three systems:

- liquid and powder
- UV gel
- fibre.

The structure of the overlay

When applying an overlay, it will help to think of the nail with its tip in terms of three different zones:

1. **Zone 1** is the free edge where the overlay needs to be thin on the edge so that the finished nail does not look artificial.
2. **Zone 2** is the area beside the smile line and onto the nail bed where maximum strength is needed. This is the area of the nail that receives the most stress. It is often called the 'stress area' and should have a highest point that is called the 'apex'. The strongest natural structure is a curve (pressure is dispersed along the curve and is not concentrated over one point). The apex should be where two curves, the upper arch and the 'C' curve, come together at their highest and thickest part. This will create maximum strength for the whole nail without putting any stress on the natural nail, the nail bed, or the matrix.
3. **Zone 3** is the area near the base of the nail. Like Zone 1, this should be thin so that any ridges on the nail bed are avoided and, by being thin, it will be more flexible and able to move with the softer natural nail in this part of the nail plate.

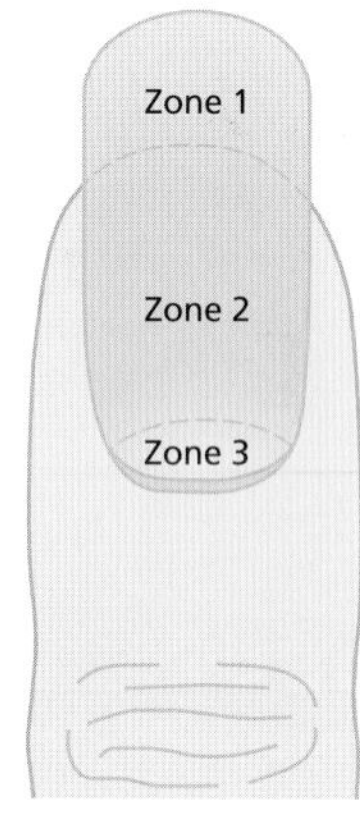

Zones of the nail

If these zones are always kept in mind when applying an overlay, the correct shape and strength will be easier to achieve.

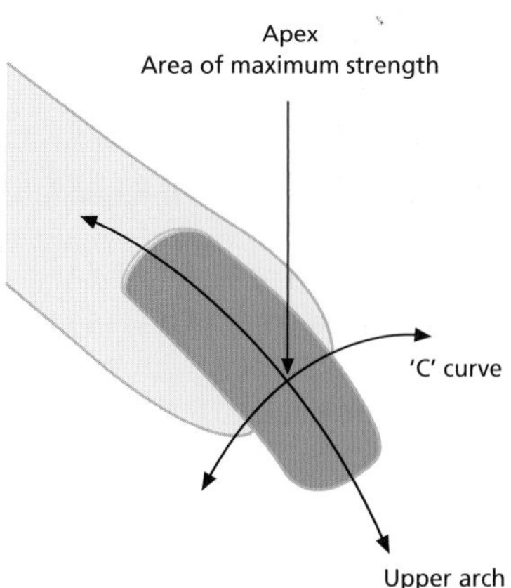

Curves of the nail

Liquid and powder

This system (usually referred to as L&P) uses a liquid monomer and powder polymer that cure to form a solid polymer.

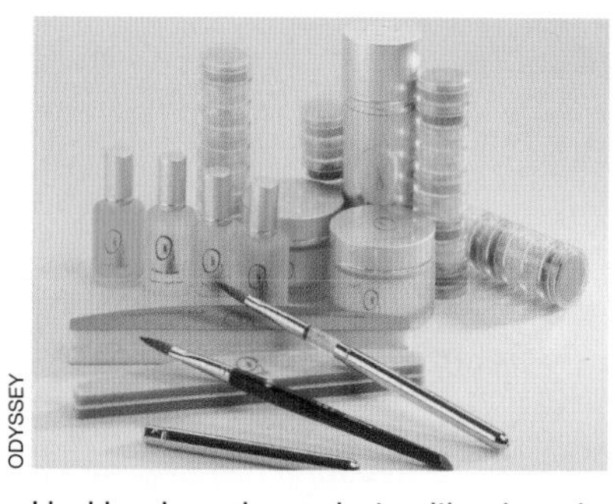

ODYSSEY

Liquid and powder products with coloured powders

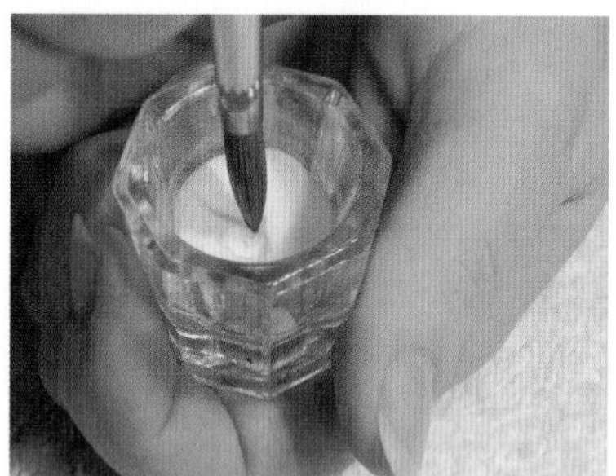

Dipping a brush in powder

KNOWLEDGE CHECK

At what angle should the nail tip be applied to the nail?

Need more time... refer to page 446 to help you.

The liquid monomer is quite volatile and has a strong odour. Working cleanly, correctly and hygienically can minimize this problem.

A version of this system is the **UV light-cured** liquid and powder system. These are applied in a very similar way to traditional acrylics; the main difference is that they do not polymerize until UV light is applied as the catalyst.

Most brands of L&P have powders in several colours. This gives the technician the ability to create very natural looking artificial nails that suit the client's preferences.

Application to the nails

The liquid and powder systems are applied with a brush made of natural hair, by dipping the tip of the brush first into the liquid monomer and then into the powder polymer where it forms a 'bead' of the material. This bead is then applied to the nail and pressed into place. Polymerization (curing) either occurs within a few minutes or when placed under a UV light if it contains a **photoinitiator.**

Picking up the product with a brush in such a way that it can be applied to a nail takes practice. The bead must be the correct consistency and size for the nail and zone of application. Some liquid and powder brands need a specific ratio of liquid to powder, others are less sensitive. The 'bead' that needs to form on the tip of the brush should look smooth and glassy.

There are different methods of picking up powder: little circles can be drawn in the surface of the powder or the brush can be drawn through in a line. It helps to tap the dish of powder on the desk to create a smooth surface.

When working, the brush should be cleaned periodically by dipping it into the liquid and taking it straight out without touching the sides of the dish and then wiping it on a disposable towel. This will remove the build-up of powder that accumulates in the hairs and then goes into the liquid. When using **white-tip powder**, the brush should be cleaned in this way after each nail.

In addition to the resources listed on pages 430–431, you will require the following products, tools and equipment for liquid and powder treatments.

PRODUCTS, TOOLS AND EQUIPMENT

ADDITIONAL EQUIPMENT FOR LIQUID AND POWDER OVERLAYS

Tissues or disposable towels To cover the work area and protect the client's clothing

Liquid monomer in a clean, covered dappen dish The volatile liquid acrylic component used in the L&P system

Powder polymer in a clean, covered dappen dish The dry powder acrylic component used in the L&P system; available in a variety of colours

Clean sable brush To apply beads of the liquid and powder to the nail

Files (240 grit) To refine and smooth the nail overlay

Nail oil To condition the nail and surrounding skin

Primer (if required) Prepares the nail for the application of the L&P system

Glosser or three-way buffer To add shine to the finished nail overlay

Step-by-step: Applying liquid and powder using white-tip powder

If the overlay is being applied without white tip, it should still be applied in zones, but it would not be necessary to create a smile line (step 6), otherwise the process is the same.

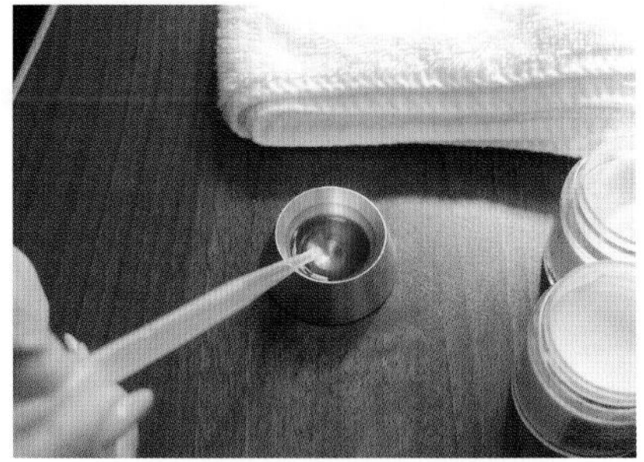

1 Nails should have the tips perfectly blended (if tips are applied), the dust removed and be clean and oil free. Using a pipette, place a small amount of monomer liquid in a dappen dish that has a lid. Do not put too much in the dish. It is easy to top up.

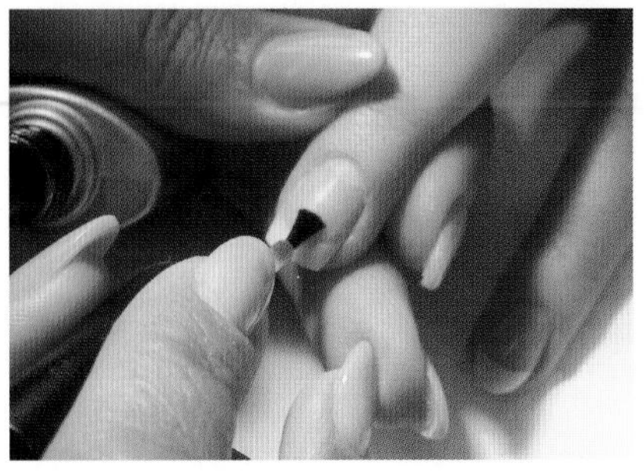

2 If necessary, apply primer (check manufacturer's instructions) sparingly around the base of the nail. Make sure the primer is dry before applying the overlay.

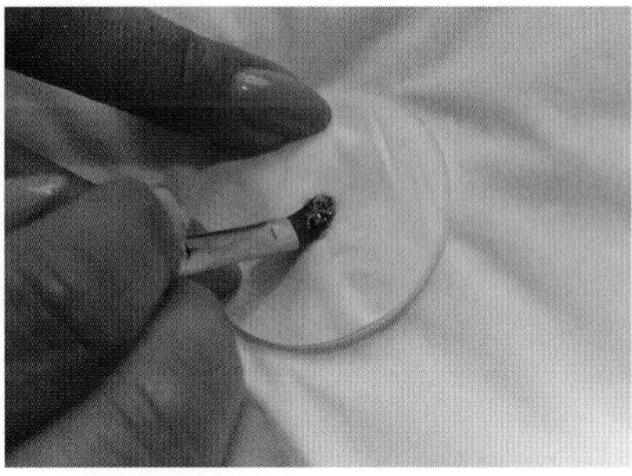

3 Clean the brush first by dipping it into the liquid monomer, taking it straight out and wiping it on disposable tissue.

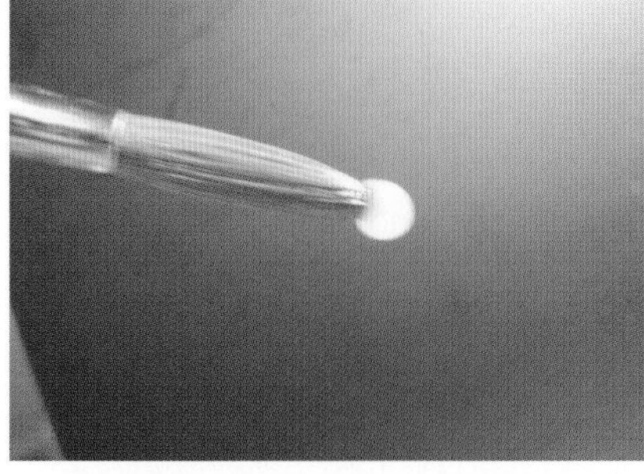

4 Dip the brush in the liquid monomer and then the powder to form a bead.

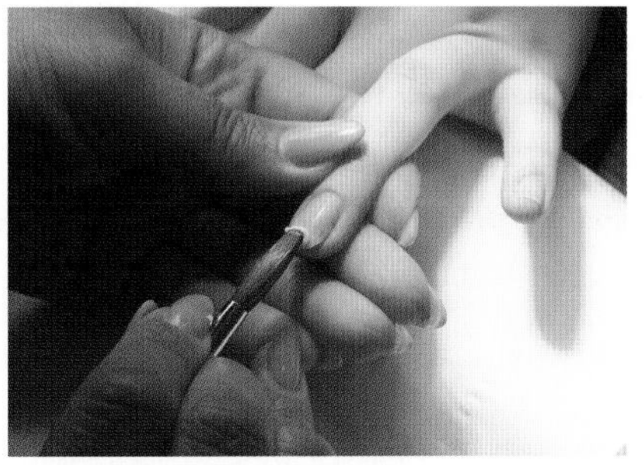

5 Place a small bead of white powder in the centre of Zone 1, closer to the smile line than the edge. Holding the brush at the same angle as the upper arch and using the tip of the brush, press the bead.

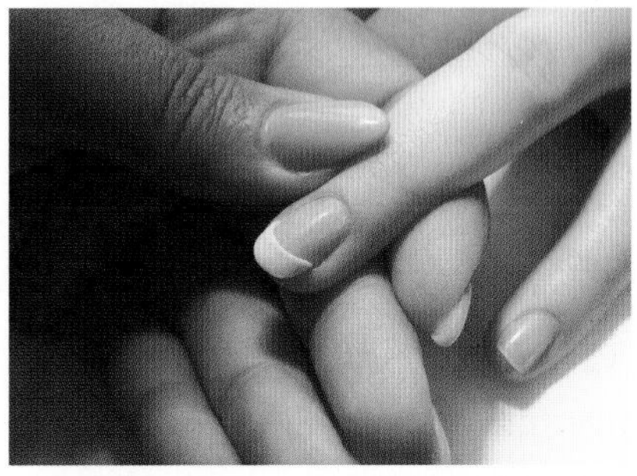

6 Using small pressing movements, take some of the bead out to one side and create a sharp smile line with a pointed 'dog ear'. Repeat the process on the other side. Make sure the 'C' curve is even and the extreme edge is thin. Tidy up the smile line if necessary.

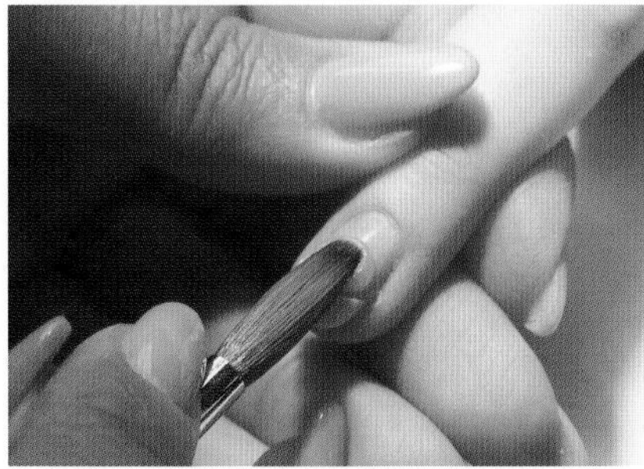

7 Pick up a medium bead of clear or pink powder and place in the centre of Zone 2 close to the smile line. Using small pressing movements take some of the bead to either side of the nail, angling the brush to create a thin and even overlay at the side walls. Blend the overlay into Zone 1 for a smooth finish. Check the 'C' curve and side view for the correct structure.

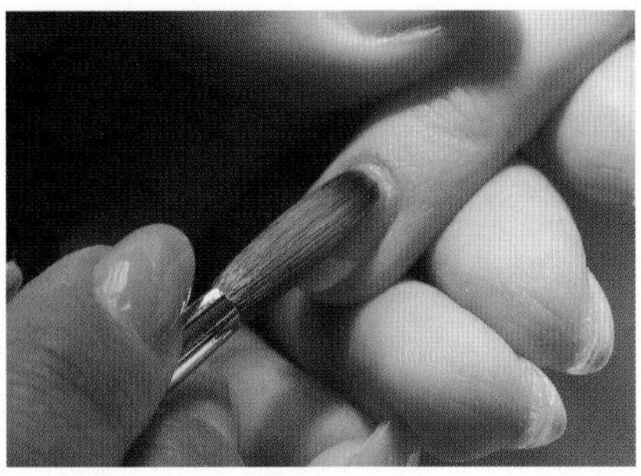

8 Pick up a small bead of clear or pink powder and place centrally in Zone 3. Angle the tip of the brush and, using gentle pressure, move the bead across Zone 3, taking care not to touch the skin. Flatten the brush against the nail, press and blend the overlay up the nail into Zone 2. Check the shape and smoothness of the overlay.

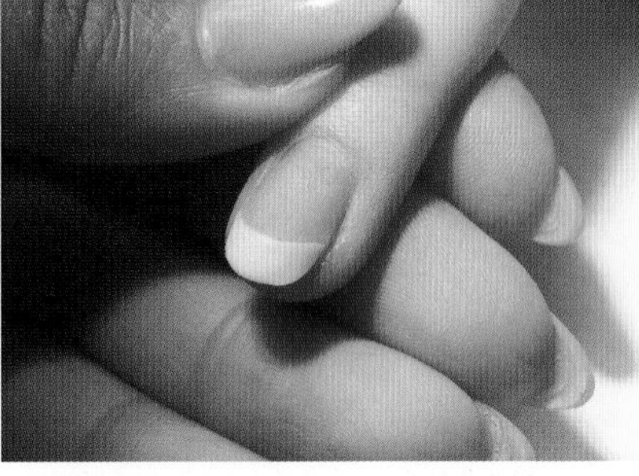

9 Repeat the process for each finger. Make sure the overlay has cured sufficiently by tapping with the handle of the brush. It should 'click' and not be a dull sound. Ideally, the nail should need minimal refining at this stage.

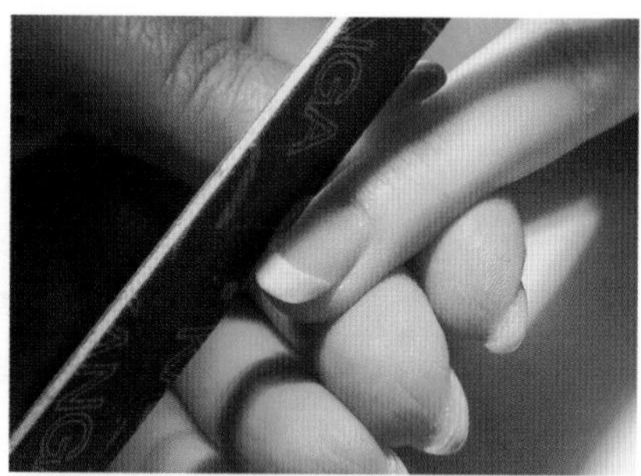

10 Using a thin file, refine the side walls. Then, with a 240 grit file, gently buff to refine and smooth the overlay. Check from all angles to make sure the structure is correct. Make sure there are no dull or flat spots.

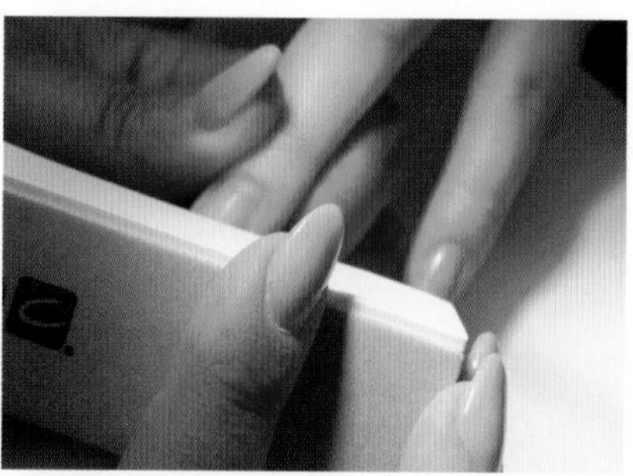

11 When the overlay is a perfect shape, use a glosser or three-way buffer to shine the surface.

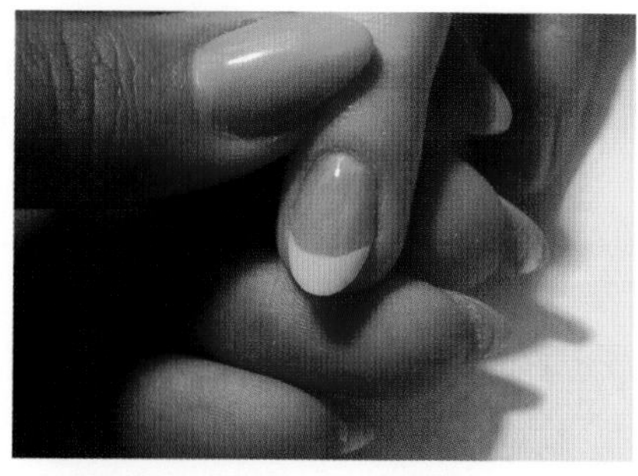

12 Massage nail oil into the nail and surrounding skin.

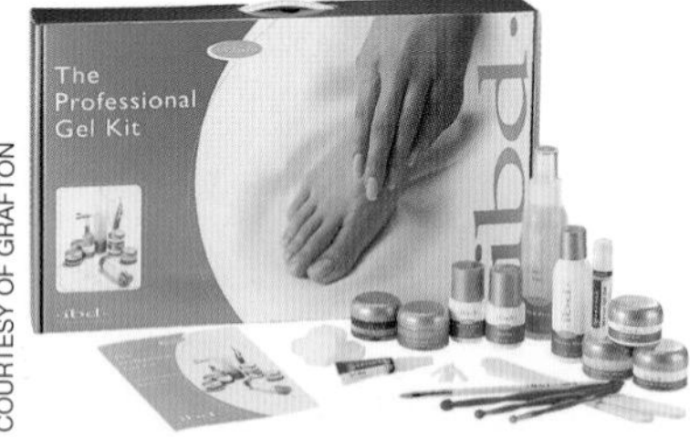

COURTESY OF GRAFTON

UV gel system products

UV gel

The UV gel system could be considered to be a 'pre-mixed' system, as there is only one material that is applied. The only other necessity is a UV light source. The gels are available in many different versions, all with different features and benefits. The main differences that will be immediately noticed by a technician is the viscosity (thickness) and how it flows. Some gels are very runny, others are very thick. Some thick gels will eventually flow, others will stay where they are put. Gels are available coloured, or clear.

Another benefit of this system is that it is virtually odour-free and therefore may be more suitable for use in areas where stronger odours are a problem. In addition, the gels can be very flexible and therefore move more with the natural nail.

The disadvantages of the UV gel system are that some gels and their application methods cannot produce an overlay that is as strong as the liquid and powder systems and are therefore suitable only for those clients who are not too hard on their nails. Many of the gels on the market can be removed only by buffing and not by soaking off with a remover. Some consider this to be a benefit, others consider it to be a disadvantage.

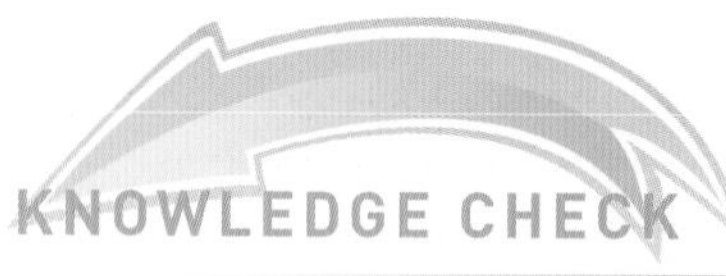

KNOWLEDGE CHECK

What are the different overlay systems available?

Need more time... refer to page 447 to help you.

Application to the nails

The gel 'system' can comprise a single component – that is, one type of gel – or it can comprise several gel components, all of which are needed to create an artificial nail.

UV gels are applied to the nail and moved around with a brush before being polymerized (cured) under a UV light source. Following cure, most gels have a sticky layer (inhibition layer) on the surface. This is uncured monomer and needs to be removed. Most brands have a specific product to do this but an alcohol-based solvent or nail polish remover can be used.

With a one-component gel system, the gel is applied to the nail in one or more layers to build up strength. In a system with two or more components, there is usually a gel that acts as a bonding layer; it is compatible with the nail plate and also with the next layer of gel; next there is a thick gel that can build an overlay with the required structure, that is curves, and then a sealer gel that provides a high-gloss shine and protection. The manufacturer's instructions should always be followed.

In addition to the resources listed on page 432, you will require the following products, tools and equipment for liquid and powder treatments.

PRODUCTS, TOOLS AND EQUIPMENT

ADDITIONAL EQUIPMENT FOR UV GEL OVERLAYS

Tissues or disposable towels To cover the work area and protect the client's clothing

Gels UV activated gels; available in a variety of colours

UV lamp To activate the polymerization process

Primer (if required) Prepares the nail for the application of the UV gel

Clean brush (either nylon or natural hair To apply the gel(s) to the nail

Files (240 grit) To refine and smooth the nail overlay

Nail oil To condition the nail and surrounding skin

Finishing wipe (if required) To remove the inhibition layer

Glosser or three-way buffer To add shine to the finished nail overlay

Step-by-step: Applying UV gel

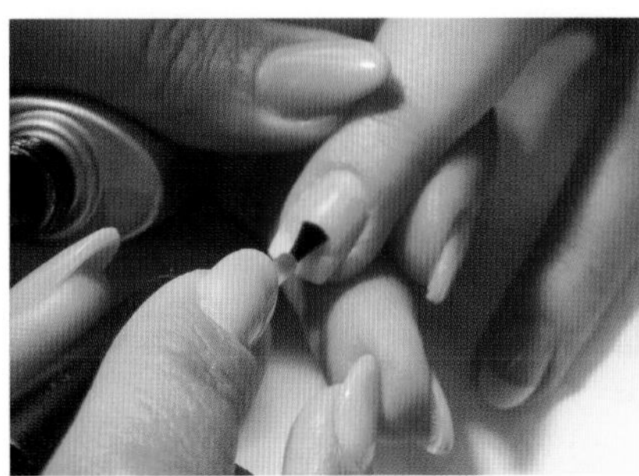

1 Most UV gel systems have a bonder layer or primer. On a nail that has had a tip applied and has been prepared, apply a very thin layer of bonder gel to each nail on the first hand making sure the whole nail is covered and the gel does not touch the skin.

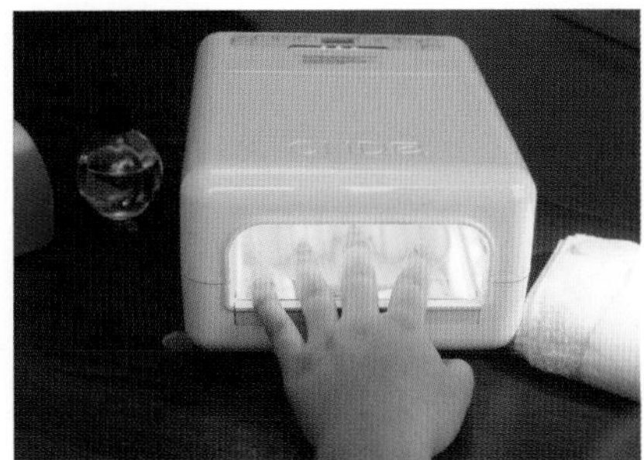

2 Cure for the manufacturer's recommended time. While the hand is in the UV lamp repeat Step 1 for the second hand. It may be necessary to cure the thumbs separately if a 'whole-hand' lamp is not being used.

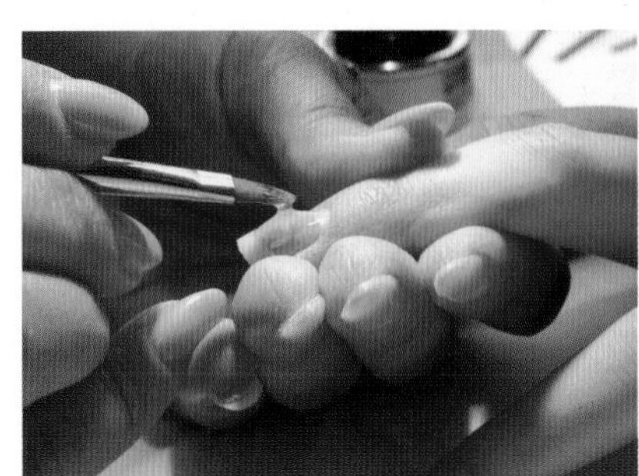

3 Apply a second layer of the builder gel. Notice how the brush is used to build an apex in the centre of the nail. At the free edge pull the brush down to seal the edge. Cure in the UV lamp for the recommended time. Depending on the viscosity of the gel, it may be necessary to 'fix' the layer on two nails at a time to prevent the gel from moving while you apply a layer to the next two nails. A third layer may be necessary if the nail are very long. Alternate the hands so one hand is always under the lamp.

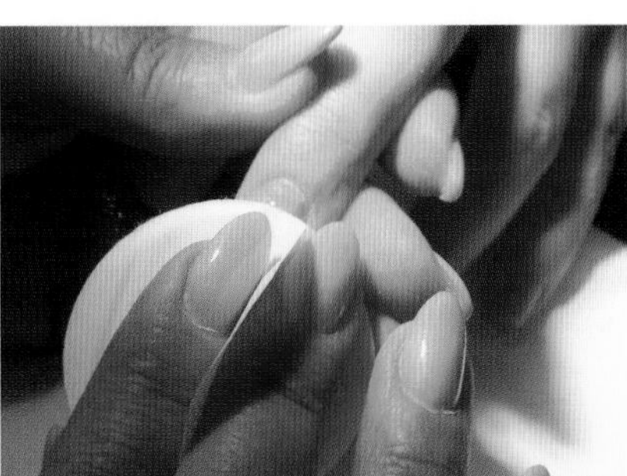

4 Using an alcohol-based product, remove the inhibition layer (the sticky surface of uncured monomer) from each nail, wiping from the cuticle to the free edge.

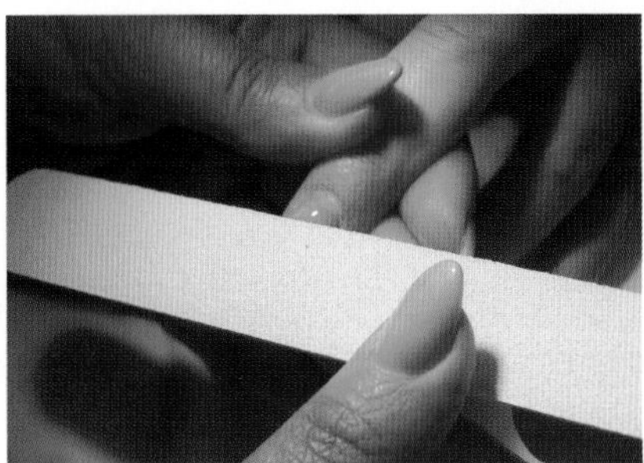

5 If necessary, use a 240 grit file to refine the shape of each nail looking at it from all angles to make sure it is even and has a good structure and a thin free edge. A three-way buffer may be used to create a shine or a further layer of gel may be applied. Remove all traces of dust with a cotton pad dampened with an alcohol-based product.

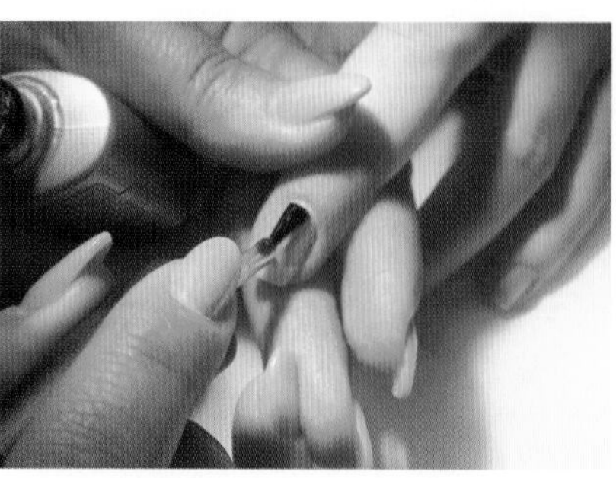

6 A thin layer of gloss top coat may be applied, making sure the whole nail is covered, the edge is sealed and the surface is smooth. Cure for the recommended time in the UV lamp.

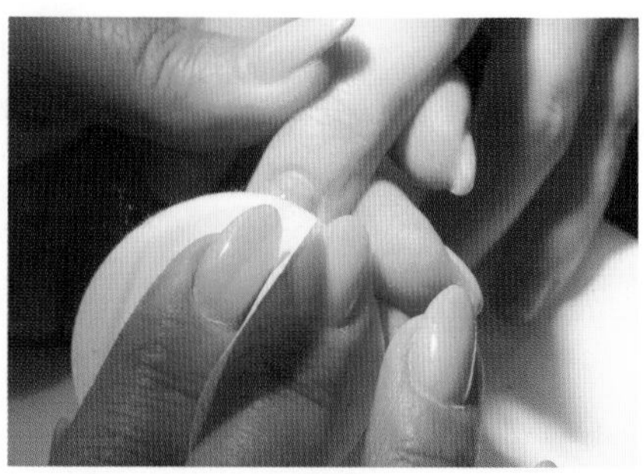

7 Remove the inhibition layer. The nails are now finished and ready for massaging in some nail oil.

Step-by-step: UV gel nails with a white tip

Follow steps 1–5 for a straightforward gel overlay. The white tip product should be applied after the nail has been refined and before the gloss top coat.

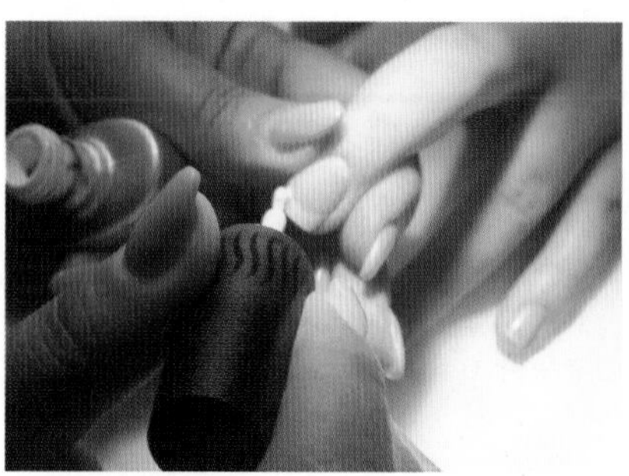

1 When all the dust has been removed from the nails, apply the white-tip product just as if painting a French manicure. The smile line can be sharpened by using a clean gel brush. Cure in the UV lamp for the recommended time. Then apply the gloss top coat.

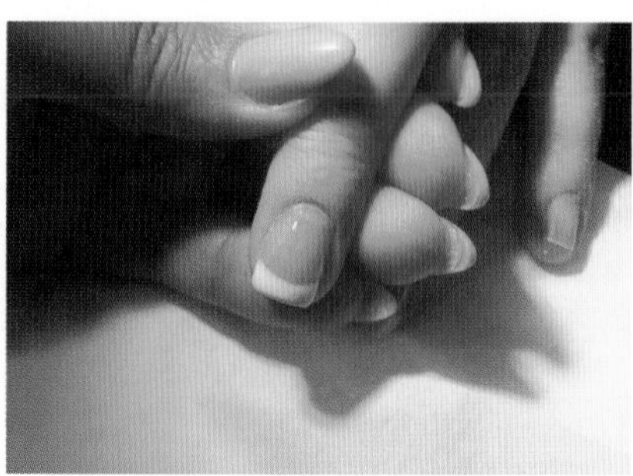

2 Finished nail.

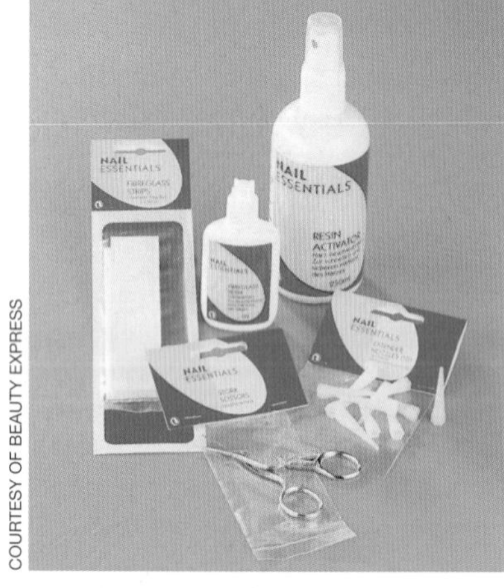

COURTESY OF BEAUTY EXPRESS

A fibre system

Fibre

The third main system involves the application of a fibre mesh (**wrap fabrics** are usually silk or fibreglass) with a cyanoacrylate resin. This is polymerized or activated with a spray or paint-on chemical. This system is quite gentle on the natural nail and odours are kept to a minimum, especially if a paint on **resin activator** is used instead of a spray.

Fibre overlays are very popular as a natural nail wrap, as it is quick and fairly easy to apply and easy to remove.

Fibre overlays are not as strong as the structured nails of other systems and some technicians find the application techniques 'fiddly'.

Application to the nails

The fibre system uses a fibre mesh with a cyanoacrylate resin which is then activated. Either silk or fibreglass can be used as the mesh. The mesh is placed on the nail and then soaked with the resin. The resin is sometimes called a no-light gel (not to be confused with a UV gel). There are two different ways of activating the resin: a spray or a brush-on activator.

Fibre overlays are not solvent resistant at all. If nail varnish is worn then a very gentle remover should be used otherwise the surface of the overlay will be destroyed.

PRODUCTS, TOOLS AND EQUIPMENT

ADDITIONAL EQUIPMENT FOR FIBRE OVERLAYS

Tissues or disposable towels To cover the work area and protect the client's clothing

Fibre mesh, silk or fibreglass To wrap around the nail as the basis of the overlay

Fibre scissors with very fine and sharp blades To cut and trim the fibre mesh to fit the nail

Resin with long nozzle To soak the fibre mesh to create the overlay

Activator, spray or brush-on To initiate the polymerization process

Files (240 grit) To refine and smooth the nail overlay

Nail oil To condition the nail and surrounding skin

Glosser or three-way buffer To add shine to the finished nail overlay

Step-by-step: Applying the fibre system

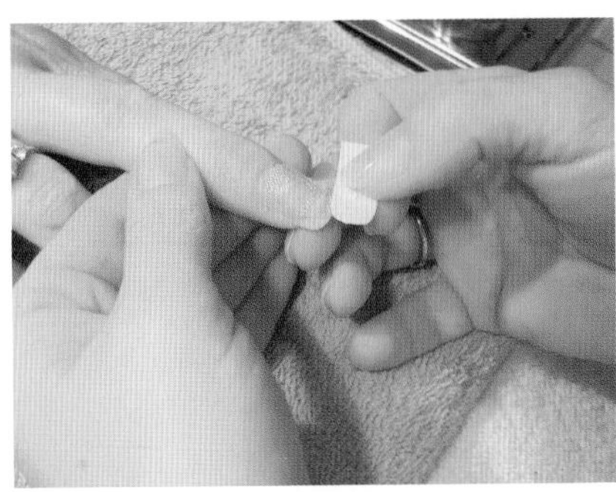

1 Using scissors and avoiding handling the fibre too much, cut a piece of fibre which is approximately the width of the nail. Remove the backing paper and place the fibre onto the nail, close to but not touching the nail fold.

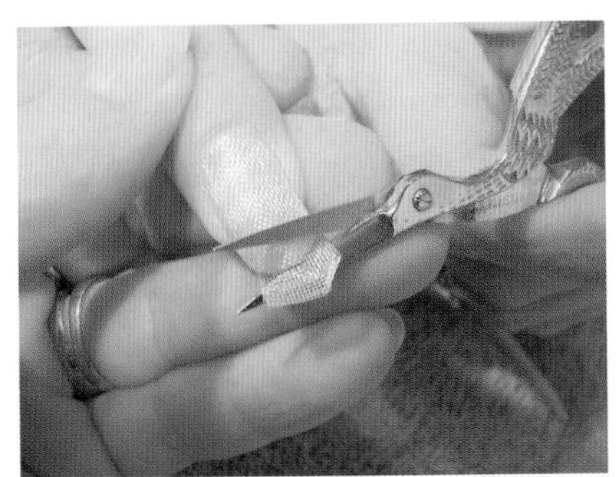

2 Trim the sides if necessary by sliding the blade of the scissors down the side wall and cutting away the excess. Trim the excess length by angling the scissors backwards on the nail tip so the fibre is slightly shorter than the tip.

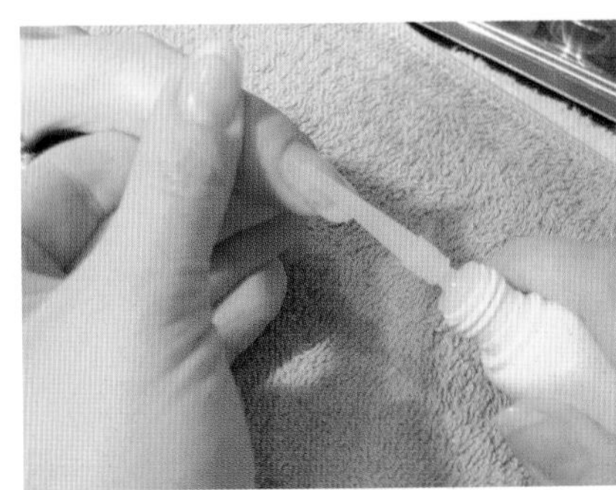

3 Apply a very small amount of resin down the centre of the nail and, with the side of the nozzle, use small circular movements to spread the resin over the nail and work it into the mesh. The mesh should be wet but visible.

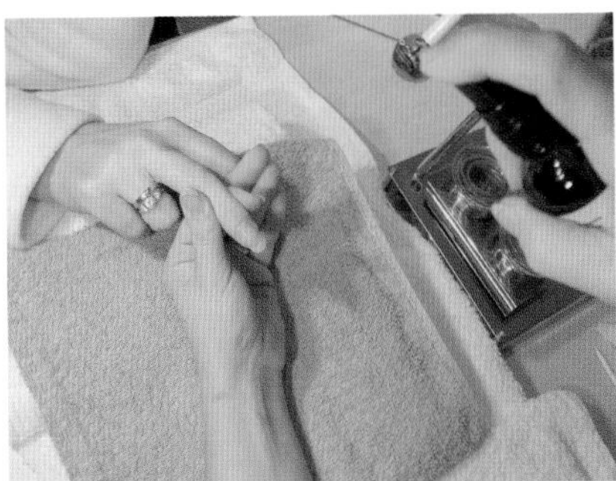

4 Apply further resin down the centre of the nail and spread using the nozzle if a brush on activator is not being used. If using spray activator, hold it at least 30 cm away from the nails and spray once.

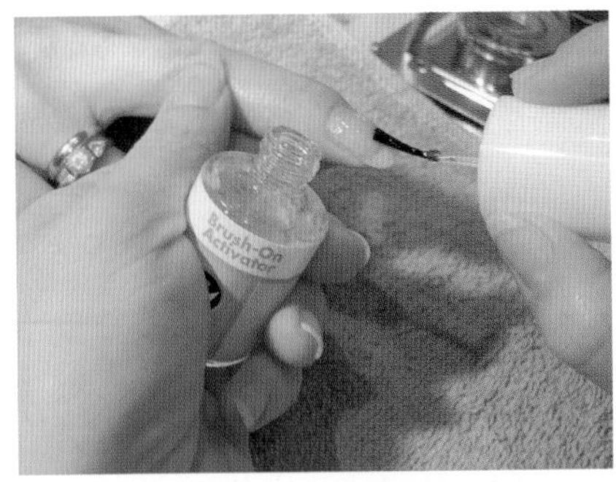

5 If using brush-on activator, have brush cleaner ready. Spread the activator over the resin with the brush to cover the nail while keeping the product off the skin and leaving a tiny margin around the edge.

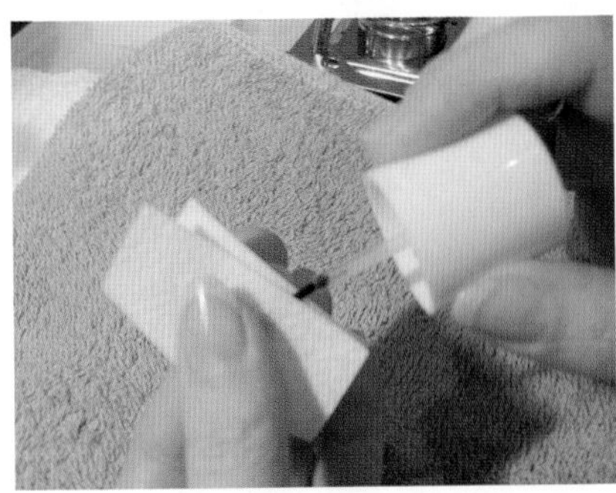

6 Clean the activator brush before replacing it in the bottle.

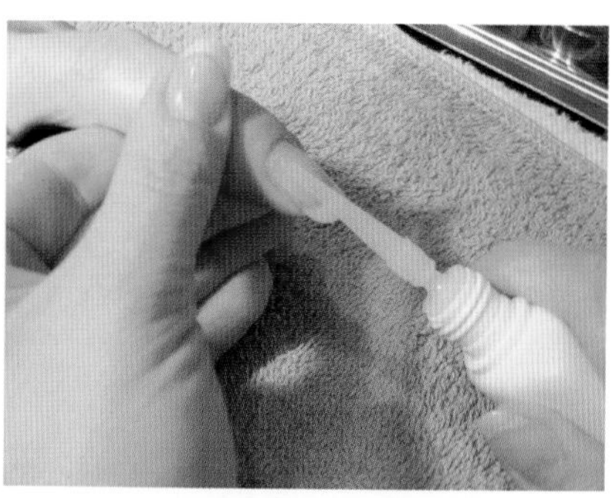

7 Apply a further layer of resin and smooth over either with the nozzle or, if using a brush-on activator, the brush.

8 Activate the same way as before.

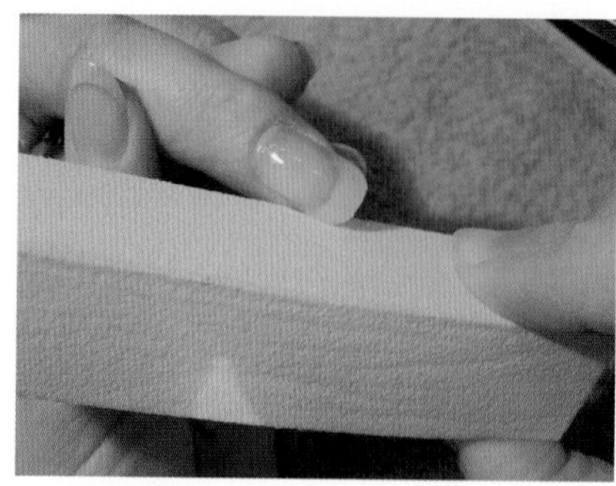

9 Refine the surface with a white block. The overlay should be relatively smooth and should need minimal buffing to refine and smooth the surface.

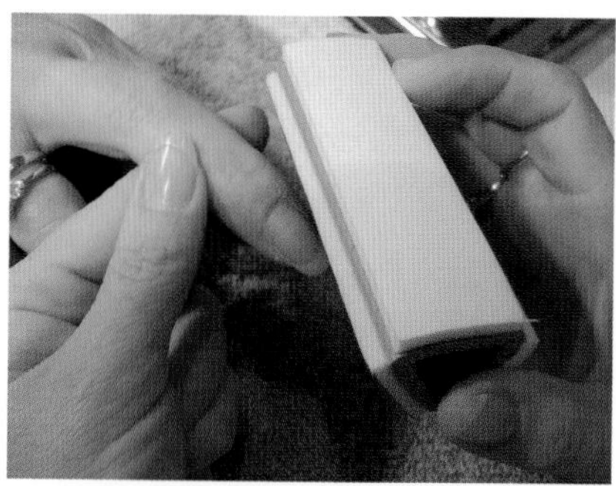

10 Bring the nails to a high shine with a three-way buffer.

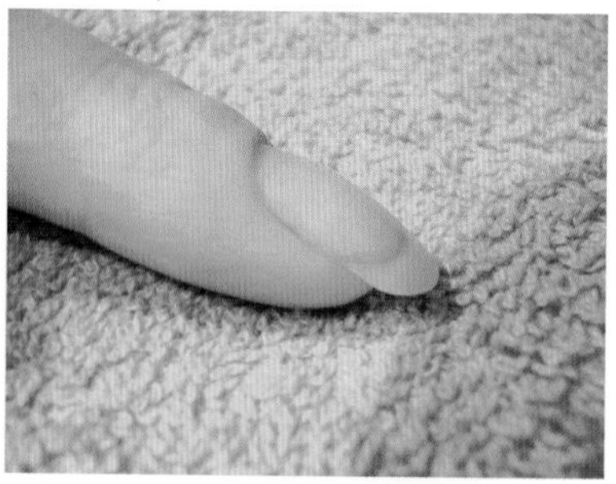

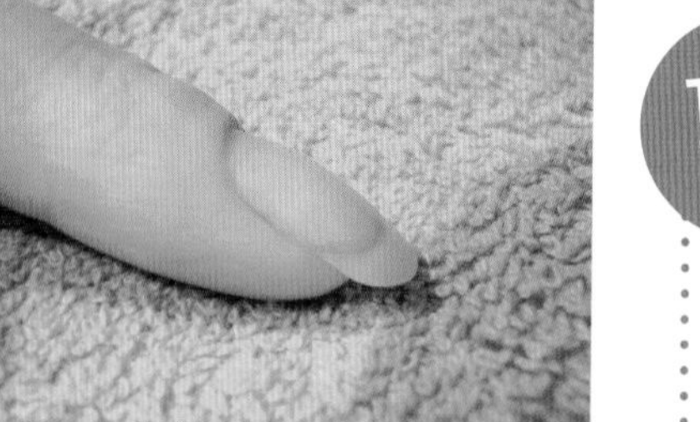

11 Remove all dust and apply oil.

TOP TIP

Fibre mesh with UV gel

Due to the nature of the resin, it is not possible to create any additional curves in the overlay, as can be done with a L&P or UV gel overlay. However, it is possible to use fibre with a UV gel to give added strength or for free-form sculpting.

Aftercare advice

The following aftercare advice should be given to clients after every artificial nail treatment:

- Return for recommended maintenance treatments.
- Keep the nails clean.
- If there appears to be discoloration under the artificial nail, return immediately.
- Do not pick off the overlay or try to remove the artificial nail product.
- Do not use nails as tools.
- Massage nail oil into the cuticle area every day.
- Do not file the surface of the nail.
- It is not advisable to shorten the nail as the thin layer at the free edge will be filed away to a thicker area.
- Use acetone-free varnish remover if necessary.
- Contact the salon of there is any sign of a contra-action including infection indicated by swelling, inflammation or discolouration this could indication a bacterial or fungal infection.

Potential retail product recommendations

- nail oil
- polish remover
- nail polish
- hand cream
- top coat

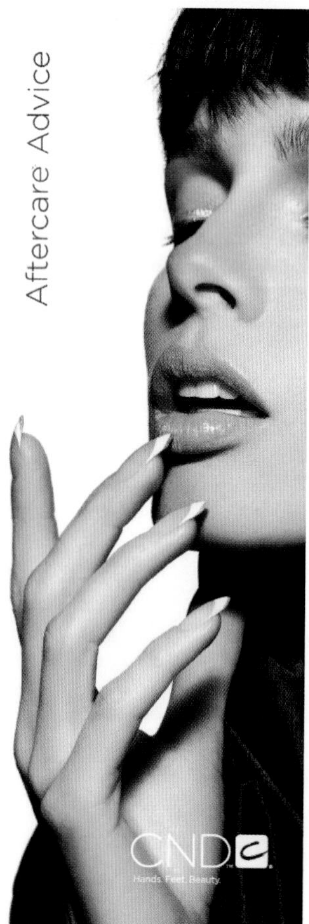

Aftercare leaflet

Maintaining artificial nails

Skilful maintenance is as important as skilful application and will keep clients returning on a regular basis.

The appearance of an outgrown artificial nail is one consideration, but there are two more important reasons for regular maintenance treatments:

1 The technician will have have explained to the client that they must watch out for any changes to the nail, and return immediately if anything is noticed. However, some slight changes may not be noticed by the client. There may be some lifting of the overlay, a slight reaction to the products or some minor nail separation. It is important that the technician monitors the heath of the nail and skin.

2 After a period of natural nail growth, the structure that was created during application with the two curves (upper arch and 'C curve) meeting at the apex or stress point of the nail to create the strongest nail possible will have moved.

The apex will have moved further away from the nail bed and could be on the free edge, making it susceptible to breakages. The smile line that was created either by the tip application or by a white tip overlay will also have moved and there will be a band of natural nail growth that will be a different colour to the tip.

KNOWLEDGE CHECK

Briefly explain the overlay application for each of the following systems:

a) liquid and powder

b) UV gel

c) fibre

Need more time... refer to pages 448–545 to help you.

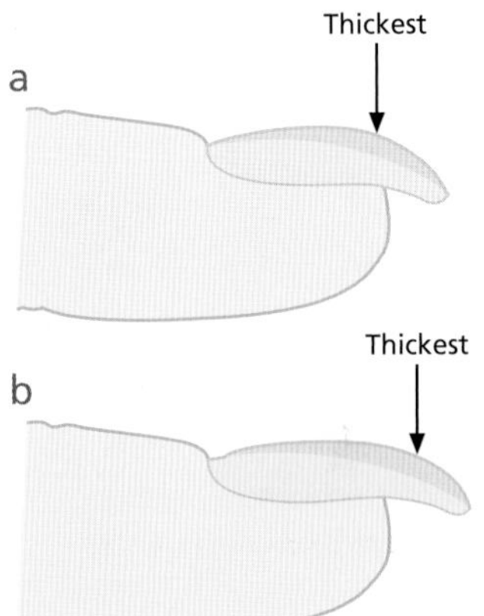

Nail growth (a) Position of overlay at application stage (b) Position of overlay at two weeks' growth

ALWAYS REMEMBER

Only maintain nails that you have applied

If you have not applied a set of nails you cannot be sure of the procedures followed, the preparation and there may be a problem that the nail is hiding. The products used previously may also not be compatible with the ones you use. Either suggest the client returns to their original technician for maintenance or, preferably, explain why you cannot provide a maintenance treatment and suggest that the nails are removed and a new set applied by you.

Maintenance treatments

Infill or rebalance?

There are two types of maintenance treatments. One, called an **infill**, is a short treatment that allows the technician to check for any problems and fill in the small area of growth to make the artificial nail look smooth without a ridge at the base (1). The other is called a **rebalance**, as it removes the apex that has moved to the wrong place and replaces it in the right place, it fills the regrowth area at the base (2) and, if required, will put the smile line back to where it should be and cover the band of natural nail growth (3).

The decision as to which treatment is needed should depend on the rate of nail growth. If growth is slow to average, it is likely that an infill will be required two weeks after the first application and a rebalance two weeks after that. These treatments can then be alternated. If nail growth is average to fast, then a full rebalance may be needed every two to three weeks.

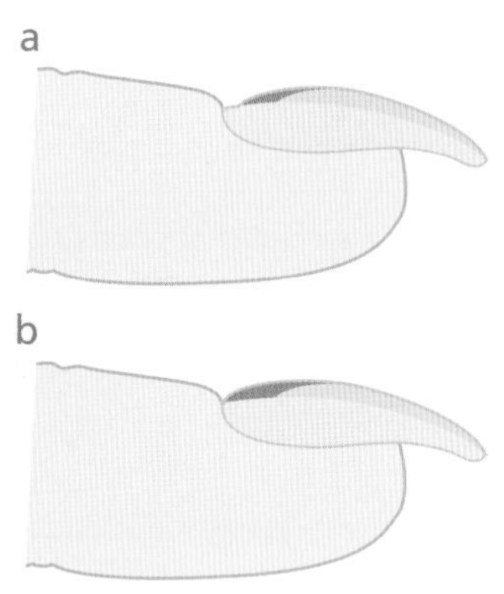

(1) Infill procedure (a) Buff overlay near cuticle (b) Replace overlay in shaded area

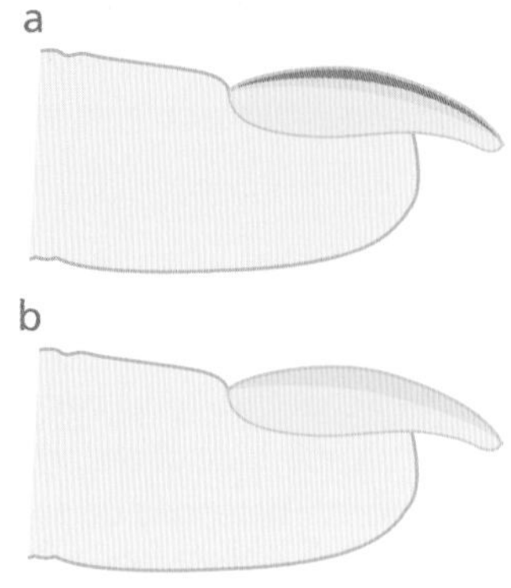

(2) Rebalance procedure (a) Remove most of overlay (b) Replace with complete overlay

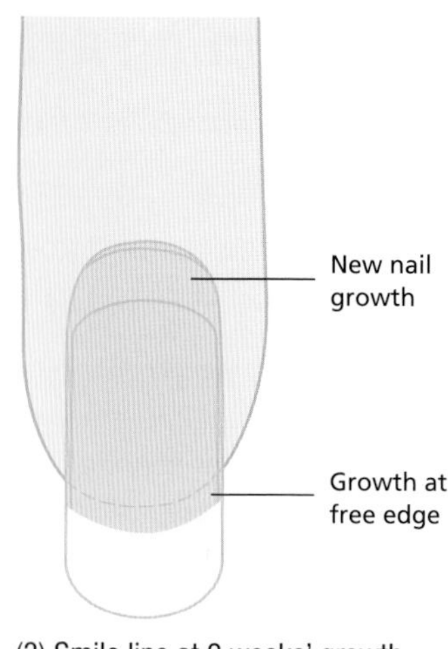

(3) Smile line at 2 weeks' growth

ACTIVITY

Maintenance – observation
When performing a first maintenance, write a log of your observations including a description of each section of each nail, including:

a. shape on looking down onto nail
b. shape from sides
c. shape of barrel
d. smile line
e. clarity of overlay
f. Zone 3
g. general.

Assessment of client's nails

Before the maintenance treatment assess the client's nails, especially on the first maintenance visit after application of a first full set.

What did the client want to achieve? When providing a maintenance treatment, always remember what the client wanted to achieve at the beginning.

Is the client happy? There should be discussion with the client as to how they are getting on and if they are happy with their nails. It may be that the original plan needs changing to achieve another goal.

Step-by-step approach At the start of each maintenance treatment, four steps should be followed, then nothing of importance will be missed out.

1 *Observation*: Look carefully at all the nails. The only difference from when they were first applied should be the natural nail growth at the cuticle, leaving a gap,

ACTIVITY

Maintenance – questioning
When performing a first maintenance, record your client's responses to the following questions:

a. How did the nails break? (If appropriate!)
b. How have you managed with them?
c. Have you followed all homecare advice?
d. If not, what has been missed?
e. Do you like the length and shape?
f. Have they caused any problem?

and at the free edge an obvious growth of natural nail. If there is anything more than this, there is a problem that needs solving and correcting and what is noticed should be noted on the client's record card.

2 *Questioning*: The client must be asked how they have managed with the nails.

3 *Diagnosing*: If the nails are less than perfect, the technician needs to decide what the possible causes of the problem may be and discuss this with the client.

4 *Treatment*: Having followed the above steps, the most appropriate treatment can be decided upon and suggested to the client.

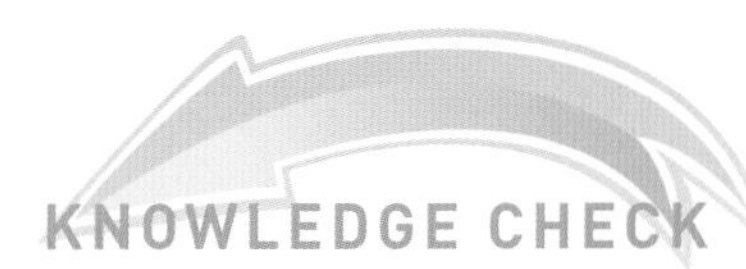

What are the main points of after-care advice to be discussed with the client?

Need more time... refer to page 454 to help you.

Contra-actions

Contra-action	Reason	Solution
Broken nails (if some product is left on the remaining nail plate)	1 Too long 2 Weak	Shorten all nails Rebuild stress area
Missing nails (nothing is left on the nail plate)	1 Oil or moisture on nail plate (If no damage to the nail plate) 2 Client picking nails (If damage to the nail plate is obvious)	Careful preparation Discussion
Lifting in Zone 3	1 Cuticle on nail 2 Oil on nail 3 Overlay too thin 4 Overlay too thick 5 Overlay touching skin	Careful preparation Careful preparation, dehydrate twice or second coat of primer (if applicable) Add slightly more Refine overlay in Zone 3 Take more care in application
Chipping at cuticle	1 Overlay too thick 2 Overlay too brittle 3 Client picking	Apply smaller beads Use wetter ratio in L&P system or less activator in fibre system Discussion

Contra-action	Reason	Solution
Chipping at free edge	1 Overlay too brittle 2 Overlay too thin	Use wetter ratio or less activator Apply more, but taper at free edge
Discolouration of overlay	1 Contamination 2 Affected by UV light 3 Coloured varnish	Use fresh product and clean tools Cover with UV-resistant sealer Use base coat under varnish
Discolouration of nail plate under overlay: yellow-green	1 Bacterial infection	If very superficial (that is very pale colour and small area) remove overlay, dehydrate, prime and re-apply; see client 1 week later. If more serious, remove overlay and refer to GP/pharmacist.
Discolouration under nail plate	1 Possible infection	Remove artificial nail and refer to GP

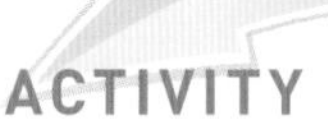

ACTIVITY

How would you deal with the following problems that may occur at a maintenance treatment:

a. shape
b. breakages
c. clarity of product
d. lifting
e. chipping
f. allergic reaction or infections

Further contra-actions

Discoloration under nail plate at free edge: white

This indicates nail separation and may be due to a number of different reasons. The correct treatment would be to remove all products and, if the condition were very minor wait and see if it improves. A pharmacist should be able to suggest what will keep the area under the nail clean.

Skin reaction If there is any irritation of the skin, such as itching, swelling, redness or a rash anywhere on the body – but especially on the hands, fingers or face – the products must be removed immediately.

A skin sensitivity patch test or a test nail should be performed to see which product or products must be avoided.

The maintenance treatment

The equipment and preparation of the work area, yourself, the client and the nails is exactly the same as for the first application. Any artificial nails that are missing will need to have a tip replaced in the same way as previously described. The step-by-steps below describe the general processes for infill and re-balance treatments across the three overlay systems (liquid and powder, UV gel and fibre); you will also need to refer back to the specific step-by-steps for each system to remind yourself of the application process. The images below show liquid and powder application.

Step-by-step: Infill treatment

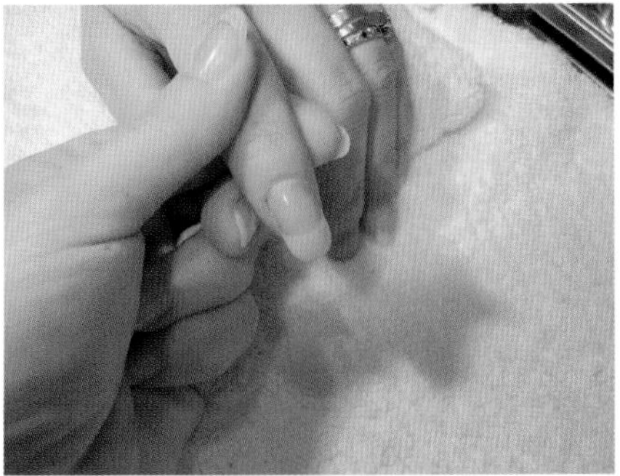

1 Assess the nails. Sanitize the hands and nails. Soften any remove any cuticle that is on the newly grown nail.

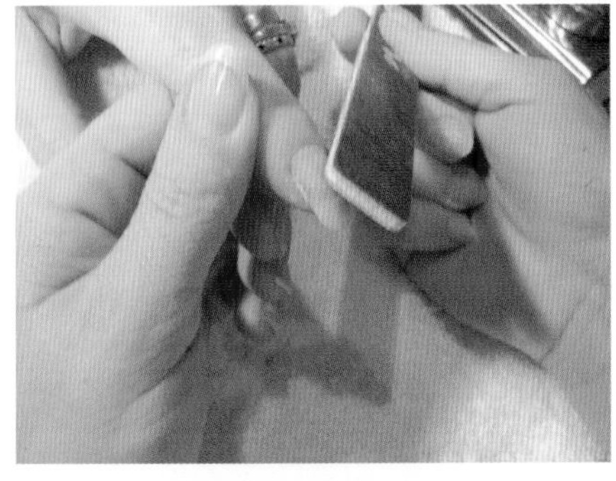

2 Using a 240 grit file, gently blend the edge of the overlay in Zone 3. This will also remove the shine. It there is any lifting in this area it will need to be buffed away, carefully without over-buffing the nail plate.

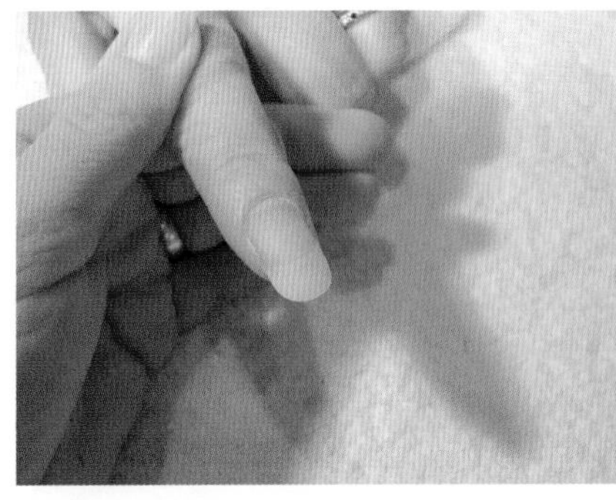

3 Remove the shine from the whole nail surface.

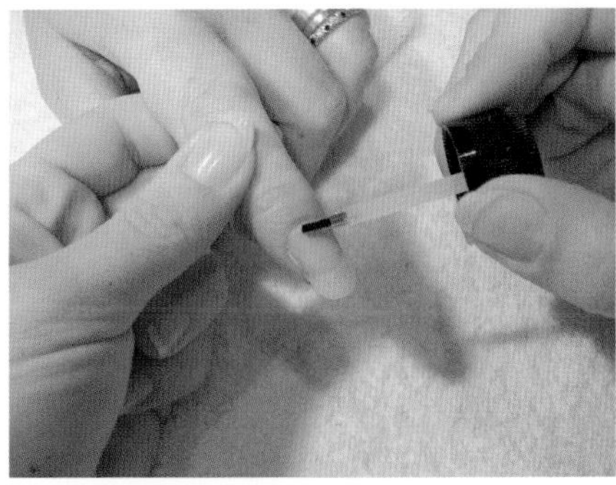

4 Remove the dust and apply dehydrator, taking care to clean around the side walls and nail fold. Apply primer if required.

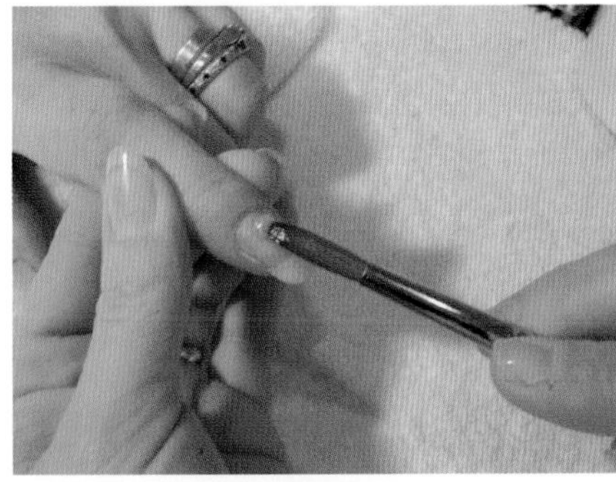

5 Apply a thin layer of product (liquid and powder, UV gel or resin) in Zone 3 as in the original application and blend with the rest of the nail. (Image shows L&P application)

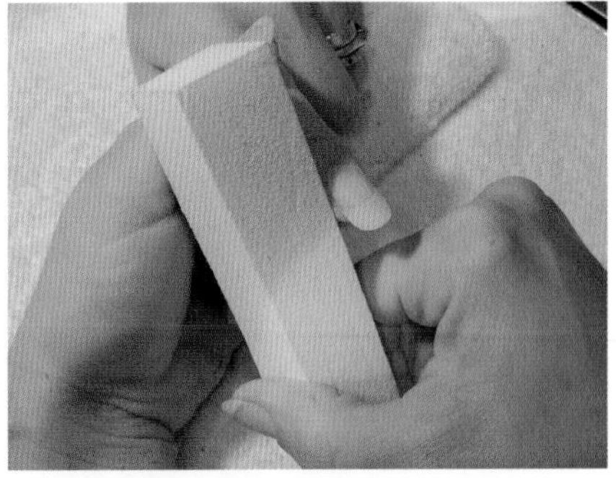

6 Refine the shape of the overlay as in the first application with a 240 grit file, checking from all angles that the structure of the curves is correct. Further refine the surface with a white block.

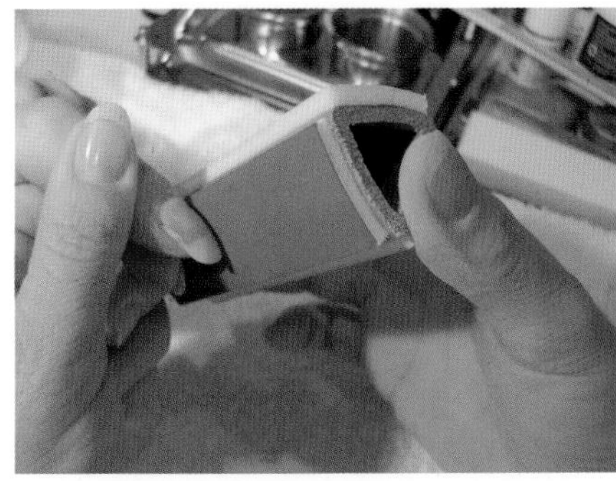

7 Finish the nail with a three-way buffer or high gloss sealant (after removing all traces of dust).

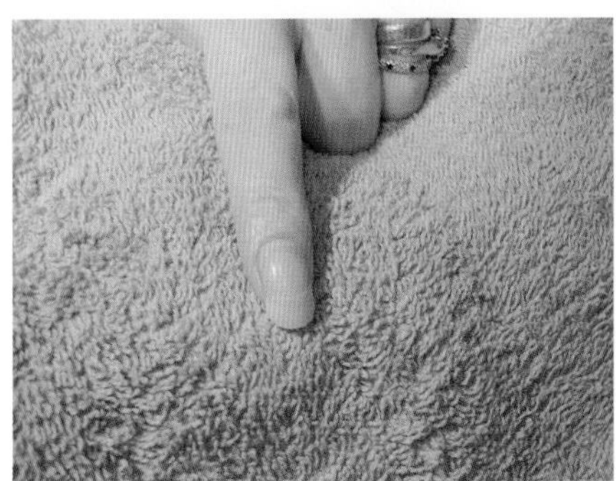

8 Apply oil to the finished nail.

Step-by-step: Re-balance treatment

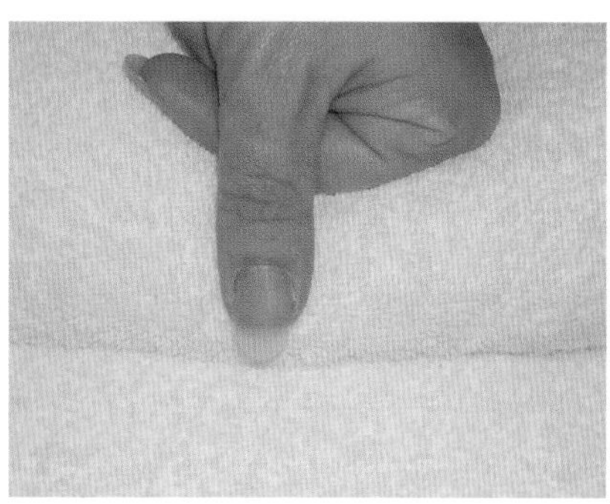

1 Assess the nails. Sanitize the hands and nails.

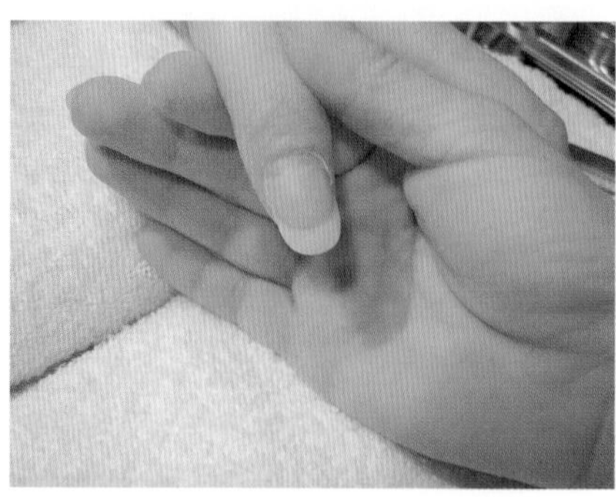

2 Shorten the length of the nail. Using a 240 grit file, thin out the whole overlay, removing the apex so that the remaining overlay is thin and even. Ensure the tip of the free edge is thinned as after shortening the nail it will be thicker than the original tip.

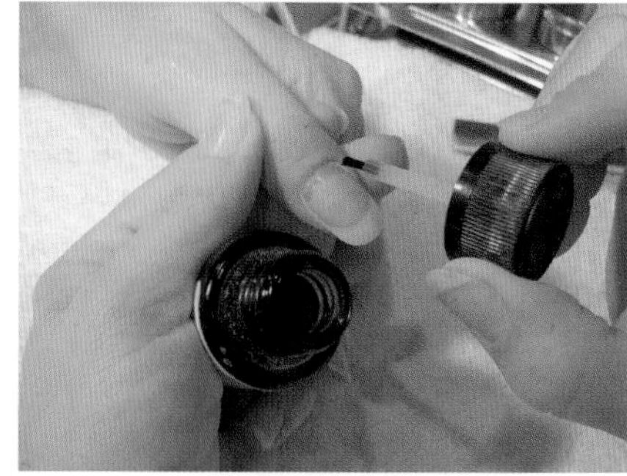

3 Remove the dust and apply dehydrator. Apply primer if required.

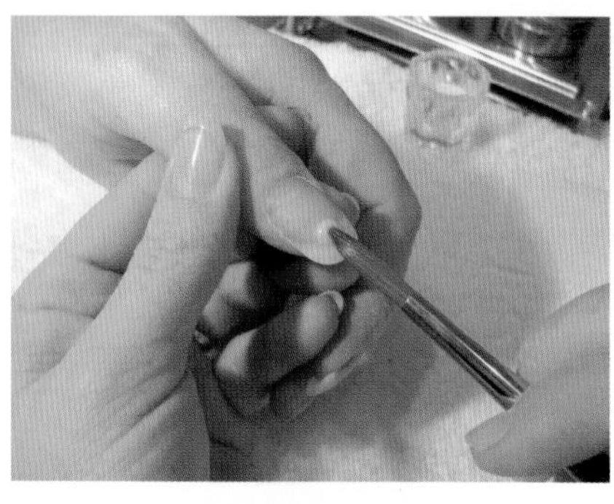

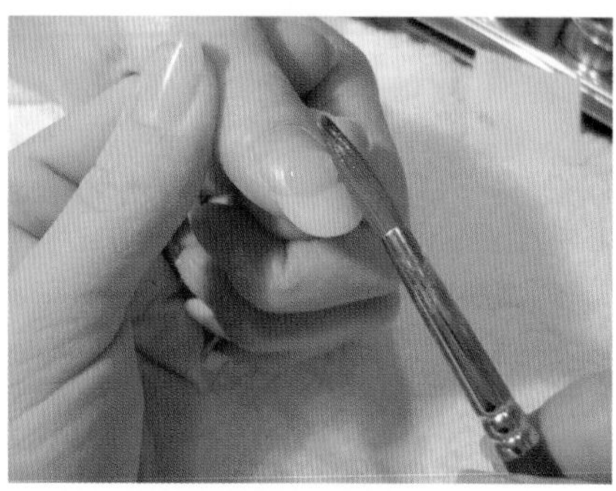

4 Apply a new overlay in exactly the same way as the original overlay. If it is a fibre system and the original fibre has not be disturbed it is not necessary to apply the fibre mesh to the whole nail as it will get too thick as time goes one. A small piece of fibre placed in Zone 3 will be sufficient. (Images show L&P application)

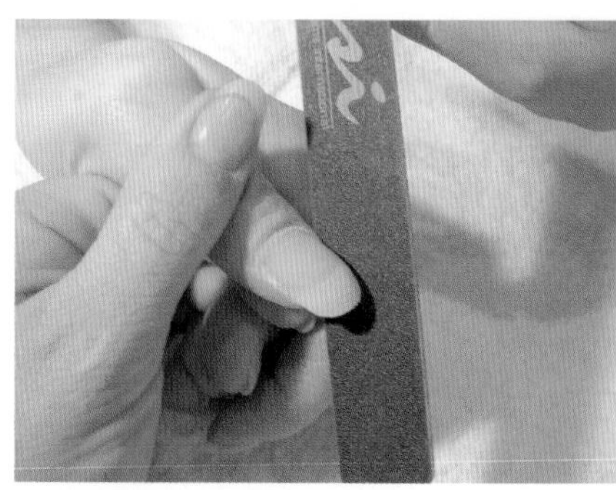

5 Refine the shape of the overlay as in the first application, checking from all angles that the structure of the curves is correct.

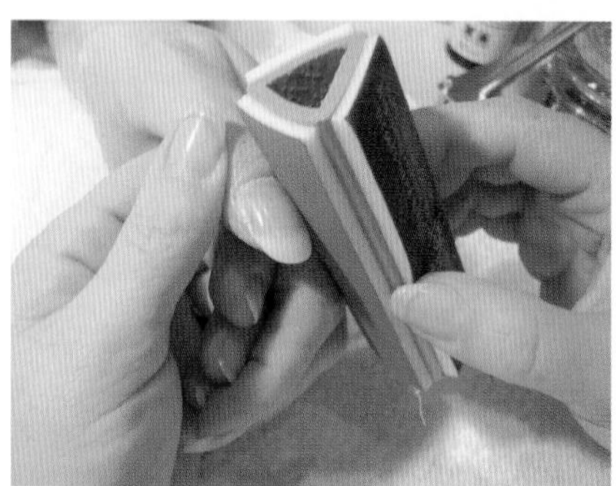

6 Finish the nail with a three-way buffer or high gloss sealant (after removing all traces of dust).

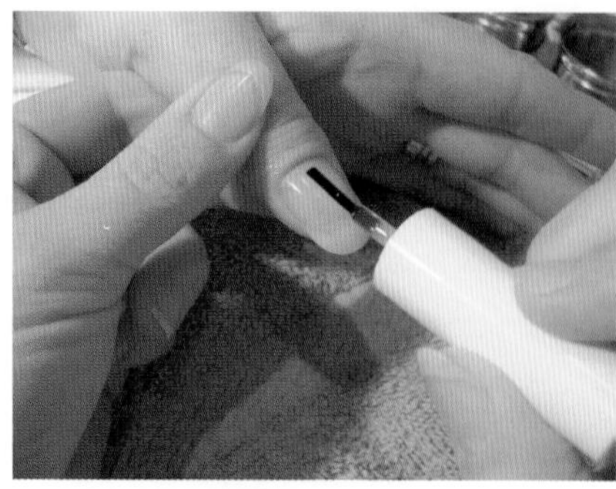

7 Apply oil to the finished nail.

Second maintenance As with the record of first maintenance, look at and ask all the same points. Compare results and determine if problems have been solved and results improved. If this is not the case, make a note of what is not right as before and complete a full self-assessment.

The removal of artificial nails

There are many occasions when it is appropriate to remove artificial nails, for example:

- the client wanted long nails for a short time only
- the natural nail has grown to a length the client is happy with
- the regular maintenance required is not possible for the client
- the client has had a set of nails applied by someone else
- there is a problem with the nails, e.g. allergic reaction, infection, etc.

TUTOR SUPPORT

Activity 9: Multiple choice quiz

Liquid and powder and fabric nails are removed in the same way:

- Remove any coloured varnish.
- Pour enough acetone into a small metal bowl (or one suitable for solvents) to just cover the nails.
- Place bowl in a larger bowl of warm (not hot) water.
- Make sure the client is seated comfortably, preferably at a desk (holding bowls of acetone on laps can result in accidents!).
- Ask the client to place their fingers in the acetone and cover the bowl and the client's hands with a towel to prevent vapours escaping.
- Liquid and powder nails will take approximately 30 minutes to come off. This time may be longer due to the thickness of the overlay and temperature. Artificial nails that have MMA as the monomer will take a lot longer.
- The resin used in the fabric system will take only 10–15 minutes.
- Do not remove the nails before the process is complete, as the product will harden immediately and then take longer.
- When all the product has gone from the nail, remove the fingers and dry them.
- Apply nail oil to the nails and fingers as they will look very white and dry.
- Buff the nails to give them a shine.
- If artificial nails have been worn for a long time, the natural nail may feel a little weak. Two or three layers of a strengthening top coat (not hardener) will help protect them until they become stronger, which will take a couple of days.

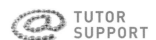

TOP TIP

Dry skin around nails

Applying oil or a barrier cream to the skin around the nails will help prevent the extreme drying effect of the acetone. This effect is very temporary and moisture will be replaced immediately but the skin does look unpleasant following the removal.

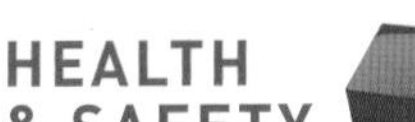

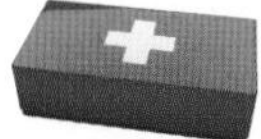

Acetone

Always dispose of the used acetone safely and always have the room well ventilated.

HEALTH & SAFETY

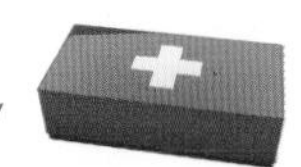

Important reminder
Always follow the manufacturer's instructions.

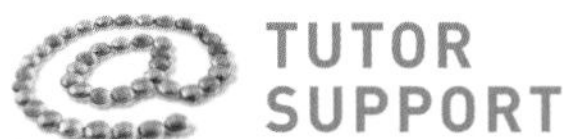

TUTOR SUPPORT

Activity 7: Recap, revision and evaluation sheet

UV gel nails are removed as follows:

- Many UV gels are resistant to acetone, so the only way to remove them is by buffing the nails off.
- Great care must be taken when doing this, as it is very easy to buff the nail plate without realizing.
- Remove any colour first.
- Using a course grit file, but taking great care when near the skin or new nail growth, remove some of the overlay.
- Before the overlay gets thin, use a fine grit file.
- When the overlay is thin, keep wiping the nail with varnish remover. This will show up overlay as shinier than natural nail and thus prevent buffing the nail.
- When the overlay and tip have gone, buff the nail for a shine and apply oil.
- The natural nail may need some protection from a nail strengthener.

If the gel used is a type that can be removed with acetone, the procedure for liquid and powder can be followed after breaking up the surface of the gel with a coarse grit file.

GLOSSARY OF KEY WORDS

Acetone a solvent commonly used as a tip remover and nail varnish remover.

Adhesive a chemical compound used to stick two surfaces together. The most common adhesive in the nail industry is cyanoacrylate.

Aftercare advice recommendations given to the client following treatment to continue the benefits of the treatment.

Allergic reaction the reaction of the body to an invasion of a chemical substance or foreign body that could be harmful or that the body has developed a sensitivity to.

Base coat a nail polish product applied to protect the natural nail.

Buffer a manicure tool with a handle made of plastic and a pad with a replaceable cover, used on the nail to give a sheen.

'C' curve the curve of the nail from side wall to side wall.

Catalyst a substance that causes or accelerates a chemical reaction.

Chemical reaction the process of two or more chemicals combining to create a different substance.

Consultation techniques assessment of client's needs using different assessment techniques, including questioning and natural observation.

Contact dermatitis a skin disorder caused by intolerance of the skin to a particular substance, or a group of substances. On exposure to the substance the skin quickly becomes irritated and an allergic reaction occurs.

Contra-action an unwanted reaction occurring during or after treatment application.

Contra-indication a problematic symptom that indicates that the treatment may not proceed.

Corrosive a substance capable of causing rapid and sometimes irreversible damage to human tissue or other surfaces.

Curing the process of polymerization.

Cuticle cream or oil a cosmetic preparation used to condition the skin of the cuticle.

Cuticle knife a metal tool used on the nail to remove excess eponychium and perionychium (the extension of the skin of the cuticle at the base of the nail).

Cuticle nippers a metal tool used to remove excess cuticle and neaten the skin around the cuticle area.

Cuticle remover a cosmetic preparation used to soften and loosen the skin cells and cuticle from the nail.

Dehydrate to remove water from the surface of the natural nail plate.

Eczema of the nail inflammation of the skin, causing changes to the nail including ridges, pitting, nail separation and nail thickening.

Fibre a nail enhancement system that combines a fibre with resin to create an artificial nail overlay.

Fibre mesh usually silk or fibreglass 'fabric' used in the fibre overlay system to provide strength.

File used to shape the free edge of the nail.

Free edge the part of the nail plate that extends past the end of the finger.

Gel a thickened liquid used as part of the UV gel system to create an artificial nail overlay.

Hangnail nail condition where small pieces of epidermal skin protrude between the nail plate and nail wall, accompanying a dry cuticle condition.

Infill a maintenance treatment than compensates for the natural nail growth after the application of artificial nails.

Ingestion one of the main routes of entry into the body; that is via the mouth.

Inhalation one of the main routes of entry into the body; that is via the lungs.

Irritant substances capable of causing inflammation of the skin, eyes, nose, throat or lungs.

Leuconychia nail condition where white spots or marks appear on the nail plate.

Lifting the separation of an artificial nail from the nail plate.

Liquid and powder a nail enhancement system that combines a liquid monomer with a powder polymer to create an artificial nail overlay.

Longitudinal ridges nail condition where grooves appear in the nail plate, running along the length of the nail from the cuticle to the free edge.

Lower arch the curve of the lower part of the free edge when viewed from the side.

Monomer a chemical compound that can be bonded to other molecules to form a polymer.

Nail plate the layers of keratinized skin cells that form a hard plate on the end of each finger and toe.

Nail polish a clear or coloured nail product that adds colour/protection to the nail. Cream polish has a matt finish and requires a top coat application. Pearlized polish produces a frosted, shimmery appearance and top coat is not required.

Nail polish remover a solvent used to remove nail polish and grease from the nails prior to applying polish.

Nail strengthener a nail polish product that strengthens the nail plate, which has a tendency to split.

Nail wrap an overlay applied to the natural nail; the fibre system is most commonly used.

Necessary action the appropriate action to take in the case of a contra-action or contra-indication to ensure the welfare of the client.

Onycholysis nail condition where the nail plate separates from the nail bed.

Onychophagy nail condition where a person bites their nails excessively.

Onychorrhexis nail condition where the person has split, flaking nails.

Orange stick a disposable wooden tool used around the cuticle and free edge of the nail and to apply products to the nail.

Overlay a coating applied to the natural nail or over a plastic tip that has been blended with the natural nail.

Paronychia bacterial infection where swelling, redness and pus appear in the cuticle area of the nail wall.

Photoinitiator a substance that responds to specific types of light to start a chemical reaction e.g. UV light.

Polymer a long chain or chemically bonded monomers e.g. the acrylics used in nail enhancement systems.

Polymerization the chemical reaction that creates polymer chains from monomer compounds.

Primer a substance used to improve the adhesion between the nail plate and artificial products.

Psoriasis of the nail an inflammatory condition where there is an increased production of cells in the upper part of the skin. Pitting occurs on the surface of the nail.

Pterygium a nail condition where the cuticle is thickened and overgrown.

Re-balance a maintenance treatment that corrects the position of the apex when it has moved because of natural nail growth.

Resin in relation to nail enhancements, a type of cyanoacrylate used in the fibre nail enhancement system.

Resin activator in relation to nail enhancements, a product that speeds up the cure time of cyanoacrylate resin.

Scissors nail tools used for cutting nails, artificial tips and fibre mesh for fibre overlays.

Sensitization the biological process of becoming sensitive to a substance that can then cause an allergic reaction.

Smile line also called the onychodermal band; the curved line that is created naturally by the hyponychium or artificially with a coloured overlay.

Stop point the part of the plastic tips that fits against the free edge of the natural nail.

System in relation to nail enhancements, the type of nail enhancement used to overlay the natural nail or plastic tip e.g. acrylic, UV gel, fibre.

Tinea unguium fungal infection of the nails. The nail is yellowish-grey in colour.

Top coat a nail polish product applied over another nail polish to provide additional strength and durability to the finish.

Transverse furrows nail condition where grooves appear on the nail, running from side to side.

Treatment plan after the consultation, suitable treatment objectives are established to treat the client's conditions and needs.

Ultraviolet (UV) light an invisible part of the spectrum above the colour violet in the visible light bands.

UV gel a nail enhancement system that uses UV light to initiate polymerization in a pre-mixed gel to create an artificial nail overlay.

UV light cured the process of polymerization (curing) using a photoiniator, in this case UV light, to start the chemical reaction.

Vapour molecules of a chemical in the air, created by evaporation of the chemical.

Verruca or wart a viral infection where small epidermal skin growths appear, either raised or flat depending upon their location, and have a rough surface.

White tip powder a white acrylic powder used to create a white free edge on an artificial nail.

Wrap fabrics material used in nail enhancements to overlay the natural nail to provide strength e.g. fibreglass, silk.

Zones in relation to nail enhancements, the three areas of the artificial nail referred to when creating the correct artificial structure.

ASSESSMENT OF KNOWLEDGE AND UNDERSTANDING

You have now learnt about providing and maintaining nail enhancements in the beauty therapy workplace. To test your level of knowledge, answer the following short questions. These will prepare you for your summative (final) assessment.

1. Nail __________ removes surface moisture and tiny amounts of oil left on the natural nail.
   a. primer
   b. dehydrator
   c. adhesive
   d. abrasive

2. A disease that is communicable or easily spread by contact is a __________ disease.
   a. contaminant
   b. contagious
   c. infection
   d. allergy

3. The portion of the skin that supports the nail plate as it grows toward the free edge is the nail:
   a. groove
   b. fold
   c. plate
   d. bed

4. Visible ridges running across the width of the natural nail plate are:
   a. ridges
   b. leukonychia
   c. melanonychia
   d. Beau's lines

5. Nail __________ is used for securing nail tips to the natural nails.
   a. primer
   b. dehydrator
   c. adhesive
   d. abrasive

6. How often should a client receive nail maintenance treatments?
   a. when the client feels it is necessary
   b. once a week
   c. every two weeks
   d. once a month

7. What is applied at the end of every nail enhancement treatment?
   a. cuticle oil
   b. cuticle remover
   c. cuticle cream
   d. hand cream

8. The maintenance procedure that removes the apex, restores and corrects it is a:
   a. re-balance
   b. infill

9. To remove liquid and powder or fibre artificial nails you can use:
   a. acetate
   b. acetone
   c. dehydrator
   d. acrylic

10. When applying overlay, the area behind the smile line where maximum strength is needed is which zone?

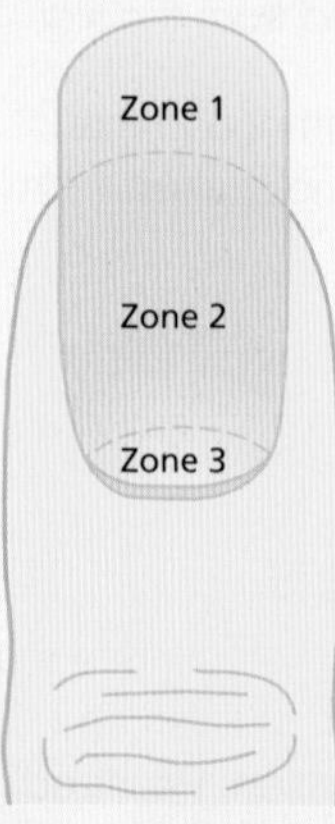

Zones of the nail

14 Nail Art

Learning Objectives

This chapter covers **VRQ Unit Provide nail art.**

This unit is about how to provide nail art. Nail art is an exciting and elaborate form of nail decoration, which may be applied to the hands and feet. There are a variety of nail art techniques which are limited only by imagination and creativity. It can be as simple as a single stripe across the nail or as intricate as a desert island.

There are **two** learning outcomes for this unit which you must achieve:

1 Be able to prepare for nail art service

2 Be able to provide nail art service

From the range statement, you must show that you can:

- use **consultation techniques** to identify the treatment objectives
- use all listed **products, tools and equipment and techniques** as appropriate
- identify **nail conditions**
- ensure that the **environmental conditions** are suitable
- complete a consultation and skin inspection to identify any **contra-indications**
- **communicate and behave** in an appropriate and professional manner
- follow all **health and safety working practices**
- provide relevant **aftercare** and **contra-action advice**

You must be able to show you have the necessary practical skills and underpinning knowledge to provide nail art.

This unit is linked to the Beauty Therapy NOS **Unit N4.**

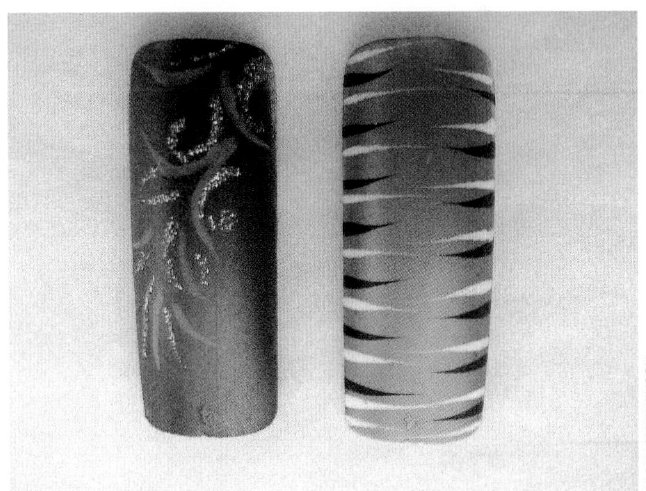

TRACEY STEPHENSON

Freehand painted designs

TOP TIP

Looking for inspiration

Nail trade magazines and websites are extremely useful to keep you updated on the latest colours, nail products and designs, as many nails artists display their designs.

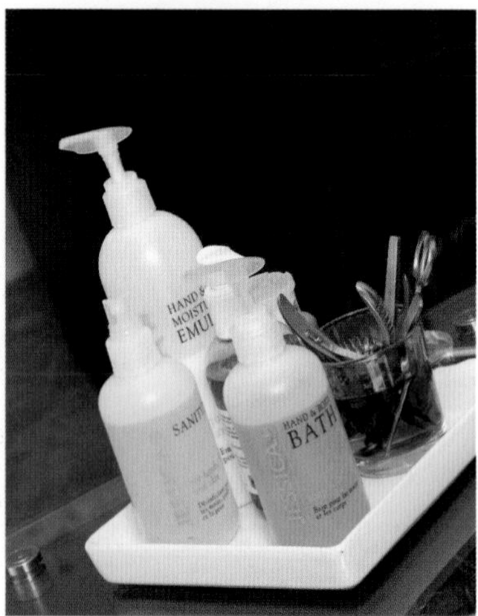

Tidy the nails with basic nail care before nail art

Essential anatomy and physiology knowledge requirements for this chapter are identified on the checklist chart on page 27.

Nail art

Nail art is a skill and takes practice and requires a very good eye for detail.

The nail art skill starts when a 'French manicure' is applied, demonstrated in Chapter 11 Manicure Treatments, as this is actually two colours which need to be painted very accurately. The skill becomes even more advanced when other colours and actual designs are incorporated. You do not need to be a great artist in order to create quite stunning and very commercially acceptable designs. There are many easy **nail art techniques** and products that allow even the most 'artistically challenged' to produce some stunning designs!

There are many products available on the market today that, with a few guidelines and hints, can create stunning 'masterpieces' at minimal cost and effort. The real effort is practising! Nail art is visual and there are a relatively small number of basic **painting techniques** that, using readily available products, can be demonstrated in a few step-by-step pictures. Every newcomer to nail art will find that, with the right direction and range of products, a few initial ideas will lead on to many, many more.

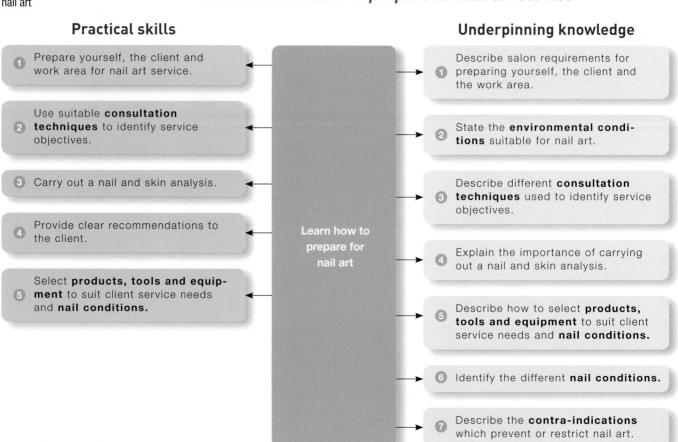

Although some more unusual designs are included, the aim of this chapter is to provide the underpinning knowledge and practical skills of the various techniques of nail art which are practical to carryout in a commercial salon or freelance situation.

Preparing for nail art

Outcome 1: Be able to prepare for nail art service

Learn how to prepare for nail art

Practical skills

1. Prepare yourself, the client and work area for nail art service.
2. Use suitable **consultation techniques** to identify service objectives.
3. Carry out a nail and skin analysis.
4. Provide clear recommendations to the client.
5. Select **products, tools and equipment** to suit client service needs and **nail conditions.**

Underpinning knowledge

1. Describe salon requirements for preparing yourself, the client and the work area.
2. State the **environmental conditions** suitable for nail art.
3. Describe different **consultation techniques** used to identify service objectives.
4. Explain the importance of carrying out a nail and skin analysis.
5. Describe how to select **products, tools and equipment** to suit client service needs and **nail conditions.**
6. Identify the different **nail conditions.**
7. Describe the **contra-indications** which prevent or restrict nail art.

Preparing the work area

Prepare the work area to meet all health and safety legislation requirements. The work surface must be stable to avoid products being knocked over or spilt. The area must be free of any other previously used materials and debris, such as dust created from the application of artificial nails. Dust can spoil the effect of a client's newly painted nails. Lighting must be good to enable you to avoid eyestrain, especially when performing intricate artwork. It is a good idea to use a magnifying lamp.

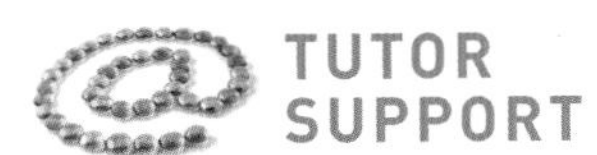

TUTOR SUPPORT

Activity 2: Design a promotional poster

All the health and safety rules and legislation that you learnt in Chapter 3 Health and Safety, Chapter 11 Manicure Treatments and Chapter 12 Pedicure Treatments must be followed.

Ensure all tools and equipment are clean, sterilized and disinfected as appropriate and are neatly organized on the nail work station. Before beginning nail art service check you have all the necessary products, tools and equipment to hand and that they meet all legal hygiene and industry requirements for nail services.

PRODUCTS, TOOLS AND EQUIPMENT

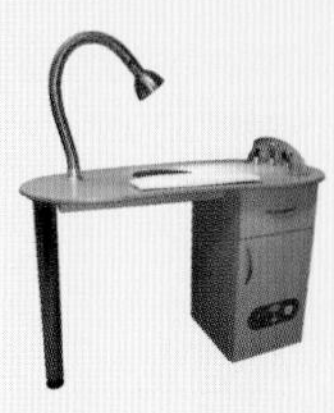

Nail work station
On which to place everything. You will require manicure tools and equipment to prepare the nails for nail art.
A light is useful when carrying out detailed techniques.

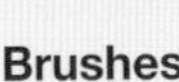

Brushes
A variety of shapes and sizes of brushes for free-hand painting including **detail brush, striping brush, flat brush** and **fan brush**

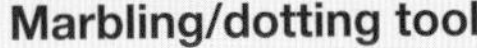

Marbling/dotting tool
For creating 'marbling' or 'dotting' designs with the paint

NAIL DELIGHTS

Foils/transfers/tapes/stencils
A variety of materials for creating designs

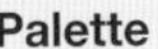

Palette
For placing nail art paints on for use or mixing

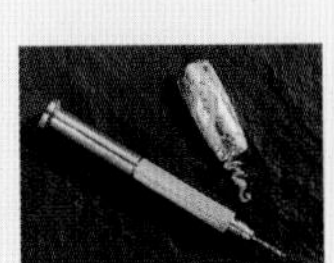

Nail piercing tool
For making small holes in the nail for jewellery attachments

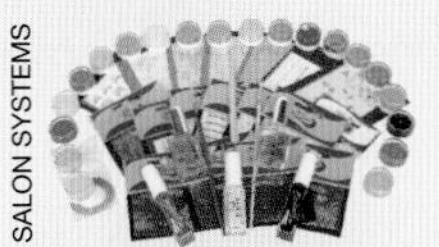

SALON SYSTEMS

Nail art paints
Specialized water-based acrylic paints for nail art

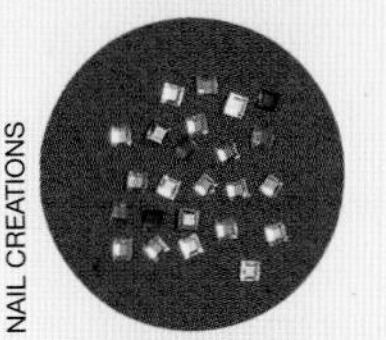

NAIL CREATIONS

Polish secures
Small stones or shapes for attaching to the nail as part of the design

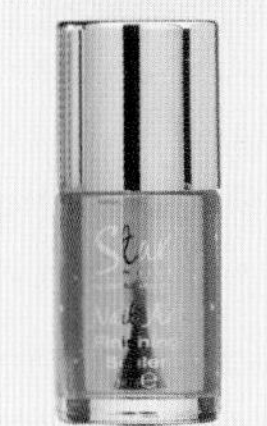

Specialized nail art sealer/top coat
For sealing the design once the paint is dry

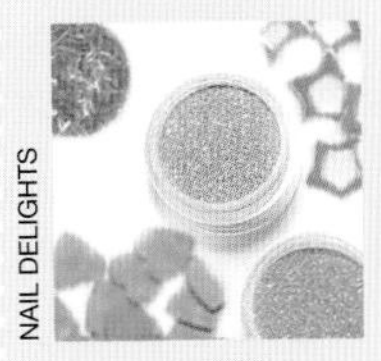

NAIL DELIGHTS

Glitter polishes/dusts
Can be used to create or enhance nail art designs

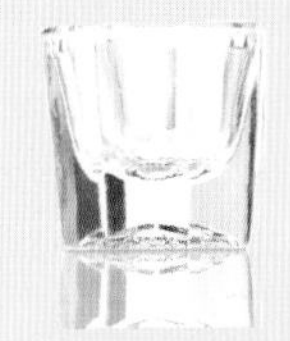

Dappen dishes
For keeping polish secures or glitter in

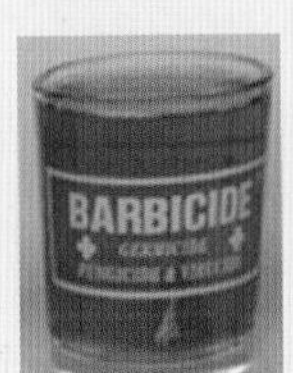

Disinfectant solution
To store small stainless steel sterilized tools

YOU WILL ALSO NEED:

Nail polish remover to remove nail polish/products as required

Nail polishes including base coat and a range of colored polishes

Medium sized towels (3) To dry the skin, nails, etc. and protect the client's clothing

Water spray For re-wetting the nail art paints when they start to dry out

Skin disinfectant To cleanse and disinfect the client's skin and nails

Waste container This should be a lined metal bin with a lid to contain vapours from solvents

Tissues or disposal towels To cover the work area when using paints and protect the client's clothing

Cotton buds A damp cotton bud can be used to remove mistakes made with nail art paint

Client record card To record the client's personal details, products used and details of the service

Sterilization and disinfection

Hygiene must be maintained in a number of ways to prevent secondary and cross-infection:

- ensure that tools and equipment are clean and where applicable sterile before use
- disinfect work surfaces after each client
- always follow hygienic practices
- clear discarded waste after each client
- maintain a high standard of personal hygiene.

TOP TIP

Spoilt polish

It is a good idea for the client to pay before the service to prevent spoiling the nail art.

Reception

Nail art should be priced as a stand alone service, not just included in the cost of a manicure, pedicure or nail extension service. When a client makes an appointment for nail art discuss the cost of the service; prices will vary depending on the products and materials used, or the time involved to create the design.

Some designs are very quick and use little product, for example a flick of paint with a nail art brush or a simple **marbling** technique. Other designs are very quick but use more costly products, for example polish secures that are fast to apply, but cost much more than a flick of nail art paint or a couple of 'blobs' of nail polish.

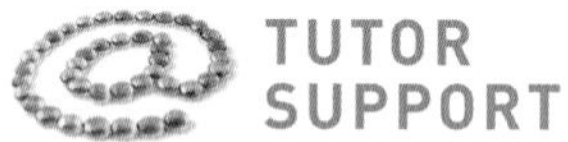

Activity 3: Nail art wordsearch 1

Nail art is very tricky to price. If it costs too much clients are unlikely to want it as it will only last a short time. However, you must be realistic in your pricing and the most popular designs are bound to be those that are quick to apply but look stunning. The simplest designs are often the most effective and may appeal to a wider client base.

If the client's natural nails are in poor condition it will be necessary to allow extra time to perform a simple nail treatment, to improve the nails' appearance, and facilitate application. The client must be aware that it may take time for the nail products to harden.

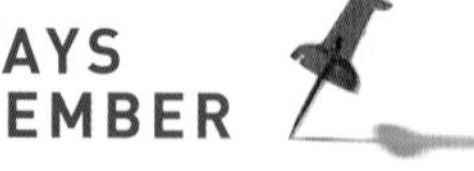

Be realistic

Although designs look effective displayed on quite large plastic tips, remember that the design will look very different on a much smaller nail on a finger and some designs are much easier to apply on a tip than a real nail as the surrounding skin can get in the way!

Commercial timing

Allow 30 minutes for nail art application.

Consultation

If a client shows an interest in nail art, the next step is careful questioning. Find out at the **consultation**, the client's likes and dislikes and how adventurous they are; do they have a specific idea for a design or are they prepared to give you free rein? Make sure you understand what your client is saying and that you are clear about the degree of 'statement' she is interested in making with her nails. For example, a client usually known for her conservative taste in clothes and natural nails with sheer or delicate colours, who is interested in nail art for a special occasion, is only likely to be interested in a very subtle design. Alternatively, a client who likes to try out new ideas, such as the latest fashion trends, may be open to a more interesting suggestion such as rhinestones or an unusual nail polish application technique.

It is a good idea to prepare a number of nail art designs to show the client. These may be applied to artificial nails, or they may be images of nail art designs that you have created and photographed. On your display have designs in two or three colour ways to demonstrate that a design can be customized to suit the client and show how different colour combinations can change the design dramatically. Start the display with the simpler and less expensive designs and progress to the more elaborate and more involved designs.

Assess the condition of the client's nails and cuticles before the service. If the client's expectations are unsuitable because of the client's natural nail shape or size or condition of the nail, offer a suitable alternative. For example, if the client's nails were too short, if qualified, you could apply tips to the natural nail, blend and paint these. Decide upon the nail shape and length. It is important the at the nail shape and length selected suits the clients hands and fingers. Refer to pages 377–378 for further guidance on preparing the natural nail.

TOP TIP

Nail art display

A display can look more realistic to clients if the tips are the commercial 'stick-ons' as they are closer to the size and shape of most clients' nails.

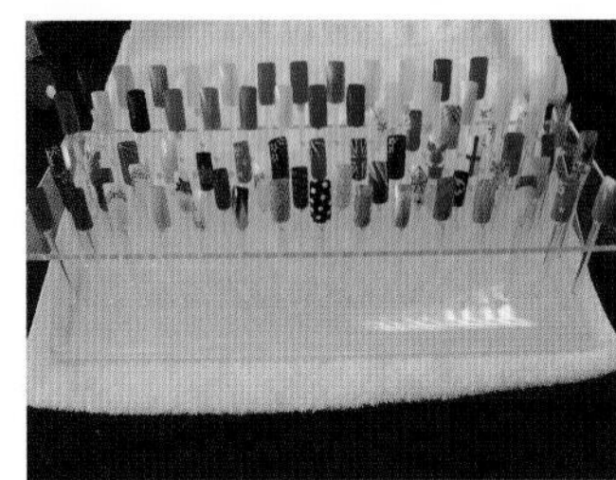

Great way to display nail art

ACTIVITY

Questioning for client satisfaction

Think of questions you could ask the client the ensure that they will be happy with the final nail art result. Examples include:

- What type of result do they wish to achieve?
- Are the nails to match a special outfit?
- What colour would be most suitable? Or if for a special occasion is the nail art to match a theme?

TOP TIP

Promotion

One of the best forms of promoting the nail art service is by wearing it.

Contra-indications

Whilst assessing the client's hands/feet you should be looking for any **contra-indications** to nail art. Contra-indications are the same as for any other nail service (see pages 362–367). If the client has a disease or disorder of the hand or nail it is in the interest of the client and therapist not to proceed with the nail art service. Treating a client with a contra-indication may lead to cross-infection or a worsening of the client's condition. It is important to advise the client to seek medical advice to ensure a correct diagnosis and treatment for their condition. Some conditions will require restriction and adaption of the nail art service.

KNOWLEDGE CHECK

What are the different nail shapes?

Need more time... refer to page 377 to help you.

Contra-actions

Certain cosmetic ingredients are known to cause allergic reactions in some people. These substances are known as allergens and may cause irritation, excessive erythema, inflammation and swelling. This is known as a **contra-action**. This may occur during or following service.

The client may at any time develop an allergy to a nail art product that has been successfully used previously. This could be for a number of reasons, such as new medication being taken or illness. If an allergic reaction occurs remove the product immediately and a soothing substance may be applied. This product should not be used again. See page 368 for more information on contra-actions.

As with all treatments, accurate **client record cards** must be kept for clients receiving nail art services. If the client has received nail art services before, consult the record card

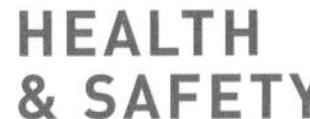

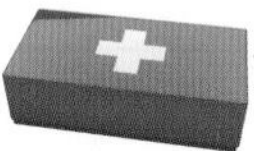

HEALTH & SAFETY

Dealing with a contra-indication

Remember never advise the client as to what the contra-indication may be; you are not qualified to do so. Always refer the client to their GP if you are at all unsure. Do not treat the client.

TOP TIP

Costing

When allowing for time in costing a design, use an average time that the design would take. Initially when inexperienced it will take you longer to achieve the finished nail art but you shouldn't be charging the client extra for that time.

HEALTH & SAFETY

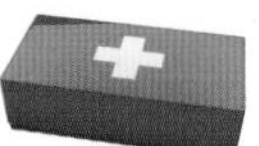

Avoiding a contra-action

Always check at the consultation for any known allergies to substances or ingredients. Formaldehyde is used in some base coats to strengthen the nail plate and it can cause an allergic reaction in some people. Always follow the manufacturers' instructions to ensure that products are used correctly and safely.

ACTIVITY

Practice some designs on a nail tip and then a real finger. You will notice the appearance and application are different.

KNOWLEDGE CHECK

Name three contra-indications observed at consultation that would prevent treatment being carried out. This can apply to the nails of the hands or feet.

Need more time... refer to pages 362–367 to help you.

and review the success and satisfaction of this with the client. Details of the products used should be recorded on the client record card. This is useful if the client returns for this service, also it is important in the event of a contra-action such as an allergic reaction.

Preparation of the nail technician

Sitting properly is important. Ideally sit on a properly designed manicure stool or chair which offers adequate back support. When completing nail art it is important to sit upright with both feet flat on the floor.

Preparation of the client

Ensure that the client is warm and comfortable when preparing them for nail art.

- Confirm the clients choice of nail art.
- File the nails to achieve the desired shape and length.
- Ensure the free edge is clean.
- The cuticles should be neat and smooth.
- Use the cuticle nippers to trim uneven, excess cuticle.
- Ensure the surface of the nail plate is clean and grease free.
- Wipe with a non-acetone polish remover to prepare the nail. Use a lint free pad as cotton wool may leave fibres, which may spoil the application of nail polish/paint.
- Apply the required nail art base (usually a good quality base coat).

Basic nail art techniques

All the basic techniques are easy! All they need is some ideas, a bit of imagination and the right products, tools and equipment.

The paints used are different from nail polishes. They are usually water-based acrylic artists' paint, as this gives a very dense colour, can be mixed and is easier to use for fine detail. There are lots of effects that can be achieved with paints, a selection of nail art brushes and a 'marbling tool'.

Nails need to be painted with a base colour that will be part of or enhance the finished design. This is usually a nail polish that should be touch dry before painting any designs.

- Very simple but effective designs can be achieved by placing dots of colour. Use either a very small round brush or a 'marbling or dotting tool' to apply the dots (1). Care needs to be taken on the size and regularity of the dots as this can spoil a good design.
- A very long, thin brush referred to as a 'striping' brush dipped in paint can achieve fine stripes and create quite sophisticated designs (2).

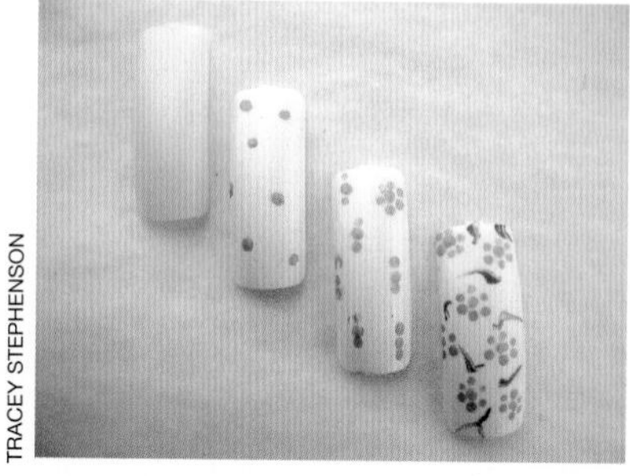

TRACEY STEPHENSON

(1) Steps: Base colour, flower centres, flower petals, finished design with stems added

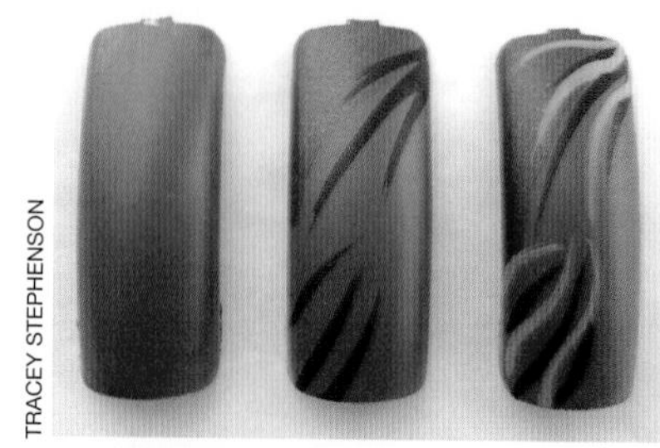

TRACEY STEPHENSON

(2) Steps: Base colour and stripes

Outcome 2: Be able to provide nail art service

Learn how to provide nail art

Practical skills

1. **Communicate and behave** in a professional manner.
2. Follow **health and safety working practices.**
3. Position yourself and client correctly throughout the service.
4. Use **products, tools, equipment and techniques** to suit clients service needs and nail conditions.
5. Complete the service to the satisfaction of the client.
6. Record the results of the service.
7. Provide suitable **aftercare advice.**

Underpinning knowledge

1. State how to **communicate and behave** in a professional manner.
2. Describe **health and safety working practices.**
3. State the importance of positioning yourself and the client correctly throughout the treatment.
4. State the importance of using **products, tools, equipment** and techniques to suit clients treatment needs and **nail conditions.**
5. Describe how treatments can be adapted to suit client treatment needs and **nail conditions.**
6. State the **contra-actions** that may occur during and following services and how to respond.
7. State the importance of completing the treatment to the satisfaction of the client.
8. State the importance of completing treatment records.
9. State the **aftercare advice** that should be provided.
10. Describe diseases and disorders of the nail.
11. Describe the structure and functions of the nail.

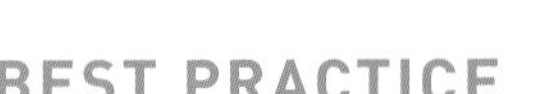

BEST PRACTICE

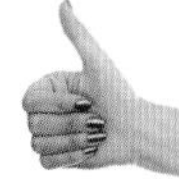

Nail polish storage

Store nail polish stock in a cool, dark place to avoid separation and fading. Use good stock control, FIFO – First In, First Out, to ensure optimum quality of resources.

HEALTH & SAFETY

Legislation

It is important that you comply with all relevant health and safety legislation while performing nail art

Examples include:

- Control of Substances Hazardous to Health Regulations (COSHH) (2002)
- Personal Protective Equipment (PPE) at Work Regulations (1992)

Remember to use the underpinning knowledge and practical skills you have learnt in **Chapter 2 Health and Safety; Chapter 11 Manicure Treatments and Chapter 12 Pedicure Treatments.**

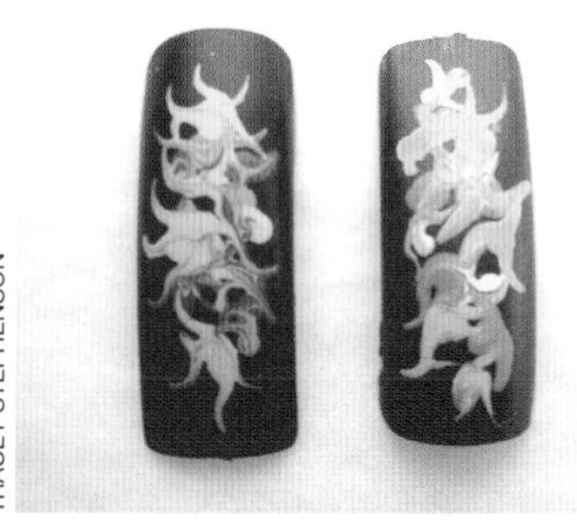
TRACEY STEPHENSON

Designs using marbling

Abstract patterns or marbling can look stunning with a good choice of colour combinations. Flicking the colour from side to side with a fine brush or placing spots of colour on the nail and mixing them together with the 'marbling tool' achieves this effect.

- Those who are not so good at hand painting designs can use stencils. The types that are readily available have a sticky back to keep them in place. These are applied to a dry nail and painted over. When the nail paint is completely dry they are removed, leaving the chosen design behind.

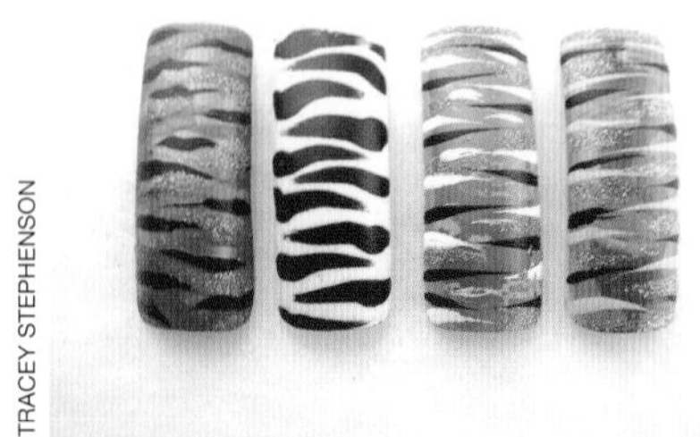
TRACEY STEPHENSON

Designs achieved with brushes

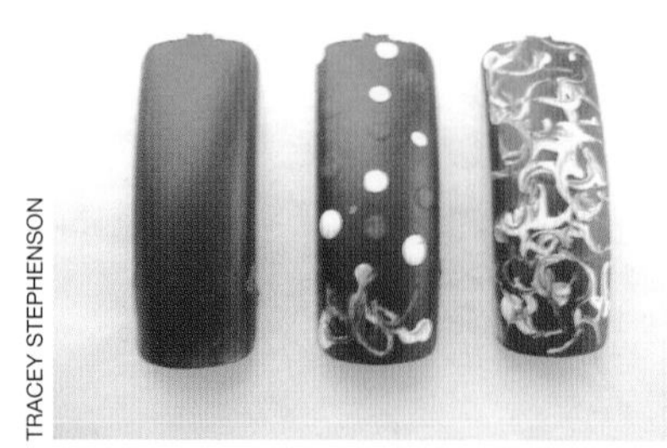
TRACEY STEPHENSON

Steps: Base colour, add two or more different coloured dots, swirl together

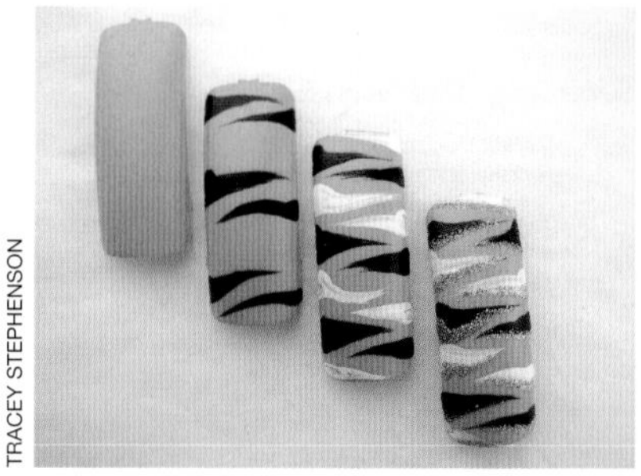
TRACEY STEPHENSON

Steps: Base colour, hand painted stripes

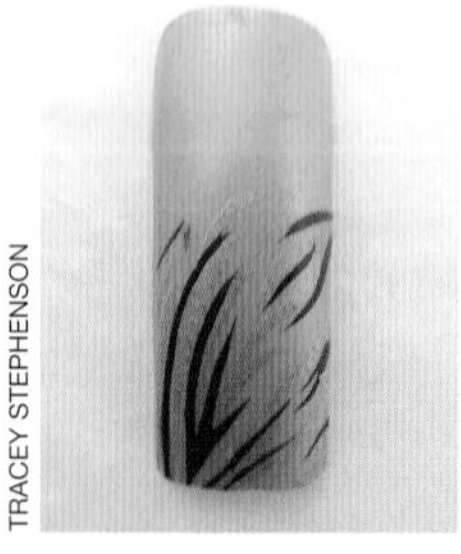
TRACEY STEPHENSON

A design achieved with brushes

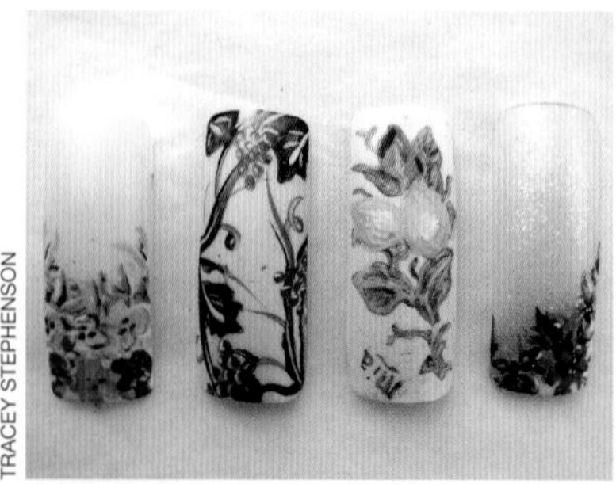
TRACEY STEPHENSON

Designs using brush techniques

- Pictures of all sorts can be painted on a nail with a steady hand, a good imagination' or an easy picture to copy. (Most nail artists keep large numbers of pictures to copy onto a nail or just to give them inspiration to create an original design.)
- Buy or find a palette. This can be any plastic surface that can be easily cleaned with water. This can be used to place nail art paints on for use or mixing. Have a small water spray to hand then, if your paints start drying out, give a small spray of distilled water to keep them workable.

Nail art paint is water-based and any mistakes can be easily removed with a wet nail wipe, or a cotton bud will remove a small part.

In all nail art, sealing the design is very important and, when the paint is dry, a sealer or top coat must be applied to fix the paint and also bring out the colour. The manufacturer's recommended sealer should be used, as some top coats may react to the paints. Clients should be advised to re-seal the nails every couple of days to keep them fresh-looking and avoid any chips.

Nail art brushes

There are many brushes specifically sold for nail art purposes but also remember that art shops sell many shapes and sizes too. A small collection of brushes is necessary to the technician in order to create a wide range of styles and these can be purchased relatively cheaply from suppliers and, with care, will last a long time.

- *Detail brush*. This is the smallest brush and is used for hand painting details or placing dots.

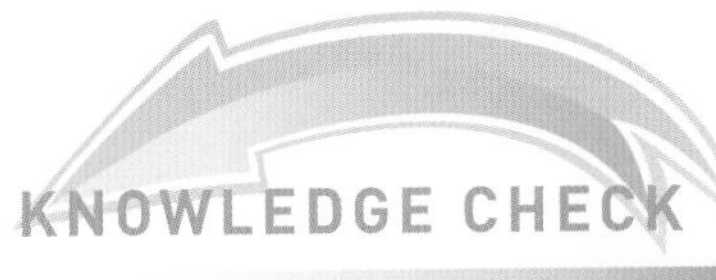

KNOWLEDGE CHECK

How would you decide upon the recommended nail art for a client?

Need more time... refer to pages 470–472 to help you.

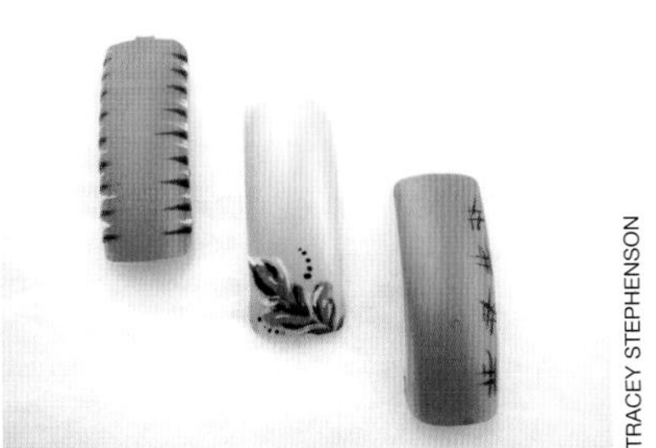

TRACEY STEPHENSON

Hand painted designs

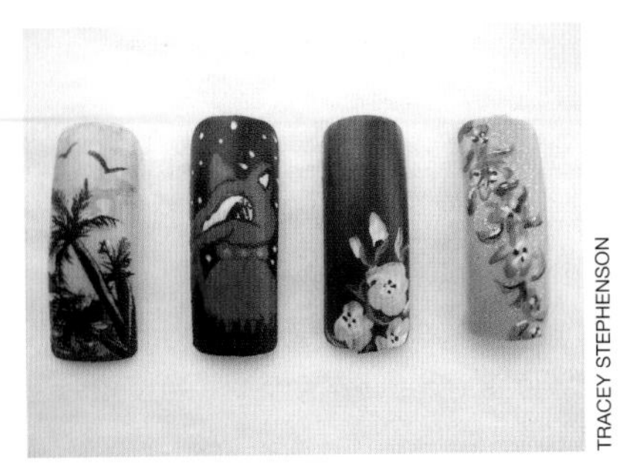

TRACEY STEPHENSON

Hand painted designs

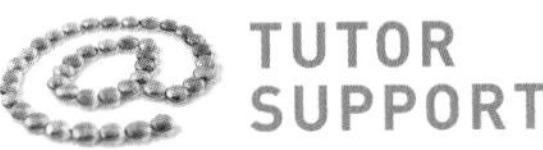

TUTOR SUPPORT

Activity 5: Develop a 'nail file'

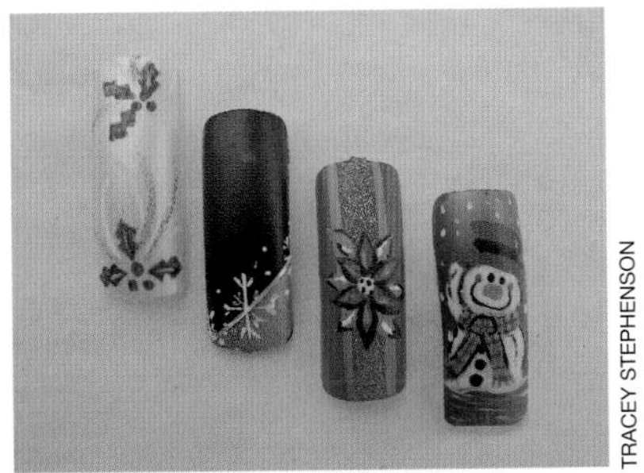

TRACEY STEPHENSON

Hand painting with a theme

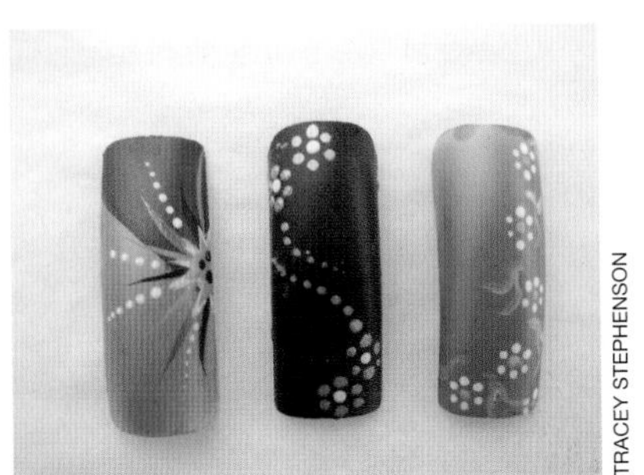

TRACEY STEPHENSON

Hand painted designs using dotting and striping

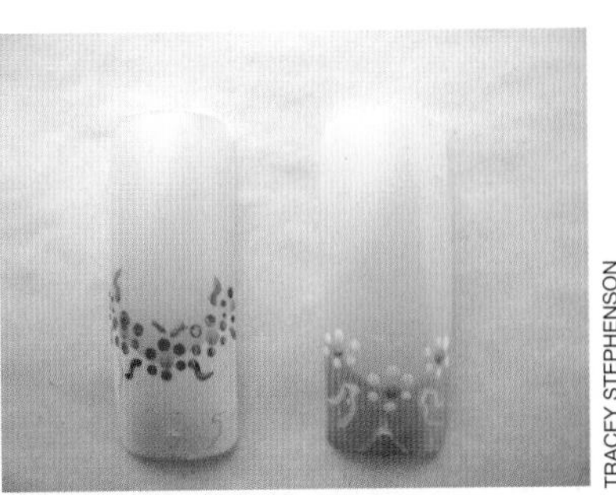

TRACEY STEPHENSON

Designs with French manicure style and dots

- *Striping brushes*. These are available in different sizes. Their length and the number of hairs are relevant. A shorter brush with several hairs will produce lines that are thick. The longer and thinner the brush, the finer and longer the line they produce. It is worth having at least two of these: a medium one for lines and flicks and a very long one for fine stripes.

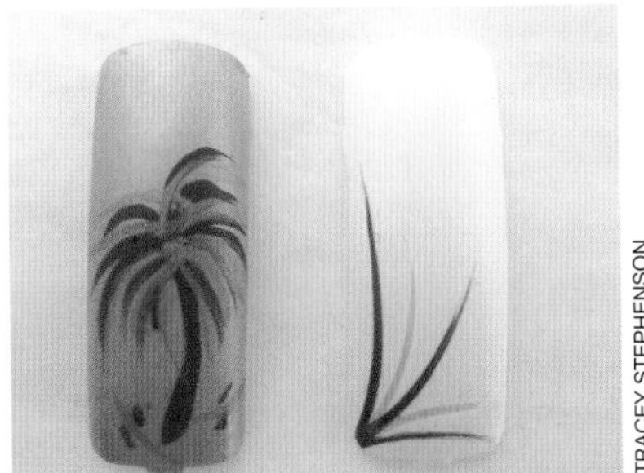

TRACEY STEPHENSON

Designs using striping

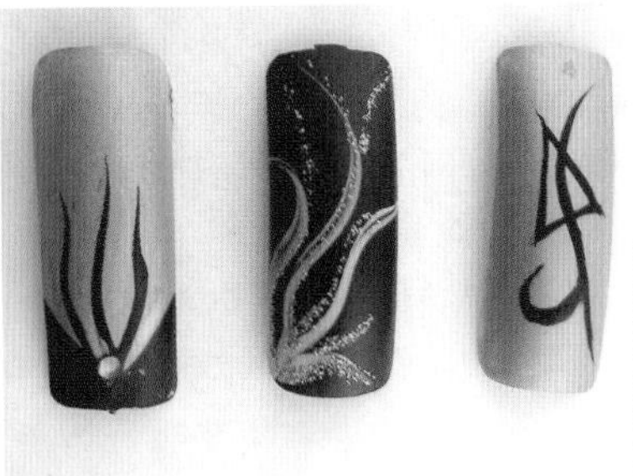

TRACEY STEPHENSON

Designs using striping

- *Flat brush*. This is a brush with a small flat head that can create several effects and is used to fill in colours. It can shade and smudge and create swirls.
- *Fan brush*. This brush can create texture and blend colours together. It is probably not as versatile as the others but worth having.

TOP TIP

Brush techniques

If you have a very long striping brush, try placing three or four dots of different coloured paint next to each other on a plastic palette (or similar). Lay the brush in the dots and turn it so all the hairs are coated. Then lay the brush on the nail and lift off. An attractive multi-coloured stripe will be left behind. Try different colours and techniques of applying to the nail and see what happens.

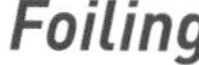

TOP TIP

Experimental techniques

Put dots of two different colours on your palette. Dip one corner of a flat brush in one colour and the other corner of the brush in the other colour. Then apply to the nail turning the brush in a circular motion. See what happens!

Foiling

Foiling is another very easy technique that uses various designs of a foil supplied on a roll. This is almost instant nail art, as some foils have designs on them and just need applying to a painted nail.

- Nails should be painted before using foils. They can be painted with a base coat, but it is worth spending the extra time to paint a colour, as this will enhance the effect.
- Foils are supplied with a special adhesive that should be painted onto the nail in a very thin coat. The adhesive is usually white and needs to turn clear before the foil is applied; this takes a very short time. The foil is then applied to the tacky adhesive, pattern side uppermost, gently pressed onto the nail with either a finger or a cotton bud and the backing pulled off leaving the foil behind. It is not necessary to cut any foil from the roll, as it will only stick to where the adhesive is.
- This is an amazingly quick process that can have spectacular results. As the foil only sticks to where the adhesive has been applied, patterns or pictures can be drawn with the adhesive. The foil needs a special sealer, as most topcoats will destroy the delicate layer. Several layers of sealer are also needed, as with all nail art, to keep it intact.

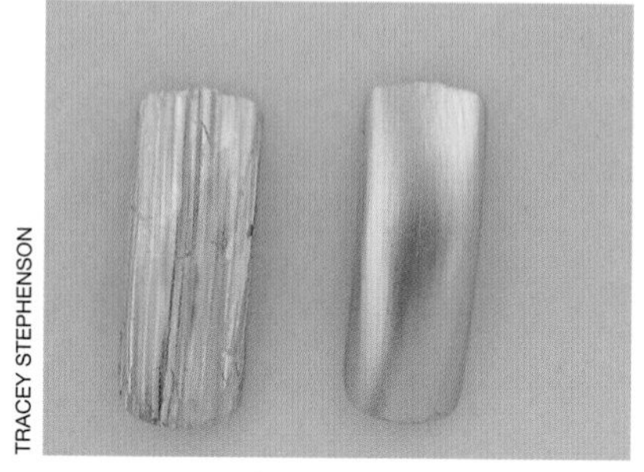

TRACEY STEPHENSON

Foiled nail

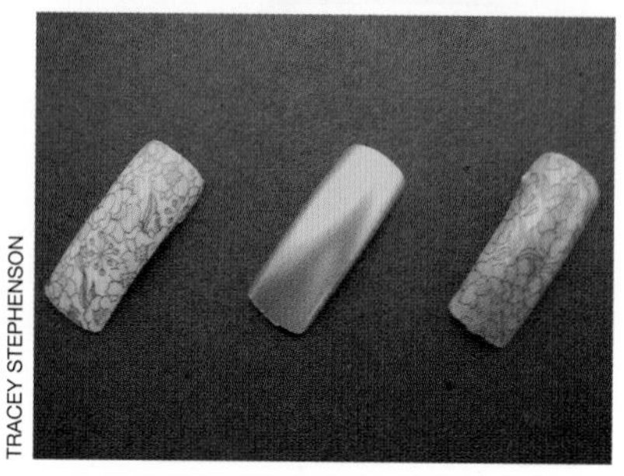

TRACEY STEPHENSON

Same foil but silver polish under one

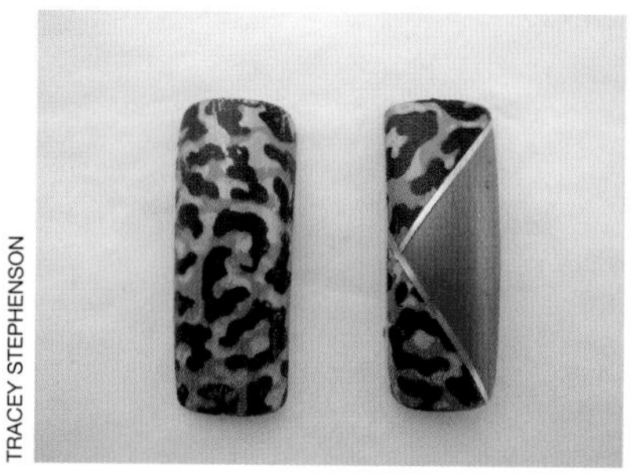

TRACEY STEPHENSON

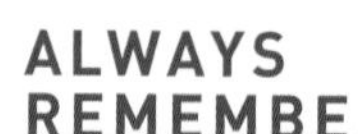

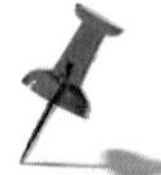

ALWAYS REMEMBER

Maintaining your nail art brushes

- Clean your brushes thoroughly after use
- Nylon brushes may be cleaned safely in acetone or washed in detergents as applicable.
- Brushes should be cleaned to remove nail art material used.
- Brushes made of animal hair are delicate so harsh detergents and acetone should be avoided. Clean in water temperatures 45–55°C.
- Always reshape the brushes when drying at room temperature.
- Dry upright to retain the brush shape.
- Only use brushes for their intended use.
- Replace brushes when quality deteriorates: poor quality brushes will affect the end result!

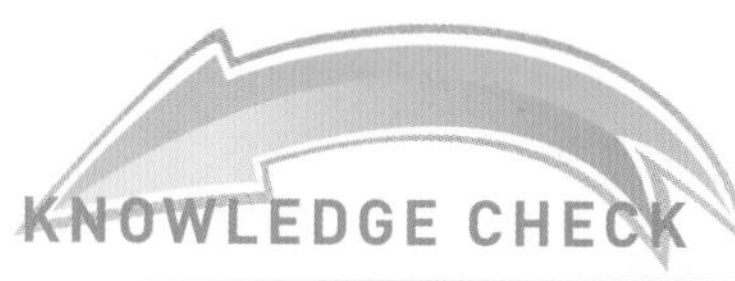

KNOWLEDGE CHECK

What different brushes are available for nail art? When are each used?

Need more time... refer to pages 472–473 to help you.

Polish secures

As the name suggests, this technique requires polish to secure the design. Many different products are available for this easy technique. **Polish secures** are the term for small stones or shapes with a flat back that are placed into the wet nail varnish and held secure when it dries. The products that fall into this category sometimes have different brand names. Most of them are available in different sizes and, although it depends on the design, the smaller versions are usually the most effective.

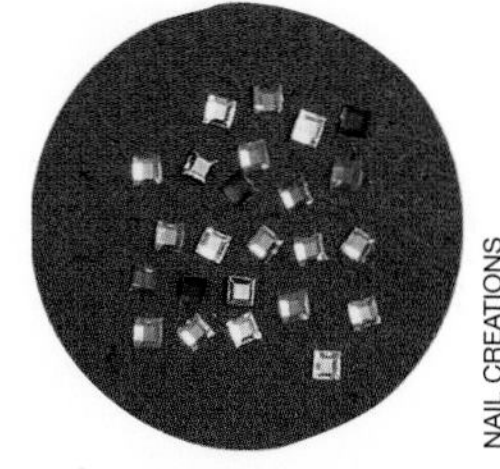
NAIL CREATIONS

Polish secures – square rhinestones

- *Rhinestones* (*or diamantes*). These are clear or coloured stones that look like precious or semi-precious stones. They are usually made of glass or crystal and cut with facets to reflect light. They can be used to encrust a design or a judiciously placed single stone can bring a simple design to life. In relative terms they are not cheap and the designs using them should reflect this cost. Good quality rhinestones will not dull or lose their sparkle if sealed with a top coat and this will ensure they stay on the nail for the maximum time, especially if the client reapplies a top coat. Although stunning, even the smallest rhinestone stands quite proud from the nail.
- *Flat backed beads*. These, like rhinestones are usually coloured glass but they are rounded rather than cut with facets. Applied in the same way to wet polish, they look like beads on the nails.

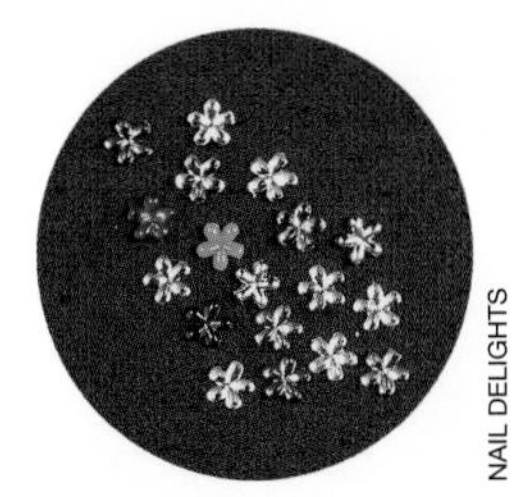
NAIL DELIGHTS

Polish secures – flower beads

- *Flatstones*. These are a less expensive version of rhinestones. As the name suggests, they are quite flat and usually very small, but they sparkle well. They can, however, lose their sparkle under a top coat. If this is the case, then apply a thicker layer of top coat than usual and push the stones into the wet polish. This should hold them in place without the need to seal them.
- *Pearls*. These are flat backed plastic shapes coloured to look like pearls. Although white is the obvious colour, they can be obtained in pastel colours, such as pink or lilac. They can look very pretty, especially in a design for a bride. Again, take account of their size.

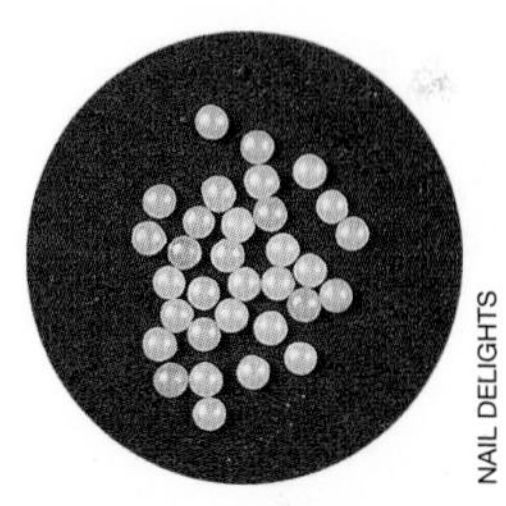
NAIL DELIGHTS

Polish secures – pearls

- *Stone shapes*. There are some interesting shapes available now, such as flower made of coloured glass.
- *Foil shapes*. These are tiny pieces of shiny or holographic plastic cut into different shapes that can look very effective incorporated into a design. The shapes may be circular, stars, moons, hexagons, even tiny hands and dolphins! These are applied in the same way, but care must be taken with the top coat. They need to be sealed, as edges that are not covered by top coat can catch and be pulled off, although some top coat have a solvent that is too strong. This will cause the colour to be affected and it will often streak.

KNOWLEDGE CHECK

How should nails be prepared for nail art?

Need more time... refer to page 470 to help you.

ACTIVITY

Nail conditions

Identify the cause of the nail conditions below and what salon service and home care/action you would recommend for a client who wished to receive nail art and to improve the appearance/condition of the nail.

- pterygium
- onychopagy
- weak, dry, brittle and split nails
- hang nails
- longitudinal or horizontal ridges
- allergies to products.

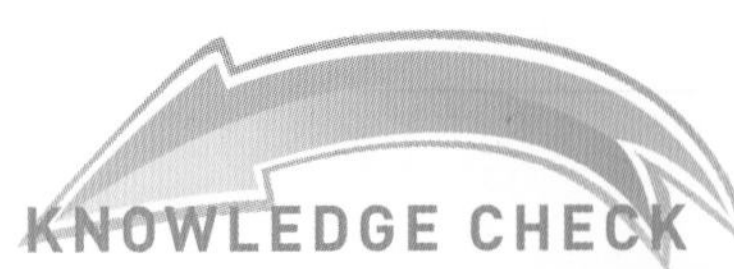

KNOWLEDGE CHECK

What is the purpose of a marbling tool?

Need more time... refer to pages 471–472 to help you.

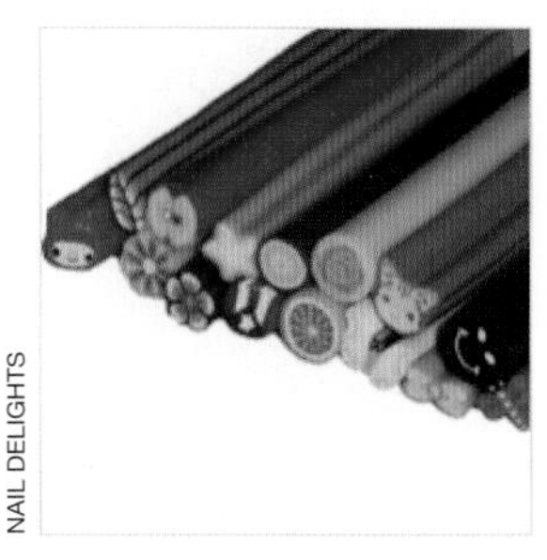

NAIL DELIGHTS

Fimo canes

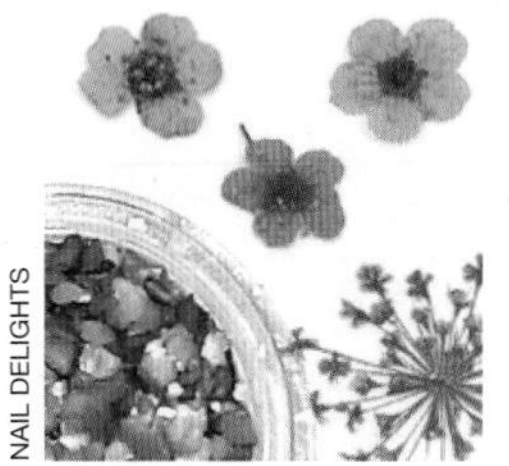

NAIL DELIGHTS

Flowers and shells

- *Metal studs*. A very effective and less 'glitzy' polish secure are metal studs. These are available in gold or silver colours and different sizes.
- *Fimo canes*. These can be bought in ready cut or in long 'canes'. There is a vast variety of designs that can be laid on the nail once a very thin 'slice' has been cut. Some of these can be partially transparent.
- *Crushed shells*. These are available in many colours and can be applied as a base for other decorations to go on top or can be used alone or with colour variations. They have an opalescence that can look spectacular.
- *Dried flowers*. Various tiny dried real flowers and leaves are available and applied in the same way.

After the base colour has been applied (or other design) a top coat or sealer must be painted. While this is still wet, the 'secures' can be placed on it. The easiest way to pick up 'secures' is with a wet orange stick or with a small piece of Blu-Tack® on the end of an orange stick. The Blu-Tack® can be shaped into a point to make picking up the tiny shapes easier.

When all the shapes have been placed, the whole nail needs to be sealed with a thick coat of sealer or top coat. Make sure your top coat does not affect the colour of foil shapes.

Recommend to your client that they re-apply a top coat every 2 to 3 days to keep the design fresh and avoid damage to or loss of stones.

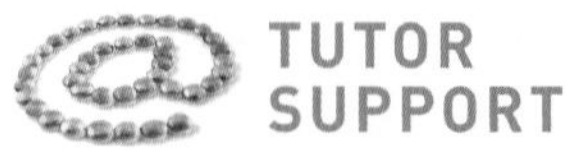

TUTOR SUPPORT

Activity 6: Develop themed nail boards

Alternative application methods:

1. Use a spot of nail adhesive to place the decoration on the nail.
2. Embed in a UV gel top coat before curing.
3. Place on the nail and apply a layer of clear L&P (liquid and powder) or UV gel over the whole design.

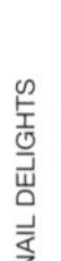
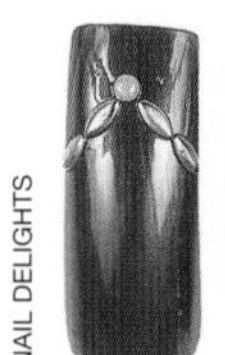
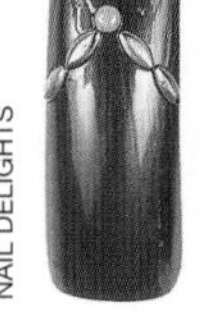
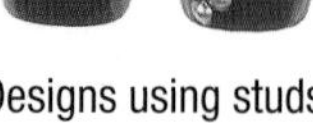
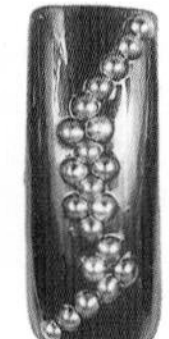
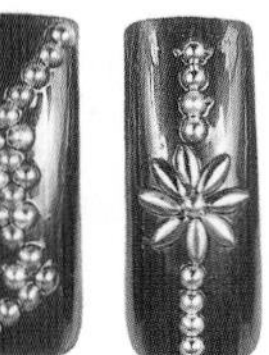
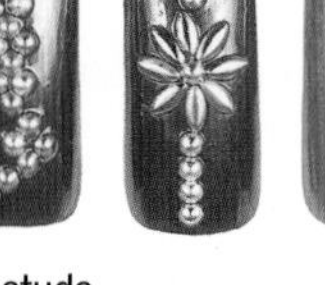
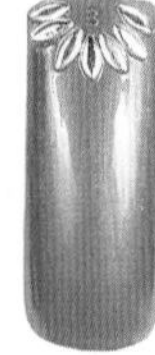
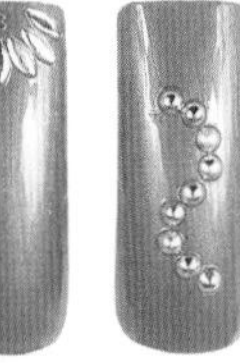
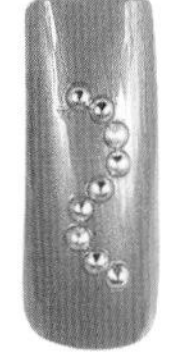

NAIL DELIGHTS

Designs using studs

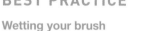

TRACEY STEPHENSON

Steps: Base colour, apply secures

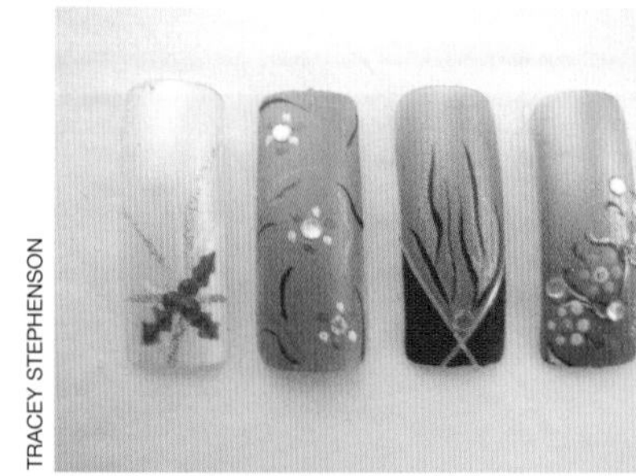

TRACEY STEPHENSON

Designs using mixed techniques

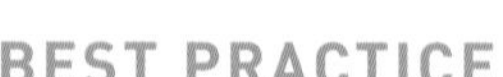

BEST PRACTICE

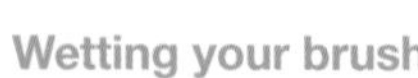

Wetting your brush

Never put an orange stick in your mouth to wet it! If Blu-Tack® is not available, dip the stick into varnish remover or a small dish of water to wet it.

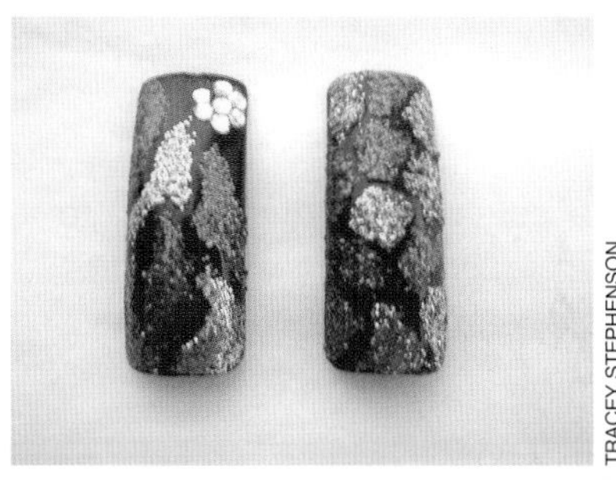
TRACEY STEPHENSON

Designs using glitter dusts

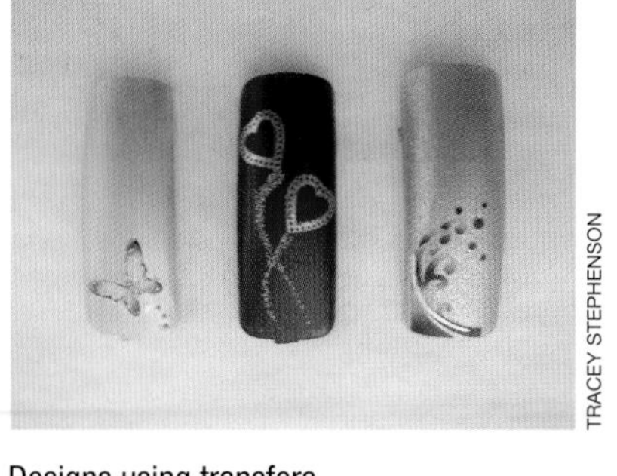
TRACEY STEPHENSON

Designs using transfers

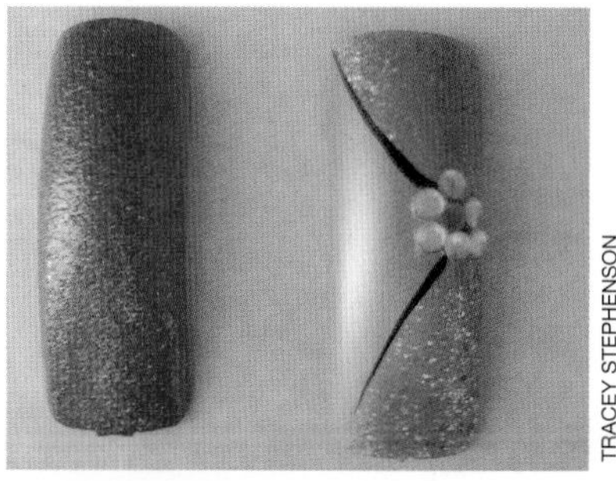
TRACEY STEPHENSON

Designs using glitter polish

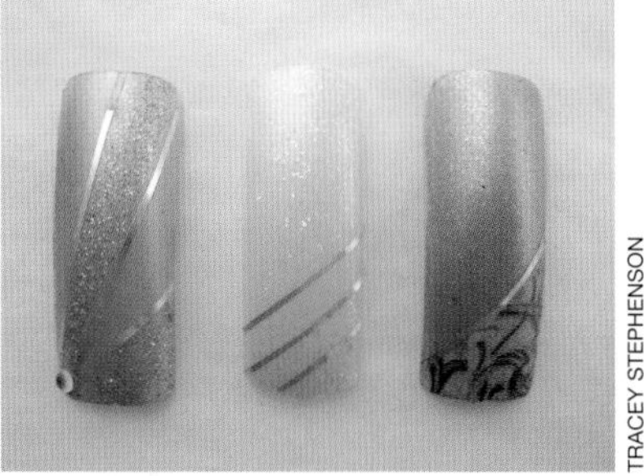
TRACEY STEPHENSON

Designs using striping tape

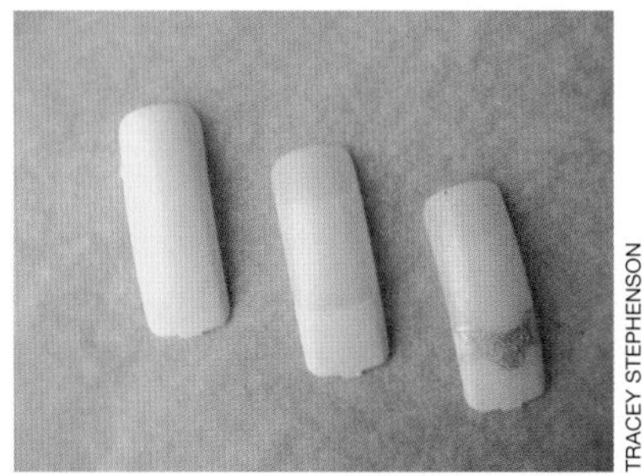
TRACEY STEPHENSON

Steps: French with a transfer

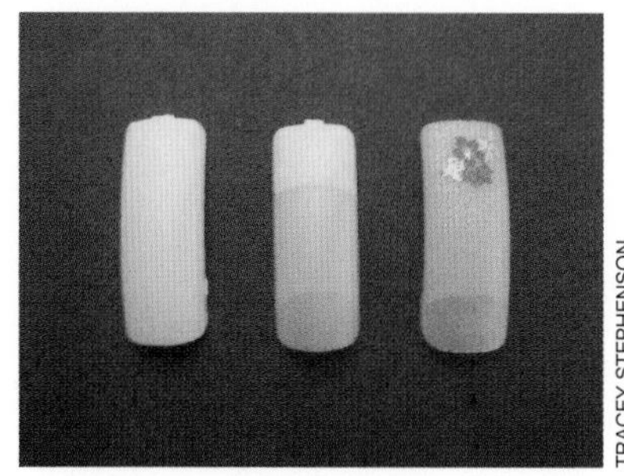
TRACEY STEPHENSON

Steps: French with a transfer

Glitter dusts

Glitter polishes and glitter dusts are a very versatile range of products to create or enhance nail art. Obviously, glitter can be applied to the whole nail, but it can also be used to make patterns or designs; a well-placed highlight on a painted or airbrushed design can make a simple piece of nail art spectacular.

- Glitter polishes can be painted straight from the bottle with either the brush supplied or a fine nail art brush. Glitter dusts can be used to create more specific designs by picking up the dust with a brush dipped in sealer, as this will give an effect that is denser than glitter polish. The dust will also stick to wet sealer, so the tip of a nail dipped into the pot will collect the dust on the tip only or where the sealer is wet.
- Like all nail art, glitter dusts need sealing. The sealer must be painted on thickly and gently to avoid moving the dust.

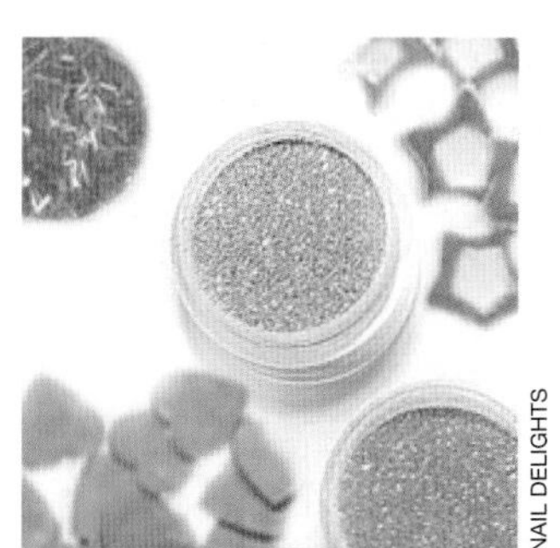
NAIL DELIGHTS

Glitter and shapes

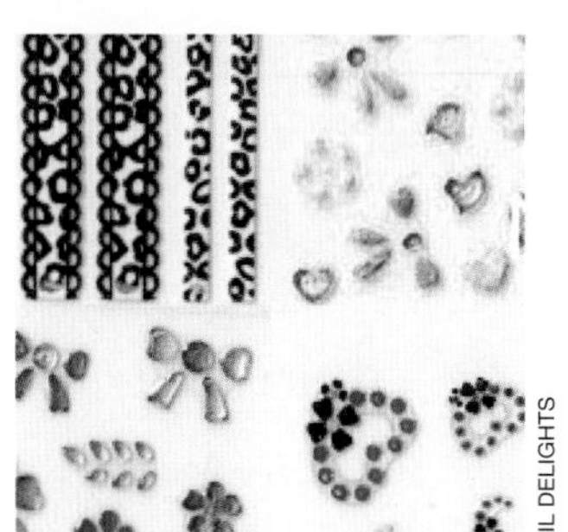
NAIL DELIGHTS

Stickers

Transfers and tapes

There are many transfers are available to apply to nails. These are ready-made nail art and can be very effective. Some need to be soaked off their backing with water (place a few drops onto the backing paper to soak through and then the transfer slides off) or they peel off their backing and stick straight on to the nail.

Tapes are also available in many plain colours and patterns. They have a sticky back and must be placed on the nail and then trimmed with a small pair of very sharp scissors.

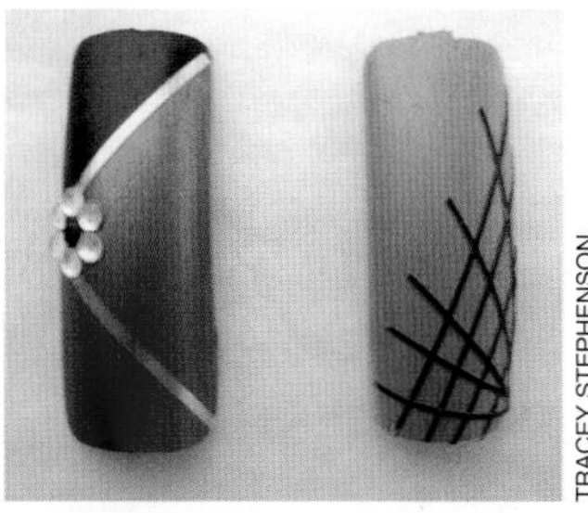
TRACEY STEPHENSON

Designs using striping tape

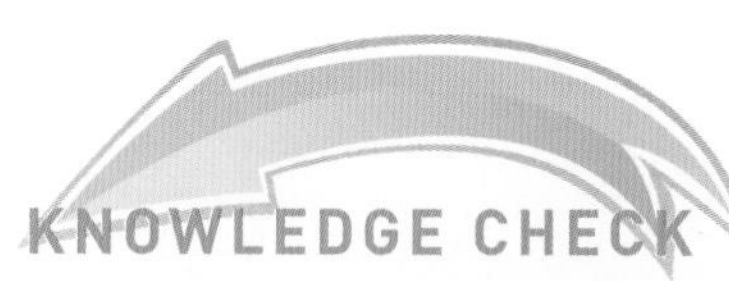

Question

How does the condition of the client's nails influence timing and choice of nail art?

Need more time... refer to page 469 to help you.

Nail jewellery

Many different types of nail jewellery are available.

- Some of the designs are applied to the nail as a 'polish secure', that is stuck to wet varnish. These can only be very light and small. Larger designs can be applied to the nail with nail glue. Both of these are reusable, as they can be removed with nail varnish remover.
- Other types of nail jewellery involve making a small hole in the free edge of the nail. This can be done with ease using a specially made tool that has a very sharp but tiny drill. There is no problem at all piercing an artificial nail, but care must be taken when piercing a natural nail:
  - A natural nail should be strengthened with a coating of resin as used in a fibre system.
  - The free edge must be long enough to provide a space for the hole without being too close to the hyponychium. If the hole is made on a nail that is too short the seal at the hyponychium could be damaged.
- There are two types of jewellery that require a pierced nail. One has a post that is put through the hole and secured with a tiny nut on the underside. The piercing tool has both the drill and the socket to tighten the nut. The other type has a clasp or ring that is attached to the nail through the hole. The first type usually sits on top of the nail plate and the second hangs from the edge.

To pierce the nail:

1. Make sure there is sufficient free edge to safely pierce.
2. Turn the finger over so that the underside of the nail is visible and the nail and finger are resting on a soft surface, for example, a piece of cork or several layers of tissues.
3. Place the tip of the drill on the nail, not too near the edge but also in the right place for the jewellery to fit on the nail (not too far away from the free edge for a pendant or ring).
4. Gently turn the drill until a neat hole is made; withdraw the drill by turning in the opposite direction.
5. Turn the finger over and smooth the surface of the nail with a white block.
6. Apply the nail jewellery.
7. If a pendant has been applied, advise the client to remove it while dressing, doing housework, washing hair, etc., as it is possible to catch it and split the nail.

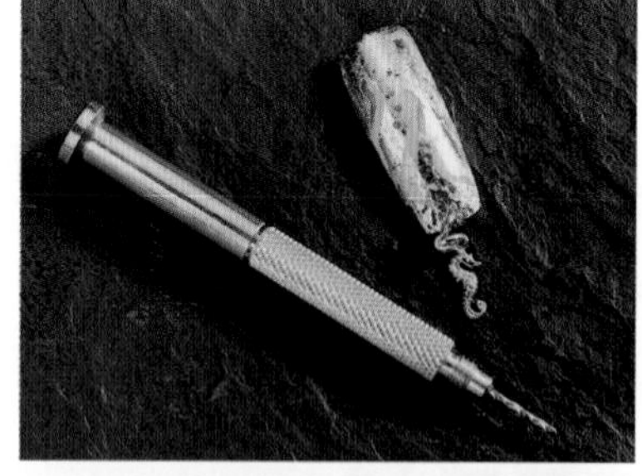

Nail piercing tool and nail pedant attached

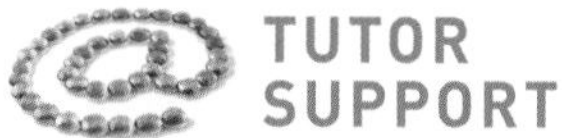

Activity 7: Recap, revision and evaluation sheet

These are some basic instructions for starting off in the realms of nail art. All the various techniques can be mixed and matched. Foil can be mixed with polish secures, paint mixed with glitter. The possibilities are endless and the only limit is imagination.

Aftercare advice

Confirm with the client that the finished result is to their satisfaction. Complete details of the nail art service on the client record card. Clear instructions should be provided on how to care for their nails and also what action to take in the event of a contra-action.

Aftercare advice will differ for each client according to their individual needs, but generally it will be as manicure aftercare advice: see pages 390–391.

Name four nail art techniques.

Need more time... refer to page 475 to help you.

When giving aftercare advice, it is a good opportunity to recommend retail products, such as nail polish or hand cream, thereby enhancing retail sales and the salon profits. It is a good idea to have the nail polish colours that you have used available for sale. The client can then touch up any accidental chips. Recommend the use of a top coat applied every three–four days to protect the nail art, increase its durability and impart shine.

Nail art will last approximately ten days, so recommend the client books their next appointment after this. Ideally, the client should return to the salon to have their nail art removed. However, nail art can usually be removed with nail polish remover. Care should be taken to remove attachments such as polish secures and nail jewellery.

KNOWLEDGE CHECK

What is a contra-action? What could be a contra-action to a nail art service?

Need more time... refer to page 469 to help you.

Contra-actions

A contra-action is an unwanted reaction to the service. An unwanted reaction to the nail art service might include an allergic reaction. This occurs when a person becomes sensitized to a product ingredient. It is possible to become allergic to a product after having been in contact with it for years. The reaction would be recognized if the skin becomes red, itchy and inflamed.

Advise the client that if an allergic reaction occurs, all nail products should be removed and a cool compress and soothing agent applied to the skin to reduce redness and irritation.

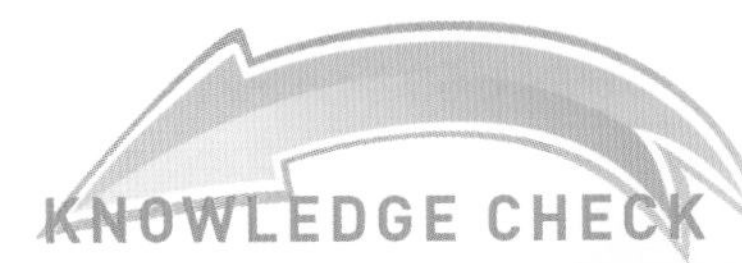

KNOWLEDGE CHECK

What aftercare advice should be given to a client following nail art service?

Need more time... refer to page 478 to help you and remember also to look at Chapter 11 Manicure Treatments and Chapter 12 Pedicure Treatments.

ACTIVITY

Create a design plan for each of the following, include the created design on a nail tip or a photograph(s) of your nail art.

1. A design plan for a photographic shot using a fantasy image. The image is to appear on the CD cover of a girl group called 'Heavenly'.
2. A design to be used on all the female models of a bridal fashion show.
3. A design for a client who is going to a Christmas party. She has asked for you to create a design that includes snow!
4. A design for a mature client who will be celebrating her golden wedding with a big family party.

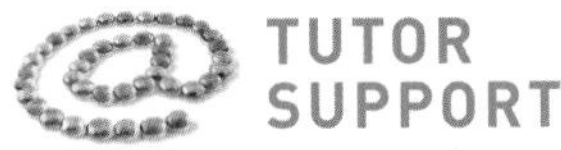

TUTOR SUPPORT

Activity 8: Evaluation task

GLOSSARY OF KEY WORDS

Client record card confidential card recording the personal details of each client registered at the business. This information may be stored electronically on the salon's computer.

Consultation assessment of the client's treatment objectives using different techniques, including questioning and natural observation.

Contra-action an unwanted reaction occurring during or after service application.

Contra-indication a problematic symptom that indicates that the service may not proceed or may restrict service application.

Foiling a technique used in nail art that uses a foil to decorate the nails.

Marbling a technique used in nail art that mixes two or more colours together to form a design feature.

Nail art nail decoration using a variety of techniques and materials.

Nail art techniques application styles used to create different effects including dotting, striping, marbling, enamelling, foiling and blending.

Nail polish a clear or coloured nail product that adds colour/protection to the nail.

Painting techniques nail art techniques using specialized paints, tools and brushes to create different effects e.g. free hand, striping, dotting and marbling.

Polish secures accessorises in nail art that stick to the nail using nail polish.

ASSESSMENT OF KNOWLEDGE AND UNDERSTANDING

You have now learnt about the underpinning knowledge and practical skills for providing nail art for the beauty therapy workplace. To test your level of knowledge, answer the following short questions. These will prepare you for your summative (final) assessment.

1. Pterygium is a nail condition recognized by:
   a. overgrown thickened cuticles
   b. pitting of the nail plate
   c. grooves in the nail plate
   d. swelling, redness and pus appearing in the cuticle area of the skin of the nail wall
2. When storing nail products, which legislation acronym applies?
   a. PPE
   b. PUWER
   c. COSHH
   d. RIDDOR
3. A marbling tool can be used:
   a. for creating thick, straight lines
   b. where detail is required
   c. to sweep products across the nail
   d. to apply dots
4. A contra-action allergy will normally affect:
   a. the nail plate
   b. the nail bed
   c. the free edge
   d. the cuticle
5. A *squoval* nail shape is a:
   a. combination of square and oval shape free edge
   b. rounded free edge
   c. square shape free edge
   d. nail plate that becomes broader at the free edge
6. Foil is applied to the nail
   a. pattern side upper most
   b. pattern side facing down
7. Polish secures 'cut with facets to reflect light' are referred to as:
   a. flatstones
   b. rhinestones
   c. stone shapes
   d. flat backed beads
8. The crescent shaped part of the nail which can be defined when painting the nails is called the:
   a. lunula
   b. mantle
   c. leuconychia
   d. free edge
9. To maintain the appearance of the nail art, what should the client apply at home?
   a. base coat
   b. top coat
10. Which of the following conditions would prevent nail art from proceeding?
   a. diabetes
   b. product allergies
   c. scar tissue
   d. severe onycholysis

15 Waxing Treatments

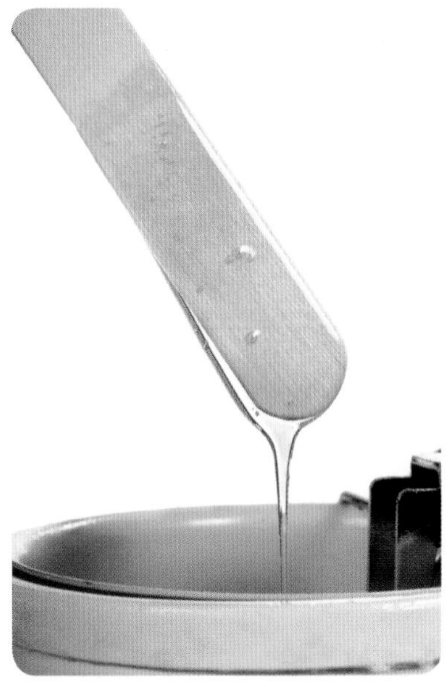

Learning Objectives

This chapter covers **VRQ Unit Remove hair using waxing techniques**.

This unit is all about how to remove facial and body hair temporarily using appropriate wax removal techniques for the hair type and area including hot wax, warm wax and roller methods. Aftercare advice is an important part of this treatment to promote skin healing and prevent possible infection.

There are **two** learning outcomes for this unit which you must achieve:

1 Be able to prepare for waxing treatments

2 Be able to provide waxing treatments

From the range statement you must show you can:

- use **consultation techniques** to identify the treatment **objectives**
- carry out the necessary **tests** before treatment
- use all the listed **products, tools and equipment** as appropriate
- ensure the **environmental conditions** are suitable
- use hot, warm and roller wax hair removal methods
- describe **alternative methods of hair removal** and their **effects** on the skin
- complete a consultation and skin inspection to identify any **contra-indications**

(continued on the next page)

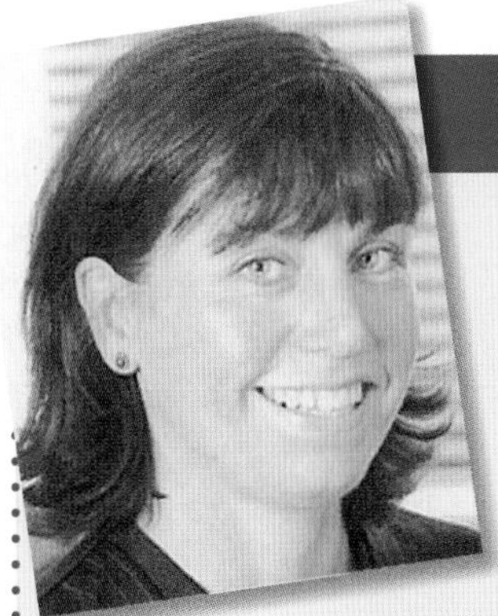

ROLE MODEL

Janice Brown

Director of HOF Beauty (House of Famuir Ltd)

“My career journey has taken me from working in and later managing a group of salons, through sales, teaching, training, research and development and I am currently director of HOF Beauty Ltd. Along the way I have specialized in electrolysis and hair removal. I am the co-author of *Practical Electrolysis: The Official Guide to Electro-epilation* along with Gill Morris. I am proud to say that I have been able to make a real difference to people's lives by helping to correct skin, body and hair growth issues. I hope I have also been able to inspire and encourage fellow beauty therapists through the training I have provided. In the course of my career I have been fortunate enough to travel the world and work with wonderful people. Beauty therapy for me is not only a career but is a true passion.

KNOWLEDGE CHECK

What are the three stages of the hair cycle? Briefly explains what happens to the hair at each stage.

Need more time... refer to pages 57–58 to help you.

- **communicate and behave** in an appropriate and professional manner
- follow all **health and safety working practices**
- adapted treatments to suit all **skin types and conditions**
- provide relevant **aftercare** and **contra-action advice**

You must be able to show you have the necessary practical skills and underpinning knowledge to remove hair using waxing techniques.

This unit is linked to the Beauty Therapy NOS **Unit B6**.

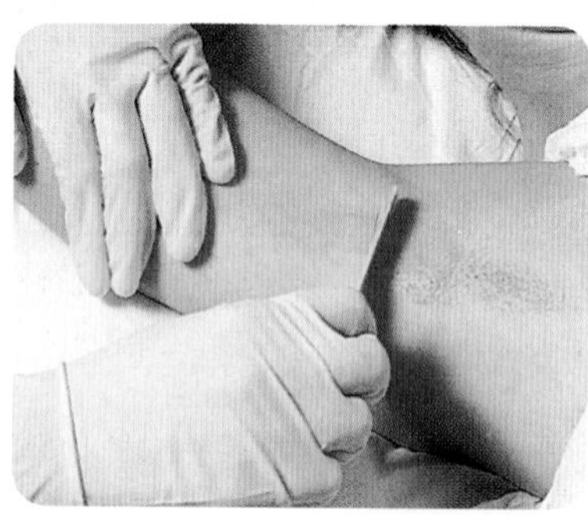

Underarm hair removal

Essential anatomy and physiology knowledge requirements for this unit are identified in the checklist on page 27.

Hair removal methods

Hair removal is a popular treatment in the beauty salon, where both temporary and permanent methods of removal are usually available. Temporary removal must be repeated regularly, as the removed hair will regrow. With permanent methods, the client needs to visit the salon regularly initially to have the hair removed; thereafter, the part of the hair responsible for its growth has been destroyed and the hair will not grow again (see the hair growth diagram on page 58).

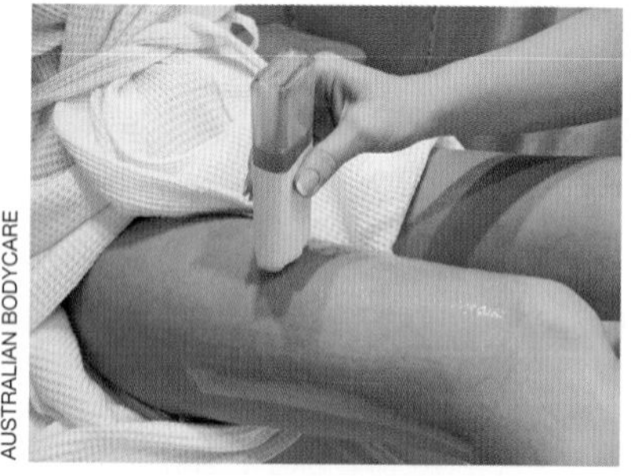

AUSTRALIAN BODYCARE

Depilatory waxing using roller wax method

Temporary methods of hair removal

Depilatory waxing Wax depilation, using a warm wax, hot wax or cold wax, involves applying wax to the treatment area and embedding the hairs in it. When the wax is removed from the area, the hairs are removed at their roots so the regrowth is of completely new hairs with soft, fine-tapered tips. They grow again in approximately four weeks.

Plucking Plucking or tweezing uses a pair of tweezers to remove the hair. These grasp the hair near the surface of the skin, and the hair is then plucked in the direction of growth, again removing it at its root. The hair grows again in approximately four weeks.

Due to the sensitive nature of the eye tissue, tweezing is often considered the most suitable choice for temporary hair removal from eyebrows.

Plucking may be used after waxing to remove those hair too short for the wax to remove or to remove specific hairs i.e. to define the final brow shape following eyebrow wax hair removal.

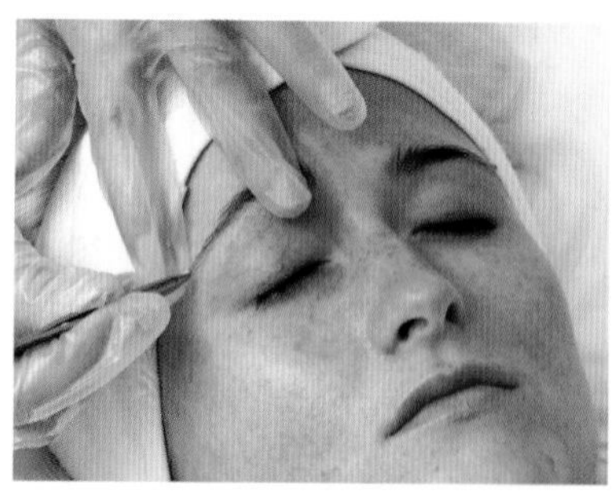

Plucking eyebrow hair

ACTIVITY

Hair removal

Make short notes on the advantages and disadvantages of the different methods of hair removal available.

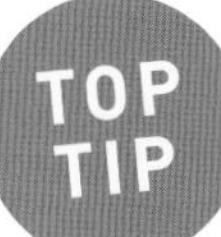

Eyebrow shaping

When carrying out eyebrow hair removal using waxing techniques refer to Chapter 8 Eyelash and Brow Treatments to inform you of eyebrow shaping procedures to consider to ensure that the finished brow shape will be to the client's satisfaction.

Some clients may use an electrical depilatory device, which performs the function of mass plucking. As the device is moved over the skin's surface hairs are grasped and removed. This does not consider the way the hair grows and therefore can be problematic when the hair regrows as it can lead to distortion of the **hair follicle** affecting the way the hairs lie when they regrow, hair breakage and ingrowing hairs may also occur.

Threading Threading involves the use of a thread of twisted cotton, which is rolled over the area from which the hair is to be removed: the hairs catch in the cotton, and are pulled out. This skill is frequently practised by people of Asian or Mediterranean origin. Please see Chapter 9, for more information on this technique.

Waxing, plucking and threading removes the entire hair, including the visible hair above the skin's surface (the hair shaft) and the part that cannot be seen in the hair follicle.

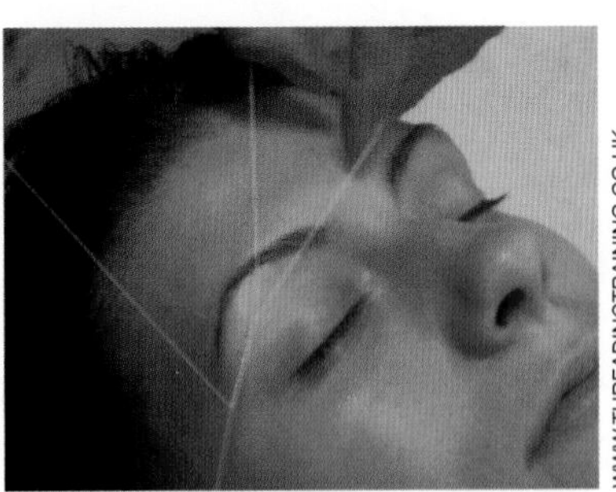

WWW.THREADINGTRAINING.CO.UK

Threading eyebrow hair

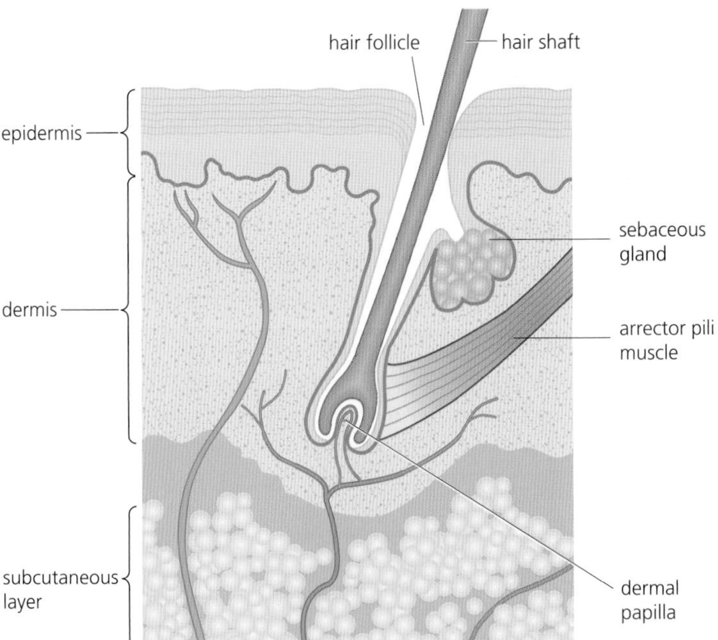

The hair in its follicle

Permanent methods of hair removal

Electrical current methods **Galvanic electrolysis, electrical epilation** and the **blend epilation technique** are all techniques that use an electrical current. The current is passed to the hair root via a fine needle inserted into the hair follicle. The current destroys the hair root, preventing hair regrowth.

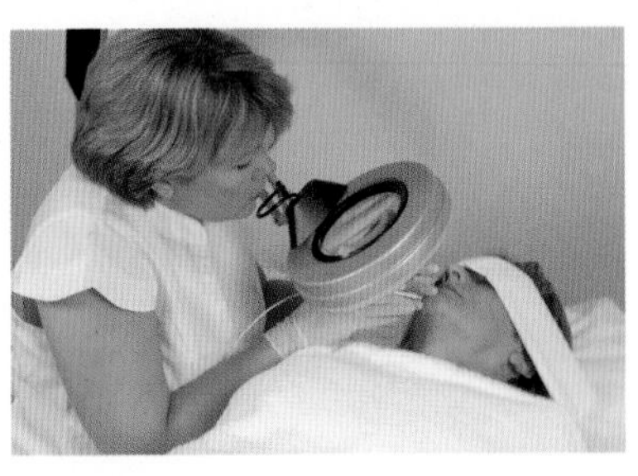

Electrolysis

HEALTH & SAFETY

Laser hair removal

Registration with the Care Quality Commission (CQC – www.cqc.org.uk) is a requirement to practise laser hair removal.

Part of their remit is to drive up quality of health care and they have a wide range of enforcement powers.

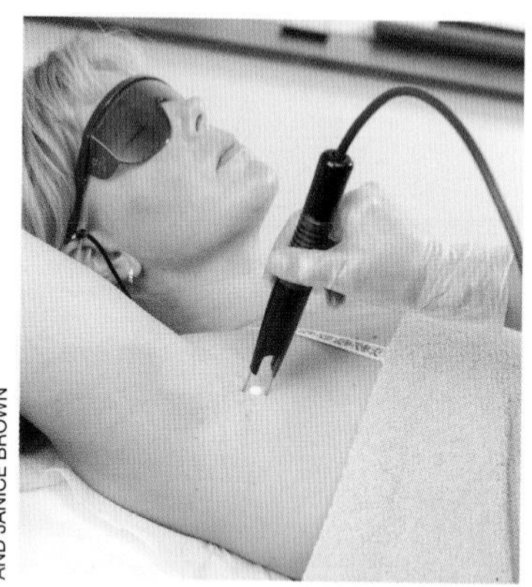

ENCYCLOPAEDIA OF HAIR REMOVAL, GILL MORRIS AND JANICE BROWN

Laser hair removal

Laser hair removal Laser energy works by producing light at various wave lengths, energy output and pulse widths. It is passed through the epidermis of the skin, which stops the activity of the hair follicle creating hair growth through a process called photothermolysis. The melanin pigment that provides hair colour absorbs the laser energy that is converted to heat, which at a sufficient temperature destroys the part of the hair follicle where the cells divide to create the hair.

The more melanin, the more destruction occurs. Therefore, generally laser hair removal works best for light-skinned people with dark hair.

A course of laser treatments is required. Treatment length will depend on the coarseness of the hair type and the size of the hair follicle. The treatment is most effective when the hair is in the anagen (growth) stage of the hair growth cycle. Subsequent treatments therefore target different hairs in their anagen stage of growth until all hairs cease to grow.

The client needs to understand that the hair will never grow back if effectively treated with any of the above permanent methods. This is an important consideration when treating the brow hair, as the desired shape and thickness of the brows change frequently under the influence of fashion.

Intensed pulsed light Intensed pulsed light (IPL) systems work on the same principle as laser; that of absorption of light energy into melanin in the skin and hair. The light energy is converted to heat energy, which causes damage to the specific target area. There are two beams of light, one yellow and one red, which together affect both the existing hair and the follicles where the hair grows. The high-energy light pulses remove the hair.

IPL systems differ to laser in that they can deliver hundreds of wave lengths of light in each burst of light instead of just one wave length, increasing the area of skin that can be treated. Certain filters are used that target these flashes of light so that they can work in a similar way to lasers.

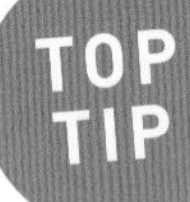

IPL

IPL produces better results in people with darker hair colour and lighter skin colour. It is less effective or ineffective where there is no pigment, e.g. grey and white hair.

Other methods of hair removal

There are other methods of hair removal that the client may have used at home previously. At the client consultation it is important to find out which method of hair removal the client has used previously and discuss suitability. If a client chooses to adopt waxing as their preferred hair removal method, temporary methods such as those discussed below should cease to be used.

- ***Cutting the hairs with scissors*** Scissors are used to trim the hair close to the skin's surface. This does not affect hair growth as only the dead hair above the skin's surface, the hair shaft is removed. The hair, however, is left with a blunt end and feels stubbly. This leaves the skin hair free for a very short time, usually only 1–2 days, dependant upon the client's hair growth.
- ***Shaving*** A razor blade is stroked over the skin, against the natural hair growth after the skin has been prepared with a suitable skin lubricant such as shaving foam or oil. This removes the hair at the skin's surface. This leaves the skin hair free for a very short time, usually only 1–2 days, dependant upon the client's hair growth. The hair feels sharp as it grows because the hair is left with a blunt end.
- ***Depilatory cream*** A strong alkaline chemical cream containing ammonium thioglycollate is applied to the hair, and removed after five to ten minutes: the hair will have been dissolved at the skin's surface. As the chemical is strong enough to dissolve the hair protein keratin, it can sometimes cause skin irritation as the skin contains keratin too.
- ***Abrasive mitt*** An abrasive glove is rubbed against the skin and the hair is broken off at the skin's surface. The result and its effectiveness are similar to shaving and is unsuitable for a sensitive skin as the skin can become reddened quickly.

For waxing treatments, it is important to keep your client warm. If your client becomes cold, the hair follicle will tighten around the hair, making the treatment more uncomfortable and the hair difficult to remove.

If it's a very cold day, at the skin preparation stage briskly rub or massage your client's skin with the preparatory products as this will increase blood supply thereby increasing skin temperature.

Janice Brown

ACTIVITY

Methods of hair removal

As well at the professional use of depilatory waxing, threading and plucking, other methods of temporary hair removal include the home use of plucking, cold wax using ready-waxed strips, sugaring, electrical devices, chemical depilatory creams, shaving and pumice powder. Find out how each method works and assess its effectiveness. Are any of them potentially hazardous?

Hair regrowth

Because of the cyclical nature of hair growth and the fact that follicles will be at different stages of their growth cycle when the hair is removed, the hair will not all grow back at the same time. Waxing, along with threading and plucking, can therefore appear to reduce

ALWAYS REMEMBER

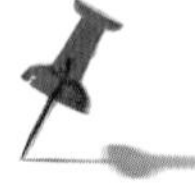

Waxing treatment legal requirements

Habia have provided a Code of Practice for Waxing. This should be referred to ensuring that you are complying with your responsibilities under relevant health and safety.

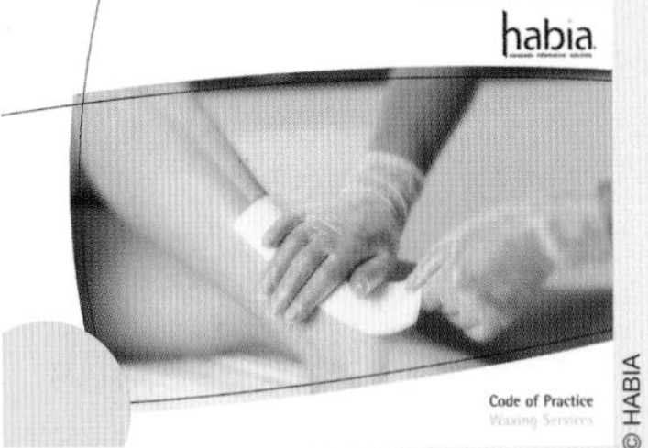

Habia Code of Practice for waxing

HEALTH & SAFETY

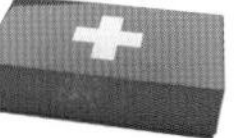

Sensitive skin

Increasingly products are being formulated which contain only natural ingredients which can reduce skin irritation. Ingredients include sugar and plant extracts such as chamomile and lavender to soothe the skin.

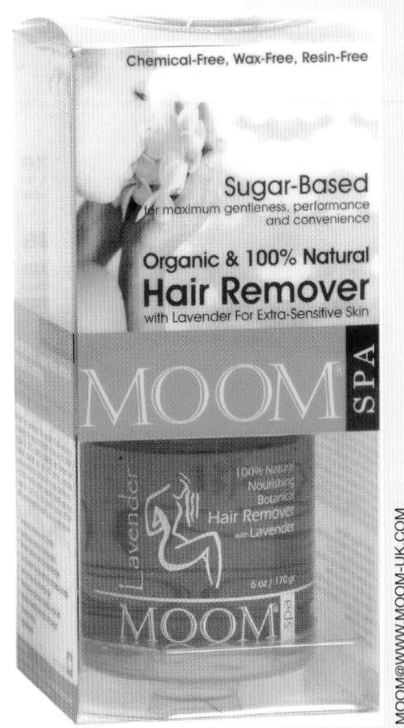

Organic sugar-based hair remover

the *quantity* of hair growth. This is not so, however, and the hair will all grow back eventually: waxing is therefore classed as a temporary form of hair removal.

Nevertheless, certain bodily changes (such as ageing), when *combined* with waxing, can result in permanent hair removal. This effect is so erratic and unpredictable, though, that waxing cannot reliably be sold as a permanent method of hair removal. Occasionally hair re-growth will increase, which is not a normal reaction and may be related to medication being taken or the medical health of the client. That is why it is important to carry out a thorough consultation before waxing treatment is provided. Waxing is unsuitable as a hair removal method in this instance.

Preparing for waxing

Outcome 1: Be able to prepare for waxing treatments

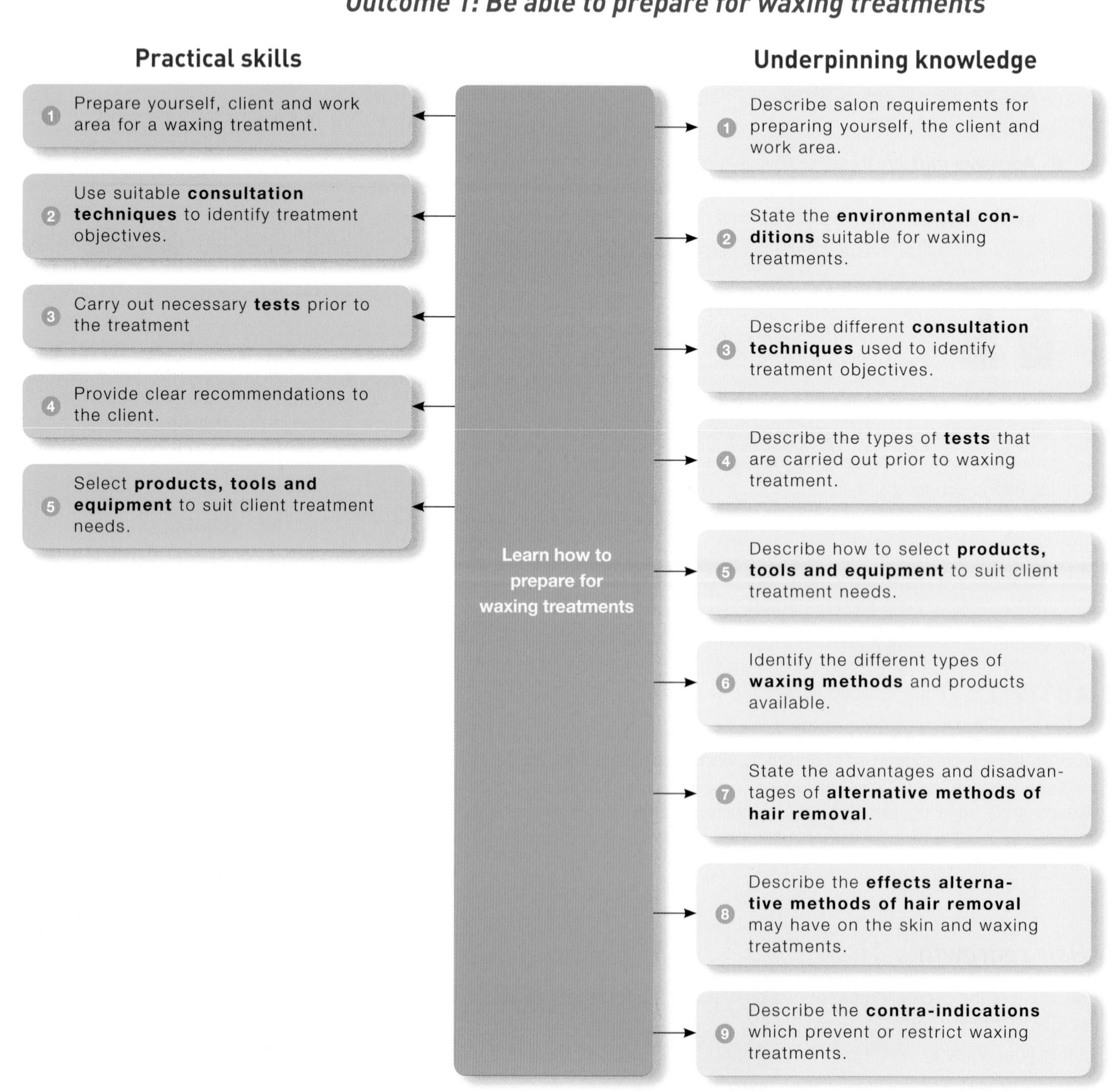

Practical skills
1 Prepare yourself, client and work area for a waxing treatment.
2 Use suitable consultation techniques to identify treatment objectives.
3 Carry out necessary tests prior to the treatment
4 Provide clear recommendations to the client.
5 Select products, tools and equipment to suit client treatment needs.
Learn how to prepare for waxing treatments
Underpinning knowledge
1 Describe salon requirements for preparing yourself, the client and work area.
2 State the environmental conditions suitable for waxing treatments.
3 Describe different consultation techniques used to identify treatment objectives.
4 Describe the types of tests that are carried out prior to waxing treatment.
5 Describe how to select products, tools and equipment to suit client treatment needs.
6 Identify the different types of waxing methods and products available.
7 State the advantages and disadvantages of alternative methods of hair removal.
8 Describe the effects alternative methods of hair removal may have on the skin and waxing treatments.
9 Describe the contra-indications which prevent or restrict waxing treatments.

Preparing the work area

Check the suitability of the environmental conditions.

To enable the hairs to be removed effectively, the treatment area should be well lit; a magnifying lamp may be available to assist observation of the area. It must also be warm, as the client must be made as comfortable as possible when performing the treatment. If the client is cold, the follicles will restrict, making hair removal more difficult. Ensure ventilation is adequate to remove odours and remove humid air, providing sufficient air movement to keep the air fresh.

Before the client is shown through, the work area its contents should be checked to ensure that they are clean and tidy. The bins should have been emptied since the previous client.

Check the trolley to ensure that you have all that you need for carrying out the treatment and that it is suitably positioned to prevent unnecessary stretching or walking which will affect commercial timing and could cause repetitive strain injury. The wax should be of a suitable consistency, i.e. ready for application.

The plastic-covered couch should be clean, having previously been washed with hot soapy water and wiped thoroughly with a disinfectant which is bactericidal, fungicidal and virucidal. The use of an additional heavy-duty plastic sheet is recommended: this is easier to wipe than the couch, and can be replaced if damaged.

All disinfectable surfaces must be disinfected after thorough cleaning between treatments.

The couch should then be covered and protected with a long strip of paper-tissue bedroll. Place a towel(s) neatly on the couch, ready to protect the client's clothing and to cover them, protecting modesty, when they have undressed. These tend to be of a medium size as large towels can make the client too warm. The tissue should be disposed of after use, and the towel freshly laundered for each client.

The couch should be in the sit-up position, unless the client is only having their bikini line or underarm areas waxed, in which case it should be flat.

Before beginning the waxing treatment, check that you have the necessary products, tools and equipment to hand and that they meet legal hygiene and industry requirements. Metal tools such as scissors and tweezers should be sterilized in an autoclave prior to use.

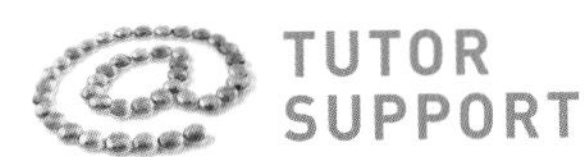

Activity 1: Hair removal research task

> "Waxing is one of, if not the most popular treatment on offer for beauty professionals. Clients therefore have a vast choice. By creating the right atmosphere, giving excellent service and paying attention to details you will encourage the client to return to *you* for their waxing treatment.
>
> **Janice Brown**

Types of wax product

Warm wax This first became available in 1975 and is now the market leader for hair removal. It is clean and easy to use.

Warm wax is used at a low temperature, around 43°C, so there is little risk of skin burning, and in less sensitive areas the wax can be re-applied once or even twice if necessary.

Warm wax does not set but remains soft at body temperature. It adheres efficiently to hairs and is quick to use; treatment is relatively pain-free. It can remove even very short hairs (2.5mm) from legs, arms, underarms, the bikini line, the torso, the face and the neck.

Warm waxes are frequently made of mixtures of glucose syrup, resin to help the wax stick, oil to help removal (e.g. almond oil), water and fragrances. Honey (fructose syrup) can be used instead of glucose syrup and this formulation is often called **honey wax**. Zinc oxide is added to **cream wax** to provide an opaque colour. This type of warm wax is capable of providing a thin, liquid consistency at lower temperatures making it less sensitizing to the skin.

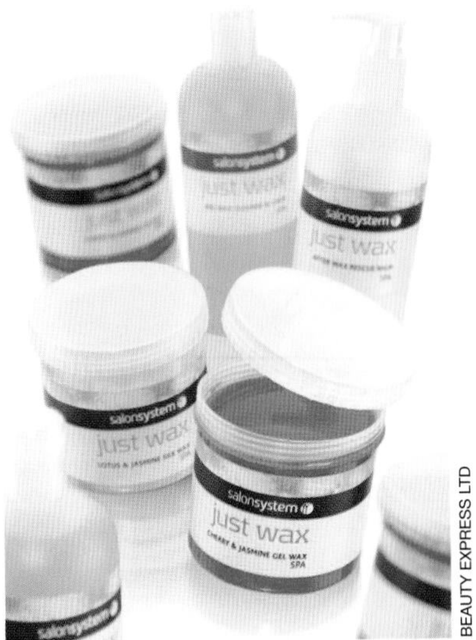

Warm wax

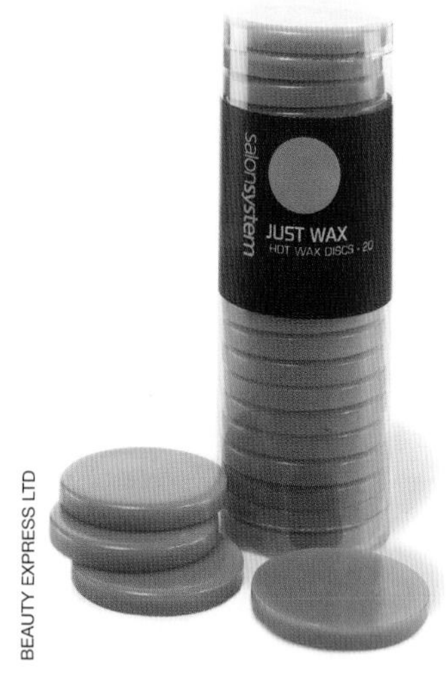

BEAUTY EXPRESS LTD

Hot wax (discs)

Hot wax This takes longer to heat than warm wax, and is relatively slow to use, taking approximately double the time of a warm waxing. This time reduces when skill is attained.

As hot wax is used at quite a high temperature, 50°C, extra care must be taken to avoid accidental **burns**. Because of this risk, hot wax cannot be re-applied to already treated areas.

Hot wax cools on contact with the skin. It contracts around the hair shaft, gripping it firmly. This makes it ideal for use on stronger, short hairs.

Hot waxes for hair removal need to be a blend of waxes and resins so that they stay reasonably flexible when cool. **Beeswax** is a desirable ingredient, and often comprises 25–60 per cent of the finished product.

Cetiol, azulene and vitamin E are often added to wax preparations to soothe the skin and minimize possible skin reactions.

Cold wax This is already applied to a strip. The pre-coated strip is applied firmly to the area of skin for hair removal and then removed quickly against hair growth. The hair sticks to the wax and is removed as the wax strip is removed, against hair growth.

Sugar wax There are two methods of sugar wax hair removal – **sugar paste** and **strip sugar**.

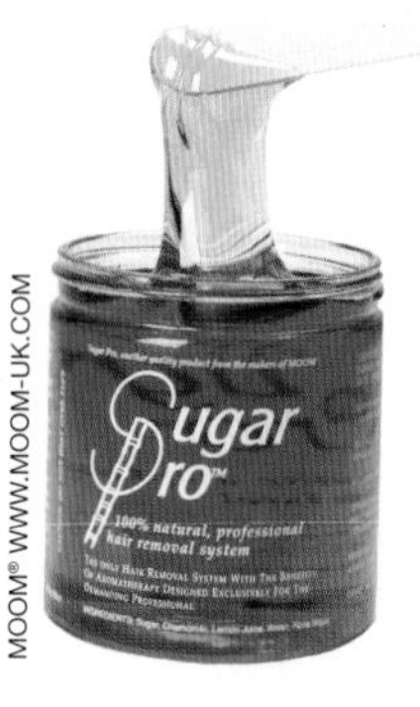

MOOM® WWW.MOOM-UK.COM

Sugar paste is applied to the skin, using the hands, in the direction of hair growth. The hairs embed in the wax, which is then removed swiftly against hair growth, removing the hairs. This method is ideal for a sensitive skin as the wax does not stick tightly to the skin. On removal it will remove surface loose skin cells with the hair. Improving overall skin appearance.

Strip sugar is similar in application and removal to warm wax and requires a wax removal strip to remove the wax, against hair growth. Sugar wax has pure sugar as the main ingredient, plus other natural ingredients such as lemon. Resins may be added to help skin adherance.

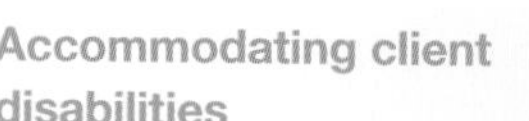

BEST PRACTICE

Accommodating client disabilities

Hydraulic couches are effective as they enable clients with mobility problems easier access on to the couch.

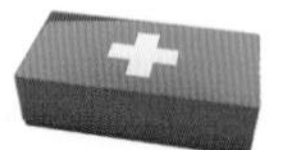

HEALTH & SAFETY

Storage of products

All products should be stored as guided by the material safety data sheets (MSDS) in compliance with COSHH Regulations (2002).

ACTIVITY

Wax heaters

Look in current beauty magazines for the different types of wax heater and applicators. Try to see demonstrations of them working. Discuss size, cleaning, safety, hygiene and any other points that you think are important. Which heater would you choose, and why?

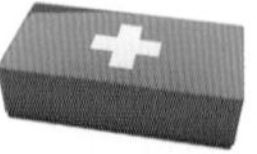

HEALTH & SAFETY

Wax and related product use

All products used in the waxing treatment should be used in accordance with the Cosmetic Regulations (2003).

Personal Protective Equipment Act (PPE) at Work Regulations (1992)

Waxing is a treatment where there is a risk of contamination and cross-infection, therefore protective equipment such as gloves and an apron should be available and worn.

PRODUCTS, TOOLS AND EQUIPMENT

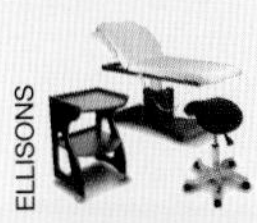

Couch
With sit-up and lie-down positions and an easy-to-clean surface

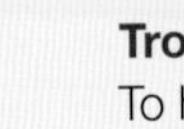

Trolley
To hold all the necessary products, tools and equipment

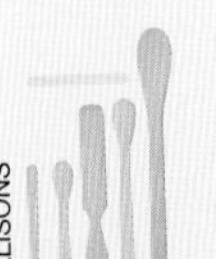

Disposable wooden spatulas (a selection of differing sizes)
For use on different body areas

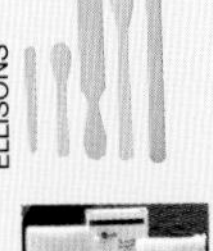

Wax-removal strips
Thick enough that the wax does not soak through, but flexible enough for ease of work. These strips should be cut to size and placed ready in a container. These may be paper or muslin

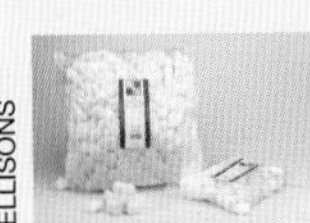

Cotton wool
For cleaning equipment and applying various skin soothing/cleansing preparations

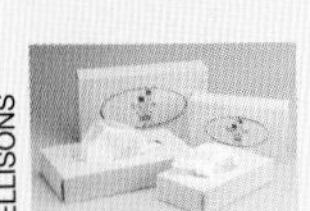

Tissues (white)
For blotting skin dry and protecting the client's clothing in the area

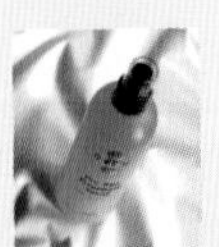

Anti-bacterial skin cleanser
(Also known as pre-wax lotion) or professional antiseptic wipes

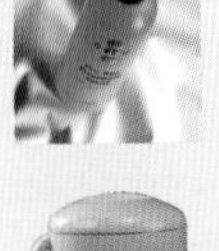

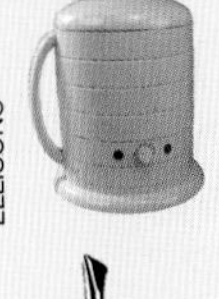

Wax heater
With a thermostatic control, a lid and a central bar for spatula methods

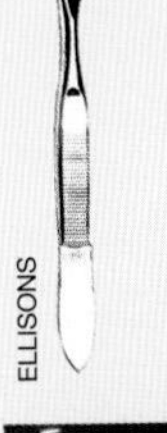

Tweezers
For removing stray hairs following wax depilation or defining the brow shape following a brow waxing treatment

Single-use disposable synthetic powder free gloves
To comply with Personal Protective Equipment (PPE) at Work regulations and ensure a high standard of hygiene and to reduce the possibility of contamination

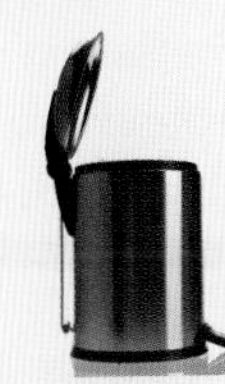

Waste container
This should be a lined metal bin with a lid. Specific disposable bags may be required for contaminated waste

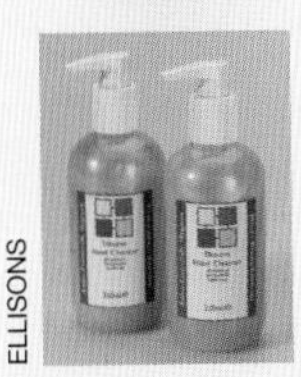

Hand disinfectant
To clean hands before each waxing treatment

YOU WILL ALSO NEED:

Magnifying lamp To provide additional assistance when observing the area of hair removal

Disposable tissue couch roll Disposable consumable placed over the couch cover prior to each treatment to prevent the client sticking to the couch cover and for reasons of hygiene

Protective plastic couch cover A durable covering which can be cleaned with a disinfectant agent before each client treatment. It is then covered with disposable tissue roll

Professional talcum powder Or alternative talc free powder formulation to avoid allergic responses in some clients. To absorb body perspiration and to facilitate hair removal

Disposable panties These may be provided when carrying out bikini waxing

Surgical spirit Or a commercial cleaner designed for cleaning waxing equipment

Towels (medium-sized) For draping around the client

Small scissors For trimming over-long hairs

Disinfecting solution In which to immerse small metal tools following sterilization in the autoclave. This must be changed regularly as stated in manufacturers' instructions

Wax A choice to suit skin types and conditions and hair types

After-wax lotion With soothing, healing and antiseptic qualities

Mirror (clean) For facial waxing treatments

Apron To comply with Personal Protective Equipment (PPE) at Work regulations and protect work wear from spillages

Client record card Confidential card recording details of each client registered at the salon to record the client's personal details, products used and details of the treatment

Aftercare leaflets Recommended advice for the client to refer to following treatment

TOP TIP

After-wax lotion

After-wax lotions reduce redness and promote skin healing. They contain ingredients such as tea tree, aloe vera, azulene and witch-hazel. These are an ideal retail product to recommend to your client to ensure effective skin healing.

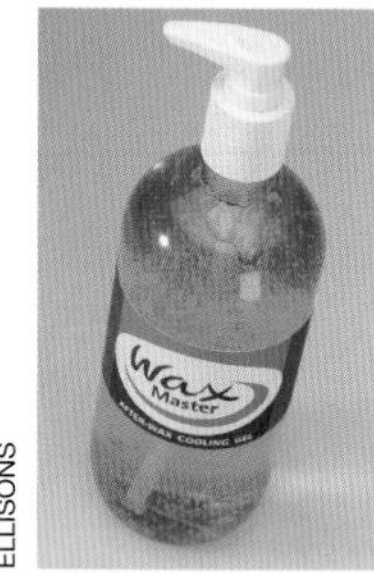

ELLISONS

After-wax cooling gel

> Selling is a vital part of the role of a therapist. It is important that the client gets the right treatment and products in order to get the results they are after. Clients do not buy our treatments or products, they buy the benefits and results. It is your job to help them imagine how using the products and treatments will make them look and feel. Remember that we all hate to be sold to but love to buy; so practise and perfect your selling skills.
>
> **Janice Brown**

ACTIVITY

Electrical testing

How can you ensure that your wax heater is safe to use?

How can you ensure you comply with the Electricity at Work Regulations (1989)?

What actions must you ensure are taken?

ACTIVITY

Safe storage

How should flammable products used in the waxing treatment be stored? Consider the environmental conditions also.

When choosing a wax, select one with the following qualities:

- It should be easy to remove from equipment.
- It should be able to remove short, strong hairs (25mm).
- It should have a pleasant fragrance or no smell.
- It should not stick to the skin, but only to the hair.

HEALTH & SAFETY

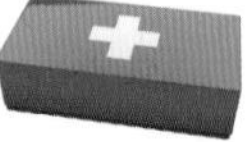

Avoiding cross-infection

Never filter hot wax after use: it cannot be used again as it will be contaminated with skin cells, tissue fluid, and perhaps even blood.

Sterilization and disinfection

Disposable waste from waxing may have body fluids on it: potentially it is a health risk. It must be handled, collected and disposed of according to the local environmental health regulations. It is a requirement to wear disposable gloves while carrying out bikini and underarm wax treatments, to protect yourself from body fluids and the client from contamination. These too should be disposed of after each waxing treatment. Wash your hands regularly with anti-bacterial soap, before and after preparing the work area and before application of the disposable gloves. This shows the client that you have a high standard of hygiene.

An apron should be worn to protect work wear from wax spillage.

HEALTH & SAFETY

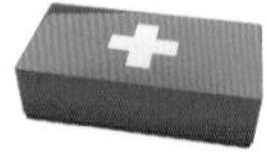

Contaminated waste

Any wax waste that contains bodily fluids should be bagged separately from other regular waste and special arrangements made for its disposal by a registered waste carrier in an approved incinerator in accordance with the Controlled Waste Regulations (1992). This may include spatulas, wax strips and wax waste, consumables such as tissues and cotton wool, disposable underwear, aprons and tissue couch roll.

All metal tools should be sterilized in the autoclave before use. This includes tweezers and scissors.

After the waxing treatment they must be replaced and resterilized.

Increasingly systems which minimize the risk of cross-infection are being adopted. These include single use tubes, cartridges using **disposable applicator** heads.

TOP TIP

Habia guidance

See the Habia *Hygiene in Beauty Therapy* booklet for further guidance to hygiene best practice. Also check Habia website for specifications and updates.

ACTIVITY

Maintaining hygiene

Spreading wax on the client and dipping the used spatula back into the tub with the spatula method creates the possibility of cross-infection between clients. How can cross-infection be avoided, with this method and the use of roll-on wax applicators?

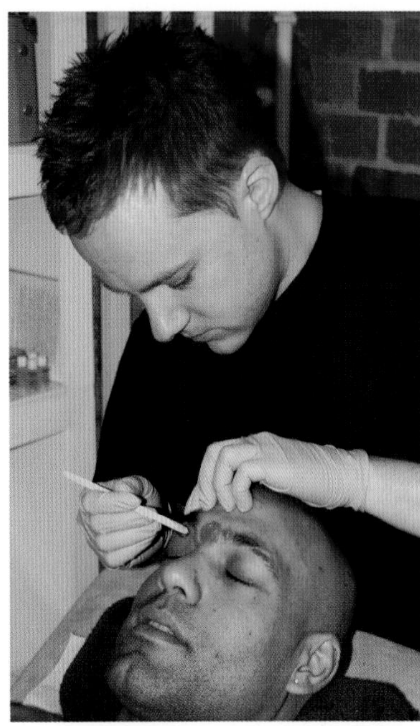

Wear disposable gloves when carrying out waxing treatments

Reception

When the client is booking their treatment they should be asked whether they have had a wax treatment before in the salon. If they have not, a small area of waxing should be carried out as a skin sensitivity patch test, to ensure that the client is not sensitive to the technique or allergic to any of the products used. If the **sensitivity test** causes an unwanted reaction within 48 hours, then the treatment must not be undertaken. Unwanted reactions include excessive redness, irritation and swelling, referred to as contra-actions.

Treatment	Warm waxing (minutes)	Hot waxing (minutes)
Half leg	20–30	30
Half leg and bikini	30	45
Full leg	50	60
Full leg and bikini	60	60–70
Bikini	15	15–20
Underarm	10–15	15–20
Half arm	10–15	15–20
Full arm	20–30	20–30
Top lip	5	5–10
Chin and throat	10	15–20
Top lip and chin	15	15–20
Eyebrows	10–15	15

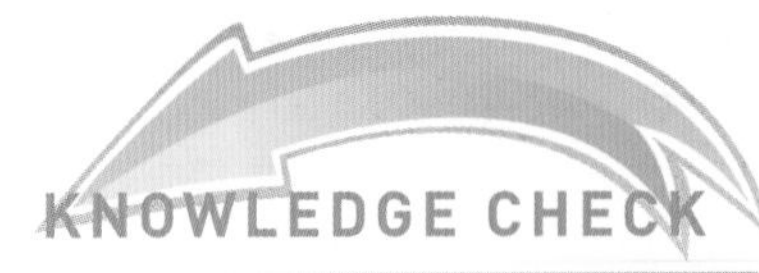

KNOWLEDGE CHECK

Following waxing treatment how should the waste be disposed of?

Need more time... refer to page 490 to help you.

HEALTH & SAFETY

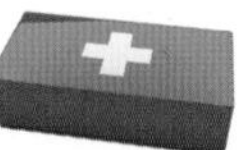

Couch covers

If the salon chooses to use stretch-towelling couch covers or additional towels to provide extra comfort, these must be provided clean for each client and laundered in hot soapy water at a temperature of 60°C after use.

HEALTH & SAFETY

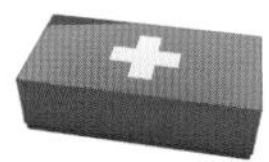

Client sensitivity: Plasters

If a client is allergic to plasters they may possibly be allergic to wax as it may contain resin a substance that is found in plasters.

Always perform a skin sensitivity test in this case.

ALWAYS REMEMBER

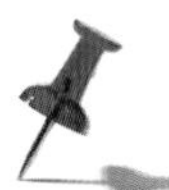

Client record card

Accurately record your client's answers to necessary questions to be asked at consultation on the record card. This is necessary for future reference.

"Consultation is the key to a successful treatment. You may be asking yourself why you need to consult your client, you may feel you already know what they want, or see it as a card filling exercise, so you should just get them on the couch and get started. However, you'd be wrong. Consultation is your opportunity and to gain the information you need to enable you to give a safe effective treatment. Learn exactly what your client wants and needs, in order to sell them the suitable products and treatments. It is also your opportunity to impress potential clients with your knowledge and professionalism to ensure they build a trust in you and become a regular customer.

Janice Brown

ALWAYS REMEMBER

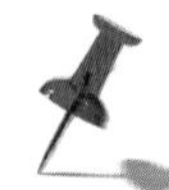

Treatment of minors

Check the salon's insurance guidelines relating to age restrictions for waxing treatment. Check age restrictions in your area (note that in England a minor is under 18, whereas in Scotland it is 16) – refer to current guidance.

Advise the client not to apply any lotions or oils to the area on the day of the treatment – these could prevent the adhesion of the wax to the hairs being removed. Ask them also to allow at least one week, and preferably two, between any home shaving or other depilatory treatment and a salon waxing treatment. This is to let the hairs grow to a length sufficient to be waxed.

When a client makes an appointment for a wax depilation treatment, the receptionist should advise the client how long the treatment will take.

It is important to complete the treatment in the time allowed in order to be efficient in treatment application and to ensure the appointment schedule runs smoothly and clients are not kept waiting.

Inform them briefly what the waxing treatment will entail so that they have an understanding of what will be required from them. This will help clients who have not received the more intimate wax removal treatments, i.e. to the underarms and bikini area, to relax.

Allow a four- to six-week interval between successive wax depilation appointments. Following set intervals between waxing treatments will improve the effectiveness of the treatment as this will follow the hair growth cycle. The times to be allowed for wax treatments are as shown in the table on the previous page. However, repeat bookings vary according to the natural hair regrowth and client requirements.

All staff, especially the staff communicating with clients at reception should be familiar with the different pricing structures for the range of waxing treatments and products available for retail.

Minors (clients under 18 years of age in England; 16 in Scotland) must be accompanied by a parent/guardian who will be required to sign a consent form for treatment to proceed.

Consultation

A **consultation** must be performed for all clients who have not received the treatment before or are new clients to you. Discuss what methods of hair removal have been used before and when they were last used. Discuss the known sensitivity of the client's skin. If the client is taking any medication that causes skin thinning, such as tetracycline, or has received facial chemical peels or retin-A, skin lifting may occur because the wax is designed to stick to the skin before removal. This will result in skin damage so waxing must not be performed. If necessary a skin sensitivity patch test should be provided to assess tolerance. A positive reaction where there is redness, irritation or swelling means that the treatment cannot proceed. A positive reaction means that it can. Maintain client privacy at all times during the consultation. Explain what is involved with the method of hair removal technique to be used, the expected costs, sensations, treatment reactions and aftercare requirements.

It is a good idea to discuss the hair growth cycle with the client using a visual aid. This will help the client to understand that hairs that grow through following hair removal were at a different stage of the hair growth cycle and were below the skin's surface at the time of the treatment. It also is beneficial to support the need for regular intervals between waxing appointments as hairs will be at a similar hair growth pattern.

Immediately following hair removal, the skin becomes slightly red around the follicle where the hair has been removed. There may also be slight swelling of the skin in the area. This will soon disappear following treatment but this will vary according to skin sensitivity and hair strength and the quantity of hair that has been removed. Occasionally spot bleeding may occur where a particularly strong hair has been removed usually when in the anagen stage where it is receiving blood from the dermal papilla resulting in capillary damage. This too may be explained at consultation.

Invite the client to ask questions. It is important that they understand fully what the treatment includes.

Advise the client following the consultation and completion of the record card of the most appropriate method of waxing temporary hair removal having considered the type of hair (vellus/terminal) and amount and the sensitivity of the skin.

TOP TIP

Describing the sensation

Here are some useful explanatory phrases: "It's a bit like ripping a plaster off and taking the hairs with it. It isn't so bad, or so many people wouldn't have it done time and time again!"

Contra-indications

When a client attends for a wax depilation treatment, the therapist should always check that there are no contra-indications that might prevent treatment.

Certain medical conditions or medications and hormonal changes in the body such as those that occur at pregnancy, puberty and menopause can affect hair growth, causing an increase, so it is important to discuss the hair growth observed in the area to be removed with the client. This will confirm client suitability for treatment. Types of hair growth and factors affecting hair growth are discussed on page 59.

If the client has any of the following, wax depilation must not be carried out:

- ***skin conditions*** such as thin and fragile skin
- ***skin disorders*** such as severe eczema or psoriasis
- ***eye disorders*** such as conjunctivitis when treating the face
- ***swellings*** – the cause may be medical
- ***diabetes*** – a client with this condition is vulnerable to infection as they have slow skin healing
- ***defective circulation*** – poor skin healing burning and infection may occur. This may be a symptom of conditions such as diabetes, heart disease and multiple sclerosis.
- ***recent scar tissue (under six months old)*** – the skin lacks elasticity
- ***broken bones***
- ***fractures or sprains*** – discomfort may occur
- ***phlebitis*** – an inflammatory condition of the vein.

TOP TIP

Examples of waxing treatment modification

- **hair removal around contra-indications that restrict treatment (such as hairy moles and skin tags)**
- **altering the choice of wax to suit skin sensitivity and hair type**

HEALTH & SAFETY

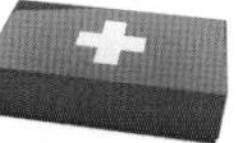

Diabetes

Clients who have the medical condition diabetes should be treated with care. This is because diabetics generally have poor circulation and are slow to heal. As there is some tissue damage to the skin during wax depilation when the hair is removed from the follicle, secondary infection could occur. Approval to treat should be obtained by the client from their GP before temporary hair removal treatment.

HEALTH & SAFETY

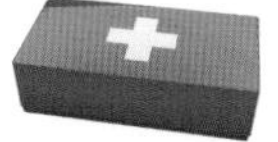

Venous problems

Venous problems can lead to vein inflammation and skin ulceration. If a vein becomes inflamed a blood clot commonly forms inside the inflamed area. **Deep vein thrombosis** results in a blood clot moving through the bloodstream, causing a blockage elsewhere which could prove fatal!

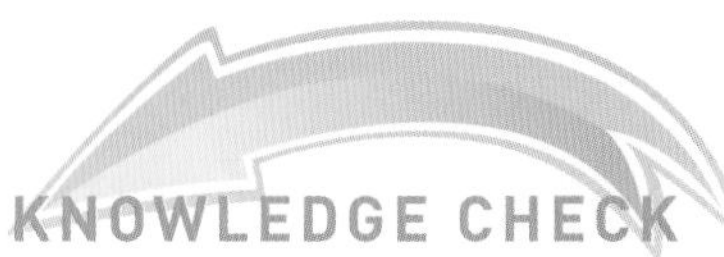

KNOWLEDGE CHECK

To assist communication, why would you use a visual aid at consultation when explaining hair growth cycle and how this may effect the 'hair free' period?

Need more time... refer to pages 492–493 to help you.

ALWAYS REMEMBER

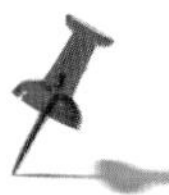

Client record card

The client record card should be updated signed and dated at every visit and stored securely in compliance with the Data Protection Act (1998). Non-compliance may invalidate insurance.

HEALTH & SAFETY

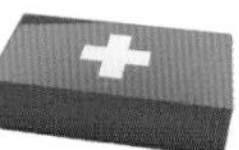

Precaution if there is a restrictive contra-indication present

If there is a hairy mole or small abrasion you may apply petroleum jelly to avoid wax adherence.

BEST PRACTICE

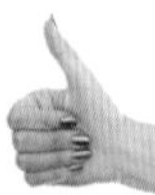

Tanned clients

Waxing a client with a recent well-established suntan may cause the loose sun-damaged epidermis to peel and be lost, along with the hair. Inform the client of this at consultation.

KNOWLEDGE CHECK

What are the necessary environmental conditions required for waxing? Consider lighting, heating and ventilation in your answer.

Need more time... refer to page 487 to help you.

- ***retin-A, Tetracycline medication*** as the skin is more sensitive, delicate and prone to skin irritation and tearing
- ***recent exfoliation treatments*** including micro-dermabrasion
- ***loss of skin sensation*** – the client would be unable to identify if the wax was too hot
- ***scar tissue*** – under six months old
- ***allergies to products*** – such as the ingredient resin, an ingredient found in wax

ALWAYS REMEMBER

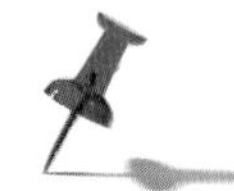

Areas to avoid

Never wax the areas inside the ears or nose or around the areola of the breast or eye lid area.

Further contra-indications that prevent waxing treatment

Name	Description
Bruising WELLCOME PHOTO LIBRARY	Injury to an area causes blood to leak from damaged blood vessels. Bruises may swell, appearing dark purple or blue at first and then turn, brown, green or yellow as they fade.
Folliculitis 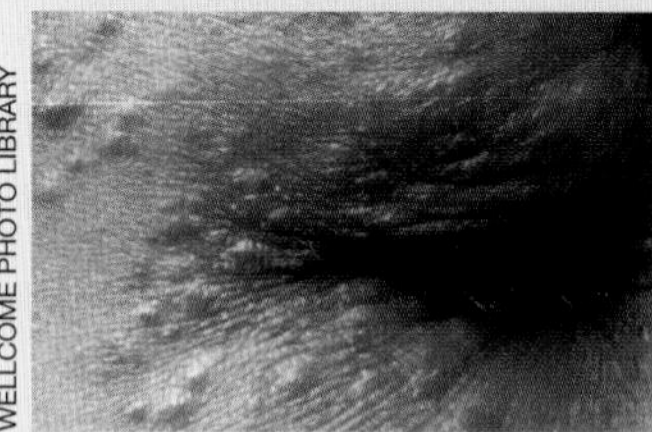 WELLCOME PHOTO LIBRARY	A bacterial infection where pustules develop in the skin tissue around the hair follicle.
Severe varicose veins 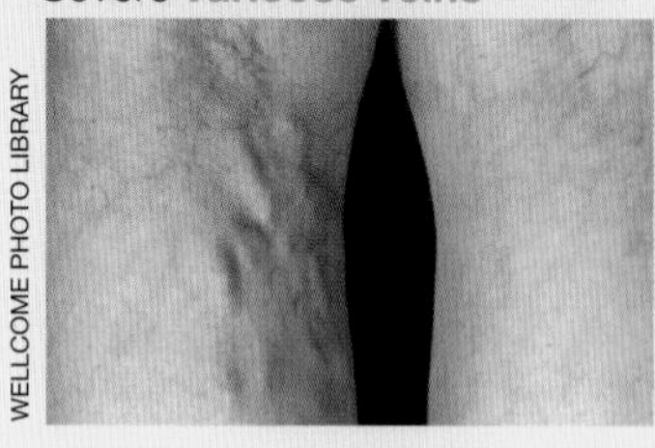 WELLCOME PHOTO LIBRARY	Veins are vessels that carry blood away from the body tissues and back to the heart. Veins have valves to prevent backflow as they carry blood under low blood pressure back towards the heart. If valves become weak and their elasticity is lost, it becomes a *varicose vein*. The area appears knotted, swollen and bluish-purple in colour.

Certain contra-indications restrict treatment application. This may mean that the treatment has to be adapted for the client. For example, in the case of a small, localized bruise the area could be avoided.

Other contra-indications that restrict treatment include:

- ***cuts*** – secondary infection could occur
- ***mild skin disorders*** such as psoriasis or eczema and skin tags
- ***abrasions*** – secondary infection could occur

- ***self tan*** – waxing will remove the surface skin cells and the chemically tanned skin
- ***bruises*** – client discomfort may be caused and the condition made worse
- ***sunburn*** – the skin is damaged and there is excessive heat in the area due to acute over-exposure to the sun
- ***varicose veins*** (non-severe) – avoid the area
- ***moles*** – avoid wax application to the area
- ***ingrowing hairs*** – the area should be avoided as the hair will not be removed; additionally, infection commonly occurs at the site of an **ingrowing hair**, leading to folliculitis

Further contra-indications that restrict waxing treatment

Name	Description
Heat rash 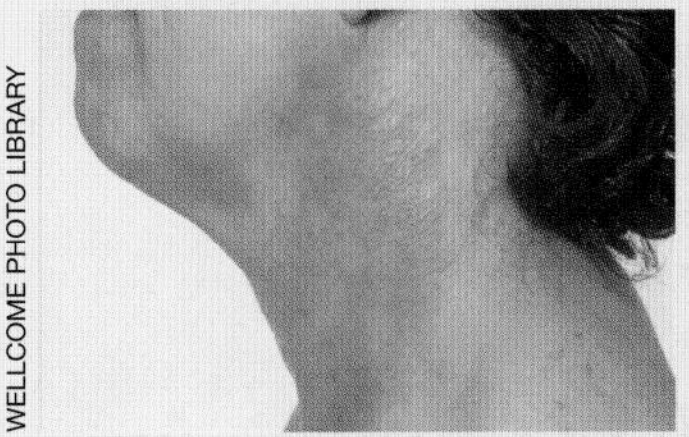 WELLCOME PHOTO LIBRARY	A reaction to heat exposure where the sweat ducts become blocked and sweat escapes into the epidermis. Red pimples occur and the skin becomes itchy.
Warts 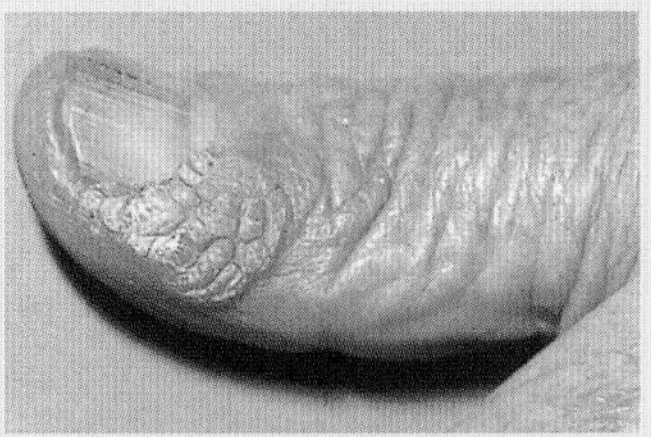 DR M H BECK	Small epidermal skin growths. Warts may be raised or flat, depending upon their position. Usually they have a rough surface and are raised.
Hairy moles 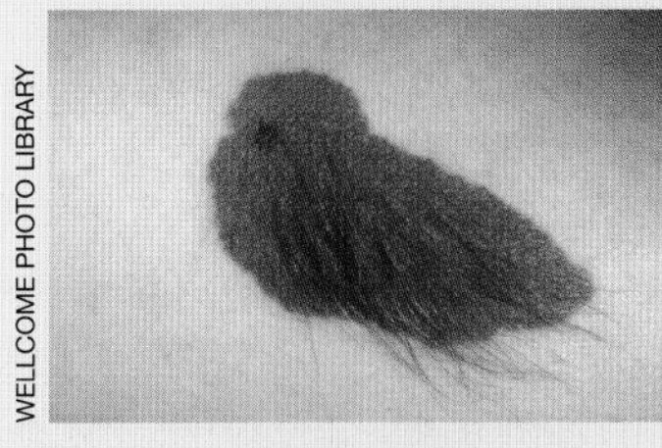 WELLCOME PHOTO LIBRARY	Models exhibiting coarse hairs from their surface. Hair growing from a mole may be cut, not plucked: if plucked, the hairs will become coarser and the growth of the hairs further stimulated.
Skin tags 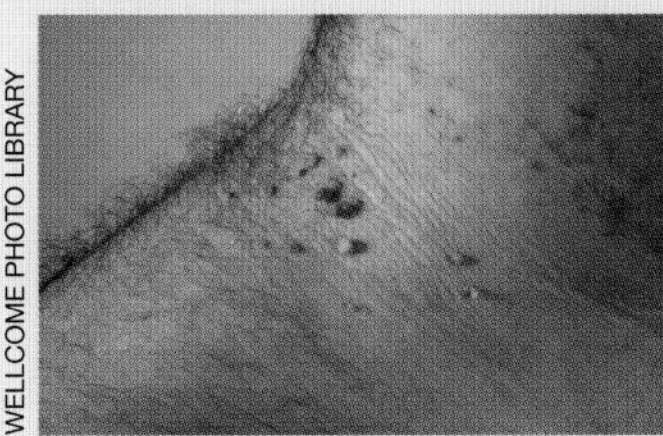 WELLCOME PHOTO LIBRARY	Skin-coloured threads of skin 3–6mm long, projecting from the skin's surface. Skin tags often occur under the arms.

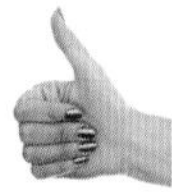

BEST PRACTICE

Bruising
If there is any bruising on the client's legs, tactfully draw their attention to these bruises, or they might later think that the treatment has caused them.

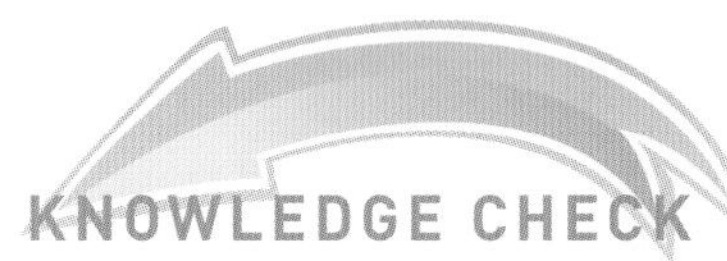

KNOWLEDGE CHECK

How often should a client have waxing treatments?

Need more time... refer to page 492 to help you.

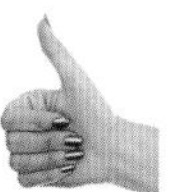

BEST PRACTICE

Habia skin safety awareness
Remember your role in helping your client stay safe by informing them of any mole that appears to have changed in size, shape or colour. See www.habia.org.

HEALTH & SAFETY

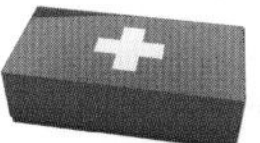

Hygiene
When carrying out any of these procedures, wear protective gloves. Both client and therapist must observe hygienic procedures; for example you should wipe over the area with a skin disinfectant before touching it.

HEALTH & SAFETY

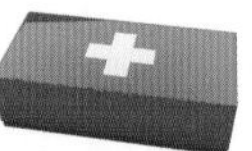

Contra-actions
If a contra-action, an unwanted reaction during treatment, occurs discontinue the treatment and provide appropriate advice.

TOP TIP

Sensitive skin
Waxing products designed for sensitive skin are available. It is a good idea to have such products available to accommodate all skin types

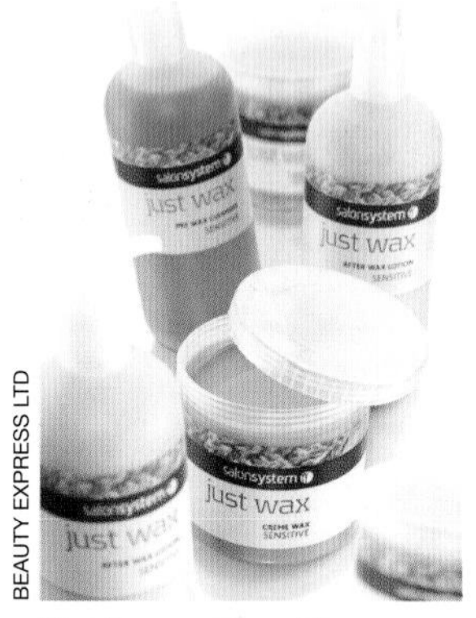

Wax for sensitive skin

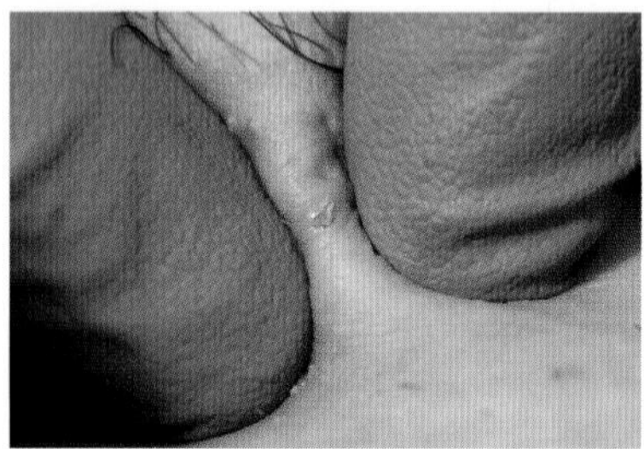

Coiled ingrowing hair

Contra-actions

Inform the client at consultation of any contra-actions that may occur and the action to take.

A contra-action is an unwanted reaction to a waxing treatment which may occur during or following the treatment.

Contra-actions which are quite common with waxing include:

- ***ingrowing hairs***
- ***removal of skin***
- ***burns*** – caused by both excessive wax temperature and friction burns
- ***excessive erythema*** – increased blood flow to the skin, causing an extreme redness

Ingrowing hairs Ingrowing hairs can arise in three ways:

- ***Over-reaction to damage*** An excessive reaction by the skin and the follicle to the 'damage' produced by depilation may cause extra cornified cells to be made. These may block the surface of the follicle, causing the newly growing hair to turn around and grow inwards.
- ***Overtight clothing*** If after the treatment the client wears clothing that is too tight, this too can block the follicle.
- ***Dry skin*** Likewise dry skin can cause blockage of the follicle.

Ingrowing hairs can usually be recognized to be one or other of three types:

- ***A hair growing along beneath the surface of the skin*** Identify the tip (the pointed end); then pierce the tissues over the root end with a sterile needle. Free the tip and leave it in place so that the follicle can heal around it.
- ***A coiled ingrowing hair*** This looks like a small black spot or dome on the skin. If this is gently squeezed and rolled between the fingertips, using a tissue, it will release the coiled ingrowing hair and some hardened sebum. If the hair does not fall out, it should be left in place (as above).
- ***An infected ingrowth*** If the trapped sebum or hair starts to decay, either of the two preceding forms can become infected or begin to display an immune response. The area first becomes red (irritation); then an infected white dome-shaped pustule develops. Release the trapped tissue (as above), and cover the affected area – which may bleed, or leak tissue fluid – with a sterile non-allergenic dressing.

Skin removal If the upper, dead, protective cornified layer of the skin is accidentally removed during a treatment – leaving the granular layer of the living, germinative layer exposed – the skin should be treated as if it has been burnt. This is often a result of poor removal techniques such as not holding the skin sufficiently taut or lifting the wax too high rather then parallel to the skin. This can also occur as a result of the client having used exfoliating skin medications, cortisone steroid medications and recent exfoliating beauty treatments such as micro-dermabrasion. Cool the area immediately by applying cold-water compresses for 10 minutes. Dry it carefully; then apply a dry, non-fluffy dressing to protect the area from infection. The dressing should be worn for three to four days, and the area then left open to the air. (Antiseptic cream by itself should be used only when the injury is very minor.) Medical attention should be sought if necessary.

Burns A burn should be treated the same as for '**skin removal**'. If blisters form, they should not be broken – they help prevent the entry of infection into the wound. Medical attention should be sought. Always remember the importance of testing the wax temperature on yourself and the client before treatment commences and make on-going checks throughout the treatment.

Erythema **Erythema** is a visible redness which is a normal reaction to skin waxing treatment. If excessive, it will be accompanied by an increase in warmth on the surface of the skin. This is created by an increased blood flow through the capillaries near the surface of the skin, caused by the **histamine** reaction after waxing. Ask the client to follow the recommended **aftercare advice**.

Certain waxing ingredients such as rosin, a resin, may cause an **allergic reaction** in some people.

The symptoms of an allergic reaction could be:

- redness of the skin (erythema)
- itching
- swelling
- blisters

Poor hygiene practice such as inadequate skin cleansing, application of aftercare lotion infecting the area of treatment and non-compliance by the client with aftercare instructions may result in bacterial infection seen as erythema and pustules in the area.

If an allergic reaction occurs during waxing application, stop treatment and remove any remaining product. Apply a cool compress and soothing agent to the area to reduce redness and irritation. Identify the possible cause of the allergic reaction. If symptoms persist, seek medical advice.

Always record any allergies on the client's record card, so that the offending product may be avoided in the future. Try an alternative **waxing products** to assess skin tolerance. In some cases the skin is too sensitive and intolerant to waxing treatment.

Always date and record any contra-actions on the client record card, with actions taken/recommendations provided and outcome.

After the record card has been completed, the client should be asked to read the list of contra-indications and sign to state that they are not suffering from any of the problems stated.

The therapist must not carry out a wax treatment immediately after a heat treatment, such as a sauna, or steam or ultra-violet treatments, as the heat-sensitized tissues may be irritated by the wax treatment.

If you are unsure if treatment may commence, tactfully refer the client to their general practitioner for permission to treat. A copy of the GP's letter on receipt should be kept with the client's record card. If the treatment cannot be carried out for any reason, always explain why, without naming a contra-indication, as you are not qualified to do so. Clients will respect your professional advice.

Following the consultation an appropriate treatment plan will be confirmed with the client. Their understanding of the treatment is important to ensure that their needs are met and that they will not be disappointed.

Record all client details accurately on the client record card. A sample record card follows.

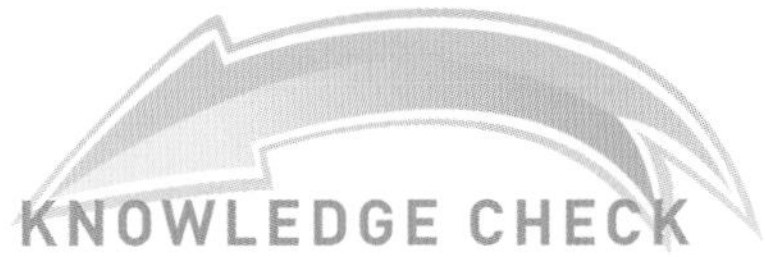

KNOWLEDGE CHECK

How can cross-infection be prevented when carrying out waxing treatments? Provide three examples.

Need more time... refer to pages 490–491 to help you.

ALWAYS REMEMBER

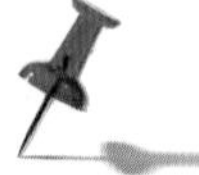

Reactions to treatment

Damage to the skin that occurs during a waxing treatment causing cells called *mast cells* to burst in the skin releasing a chemical substance called histamine. Histamine is released into the tissues causing the blood capillaries to dilate, giving the redness called erythema. The increased blood flow limits damage and begins repair. There can also be an increase in keratinised cells in the area seen as flaky patches of skin as the skin heals.

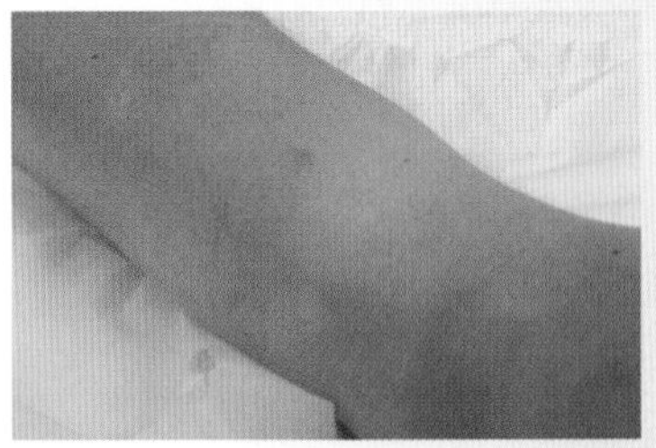

Normal erythema skin reaction

BEST PRACTICE

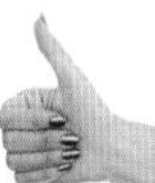

Contra-indications

While assessing the client's skin for waxing treatment, you should also be looking for contra-indications to treatment.

ACTIVITY

Ensuring client comfort

Imagine that you are a client who has never had a waxing treatment before. You are shown through to a cubicle and left to 'Get yourself ready, please'. How would you feel? What would you do? What clothing would you think it necessary to remove for each area of waxing?

If the client had mobility issues identified at consultation how could you prepare the work area to accommodate this need?

Sample client record card

Date | Beauty therapist name

Client name | Date of birth (Identifying client age group.)

Home address | Postcode

Email address | Landline phone number | Mobile phone number

Name of doctor | Doctor's address and phone number

Related medical history (Conditions that may restrict or prohibit treatment application.)

Are you taking any medication? (This may affect the sensitivity and skin reaction following treatment.)

CONTRA-INDICATIONS REQUIRING MEDICAL REFERRAL
(Preventing hair removal treatment.)

- ☐ bacterial infection (e.g. impetigo, conjunctivitis)
- ☐ viral infection (e.g. herpes simplex/warts)
- ☐ fungal infection (e.g. tinea corporis)
- ☐ severe skin conditions
- ☐ diabetes
- ☐ severe varicose veins
- ☐ phlebitis
- ☐ deep vein thrombosis
- ☐ client is undergoing chemotherapy or radiotherapy treatment

TEST CONDUCTED

☐ self ☐ client

WAX PRODUCTS

- ☐ hot wax
- ☐ warm wax – spatula method
- ☐ warm wax disposable applicator/tube/cartridge system
- ☐ strip sugar
- ☐ sugar paste

WORK TECHNIQUES

- ☐ keep the skin taut during application and removal
- ☐ speed of product removal
- ☐ direction and angle of removal
- ☐ ongoing wax product temperature checks

CONTRA-INDICATIONS WHICH RESTRICT TREATMENT
(Treatment may require adaptation.)

- ☐ cuts and abrasions
- ☐ bruising and swelling
- ☐ self tan
- ☐ skin disorders
- ☐ heat rash
- ☐ sunburn
- ☐ hairy moles
- ☐ mild eczema/psoriasis
- ☐ broken bones
- ☐ recent fractures
- ☐ recent scar tissue
- ☐ hyperkeratosis
- ☐ skin and product allergies
- ☐ circulatory conditions

AREAS TREATED FOR HAIR REMOVAL
(Treatment may require adaptation.)

- ☐ eyebrows
- ☐ face
  - ☐ upper lip
  - ☐ chin
- ☐ legs
  - ☐ full leg
  - ☐ half leg
- ☐ underarm
- ☐ bikini line

SKIN TYPE

- ☐ normal
- ☐ dry
- ☐ oily
- ☐ combination

SKIN CONDITION

☐ sensitive ☐ mature ☐ dehydrated

Beauty therapist signature (for reference)

Client signature (confirmation of details)

Sample client record card (continued)

*TREATMENT TIMINGS**

Half leg wax – *allow 30 minutes*
Full leg wax – *allow 50 minutes*
Bikini wax – *allow 15 minutes*
Underarm wax – *allow 15 minutes*

Eyebrow wax – *allow 15 minutes*
Facial wax top lip or chin – *allow 10 minutes*
top lip and chin – *allow 15 minutes*

*Waxing timings may differ according to the system used. Always allow slightly longer when using hot wax.

TREATMENT PLAN

Record relevant details of your treatment and advice provided for future reference.

Ensure the client's records are up to date, accurate and fully completed following treatment. Non-compliance may invalidate insurance.

DURING

Monitor:

- client's reaction to treatment to confirm suitability

Note:

- any adverse reaction, if any occur

AFTER

Record:

- results of treatment
- any modification to treatment application that has occurred
- what products have been used in the wax removal treatment
- the effectiveness of treatment
- any samples provided (review their success at the next appointment)

Advise on:

- use of aftercare products following wax removal treatment
- maintenance procedures
- the recommended time intervals between treatments

RETAIL OPPORTUNITIES

Advise on:

- products that would be suitable for the client to use at home to care for and maintain the treatment area (these include body exfoliation and moisturising skincare products)
- recommendations for further treatments
- further products or treatments that the client may or may not have received before

Note:

- any purchase made by the client

EVALUATION

Record:

- comments on the client's satisfaction with the treatment
- if poor results are achieved, the reasons why
- how you may alter the **treatment plan** to achieve the required treatment results in the future, if applicable

HEALTH AND SAFETY

Advise on:

- how to care for the area following treatment to avoid an unwanted reaction
- avoidance of any activities or product application that may cause a contra-action
- appropriate **necessary action** to be taken in the event of an unwanted skin or eye irritation

TOP TIP

Trimming hair

Trim long hair before waxing to avoid unnecessary client discomfort and to enable the hair growth direction to be more easily viewed.

Skin disorders such as skin tags can be hidden if the hair is too long.

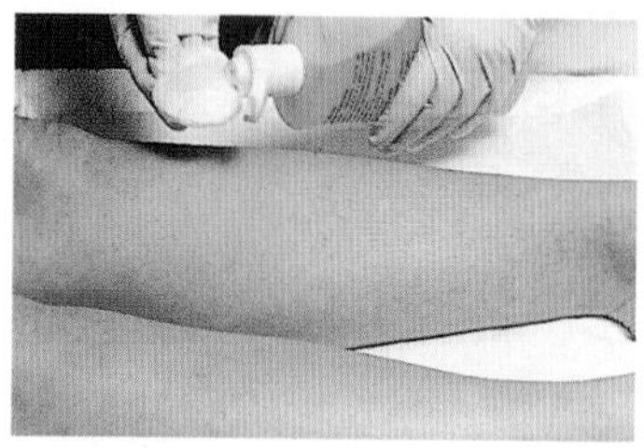

Cleansing the skin of the lower leg

TOP TIP

Time of the month

A woman's pain threshold is at its lowest immediately before and during her period. The hormones which stimulate the regrowth of hair are also at their most active during this period. For these two reasons, avoid wax depilation at this time if possible.

ALWAYS REMEMBER

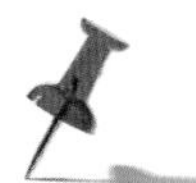

Angled follicles

An angled follicle may cause the hair to be broken off at the angle during waxing, instead of being completely pulled out with its root. If this happens, broken hairs will appear at the skin's surface within a few days.

By causing damage to the follicle and changing its shape, waxing can cause the regrowth of hairs to be frizzy or curled where previously they were straight.

ALWAYS REMEMBER

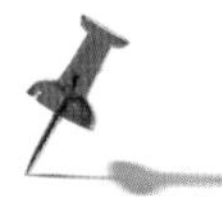

Client records

In accordance with the **Data Protection Act (1998)**, confidential information on clients should only be made available to persons to whom consent has been given. All client records should be stored securely, and be available to refer to at any time as required. They must be kept for up to three years.

Preparing the client

The client should be shown through to the treatment cubicle, and asked to remove specific items of clothing or accessories in the area as necessary so that the treatment may be carried out. Disposable briefs may be provided if a bikini wax treatment is to be received.

If it is the first time the client has had the treatment, explain to them that the treatment can be uncomfortable, but it is quick and any discomfort experienced is tolerable.

Be efficient and quick, so that the client does not have to wait. Try to get the client talking about something pleasant, such as a holiday, to take their mind off the treatment. Throughout the treatment, reassure them, praising them in order to motivate them to continue with the treatments. Do try to be sympathetic to your client's feelings, and provide support and encouragement when necessary. Waxing, although a necessity for many people, is not a particularly pleasant or relaxing treatment.

How to prepare the client for treatment

1. Use a towel to protect the client's remaining clothing. Even if performing an eyebrow wax, protect the chest area in case of wax spillage.
2. Wipe the area to be waxed with a professional antiseptic pre-wax cleansing lotion on cotton wool. This should be dispensed from a pump or spray bottle or removed with a spatula if in a container. Blot the area dry with tissues before applying the wax. While wiping the skin, look for contra-indications that restrict the treatment, e.g. varicose veins.
3. Record any bruising or contra-indications that restrict treatment on the record card to avoid potential problems later.
4. If the client's skin is very greasy (they may for example have applied oil before coming to the salon), cleanse it using an astringent lotion such as witch-hazel. Talcum powder may be applied lightly to the area to facilitate hair removal.
5. Immediately before starting the treatment, wash your hands. Apply PPE as required according to the body part being treated.
6. Perform a **thermal skin sensitivity test**: before applying the wax, check its temperature. Test the wax on yourself first, to ensure that it's not too warm; then try a little on the client on the area to be treated (to check tolerance to the heat) before spreading it on other areas.

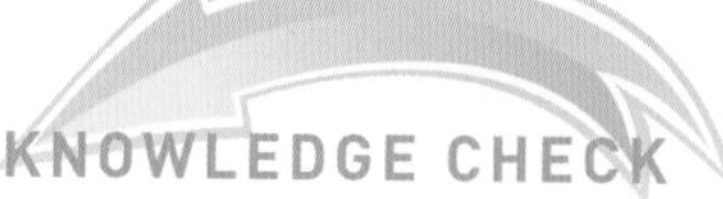

KNOWLEDGE CHECK

If the client has a sensitive or allergic skin type what must be performed in advance of the waxing treatment?

Need more time... refer to page 491 to help you.

Waxing treatments

Outcome 2: Be able to provide waxing treatments

Learn how to provide waxing treatments

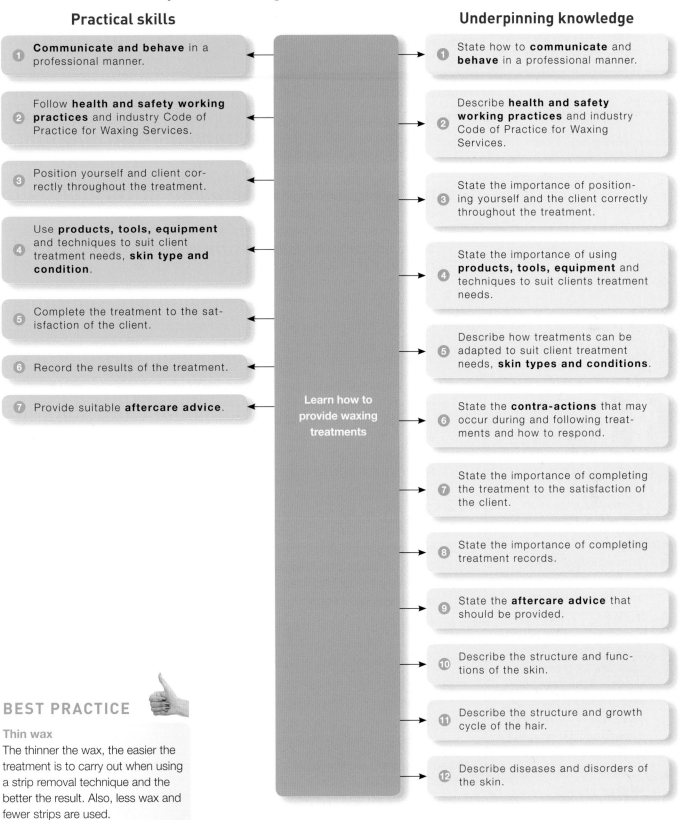

Practical skills

1. **Communicate and behave** in a professional manner.
2. Follow **health and safety working practices** and industry Code of Practice for Waxing Services.
3. Position yourself and client correctly throughout the treatment.
4. Use **products, tools, equipment** and techniques to suit client treatment needs, **skin type and condition**.
5. Complete the treatment to the satisfaction of the client.
6. Record the results of the treatment.
7. Provide suitable **aftercare advice**.

Underpinning knowledge

1. State how to **communicate** and **behave** in a professional manner.
2. Describe **health and safety working practices** and industry Code of Practice for Waxing Services.
3. State the importance of positioning yourself and the client correctly throughout the treatment.
4. State the importance of using **products, tools, equipment** and techniques to suit clients treatment needs.
5. Describe how treatments can be adapted to suit client treatment needs, **skin types and conditions**.
6. State the **contra-actions** that may occur during and following treatments and how to respond.
7. State the importance of completing the treatment to the satisfaction of the client.
8. State the importance of completing treatment records.
9. State the **aftercare advice** that should be provided.
10. Describe the structure and functions of the skin.
11. Describe the structure and growth cycle of the hair.
12. Describe diseases and disorders of the skin.

BEST PRACTICE

Thin wax

The thinner the wax, the easier the treatment is to carry out when using a strip removal technique and the better the result. Also, less wax and fewer strips are used.

HEALTH & SAFETY 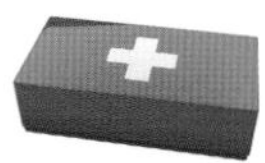

Avoid cross-contamination

It is unhygienic to return a spatula to the wax after it has been in contact with the body part. It is therefore required that a new spatula be used for each entry to the wax. This applies to warm, hot and sugar-strip wax.

"Removing the entire hair including the bulb is the aim of waxing, (though many therapists do not always achieve this goal). To ensure you always remove all the hair and so provide a lasting treatment, get two things right:

- When removing the wax, hold the skin taught this will 'open the follicles', which means you are more likely to remove the entire hair.
- Master an effective 'flicking' action when removing the wax strip; flick backwards, keeping it parallel to the skin, always against the direction of hair growth. Do not pull upwards as this is more likely to 'snap' off the hairs at the surface of the skin.

Janice Brown

Warm waxing

Warm waxing has a few basic rules which must be followed to ensure a good result.

Observe the direction of hair growth. Warm wax must always be ***applied with*** the direction of hair growth, and ***removed against*** the direction of growth. This ensures both maximum adhesion between the hair, the strip and the wax, and that the hair will be pulled back on itself in the follicle and thus removed complete with its bulb.

Spatula application technique

1. Dip the spatula into the wax. Remove the excess on the sides and tip by wiping the spatula against the metal bar or the sides of the tub. Place the strip under the spatula while transferring it to the client: this will control dripping and improve your technique.
2. Place the spatula onto the skin at a 90° angle, and push the wax along in the direction of the hair growth. Do not allow the spatula to fall forward past 45°. The objective is to coat the area with a very thin film of wax. Quite a large area can be spread with each sweep of the spatula, as warm wax does not set. Do not attempt to smooth out or go over areas on which wax has already been spread, however, as the wax will have become cooler and will not move again, but will drag painfully on the client's skin.
3. Fold back 20mm at the end of a strip and grip the flap with the thumb widthways across the strip. The flap should provide a wax-free handle throughout the treatment.
4. Place the strip at the bottom end of the wax-covered area, and make a firm bond between the wax and the strip by pressing firmly along the strip's length and width, following the direction of hair growth. If the strip is placed anywhere but at the bottom of a waxed area, the hairs at the ***bottom*** of the strip will become tangled together and held in the wax on the area below the strip: the removal of the strip will then be far more painful for the client.
5. Using the non-working hand, stretch the skin to minimize discomfort. Gripping the flap tightly, use the working hand to remove the strip against the direction of hair growth. Use a firm, steady pull. Make sure that the strip is pulled back on itself, close to the skin. (To obtain the correct angle of pull, stand at the side of the client, facing them.) Maintain this same horizontal angle of pull until the last bit of the strip has left the skin: ***do not pull the strip upwards at the end of the pull*** as this would break the hairs at the end of the strip and be very painful.
6. The strip may be used many times; in fact it works best when some wax builds up on its surface. When there is too much wax on the surface it will stop picking up more: throw it away and start with a new one.
7. Do not repeatedly spread and remove wax over one area. In particular, wax should not be spread and removed more than twice on sensitive areas such as the bikini line, the face and the underarms. Any remaining stray hairs must instead be removed using sterilized tweezers.

Alternatively, warm wax may be applied using a disposable cartridge/tube applicator system. This system is discussed on pages 515–516.

Different temperatures Summer heat and winter cold can each give rise to problems with the wax treatment. In summer, the wax stays too warm on the body, becoming sticky and difficult to work with, and tending to leave a sticky residue on the treated areas. In winter, the client's legs may be cold, causing the wax to set too quickly as you spread it, so that it becomes too thick. This prevents the efficient removal of both the wax and the hair growth.

To some extent these problems can be overcome by using thicker waxes with higher melting points in the summer, and thinner waxes with lower melting points in the winter.

TOP TIP

Take the sting out

To take the sting out of the removal, immediately place a hand or finger over the depilated area.

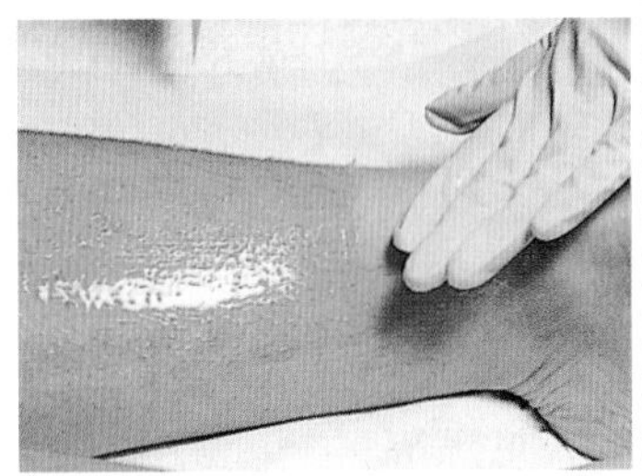

Wax removal

How to provide a half-leg wax treatment

The areas of the body where warm-wax hair removal is most frequently used are the lower legs. This is often referred to simply as a **half-leg treatment**. A 'pair of half legs' should take 20–30 minutes to treat, and use no more than three or four wax removal strips.

1. Prior to the treatment, the area to be waxed should be cleansed as previously described.
2. Sit the client on the upraised couch, with both legs straight out in front of them.
3. Spread the wax on the *front* of the leg further away from you. Use three sweeps of the spatula: each sweep should go from just below the knee to the end of hair growth at the ankle.

   Repeat this pattern of spreading on the leg nearer to you. (By spreading the further leg first, you will not have to lean over an already waxed area.)
4. Starting with the nearer leg, remove the wax using the strip. Start at the ankle and work upwards towards the knees.

   Repeat for the other leg.
5. Ask the client to bend their legs to one side. Beginning again with the further leg, spread wax on one *side* of the leg, from the knee to the ankle, using two sweeps of the spatula.

   Repeat for the nearer leg.
6. Starting with the nearer leg, remove the wax from the bottom upwards.

   Repeat for the other leg.
7. Repeat steps 5 and 6 for the other side of the legs.
8. Bend one knee. Spread the wax from just above the knee, downwards.
9. Remove this wax from the bottom upwards, remembering that strips cannot pull around corners effectively. To keep the angle of the pull horizontal, remove wax below the knee first, then that above the knee.
10. Repeat steps 8 and 9 for the other knee.
11. Lower the backrest and ask the client to turn over.

> Different brands of wax have a range of melting point temperatures so it is important to follow manufacturers' instructions regarding melting times and advised heats.
>
> **Janice Brown**

BEST PRACTICE

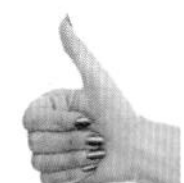

Troubleshooting

The faults most commonly seen in warm-wax depilation are these:

- spreading the wax too thickly
- placing the strip in the middle of a wax-spread area, instead of starting at the bottom and working up
- pulling the strip upwards instead of backwards, away from the leg, causing breakage of the hair
- wax left on the skin after strip removal – this may be because of poor skin preparation; the skin was damp before wax application; the skin was not held sufficiently taut on removal; insufficient pressure applied when rubbing the wax strip before removal.

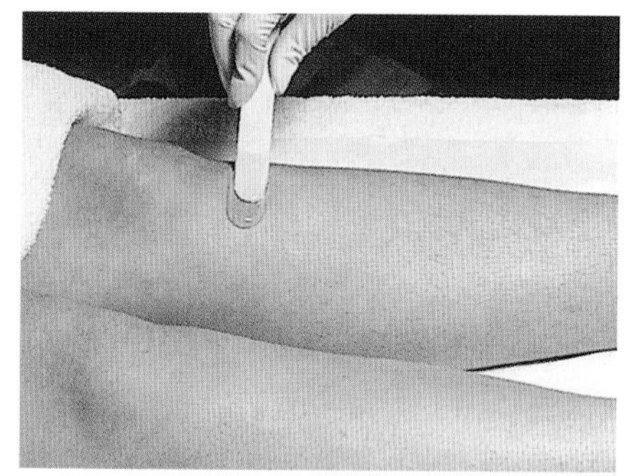
Applying warm wax to the lower leg

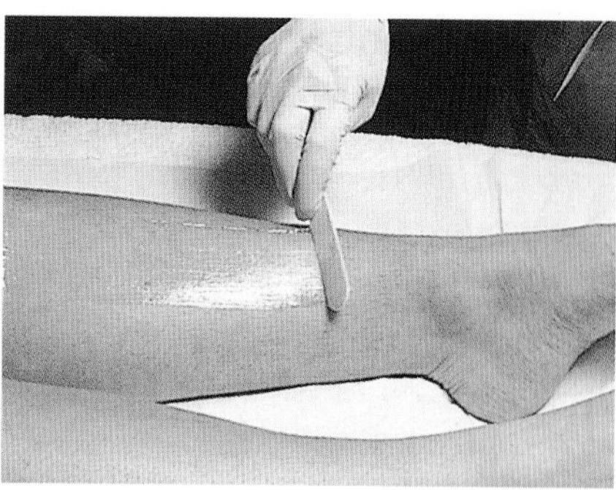
Spreading on wax (with correct spatula angle)

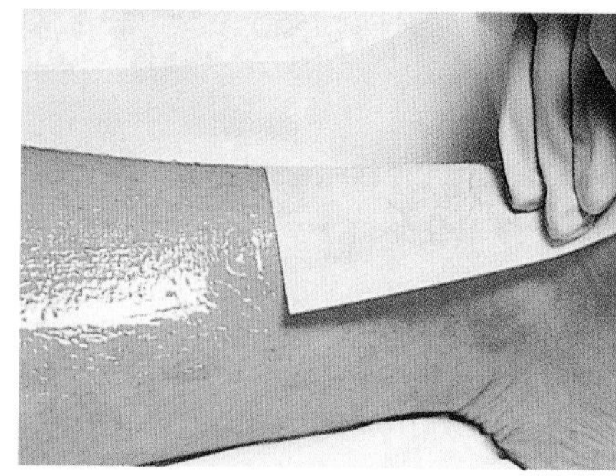
Applying a wax removal strip

KNOWLEDGE CHECK

It is necessary to consider the direction of hair growth for the different waxing hair removal techniques. Why is this?

Need more time... refer to page 500 to help you.

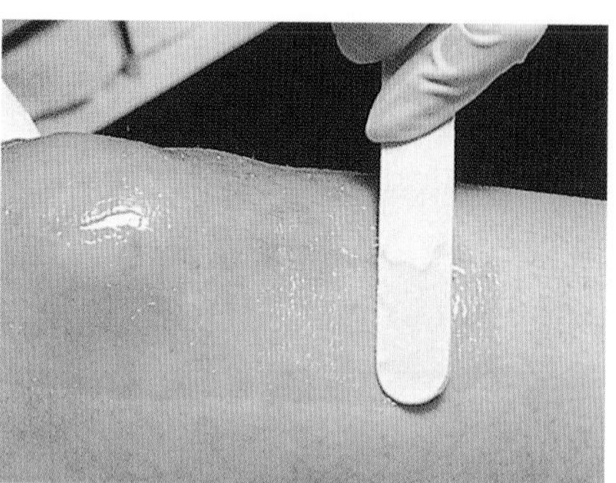
Applying warm wax to the knee

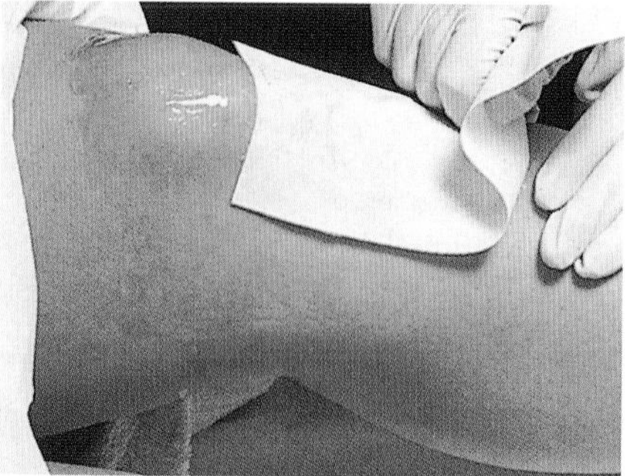
Removing the wax strip from the knee

TOP TIP

Winter and summer problems

Thick lumps of wax stuck to the legs (the winter problem) can be removed by pulling more slowly than normal, or by reversing the direction of pull on the strip. A sticky residue on the legs (the summer problem) must be removed using after-wax lotion.

HEALTH & SAFETY

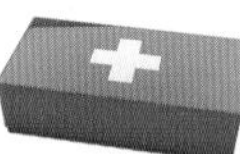

Contra-action as a result of waxing treatment

If any contra-action appears to be more than minor, advise the client to see their GP straight away after treatment.

12 On the *back* of the legs, the direction of hair growth is not from the top to the bottom but sweeping at an angle, from the outside to the inside of the calf muscle.

Starting with the further leg, spread wax following the direction of the natural hair growth.

Repeat for the nearer leg.

13 Starting with the nearer leg, remove the wax against the direction of the natural hair growth.

Repeat for the other leg.

14 Finally, apply after-wax lotion to clean cotton wool and apply this to the back of the client's legs. As you apply the lotion, check for hairs left behind: if there are any, remove them using tweezers.

Ask the client to turn over, and repeat application on the front of the legs. Remove any excess using a tissue.

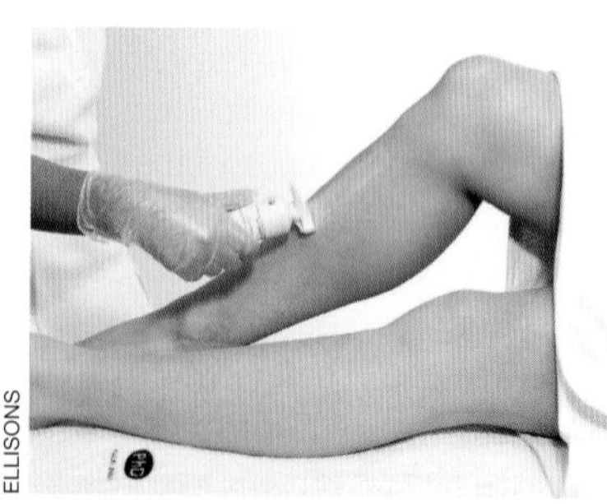
ELLISONS

Leg wax application using disposable application warm wax technique

Disposable warm wax application to leg Wax is heated in its container applied through the disposable applicator head directly to the skin area. A wax strip is used to remove the hairs from the area removing the wax strip against hair growth.

Toes Clients frequently request that their toes be waxed in conjunction with a half leg or full-leg treatment. When doing this, follow the normal guidelines for waxing, but be aware that hair may grow in many directions. Cut strips into small pieces to effectively remove hair.

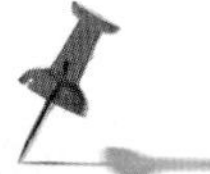

ALWAYS REMEMBER

Common faults

The most common fault seen in half-leg waxing is trying to take too big an area at once over the calf muscle and not supporting the surrounding tissues adequately. This will result in a painful treatment for the client.

Full-leg treatment

A full-leg wax should take 40–50 minutes and four to six strips should be sufficient.

When doing a full-leg wax, follow the same sequence of working as with the half leg. On the thighs, observe the direction of hair growth carefully, as the hair grows in different directions. It is best not to spread wax on too large an area at once, or you may forget the direction of growth. Each direction of hair growth should be treated as a separate area. It is of prime importance that you support the skin on the thighs as you remove the strip – the tissues in this area can bruise very easily. The two essential factors in preventing bruising, pain and hair breakage are:

- the correct angle of pull
- adequate support for the tissues

TOP TIP

Wax spills

If you spill wax on the couch cover, immediately place a quarter-width facial-sized piece of strip on top of the spill. This prevents the wax from damaging the client's clothing when they move.

How to provide a bikini-line treatment

A **bikini-line treatment** takes 10–15 minutes, and requires a new strip for each section to ensure effective hair removal from this delicate area.

1. Treat one side at a time. It is best if the client lies flat, as the skin's tissues are then pulled tighter, but the treatment can be carried out in a semi-reclining position if the client prefers. Bend the client's knee out to the side, and put their foot flat against the knee of the other leg. This is sometimes referred to as the **figure-four position**.
2. Tuck a protective tissue along and under the lower edge of the client's briefs. Raise this edge and agree with the client where they want the final line to be. Hold the briefs slightly beyond this line, and ask the client to place their hand on top of the protective tissue to hold everything in place. This leaves you with both hands free, one to pull the strip and one to support the skin.
3. Cleanse and dry the areas to be waxed.
4. Using sterilized scissors, trim both the hair to be waxed and the adjacent hairs down to about 5–12mm in length. This is essential to avoid tangling, pulling and pain, and to prevent wax going onto hair that you do not want to remove.
5. Spread and remove the wax in two or three separate and distinct areas, the number of application areas will depend on the directions of hair growth.
6. Use half of the strip length to remove the wax. Do not cover the whole area and tear it off at once! Treat the top plane of the thigh (Plane 1) and then the plane underneath this (Plane 2), see image on the next page. As soon as an area is completed, apply after-wax lotion. If necessary, use a clean tissue to remove excess lotion.

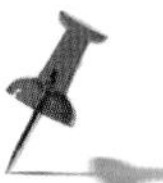

ALWAYS REMEMBER

Intimate waxing

Intimate waxing is a range of waxing techniques which remove pubic and/or anal body hair. This is an advanced waxing treatment covered at Level 3 and differs from the requirements of a bikini waxing treatment.

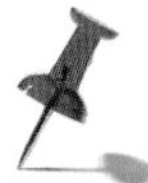

ALWAYS REMEMBER

Bruising

Bruising is neither normal nor acceptable, but a sign of faulty technique.

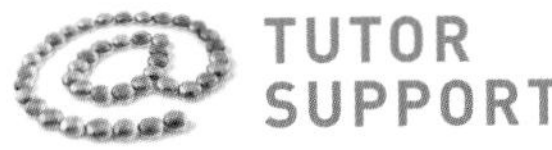

TUTOR SUPPORT

Activity 3: Treatment times

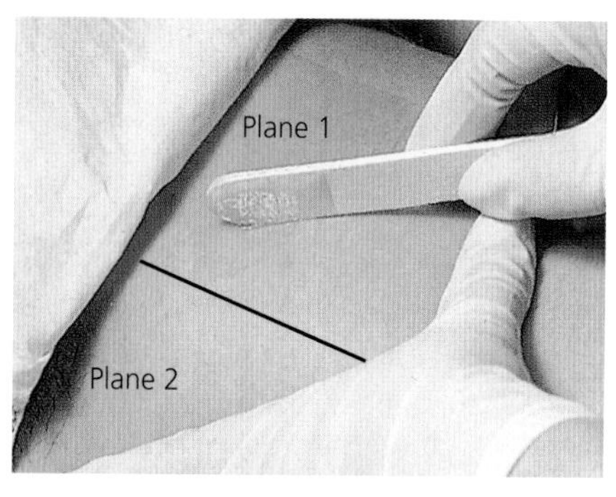

Applying warm wax to the bikini line

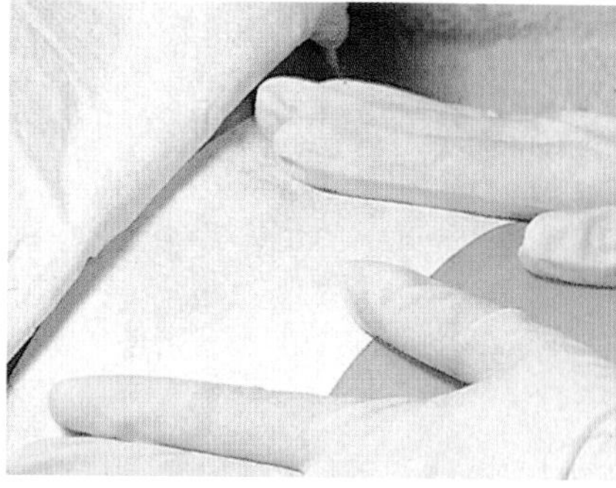

Applying a strip

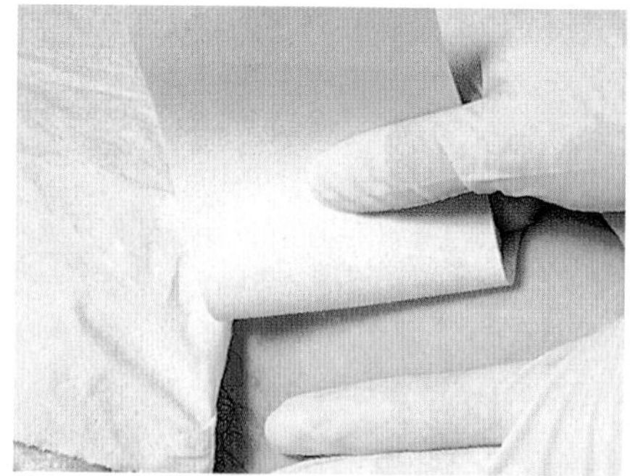

Removing the wax strip holding the skin taut

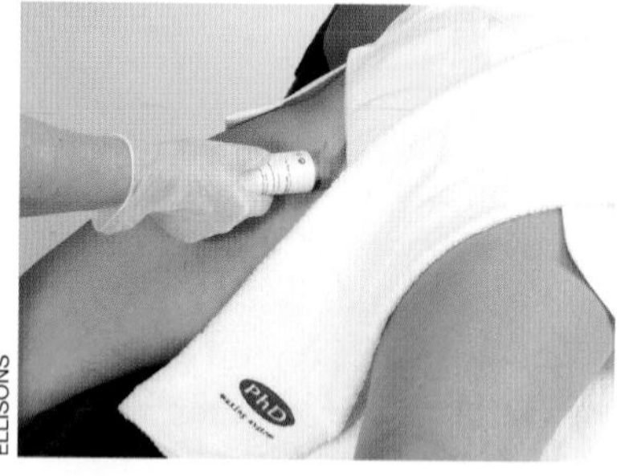

ELLISONS

Bikini wax: using disposable applicator warm wax technique

7 With both legs straight out in front on the couch, place a protective tissue along the top edge of the client's briefs, against the abdomen. Lower the briefs as necessary to expose just the hair to be removed – check this with your client. Usually the direction of hair growth here sweeps in from the sides and then up to the navel.

8 Trim the hair as before.

9 Apply and remove the wax in small sections, carefully observing hair growth. On completion, apply after-wax lotion.

Disposable warm wax application to bikini area Wax is applied in small sections through the applicator head to the skin area. A wax strip is used to remove the hairs from the area removing the wax strip against hair growth.

TOP TIP

Perspiration

If certain types of water-soluble waxes are being used, perspiration may cause problems: it may prevent the wax from gripping the hair. Bear this in mind when selecting the wax to use on areas liable to perspiration such as the underarm and the top lip.

How to provide an underarm treatment

An underarm treatment should take 5–15 minutes and two strips, one for each underarm.

1 With their bra still on, ask your client to lie flat on their back with their hands behind their head, elbows flat on the couch.

2 Cleanse both underarms with pre-wax lotion on clean cotton wool; blot with a tissue.

3 Place a protective tissue under the edge of the bra cup on the side away from you. Ask the client to bring their opposite arm down and over, and to pull the breast away from the underarm being waxed and across towards the middle of her chest. This pulls the tissues tight, making the treatment a lot more comfortable for them; it also leaves you with both hands free, one to pull and one to support.

4 Underarm hair usually grows in two main directions. Observe the directions of hair growth, then apply and remove the wax separately for each small area.

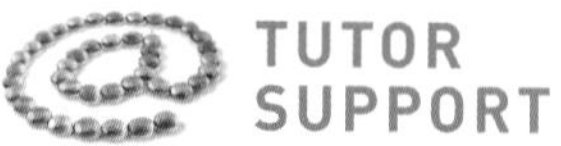

TUTOR SUPPORT

Activity 2: Aftercare leaflet design task

BEST PRACTICE

Contaminated waste

Both bikini-line and underarm waxing can be uncomfortable, especially if the hair growth is thick – always bear this in mind when carrying out the treatment. Some slight bleeding can be expected as the hairs in this area are very strong and have deep roots. Any waste contaminated by blood must be disposed of hygienically in a sealed bag.

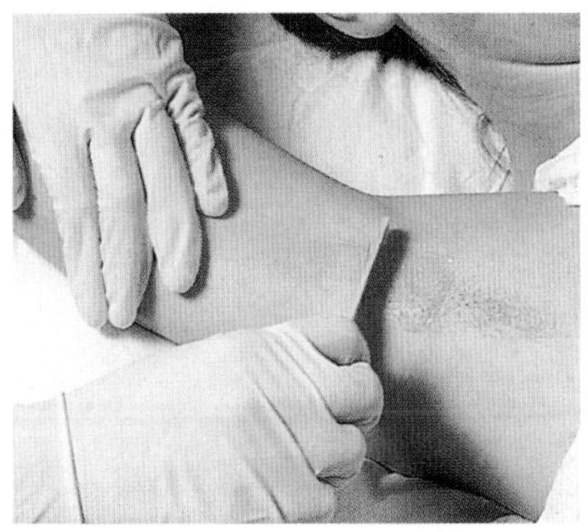

Applying warm wax to the underarm

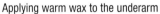

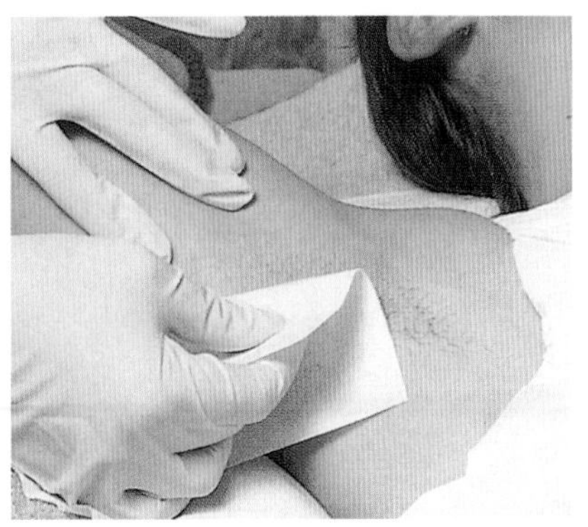
Removing the wax strip

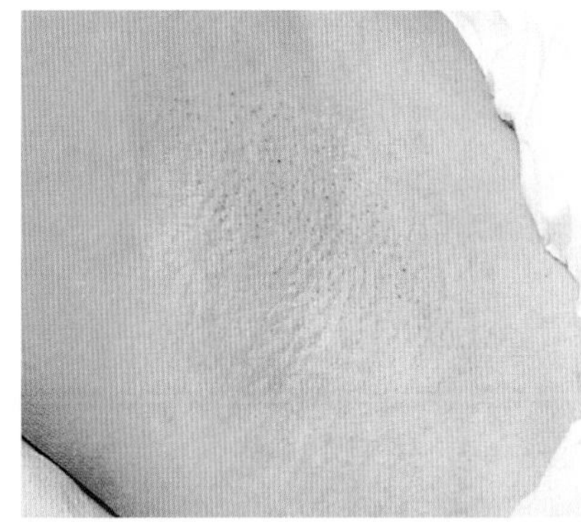
The completed area

5 Apply after-wax lotion to the treated area. Check for stray hairs; remove these with sterile tweezers.

6 Blot any excess cream with a clean tissue.

Disposable warm wax application to underarm Wax is applied in small sections through the applicator head to the skin area. A wax strip is used to remove the hair from the area, removing the wax strip against hair growth.

KNOWLEDGE CHECK

What could be three undesirable post treatment skin reactions? How would these be avoided?

Need more time... refer to pages 494–495 to help you.

Step-by-step: Arm treatment

Depilation in this area should take 10–15 minutes for a **half-arm treatment** and 20–30 minutes for a **full-arm treatment**. Half the length of the strip should be used.

Arms are usually waxed with the client in the sitting position, with their general clothing protected with a towel. Sleeve edges can be protected with tucked-in tissues; ideally, though, upper outer clothing should be removed.

The roundness of the arm means that in order to effect a horizontal pull the work must be done in short lengths. Other than this, follow the general rules for waxing.

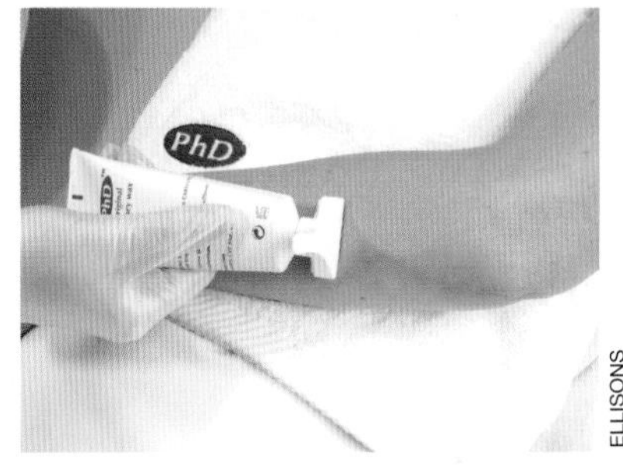

ELLISONS

Forearm wax using disposable application warm-wax technique

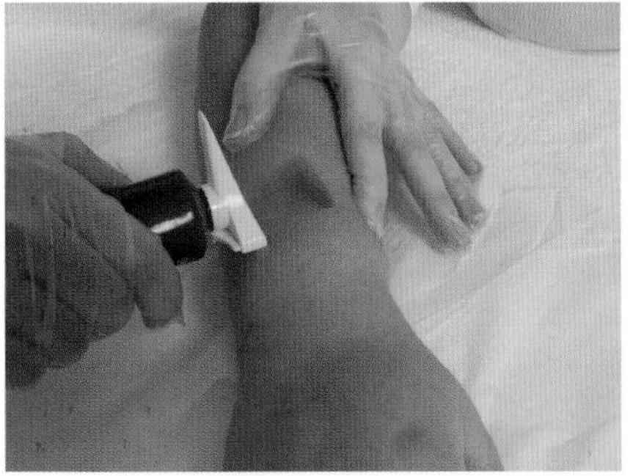
1 Wax applied in the direction of hair growth using disposable applicator warm-wax technique.

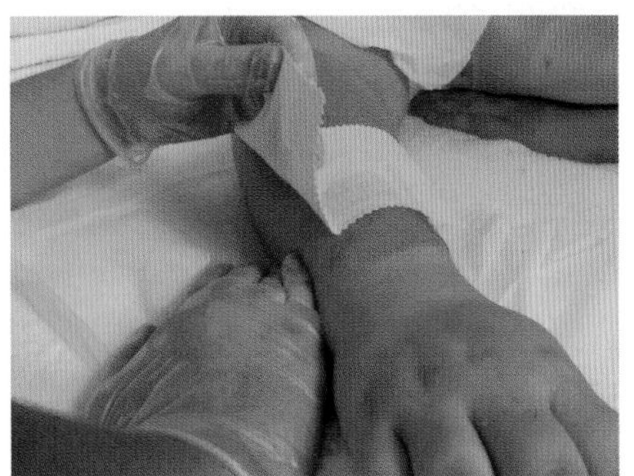
2 Wax is removed against hair growth, ensuring that the skin is held taut to minimize discomfort and ensure effective hair removal.

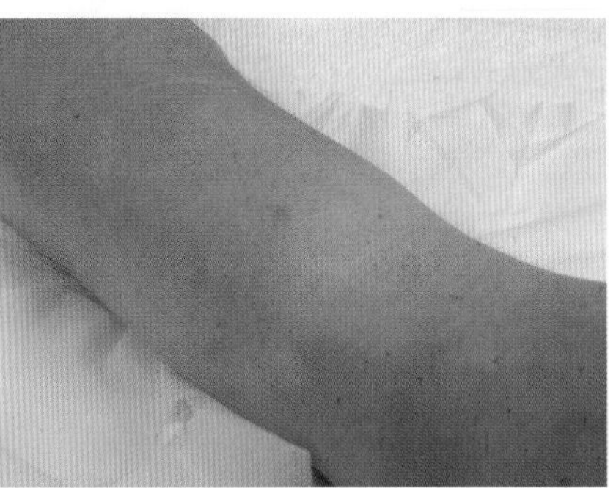
3 Mild erythema of the skin following hair removal. Check the area from all angles to ensure all hairs have been removed.

Step-by-step: Face treatment

The **face treatment** must always be approached with extra care as facial skin is more sensitive than skin elsewhere on the body. Faulty technique can result in the top layer of skin being removed. (If this happens, a scab will form after about a day and the mark will take days to heal and fade completely.)

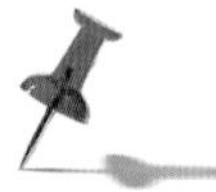

ALWAYS REMEMBER

Bleached hair
Previously bleached hair tends when waxed to break off at skin level. Clients should be told not to bleach facial hair if it is to be waxed.

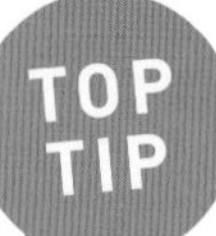

TOP TIP

Dark superfluous facial hair
Avoid obvious lines when removing facial hair. Ensure the outer border of the area treated blends into the adjacent area of skin.

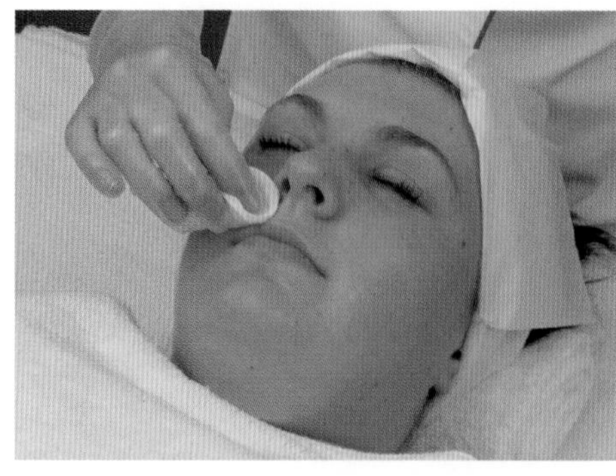

1 The client should be in a semi-reclining position, with their head supported and a clean towel draped across their shoulders to protect their clothing. A clean headband can be used to keep the hair away from the face.

2 Cleanse and wipe over the area thoroughly until the cotton wool or pre-wax cleansing wipe shows clean using an antiseptic cleansing lotion. Blot it dry with a tissue.

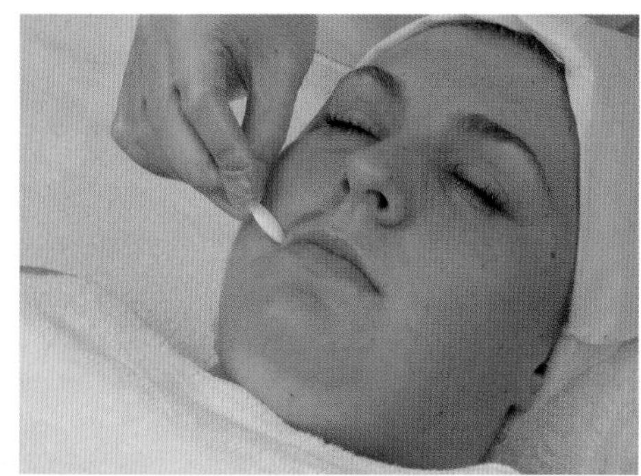

3 Application of warm wax to the upper lip using a disposable applicator, paying close attention to the direction of natural hair growth. Hair removal is only required to the outer upper lip area for this client. You might need to spread one-half of the top lip with wax; remove this in three or four narrow strips; repeat the process on the other half; and finally treat the central section immediately under the nose.

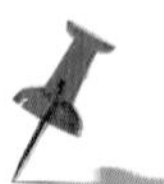

ALWAYS REMEMBER

The lips
The lips are extremely sensitive. To avoid possible irritation, do not allow the wax to come into contact with them.

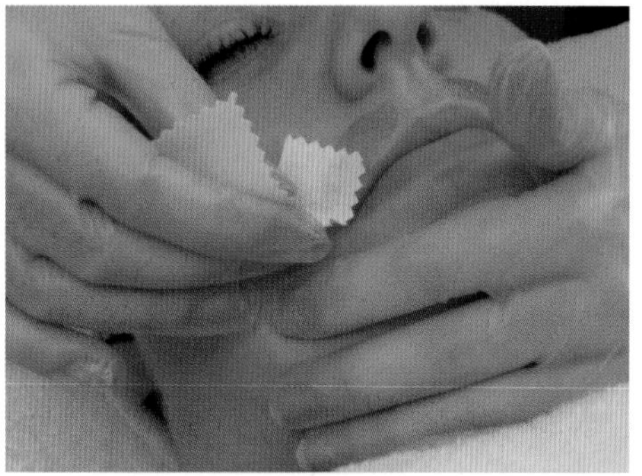

4 Removal of wax against hair growth. The area is held taut to minimize discomfort and ensure effective hair removal.

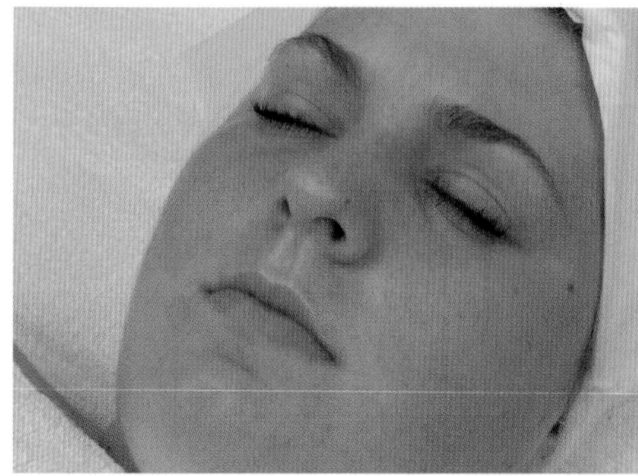

5 The completed area, free from superfluous hair.

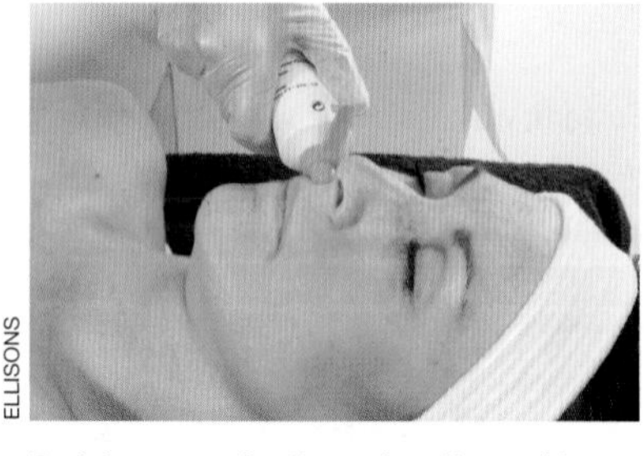

ELLISONS

Facial wax application using disposable applicator warm wax technique

A **top-lip wax** should take approximately 5 minutes, a **chin and throat wax** approximately 10 minutes, and a **lip and chin wax** approximately 15 minutes. A removal strip of no more than one-eighth normal size should be used on the face. Do not allow wax to build up on the facial wax strips – such a build-up could lead to skin removal. Use a new strip for each area.

If the chin is to be treated this area is less sensitive than the upper lip so if treating both areas complete the chin area last. Apply the wax according to the type of wax used. You may find that when treating a female client there may be small groupings of hairs and the wax may be applied to these areas only. If the client has dark superfluous facial hair it may be necessary to treat the sides of the face also.

A disposable warm wax application to facial area Wax is applied in small sections through the applicator head to the skin area. A wax strip is used to remove the hair from the area removing the wax strip against growth.

How to provide an eyebrow treatment

Eyebrows, as a part of the face, are treated accordingly (see above). An **eyebrow wax** should take approximately 10–15 minutes.

1. Study the eyebrows and decide upon their final shape and proportions.
2. Brush the eyebrows and separate the unwanted hair (**superfluous hair**) from the line of the other hairs.
3. Using a small spatula, apply a thin film of wax to the unwanted hairs in a small area. Remove the wax using a clean strip. Repeat in different areas, using a clean strip each time, until all the unwanted hairs have been removed.
4. Apply a soothing antiseptic cream and use sterile tweezers to remove any stray hairs.

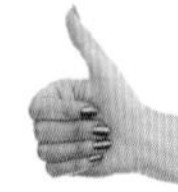

BEST PRACTICE

Protect against spillage
When performing an eyebrow wax, eyebrow hair that does not need to be removed may be protected with petroleum jelly.

Cotton wool pads may be placed over the eyes to protect the eye and eyelashes from accidental wax spillage.

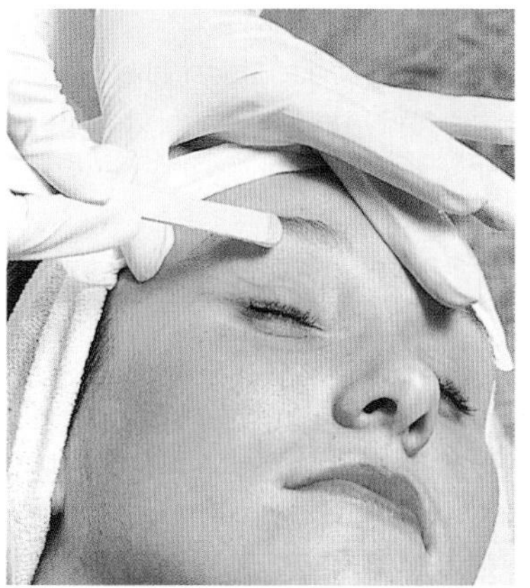

Applying warm wax to an eyebrow

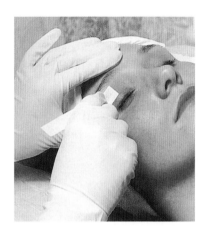

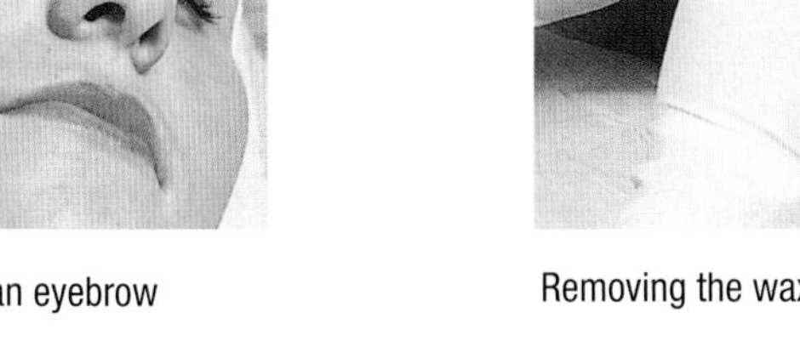

Removing the wax strip

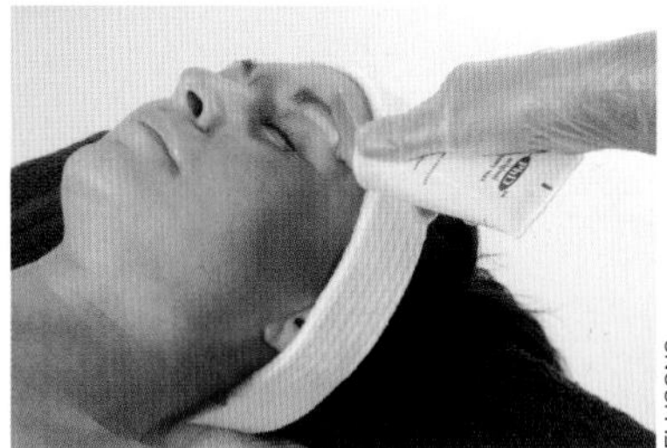

ELLISONS

Eyebrow wax application: disposable applicator technique

HEALTH & SAFETY

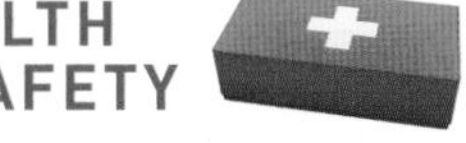

Sensitization
Under no circumstances should wax be applied to facial hair, underarm hair or bikini-line hair more than twice during any one treatment. If after this any hairs remain, they must be removed with tweezers. The delicate skin in these areas readily becomes sensitized.

A disposable warm wax application to the eyebrow area Wax is applied in small sections through the applicator head to the skin area. A wax strip is used to remove the hair from the area removing the wax strip against growth.

Aftercare and advice

The following aftercare and advice should be provided after each waxing treatment is completed to reconfirm the client's understanding of these important procedures.

TOP TIP

Waxing other areas
Other areas of the neck and face can be treated by wax depilation – for example to tidy up a haircut at the neckline, or to remove sideburns – provided that you follow the general guidelines for facial treatments.

HEALTH & SAFETY

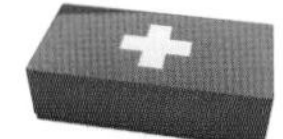

Aftercare insurance requirements
Many insurance companies require that aftercare instructions are provided in written form as well as verbally following the treatment. This will ensure that the client understands the necessity and possible consequences of not carrying these instructions out. Check your salon policy regarding this.

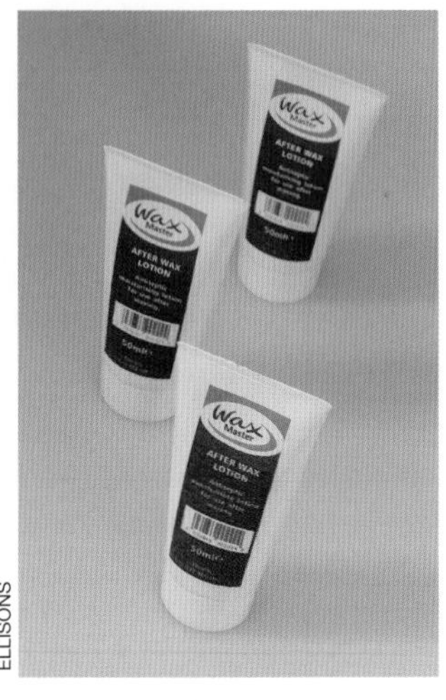
ELLISONS

After-wax products

An after-wax antiseptic, soothing lotion should be applied, using clean cotton wool, at the end of the treatment. This breaks down any wax residue, helps to guard against secondary infection and irritation, and takes away any feelings of discomfort. Encourage your client to continue with the use of such a lotion at home for up to three days: it will protect against dryness, discomfort, infection and ingrowing hairs.

BEST PRACTICE

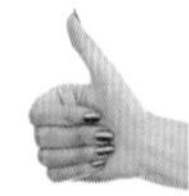

After-wax lotion

Before after-wax lotion is applied ensure that the treatment area is free of waxing product and hair and check that the finished result is to the client's satisfaction.

Any residue left will cause dirt and materials in the area to stick which could lead to secondary infection.

Products have been formulated to apply to the skin following wax depilation to slow hair re-growth. The product when entering the empty hair follicle aims to weaken the cell's matrix, slowing cell division in this area which is responsible for creating the new hair. These are available for your client to purchase as a retail product.

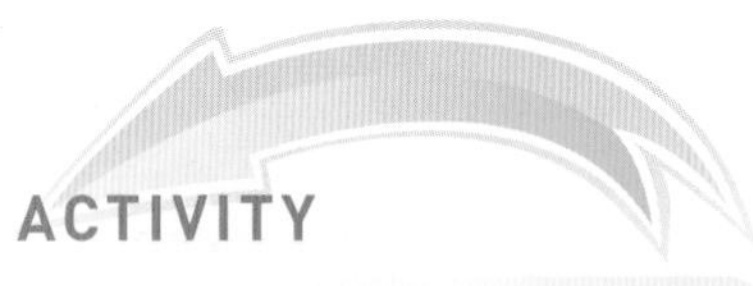

ACTIVITY

Aftercare leaflets

Discuss why aftercare leaflets should be given to clients, as well as giving them the advice verbally.

What could happen if aftercare advice is not given?

Design a suitable aftercare leaflet you could provide for your clients following waxing treatment.

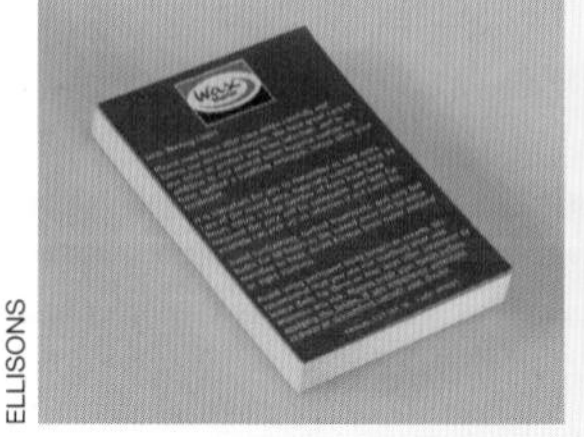
ELLISONS

Aftercare leaflet

Advise the client against wearing any tight clothing (such as tights or hosiery) over the waxed areas for the 24 hours following a treatment. Such clothing could lead to irritation and ingrowing hairs.

If the client suffers from ingrowing hairs, they should **exfoliate** their skin every four to seven days, starting two or three days after the treatment. Exfoliation prevents the build-up of dead skin cells on the surface of the skin; these would otherwise block the exit from the follicle and cause a growing hair to turn back on itself and grow inwards. Ingrowing hairs should be freed and, if possible, left in place so that the follicle exit will re-form around the hair's shaft. Demonstrate to the client the correct use and benefits of the exfoliant product.

Advise the client that for the 24 hours following their treatment they should not apply any talcum powders, deodorants, antiperspirants, perfumes, self-tanning products or make-up over the treated areas. Any of these products could block the pores or cause irritation or allergy reactions on the temporarily sensitized area. During this time they must use only plain, unperfumed soap and water on the treated area.

For the same 24-hour period they should preferably avoid exercise, especially swimming, and not apply heat or ultra-violet treatments – hot baths, for example, or the use of a sun bed or sauna – as these would add to the heat generated in the skin following the treatment and would probably cause discomfort or irritation. They must also refrain from touching or scratching the area, so as to avoid infecting the open follicles.

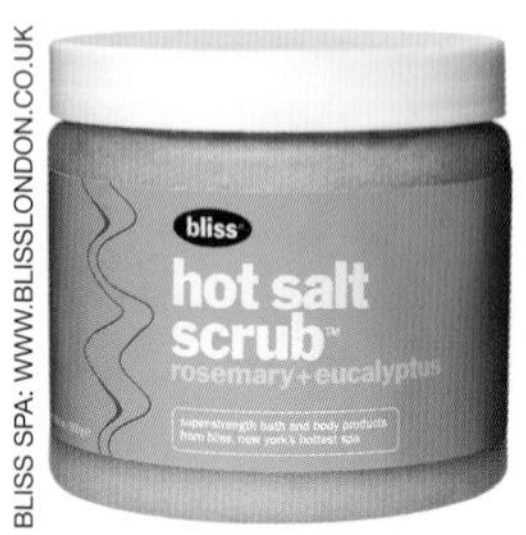

BLISS SPA: WWW.BLISSLONDON.CO.UK

Hot salt scrub exfoliant

Aftercare leaflets should contain this information: as best practice these can be given to the client at the end of the treatment to remind them what to do at home.

If there is a contra-action following treatment such as excessive redness and irritation, advise the client to apply a cool compress with soothing antiseptic lotion. If the redness does not disappear they must contact the salon. Advise the client to receive the treatment as follows: facial waxing 3–4 weeks; body waxing 4–6 weeks. Repeat bookings vary according to the natural hair regrowth and client requirements.

Ensure that the client's records are up to date, accurate and complete following the waxing treatment and provide written instructions in an aftercare leaflet.

Hot waxing

In **hot waxing**, the wax is applied at a higher temperature than warm wax. The hairs embed in the wax and are gripped tightly as the wax cools and contracts. When the wax is pulled away, it removes the hair from the base of the follicle.

Equipment and materials

The equipment and materials required for hot waxing are the same as for warm waxing (page 489), except that:

- ***a wax heater*** suitable for hot wax should be selected
- ***wax-removal*** strips are not necessary
- ***pre-wax oil*** may be applied to the skin before wax application to make wax removal easier

Some people prefer to apply the hot wax with disposable brushes rather than spatulas, but either can be used.

How to carry out the treatment

1. Ensure that the area to be waxed is clean and grease-free.
2. Apply a small amount of talc against the direction of hair growth. This will make the hairs stand on end and stick more firmly into the wax. Alternatively oil may be applied. Preparation will depend upon manufacturer's instructions.
3. Keep the same order of work as for warm waxing.
4. Apply wax in strips approximately 5cm wide and 10cm long, with about 5cm distance between the strips.
5. Carefully observe the direction of hair growth and the size of the area to be waxed.
6. Test the heat of the wax on the inside of the wrist.
7. Using either a disposable spatula or a brush, apply a layer of wax about 5cm × 10cm *against* the direction of hair growth. Apply a second layer *with* the direction of growth; and a third layer against the direction of growth. (If two or three strips are applied at the same time, you can work faster.) Keep the edges of the wax thicker than the middle, to make it easier to remove. Overlap the lower edge by about 2cm onto a hair-free area: this makes it less painful later, when you lift the edge to make a lip to pull.

   Curl up the lower end of the wax to make a lip, and press and mould the wax firmly onto the skin.
8. Leave the wax for a minute or so to cool. The wax has to cool sufficiently to grip the hairs, but not so much that the wax becomes brittle and breaks on removal. As it sets, it starts to lose its gloss: it should be removed when this happens and while it is still pliable.
9. Support the area below the wax, grasp the lip, and tear the wax off the skin *against* the direction of hair growth in one movement (as with warm-wax removal). Immediately press or firmly stroke the area with your hand: this takes away some of the discomfort.

KNOWLEDGE CHECK

If your client suffers from ingrowing hairs, what advice would you give them that could possibly prevent them recurring?

Need more time... refer to page 510 to help you.

TOP TIP

Choosing a hot wax

When selecting a hot wax, choose one that does not go brittle when cool. Wax sold as small bars is preferable as this melts quickly.

ALWAYS REMEMBER

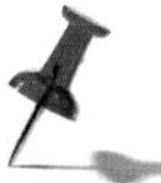

Wax temperature

If the wax is *not hot enough* when it is applied, it will not contract effectively around the hair and will therefore not grip it properly. This may result in poor depilation and possible hair breakage.

If on the other hand the wax is allowed to *overheat*, it may cause burns. Also, the quality of the wax will deteriorate and the wax will become brittle as it cools.

TOP TIP

Hot wax trouble-shooting

If the wax becomes too cool and brittle for removal, fresh hot wax may be applied with care over the area to soften it.

10 Check the area for any remaining wax and any stray hairs. Remove using tweezers. (Second applications are not advisable when using hot wax, because of the risk of burning.)

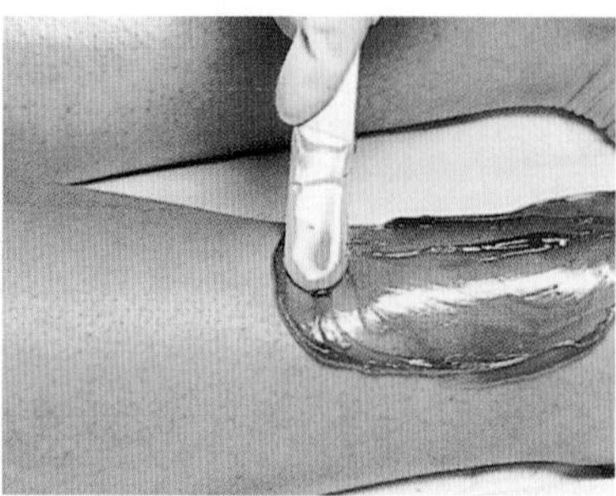
Applying hot wax to the lower leg

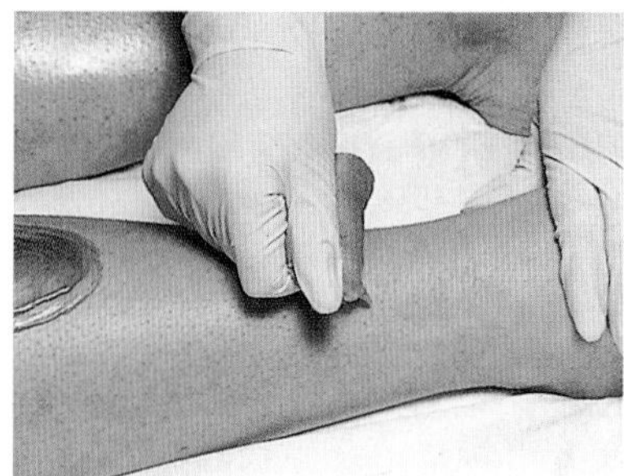
Removing the hot wax

If this general application technique is followed, any area of the body can be depilated – use the same order of work as for warm waxing: observe the direction of hair growth and take into account the body area; use smaller strips in smaller areas; support the skin; and use the correct angle of pull for removal.

Sugaring and strip sugar

Sugaring is an ancient and popular method for hair removal. The superfluous hairs become embedded in a pliable organic paste of sugar, lemon and water. The sugar paste is then removed from the skin's surface, against the hair's growth, leaving the skin hair-free.

Sugaring may be applied using a paste formulation removed with the hands, referred to as sugar paste, or in a formulation similar to warm wax, removed with material strips, referred to as strip sugar. Sugaring is effective on fine hair growth, and as it contains fewer ingredients or additives this method is less likely to cause an allergic reaction.

Reception

Re-book the client for sugaring hair removal every four to six weeks, dependent upon the hair growth rate and area. For effective hair removal, the hairs must be at least 2mm long.

ALWAYS REMEMBER 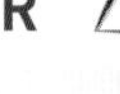

Talcum powder
Talc aids the sugaring treatment technique, by reducing stickiness when working with the paste, and by absorbing perspiration (particularly in areas such as the underarms).

Equipment and materials

The equipment and materials required for sugaring are the same as for warm waxing (page 489), except for the following differences.

Sugar paste

- ***Wax beater (with a thermostatic control) or microwave*** – to heat the paste.
- ***Sugaring paste*** – either soft or hard, depending on your personal preference and the temperature of the working environment: hard paste is a better choice in warmer temperatures and when working on coarser hair.

- ***Talc (purified)*** **to reduce stickiness and absorb perspiration** – to prevent the sugar sticking to the skin.
- ***Bowl of clean water*** – to remove the sugar paste from the hands, reducing stickiness.

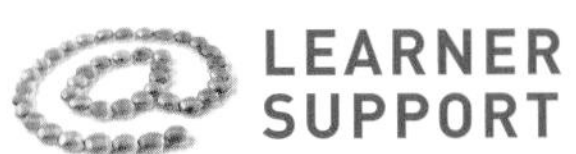

Waxing treatments fill-in-the-blanks

Strip sugar

- ***Wax heater (with a thermostatic control)*** – to heat the strip sugar.
- ***Strip sugar.***
- ***Talc (purified)*** **to reduce stickiness and absorb perspiration** – to prevent the sugar sticking to the skin.
- ***Disposable wooden spatulas*** – a selection of differing sizes, for use on different body areas.
- ***Wax-removal strips (bonded-fibre)*** – thick enough that the wax does not soak through, but flexible enough for easy working.
- ***Disposable gloves.***

Sterilization and disinfection As sugar paste is water-soluble, it is easily cleaned from any surface. However, the wax heater containing the sugar wax must be regularly disinfected.

Step-by-step: Preparing the client

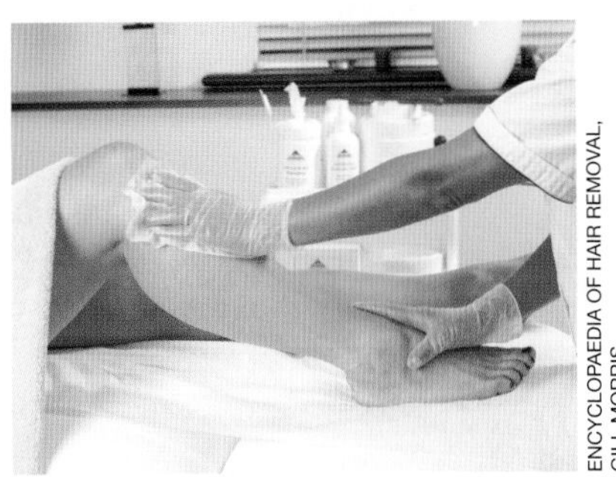

ENCYCLOPAEDIA OF HAIR REMOVAL, GILL MORRIS

Cleanse the area to be treated, using an antiseptic cleansing tissue. Blot the skin dry.

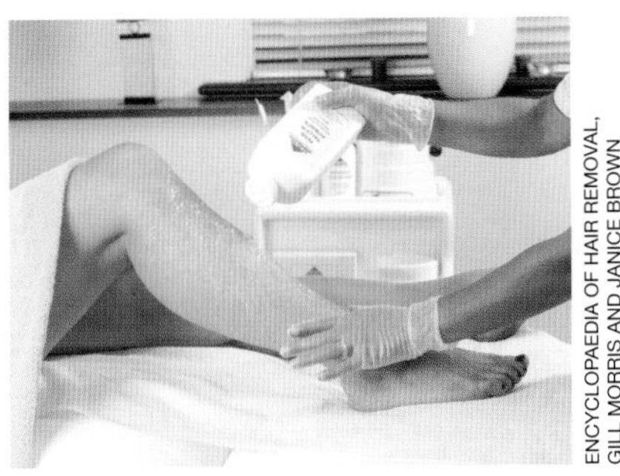

ENCYCLOPAEDIA OF HAIR REMOVAL, GILL MORRIS AND JANICE BROWN

Apply talc to cover the area: this prevents the sugar from sticking to the skin.

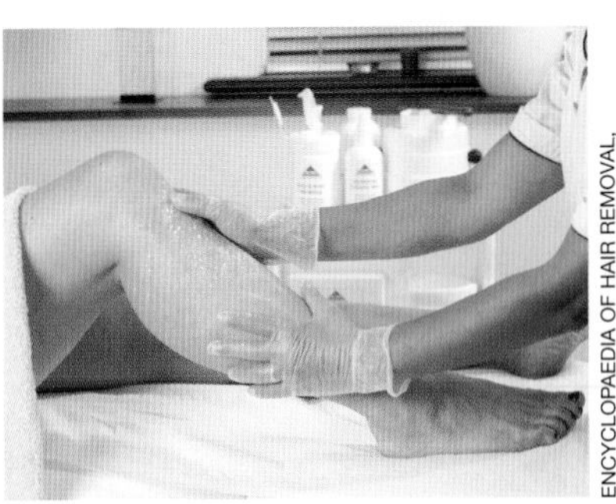

ENCYCLOPAEDIA OF HAIR REMOVAL, GILL MORRIS AND JANICE BROWN

Rubbing in the talc

How to provide a sugar paste treatment

The sugar paste adheres to the hair and not to the skin, which allows the sugar to be reapplied to a treatment area. Technique is important and it takes practice and experience to become skilled.

1. Heat the sugar gently, to soften it.
2. Apply talc to the area.
3. Apply the sugar paste to the skin by hand. Select the amount used according to the treatment area. Draw the paste over the area *in the direction* of the hair growth, embedding the hair in the paste. This can be termed 'rubbing' as it collects and embeds the hair in the wax as rubbed over skin's surface.

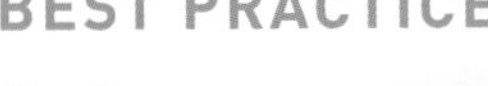

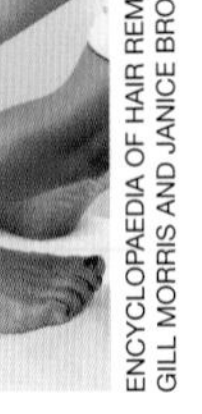

Heating sugar wax

Sugar wax – both strip and paste – may be heated in a microwave to soften it. Check guidelines set by the microwave manufacturer on power and timing.

However, also check with your salon policy as there may be potentially an increased risk of burning and the insurance may be invalid in such cases.

4 Remove it quickly *against* the hair growth.

5 If necessary, reapply the paste to the area to remove further hairs. Continue this process until no hair remains.

6 After use, discard the paste as it will be contaminated with excess hair and dead skin cells: this affects the ease of paste removal, and presents a risk of cross-infection.

7 To complete the treatment, a cooling spray may be applied to the area, followed by a soothing cream.

8 Record details of the treatment on the client's record card.

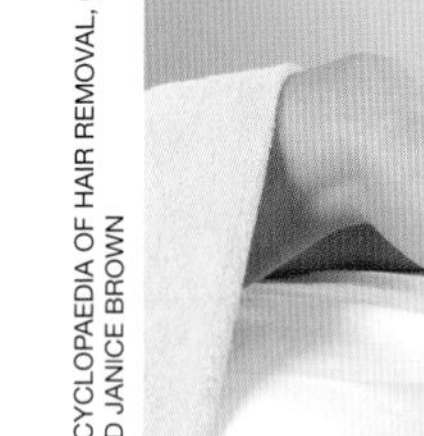

ENCYCLOPAEDIA OF HAIR REMOVAL, GILL MORRIS AND JANICE BROWN

Applying sugar paste

ENCYCLOPAEDIA OF HAIR REMOVAL, GILL MORRIS AND JANICE BROWN

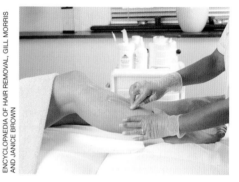

Rubbing in the sugar paste

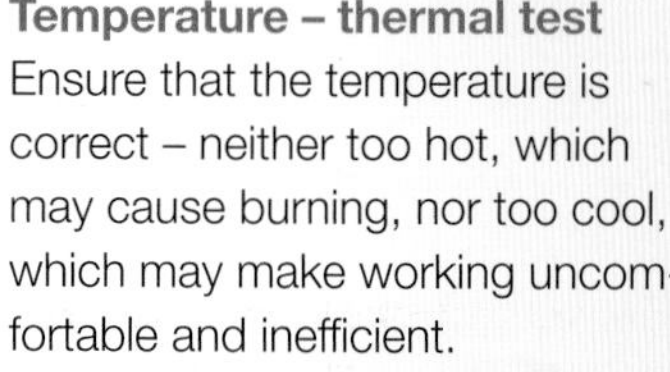

HEALTH & SAFETY

Temperature – thermal test
Ensure that the temperature is correct – neither too hot, which may cause burning, nor too cool, which may make working uncomfortable and inefficient.

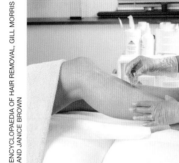

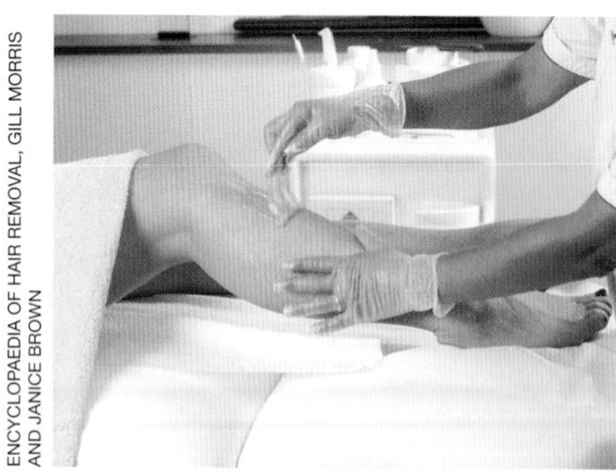

ENCYCLOPAEDIA OF HAIR REMOVAL, GILL MORRIS AND JANICE BROWN

Removing the sugar paste

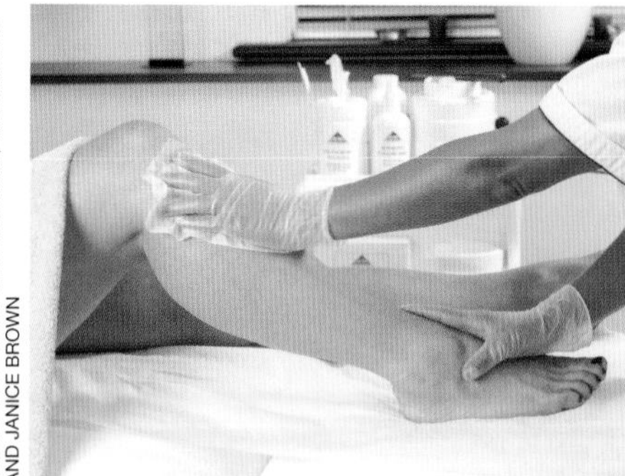

ENCYCLOPAEDIA OF HAIR REMOVAL, GILL MORRIS AND JANICE BROWN

Applying antiseptic products

How to provide a strip sugar treatment

This is similar in application and removal to warm wax.

1 The wax is gently heated following manufacturer's instructions until it is fluid.

2 Apply the wax using a spatula *in the direction of* the hair growth to cover the treatment area.

3 Remove the wax *against* the hair growth using a clean strip suitable for use with strip sugar wax.

4 To complete the treatment, a cooling spray may be applied to the area, followed by a soothing cream.

5 Record details of the treatment on the client's record card.

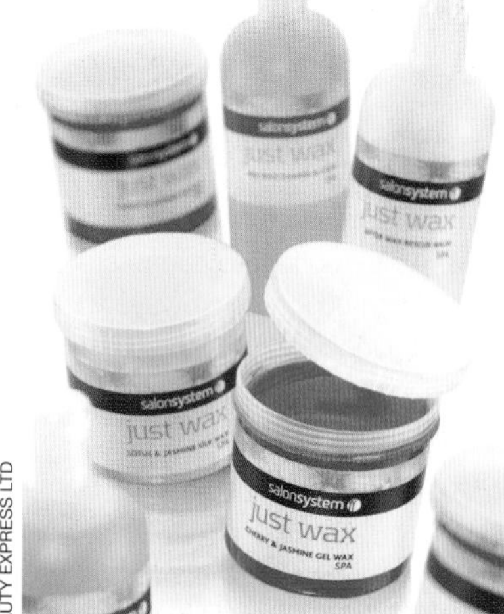

BEAUTY EXPRESS LTD

Strip sugar was removal technique

Disposable applicator roller waxing systems

Using a roller wax system is a hygienic method, using disposable applicators that are new for each client. A disposable applicator head screws onto the wax applicator tube in place of a cap. This reduces the possible risk of contamination through cross-infection. The method is less messy, as the wax is contained in the tube or cartridge and is not exposed until application.

Each tube/cartridge of wax as needed is heated to working temperature, which minimizes the risk of burning.

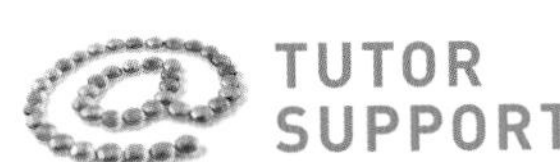

TUTOR SUPPORT

Activity 4: Wordsearch

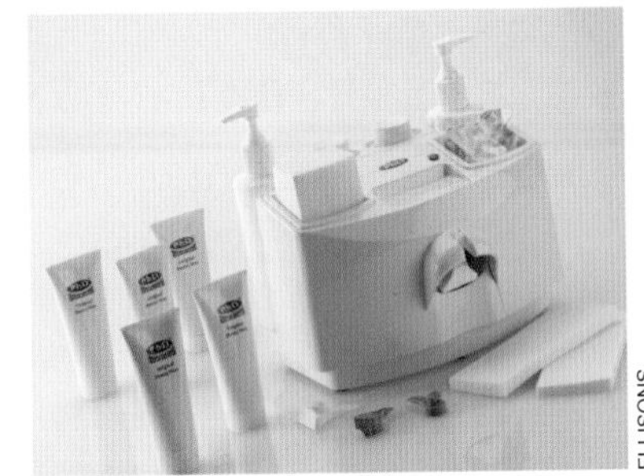

ELLISONS

Disposable applicator starter kit

Step-by-step: Waxing the legs using disposable applicator

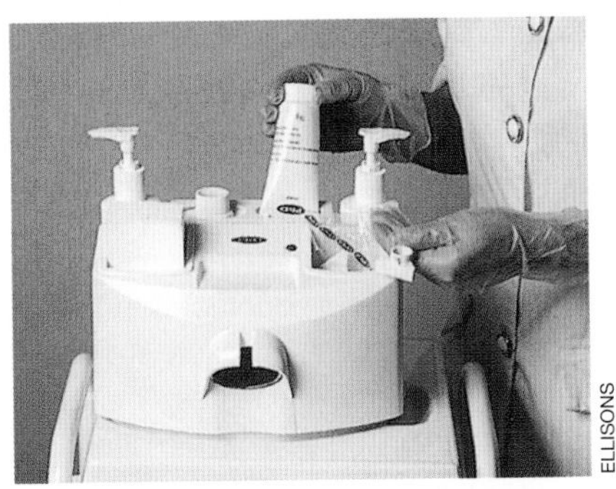

ELLISONS

1 Remove the disposable applicator from the right-hand heating and storage compartment.

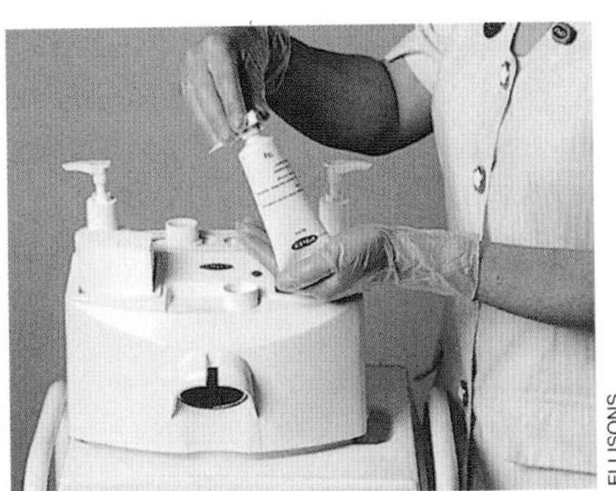

ELLISONS

2 Remove the cap from the tube of wax. Attach the applicator head to the tube.

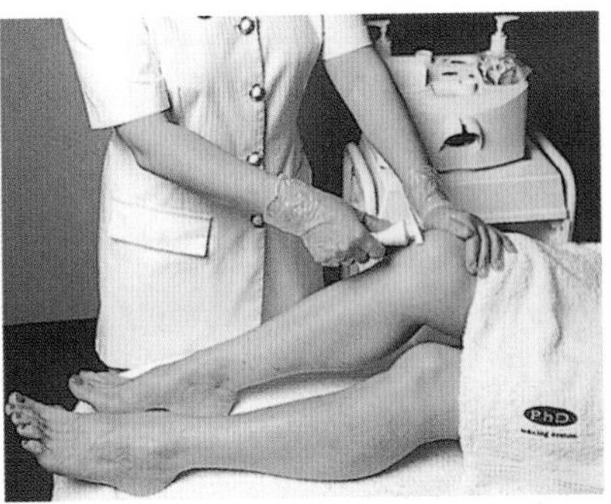

ELLISONS

3 Release the applicator by lifting the lever upwards. Squeeze until a small amount of wax appears on the front of the applicator, then apply the wax. Hold the applicator at a 45° angle to the leg, and glide it smoothly down the leg.

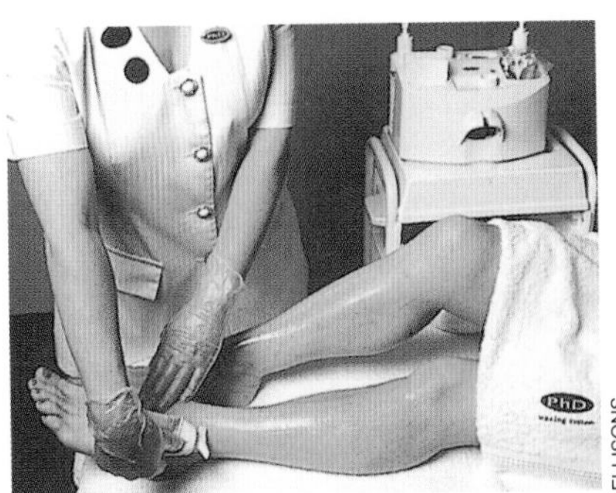

ELLISONS

4 Apply a thin film of wax to the front of both legs, then press down the closing device on the applicator to stop wax flow.

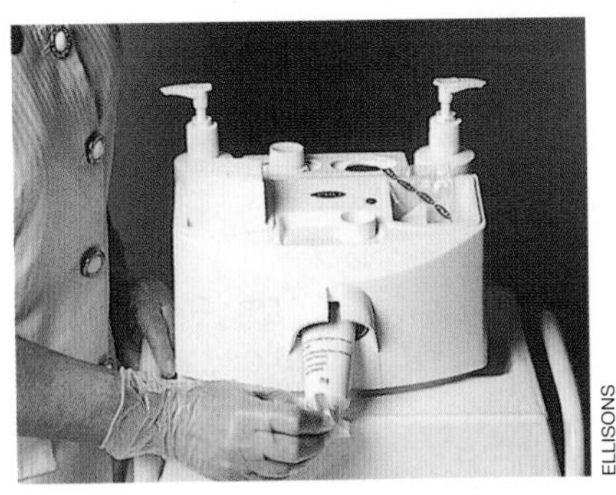

ELLISONS

5 Wipe any wax residue from the front of the applicator and return the tube to heat.

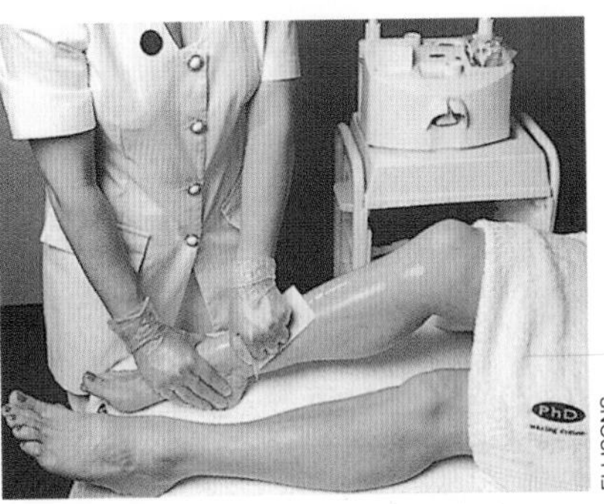

ELLISONS

6 Remove wax from the leg, starting at the ankle and working towards the knee. Support the skin with one hand, and firmly stretch it against the removal of the wax. Continue application and removal to the sides and back of the legs.

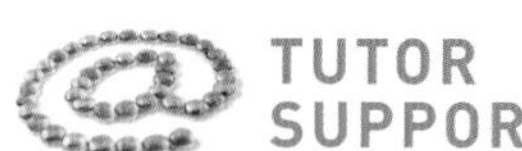

Activity 5: Re-cap, revision and evaluation

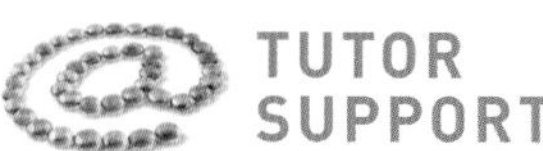

Activity 6: Multiple choice quiz

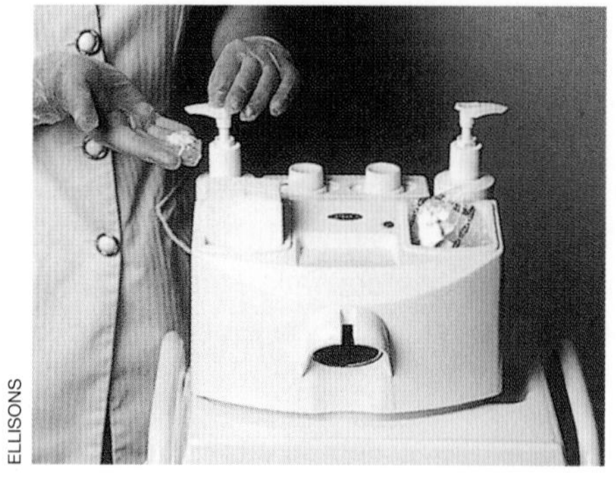
ELLISONS

7 When treatment is complete, apply antiseptic soothing lotion (shown). Record details of the treatment on the client's record card.

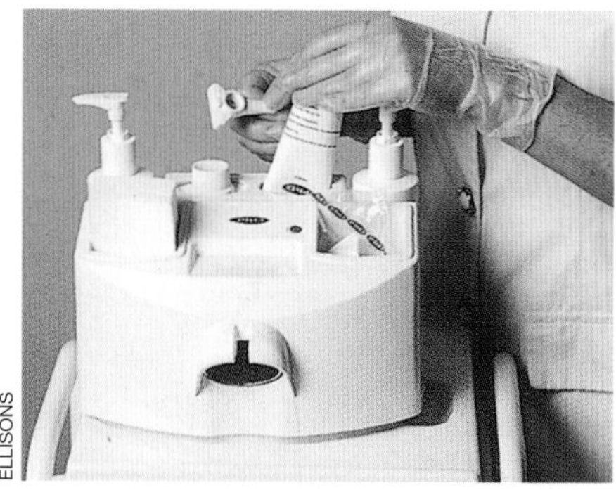
ELLISONS

8 Remove the applicator from the tube, replacing the cap and returning the tube to the heater. Dispose of the applicator head.

GLOSSARY OF KEY WORDS

Aftercare advice recommendations given to the client following treatment to continue and enhance the benefits of the treatment.

After-wax lotion a product applied to the skin following hair removal to reduce redness and promote skin healing.

Allergic reaction reaction to ingredients in a product producing symptoms including erythema, swelling, itching and bruising.

Anagen the active stage of the hair growth cycle.

Burn injury to the skin caused by excess heat; the skin appears red and may blister.

Cold wax a wax already applied to a strip and ready for use. The pre-coated strip is applied firmly to the skin and then removed quickly against hair growth, removing the hair in the area.

Consultation assessment of client's needs using different assessment techniques, including questioning and natural observation.

Contra-action an unwanted reaction occurring during or after treatment application.

Contra-indication a problematic symptom which indicates that the treatment may not proceed.

Disposable applicator used to apply wax hygienically to the area of hair removal without contaminating the wax flowing back into the tube following application. The applicator head is disposed of after each treatment.

Erythema reddening of the skin, caused by increased blood circulation to the area.

Folliculitis a bacterial infection where pustules develop in the skin tissue around the hair follicle.

Hair a long slender structure that grows out of, and is part of, the skin. Each hair is made up of dead skin cells, which contain the protein called keratin.

Hair follicle an appendage (structure) in the skin formed from epidermal tissue. Cells move up the hair follicle from the bottom (the hair bulb), changing in structure to form the hair.

Hair growth cycle the cyclical pattern of hair growth, which can be divided into three phases: anagen, catagen and telogen.

Hairy moles moles exhibiting coarse hairs from their surface.

Heat rash a reaction to heat exposure where the sweat ducts become blocked and sweat escapes into the epidermis. Red pimples occur and the skin becomes itchy.

Histamine a chemical released when the skin comes into contact with a substance that it is allergic to. Cells called 'mast cells' burst, releasing histamine into the tissues. This causes the blood capillaries to dilate, which increases blood flow to limit skin damage and begin repair.

Hot wax a system of wax depilation used to remove hair from the skin. Hot wax cools and sets on contact with the skin. They are a blend of waxes, such as beeswax and resins, which keep the wax flexible. Soothing ingredients are often included to avoid skin irritation.

Ingrowing hair a build-up of skin occurs over the hair follicle, causing the hair to grow under the skin.

Laser hair removal a technique of permanent hair removal. Laser energy is passed through the skin which stops the activity of the hair follicle creating hair growth through a process called photothermolysis.

Melanin a pigment in the skin and the hair that contributes to the skin/hair colour.

Minor a person classed as a child who requires by law to have a guardian or parent present.

Necessary action the action taken to deal safely with a contra-action or contra-indication.

Photothermolysis an effect created when using a laser for hair removal. The melanin pigment that provides hair colour absorbs the laser energy, which is converted to heat, and at a sufficient temperature destroys the part of the hair follicle where the cells divide to create the hair.

Pre-wax lotion an antibacterial skin cleanser to clean the skin before wax application.

Roller wax a warm wax used to remove hair from the skin. The wax is contained in a cartridge container with a disposable applicator, which rolls the wax onto the skin's surface. The applicator is renewed for each client.

Skin removal accidental removal of the upper, dead, protective cornified layer of the skin, leaving the granular layer exposed.

Skin sensitivity patch test a method used to assess skin tolerance, sensitivity to a particular product or treatment.

Skin tags skin-coloured threads of skin 3mm to 6mm long, projecting from the skin's surface.

Strip sugar a system of wax depilation similar to the warm-wax technique, used to remove hair from the skin. Made from sugar, lemons and water, the sugar wax is applied to the skin, and is then removed using a wax removal strip.

Sugaring an ancient popular method of hair removal using organic substances, sugar and lemon.

Sugar paste a system of wax depilation. An organic paste made from sugar, lemons and water is used to embed the hair, which is then removed by the paste from the skin.

Superfluous hair hair considered to be in excess of normal hair for the person's age, sex and therefore unwanted.

Thermal skin sensitivity test a test performed before wax application to check that the temperature of the wax is not too warm. The wax is tested by the therapist on themselves, usually on the inner wrist, and then on the client on a small visible area such as the inside of the ankle.

Treatment plan after the consultation, suitable treatment objectives are established to treat the client's conditions and needs.

Varicose veins veins whose valves have become weak and lost their elasticity. The area appears knotted, swollen and bluish/purple in colour.

Warm wax a system of wax depilation. Warm wax remains soft at body temperatures. It is frequently made of mixtures of glucose syrup and zinc oxide. Honey can be used instead of glucose syrup; this is referred to as honey wax.

Wax depilation the temporary removal of excess hair from a body part using wax.

Waxing products cosmetic preparations used with a waxing treatment which have specific benefits to cleanse the skin, assist in hair removal care and improve the appearance and healing properties of the skin following hair removal.

ASSESSMENT OF KNOWLEDGE AND UNDERSTANDING

You have now learnt about removing hair using waxing techniques treatment for the beauty therapy workplace. To test your level of knowledge, answer the following short questions. These will prepare you for your summative (final) assessment.

1. Hair removal using waxing techniques is:
   a. temporary hair removal
   b. permanent hair removal
2. The act of accurately sharing information between two people or groups of people is called:
   a. clarification
   b. communication
   c. client consultation
   d. reflective listening
3. The hair shown below is in which growth cycle stage?

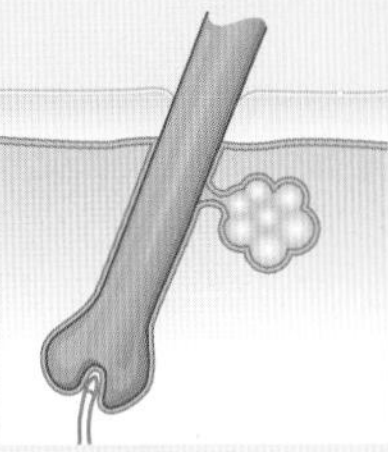

   a. catagen
   b. telogen
   c. anagen
4. Diabetes is a medical condition which if present will:
   a. prevent treatment
   b. restrict treatment
5. The part of the hair shown in the cross-section below which is not always present in vellus hair type is:

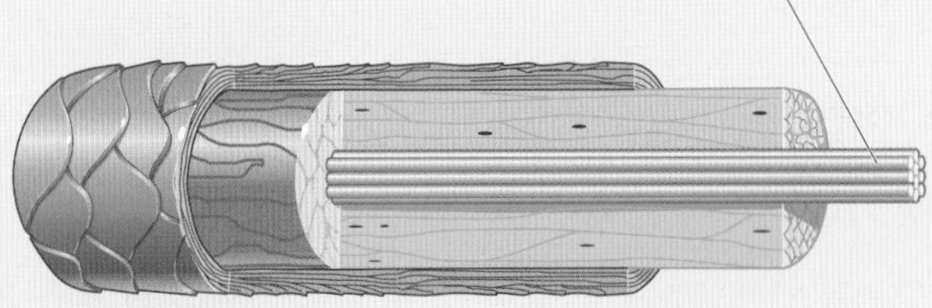

   a. cuticle
   b. cortex
   c. medulla
6. Warm wax and roller wax is applied:
   a. with the natural hair growth pattern
   b. against the natural hair growth pattern

7. When performing waxing, surface skin cells are also removed from the following layer:

a. stratum germinativum
b. stratum corneum
c. subcutaneous
d. stratum granulosum

8. Following a skin sensitivity patch test, an allergic reaction resulting in swelling and excessive erythema is referred to as:

a. a positive skin reaction
b. a negative skin reaction

9. The skin condition folliculitis is a:

a. bacterial infection
b. viral disorder
c. fungal disorder

10. Lemon can be an ingredient in formulations of:

a. hot wax
b. cold wax
c. honey wax
d. sugar wax

16 Ear Piercing

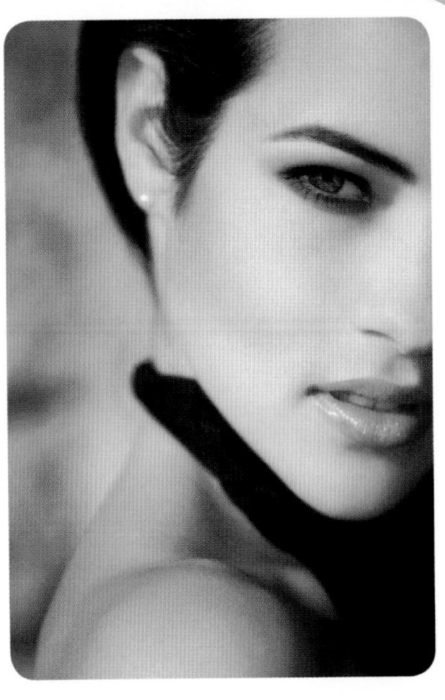

Learning Objectives

This chapter covers **VRQ Unit Provide ear piercing**.

This unit is all about providing the service skin piercing of the earlobe safely to ensure the correct placement and healing of the skin tissue avoiding any contra-action complications.

There are **two** learning outcomes for this unit which you must achieve:

1 Be able to prepare for ear piercing

2 Be able to provide ear piercing

From the range statement, you must show you can:

- use **consultation techniques** to identify the treatment **objectives**
- use the listed **products, tools and equipment** as appropriate
- ensure the **environmental conditions** are suitable
- complete a consultation and skin inspection to identify **contra-indications**
- follow all **health and safety working practices**
- provide relevant **aftercare** and **contra-action advice**

You must be able to show you have the necessary practical skills and underpinning knowledge to provide ear piercing.

This unit is linked to the Beauty Therapy NOS **Unit B7**.

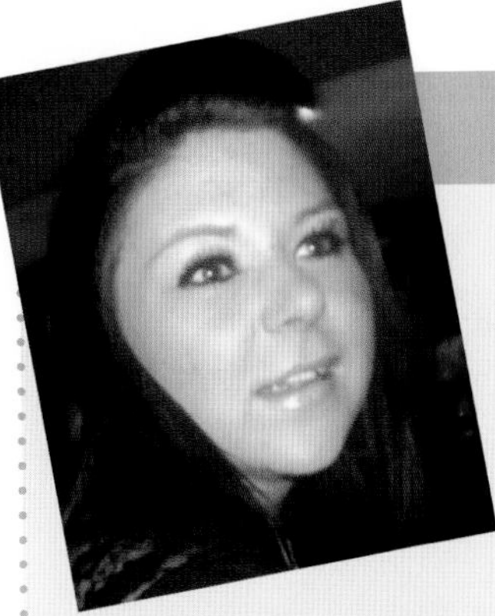

ROLE MODEL

Jade Rogers

Sales Technician

"My job is to represent Caflon Ltd within the UK. Currently 70 per cent of my time is spent training people in how to pierce ears and the remainder of the time I visit our customers throughout the UK and Ireland ensuring that they have adequate stock and answering any queries.

The role is very challenging, dealing with many differing types of people. Our customers come from the world of hair and beauty, others from the medical field and a core of clients from the jewellery industry.

Attending training in colleges, conducting seminars for our wholesale customers and one-to-one training, means that many miles are travelled throughout the year, along with exhibiting at trade shows both home and abroad.

Although it can be lonely, working at Caflon is very rewarding and I have been lucky to enjoy the ten years spent with this international organization.

I have shared important tips for my role as a sales technician, a career you may consider on qualifying.

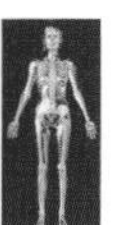

Essential anatomy and physiology for this unit is identified on the checklist on page 27.

Ear piercing is the perforation of the skin and underlying tissue of the ear to create a hole in the skin where jewellery is inserted. It is a quick, profitable and popular treatment, which also has the potential to generate further custom. This may be the client's first visit to a beauty salon, and the service they receive may encourage them to return for further treatments.

Earlobe piercing

Outcome1: Be able to prepare for ear piercing

Learn how to prepare for ear piercing

Practical skills	Underpinning knowledge
1 Prepare yourself, client and work area for ear piercing.	1 Describe the **environmental conditions** suitable for ear piercing.
2 Use suitable **consultation techniques** to identify treatment objectives.	2 Describe different **consultation techniques** used to identify treatment objectives.
3 Provide clear recommendations to the client.	3 Describe how to select **products, tools and equipment** to suit client treatment needs.
4 Select **products, tools and equipment** to suit client treatment needs.	4 Describe the **contra-indications** to ear piercing.

KNOWLEDGE CHECK

What is the helix part of the ear composed of that makes it unsuitable for piercing?

Need more time... refer to page 53 to help you.

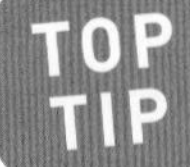

TOP TIP

Cosmetic piercing

Skin piercing of the earlobe and cosmetic body piercing are classified in the single term *cosmetic piercing*.

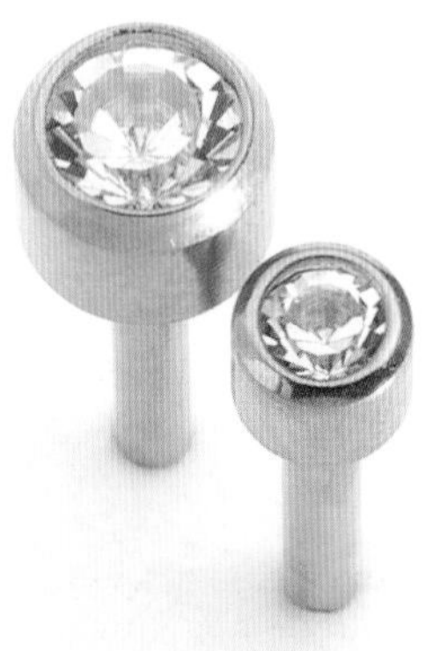

CAFLON

Studs

Preparing the work area

Ear piercing can be carried out either in a private cubicle or at reception. Use your discretion to decide which would be more appropriate.

Check the suitability of the environmental conditions. Good ventilation and lighting is important – some clients may feel faint following the service. As clients may be anxious before having their ears pierced, a calm environment should be provided, and restful, background music will help to create a relaxing environment. The client should be seated at a comfortable height for you to pierce their ears.

All furniture and fittings in the service area should be kept clean and in good repair so that they can be cleaned effectively.

The surface that the ear piercing equipment is to be placed on should be cleaned immediately prior to service with detergent and disinfectant. It should then be covered with disposable tissue roll, which is disposed of immediately following service. All work surfaces must be kept clean at all times and covered with a smooth, impervious surface.

Check that the client is positioned at a suitable height when performing the service. The earlobe should be easily accessible without risk of injury to the client. Remember, awkward positioning for the beauty therapist may result in uneven piercing and can also lead to repetitive strain injury and must be avoided.

Before carrying out the ear piercing check that you have the necessary equipment and materials to hand and that they meet legal hygiene and industry requirements for ear piercing.

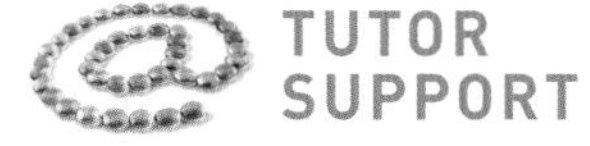

Activity 1: Label the ear structure

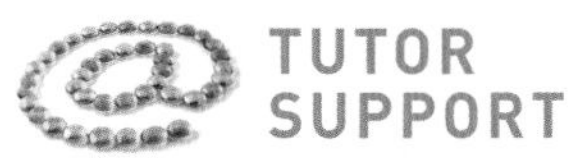

Activity 3: Equipment wordsearch

PRODUCTS, TOOLS AND EQUIPMENT

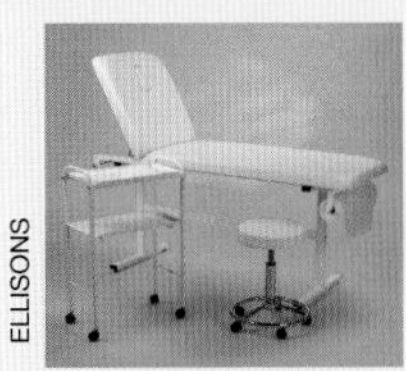
ELLISONS

Couch or chair
For client to sit on, with easy-to-clean surface

Trolley
On which to place products, tools and equipment

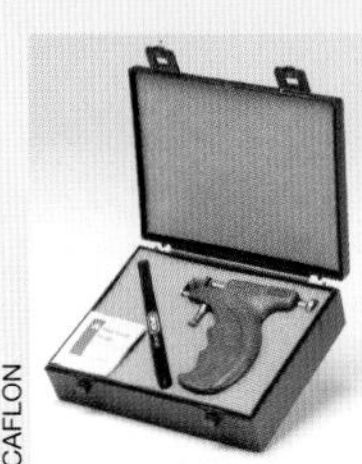
CAFLON

Ear piercing gun
Ear piercing gun that complies with current health and safety legislation

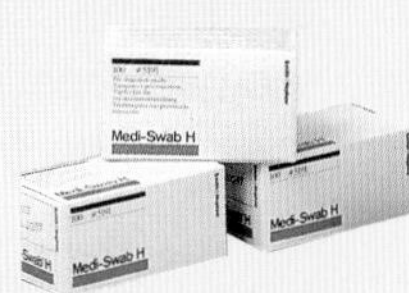

Pre-packed alcohol-based sterile cleaning tissues (2) or manufacturer's cleansing solution
Used to cleanse the ear area

YOU WILL ALSO NEED:

Studs A variety of styles and designs to accommodate differing client preferences. These must be manufactured from hypo-allergenic metal to minimize allergic reactions in people with metal allergies, e.g. nickel

Non-toxic surgical skin-marker pen To mark where the piercing will be. This is usually in gentian violet ink

Disinfectant (70 per cent alcohol) e.g. surgical spirit for cleaning the gun after use

Clean cotton wool To apply lotions/cleaning products

Single use disposable synthetic powder-free gloves To ensure a high standard of hygiene and to reduce the possibility of contamination

Disposable tissue couch roll To protect the clean work surfaces

Waste container (with yellow coloured waste liner to collect contaminated waste) This should be a lined metal bin with a lid to collect waste

Sharps box To dispose of studs when necessary

Headband (clean) or clip To hold the hair away from the ear during ear piercing

Hand mirror (clean) To show the client the proposed placement of the earrings after marking and after the completed ear piercing

Client record card For recording confidential details of each client registered at the salon, including the client's personal details, products used and details of the treatment

Aftercare solution Either to offer for sale or to include as part of the cost of the service to promote skin healing and avoid secondary infection

Aftercare instruction leaflet Instructions for the client to keep to minimize healing times and reduce the risk of secondary infection

Ultra-violet light cabinet To store the ear piercing gun between piercing services; this helps avoid the risk of contamination

Hand disinfectant Usually containing chlorhexidine to cleanse and disinfect hands

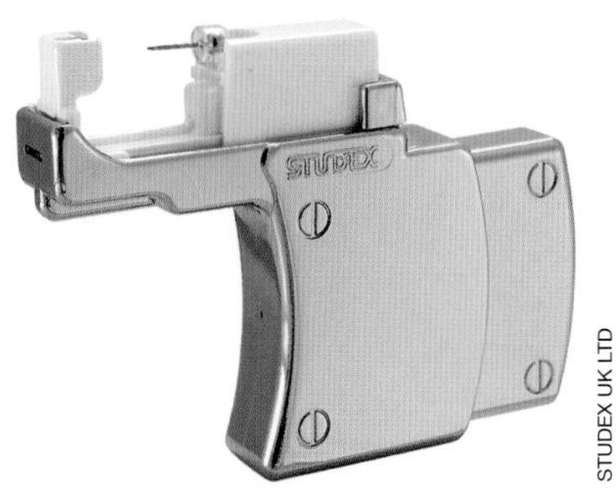

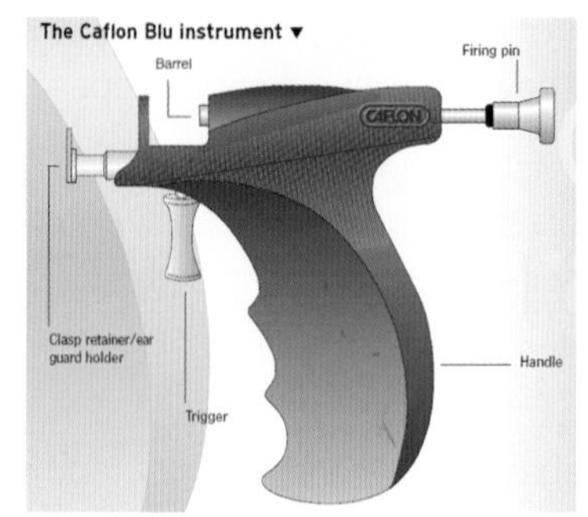

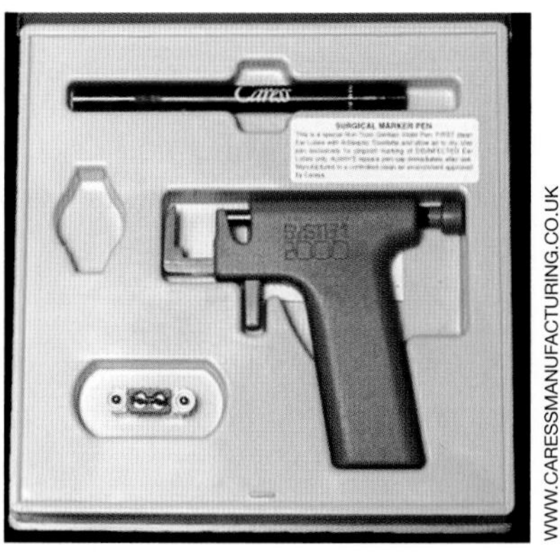

Examples of ear piercing guns

Be aware the manufacturers' systems may vary depending on the type of ear piercing gun you are using.

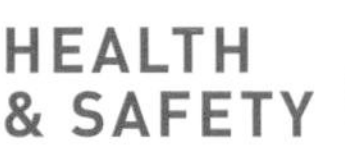

HEALTH & SAFETY

Marker pens

Keep the marker pen in a safe hygienic place – if left out, somebody might mistake it for an ordinary felt-tip pen!

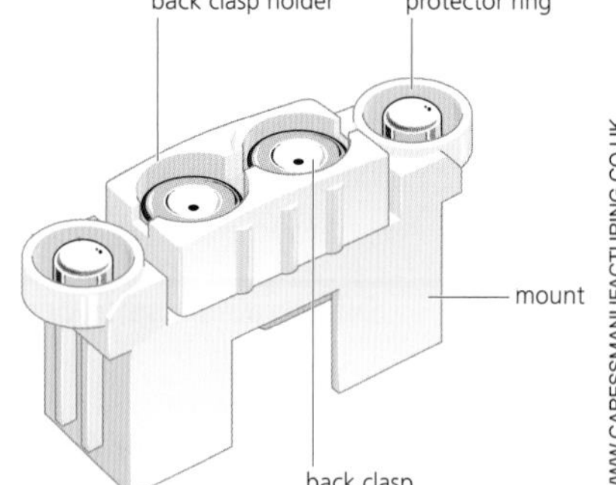

Disposable cassette

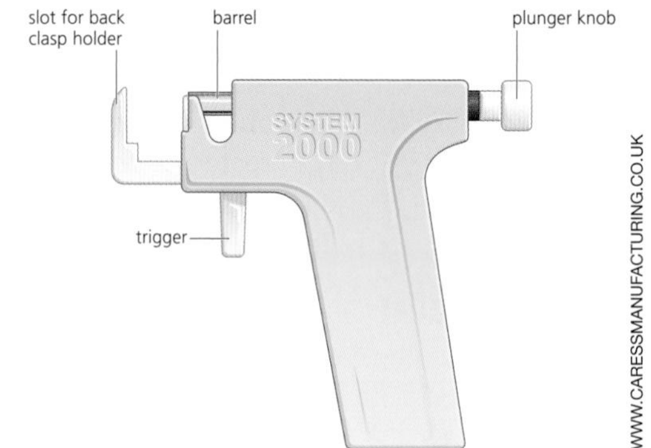

Ear piercing gun

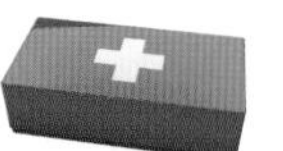

HEALTH & SAFETY

Information from Habia

See the Habia *Hygiene in Beauty Therapy* booklet for more details. It is available as a download from the Habia website www.habia.org.uk.

Sterilization and disinfection The premises should be kept clean and hygienic. The floor covering should be such that the surface can be cleaned with a disinfectant and hot soapy water; work surfaces likewise should be washed regularly with detergent and water and wiped with a disinfectant. Hypochlorite solutions (bleach) are recommended for disinfecting work surfaces. Potential hazards include skin infection and cross-infection including the transmission of blood borne viruses such as hepatitis or HIV due to poor hygiene practice to both client and beauty therapist.

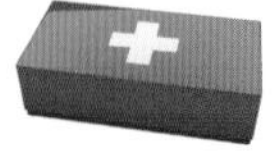

HEALTH & SAFETY

Cross-infection

If you have any cuts on your hands or fingers, these should be covered with a clean dressing before you treat the client. It is essential to wear disposable gloves.

Also, if you have an acute cold, e.g., a respiratory infection, do not perform ear piercing service. This will prevent airborne transfer of infection. A protective face mask may be worn for reasons of hygiene when working in close proximity to the client.

KNOWLEDGE CHECK

How should the client be positioned for ear piercing treatment and why is this important?

Need more time... refer to page 521 to help you.

Some salons that offer the ear piercing service also sell earrings. Those designed for pierced ears should not be tried on by a client, in the interest of health and hygiene. (Although there have been no reported cases of transmission of hepatitis B or HIV in this way, all possible risks should be avoided.) Such earrings may instead be attached to a special clear acrylic slide that can be held against the ear to assist in selection.

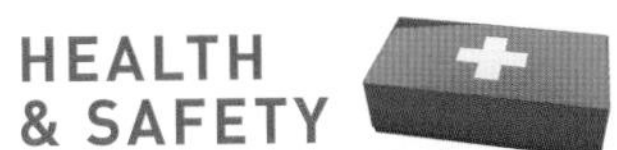

The Control of Substances Hazardous to Health (COSHH) Regulations (2002) – including biological agents

The Control of Substances Hazardous to Health (COSHH) Regulations (2002) require employers and the self-employed to prevent or control the exposure of employees and clients to hazardous substances. This includes exposure to biological agents such as bacteria, fungi and viruses and chemical cleaning/sterilizing agents. Records of the COSHH assessment must be available for inspection.

A COSHH essential information document is available for cosmetic piercers at **www.coshh-essentials.org.uk**.

The gun approved for ear piercing is designed so that it does not come into contact with the client's skin, and is used with pre-sterilized ear studs and ear clasps.

The studs are provided in sterile packs. Many give a date after which their sterility can no longer be assumed; others have a seal that changes colour when the expiry date has been reached. Only use studs that come from a sealed package, check before use that the packaging is not damaged in any way.

Ensure that all recommended skin cleansing solutions are in date and that packaging has not been damaged in any way.

The **Local Government (Miscellaneous Provisions) Act (1982)** requires that salons offering any form of skin piercing be registered with the local health authority. This registration includes both the operators who will be carrying out the service and the salon premises where the service will be carried out.

The **Local Government Act (2003) (section 120 and schedule 6)** has amended the 1982 Act to enable each local authority to regulate businesses providing differing types of cosmetic piercing and skin colouring. Each local authority can introduce its own bye-laws to set the standards as required.

Premises are inspected by a local authority enforcement officer, who checks that relevant local bye-laws are being followed. (The bye-laws are to ensure that service is carried out in a healthy, safe and hygienic manner.)

If the inspector is satisfied, the salon will be issued with a **certificate of registration**; this should be displayed in the reception area at all times. Any breach of the Act or the bye-laws could result in a fine, and permission to carry out the service could be withdrawn.

The London LAs mainly use the Greater London Council (General Powers) Act 1981 and **London Local Authorities Act (1991 and 2007)** which covers the London local authorities and enables them to regulate special treatment businesses including cosmetic piercing and micro pigmentation.

HEALTH & SAFETY

Ear piercing guidelines

The Chartered Institute of Environmental Health has developed useful best practice guidance for those employed as operators in body art, cosmetic therapies and other specialized services.

TOP TIP

Disposable ear piercing gun

Available for ear piercing is a sterile disposable ear gun. This ensures a sterile gun with preloaded ear studs and clasp.

HEALTH & SAFETY

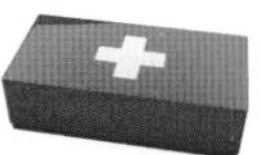

Spare studs

If only one stud of a pair is used in an ear piercing, the other stud should be discarded as it is no longer in a sterile state.

KNOWLEDGE CHECK

What environmental factors should be considered when carrying out ear piercing to ensure that the client will feel relaxed and confident in your care?

Need more time... refer to page 523 to help you.

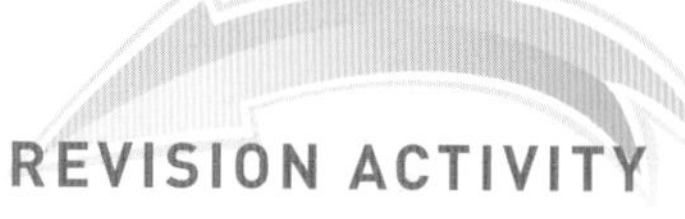

REVISION ACTIVITY

Question

Which branch of the external carotid artery supplies blood to the ear?

Need more time... refer to page 80 to help you.

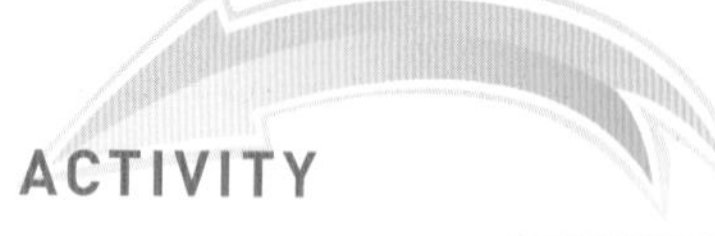

ACTIVITY

Costs

Research ear piercing service in three local salons. These may include hairdressing salons as it is a popular service to perform in the hair salon.

What is the cost of this service?

The HSE have a guidance publication for those involved in work where exposure to blood or other body fluids may occur titled *Blood-borne viruses in the workplace: Guidance for employers and employees*.

ACTIVITY

Personal cleanliness

Personal cleanliness is a fundamental requirement of the Local Government (Miscellaneous Provisions) Act (1982) and its amendments. Discuss how a high standard of personal cleanliness can be guaranteed. It is important to check any updates to the Act on a regular basis to ensure compliance.

Reception

When making an appointment for this service, allow 15 minutes. Although ear piercing is completed quickly, time must be allowed to complete the client's record card, determine the client's service plan and give clear concise aftercare instructions. Good communication is important. Speak clearly, establish what the client's requirements are and listen to ensure communication is effective and that a professional relationship is developed with the client, gaining client confidence.

A record card should be prepared for the client, recording just the information that is relevant to the ear piercing service. Record-keeping protects both the beauty therapist and client. While completing the record card you will be able to ascertain whether the client is suited to this service – if the client is under 16 years of age (a minor), for example, it may be necessary for a parent or guardian to accompany them and sign a **consent form** containing a disclaimer in the event of **contra-indications** (this is compulsory in Scotland and whilst not required by law in England, it is recommended to prevent parental complaints). These should be kept for a period of three years for inspection, enabling checks to be made on clients' ages.

Contra-indications to ear piercing should be checked for. If the area for piercing is unsuitable, politely explain to the client why this is so.

Contra-indications

In certain circumstances you should not carry out the ear piercing service. Use your professional judgement to assess the suitability of each client. The **consultation** will draw any contra-indications to your attention.

- ***If a client is particularly nervous*** it would be inadvisable to pierce their ears – they might faint or jump while the service was being carried out, causing incorrect placement of the earring.
- ***Do not pierce the ears of a client who may have allergies*** to the metal used for the jewellery stud.

If any of the following are present, do not proceed with ear piercing:

- ***Diabetes*** – the skin is very slow to heal, so infection of the area would be a strong possibility.

BEST PRACTICE

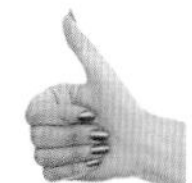

Service modification

Examples of ear piercing service modification include:

- if a second piercing is requested, ensure the first stud is placed to accommodate, leaving a 9mm distance for the second piercing.
- if the client has fat lobes, adjust the tightness following piercing to allow for swelling following the skin piercing which could cause discomfort and lead to infection.
- if 6mm or more thickness, the lobe requires a 'long post' stud.

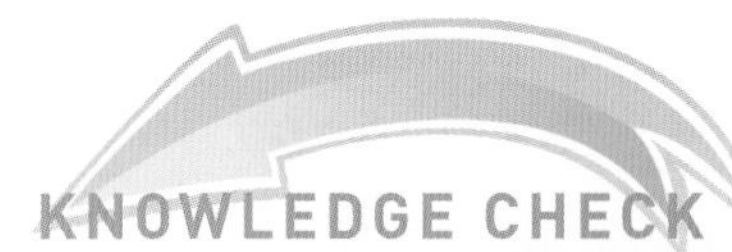

KNOWLEDGE CHECK

Provide five examples of how you can prevent infection when performing ear piercing treatment.

Need more time... refer to pages 522–523 to help you.

- ***Epilepsy*** – the stress before the service and the possible shock incurred during it might induce a fit.
- ***Skin disease or disorder***.
- ***Hepatitis B or HIV (Human Immunodeficiency Syndrome)*** – though the client may not know that they are a carrier, or may choose not to disclose the fact if they do (hygienic practice is vital, for this reason).
- ***Open wounds, cuts or abrasions*** in the area.
- ***Moles or warts*** in the area.
- ***Circulatory disorders*** such as high or low pressure.
- ***Following an operation*** – piercing must not be carried out at the site of a recent operation.
- ***Anti-coagulant drugs*** – these drugs affect blood clotting so individuals are likely to bleed persistently.
- ***Inflammation of the ear*** – the skin in the area appears red, swollen, and pus, a sign of infection, may be present.
- ***Keloid scarring*** – keloids occur following skin injury and are overgrown abnormal scar tissue which spreads, characterized by excess deposits of collagen. The skin tends to be red, raised and ridged at the site of the wound.

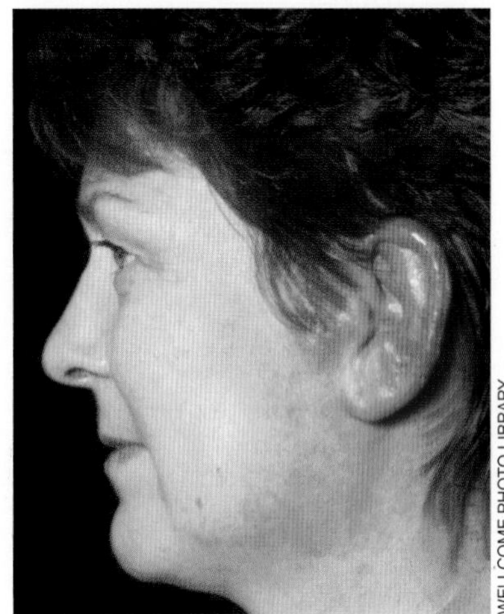

Inflammation of the ear

Where there is any contra-indication or a suspected contra-indication to ear piercing, the client must seek written permission from their GP before service can be carried out.

Feel the area to be pierced to check for cysts or keloids at consultation wearing disposable gloves for protection. Do not pierce through cysts or keloids or infection could occur.

Inform the client of possible contra-actions that could occur, especially if the correct aftercare procedures are not followed.

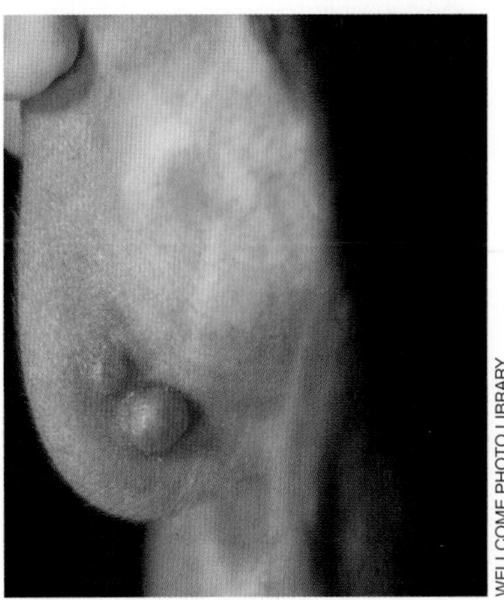

Keloid scarring of the ear

Contra-actions

- ***Infection*** – redness, swelling, inflammation and the exudation (oozing/weeping) of serum all signify that the ear is infected. If this occurs, the client should contact the salon. Depending on what they describe, it may be possible to give them adequate instructions over the telephone, or it may be necessary to make an appointment for the therapist to look at the ear. If, following action by the therapist, the infection persists, the client should be advised to contact their GP. Infection usually results from incorrect aftercare, removing the studs too early, or wearing cheap earrings.

HEALTH & SAFETY

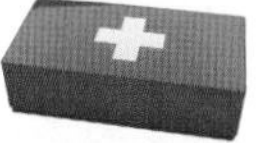

Secondary infection

If the client's ears become slightly red, indicating a possible infection, they should cleanse the area more frequently.

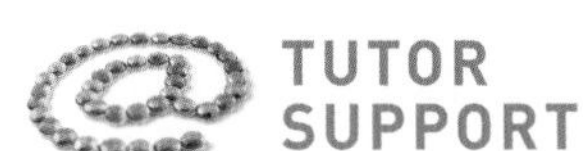

Activity 2: Aftercare leaflet design

If you suspected a client had a contagious contra-indication what actions would you take for the welfare of the client, yourself and others?

Need more time... refer to pages 524–525 to help you.

> With a diary schedule often booked eight months in advance, I have learnt how important it is to be organized and independent.
>
> **Jade Rogers**

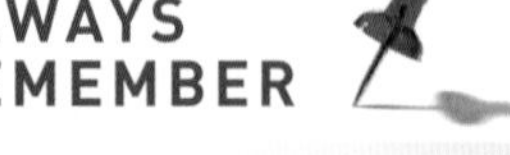

Client record card
Accurately record your client's answers to necessary questions asked at consultation on the record card.

Closed holes are caused by removing the studs too early, or by not continuing to wear earrings after the removal of the original studs.

Infections of the ear can be painful, and if ignored lead to scarring and at worst the skin tissue can die leading to disfigurement of the area.

- ***Jewellery embedding*** – this occurs when the ear jewellery descends beneath the skin's surface. This is usually a sign of infection, rejection or allergy to the ear jewellery. The client should contact the salon for advice. If, following action by the therapist, the jewellery remains embedded, the client should be advised to visit their GP.
- ***Keloids*** – overgrowths of scar tissue – sometimes occur at the site of ear piercing. If a client suffers from keloids, advise them not to have their ears pierced more than once – further keloid tissue could develop, giving an unsightly appearance.
- ***Dizziness and fainting*** – may occur if the client was particularly nervous beforehand. The shock of the ear piercing service may cause a short period of unconsciousness due to insufficient blood flow to the brain. If a client faints, loosen any restrictive clothing. Reassure the client, and position them lying flat with their feet raised higher than their head, or sat with their head bent forwards between their knees. Instruct them to breathe deeply and slowly. Increase ventilation in the area.
- ***Allergy to the aftercare lotion*** – The client may be allergic to the aftercare lotion. Check for known allergies to products at the client consultation.

All details recorded on the client record card are confidential and should be stored in a secure area following service. Access to this information will require written consent from the client. This is enforced through the Data Protection Act (1998) – legislation designed to protect the client's privacy and confidentiality. These records should be kept for at least three years, and be available for inspection as required. This may be by an authorized officer from the local health authority.

Explain the simple service procedure. Tell them that the ears will be cleansed and marked to show where the ear stud will be placed following piercing. This mark must be agreed with the client. The gun will be loaded with sterile ear studs which will enter the ear, performing the piercing. The back clasps will be fitted at the same time. A tight pinch will be experienced and some initial discomfort, with redness and slight swelling in the area which varies between clients. Most clients will be interested to know what to expect – usually the client's first question is "Will it hurt?".

Discuss aftercare. It is important to check that the client does not have any known allergies that may be contained in products to be used in the service, e.g. the aftercare lotion. Also, clients are more likely to pay attention at this stage.

Prepare the equipment required for ear piercing, and show the client the range of studs available. The stud's post has a larger diameter than regular earring posts to allow for shrinkage during the healing process; explain this to the client.

Some salon receptionists are trained to carry out this service. This is practical: many clients will be acting on impulse in deciding to have their ears pierced, and will not have made an appointment.

A sample client record card

Date | Beauty therapist name

Client name | Date of birth (Identifying client age group.)

Home address | Postcode

Email address | Landline phone number | Mobile phone number

Name of doctor | Doctor's address and phone number

Related medical history (Conditions that may restrict or prohibit service application.)

Are you taking any medication? (E.g. anti-coagulant drugs may affect the sensitivity of the skin and reaction to the service.)

CONTRA-INDICATIONS REQUIRING MEDICAL REFERRAL
(Preventing ear piercing service.)

- ☐ bacterial infection
- ☐ viral infection
- ☐ fungal infection
- ☐ severe skin conditions
- ☐ diabetes
- ☐ ear infections
- ☐ cardiovascular problems
- ☐ dysfunction of the nervous system
- ☐ allergies to metals
- ☐ epilepsy
- ☐ anti-coagulant drugs

EQUIPMENT, MATERIALS AND PRODUCTS

- ☐ ear piercing gun
- ☐ surgical skin marker pen
- ☐ sterile pre-packed alcohol skin-cleansing wipes
- ☐ personal protective equipment
- ☐ sterile pre-packed ear studs (metal type identified)
- ☐ consumables
- ☐ aftercare products
- ☐ mirror
- ☐ sharps disposal box (for use in the event of disposing of a contaminated ear stud)
- ☐ waste bin (with disposable liner)

CONTRA-INDICATIONS WHICH RESTRICT SERVICE
(Service may require adaptation.)

- ☐ cuts and abrasions
- ☐ bruising and swelling
- ☐ recent scar tissue
- ☐ skin disorders
- ☐ moles
- ☐ skin inflammation
- ☐ keloid scar tissue (piercing around the keloid permitted)

AREA TREATED

- ☐ earlobe

Beauty therapist signature (for reference)

Client signature (confirmation of details)

A sample client record card (continued)

SERVICE ADVICE
Ear piercing – *allow 15 minutes*

SERVICE PLAN
Record relevant details of your service and advice provided for future reference.
Ensure the client's records are up to date, accurate and fully completed following service. Non-compliance may invalidate insurance.

DURING
Discuss:
- details that may influence the client's ear piercing service (e.g., thickness of earlobes)

Note:
- any adverse reaction, if any occur

AFTER
Record:
- results of service
- any modification to service application that has occurred
- what type of ear studs have been used in the ear piercing service
- the effectiveness of service

Advise on:
- use of specialized aftercare products following ear piercing service for homecare use to promote skin healing and prevent contra-actions from occurring
- aftercare product application in order to gain maximum benefit from their use
- general ear piercing and maintenance advice
- the recommended time interval before removal of the stud
- the recommended time interval between ear piercing services

Provide:
- an aftercare ear piercing leaflet

RETAIL OPPORTUNITIES
Note:
- any purchases made by the client

EVALUATION
Record:
- comments on the client's satisfaction with the service
- if poor results are achieved, the reasons why
- how you may alter the service plan to achieve the required service results in the future, if applicable

HEALTH AND SAFETY
Advise on:
- how and when to turn the ear stud
- how and when to remove the ear stud
- recommended replacement of the ear stud used for piercing
- appropriate action to be taken in the event of an unwanted reaction to the service

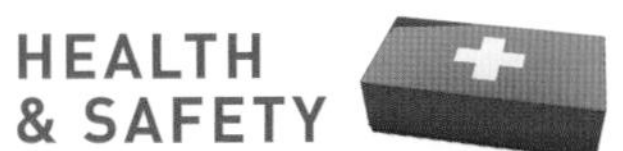

Recommended metals for ear piercing
Certain metals may cause an allergy. These include nickel, poor quality gold-plated metals and 9ct gold. The use of nickel-containing jewellery is subject to the Dangerous Substances and Preparations (Nickel) (Safety) Regulations (2005).

Recommended metals are surgical stainless steel, titanium (6AL4V) and 14ct gold.

Check what metal is used for your ear jewellery with your supplier, and that it complies with the Regulations.

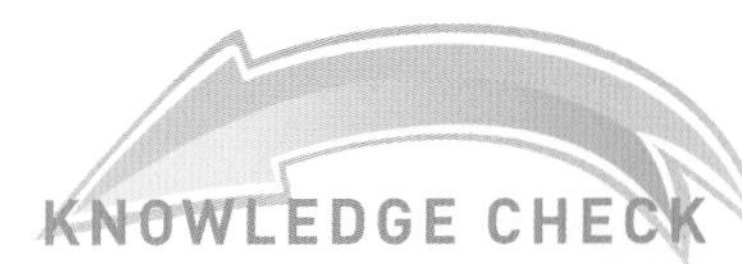

How would you describe the procedure of ear piercing to ensure a client was confident in the procedure?

Need more time... refer to page 526 to help you.

Preparation of the beauty therapist and client

If the position of the stud has not already been marked, do this now with the surgical skin-marker pen.

1. Wash your hands using a hand disinfectant that contains chlorhexidine as an active ingredient and apply a fresh pair of disposable gloves.
2. Secure the client's hair away from the treatment area. Place paper tissue roll over client's shoulder. If the client already has ear piercings, ask them to remove the existing earrings.
3. Thoroughly cleanse the back and the front of the client's earlobes using the recommended cleaning lotion. Each ear should be cleaned separately, using new, sterile cleansing lotion or alcohol-based tissues. Allow the skin to dry. (If moisture is present, the mark will blur.)
4. Holding a mirror in front of the client, discuss with them where the stud should be placed. Mark the position using the sterile pen.

Remember that the ears are not at the same level on each side of the head, and may protrude at different angles. Take time when marking the position of the studs, to ensure that the final appearance is balanced and that the client is in agreement with the proposed placing of the ear stud.

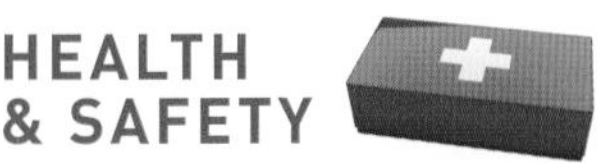

Secondary infection
As you cleanse the client's earlobes, you may notice that their skin, ear or hair is dirty. You may proceed, but when giving them the aftercare instructions politely and tactfully point out the importance of cleanliness in preventing secondary infection.

Ear studs
Studs are preferable to hooped earrings or sleepers, as dirt is less likely to cling to the stud and infect the ear. Select studs that are manufactured from hypo-allergenic material.

ALWAYS REMEMBER

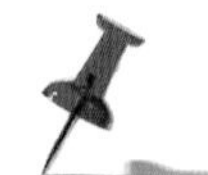

Fat lobes
If the client has fat lobes explain that the studs may feel a little tight.

Adjust tightness of stud in each ear using a clean tissue to hold the stud. Fresh disposable gloves must be worn if adjustment is necessary. Lobes more than 6mm thick need special care and may require a long post stud.

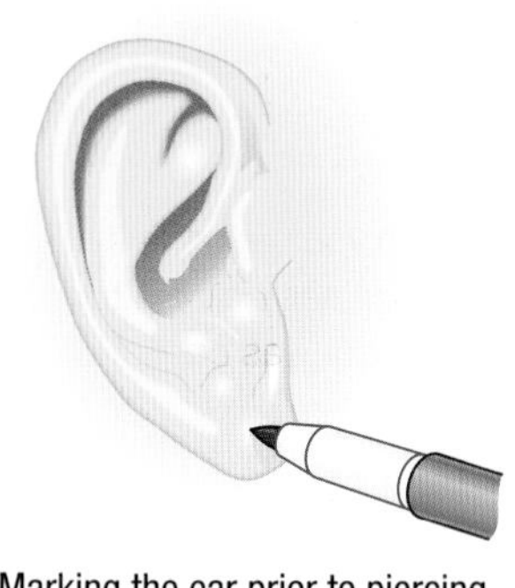

Marking the ear prior to piercing

HEALTH & SAFETY

Piercing ears

Never perform multiple piercing in each ear. The ears will swell, causing discomfort and possible infection.

When more than one hole is required in the same ear the piercing must be at least 9mm apart from the existing hole.

Piercing the ears

Outcome 2: Be able to provide ear piercing

Learn how to provide ear piercing

Practical skills

1. **Communicate and behave** in a professional manner.
2. Follow **health and safety working practices**.
3. Position yourself and the client correctly throughout the treatment.
4. Use **products, tools and equipment** and techniques to suit clients treatment needs.
5. Complete the treatment to the satisfaction of the client.
6. Record the results of the treatment.
7. Provide suitable **aftercare advice**.

Underpinning knowledge

1. State how to **communicate and behave** in a professional manner.
2. Describe **health and safety working practices**.
3. State the importance of positioning yourself and the client correctly throughout the treatment.
4. State the importance of using **products, tools and equipment** and techniques to suit clients treatment needs.
5. State the **contra-actions** that may occur during and following treatments and how to respond.
6. State the importance of completing the treatment to the satisfaction of the client.
7. State the importance of completing treatment records.
8. State the **aftercare advice** that should be provided.
9. Describe the blood and lymph supply to the ear.
10. Describe the external structure of the ear.

HEALTH & SAFETY

Hazards caused by poor practice

Medical complications can occur where conditions that are contra-indicated are not diagnosed or treated. Poor technique due to poor anatomy and physiology knowledge and understanding can cause damage to blood vessels, nerves and skin tissue, e.g. keloid scarring.

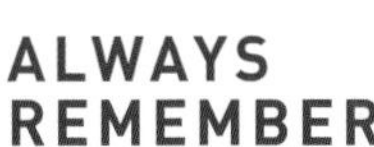

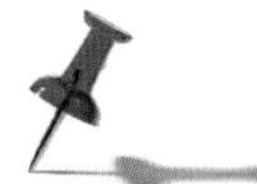

Placement

Try to aim for a central position on the earlobe – this will achieve the best result.

Step-by-step: Piercing the ears

The following procedure illustrates the general technique, with the beauty therapist wearing powder-free vinyl gloves. The details differ according to the ear piercing gun you are using. Always follow the manufacturers' instructions.

Ensure the service is cost effective and completed in a commercial time, 15 minutes.

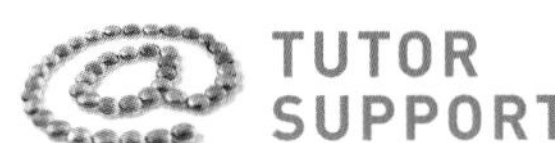

TUTOR SUPPORT

Activity 5: Client record card task

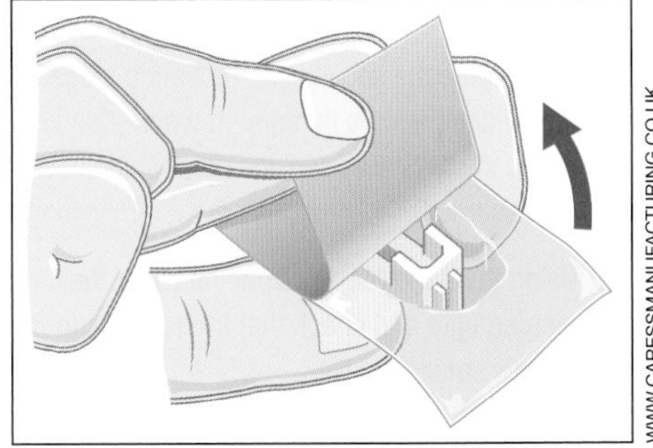

1 Holding the stud pack firmly, remove the backing paper. Take care not to drop the cartridge on the floor! (If you do drop it you will have to throw it away.)

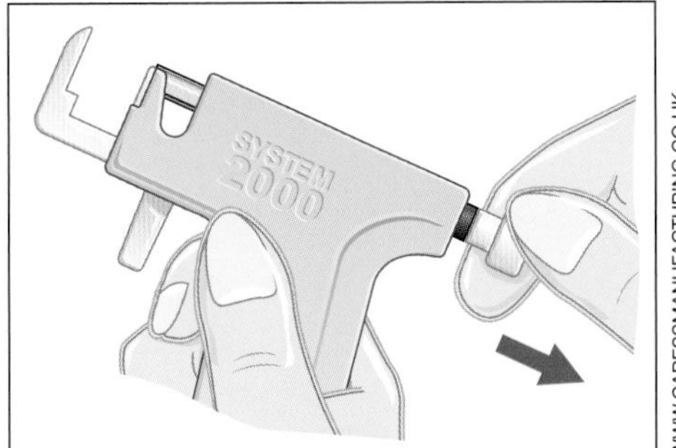

2 Pull back the plunger knob on the back of the gun, until it is fully extended – you will hear it click.

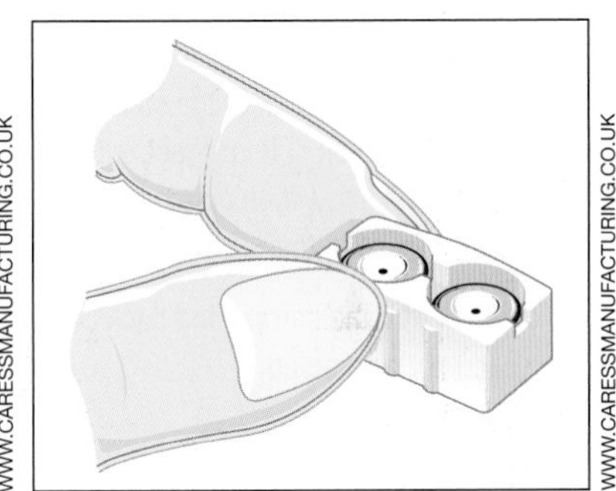

3 Remove the plastic cartridge from the package, holding it by the plastic mount. To avoid contamination, make sure that you do not touch the stud or backing clasp.

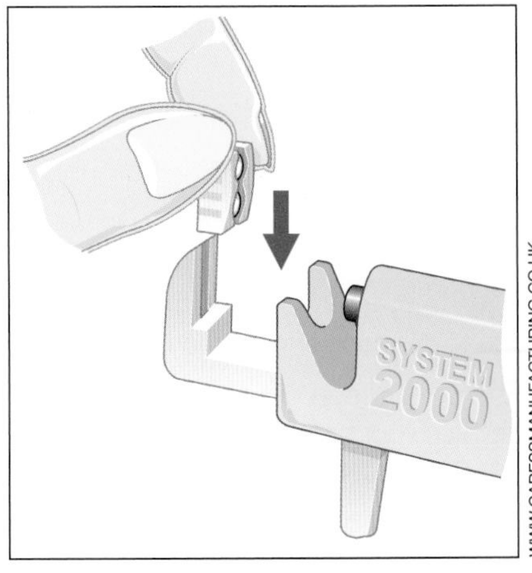

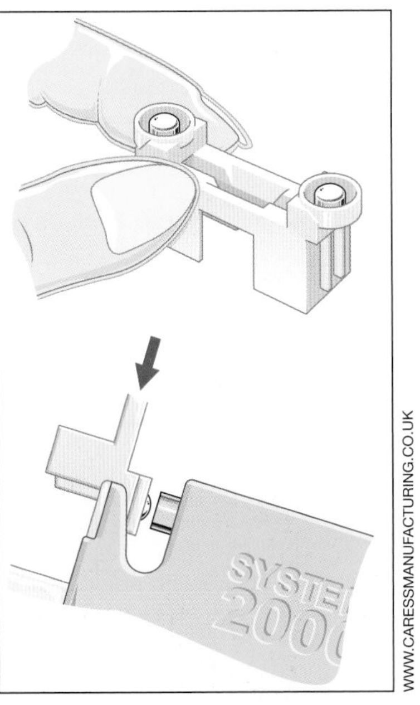

4 There are two parts, which must be separated. One part holds the back clasps: this is positioned in the slot. Push the cartridge down until it will go no further. The second holds the studs: position this against the stud barrel of the gun, which places a protective plastic ring around the barrel of the gun and stud.

5 Gently pull the holder upwards, away from the barrel: this will deposit the stud in the barrel.

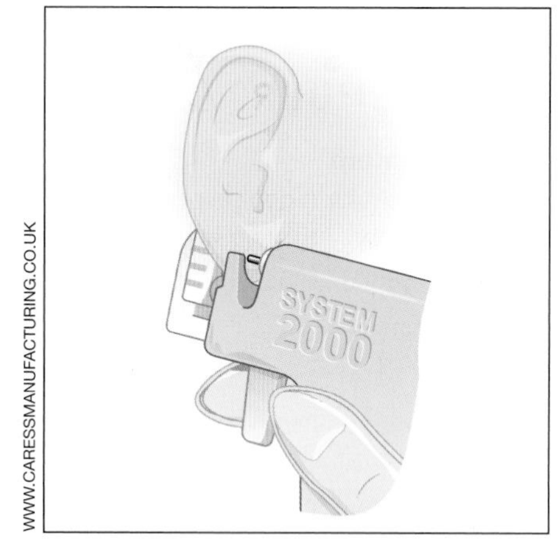

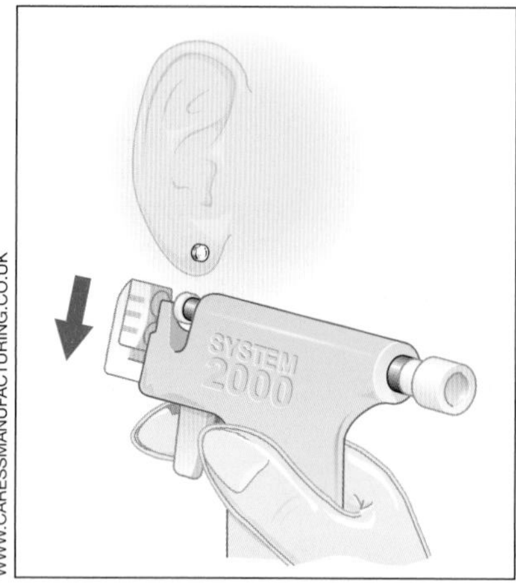

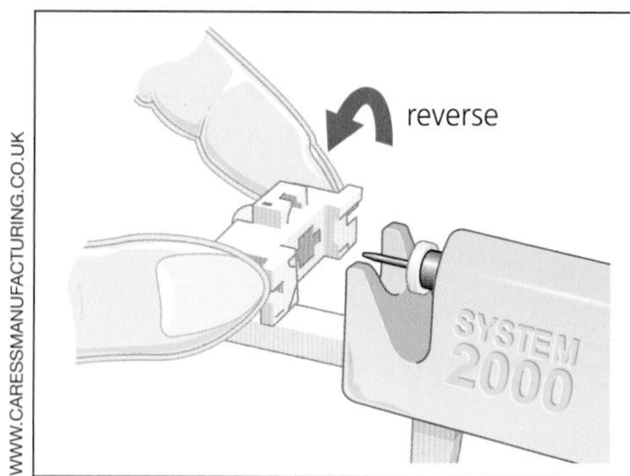

6 Holding the gun horizontally, position the stem of the stud at right angles to the ear so that it is accurately placed over the mark on the earlobe.

Gently squeeze the trigger until it stops. Check that the point of the stud is still in the correct position. If it is, squeeze the trigger again. The ear will be pierced, with the back clasp placed onto the back of the stud.

Check that the earring and back clasp are securely connected.

7 Gently, move the gun down from the lobe. Hold the gun upside down and discard the plastic ring into the waste bin. Pull back the plunger knob and insert the next stud and protective ring.

8 Holding the gun in one hand, grip the back-clasp holder (using the mount in the other hand) and remove the holder from the gun. Invert the holder and place it back into the gun, with the remaining clasp in the top position.

9 Now pierce the second ear, repeating stage 6. If only one piercing is required where double packs of studs are used, the other stud should be discarded.

10 Using the hand mirror, show the client their pierced ears and check that the result is to the client's satisfaction.

> Never become complacent with your customers, or over-familiar; we are at work and it is a business.
>
> **Jade Rogers**

HEALTH & SAFETY

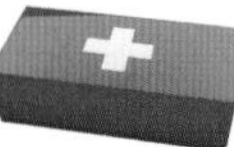

Do not handle studs with your bare hands

Follow the manufacturer's instructions for correct loading. There should not be a need to touch the studs or stud-holding devices.

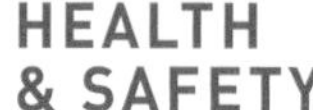

KNOWLEDGE CHECK

Why should only only one pair of studs be fitted at once?

Need more time... refer to page 530 to help you.

ALWAYS REMEMBER

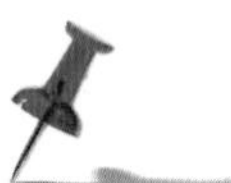

Technique

Always hold the gun either horizontally or upwards. Never point the gun downwards once it has been loaded – if you do, the studs will fall out.

ALWAYS REMEMBER

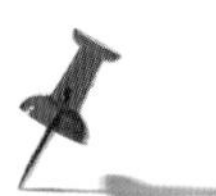

Gun malfunction

If the piercing is successful but the clasp fails to attach to the post, firmly attach this manually without causing the client unnecessary distress.

If the ear stud needs adjustment following piercing, rewash your hands and apply a fresh pair of gloves before touching the pierced ear.

BEST PRACTICE

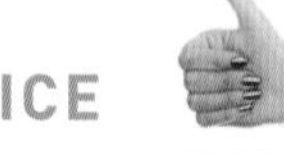

Client comfort

Allow the client to sit still for a few minutes following the service. Offer them tea or coffee. Some clients may be very anxious and need time to relax.

BEST PRACTICE

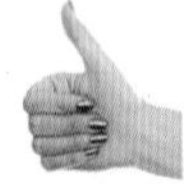

Technique

To avoid anxiety to the client, pierce the second ear without hesitation, yet safely.

How to complete the service

1 Discuss the aftercare instructions with the client (see below). Record details of the ear piercing treatment on the client's record card.

2 When the service has been completed, invert the gun, eject the protective ring, and remove the empty back-clasp holder. Dispose of the plastic cartridges into the waste bin.

3 Clean the gun using clean cotton wool and surgical spirit, and place it in the ultra-violet sterilizing cabinet. Always refer to manufacturers' instructions for guidance on hygiene maintenance of the gun.

4 Dispose of all used products in the covered lined waste bin.

BEST PRACTICE

Technique

The gun should not point down or up when piercing. If the angle of piercing is incorrect, the earring will hang forward, sideways or backwards. Hold at a right angle to the ear.

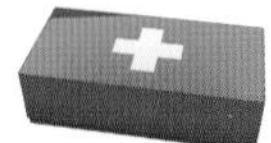

HEALTH & SAFETY

Disposal of waste

Waste from skin-piercing procedures is classed as clinical waste.

All consumable materials used during the ear piercing service should be placed in a covered, lined waste bin, and disposed of in a sealed bag.

Waste materials that have come into contact with body fluids must be collected and disposed of by special arrangement.

The disposal of clinical waste is controlled by the Environment Agency. *The Environment Protection Act (1990): Waste Management: The Duty of Care, A Code of Practice* (ISBN 011 752577 X) provides further information on this subject.

Detailed information on safe disposal of health care waste is available from the Department of Health.

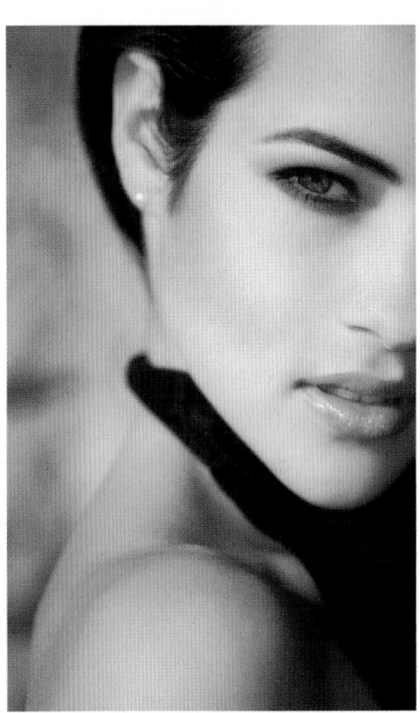

Studs can add glamour

5 Any item that is not disposable and that has been used on a client must be sterilized (or cleaned to ensure hygiene compliance for equipment such as towels) before use on another client to prevent *secondary infection*, or *cross-infection*.

Any item that has penetrated the skin (e.g., ear studs that required replacement during the procedure), must be disposed of hygienically immediately in a sharps box and should be disposed of safely in compliance with clinical waste procedures.

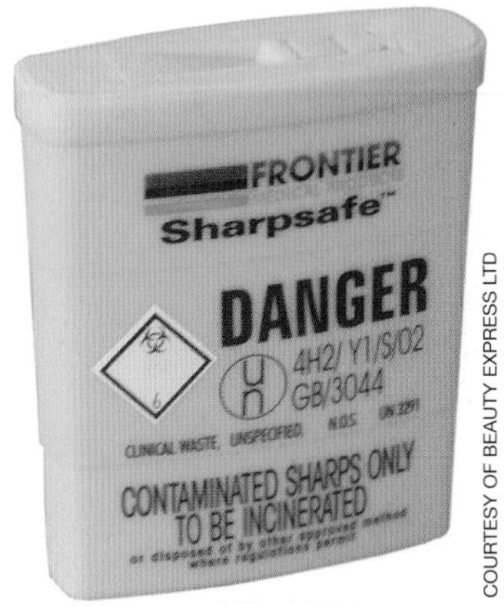

COURTESY OF BEAUTY EXPRESS LTD

Sharps box

ACTIVITY

Differing procedures

The procedure for loading the different ear piercing guns varies. The procedure given above is one example. Referring to the literature you have collected on the different guns, note ways in which the various service procedures differ.

Aftercare advice

After the ear piercing, complete details of the service on the client's record card. It is normal to experience minor pain and redness on the area following the service, explain this to the client. The client should be given clear instructions on how to care for their ears to prevent secondary infection and promote skin healing. The studs must not be removed for five to six weeks to enable effective skin healing and prevent infection. Invite the client to return to the salon after this period for you to remove the studs.

HEALTH & SAFETY 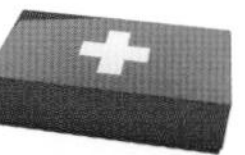

Aftercare lotion
Following an ear piercing, a professional manufacturer's aftercare lotion should be provided for each client, which is protected by the manufacturer's product liability insurance. These often contain ingredients suitable to disinfect the skin such as isopropyl alcohol.

HEALTH & SAFETY 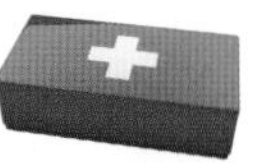

First Aid
There must be a first aid kit available that complies with the **Health and Safety (First Aid) Regulations (1981)**. It is recommended that there is a person trained in first aid holding a recognized certificate such as the SHE approved Basic First Aid Qualification.

Following ear piercing, consider the waste which will require disposal and how this waste should be disposed of.

Need more time... refer to page 533 to help you.

HEALTH & SAFETY 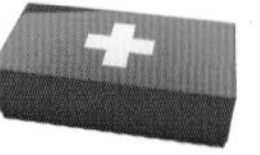

Antiseptic lotions
Remind the client that if an antiseptic lotion is applied to the ear area, it must be diluted as directed or skin burning may occur.

Remind the client always to wash their hands before cleaning the ear area. (If someone else is going to clean the ears, they also must wash their hands with soap and warm water before touching the client's ears.) The ears should be cleaned twice daily, using an aftercare lotion. The lotion must be applied as directed by the manufacturer. It should be applied to clean cotton wool, and the cotton wool squeezed to allow the lotion to run around the stud, at the front of the ear and then at the back. While the ears are being bathed with the cleansing solution, the stud should be rotated by holding it firmly at the front.

Even if the client cleanses their ears effectively, infection could still occur in other ways. These include the following:

- Long nails harbour germs. Infection of the ear can occur while the client is turning the stud.
- The client may touch the stud and ear at times other than when cleaning the ear.
- Shampoo and dirty water may collect around the ear while shampooing the hair. Remind the client to rinse the ear thoroughly with clean water after shampooing.
- The area can get wet e.g. after showering. Dry the area with a clean tissue if so.
- The client should protect their ears when applying hair lacquer or perfume, to avoid sensitizing the ear.
- Following the removal of the studs, the client should only wear gold earrings. Cheap fashion earrings should be worn only for short periods of time, or allergic reactions and ear infections may occur. Earrings must be worn to ensure the pierced hole doesn't heal following removal of the stud posts.

After oral instructions have been given, the client should be provided with an aftercare leaflet containing these instructions.

Body piercing

You may advance your piercing skills further to perform body piercing. **Body piercing** is currently very fashionable. Common areas for piercing include the nipples, the eyebrows, the nose and the navel. Note that body piercing is inappropriate for clients under 17 years of age, as the body is still growing.

Beauty therapy salons that offer ear piercing are often also asked for body piercing. Body piercing should be undertaken only if you have had thorough training, however, and only if you have the necessary specialized equipment and appropriate insurance cover.

Equipment

The equipment for piercing is either a **body piercing** gun, which inserts a hollow reed, or the **needle and clamp** method. With the latter, the clamp reduces circulation in the area, thereby anaesthetizing it, and the needle is inserted into the skin. The opening made by the needle is then filled with a ring or stud of high-quality non-reactive surgical steel or gold (above 16 carat).

Aftercare and advice

Special care should be taken of the area for one month following piercing. Ideally the jewellery must not be changed for four to six months to avoid tissue damage and possible infection. If infection occurs, causing excessive redness, swelling or a discharge, the client should return to the salon.

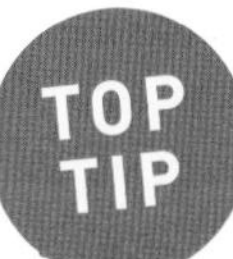

Legal requirements

Always check with your insurance company which areas of the body you are able to pierce.

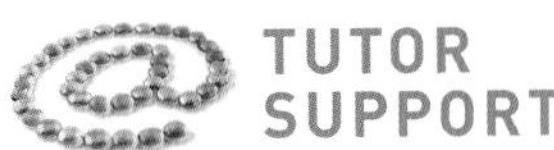

Activity 4: Re-cap, revision and evaluation

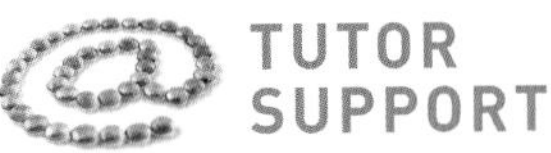

Activity 6: Multiple choice quiz

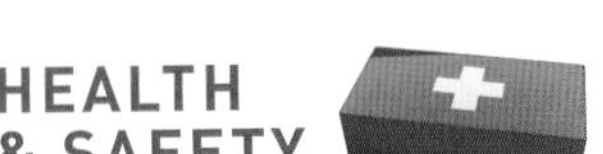

Body piercing

Before performing body piercing, approval is required from your local environmental health authority and registration is required.

Age and consent issues can be confirmed with your local authority who may have used licensing powers to impose licensing conditions relating to the age of the client.

KNOWLEDGE CHECK

What aftercare instructions should be given to a client following ear piercing?

Need more time... refer to pages 533–534 to help you.

GLOSSARY OF KEY WORDS

Aftercare advice recommendations given to the client following service to continue the benefits of the service.

Certificate of registration awarded when the premises have been successfully inspected to ensure that the local bye-laws are being followed in relation to cosmetic piercing.

Clinical waste waste from ear piercing is classed as clinical waste. The disposal of clinical waste is controlled by the Environment Agency. Waste materials that have come into contact with body fluids must be collected and disposed of by special arrangements. *The Environment Protection Act (1990): Waste Management: The Duty of Care, A Code of Practice* (ISBN 011 752577 X) provides further information on this subject.

Consent form written permission obtained from a parent or guardian to perform a service on a client under 16 years of age.

Consultation assessment of client's needs using different assessment techniques, including questioning and natural observation.

Contra-action an unwanted reaction occurring during or after service application.

Contra-indication a problematic symptom that indicates that the service may not proceed.

Control of Substances Hazardous to Health (COSHH) Regulations (2002) (Including Biological Agents) Regulations legislation that requires employers and the self-employed to prevent or control the exposure of employees and clients to hazardous substances. This includes exposure to biological agents such as bacteria, fungi and viruses and chemical cleaning/sterilizing agents. Records of the COSHH assessment must be available for inspection.

Dangerous Substances and Preparations (Nickel) (Safety) Regulations (2005) the use of nickel has been found to cause allergies. Check what metal is used for your supplier's ear piercing jewellery and that it complies with the regulations.

Ear piercing the perforation of the skin and underlying tissue of the earlobe to create a hole in the skin where jewellery is inserted.

Greater London Council (General Powers) Act (1981) this act covers the London boroughs and relates to cosmetic piercing. It provides that no person can carry out cosmetic piercing unless they and the business are registered. It also states what records are required to be kept.

Keloids overgrowths of scar tissue, occurring at the site of the ear piercing.

Local Government Act (2003) (section 120 and schedule 6) has amended the Local Government (Miscellaneous Provisions) Act (1982) to enable each authority to regulate businesses providing cosmetic body piercing. Each local authority can introduce its own bye-laws to set the standards for cosmetic piercing.

Local Government (Miscellaneous Provisions) Act (1982) requires that salons offering any form of skin piercing be registered with the local health authority. This registration includes the operators who will be carrying out the service and the salon premises where the service will be carried out.

London Local Authorities Act (1991 and 2007) this act states that no person shall carry out cosmetic piercing at an establishment without obtaining a licence from a participating council. Conditions can be attached to the licence, such as hygiene practices, age restrictions, etc.

Service plan after the consultation, suitable service objectives are established to treat the client's conditions and needs.

ASSESSMENT OF KNOWLEDGE AND UNDERSTANDING

You have now learnt about ear piercing in the beauty therapy workplace. To test your level of knowledge, answer the following short questions. These will prepare you for your summative (final) assessment.

1. The part of the ear that is recommended for ear piercing is the:
   a. helix
   b. lobule
   c. pinna
2. Which part of the ear is considered unsuitable and can result in keloid scarring?
   a. lobule
   b. helix
   c. pinna
3. What is the healing period before the removal of the initial jewellery used to pierce the ears?
   a. 6 weeks
   b. 5–6 weeks
   c. 6–8 weeks
   d. 3–4 weeks
4. The legislation that enables each local authority to regulate businesses providing cosmetic piercing is the:
   a. Control of Substances Hazardous to Health (COSHH) Regulations (2002)
   b. Management of Health and safety at Work Regulations (1999)
   c. Local Government Act (2003)
5. How often is it recommended the ear studs be rotated during the healing period?
   a. once a day
   b. twice a day
   c. three to four times a day
   d. once per week
6. The group of lymph nodes that drain the ear area are the:
   a. parotid nodes
   b. occipital nodes
   c. buccal nodes
   d. sub-mental nodes
7. Which of the following contra-indications would require to be verbally checked for?
   a. anti-coagulant drugs
   b. epilepsy
   c. diabetes
   d. all of the above
8. Disposable gloves must be worn when performing ear piercing service. Which legislation does this comply with?
9. The image below shows skin healing contra-action in the ear tissue, known as what?

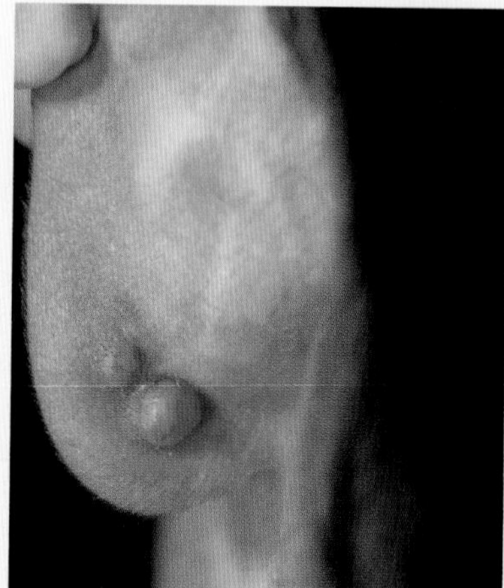

10. Poor aftercare may result in secondary infection – how would this be recognised?

17 Head Massage

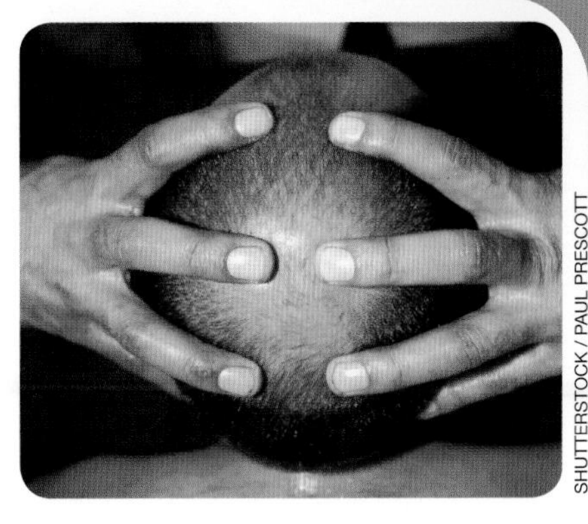
SHUTTERSTOCK / PAUL PRESCOTT

Learning Objectives

This chapter covers **VRQ Unit Head massage.**

This unit is all about how to provide head massage treatment. The massage is applied to the head, neck and scalp providing both a physiological and psychological effect. Application is modified to achieve the client's service objectives identified at consultation. This includes for the purpose of relaxation, well-being and stimulation. Oils may be used selected to enhance the treatment results, improving the condition of both the skin and hair.

There are **two** learning outcomes for this unit which you must achieve:

1 Be able to prepare for head massage

2 Be able to provide head massage

From the range statement you must show you can:

- use **consultation techniques** to identify the treatment **objectives**
- meet all preparation requirements
- carry out checks before treatment to take into account **factors** which may affect the treatment plan
- ensure the **environmental conditions** are suitable
- followed all **health and safety working practices**
- use all listed **products, tools and equipment** as appropriate

(continued on the next page)

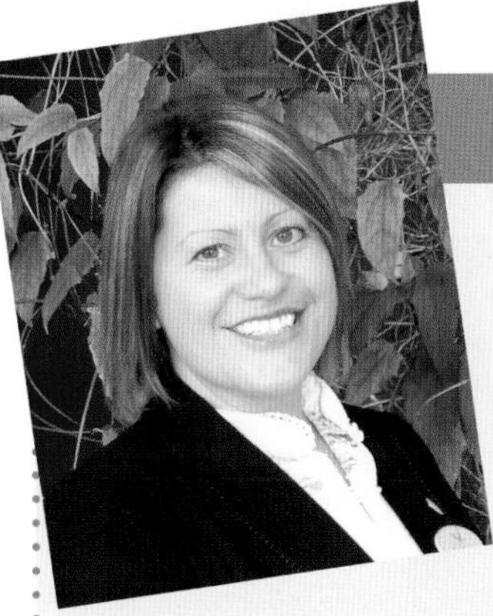

ROLE MODEL

Zoe Crowley

Aqua Sana Manager, Elveden Forest Center Parcs

"I qualified as a Beauty Therapist in 1996 and then worked for Steiner Transocean onboard cruise ships. I loved life at sea and stayed for seven contracts, working my way up from Beauty Therapist, to Senior Beauty Therapist, Assistant Spa Manager until I became Spa Director and managed my own ships. Once I returned to dry land I worked for Molton Brown in a retail store before setting up a brand new day spa in the Malmaison Hotel in Birmingham. That was a great challenge and very rewarding to see the project through from start to finish, choosing the decoration, employing the team, opening orders of stock, etc.

I then relocated and joined Center Parcs and have now been here for 5 years. I manage the Aqua Sana team of around 90 which includes beauty therapists, spa attendants, hairdressers and reception staff, I also have four assistant managers who help me with the operation.

Our facilities include 21 treatment rooms including a dry floatation room and dual treatment rooms, and over 16 experiences to try in our wonderful World of Spa including Tyrolean sauna, Turkish Hammam, Aqua Meditation room and water beds. It is a fantastic spa and no two days are ever the same.

- complete a consultation and skin inspection to identify any **contra-indications**
- **communicate and behave** in an appropriate and professional manner
- identify **contra-actions**
- provide relevant **aftercare advice**
- use different **methods of evaluation** to assess the success of the treatment, including observation, written, verbal and self evaluation

You must be able to show that you have the necessary practical skills and underpinning knowledge to provide head massage.

This unit is linked to the Beauty Therapy NOS **Unit B23**.

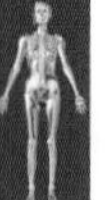

Essential anatomy and physiology knowledge requirements for this unit are identified on the checklist on page 27. This chapter also discusses anatomy and physiology specific to this unit.

Introduction

Head massage is a treatment applied to the neck and head using the hands. It helps to relieve stress and tension, and creates a feeling of well-being. Head massage combines the modern Swedish body massage techniques with the traditional techniques of Indian head massage. This unit will cover the application of massage movements effleurage, petrissage, tapotement, frictions and vibrations. These techniques can be developed further at Level 3 to provide Indian head massage treatment.

As the therapeutic effects of massage become more popular, head massage is an ideal service to offer and has many advantages that can meet the needs of different clients. It can be used to enhance other treatments such as facials e.g. you may perform a scalp and neck massage after the face mask has been applied. There is no need for the client to undress, it is relatively quick to perform, can be performed almost anywhere and does not require expensive equipment.

Oils may be incorporated into the massage to condition the skin of the scalp and hair. This also helps to induce relaxation.

The massage is adapted to the client's physiological and psychological needs. These are determined during the client consultation and are termed the objectives of the service.

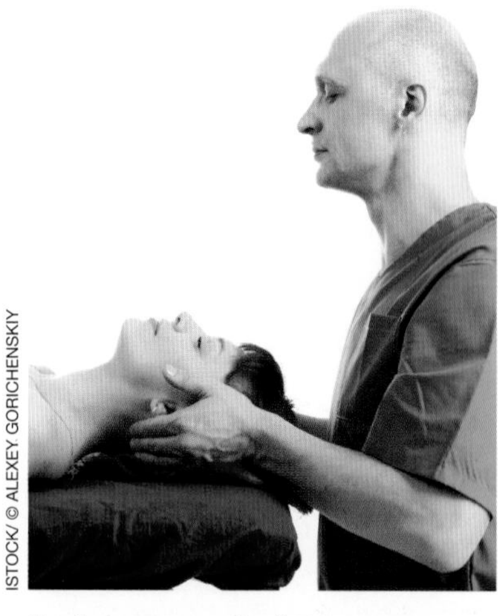

Head massage application

These objectives may include:

- relaxation
- creating and maintaining a feeling of well-being
- an uplifting or stimulating effect
- to improve the condition of the skin of the scalp and hair

Physiological effects of head massage

- The muscles receive an improved supply of oxygenated blood, essential for cell growth. The tone and strength of muscles are improved. Areas of muscular tension will become relaxed.
- Increased joint mobility in the neck area occurs through massage manipulation to the area.
- The increased blood circulation in the area warms the tissues. This induces a feeling of relaxation, which is particularly beneficial when treating tense muscles.
- As the blood capillaries dilate and bring blood to the skin's surface, the skin colour improves.
- The lymphatic circulation and the venous blood circulation increase. These changes speed up the removal of waste products and toxins. The removal of excess lymph improves the appearance of a puffy oedematous skin, it also improves production of white blood cells to fight infections.
- Sensory nerve endings can be soothed or stimulated, depending on the massage manipulations selected.
- Massage stimulates the sebaceous and sudoriferous glands and increases the production of sweat and sebum. This increases the skin's natural oil and moisture balance.
- Applying oil to the head (optional) adds moisture and improves the condition of dry hair or scalp.
- Massage to the scalp may stimulate hair growth by increasing blood supply to the hair follicle, e.g. in cases of alopecia, hair loss.

The psychological effects of massage are broad, and when performed on a regular basis, can relieve stress and tension in the client. The client may feel fresh, invigorated and healthier.

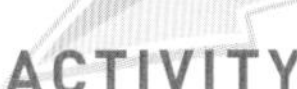

ACTIVITY

Indian head massage
Research the art of Indian head massage, with particular reference to the following:

- the history of Indian head massage
- the culture of Indian head massage
- **Ayurveda,** the 'science of life'
- the three *doshas*

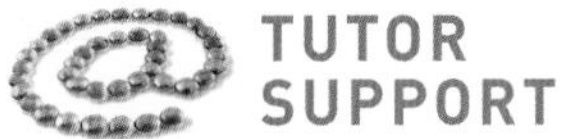

TUTOR SUPPORT

Activity 5: Promote on site/Indian head massage service

Psychological effects of head massage

- helps to improve concentration – increased oxygen to the brain
- relieves tension
- induces relaxation
- relieves stress and anxiety
- confidence-raising following the removal of tension

TOP TIP

Popularity and benefits

Head massage is increasing in popularity due to it being a relatively quick service which can be received with minimal client preparation.

Airlines are increasingly offering this to their customers as an in-flight service.

Also, it is popular in many companies who enable their employees to receive the service during work hours to relieve stress and maintain well-being.

ALWAYS REMEMBER

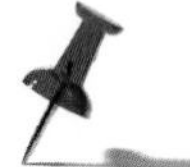

Emotional effect
Because clients relax with head massage they may then wish to talk about their problems.

If this happens, *listen* – but unless qualified you should not *counsel*.

KNOWLEDGE CHECK

Name the eight bones that form the cranium.

Need more time... refer to page 76 to help you.

Massage techniques

Head massage is based on a series of classic westernized and Indian massage movements, used to create different effects. There are six basic types of massage techniques:

- effleurage
- petrissage
- tapotement (percussion)
- frictions
- vibrations

The beauty therapist can adapt the way each of these movements is applied, according to the needs of the client. Either the *speed* of application or the *depth of pressure* can be altered.

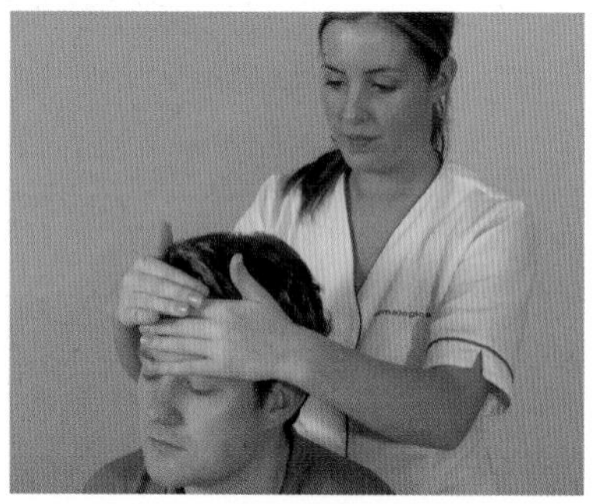

Effleurage – stroking technique to the forehead frontal bone. This technique can be used to cover the whole scalp area.

Effleurage Effleurage is a stroking movement, used to begin the massage, as a link manipulation, and to complete the massage sequence. This manipulation can be applied lightly or briskly, has an even pressure and is applied in a rhythmical, continuous manner to induce relaxation. The speed of application depends upon the effect to be achieved and according to the underlying structures and tissue type, but it must *never* be unduly heavy. Movements also include stroking. Effleurage has the following effects:

- desquamation (skin removal) is increased
- arterial blood circulation is increased, bringing fresh nutrients to the area, energizing the client and warming the tissues
- venous circulation is improved, aiding the removal of congestion from the veins
- lymphatic circulation is increased, improving the absorption of waste products and elimination of toxins from the tissues
- the underlying muscle fibres are relaxed
- relaxes and soothes sensory nerve endings

Uses in service: to relax tight and contracted muscles.

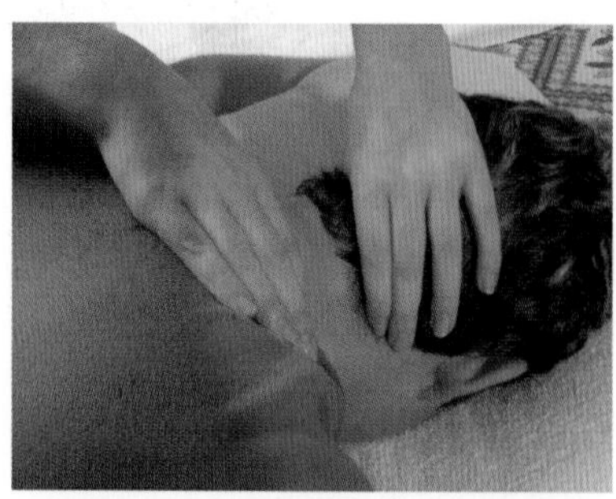

Petrissage – picking up the muscle and skin at the back of the neck

TOP TIP

Relief from tension and stress

Massaging the scalp and neck can relieve symptoms of stress such stiffness in the neck and headaches.

Petrissage Petrissage involves a series of movements in which the tissues are lifted away from the underlying structures and compressed, including kneading and squeezing and releasing the muscles along their length. The whole hands or just the fingers and thumbs may be used. Pressure is intermittent, and should be light yet firm. Petrissage has the following effects:

- improvement of muscle tone, through the compression and relaxation of muscle fibres
- improvement in blood and lymph circulation, as the application of pressure causes the vessels to empty and fill
- increased activity of the sebaceous glands, due to the stimulation effect on the skin tissues

Movements include picking up, kneading, pinching and rolling.

Uses in service: to stimulate a sluggish circulation; to increase sebaceous gland and sudoriferous gland activity when treating a dry skin condition.

Percussion **Percussion**, also known as **tapotement**, is performed in a brisk, stimulating manner. Rhythm is important as the fingers are continually breaking contact with the skin; irritation or damage can occur if this movement is performed incorrectly. Percussion has the following effects:

- stimulation of the nerves
- a fast vascular (skin reddening) reaction because of the skin's nervous response to the stimulus – this reaction, erythema, is a sign of skin stimulation
- increased blood supply, which nourishes the tissues
- improvement in skin and muscle tone in the area

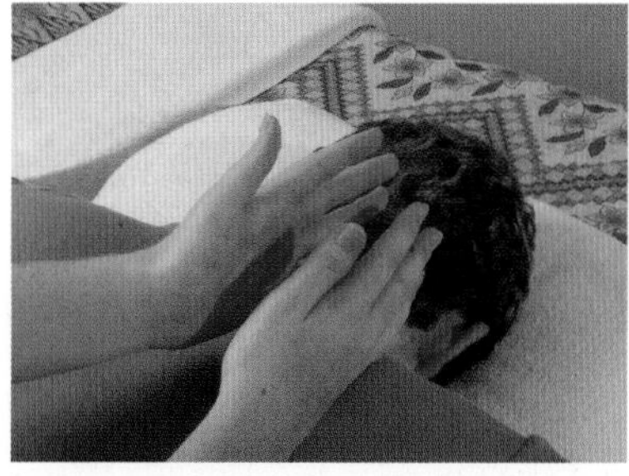

Percussion – hands positioned for hacking movement. This movement can be applied lightly to the scalp.

Movements include hacking and **tapping**. When performed on the scalp, only light pressure should be used. In facial massage only light tapping should be used.

HEALTH & SAFETY

Skin elasticity

As the skin ages it becomes thinner and less elastic. Take care when using petrissage movements to avoid skin tissue damage.

Also, any areas of scar tissue will not be as supple as normal skin, care in handling is required.

Uses in service: to tone areas of loose skin and improve circulation in the area.

Frictions Frictions cause the skin and superficial structure to move together over the underlying structures. These movements are performed with either the fingers or the thumbs and concentrated in a particular area, applied with regulated pressure. Frictions have the following effects:

- desquamation (skin removal) is increased
- gentle stimulation of the skin and superficial tissues improving functioning
- improves scar tissue by breaking down the tissue adhesions
- improved lymphatic and blood circulation
- breaks down tight nodules (tension in the muscle fibres), improving mobility

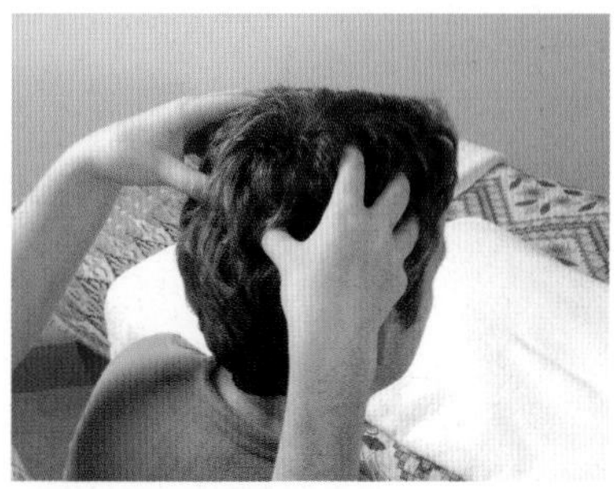

Frictions to the scalp

Uses in service: to help break down fatty deposits, fibrous thickening and the removal of non-medical oedema (fluid retention). To stimulate and improve a dry skin condition.

Vibrations Vibrations are applied on the nerve centre. They are produced by a rapid contraction and relaxation of the beauty therapist's arm, resulting in a fine trembling movement. Vibration has the following effects:

- stimulation of the nerves, inducing a feeling of well-being
- gentle stimulation of the skin

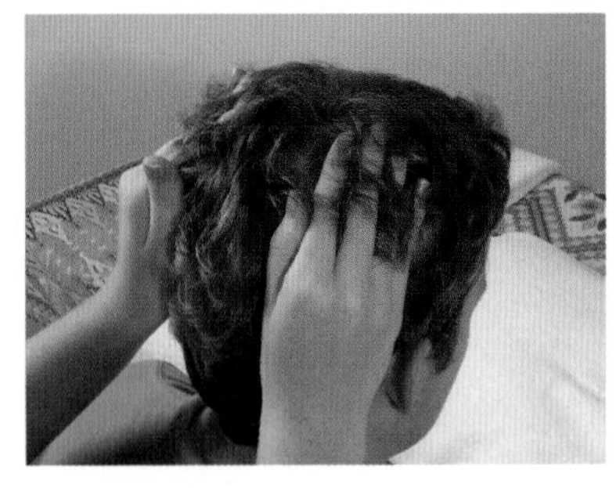

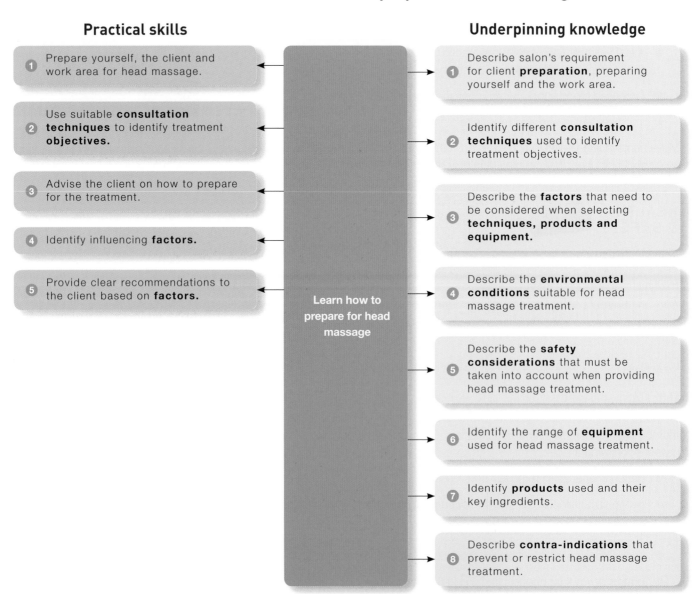

Vibrations to the scalp

Movements include *static* vibrations, in which the pads of the fingers are placed on the nerve and the vibratory effect created by the beauty therapist's arms and hands is applied in one position; and running vibrations, in which the vibratory effect is applied along a nerve path.

Uses in service: to stimulate a sensitive skin in order to improve the skin's functioning without irritating the surface blood capillaries.

Outcome 1: Be able to prepare for head massage

Learn how to prepare for head massage

Practical skills

1. Prepare yourself, the client and work area for head massage.
2. Use suitable **consultation techniques** to identify treatment **objectives.**
3. Advise the client on how to prepare for the treatment.
4. Identify influencing **factors.**
5. Provide clear recommendations to the client based on **factors.**

Underpinning knowledge

1. Describe salon's requirement for client **preparation**, preparing yourself and the work area.
2. Identify different **consultation techniques** used to identify treatment objectives.
3. Describe the **factors** that need to be considered when selecting **techniques, products and equipment.**
4. Describe the **environmental conditions** suitable for head massage treatment.
5. Describe the **safety considerations** that must be taken into account when providing head massage treatment.
6. Identify the range of **equipment** used for head massage treatment.
7. Identify **products** used and their key ingredients.
8. Describe **contra-indications** that prevent or restrict head massage treatment.

PRODUCTS, TOOLS AND EQUIPMENT

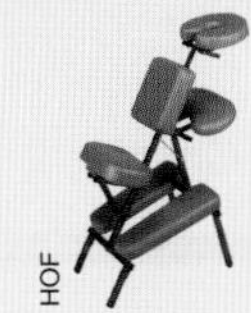

Massage chair or couch

Chair

With adjustable height, low back support without an arm rest

Specialist head and neck massage treatment chair shown.

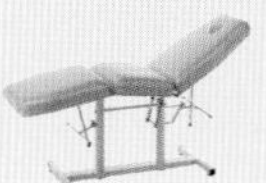

Couch

Covered with an easy-to-clean surface; it must withstand cleaning with warm water and detergent; it must have an adjustable back rest for both the comfort of the client and beauty therapist when performing different massage movements.

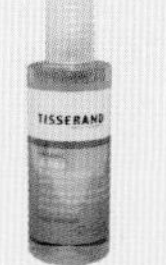

Organic massage oil

e.g. almond, olive, mustard, sesame coconut or pre-blended oil. The oil is warmed before application to aid absorption and induce relaxation

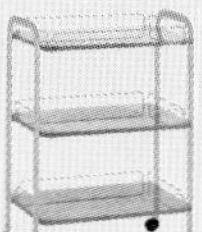

Trolley

Or other surface on which to place everything

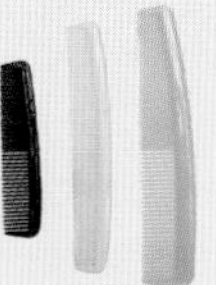

Combs

To allow the client to comb their hair following service

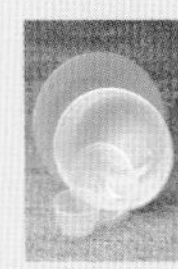

Plastic bowls

Two, to dispense products into as necessary and hold consumables

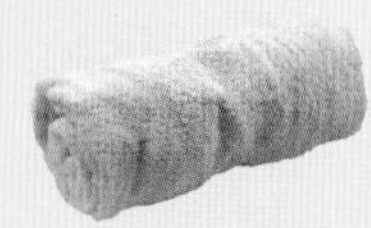

Clean towels

Freshly laundered for each client

A towel may be placed over the client's shoulders if using oils

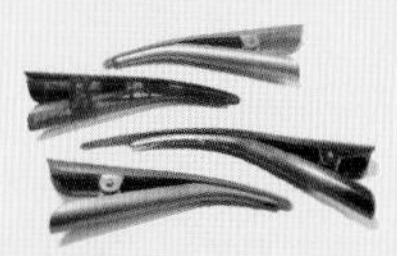

Hair clips

Used to secure long hair away from the neck area

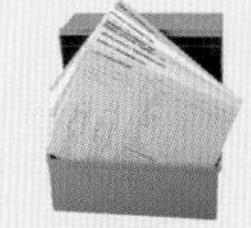

Client record card

To record confidential details of each client registered at the salon including personal details, products used and details of the treatment.

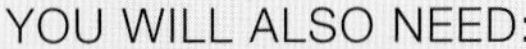

YOU WILL ALSO NEED:

Paper tissue disposable bedroll To cover the treatment couch cover if used

Dry and damp cotton wool and tissues To apply skin-cleansing agents and dry the skin

Skin cleansing agent Such as witch hazel or eau de cologne

Cosmetic cleansing preparations To remove facial make-up (as necessary)

Waste container – Metal lined bin with a disposable liner

Aftercare advice – Recommended advice for the client to refer to following the service

Plan and prepare for the treatment

Sterilization and disinfection

Prior to the head massage service, make sure that the work area is hygienic. The surface of the massage couch and the trolley surface should be wiped over with warm soapy water and disinfectant.

Plastic spatulas, if used, should be cleaned and placed in an UV cabinet prior to use to ensure they are free from bacteria.

An **aseptic** condition should be maintained, a situation where you are trying to eliminate bacteria. The treatment area should remain in a safe and hygienic state throughout the day, ready for further use. Waste at the conclusion of treatment should be disposed of in a sealed polythene bag and towels laundered.

Clean towels should be provided for each client to prevent cross-infection.

Remember to use the underpinning knowledge you learnt about in Chapter 3 Health and Safety.

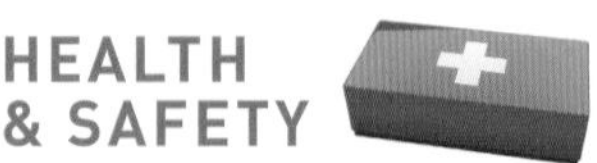

Legislation

It is important that you comply with all relevant health and safety legislation while performing head massage.

Examples include:

Workplace (Health, Safety and Welfare) Regulations (1992)

Control of Substances Hazardous to Health Regulations (COSHH) (2002)

Electricity at Work Regulations (1989)

When applying for a beauty therapy position make sure you are prepared. Research the spa or salon. Consider a 'dry run' of the journey to prevent you from being late for the interview. Remember to be yourself and show your personality.

Zoe Crowley

Preparing the work area

Prepare the work area to meet all health and safety legislation requirements.

The treatment area should be clean and at a warm, comfortable working temperature for both the client and the beauty therapist, between 18 and 21°C. Adequate ventilation should be provided to create a hygienic environment, preventing cross-infection through viral airborne spores, drowsiness through carbon dioxide-saturated air and the removal of stale smells and odours. The treatment area should make the client feel comfortable and relaxed. Lighting should be soft, the colour of the decor should be subtle and non-gender biased. Sound levels should be low and selected for relaxation. If performing the service over a couch there should be adequate support in the form of a bolster (a pillow) cushion to support the head and neck and ensure client comfort. Place all the products, tools and equipment required on the trolley prior to the treatment, to ensure that an efficient treatment is provided without unnecessary disruptions.

Before beginning the head massage treatment, check that you have the necessary products, equipment and materials to hand and that they meet the legal, hygiene and industry requirements for head massage treatment.

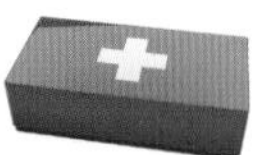

Allergies

Refer to the record card to check for any known allergies to products, which could cause a contra-action, e.g., sesame oil can cause skin irritation, where possible select an alternative such as olive oil.

Preparation of the beauty therapist

The beauty therapist should wear a professional work uniform which does not restrict movement. Full, enclosed shoes should be worn with low or medium-height heels. Optionally shoes may be removed when performing the massage to assist energy flow through the body. (Always follow your workplace policy.) Jewellery must be removed from the hands and wrists.

Before preparing the client for the treatment, wash your hands. The hands need to be flexible in order to fit the contour of the client's upper body. Shake the hands to remove any tension from the wrists and hands. Practise deep slow breathing technique before applying massage. This will help you to relax and focus your concentration on the massage service.

Collect the client's record card from reception prior to their arrival. A full client consultation should be carried out before the service commences, including a postural check of the neck area. This will help you to identify any areas of tension.

Is the neck straight or is there an exaggerated curve? Is the neck drawn towards the left or right shoulder? Does the chin poke forwards causing the neck to curve forwards? Treatment can only proceed if the reason for the curvature is non-medical and is related to tension or poor posture.

Beauty therapist's hands The beauty therapist should always sanitize their hands prior to the service. Nails should be short, to avoid scratching the client and to facilitate massage application. The hands also need to be flexible in order to fit the contours of the client's body. Mobilizing the joints of the hands and fingers will loosen the hands and facilitate good manipulations. Hand exercises should be practised on a regular basis.

> It is very important to communicate with your client at all times. Make sure you confirm the service your client is expecting, ask what your client hopes to get out of the service, check throughout the service that your client is warm enough and comfortable and that the pressure is ok for her or him.
>
> Head massage is designed to de-stress and relive tension, so make sure you do everything within your power to ensure your client leaves your room feeling better.
>
> **Zoe Crowley**

TOP TIP

Beauty therapist's hands

Mobilizing the joints of the hands and fingers will loosen the hands and facilitate good manipulations.

Hand exercises should be practised on a regular basis.

Nails should be short, to avoid scratching the client and to facilitate massage application.

BEST PRACTICE

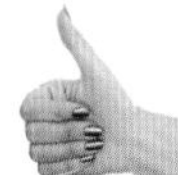

Breathing technique

Advise the client that breathing should be deep and slow, not shallow and rapid.

Before treatment encourage the client to breathe in slowly through the nose – the stomach should move out slightly – and out through the mouth.

HEALTH & SAFETY

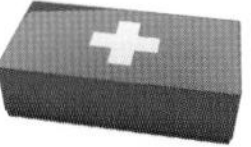

Footwear

If worn for work high heels can lead to serious foot and postural problems for the beauty therapist.

> As a beauty therapist it is important to be able to work using your own initiative but also as part of a team. Helping out colleagues, giving advice and swapping techniques will help the operation run smoothly and create a happy working environment.
>
> **Zoe Crowley**

ALWAYS REMEMBER

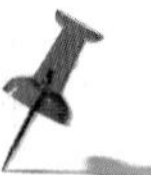

Local Authority Licensing Regulations (2003)

Massage services must apply for a license to practice from their local authority's environmental health department. Your local authority will advise you on the requirements for license and how to obtain a license.

BEST PRACTICE

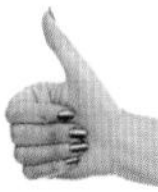

Long hair

If the client has long hair it may be necessary to secure it with a clip while performing massage to the head and neck.

Outcome 2: Be able to provide head massage

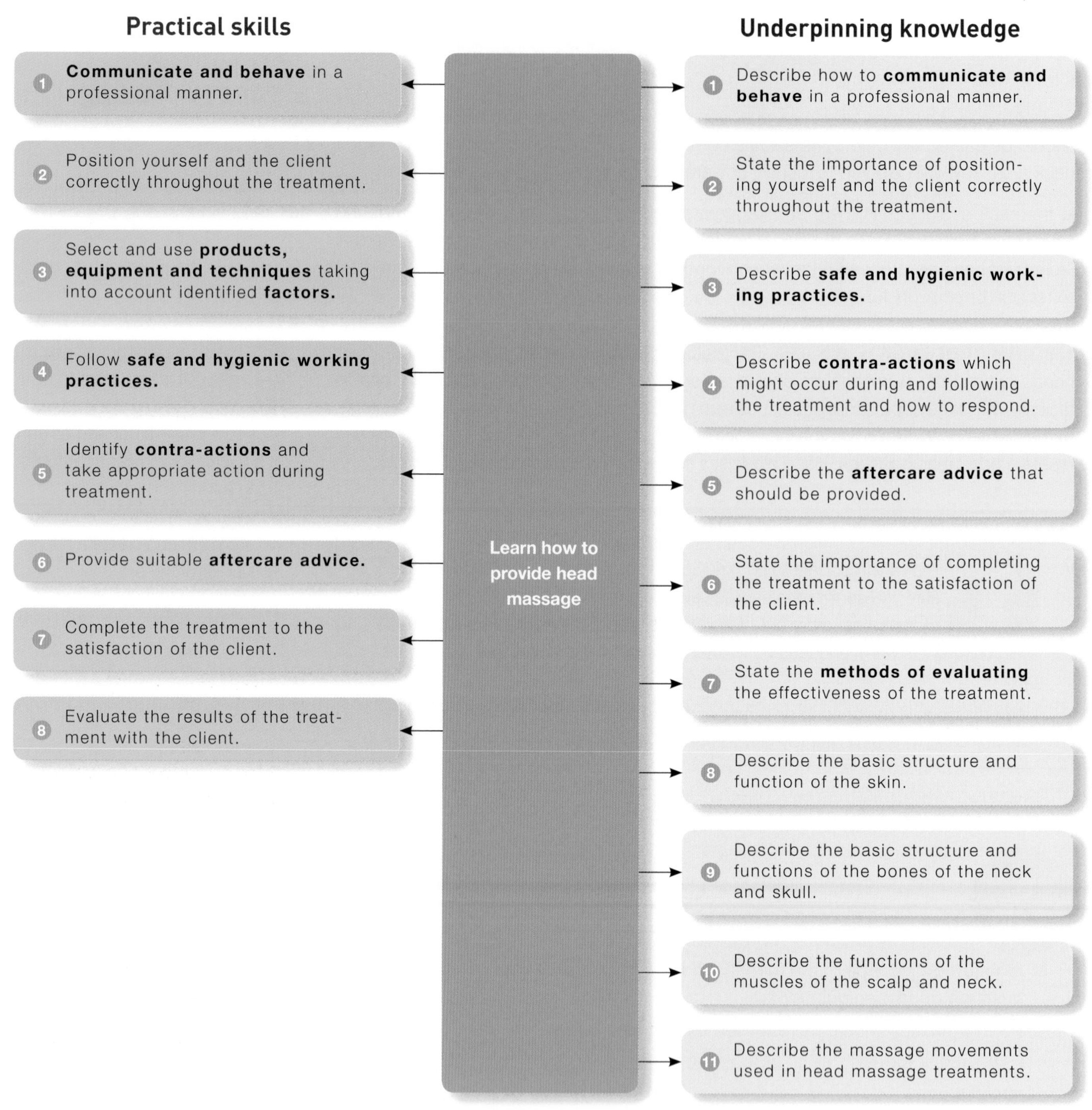
Practical skills
1 **Communicate and behave** in a professional manner.
2 Position yourself and the client correctly throughout the treatment.
3 Select and use **products, equipment and techniques** taking into account identified **factors.**
4 Follow **safe and hygienic working practices.**
5 Identify **contra-actions** and take appropriate action during treatment.
6 Provide suitable **aftercare advice.**
7 Complete the treatment to the satisfaction of the client.
8 Evaluate the results of the treatment with the client.
Learn how to provide head massage
Underpinning knowledge
1 Describe how to **communicate and behave** in a professional manner.
2 State the importance of positioning yourself and the client correctly throughout the treatment.
3 Describe **safe and hygienic working practices.**
4 Describe **contra-actions** which might occur during and following the treatment and how to respond.
5 Describe the **aftercare advice** that should be provided.
6 State the importance of completing the treatment to the satisfaction of the client.
7 State the **methods of evaluating** the effectiveness of the treatment.
8 Describe the basic structure and function of the skin.
9 Describe the basic structure and functions of the bones of the neck and skull.
10 Describe the functions of the muscles of the scalp and neck.
11 Describe the massage movements used in head massage treatments.

HEALTH & SAFETY

'Use by' dates and safe storage

Check that all products are clean and that the 'use by' date has not expired. Ensure all bottles are wiped over and lids are securely replaced after use to prevent spillage and the spread of bacteria.

To maintain the quality of organic oils they must be kept in cool dark conditions away from heat and light.

BEST PRACTICE 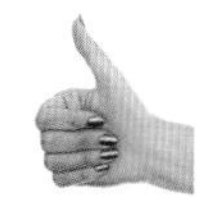

The client chair must not be on castors or they could move while the treatment is performed. The chair must support the client and the height adjustable to avoid the beauty therapist having to adopt poor posture or strain which could lead to repetitive strain injury.

Consultation

Reception

Head massage can be carried out as required, but is usually recommended once or twice a week, and preferably as a course for maximum effect. Regularity of treatments will depend upon the client's personal circumstances including their financial position and time constraints. When a client is booking for this treatment, allow 10–15 minutes (excluding consultation and preparation time), which includes consultation, practical service and aftercare advice. Warn the client that they may have a reaction after service. Symptoms can include tiredness, muscular aches, and possibly headaches. This reaction will normally subside after 24 hours. If the client is wearing a false hair piece warn them that this will have to be removed.

Discuss with the client their treatment requirements. Explain clearly to the client what the head massage treatment involves and the effects that can be gained. Treatment objectives must be realistic and achievable. Discuss the way the treatment application can be modified or adapted to meet their specific needs including the use of oil. Agree the treatment objectives with the client to meet their needs, both physically and psychologically. Allow time and invite the client to ask questions – the client should fully understand what the service involves including costs, duration, frequency recommendations including post-service reactions.

The beauty therapist needs to obtain relevant details from the client before starting the head massage treatment. The beauty therapist must ensure that their communication skills make the client feel welcome and comfortable. The client should be at ease throughout the treatment and a good, professional rapport should be built between client and beauty therapist. Personal details taken from the client are recorded on a record card. These should include medical history, doctor's details, and contra-indications that may be present.

Contra-indications

Certain contra-indications prevent or restrict head massage. These can be divided into three categories: general, local and temporary. **General** contra-indications affect the whole body or part of the body; **local** contra-indications are concentrated in a particular area; the symptoms of **temporary** contra-indications have only a short time span and clear up quite quickly. If the beauty therapist has any concern over the client's health or well-being, medical advice should be sought prior to the service. A doctor's note should be obtained before treatment is carried out.

If the client has skin sensitivity or product allergies a skin sensitivity patch test should be carried out in advance to assess their tolerance to the recommended products to be used in the treatment.

Those requiring GP referral should be tactfully and clearly discussed to ensure client understanding.

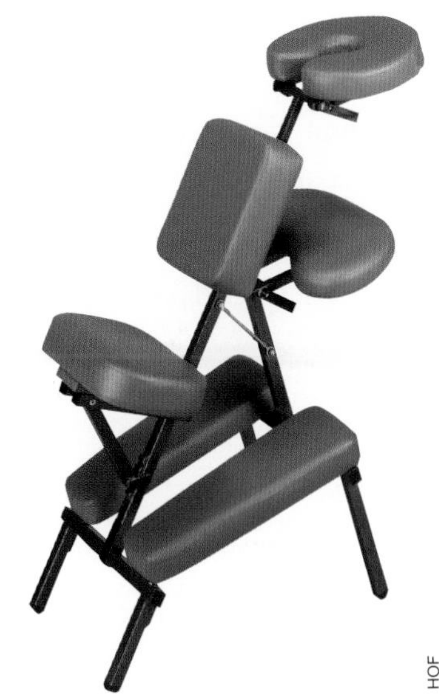

HOF

On-site massage chair

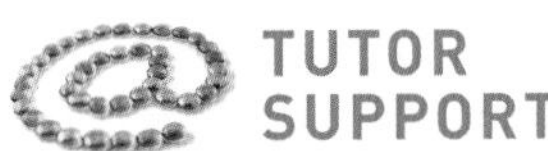

Activity 2: Consultation and planning for the treatment

ALWAYS REMEMBER 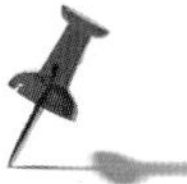

Treatment timing

It is important to complete service in the given time. This will ensure that:

- each client receives a competent service meeting their service requirements
- clients are not disadvantaged by receiving a hurried service
- a relaxing service environment in which clients are not made to feel anxious or stressed due to service delay is maintained

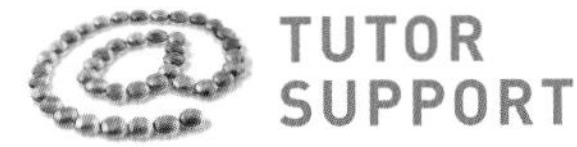

Activity 3: Contra-indications to head massage

Contra-indications

General	Local	Temporary
Heart conditions	Recent operations*	Medication
High or low blood pressure	Recent scar tissue (up to 6 months)*	Severe bruising*
Medication	Psoriasis or eczema*	Skin cuts and abrasions*
Diabetes	Skin disease	Pregnancy
Cancer	Skin disorder	Medical oedema
Rheumatism and arthritis (especially of the neck)	Recent injury*	Skin disease
Undiagnosed, lumps, bumps and swelling		Skin disorder
Loss of skin sensation		Intoxication
High temperature		Flu, cold symptoms
Migraine or severe headaches		Scalp disorders
Disorders of the nervous system		Infestations such as headlice.
		Headaches

* Only apply if located in the area.

HEALTH & SAFETY

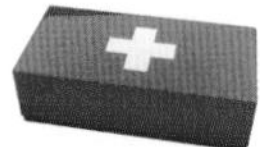

Service to minors

Anyone under 16 years of age must not receive a massage service unless accompanied by a parent or guardian who must also sign a consent form.

Follow your salon policy on supplying a service to minors.

ALWAYS REMEMBER

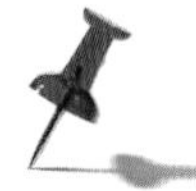

Health and well-being can be disturbed by factors such as:

- stress
- alcohol
- nicotine
- processed foods
- medication

Discuss how lifestyle change can affect health and well-being at consultation.

Check for contra-indications at the consultation, and if present do not proceed with the treatment. If in doubt as to the client's suitability for service the beauty therapist should first obtain a letter of approval from the client's doctor.

Lifestyle

It is important to find out about the lifestyle habits of the client. These include:

- *Occupation* – the client's occupation may be stressful or contribute to poor posture and muscle fatigue.
- *Family situation* – the client's domestic situation may affect their stress levels and limit their opportunities to take exercise or relax.
- *Dietary and fluid intake* – a nutritionally balanced diet is vital to the health of the body and the appearance of the skin. Lack of energy, skin allergies and disorders are, in part, the result of a poorly balanced diet. A healthy diet contains all the nutrients we need for health and growth. *Caffeine*, which is a stimulant, is found in tea, coffee and some fizzy drinks. Excessive amounts can interfere with digestion and block the absorption of vitamins and minerals. *Water* is important to avoid dehydration of the body and *at least* one litre of natural water should be drunk per day.
- *Alcohol* – alcohol is a toxin (poison) and deprives the body of vitamin reserves, especially vitamins B and C. It also causes dehydration.
- *Hobbies and interests* – these leisure activities can be a form of relaxation and method to alleviate stress.

- *Exercise taken and regularity* – a lack of exercise leads to poor lymph and blood circulation and poor muscle tone, resulting in slack contours and weight gain due to inactivity. Lack of exercise also results in lethargy.
- *Smoking habits* – smoking interferes with cell respiration and slows down the circulation. This makes it more difficult for nutrients to reach the skin cells and for waste products to be eliminated. The skin looks dull with a tendency towards open pores. Nicotine is a toxic substance.
- *Sleeping patterns* – disturbed sleeping patterns are often a result of raised stress levels. Disturbed sleep can result in exhaustion, fatigue, irritability and poor concentration.

Best practice for head massage

- Prepare your room to help the client start to relax as soon as they enter.
- Don't think of this service as for the head only, it will benefit the whole body.
- Ensure the client is seated comfortably and positioned so you can reach the head and neck easily.
- Adapt the service to suit your client's individual needs.
- Ensure you offer the client the chance to relax and unwind in an appropriate area after the service has finished.

Zoe Crowley

TOP TIP

Healthy diet

Although a healthy diet does not always guarantee a healthy hair and scalp, you are what you eat. Your body cannot produce healthy hair without the proper nutrients. The body can produce 11 of the 20 amino acids that make up hair, but the remaining nine must come from your daily diet. This is why crash dieting and anorexia can cause hair loss, lackluster hair and unhealthy scalp conditions. Proteins in meat, fish, eggs, and dairy products are good sources of these amino acids, as are food combinations such as peanut butter and bread, rice and beans, and beans and corn.

Questioning the client on expectations and outcomes ensures that the client gains satisfaction from the treatment. Listen carefully to make sure you fully understand the client's service requirements. You will need to assess the client's skin type, hair and scalp condition in order to check client suitability for treatment, plan the treatment and select suitable massage medium oils.

Retail sales are part of performing your treatments and should come naturally if you have completed your consultation. Look and listen to your client and offer solutions in their homecare programme.

Zoe Crowley

Hair analysis

Hair length If the client's hair is long it may be necessary to clip the hair away to perform certain movements. Ensure the hair is tangle free before you begin.

Hair texture The thickness or diameter of the individual hair strand. Hair texture can be classified as coarse, medium or fine. It is not uncommon for hair from different areas of the head to have different textures. Coarse hair texture has the thickest diameter and is the strongest. Care must be taken with fine hair to prevent breakage when performing movements which pull at the base of the hair. If the hair is thick in diameter it will be more difficult to access the scalp.

Hair density Relates to the amount of hair the client has on their scalp. Hair density can be classified as low, medium or high. The average hair density is about 2,200 hairs per square inch. Hair with high density (thick or dense hair) has more hairs per square inch, and hair with low density (thin hair) has fewer hairs per square inch. Density of hair will affect the quantity of oil required, if used, thick density requiring more oil. The average head of hair contains about 100,000 individual hair strands. If the hair density suddenly changes this may be related to the client's health, refer the client to their GP before treatment.

KNOWLEDGE CHECK

Why is it important to discuss the client's lifestyle?

Need more time... refer to pages 548–549 help you.

TOP TIP

The number of hairs on the head generally varies with the colour of the hair.

Hair colour	Average number of hairs on head
Blonde	140,000
Brown	110,000
Black	108,000
Red	80,000

Degree of curl This is determined by the **wave pattern** of the hair which refers to the shape of the hair shaft, and is described as straight, wavy, curly, or extremely curly. Natural wave patterns are genetic. Although there are many exceptions, as a general rule Asian hair tends to be extremely straight hair, Caucasian hair tends to be straight to wavy and African hair tends to be extremely curly. But anyone of any race, or mixed race, can have hair with varying degrees of curliness from straight to extremely curly. Care must be taken when performing head massage on extremely curly hair as it often has low elasticity, breaks easily, and has a tendency to knot, especially on the ends. It will benefit from the oil application to condition, strengthen and reduce tangling.

Hair porosity is the ability of the hair to absorb moisture. The degree of porosity is directly related to the condition of the cuticle layer. Healthy hair has a compact cuticle layer and is naturally resistant to penetration. Porous hair has a raised cuticle layer that easily absorbs moisture. Chemically treated hair is more porous and will benefit from the moisturising effect of the chosen oil. Overly porous hair is often dry, fragile, and brittle. It can also often feel rough to the touch. Care must be taken with very porous hair to avoid breakage.

Hair and scalp conditions

Dry hair and scalp Dry hair and scalp can be caused by underactive sebaceous glands, and can be made worse by excessive shampooing or exposure to dry, warm air, such as during winter. The lack of natural oils (sebum) leads to hair that appears dull, dry and lifeless. Dry hair and scalp should be treated with oils that stimulate the sebaceous gland and have an emollient effect.

Oily hair and scalp Oily hair and scalp can be caused by improper shampooing or overactive sebaceous glands, and is characterized by a greasy build up on the scalp and an oily coating on the hair. Oily hair and scalp can be improved by properly washing and rinsing the hair and using an oil regulating shampoo. A well-balanced diet, exercise, regular shampooing, and good personal hygiene are essential to controlling oily hair and scalp.

Hair loss Under normal circumstances, some hair is lost every day. Normal daily hair loss is the natural result of the three phases of the hair's growth cycle. Abnormal hair loss is called **alopecia.** Head massage must not be provided in the case of abnormal hair loss. Massage is beneficial to perform when healthy hair begins to grow back following abnormal hair loss, with GP consent. Care must be taken to avoid irritating the scalp when massaging a client with low hair density as the scalp will have less protection and may easily become sensitised.

Dandruff (Pityriasis) A scalp condition characterised by the excessive production and accumulation of skin cells and is thought to be caused by a fungus. Instead of the normal shedding of tiny individual skin cells, one at a time, dandruff results from the removal of an accumulation of large visible clumps of cells. Some individuals are more susceptible to the irritating effects of dandruff and factors such as stress, age, hormones and poor hygiene can cause dandruff symptoms to worsen. Dandruff is not contagious and may be treated when controlled by a specialist shampoo. Sometimes when not treated, scales may build up and the scalp may be itchy and irritated which should not be treated and referred to a GP.

Psoriasis A non-contagious skin condition involving abnormal cell growth (see page 50). Psoriasis can appear on the scalp. Do not treat severe psoriasis where the skin is broken as bacterial infection could occur. If there are scales present avoid these areas as bleeding can occur if these are removed whilst massaging. Only ever treat mild psoriasis where there is no risk of harm to the client or contact with tissue fluid.

Seborrheic warts Raised, pigmented rough patches of skin (see page 45). These are non-contagious and may occur on the scalp of elderly clients. Avoid massaging over the area but if unsure refer the client to their GP before treatment.

Fungal infections (tinea capitis) A fungal disease, for more information see page 44. It is characterized by itching, scales, and, sometimes, painful circular lesions. Several such patches may be present at one time. The hair can also become brittle, often breaks off, leaving only a stump, or may be shed. All forms of tinea are contagious and can be easily transmitted from one person to another. Infected skin scales or hairs that contain the fungi are known to spread the disease. A client with this condition should be referred to their GP for medical treatment.

Parasitic infestations

- **Scabies** or itch mites (sarcoptes scabiei) are highly infectious (see pages 42–43). A client with this condition should be referred to their GP for medical treatment.
- **Pediculosis capitis** A condition in which small lice parasites infest scalp hair and is highly infectious (see page 93). A client with this condition should be referred to their GP for medical treatment.

Staphylococci infections Staphylococci are harmful bacteria that can infect the skin of the scalp, for further information see page 91. The two most common types of staphylococci infections are furuncles and carbuncles (see page 41). A client with either condition must be referred to their GP for medical treatment.

Selecting massage oils

Suitable massage oils If using oils, organic oils are the most suitable oils when massaging the scalp. High in polyunsaturated fats, these fats are very soft and liquid at room temperature. They have healing benefits from their fatty acid, vitamin and nutrient content. They absorb easily through the skin, and have both an internal and external effect. Approximately 2–5 ml is required for the scalp massage, this will, of course, vary according to the length of the client's hair and condition of the scalp. The oil is applied at body temperature or 1–2 degrees above. The choice of oil depends on its texture, smell and specific properties. Popular oils are sesame, mustard, almond, olive and coconut.

HEALTH & SAFETY

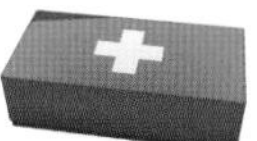

Avoid excessive use of oil which would hinder effective treatment application and possibly could enter the eyes.

ALWAYS REMEMBER

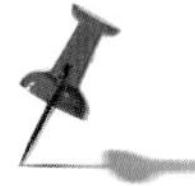

Pre-blended oils

The smell of the essential oil is picked up when inhaled by the olfactory nerve, a nerve high inside the nose and responsible for the sense of smell. The odour molecules, simple chemical units from the essential oils, dissolve in the nasal mucus. The receptor cells cause a nerve impulse to the olfactory nerves. The smell can influence the behaviour of the person causing stimulation or relaxation.

Massage oils

Name	Plant	Use
Sesame oil		This oil is high in minerals which nourish the skin and hair. Sesame oil has a high lecithin content (a fat-like substance) thought to relieve swelling and muscular pains. Sesame oil may irritate sensitive skin and scalps.
Mustard oil		A strong-smelling oil which creates an intense heating, invigorating action. Popular for use in winter due to its warming action. The increase in body heat relieves pain, swellings and relaxes stiff muscles. The skins' pores open and a cleansing action is created. Not suitable on sensitive skin and scalps as it may cause irritation.
Almond oil		A light-textured oil, it is warm pressed and good to moisturise dry skin and hair as it is high in unsaturated fatty acids (essential fats derived from food), protein and vitamins A, B, D and E.
Olive oil		Cold pressed from olives and has an emollient, healing and nourishing effect. It has a thick consistency high in unsaturated fatty acids, suitable for excessively dry hair and skin. It also creates a heating action which helps to relieve pain, swellings and relax stiff muscles.
Coconut oil		A medium-to-light oil with skin and hair conditioning and emollient properties; particularly suitable for dry, brittle, chemically-treated hair. Popular for use in summer as it induces a cooling action on the scalp.

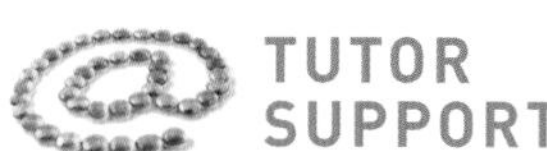

Activity 4: Consultation card for head massage treatment

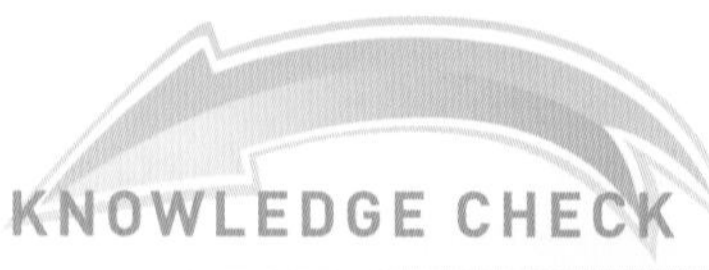

When preparing the treatment plan, how is the massage oil selected for the client?

Need more time... refer to page 551 to help you.

Pre-blended oils can also be used which are essential oils, aromatic substances which can be hazardous if applied to the skin. They are added to a vegetable oil called a carrier oil. Enabling the oils to penetrate into the skin in order to achieve different therapeutic effects dependant upon the oils chosen.

Benefits of head massage

There are many general benefits of head massage that address the symptoms of everyday working, including:

- headaches caused by stress and tension
- aches and pains caused by poor posture in the neck and shoulder area, i.e. long periods working on a computer
- poor sleeping problems are improved

Head massage treatment should be adapted in application to meet the client's needs and physiological and psychological obtained at the consultation.

Once the consultation is complete, the beauty therapist should ensure that all details are recorded accurately and that the client has signed her record card. This enables continuity of service and up-to-date tracking of the treatments received. An example of a typical record card is provided in this chapter.

ALWAYS REMEMBER

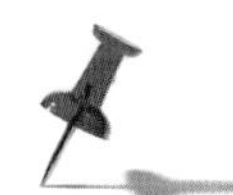

Accurately record your client's answers to necessary questions to be asked at consultation on the record card. This is important for future reference for any reason including legal requirements.

HEALTH & SAFETY

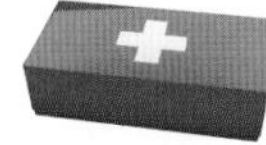

If a contra-action occurs during the service discontinue and provide appropriate action and advice.

KNOWLEDGE CHECK

Name three benefits to the skin that occur as a result of a head massage treatment.

Need more time... refer to page 552 to help you.

Contra-actions

A contra-action is an unwanted reaction to Indian head massage service which may occur during or following the service. Contra-actions to the service should be discussed at the consultation so the client would recognise symptoms if experienced.

Contra-actions occur mainly as a result of the increased circulation of waste products following the massage. Monitor the contra-action to confirm client suitability for further service.

These might include:

- nausea or headache caused by increased circulation of waste products transported in the lymphatic system.
- fainting caused by dilation of the blood capillaries, altering blood pressure levels
- tiredness
- skin reactions, such as an allergy to the massage oil
- aching muscles

If the client suffers any contra-action, you must assist the client before letting them leave the salon:

- Ensure the client can breathe properly and that the room is well ventilated.
- Offer the client a glass of water
- Remove product and apply a cold compress if a skin reaction occurs.
- Advise the client to seek medical advice if the symptoms persist.

Allow time and invite the client to ask any questions before service commences. Be honest and concise in your answers. Confirm the objectives of the service.

HEALTH & SAFETY

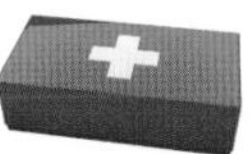

Pregnancy

It is best not to treat a client in the early stages of pregnancy, as the side-effects may include feelings of nausea. This is a common symptom in the early stages of pregnancy and could cause a client to feel worse.

> While performing Indian head massage and all services it is very important to remember the medical contra-indications and the health and safety aspects at all times.
>
> Make sure you are aware of your spa or salon's operating procedures and follow them with every service to continually provide safe services to a high standard.
>
> **Zoe Crowley**

Preparation of the client

Take the client through to the service area. Preparation will depend upon how the service is being positioned for the treatment. The client will need to remove any outdoor clothing such as a coat or jacket. Footwear may be removed and the feet placed flat on the floor.

Record card for head massage

Date | Beauty therapist name

Client name | Date of birth (Identifying client age group.)

Homé address | Postcode

Email address | Landline phone number | Mobile phone number

Name of doctor | Doctor's address and phone number

Related medical history (Conditions that may restrict or prohibit service application.)

Are you taking any medication? (i.e. if taking medication to control blood pressure, head massage will alter blood pressure temporarily.)

CONTRA-INDICATIONS REQUIRING MEDICAL REFERRAL
(Preventing Indian head massage service application.)

- ☐ bacterial infection, e.g. impetigo
- ☐ viral infection, e.g. herpes simplex
- ☐ fungal infection, e.g. tinea unguium
- ☐ skin disorders, i.e. sebaceous cyst, eczema, acne vulgaris
- ☐ skin disease
- ☐ hair and scalp disorders
- ☐ high or low blood pressure
- ☐ recent head and neck injury
- ☐ severe bruising
- ☐ severe cuts and abrasions
- ☐ hair disorders
- ☐ medical conditions
- ☐ diabetes
- ☐ recent scar tissue
- ☐ dysfunction of the nervous system
- ☐ epilepsy
- ☐ during chemotherapy and radio therapy

SERVICE AREAS

- ☐ scalp
- ☐ head
- ☐ neck

MASSAGE TECHNIQUE

- ☐ effleurage
- ☐ petrissage
- ☐ tapotement
- ☐ frictions
- ☐ vibrations

MASSAGE MEDIUM (IF USED)

- ☐ organic oil – type__________

CONTRA-INDICATIONS THAT RESTRICT SERVICE
(Service may require adaptation.)

- ☐ cuts and abrasions
- ☐ bruising and swelling
- ☐ recent injuries to the service area
- ☐ medication
- ☐ mild eczema/psoriasis
- ☐ recent scar tissue (avoid area)
- ☐ undiagnosed lumps, bumps, swellings
- ☐ migraine
- ☐ product allergies

LIFESTYLE

- ☐ occupation ____________
- ☐ family situation ____________
- ☐ dietary and fluid intake (including allergies) ____________
- ☐ hobbies, interests, means of relaxation ____________
- ☐ exercise habits ____________
- ☐ smoking habits ____________
- ☐ sleep patterns ____________

PHYSICAL CHARACTERISTICS

- ☐ posture
- ☐ hair condition
- ☐ health
- ☐ scalp condition
- ☐ muscle tone
- ☐ age
- ☐ skin condition

OBJECTIVES OF SERVICE

- ☐ relaxation
- ☐ stimulating and uplifting
- ☐ health and well-being
- ☐ improvement of hair and scalp condition

PRODUCTS, TOOLS AND EQUIPMENT

- ☐ towels
- ☐ comb
- ☐ spatulas
- ☐ protective covering
- ☐ consumables
- ☐ hair clip
- ☐ massage chair/couch

Beauty therapist signature (for reference)

Client signature (confirmation of details)

SERVICE ADVICE

Head massage service – *this service will take approximately 10–15 minutes*

SERVICE PLAN

Record relevant details of your service and advice provided for future reference. Ensure the client's records are up-to-date, accurate and fully completed following service. Non-compliance may invalidate insurance.

DURING

- explain choice of massage medium and its benefits
- explain the service procedure at each stage of the massage to meet the service needs
- explain how the massage products should be applied and removed for home use
- note any adverse reaction, if any occur, and action taken

AFTER

- record the areas treated
- record any modification to service application that has occurred
- record what products have been used in the service as appropriate
- provide postural advice
- provide hair and scalp advice
- provide advice to follow immediately following service, to include suitable rest period following service, general advice regarding food and drink intake, avoidance of stimulants
- recommended time intervals between services
- discuss the benefits of continuous services
- record the effectiveness of service
- record any samples provided (review their success at the next appointment)

RETAIL OPPORTUNITIES

- provide guidance on progression of the service plan for future appointments
- advice regarding products that would be suitable for home use and how to gain maximum benefit from their use to care for the skin and continue the service benefits
- recommendations for further services including heat services and body massage services
- advice of further products or services that you have recommended that the client may or may not have received before.
- note any purchase made by the client

EVALUATION

- record comments on the client's satisfaction with the service
- record if the service objectives were achieved, e.g. relaxation, if not, explore the reasons why not
- record how you will progress the service to maintain and advance the service results in the future

HEALTH AND SAFETY

- advise on avoidance of activities that may cause a contra-action, including strenuous exercises and stimulants such as caffeine and alcohol
- advise on appropriate necessary action to be taken in the event of an unwanted reaction (an allergy to the oil used, headaches, and aching muscles.

SERVICE MODIFICATION

Examples of massage service modification includes:

- altering the pressure or choice of manipulations during massage to suit the client's skin and muscle tone
- adapting the massage to achieve an effect of relaxation, stimulation
- altering the choice of massage medium to treat the skin/hair condition

TOP TIP

Hair products

If the client has styling/setting products on the hair, brush through as part of client preparation to ensure continuity of the service application and avoid client discomfort.

Clients can generally receive head massage through their outdoor clothing, but bulky clothing which may restrict service application should be removed. Shirt or blouse collars should be loosened to allow access to the neck region. If oil is to be used for the massage, upper clothing should be removed and the client provided with a towel. Any jewellery in the area of massage application should be removed – this includes earrings, necklaces, bracelets and watches. Other accessories such as glasses should also be removed. False hairpieces will also need to be removed before service. If you are using screens, ensure that these are fully closed to maintain the client's privacy. This will enable the client to feel more comfortable and relaxed – essential if they are to gain service benefit. Seat the client on a low-backed massage chair or alternatively they can be positioned lying on a treatment couch. If the client is in a wheelchair it may be possible to treat them while sitting in their chair, which means minimum disturbance to the client. Ensure the client is seated comfortably; correct positioning will optimise the massage treatment effects. If the client is lying down for the head massage prepare the client as if receiving a facial.

TOP TIP

Tension

Tension accumulates in the head, neck and shoulders. Through massage, pressure in these areas will be released.

Before the head massage is applied, the face may be cleansed to remove facial make-up using suitable facial products for their skin type using your regular cleansing routine. If the head massage follows a facial the skin will already have been cleansed.

After preparing the client, and before touching the skin, wash your hands again.

If your client is having a service using oils you will need to select and warm a suitable oil to use.

Place a towel over their shoulders if applying a massage oil medium.

TOP TIP

Relaxation practices

Audio tapes have been manufactured for the purpose of relaxation and these make an excellent accompaniment to create a calm environment in the service room.

Aromatherapy burners can be used to create a specific atmosphere in the service room. Essential oils which create different therapeutic effects when inhaled can be burnt.

Crystals may be placed in the work area.

Selected for their therapeutic properties, crystals mined for thousands of years have their own energy and are used to help balance the body's energy channels.

Massage position or stance

When performing the head massage it is important to position yourself correctly. Massage may be performed with the client seated or lying on the couch. This will prevent pain and fatigue while working. Working positions are *walk standing* and *stride standing*. If performing the head massage with the client seated it is important to consider your working position or stance.

KNOWLEDGE CHECK

To perform an effective consultation you need the client to feel confident about providing you with positive, honest answers to your questions.

You should have good:

a. communication skills

b. questioning techniques

c. listening skills

d. answering techniques

Give examples of what you understand by good skills and techniques for each of the above.

Need more time... refer to pages 135–137 to help you.

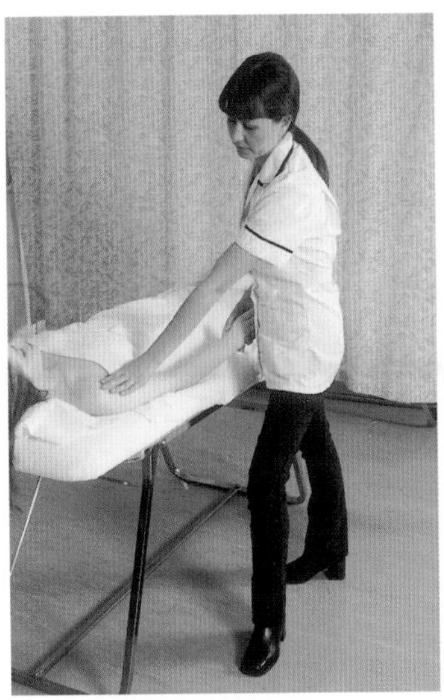

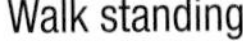
Walk standing

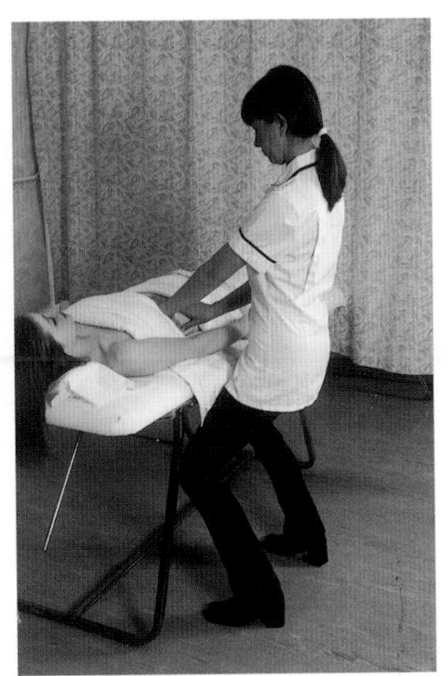

Stride standing

KNOWLEDGE CHECK

Why is the positioning of the client an important consideration when performing head massage treatment?

Need more time... refer to page 556 help you.

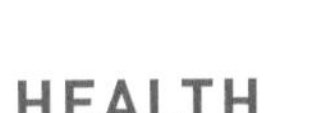

HEALTH & SAFETY

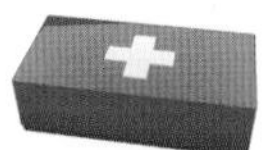

Failure to adopt the correct stance will result in the beauty therapist not being able to work a full day and eventually serious neck or back injury could occur.

Walk standing The beauty therapist stands with one foot in front of the other. This enables the beauty therapist to work longitudinally (along the length) of the body.

Stride standing The beauty therapist works transversely (across) the body. This is the most common position when performing Indian head massage services.

If performing the massage whilst the client is positioned on the treatment couch ensure good sitting posture, see page 100.

Examples of a head massage routine are provided with clients in both lying and sitting positions.

Step-by-step: Head massage with client sitting

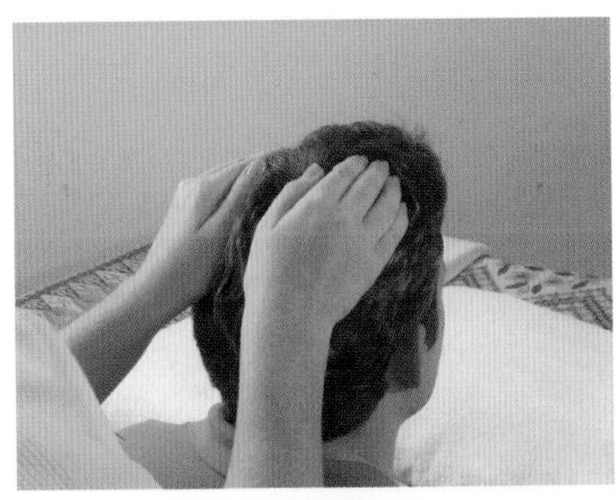

1 With both feet placed firmly on the floor, place the hands on the client's shoulders. Ask the client to close his eyes and relax.

2 Place your hands on the client's scalp on the crown area.

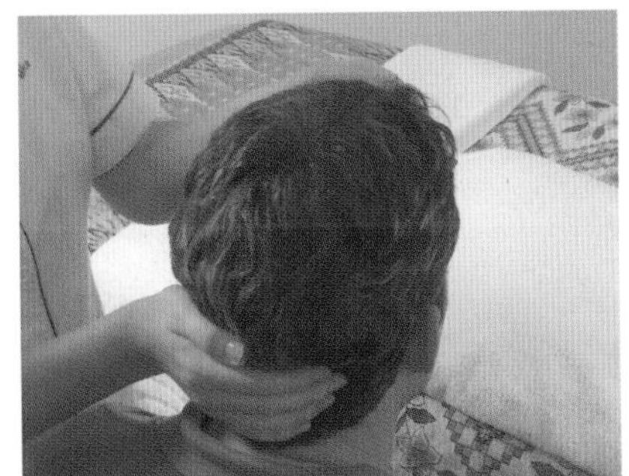

3 Then place the hands, one on the forehead and one on the occiput (anatomical term for the back part of the head), hold this position for 2 minutes.

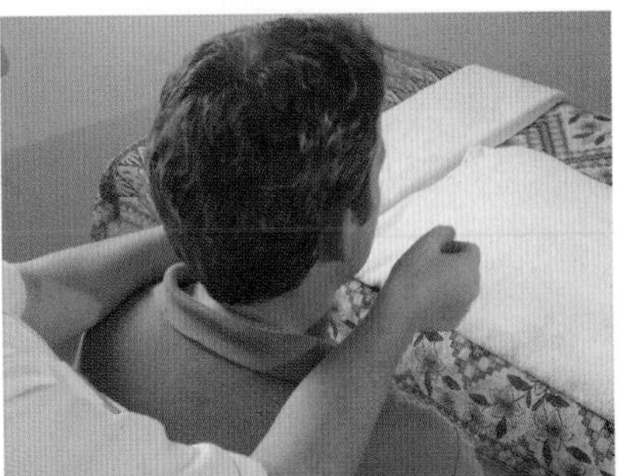

4 Rest your forearms on the client's shoulders – ask the client to slowly breathe in and then slowly breathe out. This will cause the client to relax and feel calmer. As the client breathes out apply gentle pressure with your forearms onto the client's shoulders. If oil is to be used when performing the scalp massage this is applied now, selected according to the treatment effect required. The hair is gently parted and oil is applied to the partings. Massage the oil in using the fingers with a rotary movement. Ideally apply the oil to a position between the hair line and the crown of the head.

HEALTH & SAFETY

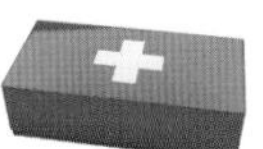

Posture

It is important to ensure that the client and beauty therapist are correctly positioned when performing the head massage. This will prevent strain and fatigue to the beauty therapist. Failure to maintain good posture may lead to serious back injury.

If the client is uncomfortable, they will be unable to relax and will not gain maximum benefit from the service. Check on client comfort during service application.

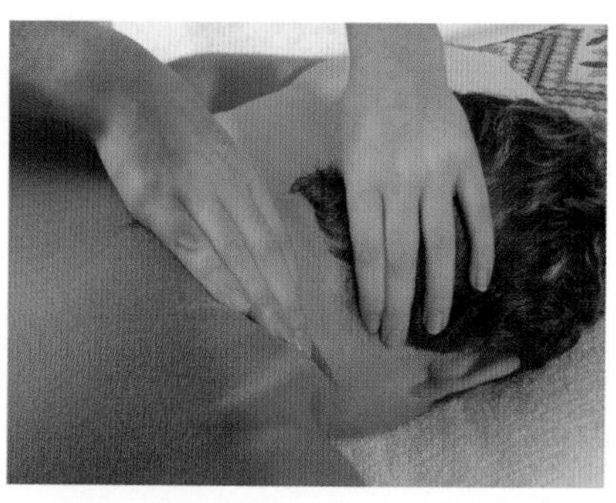

5 Pick up the muscle and skin at the back of the neck. Gently lift the tissue with each hand alternately.

6 Apply frictions under the occiput. Using both thumbs apply gentle pressure in a circular movement.

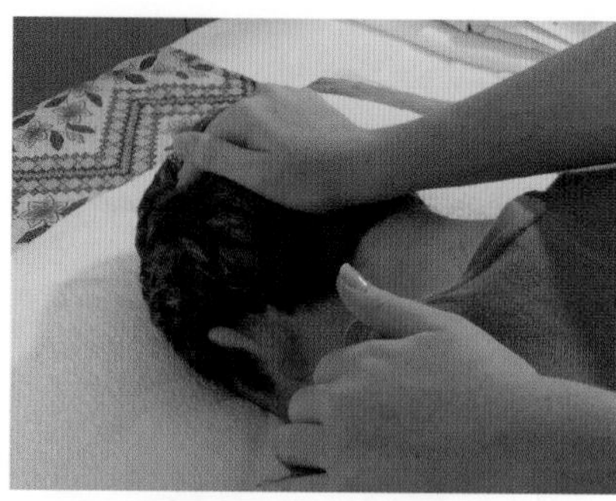

7 Apply petrissage under the occiput. Using the heel of one hand, apply a gentle circular pressure.

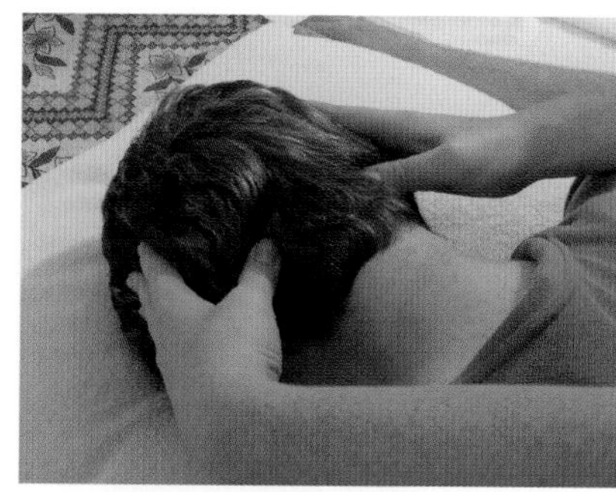

8 Apply frictions with both thumbs in a triangular movement under the occiput.

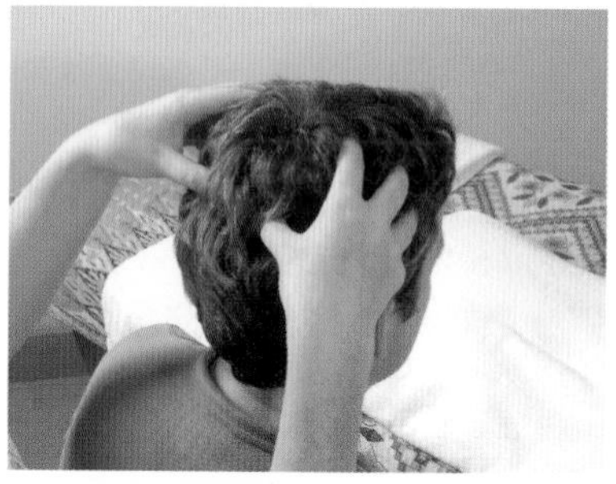

9 Apply effleurage strokes to the scalp. Place each hand alternately on the hair line and stroke hand upwards, covering the whole scalp.

10 Apply frictions to the scalp (shown) – using the pads of the fingers to apply small circular movements.

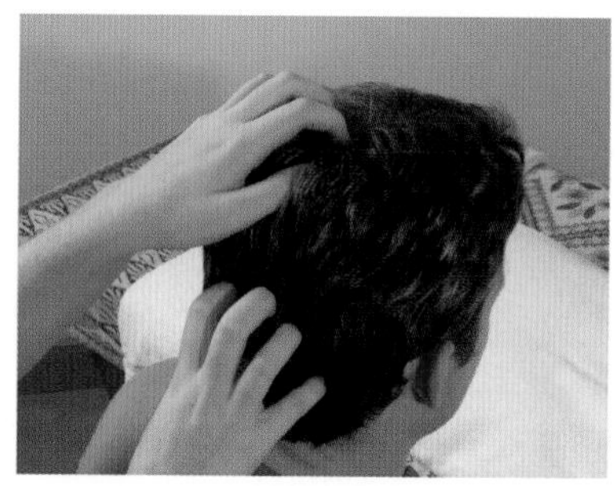

11 Apply finger stroking, place the fingertips on the hairline and draw them in a combing action through the hair.

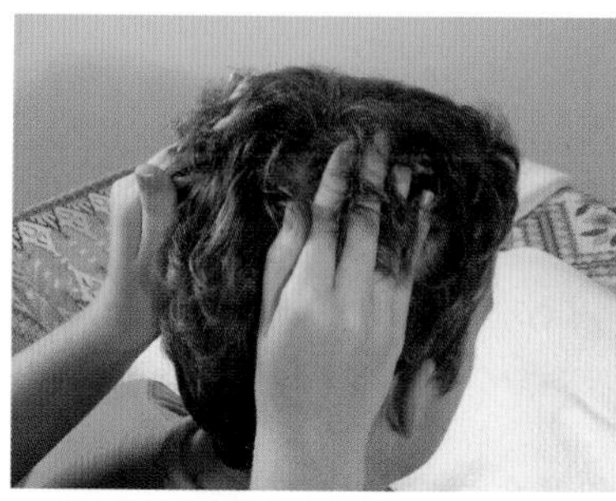

12 Apply vibrations: gently grasp the hair and pull in a vibrating manner (shown).

13 Apply light hacking using both hands to cover both sides of the head.

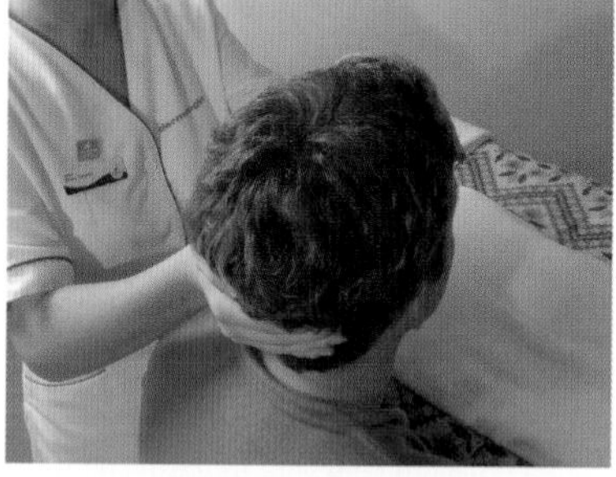

14 Using flat hands, place one hand on the forehead and the other over the occipital bone and gently lift the head. Move the hands, place one hand over the corner of the forehead the other over the corner of the back of the skull and lift. Repeat on remaining corners of the head.

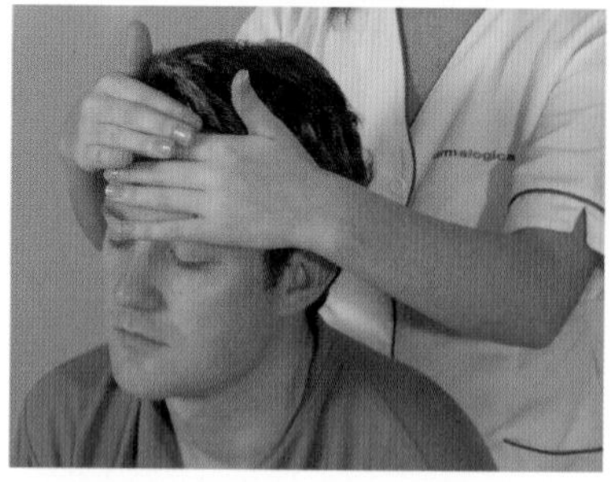

15 Stroke over the forehead using alternate hands.

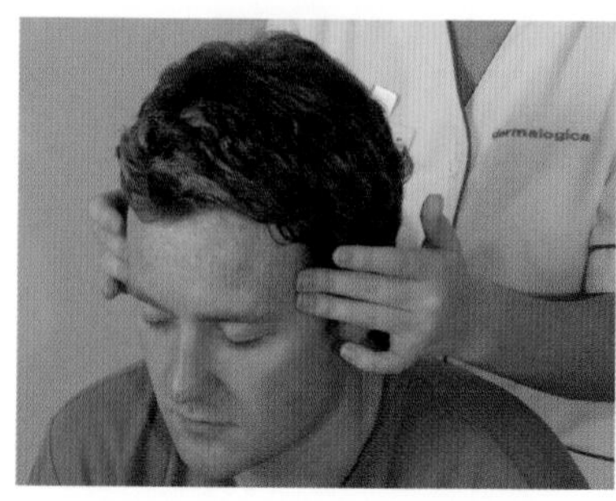

16 Apply circular pressure to the temples simultaneously using the fingertips.

17 Finally, apply effleurage to the scalp. Wash your hands. Remove excess oil if used using damp warm towelling mitts or sponges and warm water.

Step-by-step: Head massage with client lying down

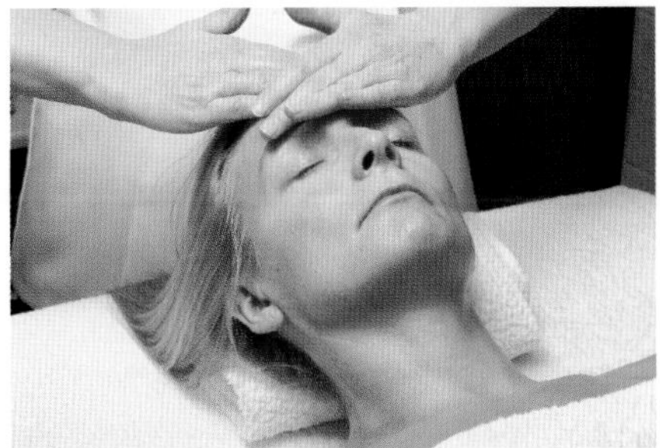

1 Apply effleurage strokes to the scalp. Place each hand alternately on the hair line and stroke hand downwards, covering the whole scalp.

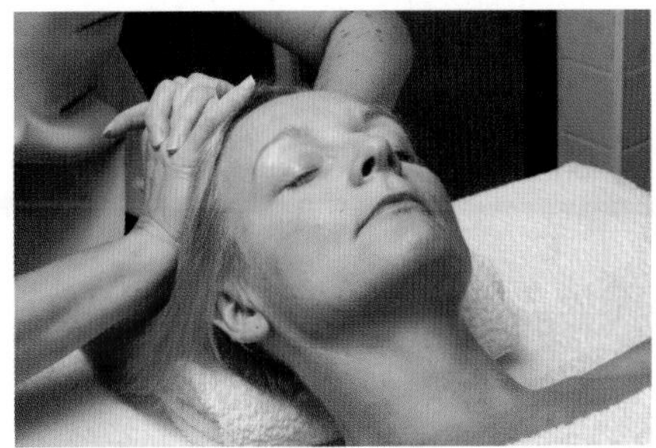

2 Interlock fingers and place joined hands above the forehead. Using the heel of the hands simultaneously perform circular, petrissage movements, moving the hands to cover the scalp.

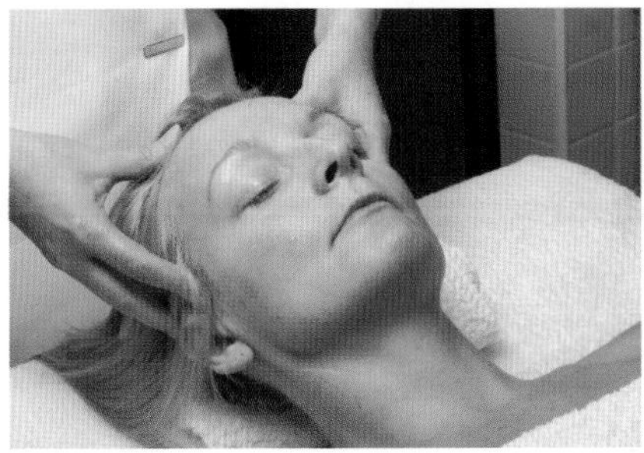

3 Place the thumbs on the scalp at the hairline and gently apply frictions. This helps to relieve stress and tension as the pressure points are on the meridians of energy pathways that connect the body. This in turn stimulates the nerve pathways, frees blockages on the meridian lines of the body and helps to balance the body.

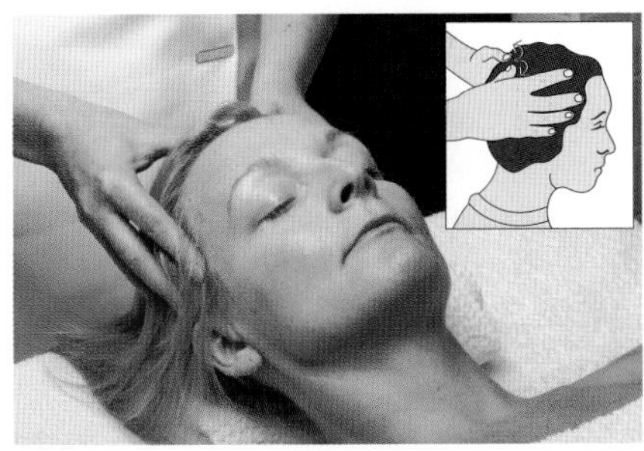

4 Place one thumb above the other. Each thumb alternately applies pressure in a 'C' shape moving from the hairline towards the crown area.

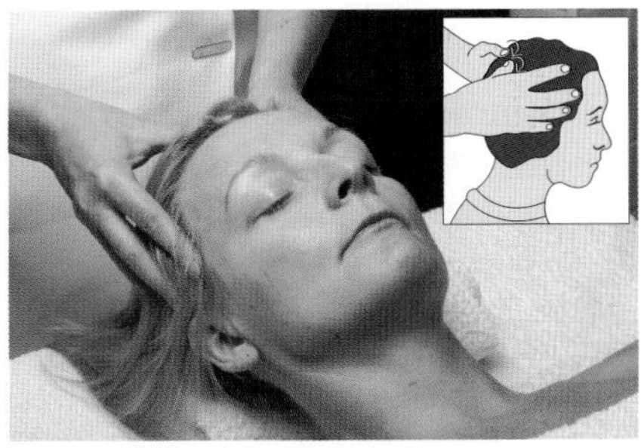

5 Position both thumbs at the crown area. Rotate both thumbs simultaneously in a clockwise direction, increasing pressure with each rotation: check pressure with client for comfort. Follow by rotating thumbs anti-clockwise, reducing pressure with each rotation.

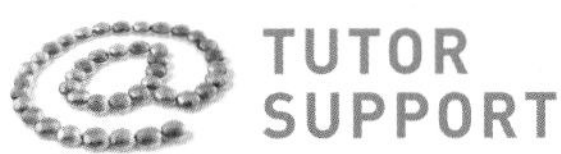

Activity 8: Crossword

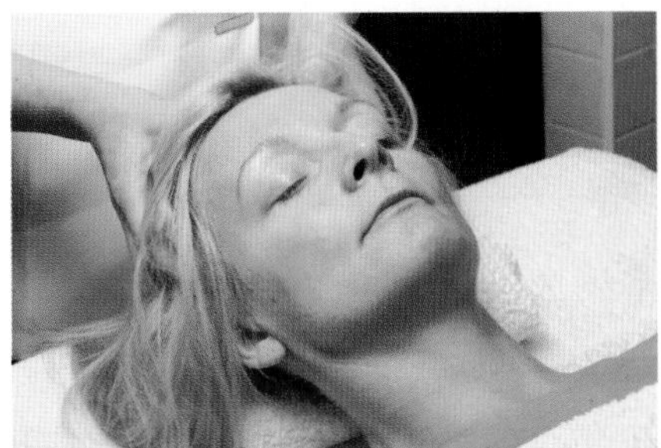

6 Apply petrissage movement over the scalp as if shampooing the scalp, using the fingertip pads to move the scalp gently.

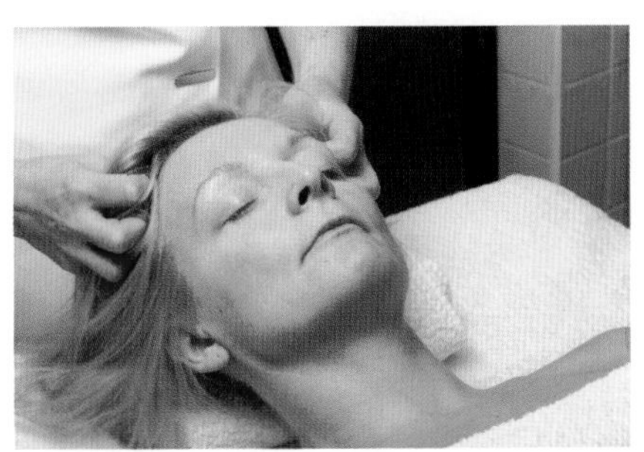

7 Place the knuckles of each hand against the scalp and apply gentle pressure, rotating the knuckles of each finger to cover the scalp.

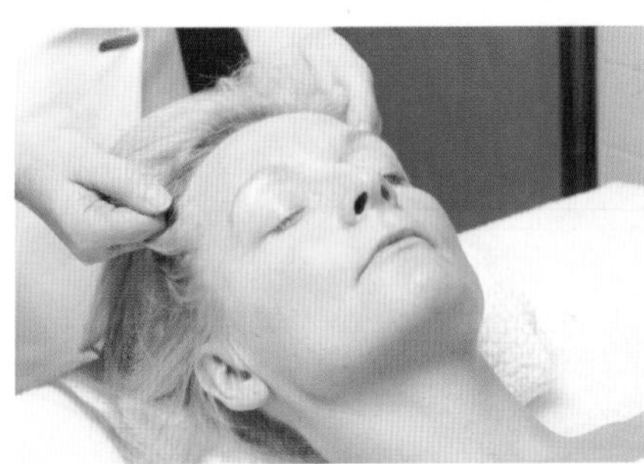

8 Grasp sections of hair between the fingers of each hand and gently pull the hair at the roots.

BEST PRACTICE 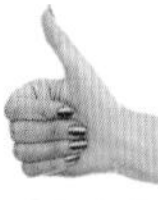

Checking body language for effectiveness

The client posture should become more relaxed during application of the service. The shoulders should drop and breathing should become deeper.

Encourage the client to relax if their shoulders appear stiff.

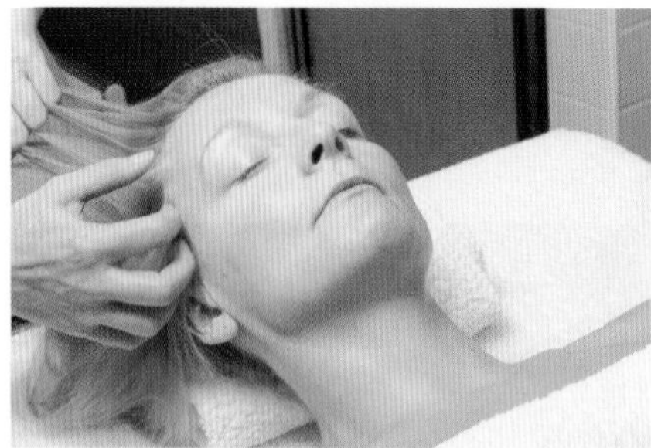

9 Alternating the fingers of each hand, use the fingers to slowly comb through the hair from the scalp to the end of the hair. Cover the scalp.

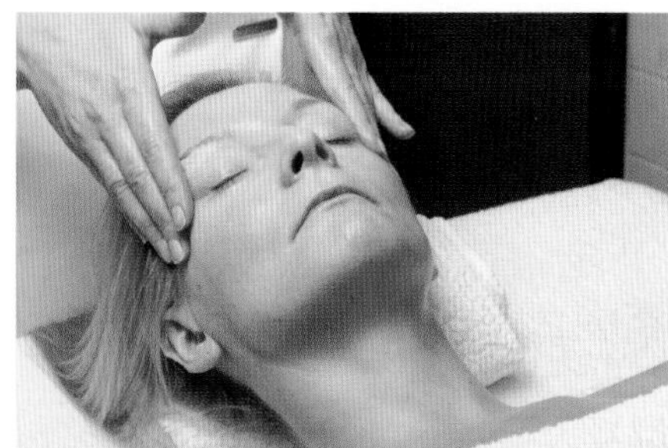

10 To complete the massage apply effleurage strokes to the scalp. Place each hand alternately on the hair line and stroke hand upwards, covering the whole scalp. Wash your hands following scalp massage.

11 Apply gentle pressure at the temples to indicate to the client that the massage routine is completed.

KNOWLEDGE CHECK

How should the massage medium be stored and why?

Need more time... refer to page 546 to help you.

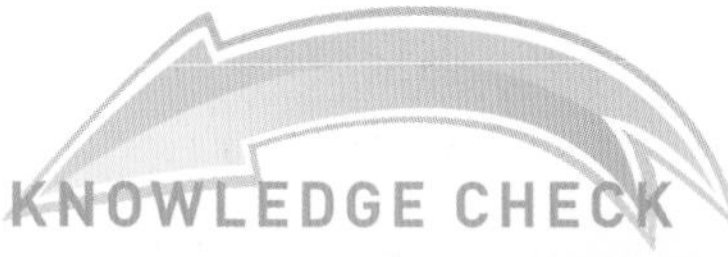

KNOWLEDGE CHECK

How should the client be advised to breathe to induce relaxation?

Need more time... refer to page 557 to help you.

TOP TIP

If the client falls asleep during the massage a benefit of relaxation technique. Awaken them in to consciousness by gently speaking to them telling them that their treatment has completed.

Adapting the massage

Relaxing massage: avoid stimulating movements and incorporate more effleurage, light petrissage movements. Pressure should be firm and rhythm slower. Concentrate massage application on areas of tension. Remember these areas may feel uncomfortable initially until the muscle warms and relaxation is induced.

Tight or contracted muscles: avoid excessive use of percussion movements. Slow, rhythmical movements should be used to stretch the muscles. Again, concentrate massage application on these areas and recommend the client has a regular massage service to gain cumulative benefits.

Slack muscles: stimulating percussion massage movements should be used to help to tone and firm the area being treated.

Massage for excess weight: incorporate stimulating movements such as hacking over fatty areas, to help mobilize adipose (fatty) tissue.

Massage for males: muscle bulk tends to be larger and firmer. The skin is thicker and generally there is less fatty tissue. The massage usually needs to be firmer.

Before the client gets up, encourage them to rest for a few minutes to allow the blood circulation to return to normal. Provide water to for hydration and to refresh the client. A relaxation massage can leave the client feeling light-headed. Sudden movement may result in a light-headed feeling as the brain is temporarily starved of blood; they may even faint. You may have a relaxation room where the client could go following service. You can also assist the client as they stand.

As the client's circulation returns to normal, the blood vessels will constrict.

BEST PRACTICE 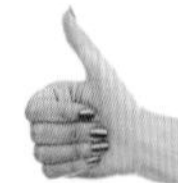

Drink and rest

Offer the client a glass of water following the service to rehydrate and allow a suitable rest period to avoid feelings of dizziness caused by changes to blood pressure.

ALWAYS REMEMBER

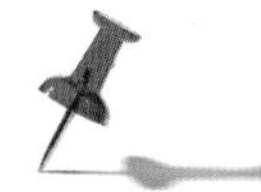

Faults during massage

- Incorrect pressure applied. If it is too light or too heavy the client will not feel the benefits.
- Avoid placing excessive pressure on top of the client's head: this can cause discomfort to the head and neck.
- Inconsistent massage movements will not relax the client and the massage will not flow.
- Ensure the client is appropriately positioned. This prevents discomfort to yourself and the client.

While resting, use the time to discuss with the client suitable aftercare and home care to complement the massage. The client will probably feel extremely relaxed at this point. It is important they do not leave the salon until they feel fully awakened.

If the massage was for relaxation, you might give advice on relaxing bath products and massage techniques that could be used at home. Recommend the client increases their water intake to help detoxification and encourage good eating habits.

Remind the client about the benefits of deep breathing. Encourage them to practise breathing exercises at home, and at any time of anxiety.

Provide hair and scalp care advice, including the avoidance of excessive chemical hair services, the importance of hair protection when exposed to UV, and the application of specialized hair/scalp service products. If the service was for alopecia to stimulate new hair growth, clients should massage their scalp gently at home between services.

For the following 24 hours avoid:

- stimulants such as caffeine or alcohol
- heavy or highly spiced meals
- strenuous exercise

For several hours:

- avoid shampooing the hair, especially if oils have been used to maximize service effects. To remove the oil advise the client to apply shampoo directly to the oil before wetting the hair, massage the shampoo into the hair and rinse, this will break down the oil.

Warn the client of post-service reactions including:

- emotional anxiety
- headaches
- aching muscles

These reactions will normally subside within 24 hours. Remind the client what action to take in the event of a contra-action previously discussed at the consultation.

Ask the client how they feel to establish if the service has achieved the outcome agreed at consultation. Explain the benefits of regular service to achieve maximum benefit.

You should complete the client's record card fully so that continuation of the service can be tracked and any adverse reactions noted for future reference.

KNOWLEDGE CHECK

How can the massage be adapted to achieve different effects?

Need more time... refer to page 560 to help you.

ACTIVITY

As part of the client's home-care programme, simple massage techniques could be taught.

Think of three simple self-massage techniques that the client could use at home.

These may also be applied to relax the face during the day if working in an office, looking at the computer screen for long periods.

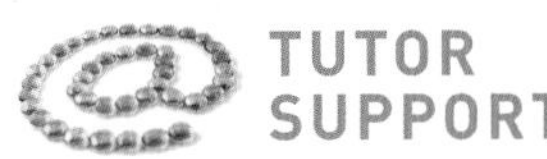

TUTOR SUPPORT

Activity 9: End Test

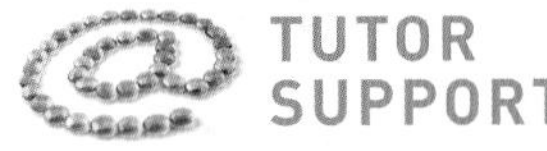

TUTOR SUPPORT

Activity 10: Re-cap, Revision and Evaluation (RRE sheet)

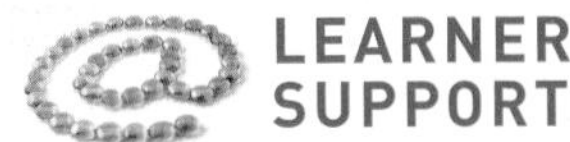

LEARNER SUPPORT

Multiple choice quiz: Indian head massage and massage using pre- blended oils

KNOWLEDGE CHECK

After the massage treatment the client should be given advice to follow to ensure that they gain maximum benefit from the treatment. Discuss the advice to be given.

Need more time... refer to pages 560–561 to help you.

GLOSSARY OF KEY WORDS

Ayurveda (art of life) a sacred Hindu text written around 1800BC. In Ayurveda life consists of body, mind and spirit – each person is different. By restoring balance and harmony of the body, mind and spirit, the health of the individual improves.

Effleurage a massage technique which has a sedating and relaxing effect; applied with the whole palm, it can be applied superficially or deeply.

Frictions a massage technique which causes the skin and superficial structure to move together over the underlying structures. These movements are performed with either the fingers or the thumbs and concentrated in a particular area, applied with regulated pressure.

Oils oils selected to use with the head massage and applied to the scalp. Usually organic they are high in polyunsaturated fats which have healing benefits from their fatty acid, vitamin and nutrient content. They absorb easily through the skin, and can have an external and internal effect.

Petrissage massage technique which apply intermittent pressure to the tissues of the skin, lifting them from the underlying structures. Petrissage improves muscle tone by the compression and relaxation of the muscle fibres.

Tapotement also known as percussion, massage movements performed in a brisk, stimulating manner to increase blood supply and improve tone of the skin and muscles. Movements include clapping and tapping.

Vibrations a vibration massage technique which involves rhythmically drumming the skin and underlying tissues to create a vibrational effect.

ASSESSMENT OF KNOWLEDGE AND UNDERSTANDING

You have now learnt about the knowledge and skills for applying head massage treatment for the beauty therapy workplace. To test your level of knowledge, answer the following short questions. These will prepare you for your summative (final) assessment.

1. Which of the following massage oils is unsuitable for sensitive skin and scalps?
   a. olive oil
   b. almond oil
   c. mustard oil
   d. coconut oil
2. Which of the following is a temporary contra-indication to head massage?
   a. heart condition
   b. scalp disorder
   c. diabetes
   d. dysfunction of the nervous system
3. Which massage oil is particularly suitable for chemically treated hair?
   a. coconut oil
   b. sesame oil
   c. almond oil
   d. olive oil
4. Does all hair on a persons head have the same texture?
5. Which of the following is not a cause of dry hair and scalp?
   a. winter weather
   b. hot, dry climate
   c. underactive sebaceous glands
   d. overactive sebaceous glands
6. Match the following scalp disorders with its definition:

1. pityriasis	a) medical term for ringworm
2. tinea	b) bacterial infection of numerous hair follicles
3. scabies	c) medical term for dandruff
4. pediculosis capitis	d) bacterial infection, with red, painful pustular lumps around the hair follicle
5. furnucle	e) the infestation of the hair and scalp with head lice
6. carbuncle	f) caused by a parasite called a 'mite'

7. Which muscle of the neck flexes, lowers and rotates the head?

8. Match the following bones of the cranium with its correct description:
   1. parietal a) forms the forehead
   2. occipital b) lower back of the cranium
   3. frontal c) form the sides of the cranium
   4. temporal d) form the sides and crown of the cranium

9. What is the term for light, continuous stroking massage movement applied with the fingers or the palms in a slow rhythmic manner?
   a. petrissage
   b. effleurage
   c. friction
   d. tapotement

10. Which layer of the skin contains numerous blood vessels, lymph vessels, nerves, sweat and oil glands and hair follicles?
   a. subcutaneous
   b. dermis
   c. adipose
   d. epidermis

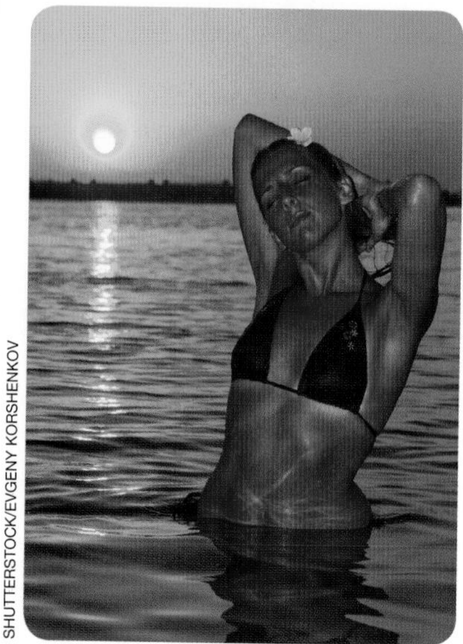

SHUTTERSTOCK/EVGENY KORSHENKOV

18 Skin Tanning

Learning Objectives

This chapter covers **VRQ Unit Apply skin tanning techniques.**

This unit is all about how to provide skin tanning treatments using self-tanning products. Application can be modified to achieve the client's treatment objectives identified at consultation. Relevant health safety and hygiene practice must be effectively implemented throughout the service.

The communication of pre and post tanning information and advice is essential to ensure the effectiveness of the treatment and client satisfaction with the result.

There are **two** learning outcomes for this unit which you must achieve:

1 Be able to prepare for self-tanning techniques

2 Be able to provide self-tanning techniques

From the range statement, you must show you can:

- use **consultation techniques** to identify the treatment objectives
- carry out client **preparation** and adapt treatment to suit different **factors,** including client's skin type and condition
- use all listed **products, tools and equipment** as appropriate
- ensure the **environmental conditions** are suitable
- demonstrate knowledge of the **benefits and effects** of tanning techniques and the product **key ingredients**

(continued on the next page)

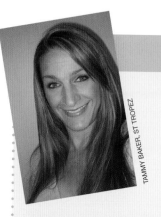

TAMMY BAKER, ST TROPEZ

ROLE MODEL

Tammy Baker

Education and Events Manager for St Tropez

" I have been involved in the beauty, hair and wellness industry for over 17 years. During this time I also competed in fitness competitions, which built the base for my career within the television industry and my being selected to participate as 'Fox' in the hit TV series 'Gladiators'. I continued studies in personal training, sports nutrition/psychology and personally trained pop star Robbie Williams, attending to his training, massage and nutritional needs. I co-published and edited a health and wellness-based publication which gave me a platform to educate the masses in related topics for total self improvement and wellness for men and women.

My role as Education and Events Manager includes the continuous improvement of teaching material, techniques and development of the Education team. I organize, attend and present business seminars, exhibitions and events related to promotion and education in tanning. I regularly train and update internal staff and deliver training to international accounts and press/TV and support the marketing department in implementing brand communication and education of new products.

I have developed my knowledge through several industry-related career choices and I have enjoyed the diversity of my career to date which includes make-up, fitness and nutrition, sales/retail and salon management through to teaching/training and development.

- complete a consultation and skin inspection to identify any **contra-indications**
- follow all **health and safety working practices** including skin sensitivity patch testing
- **communicate and behave** in an appropriate and professional manner
- identify **contra-actions** and provide relevant **aftercare advice**
- use different **methods of evaluating** the results of the treatment including observation, written and verbal
- describe the **structure and function of the skin**

You must be able show you have the necessary practical skills and underpinning knowledge to apply skin tanning techniques.

This unit is linked to the beauty therapy NOS **Unit B25.**

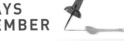

ALWAYS REMEMBER 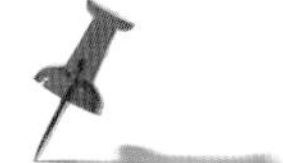

Faux tan is an alternative word for fake tan.

Essential anatomy and physiology knowledge requirements for this Unit are identified on the checklist on page 27. This chapter also discusses anatomy and physiology specific to this unit.

Self-tanning

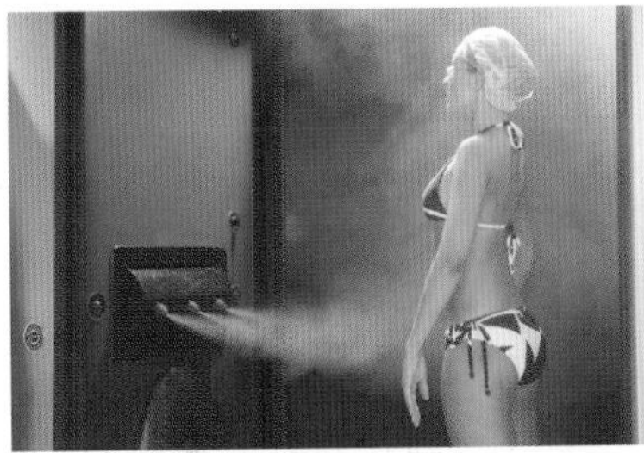

MYSTIC TAN

Self-tan applied in an automated booth

The application of self-tanning products creates a healthy, artificially tanned appearance to the skin without any of the harmful effects of UV light. UV light may be outdoor (natural sunlight) or indoor (artificially created by UV tanning equipment). Sensible UV exposure minimizes the associated risks and enables the associated benefits of tanning.

A tan is the skin's method of protecting the body from exposure to UV, where the skin darkens in order to protect itself from further sun exposure. The **melanocytes**, cells in the epidermis which create skin pigmentation, are stimulated to produce melanin.

Melanosomes are small organs called organelles found in the melanocyte cell which make and store the skin's pigment melanin. The melanocytes increase melanin production as a protective measure to absorb harmful rays of UV light. Pigmentation changes can occur in the skin due to the changes in activity and numbers of melanocytes. This can result in increased ephelides (freckles), solar lentigines or chloasma (liver spots) and irregular pigmentation. Pigmentation changes are not uncommon in Asian skin and often result in large hyper-pigmentation marks. The skin also thickens as the cells in the epidermis multiply to absorb UV and reduce its penetration.

The quantity and distribution of melanocytes differs according to race. In a white Caucasian skin the melanin tends to be destroyed when it reaches the stratum granulosum layer of the epidermis. With stimulation from UV exposure, however, melanin will also be present in the upper epidermis. In a black-skinned person, melanin is present in larger quantities throughout all the layers, a level of protection that has evolved to deal with bright UV light. The increased protection allows less UV to penetrate the dermis below. The less melanin there is in the skin the less natural protection the skin has from the harmful UV rays.

On exposure to UV the melanin that is already available will produce a tanned effect, which will quickly disappear. It can take between three and seven days before new melanin is released following UV exposure, so the tanned appearance gradually develops. The development of a gradual tan without burning should be aimed for.

Overexposure to the sun results in an erythema of the skin as the blood capillaries dilate. The skin will also feel sore as the nerve endings become stimulated. The skin may then form a blister and then form a crust as the skin begins to heal. This can lead to skin hyper-pigmentation and hypo-pigmentation. In hypo-pigmentation the skin loses colour caused by decreased melanin production and therefore has less protection.

The effect of tanned skin created by self tanning is temporary: as dead skin cells are shed, so too is the colour. This process of losing the tan usually takes 5–6 days. However, the life of the tan can be extended through client maintenance procedures following the service.

There are many different self-tan applications to choose from for professional or retail use, including self-tan tissues, mousses, **spray-gun**, airbrush, automated spray booth, cream and gel.

Formulations differ as they are often designed for different parts of the face or body, and for various skin tones – fair or dark – to achieve a realistic result. Maximum tanning effect takes between 8 to 24 hours depending upon the tanning product and the client's natural skin type/colour.

Self-tanning is ideal for clients who want an immediate colour, have fair skin with a tendency to burn in UV light or who are concerned with the associated risks of UV exposure.

HEALTH & SAFETY

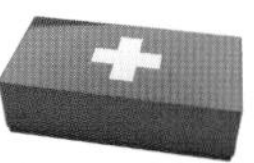

DHA

DHA is only recommended for external use to the body, so care must be taken to avoid inhaling the product, ingesting the product or contact with the eyes.

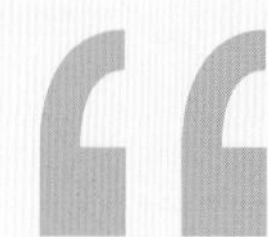

> When providing self-tanning services the beauty therapist needs to ensure that their own tan is perfect. Your appearance is a sales tool!
>
> **Tammy Baker**

HEALTH & SAFETY

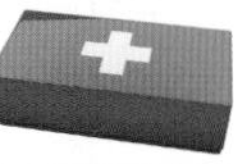

Manufacturer's guidance

The product manufacturer will guide you if SPF is required – inform the client of this requirement as necessary.

Anatomy and physiology

The active ingredient in **self-tan products** is **dihydroxyacetone** (DHA), a colourless sugar which reacts with the amino acids – proteins found in the stratum corneum, the skin's epidermal skin cells creating the pigmented, tanned look, referred to as Maillard's reaction. DHA reacts differently to the everyone's amino acids, producing different tanning colourations. DHA concentrations range from 1–15 per cent affecting the depth of colouration. A fast acting solution will be 10–12 per cent DHA.

KNOWLEDGE CHECK

Which part of the skin is affected by the dihydroxyacetone (DHA) in the self tanning treatment?

Need more time... refer to page 566 to help you.

Erythrulose may also be used, a natural based sugar similar in composition to DHA, but produces a lighter and slower developing tan taking between 24–48 hours to develop. This can be combined with DHA to enhance the overall result to create a more natural skin tone.

Some contain UV protection and have a SPF, however, the skin still requires protection.

It is essential that exfoliation is carried out before the service is performed to remove dry, flaky skin cells which would create a patchy uneven colouration.

TOP TIP

Fair-skinned clients

If the client has a fair skin, choose a self-tanning product with a low percentage DHA.

ALWAYS REMEMBER

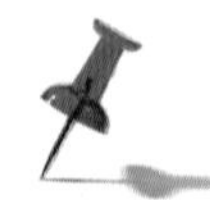

Development time

Dihydroxyacetone begins to tan the skin after 1 hour following application and continues darkening during the following 24–72 hours, depending on formulation. Explain this to the client.

Plan and prepare for the treatment

Outcome 1: Be able to prepare for self-tanning techniques

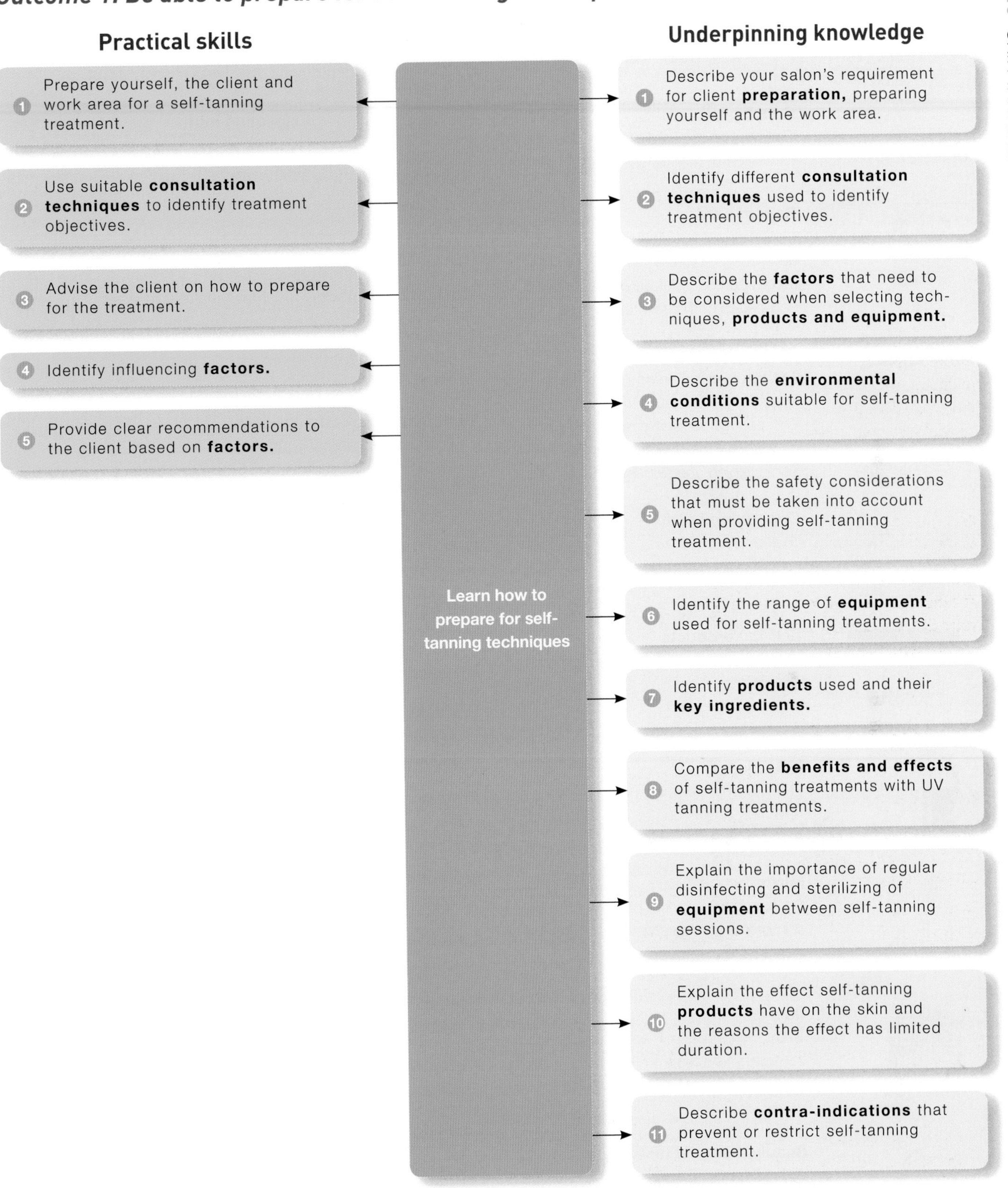

Practical skills
1 Prepare yourself, the client and work area for a self-tanning treatment.
2 Use suitable **consultation techniques** to identify treatment objectives.
3 Advise the client on how to prepare for the treatment.
4 Identify influencing **factors.**
5 Provide clear recommendations to the client based on **factors.**
Learn how to prepare for self-tanning techniques
Underpinning knowledge
1 Describe your salon's requirement for client **preparation,** preparing yourself and the work area.
2 Identify different **consultation techniques** used to identify treatment objectives.
3 Describe the **factors** that need to be considered when selecting techniques, **products and equipment.**
4 Describe the **environmental conditions** suitable for self-tanning treatment.
5 Describe the safety considerations that must be taken into account when providing self-tanning treatment.
6 Identify the range of **equipment** used for self-tanning treatments.
7 Identify **products** used and their **key ingredients.**
8 Compare the **benefits and effects** of self-tanning treatments with UV tanning treatments.
9 Explain the importance of regular disinfecting and sterilizing of **equipment** between self-tanning sessions.
10 Explain the effect self-tanning **products** have on the skin and the reasons the effect has limited duration.
11 Describe **contra-indications** that prevent or restrict self-tanning treatment.

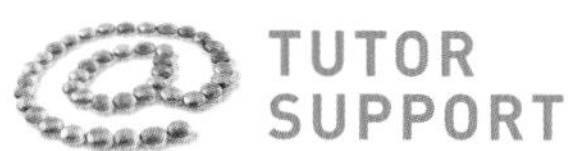

Activity 1: Self-tanning

Before beginning the self-tanning service, check that you have the necessary products, tools and equipment to hand and that they meet legal, hygiene and industry requirements for self-tanning.

PRODUCTS, TOOLS AND EQUIPMENT

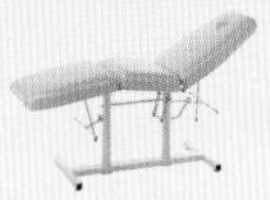

Couch
This may be required when performing exfoliation or manual skin tanning service

Record card
Confidential card recording details of each client registered at the salon to record personal details/products used and details of the service

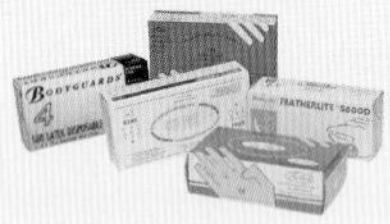

Disposable gloves
To comply with Personal Protective Equipment (PPE) at Work regulations. Thin enough to enable even application and protect the beauty therapist's hands from staining and skin irritation

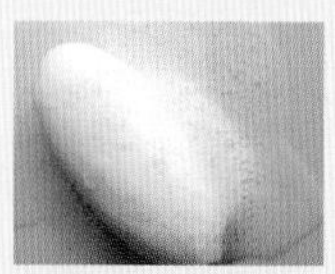

Unperfumed soap
To cleanse the skin

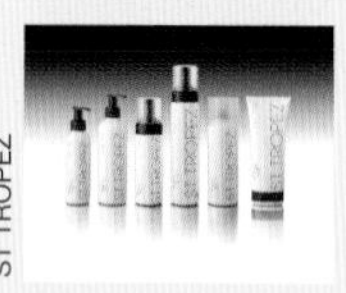

ST TROPEZ

Self-tan products
These may include gels, spray, cream and lotions

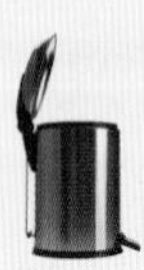

Bin
This should be a lined metal bin with a lid

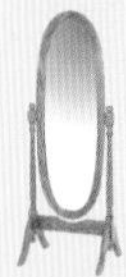

Mirror
Full length to allow the client to prepare skin before service and to view afterwards

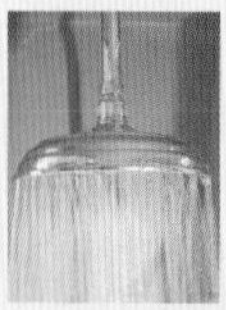

Shower
To cleanse the skin, if applicable, prior to the self-tan system

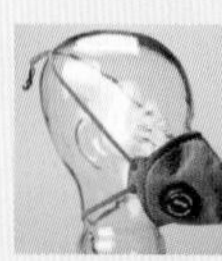

Beauty therapist face mask
With carbon filter to filter out any excess airborne particles

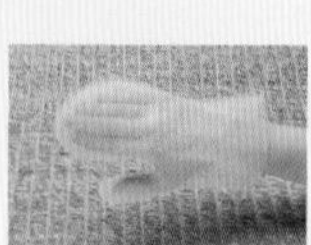

Exfoliating mitt
Used to remove dead skin before self-tanning application

YOU WILL ALSO NEED:

Cosmetic cleansers To remove make-up if worn

Cleansing wipe Used following tanning application to remove product from the eyebrows, fingers, toe nails and palms of the hand.

Buffing mitt To remove excess tanning product during manually-applied self-tan

Self-tanning guidance instructions If using the spray booth system

Barrier cream/oil For the palms of the hands, soles of the feet and any area of dry skin, i.e. ankle area

Self-tan equipment As appropriate, e.g. spray-gun and compressor

Disposable briefs (If required)

Protective nose filters or mask For client to use to avoid inhalation of airborne particles during spray-tanning techniques

Protective apron To protect work-wear from spillages

Protective hair covering To prevent hair staining

Protective eyewear To avoid eye irritation during spray-tanning application techniques

Cotton wool and buds To remove self-tan from parts not required and to remove cleansing preparations

Tissues To protect against staining and for removing cleansing preparations and self-tan product

Protective disposable coverings A paper bedroll for trolley surfaces and flooring and for cleaning the area

Cleaning agents To clean equipment and work area

Aftercare advice Recommended advice for the client to refer to following the service

TOP TIP

Self-tanning preparations

There is an extensive range of self-tanning products available for both manual and spray-tanning techniques taking into consideration skin colour and skin type.

Skin colours range from fair to medium and medium to dark. Ingredients which enhance the cosmetic effect such as metallic, sparkly finishes should be avoided on coarse, uneven skin textures and mature skin types.

Sterilization and disinfection

The beauty therapist's hands should be protected with disposable gloves. Regular exposure of the skin to self-tanning preparations without protection may lead to contact dermatitis. Contact dermatitis is a skin problem caused by intolerance of the skin to a particular substance or a group of substances. On exposure to the substance the skin quickly becomes irritated and an allergic reaction occurs. This may occur when a beauty therapist's skin is exposed to self-tanning chemicals on a regular basis. It is recommended that the beauty therapist wears additional personal protective equipment such as a protective apron to protect work-wear from staining, especially during manual application technique. A face mask can be worn to filter excess airborne particles that are transient in the tanning mist created. A charcoal filter may be fitted in the face mask to remove the perfume component of the self-tanning product. Long hair should be tied back. The hands should be disinfected before the protective gloves are applied.

The shower if used must be cleaned after each client to avoid cross-infection. The service floor where the client stands during service application must be cleaned with a disinfectant cleaning agent and protected as appropriate using a disposable non-slip covering. The self-tan liquid used in spray systems is a hazard if not adequately removed through ventilation systems and could cause slippage if not removed with cleaning.

An automatic wash cycle cleans the automated spray-tanning booth after each use. Waste is collected in floor filters which will require regular cleaning.

Spray-tan extraction booths require cleaning and have filters which may be disposable or can be cleaned. Follow your manufacturer's instructions.

Airbrush spray-tanning has less opportunity for cross-infection in application as there is no direct contact apart from with the floor, and sole protectors should be worn.

Waste bins in the area should be emptied after each client.

Waste generated from automated spray-tan systems is classed as trade effluent requiring a trade effluent license. Check your responsibilities with the local water authority.

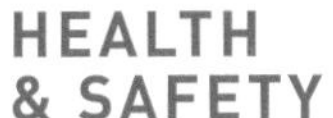

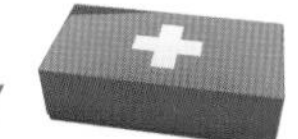

COSHH assessment

The safety of the selected tanning product should be assessed by obtaining a Material Safety Data Sheet (MSDS) to learn the safe use and handling of the product. Obtain this from the product supplier.

BEST PRACTICE

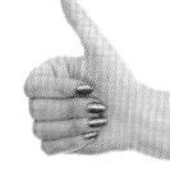

Products

Check that all products are kept clean and airtight. Check the 'use by' date has not expired.

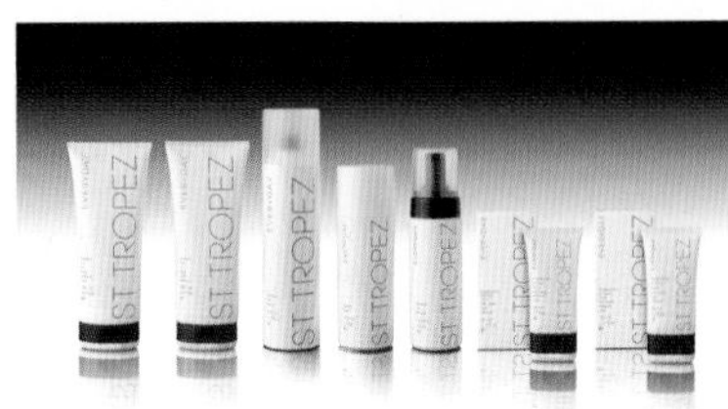

St Tropez tan range

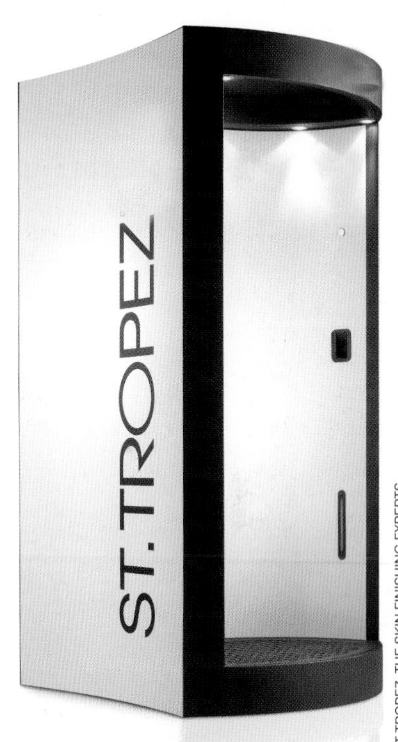

ST TROPEZ, THE SKIN FINISHING EXPERTS

St Tropez Elegance spray booth

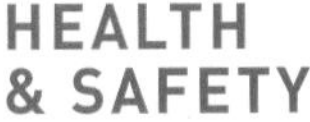

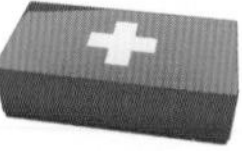

Occupational exposure limit (OEL)

Each self-tanning product contains different ingredients. Check with your supplier the ventilation/ extraction requirements for the tanning system.

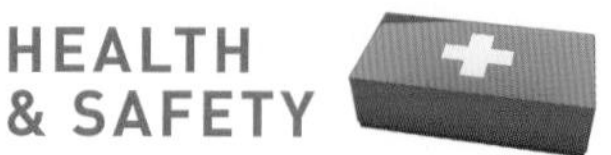

Compressors

The automated spray booth and spray-gun tanning systems use a compressor to apply the tanning product.

The use and system must comply with the Pressure Safety Regulations (2000).

A pressure system is a piece of equipment containing a fluid under pressure.

As water is held in small holding tanks in automated spray booths it is necessary to carry out a risk assessment of the safety levels of bacteria and possible legionnella bacteria which can lead to legionnaires' disease by inhaling small droplets of water suspended in the air, which contain the bacteria.

Remember to use the underpinning knowledge you learnt in Chapter 3 Health and Safety.

Preparation of the work area

Floors in the work area should be non-slip and easy to clean.

Ensure that tanning equipment is serviced regularly as per the manufacturer's instructions.

Some compressors are noisy, so this should be considered when choosing where the treatment is carried out.

For the spray-tan automated application technique a cold water supply and waste pipe for drainage is required. It is essential that spray-tan booths are sealed adequately to prevent chemical leakage into the atmosphere. Ventilation must also be adequate to avoid excessive chemical fumes and extraction of airborne particles. Filters and extraction systems should be checked for efficiency.

Ensure there is sufficient tanning product to operate the spray-tanning systems.

For automated booth spray systems check pressure gauges and fluid tank levels.

There must be sufficient room in the working area to adequately perform the service.

Ensure there is adequate lighting when applying self-tan manually to ensure an even application.

Any equipment that comes into contact with clients should be cleaned immediately after use, to prevent cross-infection, using cleaning materials specified by the manufacturer.

Trolley surfaces should be protected against accidental spillage of self-tan product from manual and spray-tan techniques.

HEALTH & SAFETY

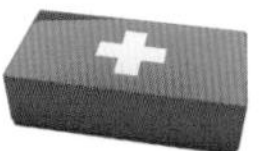

Gloves

Gloves should be powder-free nitrile gloves or powder-free vinyl gloves to avoid possible allergic reaction to known allergens such as latex.

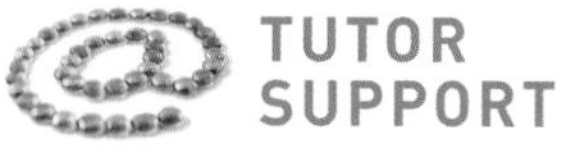

Activity 2: Methods of self-tanning

TOP TIP

Self-tan products

Some self-tan products contain alpha hydroxy acids (AHA) which continue to gently remove dead skin cells, aiming to produce a more even colour as the product achieves the skin's colour change.

Some products contain ingredients to achieve a sparkly finished effect.

Disposable floor coverings or sole protectors should be provided if providing spray-tanning technique.

Service couches required for the application of manual self-tan applications must be adequately protected with disposable coverings to prevent staining and cross-infection.

> Always describe the features, advantages and benefits of a product and allow your client to feel, smell and experience the products you are recommending.
>
> Tammy Baker

Reception

Preparation procedures should be given in advance of the service where possible so that the client's skin is compatible with effective tanning. A skin preparation information sheet is a good idea to give your client when booking the appointment which can detail all aspects of the service including aftercare requirements.

If the client has hypersensitive skin or known allergies, a skin sensitivity patch test should be performed to assess skin suitability. This should test the product(s) to be used in the self-tanning treatment. The self-tanning application can only proceed if the client has a negative skin reaction – no skin reaction.

Depending on the system used, time should be allowed when booking the service for client preparation, self-tan application and drying off.

Advise the client as it may be necessary to wear disposable underwear which will be provided which is costed into the service. Some clients, however, will be happy not to wear any underwear (follow your workplace policy). Also ideally loose, dark coloured clothing should be worn to avoid removal of product and staining following the service.

Waxing, shaving, electrical epilation or injectable services such as Botox® injections should be carried out 24-hours prior to service to avoid skin irritation.

Body lotions, especially those containing therapeutic/perfumed ingredients should not be applied to the skin on the day of self-tan application as this may affect the result obtained.

Beauty therapy services where therapeutic products are applied to the skin or remove the surface skin cells should not be performed before or after the service, such as galvanic therapy, micro-dermabrasion or massage using pre-blended aromatherapy oils.

Where you require the client to shower and exfoliate before the service, explain this when they book. An oil free exfoliating, shower or bath product should be used. Attention should be given to the ankles, elbows and knees to remove dead skin to ensure even tanning. Inform the client not to apply deodorant or body lotions following showering which can cause uneven skin tanning.

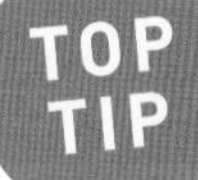

TOP TIP

Link selling

It is a good idea for clients to receive an exfoliation service professionally applied before their service. This must be compatible with the self-tanning product or the final tan colour may be affected and the desired colour not achieved.

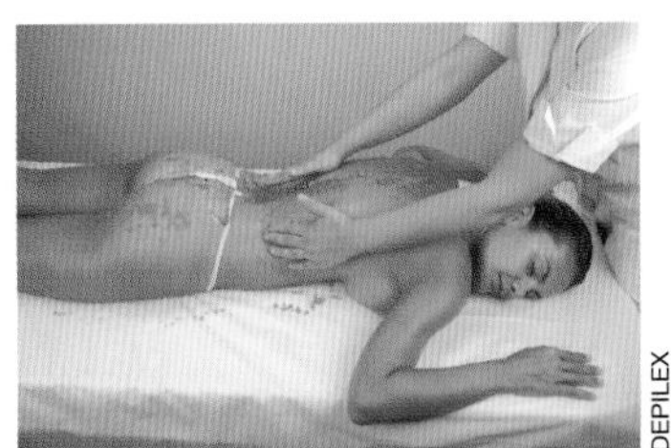

DEPILEX

Depilex exfoliating service

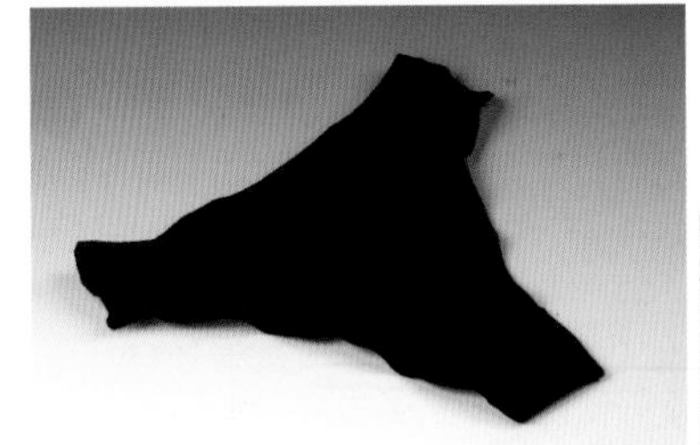

BEAUTY EXPRESS LTD

Disposable underwear

TOP TIP

Avoid staining

Recommend the client avoids wearing silk or leather clothing as the pigment can cause staining.

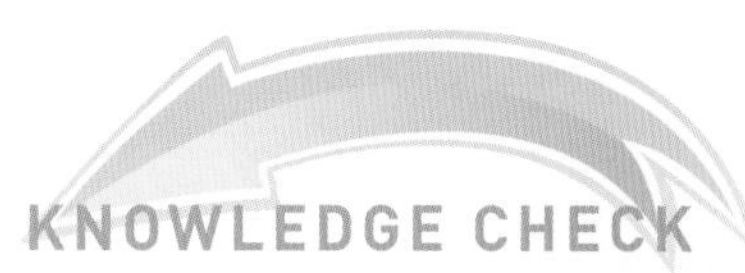

How can a hygienic environment be maintained when providing self-tanning services? Give five examples of necessary cleaning regimes.

Need more time... refer to pages 570–571 to help you.

> To ensure that your client's tan fades evenly it is crucial to recommend aftercare advice. Simple tips include polishing every two to three days to remove dead skin cells to help the tan fade evenly and to moisturise the skin every day to maintain hydration to help the tan last longer.
>
> **Tammy Baker**

> Customers generally fall into two categories: those who think and behave similarly to you, and those who don't. The most successful service providers have learned how to work with both groups. When you are able to speak another person's language, it becomes easier to understand – and be understood – by them. Being able to adapt to various personalities will create and build strong relationships.
>
> **Tammy Baker**

Consultation

On arrival, complete the client's personal details on the client record card. Question the client to check for suitability and for possible contra-indications. If contra-indications are present do not proceed with the service. Carry out a client consultation to assess the client's treatment objectives and expectations.

HEALTH & SAFETY

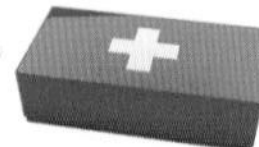

Skin sensitivity patch test

In order to assess skin tolerance to the self-tan product, a skin test may be performed on a small area of skin. This is usually done in the crook of the elbow or behind the ear. This must be completed a minimum 12–24 hours before treatment application dependant upon manufacturer recommendations.

Some products contain 'walnut oil' which creates a dark toned effect. This may be unsuitable for use on a client with nut allergies.

Storage

Ensure all products are clearly labelled and stored at room temperature away from heat and sunlight, ideally in a cupboard.

Temperatures in excess of 40°C should be avoided as this will affect the quality and effectiveness of the product.

If the client has stretch marks or recently healed skin, the colour result will differ. Inform the client of this.

If the client is a minor under the age of 16 years of age, it is necessary to obtain parent/guardian permission for service. The parent/guardian will also have to be present when the service is received.

Explain what is involved in the different self-tanning services, timing, how long the effect will last and costs – a choice will then be able to be agreed on the most suitable technique.

Agree with the client the colour required and what can be achieved with the chosen tanning system. Consider the client's natural skin colouring. Ideally the colour should be two to three shades darker. A fair skinned client will not achieve the possible dark tanning of a darker skinned client. The tan may initially appear too dark for a fair skinned client as they do not usually tan, explain this, but cautiously apply a lighter application of tan if spray-tanning using a spray-gun on a client's first service.

Explain how the client will be prepared for the service and how long the service will take.

If the client is receiving an automated spray-tan booths application they will need to be instructed to adopt typically four different poses between each spray application exposure. For some clients with mobility issues these may be difficult to adopt and they should be advised accordingly. For clients who suffer from claustrophobia this method of self-tanning service may be an unsuitable choice.

Discuss the expected skin colour, expected skin reactions following service and aftercare requirements. If the client has a tattoo it will appear faded when the tan is initially applied.

Once the consultation is complete, the beauty therapist should ensure that all details are recorded accurately and that the client has signed their record card. This enables reference for future services and up-to-date tracking of services received. A sample record card is shown on the following page.

Invite the client to ask questions, the client should fully understand what the service involves.

ST.TROPEZ

TANNING TREATMENT CONSULTATION

	YES	NO
Have you used self-tanning products before?	☐	☐
How were the results? POOR ☐	AVE ☐	GOOD ☐
Have you had a St.Tropez tan before?	☐	☐
If yes, were you pleased with the results?	☐	☐
Do you require an all over tan?	☐	☐
Is the tan for a special occasion?	☐	☐
Are you going on holiday?	☐	☐
Is your skin free from SPF and salt water?	☐	☐
Have you removed all deodorant/perfume/make-up?	☐	☐
Have you shaved or waxed less than 24 hours ago?	☐	☐
Do you have bleached hair or eyebrows?	☐	☐
Are you on any medication?	☐	☐
Have you recently had a course of antibiotics or chemotherapy?	☐	☐
Have you any known allergies?	☐	☐
Have you any open cuts, wounds, rashes or grazes?	☐	☐
Do you suffer from any skin disorders?	☐	☐
Do you have any pigmentation patches or pigmentary disorders?	☐	☐
Would you describe your skin as hyper-sensitive?	☐	☐
Do you suffer from any respiratory problems?	☐	☐
Are you pregnant or breastfeeding?	☐	☐
Have you recently had any body piercings or tattoos?	☐	☐
Have you received a pre-treatment advice slip?	☐	☐
Have you any queries from this advice or any other questions?	☐	☐

How will you maintain your tan?

What concerns do you have with home tanning?

PATCH TEST

We recommend that you have a patch test prior to every treatment.	YES	NO
Have you taken the patch test?	☐	☐
If no, are you happy to receive a tan without a patch test?	☐	☐

DETAILS

Name: ....

Address: ....

....

....

Date of Birth: ....

Telephone: ....

E-mail: ....

....

INDEMNITY

I have read and understood the recommendations.
To the best of my knowledge, there is no reason why I should not tan.

Signed: ....

St.Tropez and its agents would like to be able to advise you of products, services and special promotions in the future. If you do not wish to receive further communications, please tick the box ☐

ST.TROPEZ

DATE	TREATMENT/COMMENTS	INITIALS

ST TROPEZ, THE SKIN FINISHING EXPERTS

Record card for self-tanning

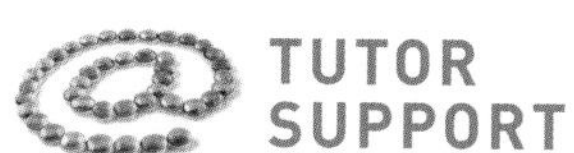
TUTOR SUPPORT

Activity 4: Contra-indications to self-tanning services

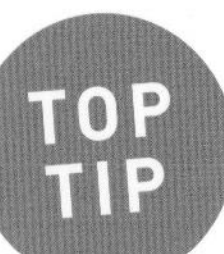
TOP TIP

Vitiligo

Vitiligo skin cannot be effectively treated with self-tan as the melanin is not present. A skin coloured make-up camouflage application can help disguise the appearance of the skin condition vitiligo (lack of skin pigment), especially when applied specifically to one area, e.g. using spray-tan airbrush technique. Choose a colour close to the client's natural skin tone.

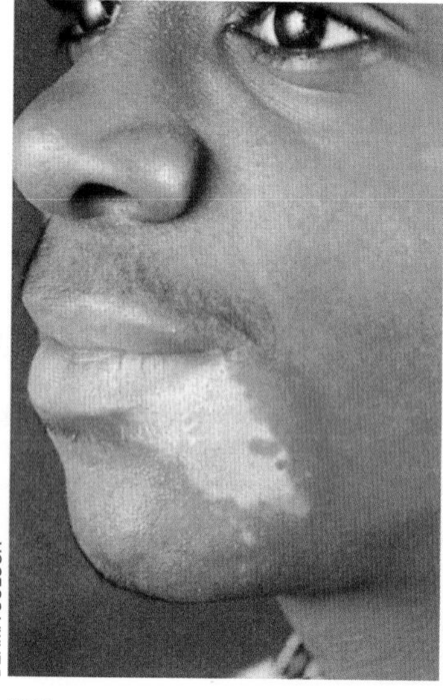
DERMA COLOUR

Vitiligo

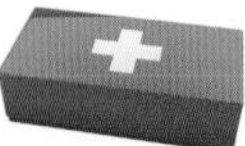
HEALTH & SAFETY

Respiratory contra-indications
Severe asthma is unsuitable for exposure to spray-tanning. An alternative would be manual application technique.

Contra-indications

Certain contra-indications prevent a self-tanning service. If there is any concern over the client's suitability, medical advice should be sought before the service proceeds.

During the client consultation, if you find any of the following, self-tan service must not be recommended or carried out.

- Pregnancy – due to the hormonal changes in the body, the colour result may change. There is also an insurance implication as no body services should be carried out in the first three months of pregnancy (often referred to as the first trimester).
- Hypersensitive, allergenic skins – an allergic reaction can occur caused by the ingredients in the self-tan product.
- The client is undergoing chemotherapy or radiotherapy treatment which can affect cell renewal and the production of melanin and may result in uneven tanning.
- Infectious skin conditions – fungal, viral or bacterial.
- Cuts and abrasions in the area – skin irritation and secondary infection could occur.
- Recent tattoo, as scar tissue will not tan evenly and there may be a risk of bacterial infection.
- Recent piercings must be covered to prevent skin irritation and bacterial infection. It is best not to treat an area where the piercing is less than six weeks old.
- Immediately after other heat or sensitizing services such as waxing hair removal, electrolysis or sauna. Again, skin irritation and secondary infection can occur if the skin has been damaged.
- Contact lenses, unless removed – to avoid eye irritation.
- Respiratory conditions – these may be aggravated by the chemical fumes with spray-tan technique.
- Skin conditions where the skin is thickened and broken such as psoriasis, eczema and dermatitis. Excessive skin plaques will also result in uneven tanning. A barrier cream should be applied to minor areas of eczema and psoriasis.
- Positive (allergic) reaction to a skin sensitivity patch test.
- Skin erythema – the skin is already sensitized.

Those requiring GP referral should be tactfully and clearly discussed to ensure client understanding. Never attempt to diagnose a condition as you are not qualified to do so and could cause the client unnecessary concern.

Inform the client at consultation of any relevant contra-actions that may occur and the action to take.

Contra-actions

- **Erythema** (reddening of the skin) **irritation, burning** sensation and **swelling** caused by an allergic reaction to the self-tanning product used. The allergic reaction is rarely to DHA but other ingredients such as perfume and preservatives. If this occurs, advise that the client showers to remove the product, apply a cool compress with cold water and make a record of this skin response on the client's **record card**. If the redness does not reduce, the client may require to seek medical attention.

A skin sensitivity patch test may take place in the future using a different skin self-tanning product to assess skin tolerance.

- **Respiratory problems** due to inhalation of airborne self-tanning particles or inadequate ventilation leading to shortening of breath and tightening of the chest.
- Respiratory problems should be checked for at consultation and appropriate action taken. A mask or nose filters may be provided for client use and used as a precautionary measure.
- **Watery eyes** caused by an irritant effect to the self-tanning product. Protective eyewear is available for use as a precautionary measure.
- **Fainting** may occur if standing during spray-gun tan applications. Check client comfort during application. Have water available to ensure client hydration. Ensure the work area is free from obstacles that could harm the client if they fainted. Have an awareness of what action to take if a client fainted.
- **Nausea** ingestion of the self-tanning product can occur when using spray systems which may cause nausea. Discuss the procedure at consultation to avoid unnecessary ingestion.
- **Undesirable hair colouration** caused by inadequate protection and contact with the self-tanning product this may include facial and scalp hair.
- **Undesirable skin colouration** caused by poor preparation, consultation, choice of product, application techniques and non-adherence by the client with aftercare advice. This is discussed in more detail on page 582.

Have tanning instructions clearly displayed for use with automated spray-tanning systems.

TOP TIP

Hair protection

Ensure clients with bleached, fair or white hair adequately protect their hair when receiving spray-tanning or the hair may become discoloured where not protected.

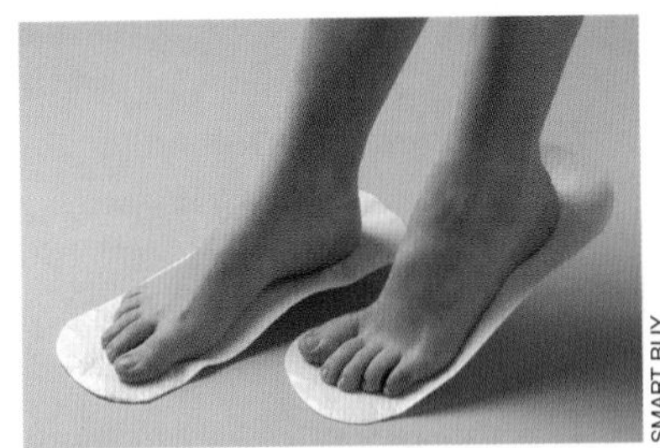

Disposable sole protectors

KNOWLEDGE CHECK

State the skin care instructions a client should follow to ensure that an optimum result is achieved from the self tan.

Need more time... refer to page 571 and 575 to help you.

Preparation of the client

Choose the correct shade for the skin colour – light, medium or dark. Some manufacturers provide shade charts to enable the client to identify the colour. If an automated spray-tan booth is used this cannot be accommodated for. The service cannot be personalized. The client must be confident of the poses to adopt during spray-tan application and the service sensations.

Best results are achieved on clean skin which has been cleansed and exfoliated to remove skin lotions, sebum and dead skin cells, all of which will act as a barrier. This type of cleansing enables an even application, although not all tanning systems require this.

Poor skin preparation can result in streaking, darker uneven patches or a lack of colour development.

For automated booth spray systems check pressure gauges and fluid tank levels.

Exfoliation may be performed in the salon or by the client at home, depending on the self-tan product. Areas requiring exfoliation attention by the client or beauty therapist are the elbows, knees and ankles, where dead skin cells build up.

TOP TIP

Exfoliation

Dry exfoliation can be performed using an exfoliating mitt before the service.

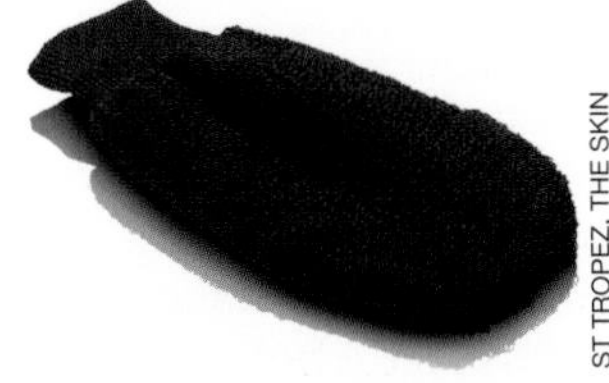

ST TROPEZ, THE SKIN FINISHING EXPERTS

Buffing/exfoliating dual purpose mitt

Why is it important not to name specific contra-indications when encouraging clients to seek medical advice before service?

Need more time... refer to page 574 to help you.

TOP TIP

Avoid stained nails

If the client has long nails, barrier cream may be applied under the free edge to avoid staining.

A lip balm may be applied before spray-tanning technique to avoid skin staining. Glasses and jewellery should be removed from the treatment area to ensure an even application, and make-up should be removed.

It is recommended to provide paper underwear to prevent staining the client's underwear. It is the client's choice if worn.

In the self-tan spray techniques a barrier cream is applied to the palms of the hands, soles of the feet, ankles and nails of the client to prevent staining. Disposable sole protectors may be used. Ask the client to step firmly onto the adhesive surface.

A protective cap is worn to cover the hair. This is lifted at the hairline to expose the ears. Ensure this is not too low on the forehead or a demarcation line will occur. The eyebrow hair may also be protected with a barrier cream.

Remind the client of the procedure and sensations. Invite any questions from the client to confirm understanding. It is a good idea if you ask them to signal to you if you need to stop for any reason during spray-tan manual application.

If using an automated tanning booth, ensure the client is confident on the procedure to ensure their safety and efficiency of the tanning application. Have instructions clearly placed for the client to refer to.

Provide self-tanning treatments

Outcome 2: Be able to provide self-tanning techniques

Learn how to provide self-tanning techniques

Practical skills

1. **Communicate and behave** in a professional manner.
2. Position yourself and the client correctly throughout the treatment.
3. Select and use **products and equipment** taking into account identified **factors.**
4. Follow **safe and hygienic working practices.**
5. Identify **contra-actions** and take appropriate action during treatment.
6. Provide suitable **aftercare advice.**
7. Complete the treatment to the satisfaction of the client.
8. Evaluate the results of the treatment with the client.

Underpinning knowledge

1. Describe how to **communicate and behave** in a professional manner.
2. State the importance of positioning yourself and the client correctly throughout the treatment.
3. Describe **safe and hygienic working practices.**
4. Describe **contra-actions** which might occur during and following the treatment and how to respond.
5. Describe the **aftercare advice** that should be provided.
6. State the importance of completing the treatment to the satisfaction of the client.
7. State the **methods of evaluating** the effectiveness of the treatment.
8. Describe the **structure and function of the skin.**

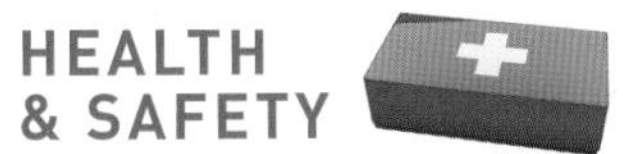

HEALTH & SAFETY

When performing a self-tanning service consider your responsibilities under the following legislation at all times:

- **Health and Safety at Work Act (1974)**
- **Control of Substances Hazardous to Health Regulations (2002)**
- Pressure Systems Safety Regulations (2000)
- **Workplace (Health Safety and Welfare) Regulations (1992)**
- **Management of Health and Safety at Work Regulations (1999)**

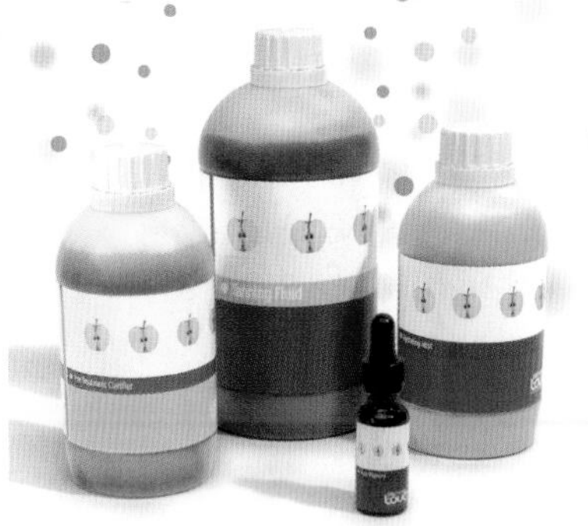

ST TROPEZ, THE SKIN FINISHING EXPERTS

Self-tanning products – pre-service clarifier, tanning fluid, pure pigment, hydrating mist

How to apply self-tanning products

The following tanning systems application techniques are discussed: automated spray booth, spray-tan using an airbrush or gun and manual hand-applied technique. Always follow the manufacturer's instructions to ensure the optimum effect is achieved.

When applying self-tan to the face, the eyes should be closed or protected as per the manufacturer's instructions and system used. Hair should be protected and covered. Nose filters should be provided to prevent inhalation of tanning particles if using spray systems.

> It is important to be self-motivated, but you must be able to work equally well as part of a team. Nominating a 'St Tropez specialist' within your team will ensure that one person is solely responsible for updating the team on new product releases and tanning techniques to ensure you are all offering the ultimate service.
>
> **Tammy Baker**

BEST PRACTICE

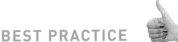

Spray booths
Spray booths provide privacy during application of the spray-tan. The booth features fans to clean the air following application and a protective floor cover.

How to apply self-tan using spray-tan automated booth application technique

1. The client and their skin are prepared for spray application.
2. A large air compressor sprays liquid product in a mist evenly all over the client's skin from a set of spray nozzles in a large self-contained booth constructed from fibreglass, acrylic or aluminium. The booth contains filters to remove chemical particles from the air. Some systems also have inbuilt heaters so that the environment is temperature regulated to prevent the skin drying too quickly.
3. The client stands in the cubicle in front of the nozzles where, after operating a start button, the front and then the back of the body are sprayed with self-tan. Different positions are adopted by the client, usually four simple standing positions to ensure even application. The client then strokes the product over the skin until it has dried. Excess product should be removed with a paper towel, including the palms of the hands and soles of the feet. This system offers additional privacy for the client.

   Application and drying time: *5–10 minutes depending on the system.*
4. If required, a second application may be given when the skin has dried. An immediate colour is achieved and then the tan continues to develop.
5. Ensure the client is satisfied with the finished result and understands how the finished result will appear.

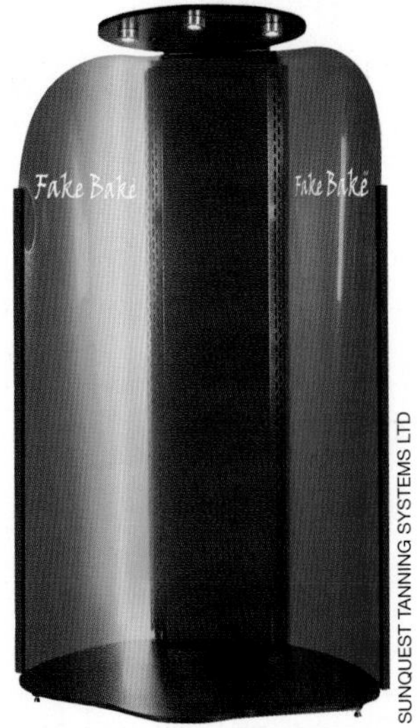

SUNQUEST TANNING SYSTEMS LTD

Spray-tanning booth

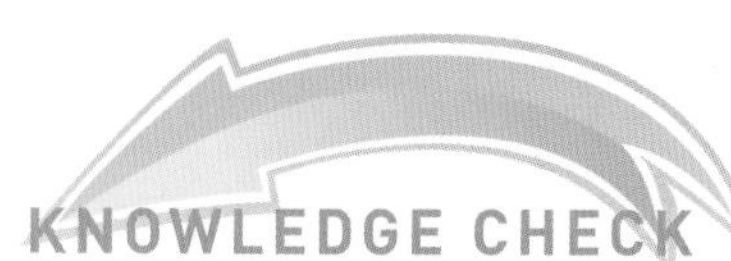

KNOWLEDGE CHECK

How is the choice of self-tan product and colour selected?

Need more time... refer to page 572 to help you.

TOP TIP

Avoid stained hands

When removing the protective hair covering, advise the client to use a paper towel to avoid contact with the skin of the hand, which could lead to skin staining.

KNOWLEDGE CHECK

Why should a skin sensitivity test be performed before each self-tanning service? How is this performed?

Need more time... refer to page 572 to help you.

HEALTH & SAFETY

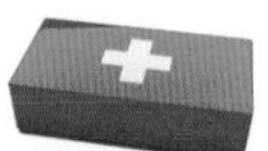

Spillages

If product is spilt during application, soak up excess liquid with tissue while wearing hand protection and dispose of in accordance with Waste Regulations.

A disadvantage of the automated systems is that you cannot control where the product is applied by taking into consideration the size, shape and skin condition of the client which can be achieved with a personal manual application.

Automated spray-tanning has the following benefits:

- it is the quickest self-tanning service
- there is little time required as a resource for the beauty therapist
- it offers the client total privacy

How to apply self-tan using spray-gun application technique This technique uses a compressor, which generates pulses of air pressure producing a stream of compressed air, to power an airbrush that directs a fine mist of self-tan product onto the skin through a flexible hose and a spray-gun nozzle.

Normally two full body applications will be given during the service but only one application to the hands and feet, at the end of the service.

- The client and their skin are prepared for application. Explain to the client the service sensation of a cool mist of moisture.
- The client stands in a booth or working area protected from spray, while the beauty therapist applies self-tan with an air gun. It is important that the client does not touch the skin during application to avoid uneven coverage.
- The client should stand upright with legs apart facing the beauty therapist with arms relaxed at their side. It is important to explain throughout the application how you want them to stand and move different parts of their body.
- Start spraying the body starting at the face and working your way down.
- When spraying the face the client should be advised to hold their breath and close their eyes.
- Overlap each stroke as you work down the body, keeping the spray-gun level.
- Ensure that you spray underneath the breasts, this will be achieved by asking the client to raise their arms to the sides of the body.
- Hold and rotate the arms spraying down towards the hand (without spraying the hands) spraying the inside and side of each arm.
- Spray down each leg (without spraying the feet) and release the trigger on the gun as you reach the ankles. A lighter application is required over the knees where the area is drier.
- Ask the client to turn around and face the back of the booth.
- The client should tilt their head forward while you spray the neck. Work your way down the body, spraying over the shoulders and back.
- Ask the client to point their hands towards the back of the booth with palms facing down and arms held slightly away from their trunk while you spray the back of the arms.
- Continue spraying down the body, the client may bend forward slightly when spraying over the buttocks in order to tan the crease underneath the buttocks or a lighter line will result in this area. Spray the outside to inside of one leg and the inside to outside of the other. Stop at the ankle.
- Spray the sides of the body asking the client to turn to one side so that they are facing side on to you. This will require the client to position themselves with one

leg in front of the other and one arm raised above their head and elbow pointed back. Spray the sides of the breast and trunk.

- Spray down the inside of the back leg and then the outside. Repeat this application to the other side of the body which will require the client to alter the position and raise the other arm.
- Repeat the spray application again.
- Finally increase the distance from the client and lightly spray each foot and hand. The hands will require the client to move their hands into different positions in order to cover the backs and sides of their hands effectively.
- Apply the tan in a specific sequence to ensure even coverage. Adjust pressure according to the effect required. Follow your manufacturer's application, including vertical, horizontal and circular spray patterns. Always try to use the lowest pressure as less fumes will be created and a good coverage achieved.
- Any area which appears wet should be gently patted dry.
- A cleansing wipe can be used following application to remove product from the fingers, toenails and palms of the hand.
- Ensure the client is satisfied with the finished result and understands how the finished result will appear. Advise the client to allow the product to dry for approximately 5–10 minutes before dressing.
- Body moisturiser may be applied to areas that typically can crease and stain such as the wrists, knees and ankles.
- Following application the client stands in the booth to allow the warm air to dry the skin.
- The sole protectors are removed and any sticky residue may be removed with a cleansing tissue.
- Clean the work area and dispose of waste.

Application and drying time: *20–30 minutes*.

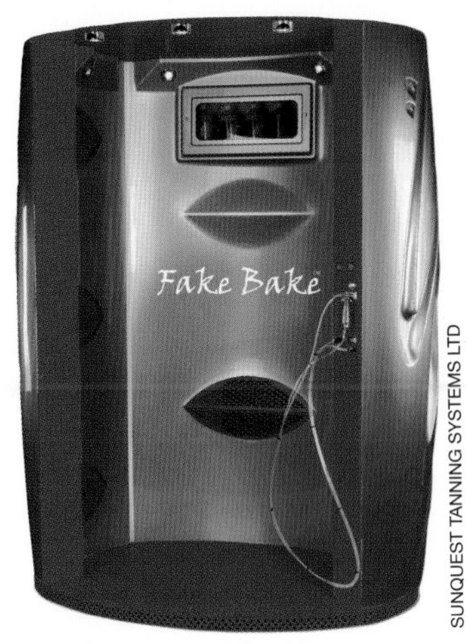

Airbrush spray booth

TOP TIP

Spray booth

Spray booths provide privacy during application of the spray tan. The booth features fans to clean the air following application and a protective floor cover.

Spray-gun tanning application technique To ensure even application a small rotating platform, which the client stands on, can be used to facilitate application.

- To create a more natural, lighter result reduce pressure and increase the distance.
- Start moving the air gun before you start spraying to avoid darker areas of application.
- Ensure no body parts are missed, e.g. under the chin!
- Wipe over fair brow hair to avoid staining, following face application.
- If application is excessive, blot the area to avoid too dark a colour developing.
- Keep the airbrush at 90 degrees and move at all times to ensure even application. A repetitive finger, hand and arm movement is required. Safe working must be considered to prevent repetitive strain injury.
- Spray the legs first as they take the longest to dry.
- Do not over-wet the skin.
- If the client has any folds of skin e.g. on the back, it will be necessary for them to stretch while these body parts are sprayed.

ACTIVITY

PSI is often referred to as a feature in the sale of spray-guns. This means pounds per square inch and refers to the pressure of the air generated by the compressor. This requires adjustment of the pressure to create the result required.

Research different spray-gun tan systems and identify their PSI and other technology features.

Remember, technology advances all the time and it is important to be using the equipment that will give your clients the best result wherever possible.

- When spraying the face, ask the client to inhale through the nose and as they exhale through the mouth spray the face from the chin to forehead to avoid inhalation of the spray. The client's eyes are closed at all times.
- Blemished areas, and areas of dry skin absorb more colour and lighter application is required over such areas.

Step-by-step: Airbrush tanning application techniques

A small pen-like spray-gun applicator atomises the spray-tan liquid into tiny particles. Again, operated by a compressor. This is useful for performing corrective work, i.e. concealment of vitiligo.

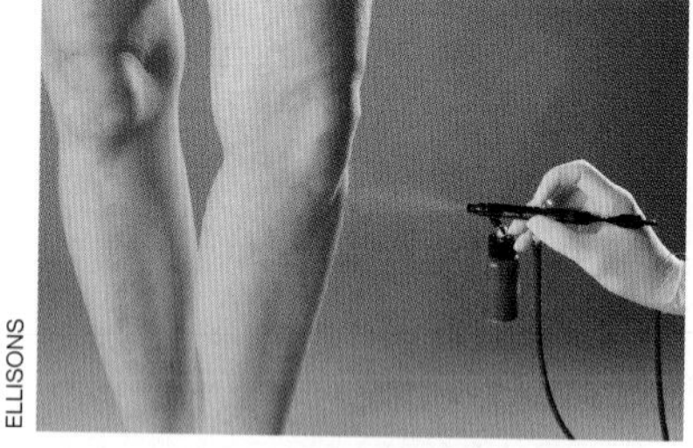

ELLISONS

1 Switch on the compressor and adjust the pressure to create the desired result. Leg application – apply tan to the client's legs as these take the longest to dry. Work down the leg at a distance of 13–21 cm to ensure full, even coverage.

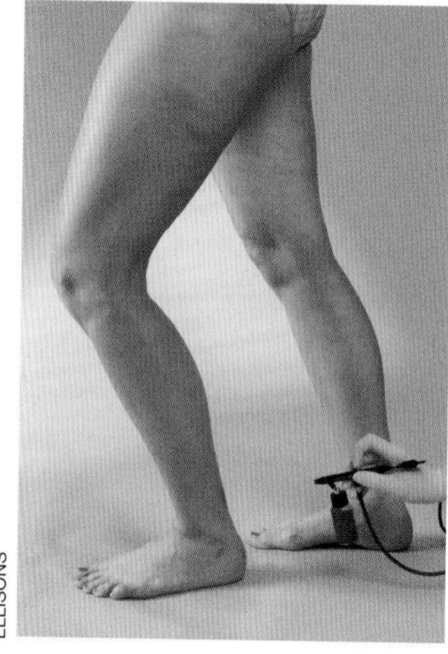

ELLISONS

2 Ankle application – this area can be dry, creating a darker effect, so a lighter application is required. Lightly spray the tops of the feet. Increase distance and reduce pressure. Advise the client to lean forward to stretch the skin in this area. Continue to apply tan to the upper body front and back by applying tan in a downwards direction until the area is evenly covered. Ask the client to move their body as required to facilitate application.

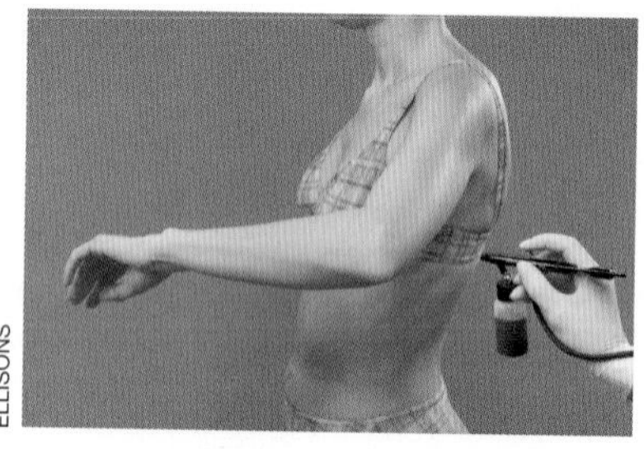

ELLISONS

3 Arm application – apply tan to the client with their arm raised, working from the wrist down the arm and then apply to the rest of the arm, asking the client to move their arms as required to ensure full, even coverage.

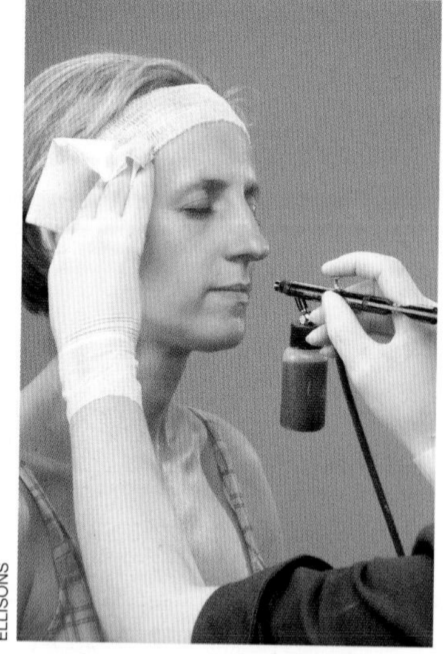

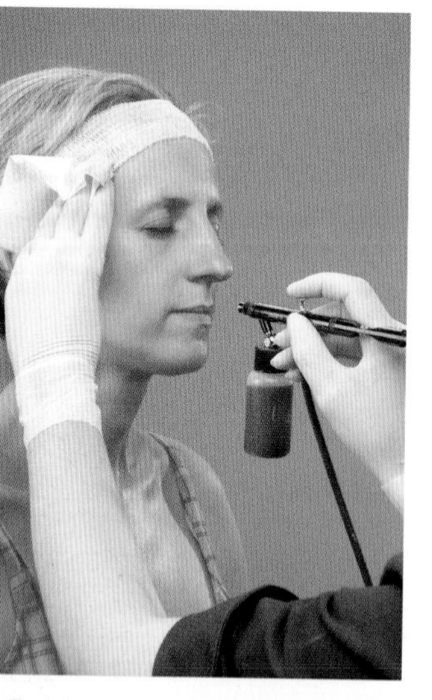

ELLISONS

4 Facial application – protect the hair (including brow hair) to prevent staining. Ask the client to close their eyes and take a deep breath while you apply tan to the face. Include the ears, around the ears and the neck area.

ELLISONS

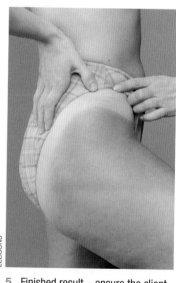

5 Finished result – ensure the client is satisfied with the finished result and that the application is even. Re-apply to any lighter areas.

Rinse the air gun immediately with warm clean water to prevent clogging with dried product. Tanning product is water-based.

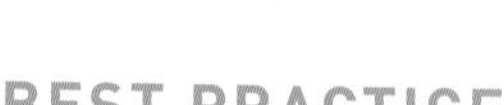

BEST PRACTICE

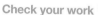

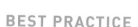

Check your work

Check your application of the product as you are working. The skin should look initially as if it has a fine mist on its surface which dries quickly. If it is too wet it will run resulting in streaking.

ALWAYS REMEMBER 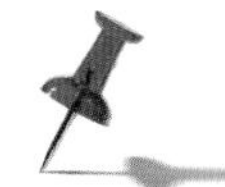

Care of the air gun

Temporarily between use, store the air gun in water to prevent clogging.

When not in use, store the air gun in an air gun holder.

If clogged, the air gun will not apply the product evenly and will spit the product.

TOP TIP

Uneven application

If you make a mistake during application, pat the area dry, do not rub the skin as this will lead to uneven patchy colouration.

You can always apply a further application to produce an even result.

> The most common cause of a patchy tan is dry skin, so it is crucial to polish the entire body and moisturise problem areas such as hands, elbows, knees and feet prior to self-tan applications.
>
> Tammy Baker

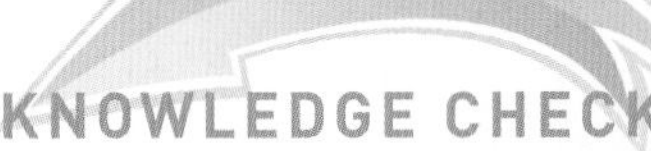

KNOWLEDGE CHECK

What is the meaning of the term PSI, and which self-tanning system does this relate to?

Need more time... refer to page 579 to help you.

How to apply self-tan using manual hand-applied application technique This is a luxurious service which is recommended if the client would like to benefit from a relaxing massage to the skin's surface

1. The client should be dressed in disposable underwear, hair secured from the face and covered on the couch with towels for modesty and to keep warm. The client and their skin are prepared for self-tan application. This usually requires showering and the application of an exfoliant.
2. Moisturiser may be applied to the elbows, knees, ankles and feet. Adding moisturiser lightens the result but should only be used if recommended by the manufacturer as it can also create a barrier if too much is used.
3. The self-tan product is applied over the body following the manufacturer's guidelines for application using the hands, which are usually protected with gloves to prevent staining.
4. Service must be methodical to ensure no body parts are missed and that an even coverage is obtained.
5. Product should be removed immediately during application, using a clean tissue, from the palms of the hands, toes and fingernails to prevent staining.
6. Time should be allowed for the product to dry, *approximately 10 minutes*.
7. The skin is then buffed to remove excess product, avoid rubbing the skin which could result in uneven colouration. Pay particular attention to areas where the skin is drier, i.e. ankles and wrists.
8. Ensure the client is satisfied and understands how the finished result will appear. Application and drying time: *Approximately 1 hour 20 minutes* including pre-exfoliation and post skin buffing.

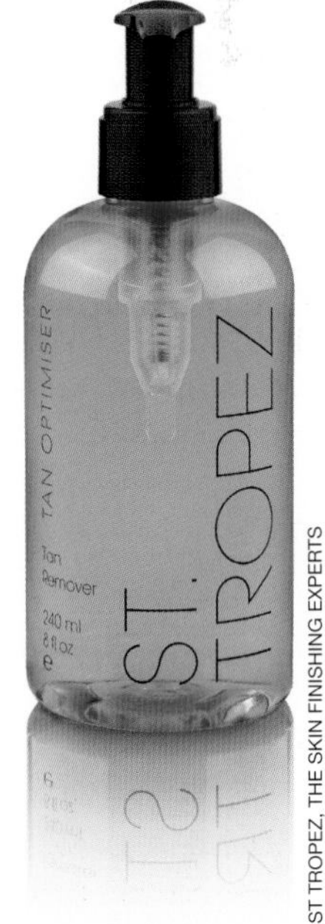

ST TROPEZ, THE SKIN FINISHING EXPERTS

Tan remover (corrective) lotion

TOP TIP

Protecting the hands

The hands have more pores than other body areas and will soon tan. To prevent staining wear thin gloves during application.

KNOWLEDGE CHECK

If the client experienced an allergic reaction following the self-tanning treatment, what action would the client have been advised to take at consultation?

Need more time... refer to page 574 to help you.

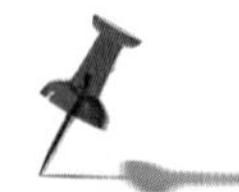

ALWAYS REMEMBER

Medication

Some forms of medication can affect how the skin responds to self-tanning product.

Poor tanning results These are commonly caused by the beauty therapist and their choice and application of products, or the client not following the necessary skin preparation/aftercare instructions.

- **Tan too light in colour**: incorrect colour shade selected. Insufficient application of product to area if using spray-gun tanning, the pressure may have been too low or distance too far away. The addition of too much moisturiser to the tanning product during manual hand application technique.
- **Tan too dark**: incorrect colour shade selected. Incorrect formulation, percentage of DHA too high for skin colouring. If using spray-gun tanning the pressure used was too high or application distance too near the client.
- **Uneven application**: the client may have products on the skin which have not been effectively removed before tanning. Insufficient exfoliation and moisturising of the skin before service.
- **Incorrect application technique**: this must be methodical to avoid missing areas of skin. Excessively dry skin conditions can result in a patchy uneven result. Not allowing the skin to dry properly before dressing can result in removal of some of the product. There may be a problem with the quality of the product, if it happens again contact the supplier for guidance.
- **Tan corrector products**: used with leading tanning manufacturer products usually within five hours of application to correct streaking. Alternatively, an exfoliant may be used. Self-tan can be reapplied to the area to even the result, the application may be modified to create the necessary result, i.e. darker or lighter.
- **Orange or ashy cast to the skin**: caused by over-application or incorrect choice of formulation for the client's skin colour. There may be alkaline products on the skin which will create an orange colour to the skin.

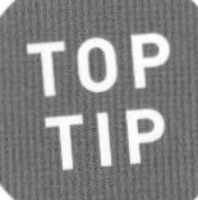

TOP TIP

Lightening the result

Moisturiser may be used to lighten the result for the areas: face, hairline, inner arm. underarm, hands, ankles, knees and feet.

TOP TIP

Removing unwanted product

Any product applied to unwanted areas should be removed with cotton wool during the application.

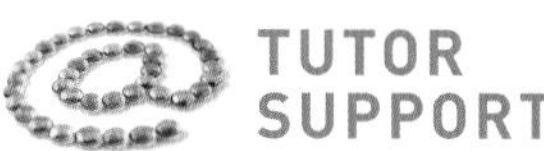

TUTOR SUPPORT

Activity 3: Self-tanning – comparison of costs

"Self-tan and gradual tan can stain blonde or bleached hair. Put a little extra moisturiser on the eyebrows and the hairline prior to application.

Tammy Baker

"Excellent customer service and product knowledge will result in an increase in sales revenue, repeat business and customer retention. With the ultimate consultation the customer/client will receive the correct advice to follow up any professional service with the best product choices and achieve the best results.

Tammy Baker

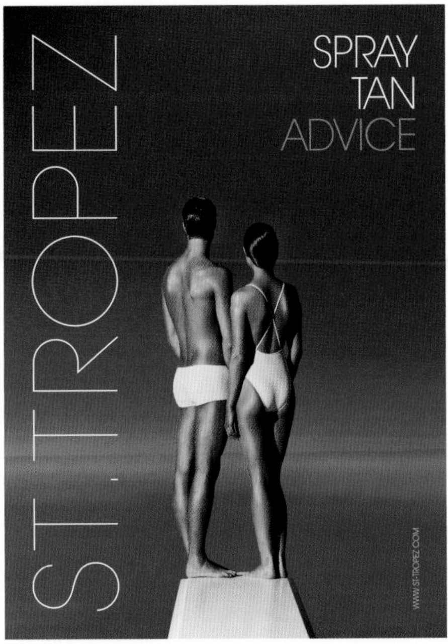

SPRAY TAN ADVICE

A St.Tropez Spray Tan Treatment gives you a fast, flawless tan in a controlled environment. Now with Aromaguard™ fragrance technology which eliminates the tell-tale self tan aroma by a minimum of 70%. The tan is applied and tailored by an expert and takes no more than 15 minutes. You need to allow some time to prepare and dress.

To ensure your tan is flawless and even, please follow this simple guide:

Before Treatment Advice

- It is preferable not to apply any type of perfume, deodorant or aromatherapy oils on the day of your treatment as these reduce the results.
- Waxing or shaving should be completed at least 24 hours prior to the treatment to reduce sensitivity.
- The evening before or morning of your treatment, exfoliate your entire body using St.Tropez Body Polish. Pay special attention to dry areas of your body such as hands, elbows, knees and feet.
- Wear dark, loose fitting clothing with a dark coloured bra or preferably no bra at all. Please be aware the guide colour can stain light hair, man-made fibres and wool.
- We recommend you have a patch test prior to every St.Tropez Spray Tan Treatment.

The Treatment

The application takes up to 15 minutes to cover the whole body. The Bronzing Mist will dry on your skin in just a few minutes so you can dress straight after the treatment. Avoid touching or rubbing the applied tan once the treatment is completed.

- For the short period that your face is sprayed, close your eyes and do not inhale. If you suffer from respiratory problems, please contact your doctor before having a treatment.

After Treatment Advice

Your tan will begin to develop immediately after your treatment.

- Do not shower or bathe for a minimum of 4 hours after your treatment.
- Do not participate in any activity which may cause perspiration for at least 12 hours after the treatment.
- It is fine to leave the guide colour on overnight and wash in the morning. Some guide colour may transfer to bed linen. This will wash out of cotton but not so easily from man-made fibres or wool.

Tan Maintenance Tips

With the correct aftercare your tan will last longer.

- Apply St.Tropez Body Moisturiser or NEW St.Tropez Body Butter daily in between self tan applications to maintain your tan for longer and to ensure even fading.
- Exfoliate your skin with St.Tropez Body Polish every 3 days to ensure your tan fades evenly.
- Do not rub, but pat your skin dry after showering or bathing.
- Avoid swimming pools as chlorine can bleach the tan.

WARNING St.Tropez products do not contain a sunscreen and do not protect against sunburn. Repeated exposure of unprotected skin while tanning may increase the risk of skin ageing, skin cancer and other harmful effects to the skin, even if you do not usually burn.

ST TROPEZ, THE SKIN FINISHING EXPERTS

Aftercare leaflet

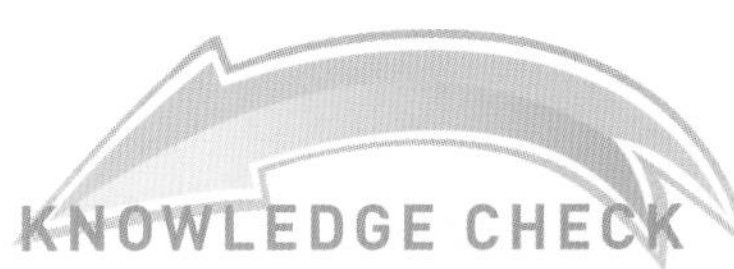

Describe three results that could occur if the client did not follow the pre- and post-treatment self-tanning instructions.

Need more time... refer to page 582 to help you.

Aftercare advice

- Details of the service should be entered on the record card, to include date, colour, result, any adverse skin reaction. To ensure effective tan development, avoid streaking and to maintain the result:
  - Avoid anything that will make you sweat immediately following service as this will dilute the product, disturb application affecting the finished effect. Therefore no strenuous exercise for approximately 6–8 hours.
  - Cosmetic products which remove the surface cells such as facial peeling masks should be avoided.
  - Avoid tight clothing or friction with any body part immediately following application to avoid product removal.
  - Do not bath/shower for at least 8 hours following service application. Care should be taken when washing the hands to avoid product removal following service.
  - Avoid chlorinated pools, excessive bathing and heat services such as sauna as they encourage fading. Avoid long baths and showers as they will encourage exfoliation.
  - On showering, excess self-tanning product will be removed making the water appear brown. The skin should be gently patted dry with a soft towel.
- Encourage the retail of self-tanning preparations. Tinted products are useful as this assists in even application. They often contain ingredients, such as vitamins and plant extracts, to keep the skin moisturised.
- Other relevant products are exfoliators, which can be used between services as advised by the beauty therapist and to prepare the skin for future self-tan applications. These must be used cautiously as they will reduce the life of the tan if used incorrectly or too often.

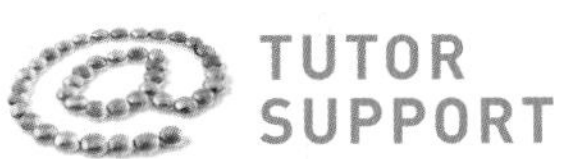

Activity 5: Self-tanning promotional leaflet

TOP TIP

Retail opportunities

Many self-tanning product suppliers have extensive retail ranges to care for and enhance the tanned skin.

TOP TIP

Oily skin

The result will be better on a client with an oily skin, however, all skin will require moisturising to avoid dry, uneven, flaky patches, resulting in uneven desquamation.

- Moisturiser should be applied daily to prevent the skin becoming dry and to keep the skin hydrated. Avoid the use of AHA products, which will encourage skin removal and loss of skin colour.
- Encourage the client to use a tan enhancer to maintain and enhance the result.
- If a contra-action occurs, follow advice provided and contact the salon for professional advice.
- Encourage a repeat appointment booking, usually every two weeks as the tan fades. A client, however, requiring a deeper tan could return in 48 hours for a second application if suitable.
- Sun protection is necessary on exposure to UV.

> The tan will not deepen the longer it is left on. Once it has been left on for the required amount of time, generally 4–12 hours, it will have developed into a natural looking golden tan. For a deeper tan you should re-apply on 2 successive days which is known as a 'Double Dip' and will result in a really deep, rich bronze tan.
>
> **Tammy Baker**

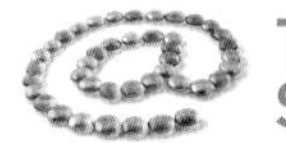

TUTOR SUPPORT

Activity 6: Re-cap, Revision and Evaluation (RRE sheet)

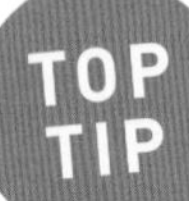

TOP TIP

Tan enhancer

The use of tan enhancer will extend the life of the tan as it will keep the skin moisturised and has a small amount of self-tan in its formulation.

GLOSSARY OF KEY WORDS

Compressor a piece of equipment used to compress air. The air pressure is then regulated by the attachment of a regulator. It is used in the application of make-up, nail art, airbrushing and self-tan.

Control of Substances Hazardous to Health Regulations (2002) these regulations require employers to identify all hazardous substances used in the workplace and state how they should be stored and handled.

Dihydroxyacetone (DHA) the active ingredient in self-tan products. A colourless sugar which reacts with amino acids in the skin creating the pigmented look.

Erythema reddening of the skin.

Exfoliation a cosmetic service used to remove dead skin cells from the skin's surface and accelerate the process of natural skin loss – called desquamation.

Faux tan alternative term for fake tan.

Health and Safety at Work Act (1974) legislation which lays down the minimum standards of health, safety and welfare requirements in each area of the workplace.

Management of Health and Safety at Work Regulations (1999) this legislation requires the employer to make formal arrangements for maintaining a safe, secure working environment under the Health and Safety at Work Act. This includes staff training for competently monitoring risk in the workplace, known as a risk assessment.

Melanin a pigment in the skin and hair created by cells called melanocytes. Melanin contributes to the colour of the skin and hair and helps to protect the lower layers of skin from ultra-violet damage.

PSI Pounds per square inch. Often used in relation to spray-tan guns, meaning the pressure of the air generated by the compressor. This can usually be adjusted to created the required result.

Self-tan products cosmetic products containing an ingredient which gives a healthy, tanned appearance to the skin. Different methods can be used to apply self-tan products including spray, manual and airbrush application.

Spray-gun equipment used to apply liquid self-tanning product to the skin.

Workplace (Health, Safety and Welfare) Regulations (1992) these regulations ensure the workplace is a safe, healthy and secure working environment meeting the needs of all employees.

ASSESSMENT OF KNOWLEDGE AND UNDERSTANDING

You have now learnt about the knowledge and skills for applying skin tanning techniques treatment for the beauty therapy workplace. To test your level of knowledge, answer the following short questions. These will prepare you for your summative (final) assessment.

1. The active ingredient in self-tan products is:
   a. amino acetone
   b. hydroxydiacetone
   c. dihydroxyacetone
   d. diacetone–hydroxide
2. The active ingredient in self-tan product is a sugar that reacts with:
   a. amino acids (proteins) in the stratum granulosum
   b. fatty acids in the stratum lucidum
   c. glucose in the stratum spinosum
   d. amino acids (proteins) in the stratum corneum
3. If a client is fair skinned choose a product with:
   a. a higher percentage of DHA
   b. no DHA in it at all
   c. a lower percentage of DHA
   d. the very strongest DHA percentage available
4. The skin condition which is unsuitable for self-tanning as the skin lacks pigment is called:
   a. ephelides
   b. vitiligo
   c. dermatitis
   d. leuconychia
5. A self-tan service/treatment can be carried out immediately after:
   a. micro-dermabrasion
   b. waxing
   c. electrical epilation
   d. none of the above
6. To lighten the tanning effect, mix the self-tanning product with a small amount if recommended:
   a. cleanser
   b. moisturiser
   c. massage cream
   d. witch hazel
7. Which health and safety legislation should be considered when applying self tanning techniques?
   a. Health and Safety at Work Act (1974)
   b. Control of Substances Hazardous to Health Regulations (2002)
   c. Workplace (Health Safety and Welfare) Regulations (1992)
   d. all of the above
8. What time intervals would you advise a client between each self-tanning treatment?
   a. every 5 days
   b. every 7 days
   c. every 10 days
   d. every month
9. The skin must be exfoliated to remove dead skin cells before the tanning treatment. Which epidermal layer are the cells removed from?
   a. stratum corneum
   b. stratum lucidum
   c. stratum granulosum
   d. subcutaneous layer
10. Melanin is the skin's natural pigment, exposure to ultra-violet stimulates the following cells to produce melanin as a protective function:
    a. erythrocytes
    b. leucocytes
    c. melanocytes
    d. pheo-melanin

Glossary

Accident book health and safety legislation requires that a written record is kept of any reportable injury, disease or dangerous occurrence in the workplace. This can be recorded in an accident book. Incidents in the accident book should be reviewed to see where improvements to safe working practice could be made.

Accident form a detailed report form to be completed following any accident in the workplace.

Acetone a solvent commonly used as a tip remover and nail varnish remover.

Acid mantle the combination of sweat and sebum on the skin's surface, creating an acid film. The acid mantle is protective and discourages the growth of bacteria and fungi. The pH scale is used to measure the acidity or alkalinity of a substance using a numbered scale. The skin's pH is acid at 5.5-5.6.

Additional products and services products and services offered by your workplace which a client may receive or purchase to enhance their service or treatment benefits.

Adhesive a chemical compound used to stick two surfaces together, such as the glue used to attach artificial eyelashes to the natural lashes or the glue used to attached nail tips to the natural nail.

Aftercare advice recommendations given to the client following a service to maintain the finished result and enable the benefits to be continued at home.

After-wax lotion a product applied to the skin following hair removal to reduce redness and promote skin healing.

Age groups the different classification of age groups to be covered e.g. 16–30, 31–50 and over 50 years.

Allergic reaction the reaction of the body to a substance or material that could be harmful or that the body has developed a sensitivity to. It produces symptoms including erythema, swelling, itching and bruising.

Anagen the active growth stage of the hair growth cycle.

Antioxidant a molecule found in some foods that maintains the health of the skin by fighting the damaging effects of free radicals (unstable molecules which can cause skin cells to degenerate). Antioxidant ingredients are increasingly being included in skincare preparations to neutralize free radicals or repel them from the skin.

Antiseptic a chemical agent that prevents the multiplication of microorganisms. It has limited action and does not kill all microorganisms.

Apocrine gland sweat gland found in the armpit, nipple and groin area. Larger than the eccrine sweat gland and attached to the hair follicle. These sweat glands are controlled by hormones and become active at puberty.

Appointment an arrangement made for a client to receive a service on a particular date and time.

Arrector pili muscle a small muscle attached to the hair follicle and base of the epidermis. When the muscle contracts (shortens) it causes the hair to stand upright in the hair follicle.

Artificial lashes threads of nylon fibre which are attached to the natural hair. These are referred to as strip lashes, individual artificial lashes or single lash extensions.

Aseptic the process of implementing disinfection and sterilization procedures to prevent contamination of tools and equipment which could lead to cross-infection.

Assistance the act of providing help or support.

Autoclave an effective method of sterilization, suitable for small metal objects and beauty therapy tools. Water is boiled under increased pressure and reaches temperatures of 121–134°C.

Ayuveda (art of life) a sacred Hindu text written around 1800BC. In Avuyeda life consists of body, mind and spirit – each person is different. By restoring balance and harmony of the body, mind and spirit, the health of the individual improves.

Bacteria minute, single-celled organisms of various shapes. Large numbers live on the skin's surface and are not harmful (they are non-pathogenic); others, however, are harmful (pathogenic) and can cause disease.

Base coat a nail polish product applied to protect the natural nail and prevent staining from coloured nail polish.

Behaviour this refers to how we conduct ourselves in the workplace. It is important to be polite and friendly at all times, work cooperatively with others and conform with all workplace policies and procedures.

Benefit the gain to be made from using a product or service.

Bevelling a nail filing technique used at the free edge of the nail to ensure it is smooth.

Blepharitis inflammation of the eyelid caused by an infection or an allergic reaction.

Blood nutritive liquid circulating through the blood vessels. It transports essential nutrients and other important substances, such as oxygen and hormones, and removes waste products.

Blood vessel part of the circulatory system that carries blood around the body. There are three main types of blood vessel; arteries, veins and capillaries, which differ in their structure and role in blood transportation.

Blue nail nail condition where the nail bed has a blue tinge rather than a healthy pink colour due to poor blood circulation in the area.

Blusher a make-up product applied to add warmth to the face and emphasize the facial contours and draw attention to the cheekbones.

Body language communication involving the body rather than speech, including facial expressions and hand gestures.

Bone a specialized form of connective, structural tissue that supports, surrounds and connects different parts of the body. Bones support and protect the underlying structures, give shape to the body and provide an attachment point for muscles.

Bones of the chest a group of bones, including the sternum and the ribs, that protect the inner organs and provide a surface for muscle attachment that allows movement.

Bones of the foot and lower leg these include the tarsals, metatarsals and phalanxes in the foot and the tibia and fibula in the lower leg.

Bones of the lower arm and hand these include the carpals, metacarpals and phalanges in the hand and the radius and ulna in the lower arm.

Bones of the neck a group of bones that support the skull and form the neck. The bones in the neck include the cervical vertebrae.

Bronzing products make-up products applied to create a healthy, natural or subtle tanned look. They are formulated to create a matt or shimmer effect and are also suitable as a highlighting contouring product.

Bruised nail a nail condition where the nail appears blue/black in colour where bleeding has occurred on the nail bed following injury.

Buffer a manicure tool with a pad with a replaceable cover, used on the nail to give a sheen, increase blood supply to the area and, if used with the gritty cream buffing paste, to help smooth out nail surface irregularities.

Bunion a foot condition. The large joint at the base of the big toe protrudes, forcing the big toe inwards towards the other toes.

Burn injury to the skin caused by excess heat; the skin appears red and may blister.

'C' curve the curve of the nail from side wall to side wall.

Callus a foot condition, displaying thick, yellowish hardened skin, usually found on prominent areas of the foot such as the heel.

Camouflage products cosmetic make-up products designed to conceal skin imperfections including creams, powders and setting products for the face and body.

Catagen the stage of the hair growth cycle where the hair becomes detached from its source of nourishment, the dermal papilla, and stops growing.

Catalyst a substance that causes or accelerates a chemical reaction.

Cell basic units of life which specialize in carrying out particular functions in the body. Groups of cells which share function, shape, size or structure are called tissues. The human body consists of trillions of cells.

Certificate of registration awarded when the premises have been successfully inspected to ensure that the local bye-laws are being followed in relation to cosmetic piercing.

Charge card an alternative form of payment where the complete amount of credit spent must be repaid by the cardholder each month to the card company.

Chemical reaction the process of two or more chemicals combining to create a different substance.

Cheque an alternative form of payment to that of using cash. A cheque must be accompanied by a cheque guarantee card.

Chilblains poor blood supply where the toes become red, blue or purple in colour and the area may become painful and itchy; aggravated in cold weather.

Chiropodist a person who is trained and qualified to treat minor foot complaints.

Circulatory system the system that controls blood and lymph flow and transports material around the body. It supplies cells with oxygen and nutrients and carries away waste products.

Cleanser a skincare preparation that removes dead skin cells, excess sweat and sebum, make-up and dirt from the skin's surface to maintain a healthy skin complexion. These are formulated to treat the different skin types, skin characteristics and facial areas.

Client record cards confidential cards recording the personal details of each client registered at the business. This information may be stored electronically on the salon's computer.

Clinical waste waste from ear-piercing is classed as clinical waste. The disposal of clinical waste is controlled by the Environment Agency. Waste materials that have come into contact with body fluids must be collected and disposed of by special arrangements. The Environment Protection Act (1990): Waste Management: The Duty of Care, A Code of Practice (ISBN 011 752577 X) provides further information on this subject.

Code of conduct workplace service standards with regard to appearance and behaviour while in the working environment.

Code of practice the expected standards and behaviour for the professional beauty therapist to follow, which will uphold the reputation of the industry and ensure best working practice for the industry and protect members of the public.

Beauty therapy professional bodies produce codes of practice for their members. A business may have its own code of practice.

Cold wax a wax already applied to a strip and ready for use. The pre-coated strip is applied firmly to the skin and then removed quickly against hair growth, removing the hair in the area.

Collagen a protein fibre found in the dermis of the skin that provides strength to the skin and other types of connective tissue.

Colour corrector a make-up product applied to target problem areas. It contains pigments which balance skin tone.

Colouring characteristics identified through consultation with the client and by examining the client's natural hair colouring (e.g. fair, red, dark or white) to determine the correct service plan e.g. selecting the appropriate tint colour for permanent tinting treatment.

Comedone removal facial techniques used to extract comedones (blackheads) from the skin. A small tool called a comedone extractor is used for this purpose.

Communication the exchange of information and the establishment of understanding between people.

Complaints procedure a formal, standardized approach adopted by the organization to handle any complaints.

Compressor a piece of equipment used to compress air. The air pressure is then regulated by the attachment of a regulator. It is used in the application of make-up, nail art, airbrushing and self-tan.

Concealer cosmetic product used to disguise minor skin imperfections such as blemishes, uneven skin colour or shadows.

Confidentiality keeping information or data private. In order to gain trust between yourself and your client it is important to keep client information confidential. This may also be a legal requirement stipulated by the Data Protection Act.

Conjunctivitis a bacterial infection. Inflammation of the mucous membrane that covers the eye and lines the eyelid. The skin of the inner conjunctiva of the eye becomes inflamed, the eye becomes very red, itchy and sore, and pus may exude from the eye area.

Consent form written permission obtained from a parent or guardian to perform a service on a minor.

Consultation assessment of client needs using different assessment techniques including questioning and natural observation.

Consultation techniques methods used to identify the client's needs using differing assessment techniques, including questioning, manual and natural observation.

Consumer Protection Act (1987) this act follows European Union directives to protect the customer from unsafe, defective services and products that do not reach safety standards.

Consumer Protection (Distance Selling) Regulations (2000) these Regulations as amended by the Consumer Protection (Distance Selling) (Amendment) Regulations (2005), are derived from a European Union directive and cover the supply of goods/services made between suppliers acting in a commercial capacity and consumers. They are concerned with purchases made by telephone, fax, internet, digital television and mail order.

Consumer Safety Act (1978) this act aims to reduce risks to consumers from potentially dangerous products.

Contact dermatitis a skin disorder caused by intolerance of the skin to a particular substance, or a group of substances. On exposure to the substance the skin quickly becomes irritated and an allergic reaction occurs.

Continuous professional development (CPD) activities undertaken to develop technical skill and expertise to ensure current, professional experience in the beauty industry is maintained.

Contour cosmetics make-up products applied to change the shape of the face and the facial features. These cosmetics draw attention either towards or away from the shape of the face or specific facial features, helping to create the optical illusion of balance and perfection.

Contra-action an adverse or unwanted reaction occurring during or after service application.

Contra-action advice recommended action to be taken to correct an adverse or unwanted reaction.

Contra-indication a problematic symptom that indicates that the service may not proceed or may restrict service application.

Control of risk the means by which risks identified are removed or reduced to acceptable levels.

Control of Substances Hazardous to Health (COSHH) Regulations (2002) (including Biological Agents Regulations) legislation that requires employers and the self-employed prevent or control the exposure of employees and clients to hazardous substances.

Controlled Waste Regulations (1992) categorizes waste types. The Local Authority provides advice on how to dispose of waste types in compliance with the law.

Corn a small area of thickened skin on the foot. Often white in appearance.

Corrosive a substance capable of causing rapid and sometimes irreversible damage to human tissue or other surfaces.

Cortex the thickest layer of the hair structure.

Cosmetic Products (Safety) Regulations (2008) part of consumer protection legislation that requires that cosmetics and toiletries are safe in their formulation and are safe for use for their intended purpose as a cosmetic and comply with labelling requirements.

Credit card an alternative form of payment to that of using cash. These cards are held by those who have a credit account, where there is a pre-arranged borrowing limit. These can only be used if your business has an arrangement to deal with the relevant credit card company.

Cross contamination transfer of an infection directly from one person to another or indirectly from one person to a second person via an object.

Cross-infection the transfer of contagious microorganisms by direct contact with another person or indirectly by contact with an infected object.

Cure an another word for polymerization; when a liquid turns into a solid structure.

Curing the process of polymerization.

Customer care statement defined customer service standards that are expected.

Cuticle (hair) the protective outer layer of the hair composed of thin, unpigmented, flat, scale-like cells. These cells contain hard keratin and overlap each other from the base to the tip of the hair.

Cuticle (nail) The overlapping epidermis around and extending onto the base of the nail, developing from the stratum corneum.

Cuticle cream or oil a cosmetic preparation used to condition the skin of the cuticle.

Cuticle knife a metal tool used on the nail to remove excess eponychium and perionychium (the extension of the skin of the cuticle at the base of the nail).

Cuticle nippers a metal tool used to remove excess cuticle and neaten the skin around the cuticle area.

Cuticle remover a cosmetic preparation used to soften and loosen the skin cells and cuticle from the nail.

Cyclical pattern of growth the hair growth cycle, which can be divided into three phases: anagen, catagen and telegen.

Cyst a localized pocket of sebum that forms in the hair follicle or under the sebaceous glands in the skin. Semi-globular in shape, either raised or flat, and hard or soft. Cysts are the same colour as the skin, or red if bacterial infection occurs.

Dangerous Substances and Preparations (Nickel) (Safety) Regulations (2005) the use of nickel has been found to cause allergies. Check what metal is used for your supplier's ear-piercing jewellery and that it complies with the regulations.

Data Protection Act (1998) legislation designed to protect client privacy and confidentiality.

Debit card a method of payment where the card authorizes immediate transfer of the cash amount from the client's account.

Dehydrate to remove water from the surface of the natural nail plate.

Dermal papilla an organ that provides the hair follicle with blood, necessary for hair growth.

Dermatitis an inflammatory skin disorder where the skin becomes red, itchy and swollen.

Dermis the inner portion of skin situated underneath the epidermis.

Diabetes a disease that prevents sufferers breaking down glucose in their cells. Insulin, a hormone produced by the pancreas organ, is not produced in sufficient quantities to regulate the sugars and carbohydrates, resulting in excess sugar in the blood.

Dihydroxyacetone (DHA) the active ingredient in self-tan products. A colourless sugar which reacts with amino acids in the skin creating the pigmented look.

Disability Discrimination Act (1996) implemented to prevent disabled persons being discriminated against. Employers have a responsibility to remove physical barriers and to adjust working conditions to prevent discrimination on the basis of having a disability.

Discrepancy a disagreement over amounts of money etc. This is referred to in instances where a client disagrees with what they are being asked to pay or the amount of change received.

Disinfectant a chemical agent that destroys most microorganisms.

Disposable applicator a piece of equipment used to apply wax hygienically to the area of hair removal without contaminating the wax flowing back into the tube following application. The applicator head is disposed of after each treatment.

Ear the external or outer part of the ear collects sound waves and directs these to the inner ear. This part of the ear that stands out at the side of the head is called the pinna, which comprizes of the helix and lobule.

Ear piercing the perforation of the skin and underlying tissue of the earlobe to create a hole in the skin where jewellery is inserted.

Eccrine gland simple sweat producing gland responsive to heat, appearing as tiny tubes which are straight in the epidermis, and coiled in the dermis. Its function is to maintain the body temperature by sweating.

Eczema a skin condition which appears as a reddening of the skin accompanied by itching and sometimes blisters. The blisters can leak tissue fluid which later hardens, forming scabs.

Eczema of the nail a skin condition affecting the nail, resulting in changes to the nail including ridges, pitting, nail separation and nail thickening.

Effleurage a stroking massage manipulation used to begin the massage, as a link manipulation, and to complete the massage sequence. Applied in a rhythmic, continuous manner, it induces relaxation.

Eggshell nail a nail condition where thin, fragile white nails curve under at the free edge.

Elastin a protein fibre found in the dermis of the skin that helps the skin maintain its elastic properties and return to shape.

Electricity at Work Regulations (1989) these regulations state that electrical equipment in the workplace should be tested every 12 months, by a qualified electrician. The employer must keep records of the equipment tested and the date it was checked.

Emery board a nail file used to shape the free edge of the nail.

Employers' Liability (Compulsory Insurance) Act (1969) this provides financial compensation to an employee should they be injured as a result of an accident in the workplace. A certificate indicating that a policy of insurance has been purchased should be displayed.

Enquiries questions presented by clients or business contacts to find out more information.

Environmental conditions this includes heating, lighting, ventilation and general comfort requirements for the workplace or service.

Epidermis the outer layer of the skin located directly above the dermis. The epidermis is composed of five layers with the surface layer forming the outer skin which has a protective function.

Equal opportunity non-discrimination on the basis of sex, race, disability, age, etc.

Equipment and tools used within a service that enable the service to be completed competently.

Erythema reddening of the skin, caused by increased blood circulation to the area.

Evaluation method used which measures the value of the instructional activity.

Exfoliant a service used to remove excess dead skin cells from the surface of the skin, which has a skin cleansing, cell rejuvenating action. This process can be achieved using a specialized cosmetic, or mechanically by using facial equipment where a brush is rotated over the skin's surface.

Exfoliation a cosmetic service used to remove dead skin cells from the skin's surface and accelerate the process of natural skin loss – called desquamation.

External ear structure the visible, outer part of the ear which funnels sound waves into the ear to enable hearing. It comprises the pinna, lobe, cartilage and cartilaginous tissue.

Eye shadow a cosmetic product applied to the eye to complement the natural eye colour, to give definition to the eye area and enhance the natural shape of the eye.

Eyebrow colour a cosmetic product applied to emphasize the eyebrows, alter their shape, and which can make sparse eyebrows look thicker.

Eyebrow shaping the removal of eyebrow hair to create a new shape (reshape) or to remove stray hairs to maintain the existing brow shape (maintenance). Shaping treatments can be performed with tweezers, threading or waxing, or a combination of techniques.

Eyelash adhesive a specialized glue used to apply artificial strip eyelashes and individual artificial eyelashes to the natural eyelashes.

Eyelash and eyebrow tinting the permanent colouring of the eyelash or eyebrow hair to enhance and define their appearance by applying specialized dye formulated for use around the delicate eye area.

Eyelash curlers small flexible rods around which the natural eyelashes are curled during eyelash perming treatment.

Eyelash perming a chemical treatment applied to the eyelashes to permanently curl the lashes, enhancing the appearance of the eyes.

Eyeliner a cosmetic product applied to define and emphasize the eyelid area directly above or below the eyelash hair.

Face shape the size and shape of the facial bone structure. Face shapes include oval, round, square, heart, diamond, oblong and pear.

Facial a service to improve the appearance, condition and functioning of the skin and underlying structures.

Facial bones a type of connective tissue forming a hard structure that forms the face and forms an attachment point for muscles. These include the zygomatic, mandible, maxilla, nasal, vomer, turbinate, lacrimal and palatine.

Facial features the size of a person's nose, eyes, forehead, chin, neck, etc. When applying make-up products, make-up application can emphasize or minimize the appearance of facial features.

Facial products skincare used with a facial service which have specific benefits to care for and improve the function and appearance of the skin.

False eyelashes threads of nylon fibre or real hair attached to the natural eyelash hair. There are two main types: individual or strip.

Faux tan alternative term for fake tan.

Feature a unique or defining characteristic of a product or service.

Fibre a nail enhancement system that combines a fibre with resin to create an artificial nail overlay.

Fibre mesh usually silk or fibreglass 'fabric' used in the fibre overlay system to provide strength.

File used to shape the free edge of the nail.

Fire Precautions Act (1971) legislation that states that all staff must be familiar with, and trained in fire, and emergency evacuation procedures for their workplace.

Fitzpatrick Classification System a scale developed to assess the amount of melanin pigment in the skin providing your skin colour and how your skin will react to sun without protection (photo-sensitivity). There are six skin type classifications from Caucasian (skin type I) to African-Caribbean (skin type VI).

Foiling a technique used in nail art that uses a foil to decorate the nails.

Folliculitis a bacterial infection where pustules develop in the skin tissue around the hair follicle.

Foot and nail services specialized products and equipment designed to improve the condition and appearance of different nail and skin conditions.

Foot cream lotion/oil a cosmetic mixture of waxes and oils applied to soften the skin of the feet and cuticles.

Foot rasp a pedicure tool used to remove excess dead skin from the foot.

Foot spa a foot bath incorporating massage and water aeration, creating a bubbling effect to cleanse and relax the feet.

Foundation a make-up product applied to produce an even skin tone, to disguise minor skin blemishes and as a contour cosmetic.

Free edge the part of the nail plate that extends past the end of the finger.

Frictions massage technique using small circular massage movements using the pads of the fingers or thumbs. The skin and muscle below is massaged against the underlying bone. This can be used to loosen any adhesions in the tissues.

Fungus (fungi) a microorganism that can cause fungal diseases of the skin and feed off the waste products of the skin. They are found on the skin's surface or they can attack deeper tissues.

Gel a thickened liquid used as part of the UV gel system to create an artificial nail overlay.

Gift voucher a pre-payment method for beauty therapy services or retail sales.

Greater London Council (General Powers) Act (1981) this act covers the London boroughs and relates to cosmetic piercing. It provides that no person can carry out cosmetic piercing unless they and the business are registered. It also states what records are required to be kept.

Grievance a cause for concern or complaint.

Grit the measure of abrasiveness of nail files and buffers. The higher the number, the finer the abrasive. A level of no less than 240 grit should be used on the natural nail.

Habia the Hairdressing and Beauty Industry Authority; the government appointed standards setting organization for the hair and beauty sector.

Hair a long slender structure that grows out of, and is part of the skin. Each hair is made up of dead skin cells, which contain the protein called keratin.

Hair follicle an appendage (structure) in the skin formed from epidermal tissue. Cells move up the hair follicle from the bottom (the hair bulb), changing in structure, to form the hair.

Hair growth cycle the cyclical pattern of hair growth, which can be divided into three phases: anagen, catagen and telogen.

Hair shaft the part of the hair that can be seen above the skin's surface, extending from the hair follicle.

Hairy moles moles exhibiting coarse hairs from their surface.

Hand and nail treatments specialized products and equipment designed to improve the condition and appearance of different nail and skin conditions.

Hand cream/oil a cosmetic mixture of waxes and oils applied to soften the skin of the hands and cuticles.

Hand technique threading hair removal using thread held and looped between both hands. This technique is also known as cat's cradle, double looped or self technique.

Hangnail nail condition where small pieces of epidermal skin protrude between the nail plate and nail wall, accompanying a dry cuticle condition.

Hazard a hazard is something with potential to cause harm.

Health and Safety (Display Screen Equipment) Regulations (1992) these regulations cover the use of visual display units (VDUs) and computer screens. They specify acceptable levels of radiation emissions from the screen and identify correct working posture, seating position, permitted working heights and rest periods.

Health and Safety (First Aid) Regulations (1981) legislation that states that workplaces must have appropriate and adequate first aid provision.

Health and Safety at Work Act (1974) legislation that lays down the minimum standards of health safety and welfare requirements in all workplaces.

Health and Safety policy each employer of more than five employees must have a written health and safety policy issued to their employees outlining their health and safety responsibilities.

Heat rash a reaction to heat exposure where the sweat ducts become blocked and sweat escapes into the epidermis. Red pimples occur and the skin becomes itchy.

Highlighter a make-up product that draws attention to and emphasizes features.

Histamine a chemical released when the skin comes into contact with a substance that it is allergic to. Cells called 'mast cells' burst, releasing histamine into the tissues. This causes the blood capillaries to dilate, which increases blood flow to limit skin damage and begin repair.

Hoof stick a nail tool used to gently push back the softened cuticles.

Hospitality this covers welcoming the client, being helpful and offering refreshments and magazines, and ensuring the client is comfortable while at reception.

Hot wax a system of wax depilation used to remove hair from the skin. Hot wax cools and sets on contact with the skin. They are a blend of waxes, such as beeswax and resins, which keep the wax flexible. Soothing ingredients are often included to avoid skin irritation.

Hydrogen peroxide (H_2O_2) an oxidant, a chemical that contains available oxygen atoms and encourages chemical reactions.

Hygiene requirements the expected standards as required by law, industry codes of practice or written procedures specified by the workplace.

Hyperpigmentation increased pigment production.

Hypopigmentation loss of pigmentation.

Induction an introductory activity delivered when you start or progress into a new job role. Its aim is to provide you with general and essential information related to the work environment, welfare and your job roles and responsibilities.

Industry Code of Practice a set of guidelines written by the industry to provide a framework for good practice and minimum standards.

Infection the communication of disease from one body to another. An infection is the colonization of a host organism by parasite species. If a client has an infection, do not treat the client.

Infestation a condition where animal parasites live off and invade a host.

Infill a maintenance treatment than compensates for the natural nail growth after the application of artificial nails.

Ingestion one of the main routes of entry into the body; that is via the mouth.

Ingrowing hair a build-up of skin occurs over the hair follicle, causing the hair to grow under the skin.

Ingrowing toenails nail condition where the side of the nail penetrates the nail wall; redness, inflammation and pus may be present.

Inhalation one of the main routes of entry into the body; that is via the lungs.

Irritant substances capable of causing inflammation of the skin, eyes, nose, throat or lungs.

Job description written details of a person's specific work role, duties and responsibilities.

Joint manipulations massage technique where the joints of the hand are manipulated through their range of movement dependant upon the type of joint.

Keloids overgrowths of scar tissue, occurring at the site of the ear-piercing.

Keratin a protein produced by cells in the epidermis called keratinocytes. Keratin makes the skin tough and reduces the passage of substances into our bodies. Each hair and nail contains keratin.

Laser hair removal a technique of permanent hair removal. Laser energy is passed through the skin which stops the activity of the hair follicle creating hair growth through a process called photothermolysis.

Legislation laws affecting the beauty therapy business relating to products and services, the business premises and environmental conditions, working practices and those employed.

Leuconychia nail condition where white spots or marks appear on the nail plate.

Lifting the separation of an artificial nail from the nail plate.

Limits of own authority the extent of your responsibility as determined by your own job description and workplace policies.

Lip balm a lip moisturiser which may contain pigment.

Lip gloss cosmetic applied to the lips to provide a moist, shiny look.

Lip liner cosmetic used to define the lips, creating a perfectly symmetrical outline.

Lip stain make-up product which adds intense colour to the lips.

Lipstick cosmetic applied to the lips to add colour and keep the lips soft and supple.

Liquid and powder a nail enhancement system that combines a liquid monomer with a powder polymer to create an artificial nail overlay.

Local Government (Miscellaneous Provisions) Act (1982) legislation that requires that salons offering any form of skin piercing be registered with the local health authority. This registration includes both the operators who will be carrying out the service and the salon premises where the service will be carried out.

Local Government Act (2003) (section 120 and schedule 6) an amendment to the Local Government (Miscellaneous Provisions) Act (1982) to enable each authority to regulate businesses providing cosmetic body piercing. Each local authority can introduce its own bye-laws to set the standards for cosmetic piercing.

London Local Authorities Act (1991 and 2007) this act states that no person shall carry out cosmetic piercing at an establishment without obtaining a licence from a participating council. Conditions can be attached to the licence, such as hygiene practices, age restrictions, etc.

Longitudinal ridges nail condition where grooves appear in the nail plate, running along the length of the nail from the cuticle to the free edge.

Lower arch the curve of the lower part of the free edge when viewed from the side.

Lymph a clear, straw-coloured liquid circulating in the lymph vessels and lymphatics of the body, filtered out of the blood plasma.

Lymph vessel referred to as lymphatics. They transport lymph a watery fluid that flows through the lymphatic system from the tissues to the blood.

Lymphatic system closely connected to the blood system. Its primary function is defensive: to remove bacteria and foreign materials to prevent infection.

Make-up cosmetics applied to the skin of the face to enhance and accentuate, or to minimize facial features. Make-up products create balance in the face.

Make-up products different cosmetics available to suit skin type, colour and condition, i.e. sensitive or mature. Make-up products include concealing and contour cosmetics, foundations, translucent powders, eye shadows, eyeliners, brow liners, mascaras, lipsticks, lip glosses, lip liners, etc.

Management of Health and Safety at Work Regulations (1999) this legislation provides the employer with an approved code of practice for maintaining a safe, secure working environment.

Manicure a service to care for and improve the condition and appearance of the hands and nails.

Manual Handling Operations Regulations (1992) legislation that requires the employer to carry out a risk assessment of all activities undertaken which involve manual handling (lifting and moving objects).

Marbling a technique used in nail art that mixes two or more colours together to form a design feature.

Mascara cosmetic that enhances the natural eyelashes, making them appear longer, changed in colour and/or thicker.

Mask a service mask applied to the skin of the feet to treat and improve the condition of the skin; this may include stimulating, rejuvenating or moisturising properties.

Massage manipulation of the soft tissues of the body, producing heat and stimulating the muscular, circulatory and nervous systems.

Massage manipulations movements which are selected and applied according to the desired effect, and which may be stimulating, relaxing or toning. Massage manipulations include effleurage, petrissage, percussion (also known as tapotement) and vibrations.

Massage medium a skincare product which acts as a lubricant to allow sufficient slip over the skin's surface while performing massage.

Melanin a pigment in the skin and hair created by cells called melanocytes. Melanin contributes to the colour of the skin and hair and helps to protect the lower layers of skin from ultra-violet damage.

Melanocytes cells that produce the skin pigment melanin that contributes to skin and hair colour.

Messages communication of information to another person in written, electronic or verbal form.

Method of payment different forms of payment that may be accepted to pay for a product or service including cash, cash equivalents, cheque and payment cards.

Milium extraction skincare technique used to extract milia (whiteheads) from the skin. A small tool called a milia extractor is used for this purpose, which superficially pierces the epidermis, allowing effective removal of the milia.

Mineral make-up created from finely ground minerals (a process called micronization). It is used in the formulation of different make-up products.

Minor a person classed as a child who requires by law to have a guardian or parent present.

Moisturiser a skincare preparation whose formulation of oil and water helps maintain the skin's natural moisture by locking moisture into the skin, offering protection and hydration. The formulation is selected to suit the skin type, facial characteristics and facial area.

Molecule an arrangement of two or more atoms to create specific chemical compound.

Monomer a chemical compound that can be bonded to other molecules to form a polymer.

Mood board a collation or collage of images which have inspired or instigated innovation and creativity used to express your overall ideas. A mood board may include objects such as photographs, fabric swatches, make-up colour samples or anything else that has progressed your ideas.

Mouth technique threading hair removal where one part of the thread is anchored in the mouth and the other part is looped in the hands.

Muscle contractile tissue responsible for movement of the body.

Muscle tone the normal degree of tension in healthy muscle.

Muscles of facial expression muscles which when contracted, pull the facial skin in a particular way and create facial expressions. These include the frontalis, corrugators, temporalis, orbicularis oculi, levator labii, orbicularis oris, buccinators, risorius, mentalis, zygomaticus, masseter, depressor labii.

Muscles of the foot and lower leg the muscles of the foot work together to help move the body. The foot is moved by muscles in the lower leg which pull on tendons that attach the muscle to the bone.

Muscles of the lower arm and hand the hands and fingers are moved by muscles and tendons. The muscles that bend the wrist in towards the forearm are flexors; the extensors straighten the wrist and hand.

Muscles of the upper body these move the arm and include pectoralis and deltoid.

Muscles that move the neck these include sternocleido mastoid, platysma, trapezius.

Nail the structure on the end of each finger and toe formed from hard, horny, epidermal cells that protect the living nail bed of the fingers and toes.

Nail art nail decoration using a variety of techniques and materials.

Nail art techniques application styles used to create different effects including dotting, striping, marbling, enamelling, foiling and blending.

Nail bed the area of skin that lies directly under the nail and is protected by the nail plate.

Nail finish the product finally applied to the natural nail to enhance its appearance, e.g. choice of polish application.

Nail growth cells divide in the matrix and the nails grow forward over the nail bed until they reach the end of the finger. The nail cells harden as they grow through a process called keratinization.

Nail plate a tough hard covering on top of the nail bed, composed of keratinized skin cells.

Nail polish a clear or coloured nail product that adds colour/protection to the nail. Cream polish has a matt finish and requires a top coat application. Pearlized polish produces a frosted, shimmery appearance and top coat is not required. Nail polish is also referred to as nail varnish and enamel.

Nail polish drier an aerosol or oil preparation applied following nail polish application to increase the speed at which the polish hardens.

Nail polish remover a solvent used to remove nail polish and grease from the nails prior to applying polish.

Nail polish solvent used to thin nail polish and restore its consistency.

Nail strengthener a nail polish product that strengthens the nail plate, which has a tendency to split.

Nail structure composed for protection the nail is made up of the following parts: nail plate, nail bed, matrix, cuticle, lunula, hyponychium, eponychium, nail wall, free edge, lateral nail fold.

Nail wrap an overlay applied to the natural nail; the fibre system is most commonly used.

National Occupational Standards for Beauty Therapy standards that set the relevant performance objectives, range statements and knowledge specifications to support performance. These can be obtained from the Hairdressing and Beauty Industry Authority (Habia) website: www.habia .org.uk.

Necessary action the action taken or service modification required to deal safely with a contra-action or contra-indication.

Neck technique threading hair removal where one part of the thread is anchored around the neck and the other part is looped in the hands.

Negative skin sensitivity test a test where result produces no skin reaction. in this case you may proceed with the service.

Nerve a collection of single neurones surrounded by a protective sheath through which impulses are transmitted between the brain or spinal cord and another part of the body.

Nervous system co-ordinates the activities of the body by responding to stimuli received by sense organs.

Neurones nerve cells which make up nervous tissue.

Non-verbal communication communicating using body language, i.e. using your eyes, face and body to transmit your feelings.

Nutrition the nourishment derived from food, required for the body's growth, energy, repair and production.

Oedema extra fluid in an area, causing swelling.

Oils oils selected to use with the head massage and applied to the scalp. Usually organic they are high in polyunsaturated fats which have healing benefits from their fatty acid, vitamin and nutrient content. They absorb easily through the skin, and can have an external and internal effect.

Onycholysis nail condition where the nail plate separates from the nail bed.

Onychophagy nail condition where a person bites their nails excessively.

Onychorrhexis nail condition where the person has split, flaking nails.

Orange stick a disposable wooden tool used around the cuticle and free edge of the nail and to apply products to the nail.

Organizational requirements beauty therapy procedures or work rules provided by the workplace management.

Overlay a coating applied to the natural nail or over a plastic tip that has been blended with the natural nail.

Painting techniques nail art techniques using specialized paints, tools and brushes to create different effects e.g. free hand, striping, dotting and marbling.

Paraffin wax this is heated and applied to the skin of the feet to provide a heating effect. This improves skin functioning, aids the absorption of service products and is beneficial to ease the discomfort of arthritic and rheumatic conditions.

Perm solution usually contains 6% thioglycollate, which when applied to eyelash hair softens and curls the hair into its new shape.

Paronychia bacterial infection where swelling, redness and pus appear in the cuticle area of the nail wall.

Pedicure a service to care for and improve the condition and appearance of the skin and nails of the feet.

Personal Protective Equipment (PPE) at Work Regulations (1992) this legislation requires employers to identify through risk assessment those activities that require special protective equipment to be worn.

Personal space the space around a person that they see as theirs. Invasion of this can make them feel uncomfortable.

Petrissage massage movements, including kneading, where the tissues are lifted away from the underlying structures and compressed. Pressure is intermittent, and should be light yet firm.

pH scale a scale from 0–14 used to measure the level of acidity or alkalinity of a substance. In the range of 0–6.9, the lower the pH value, the greater the acidity; 1 being the most acidic. In the range 7+, the greater the pH value, the greater the alkalinity; 14 being the most alkaline. A pH of 7 is neutral, meaning it is neither acid nor alkaline.

Phlebitis recognized by swelling and pain in the leg caused by inflammation of the vein wall (veins transport blood from the tissues back towards the heart).

Photoinitiator a substance that responds to specific types of light to start a chemical reaction e.g. UV light.

Photothermolysis an effect created when using a laser for hair removal. The melanin pigment that provides hair colour absorbs the laser energy, which is converted to heat, and at a sufficient temperature destroys the part of the hair follicle where the cells divide to create the hair.

Pigment the colour of skin and hair, called melanin. The amount of pigment varies for each client, resulting in different skin and hair colour.

Pilo-sebaceous unit the structure in the skin's epidermis and dermis consisting of the hair follicle and its associated sebaceous gland.

Polish secures accessorises in nail art that stick to the nail using nail polish.

Polymer a long chain or chemically bonded monomers e.g. the acrylics used in nail enhancement systems.

Polymerization the chemical reaction that creates polymer chains from monomer compounds.

Positive skin sensitivity test an allergic reaction to the skin test. The skin appears red, swollen and feels itchy.

Posture the position of the body, which varies from person to person. Good posture is when the body is in alignment. Correct posture enables you to work longer without becoming tired; it prevents muscle fatigue and stiff joints.

Powder cosmetic applied to set the foundation, disguise minor skin blemishes and make the skin appear smoother and oil-free.

Pre-wax lotion an antibacterial skin cleanser to clean the skin before wax application.

Prices Act (1974) this act states that the price of products has to be displayed in order to prevent the buyer being misguided.

Primer provides a base for make-up and acts as a barrier preventing absorption of the make-up products into the skin.

Promotion ways of communicating products or services to clients to increase sales.

Provision and Use of Work Equipment Regulations (PUWER) (1998) this regulation lays down important health and safety controls on the provision and use of equipment.

PSI pounds per square inch. Often used in relation to spray-tan guns, meaning the pressure of the air generated by the compressor. This can usually be adjusted to created the required result.

Psorasis an inflammatory, noncontagious skin disorder where there is an increased production of cells in the upper part of the skin, appearing as patches of itchy, red, flaky skin on the body.

Psoriasis of the nail an inflammatory condition where there is an increased production of cells in the upper part of the skin. Pitting occurs on the surface of the nail plate.

Pterygium nail condition where the cuticle is thickened and overgrown.

Public liability insurance protects employers and employees against the consequences of death or injury to a third party while on the premises.

Punctual arriving at the correct time.

Re-balance a maintenance treatment that corrects the position of the apex when it has moved because of natural nail growth.

Reception the area where clients are received.

Receptionist person responsible for maintaining the reception area, scheduling appointments and handling payments.

Record cards confidential cards recording the personal details of each client registered at the business. This information may be stored electronically on the salon's computer.

Regulatory Reform (Fire Safety) Order (2005) this legislation requires that the employer or designated 'responsible person' must carry out a risk assessment for the premises in relation to fire evacuation practice and procedures.

Relevant person the person (or persons) at work to whom you should report any issues which are not within the limits of your own authority e.g. manager, receptionist, senior therapist/nail technician, so they can resolve the problem.

Reporting of Injuries, Diseases and Dangerous Occurrences Regulations (RIDDOR) (1995) these regulations require the employer to notify the local enforcement officer in writing, in cases where employees or trainees suffer personal injury at work.

Resale Prices Acts (1964 and 1976) this act states that the manufacturer can supply a recommended price (MRRP), but the seller is not obliged to sell at the recommended price.

Resin in relation to nail enhancements, a type of cyanoacrylate used in the fibre nail enhancement system.

Resin activator in relation to nail enhancements, a product that speeds up the cure time of cyanoacrylate resin.

Resources the different products, equipment and other things needed to complete an activity.

Responsible persons this term is used in the Health and Safety unit to mean the person or persons at work to whom you should report any issues, problems or hazards. This could be a supervisor, line manager or your employer.

Restriction something that limits you. Certain contra-indications do not prevent a service completely but they restrict how the service is carried out.

Retail the selling of goods e.g. products for clients to use at home.

Ridge-filler a nail product used on ridged nails that improves the nail's appearance and provides a more even surface.

Risk the likelihood of a hazard's potential being recognized.

Roller wax a warm wax used to remove hair from the skin. The wax is contained in a cartridge container with a disposable applicator, which rolls the wax onto the skin's surface. The applicator is renewed for each client.

Sale and Supply of Goods Act (1994) goods must be as described, of merchantable, satisfactory quality and fit for their intended purpose.

Salon requirements workplace procedures that ensure the smooth running of the business and compliance with any legislation, codes of practices etc.

Salon services a general term, covering all of the treatments and services offered in a salon or workplace.

Scissors nail tools used to shorten the length of the nail before filing.

Sculptured nails artificial nails created by building the overlay onto the natural nail and extending it over a form rather than a plastic tip.

Sebaceous gland a minute sac-like organ usually associated with the hair follicle. The cells of the gland decompose and produce the skin's natural oil sebum. Found all over the body, except for the soles of the feet and the palms of the hands.

Sebum the skin's natural oil that keeps the skin supple.

Secondary infection bacterial penetration into the skin, causing infection.

Self-tan products cosmetic products containing an ingredient which gives a healthy, tanned appearance to the skin. Different methods can be used to apply self-tan products including spray, manual and airbrush application.

Sensitization the biological process of becoming sensitive to a substance that can then cause an allergic reaction.

Sensory nerve endings these nerves receive information and relay this to the brain. They are found near the skin's surface and respond to touch, pressure, temperature and pain.

Service/treatment plan after the consultation, suitable service objectives are established to treat the client's conditions and needs.

Shader a make-up product that draws attention away from and minimizes certain facial features.

Shoulder girdle bones a type of connective tissue that provides attachment for the muscles which move the arms, and includes the clavicle and scapula.

Skin allergy if the skin is sensitive to a particular substance, an allergic skin reaction will occur. This is recognized by irritation, swelling and inflammation.

Skin analysis assessment of the client's skin type and condition.

Skin appendages structures within the skin including sweat glands (that excrete sweat), hair follicles (that produce hair), sebaceous glands (produce the skin's natural oil, sebum) and nails (a horny substance that protects the ends of the fingers/toes).

Skin characteristics while looking at the skin type, additional characteristics may be seen. These include skin that may be sensitive, dehydrated, moist or oedematous (puffy), in addition to dry, oily or combination.

Skin condition while looking at the skin type, additional characteristics may be seen that indicate its condition. These include skin that may be sensitive, dehydrated or mature.

Skin removal accidental removal of the upper, dead, protective cornified layer of the skin, leaving the granular layer exposed.

Skin sensitivity patch test a method used to assess skin tolerance/sensitivity to a particular product or service.

Skin tags skin-coloured threads of skin 3mm to 6mm long, projecting from the skin's surface.

Skin tone the strength and elasticity of the skin.

Skin type the different physiological functioning of each person's skin dictates their skin type. There are four main skin types: normal (balanced), dry (lacking in oil), oily (excessive oil) and combination (a mixture of two skin types, e.g., dry and oily).

Skull bones a type of connective tissue forming a hard structure. It surrounds and protects the brain and forms an attachment point for muscles. These include the occipital, frontal, parietal, temporal, sphenoid and ethmoid.

Smile line also called the onychodermal band; the curved line that is created naturally by the hyponychium or artificially with a coloured overlay.

Solvent a product designed to remove and clean artificial lashes without causing eye irritation.

Specialist skincare service products additional skincare preparations available to target improvement. These products include eye gels, throat creams and ampoule services.

Spray-gun equipment used to apply liquid self-tanning product to the skin.

Steam service a warming effect created by boiling water, which is then vaporized and used on the skin to achieve both cleansing and stimulation.

Sterilization the total destruction of all microorganisms in metal tools and equipment.

Stock-keeping maintenance of stock levels to anticipate needs. Stock records note how much stock has been used and when a new order is needed. This may be achieved using a manual or computerized system.

Stop point the part of the plastic tips that fits against the free edge of the natural nail.

Strip sugar a system of wax depilation similar to the warm-wax technique, used to remove hair from the skin. The sugar wax is applied to the skin, and is then removed using a wax removal strip.

Stye bacterial infection. Infection of the sebaceous glands of the eyelash hair follicles. Small lumps appear on the inner rim of the eyelid and contain pus.

Subcutaneous layer a layer of fatty tissue situated below the epidermis and dermis.

Sugar paste a system of wax depilation. An organic paste made from sugar, lemons and water is used to embed the hair, which is then removed by the paste from the skin.

Sugaring an ancient popular method of hair removal using organic substances, sugar and lemon.

Superfluous hair hair considered to be in excess of normal hair for the person's age, sex and therefore unwanted.

Sweat gland or sudoriferous gland is composed of a specialized lining tissue called epithelial tissue. Its function is to control body temperature through the evaporation of sweat from the surface of the skin.

System in relation to nail enhancements, the type of nail enhancement used to overlay the natural nail or plastic tip e.g. acrylic, UV gel, fibre.

Systemic medical condition a medical condition caused by a defect in one of the body's organs, e.g. the heart.

Tapotement, also known as percussion, massage movements performed in a brisk, stimulating manner to increase blood supply and improve tone of the skin and muscles. Movements include clapping and tapping.

Targets goals or objectives to achieve, usually set within a timescale.

Teamwork supportive work by a team.

Telogen the resting stage of the hair growth cycle, when the hair is finally shed.

Terminal hair deep-rooted, thick, coarse, pigmented hair found on the scalp, underarms, pubic region, eyelash and brow areas.

Thermal booties electrically heated boots in which the feet are placed following the application of a skin service product such as a mask. The heat aids the absorption of the product and improves skin functioning.

Thermal mitts electrically heated gloves in which the hands are placed following the application of a skin service product such as a mask. The heat aids the absorption of the product and improves skin functioning.

Thermal sensitivity test a test performed before wax application to check that the temperature of the wax is not too warm. The wax is tested by the therapist on themself, usually on the inner wrist, and then on the client on a small visible area such as the inside of the ankle.

Thermometer equipment used to measure temperature.

Thioglycollate the active ingredient in perm solution.

Threading hair removal using a length of thread which is moved over the skin's surface, gripping hairs and removing them from the skin against hair growth.

Thrombophlebitis inflammation of a vein related to a blood clot (see **phlebitis**).

Tinea corporis or body ringworm fungal infection of the skin where small scaly red patches, which spread outwards and then heal from the centre, leave a ring.

Tinea pedis or athlete's foot fungal infection of the foot occurring in the webs of the skin between the toes. Small blisters form, which later burst. The skin in the area can become dry with a scaly appearance.

Tinea unguium fungal infection of the nails. The nail is yellowish-grey in colour.

Tissues cells in the body which specialize in carrying out particular functions. These include epithelial, connective, muscular and nervous tissue.

Toluenediamine small molecules of permanent dye used in tinting service.

Toning lotion a skincare preparation formulated to treat the different skin types and facial characteristics. It is applied to remove all traces of cleanser from the skin. It produces a cooling effect on the skin and has a skin-tightening effect.

Top coat a nail polish product applied over another nail polish to provide additional strength and durability to the finish.

Towel steaming an alternative to facial steaming using an electrical vapour unit. Small, clean facial towels are heated in a bowl of warm water or specialized heater before application to the face to warm, cleanse and stimulate the skin.

Trade Descriptions Acts (1968 and 1972) legislation that states that information when selling products both in written and verbal form should be accurate.

Transverse furrows nail condition where grooves appear on the nail, running from side to side.

Travellers' cheques alternative form of payment used when travelling abroad and must be compared with the client's passport.

Treatment plan the stages or process you intend to follow when carrying out a particular treatment or series of treatments to meet the agreed objectives following a consultation and diagnostic procedure.

Tweezers small metal tools used to remove body hair by pulling it from the bottom of the hair follicle (small opening in the skin where the hair grows from). There are two types: automatic – designed to remove the bulk of the hair and manual – designed to remove the stray hairs.

Ultraviolet (UV) light an invisible part of the spectrum above the colour violet in the visible light bands.

UV gel a nail enhancement system that uses UV light to initiate polymerization in a pre-mixed gel to create an artificial nail overlay.

UV light cured the process of polymerization (curing) using a photoiniator, in this case UV light, to start the chemical reaction.

Vapour molecules of a chemical in the air, created by evaporation of the chemical.

Vapour unit an electrical appliance that heats water to produce steam which is applied to the skin of the face and neck, to warm, cleanse and stimulate the skin. Also referred to as a steamer.

Varicose veins veins whose valves have become weak and lost their elasticity. The area appears knotted, swollen and bluish/purple in colour.

Vellus hair fine, downy and soft hair – found on the face and body.

Ventilation the transport of fresh air into an area. The spa pool will create heat, humidity and chemical smells. Adequate ventilation is necessary.

Verbal communication occurs when you talk directly to another person either face to face or over the telephone.

Verruca or plantar wart a viral infection where small epidermal skin growths appear, either raised or flat depending upon their location, and have a rough surface.

Vibrations massage manipulations applied on the nerve centre. They stimulate the nerves to induce a feeling of wellbeing and to provide gentle stimulation of the skin.

Viruses the smallest living bodies, too small to see under an ordinary microscope. Viruses invade healthy body cells and multiply within the cell. Eventually the cell walls break down and the virus particles are freed to attack further cells.

Vitamin D a fatty substance in the skin converted to vitamin D with UV light from the sun. This circulates in the blood and with the mineral salts calcium and phosphorus helps the formation and maintenance of the health of the body's bones.

Warm wax a system of wax depilation. Warm wax remains soft at body temperatures. It is frequently made of mixtures of glucose syrup and zinc oxide. Honey can be used instead of glucose syrup; this is referred to as honey wax.

Warm-oil service involves gently heating a small amount of oil and soaking the nails and cuticles in it to nourish the nails and soften the cuticles and surrounding skin.

Waste items, substances and materials requiring disposal following a service. Waste must be disposed of safely and in accordance with legal and salon requirements.

Watery eye over-secretion of tears from the eyes, which would normally drain into the nasal cavity.

Wax depilation the temporary removal of excess hair from a body part using wax.

Waxing products cosmetic preparations used with a waxing service which have specific benefits to cleanse the skin, assist in hair removal care and improve the appearance and healing properties of the skin following hair removal.

White tip powder a white acrylic powder used to create a white free edge on an artificial nail.

Work techniques the methods you use to carry out waxing services.

Workplace (Health Safety and Welfare) Regulations (1992) these regulations provide the employer with an approved code of practice for maintaining a safe, secure working environment.

Workplace policies this covers the documentation prepared by your employer on the procedures to be followed in your workplace. Examples are your employer's safety policy statement, or general health and safety statements and written safety procedures covering aspects of the workplace that should be drawn to the employees' (and "other persons'") attention, pricing policies and customer service policies.

Workplace practices any activities, procedures, use of materials or equipment and working techniques used in carrying out your job. Lifting techniques and maintaining good posture whilst working are also included.

Wrap fabrics material used in nail enhancements to overlay the natural nail to provide strength e.g. fibreglass, silk.

Zones in relation to nail enhancements, the three areas of the artificial nail referred to when creating the correct artificial structure.

Index